BOWES & CHURCH'S
FOOD VALUES
OF PORTIONS COMMONLY USED

BOWES & CHURCH'S FOOD VALUES OF PORTIONS COMMONLY USED

EIGHTEENTH EDITION

Jean A.T. Pennington, PhD, RD & Judith Spungen Douglass, MS, RD

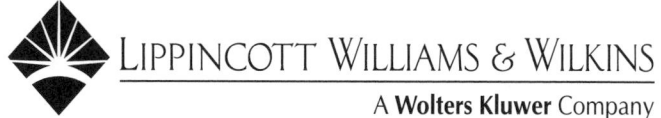

LIPPINCOTT WILLIAMS & WILKINS
A **Wolters Kluwer** Company

Philadelphia · Baltimore · New York · London
Buenos Aires · Hong Kong · Sydney · Tokyo

Executive Editor: David Troy
Managing Editor: Matt Hauber
Senior Project Editor: Karen Ruppert
Marketing Manager: Samantha Smith
Designer: Risa Clow
Compositor: Maryland Composition
Printer: Quebecor

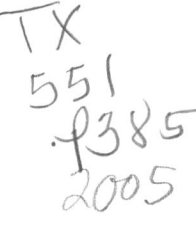

351 West Camden Street
Baltimore, MD 21201

530 Walnut St.
Philadelphia, PA 19106

The information provided in this book should be used by the healthcare practitioner under appropriate supervision in accordance with professional standards of care with regard to the unique circumstances that apply in each practice situation. Care has been taken to confirm the accuracy of information presented. The authors, editors, and publisher cannot accept any responsibility for errors or omissions or for any consequences from application of the information in this book and make no warranty, express or implied, with respect to the contents of the book.

The authors have attempted to provide readers with the most accurate food composition data available as of the date of manuscript submission. However, the field of food composition is a dynamic one. The nutrient composition of foods varies because of food sampling designs; advances in analytical methods; genetic, environmental, and processing variables; and changes in product formulations and package sizes. The information in these tables should be used as reasonable approximations of the nutrient composition of foods. Individuals who are on therapeutic diets for medical purposes may need to contact food manufacturers for more specific information.

Printed in the United States of America

Library of Congress Cataloging-in-Publication Data
Pennington, Jean A. Thompson.
  Bowes & Church's food values of portions commonly used/Jean A.T. Pennington & Judith S. Douglass.—18th ed.
    p. cm.
  Includes bibliographical references and index.
  ISBN 0-7817-4429-6
    1. Nutrition—Tables. 2. Food—Composition—Tables. I. Douglass, Judith Spungen. II. Title.

TX551.P385 2004
613.2′8—dc22

2003066133

The publishers have made every effort to trace the copyright holders for borrowed material. If they have inadvertently overlooked any, they will be pleased to make the necessary arrangements at the first opportunity.

To purchase additional copies of this book, call our customer service department at **(800) 638-3030** or fax orders to **(301) 824-7390**. International customers should call **(301) 714-2324**.

Visit Lippincott Williams & Wilkins on the Internet: http://www.LWW.com. Lippincott Williams & Wilkins customer service representatives are available from 8:30 am to 6:00 pm, EST.

05 06 07 08 09
1 2 3 4 5 6 7 8 9 10

Dedication

The Eighteenth Edition of *Bowes and Church's Food Values of Portions Commonly Used* is dedicated to the authors of previous editions:

Anna dePlanter Bowes, MA
Charles F. Church, MD
Helen Nichols Church, BA, RD

Ms. Anna dePlanter Bowes and Dr. Charles F. Church developed the first edition of *Food Values* in 1937 and made it available as a private publication in Philadelphia, Pennsylvania. Ms. Bowes completed editions two through eight, published in 1939, 1940, 1942, 1944, 1946, 1951, and 1956, respectively, as private publications in Philadelphia. Dr. Church and his wife, Ms. Helen Nichols Church, worked together on editions nine through twelve (1963, 1966, 1970, and 1975), which were published by the Lippincott Publishing Company in Philadelphia. To all three previous authors of *Food Values* we express our gratitude for their devotion to the quality of this reference textbook. We hope that we have carried it forward in their tradition.

Preface to the First Edition

The purpose of this book is to supply authoritative data on the nutritional values of foods in a form for quick and easy reference. In teaching nutrition to students of medicine, dentistry, dental hygiene, and public health nursing, food values based on common measures of portions frequently served have been found most useful. This basis of calculation is particularly well suited to the practical study of comparative food values, as well as to the approximate analysis of diets from records of daily food intake. For calculations of diets from weighed portions, the actual weight of each food is given in grams or ounces.

Anna dePlanter Bowes
Charles F. Church
November 1937
Philadelphia, PA

Preface to the Eighteenth Edition

Bowes and Church's Food Values of Portions Commonly Used is a reference food composition database intended "to supply authoritative data on the nutritional values of food in a form for quick and easy reference." This was the goal established for the first edition by Ms. Anna dePlanter Bowes and Dr. Charles F. Church in 1937 and has remained the goal for all subsequent editions. The preface to the first edition placed an emphasis on providing nutrient values per typical serving portion (as opposed to 100 grams or 1 pound as purchased), and indeed, the Bowes & Church book was the first food composition book in the United States to do this.

The database and accompanying information for this eighteenth edition are intended to assist dietitians and nutritionists in providing dietary information to their patients and clients. The information in this book may also be of use to research nutritionists, students of nutrition and dietetics, and individuals who are on special diets or who want to know more about the composition of foods.

The contents of this publication are identified in the *Features of the Eighteenth Edition*. We have attempted to provide current information for a wide range of commonly consumed foods as well as various foods of interest and curiosity. We gratefully acknowledge the expert review of this edition provided by Ms. Sally Schakel, RD, and Mary Murphy, MS, RD; the industry nutritionists and representatives who responded to our requests for food composition data; and the editorial assistance provided by Mr. David Troy and Mr. Matt Hauber at Lippincott Williams & Wilkins in Baltimore, Maryland.

Jean A.T. Pennington, PhD, RD
Judith Spungen Douglass, MS, RD
June 2003
Chevy Chase MD and Reston VA

Contents

SUPPLEMENTARY TABLES FOR THE NUTRIENT CONTENT OF FOODS

Features of the Eighteenth Edition

FRONT MATERIAL

The front material provides information on standards for the dietary intake of food components in the United States (US). The standards for macronutrients, vitamins, minerals, and energy are those established by the Food and Nutrition Board of the National Academy of Sciences (NAS). The standards for the nutrition labeling of food are those developed by the US Food and Drug Administration (FDA). Also provided are food component definitions; abbreviations and symbols used in the text; reference codes that identify the data sources used in this edition; conversion tables for measures of heat, weight, and volume; and a table of gram-ounce equivalents.

MAIN TABLES

The main food composition table in this database, entitled *Nutrient Content of Foods*, provides values for 30 nutrients in approximately 8,000 foods. The foods are grouped into 32 sections on the basis of food type with considerations for common usage. The foods within each of the 32 sections are arranged in a hierarchical structure and are listed alphabetically. The two-line heading at the top of each page of the main table indicates the nutrients and units of measurement for the numerical values listed in the two lines of nutrient values for each food. For Section 32, Special Dietary Foods, there are four lines of nutrient data per food to include the complete nutrient profiles that were available for these formulated products. This section includes infant formulas, formulated products used for medical purposes, and meal replacement or enhancement products described as sport, energy, or weight reduction products.

With regard to food names, upper case is used for brand and trademark names; lower case is otherwise used for food names and for proper nouns and adjectives (e.g., french fries, danish pastry, brussels sprouts, and chinese cabbage). Each food is identified by name, description (e.g., color, maturity, preservation method, and cooking method), brand name (if applicable), and serving portion. The individual food names are bolded, while the descriptive terms are printed in regular type. Some foods are listed several times with different descriptors. In these cases, the food name is listed once in bold, and its subsequent entries provide only the descriptive terms in regular type. Abbreviations are used to provide as complete a description as is possible for each food within the space limitations. The abbreviated words and symbols used with the food names and descriptors are listed in the section *Abbreviations and Symbols.*

Foods are presented primarily in their *as consumed* form, although ingredient items (e.g., flour, baking soda, herbs) are also listed in the database. Where available, brand names are used to help identify commercial products such as ready-to-eat breakfast cereals, desserts, candy bars, soups, and entrees. The serving portions are those provided by food companies or the USDA food composition database. Each food is listed only once, although some foods may be applicable to several food group sections. The index may be used to locate foods for which classification may not be apparent, and the section *Food Name Synonyms and Cross-References* provides a means to locate foods known by several different names. Nutrient values for different flavors of some foods (e.g., gelatin desserts, icings, puddings, granola bars, ice cream) may reflect a specific flavor, as indicated in the description, or may be averages for different flavors, as indicated in the footnotes. The nutrient values were averaged if the different flavored items had similar profiles; listing the food only once saved space by allowing one food entry to represent similar foods.

SUPPLEMENTARY TABLES

The supplementary tables, which follow the main table, provide information on the levels of ethyl alcohol, amines, amino acids, caffeine, carotenoids, dietary fiber fractions, gluten, omega-3 and trans fatty acids, flavonoids, glutathione, two additional minerals, plant acids, plant sterols, purines, starch and sugars, and four additional vitamins. The supplementary tables provide information on food components for which there were not sufficient data to warrant a listing in the main table. The foods in the supplementary tables are generally listed by the major food groupings used for the main table. All of the foods in the amino acid supplementary table are listed in the main table and are identified by USDA code numbers. Many of the foods in the other supplementary tables are also listed in the main table and the serving portions, if used, are usually consistent. Foods in some of the supplementary tables are also identified by code numbers to link them to foods in the main table.

Food components in the supplementary tables are listed per 100 grams of food and/or per serving portions. Much of the information in the supplementary tables was obtained through computer searches of published literature. The information should be used with discretion, as some of it is from older papers and some is from foods produced and analyzed in countries other than the US. Thus, the values may reflect foods that are different than those on the US market and may reflect analytical methods not currently in use in the US.

DATA SOURCES

The nutrient values included in the main and supplementary tables have been obtained directly from the USDA Database for Standard Reference, Release 15 (2002) (SR15); food companies; food labels; food company websites; and the scientific literature. The data sources for the main table are indicated by the Reference Code in the lower left-hand location of the two lines of data for each food. The data sources for the supplementary tables are indicated in or at the end of each table. The data provided by most food companies were in the form of nutrition labeling data. Labeling values are usually derived from analytical data and are rounded and adjusted to be in compliance with government labeling regulations. Labeling values are therefore not as precise as the original analytical data but are sufficient for most dietary purposes. The values for vitamins and minerals, provided as percent daily values (DV), were back-calculated to obtain weight values. (See the section on *Daily Values (DV) for Nutrition Labeling*.)

The DVs for folic acid provided as nutrition labeling data were back-calculated to micrograms of folic acid rather than to micrograms of dietary folate equivalents. It was not possible to determine how much of the folic acid in the foods was naturally occurring versus that added by the manufacturer. Therefore, it is possible that some of the listed folic acid values may underestimate the available folic acid.

Labeling information for vitamin E was provided as percent DV or international units (IU) of vitamin E. IUs of vitamin E were converted to milligrams of alpha-tocopherol equivalents (ATE) assuming that 1.5 IU of vitamin E is equivalent to 1 milligram of ATE. Although alpha-tocopherol is the primary form of vitamin E, the main table lists ATE because more data were available in this form and it is closer to the data provided by food companies.

For some food products, the serving size provided by the original source was specified only as a volume measure (fluid ounces, cups) or approximate measure (slice, piece, medium, large, small) rather than as a weight unit (grams or ounces). The gram weights for these foods were estimated. Some of the foods were purchased and weighed; the gram weights of some of the foods were estimated by considering the weight of the proximate nutrients (water, protein, fat, and carbohydrate). In cases wherein the water weight was not provided, it was esti-mated from the percent water content of similar foods. For foods wherein the portion size was provided in fluid ounces without an equivalent weight unit, the gram weight was estimated from the fluid ounce-gram weight equivalent of a similar food. (See *Heat, Weight, & Volume Conversions* and *Gram-Ounce Equivalents*.)

BACK MATERIAL

The back material includes the scientific names for plants and animals, food name synonyms and cross-references, a bibliography of publications on the composition of foods, and an index. The list of food name synonyms and cross references is included to assist users in locating foods with various names (including regional names) or various arrangements of the same name (e.g., lima beans vs. beans, lima vs. butter beans).

The bibliography includes papers concerning food composition that were published between February 1997 (when the seventeenth edition of *Food Values* was submitted to the publisher) and June 2003 (when the eighteenth edition was submitted to the publisher). The references are listed alphabetically by the first authors' last names. Key words are listed in bold to identify the foods and food components that are discussed in these papers.

CAUTIONARY NOTES

The precision and accuracy of the data and the level of detail of food descriptions and serving sizes are limited to that provided by the sources. The collection and aggregation of data from various sources invariably results in some unevenness in food descriptions and some apparent inconsistencies of food component values and serving sizes. The attempt to aggregate generic and brand-specific products causes some unevenness because descriptions for generic foods tend to be less precise, and the foods may not be recognized by data users. Likewise, data for commercial products identified only by brand or trademark names are only useful for database users who are familiar with the products.

Those unfamiliar with the use of food composition tables are requested to note the following:

- These tables should be used as approximate guides to the nutrient content of foods. Persons on special diets for various medical conditions may require more specific nutrient composition data from food manufacturers.
- Blank spaces indicate a lack of data from the original source. Blank spaces should not be assumed to be zeros, as this could underestimate the dietary intake of various food components.
- The food component values presented here are mean values or values used for nutrition labeling. Some of the values have large standard deviations and wide ranges. Causes of nutrient variations in

foods include soil type, season, geography, genetics, animal diets, processing, method of preparation, changes in product formulations, sampling designs, and methods of analysis.

- Because of nutrient variation and the fact that the data are collected from various sources (i.e., USDA, food companies, food labels, websites, and the scientific literature), apparent inconsistencies may occur. For example, portion sizes, gram weights of similar foods, and food component values may vary among sources.
- The values presented here may not be representative of the entire US food supply. Representativeness depends on the sampling designs and on the number of samples collected and analyzed.
- The mineral content of water varies from one geographic location to another. The mineral content of beverages made by addition of water to powders or frozen concentrates and of foods cooked in water (e.g., rice, oatmeal, pasta, and vegetables) may vary depending on the mineral content of the water used. Likewise, the mineral content of commercial beverages (e.g., beer, carbonated sodas, and juice drinks) depends on the mineral content of the water in the area where the beverages are bottled. Individuals on therapeutic diets may need to obtain information on the mineral content of their home tap water and on the mineral content of the specific beverage they consume.

- Information presented in these tables may not be the same as that provided on food labels because of industry changes in serving sizes or industry product reformulation with different ingredients or different proportions of ingredients.
- As noted above, some of the data in the supplementary tables are old and from countries other than the US. They are provided here for information purposes but should be used with caution, as they may not reflect foods available from the US market or current analytical methods.

Dietary Reference Intakes (DRIs)—Recommended Intakes for Macronutrients[1]

Life Stage Group	Carbohydrate (g/day)	Total Fiber (g/day)	Fat (g/day)	n-6 PUFA[2] (g/day)	n-3 PUFA[3] (g/day)	Protein[4] (g/day)
INFANTS						
0–6 mo	60	ND	31	4.4	0.5	9.1
7–12 mo	95	ND	30	4.6	0.5	**13.5**
CHILDREN						
1–3 yr	**130**	19	ND	7	0.7	**13**
4–8 yr	**130**	25	ND	10	0.9	**19**
MALES						
9–13 yr	**130**	31	ND	12	1.2	**34**
14–18 yr	**130**	38	ND	16	1.6	**52**
19–30 yr	**130**	38	ND	17	1.6	**56**
31–50 yr	**130**	38	ND	17	1.6	**56**
51–70 yr	**130**	30	ND	14	1.6	**56**
>70 yr	**130**	30	ND	14	1.6	**56**
FEMALES						
9–13 yr	**130**	26	ND	10	1.0	**34**
14–18 yr	**130**	26	ND	11	1.1	**46**
19–30 yr	**130**	25	ND	12	1.1	**46**
31–50 yr	**130**	25	ND	12	1.1	**46**
51–70 yr	**130**	21	ND	11	1.1	**46**
>70 yr	**130**	21	ND	11	1.1	**46**
PREGNANCY						
14–18 yr	**175**	28	ND	13	1.4	**71**
19–30 yr	**175**	28	ND	13	1.4	**71**
31–50 yr	**175**	28	ND	13	1.4	**71**
LACTATION						
14–18 yr	**210**	29	ND	13	1.3	**71**
19–30 yr	**210**	29	ND	13	1.3	**71**
31–50 yr	**210**	29	ND	13	1.3	**71**

[1] This table presents Recommended Dietary Allowances (RDAs) in **bold type** and Adequate Intakes (AIs) in unbolded type. Both RDAs and AIs may be used as goals for individual intake. RDAs are set to meet the needs of almost all (97 to 98%) individuals within a life stage group. For healthy breastfed infants, the AI is the mean intake. The AI for other life stages is believed to cover the needs of all individuals within the group, but lack of data or uncertainty in the data prevent confidence in the percent of individuals covered by this intake.

[2] Primarily linoleic acid; however, approximately 10% of the total n-6 polyunsaturated fatty acids (PUFA) may come from longer-chain n-6 fatty acids.

[3] Primarily alpha-linolenic acid; however, approximately 10% of the total n-3 polyunsaturated fatty acids (PUFA) may come from longer-chain n-3 fatty acids.

[4] Based on 0.8 grams protein/kg body weight for reference body weight.

Source:
National Academy of Sciences. *Dietary Reference Intakes for Energy, Carbohydrate, Fiber, Fat, Fatty Acids, Cholesterol, Protein, and Amino Acids.* National Academy Press, Washington DC. 2002. Available at www.nap.edu.

Dietary Reference Intakes (DRIs)—Recommended Intakes for Amino Acids[1]

Amino Acid	AI[2] 0–6 mo (mg/kg/ day)	EAR/RDA 7–12 mo (mg/kg/day)	EAR/RDA 1–3 yr (mg/kg/day)	EAR/RDA 4–8 yr (mg/kg/day)	EAR/RDA 9–13 boys (mg/kg/day)	EAR/RDA 9–13 girls (mg/kg/day)
Histidine	23	22/32	16/21	13/16	13/17	12/15
Isoleucine	88	30/43	22/28	18/22	18/22	17/21
Leucine	156	65/93	48/63	40/49	40/49	38/47
Lysine	107	62/89	45/58	37/46	37/46	35/43
Methionine + Cysteine	59	30/43	22/28	18/22	18/22	17/21
Phenylalanine + Tyrosine	135	58/84	41/54	33/41	33/41	31/38
Threonine	73	34/49	24/32	19/24	19/24	18/22
Tryptophan	28	9/13	6/8	5/6	5/6	5/6
Valine	87	39/58	28/37	23/28	23/28	22/27

Amino Acid	EAR/RDA 14–18 yr boys (mg/kg/day)	EAR/RDA 14–18 yr girls (mg/kg/day)	EAR/RDA ≥19 yr adults (mg/kg/day)	EAR/RDA pregnancy (mg/kg/day)	EAR/RDA lactation (mg/kg/day)
Histidine	12/15	12/14	11/14	15/18	15/19
Isoleucine	17/21	16/19	15/19	20/25	24/30
Leucine	38/47	35/44	34/42	45/56	50/62
Lysine	35/43	32/40	31/38	41/51	42/52
Methionine + Cysteine	17/21	16/19	15/19	20/25	21/26
Phenylalanine + Tyrosine	31/38	28/35	27/33	36/44	41/51
Threonine	18/22	17/21	16/20	21/26	24/30
Tryptophan	5/6	4/5	4/5	5/7	7/9
Valine	22/27	20/24	19/24	25/31	28/35

[1] AI = Adequate Intake; EAR = Estimated Average Requirement; RDA = Recommended Dietary Allowance.
[2] In mg/day, the AIs for 0–6 month-old infants are 214 for histidine, 529 for isoleucine, 938 for leucine, 640 for lysine, 353 for methionine + cysteine, 807 for phenylalanine + tyrosine, 436 for threonine, 167 for tryptophan, and 519 for valine.

Source:
National Academy of Sciences. *Dietary Reference Intakes for Energy, Carbohydrate, Fiber, Fat, Fatty Acids, Cholesterol, Protein, and Amino Acids.* National Academy Press, Washington DC. 2002. Available at www.nap.edu.

Dietary Reference Intakes (DRIs)—Recommended Intakes for Vitamins[1]

Life Stage Group	Vit A[2] (mcg/day)	Vit C (mg/day)	Vit D[3] (mcg/day)	Vit E[4] (mg/day)	Vit K (mcg/day)	Thiamin (mg/day)	Riboflavin (mg/day)
INFANTS							
0–6 mo	400	40	5	4	2.0	0.2	0.3
7–12 mo	500	50	5	5	2.5	0.3	0.4
CHILDREN							
1–3 yr	**300**	**15**	5	**6**	30	**0.5**	**0.5**
4–8 yr	**400**	**25**	5	**7**	55	**0.6**	**0.6**
MALES							
9–13 yr	**600**	**45**	5	**11**	60	**0.9**	**0.9**
14–18 yr	**900**	**75**	5	**15**	75	**1.2**	**1.3**
19–30 yr	**900**	**90**	5	**15**	120	**1.2**	**1.3**
31–50 yr	**900**	**90**	5	**15**	120	**1.2**	**1.3**
51–70 yr	**900**	**90**	10	**15**	120	**1.2**	**1.3**
>70 yr	**900**	**90**	15	**15**	120	**1.2**	**1.3**
FEMALES							
9–13 yr	**600**	**45**	5	**11**	60	**0.9**	**0.9**
14–18 yr	**700**	**65**	5	**15**	75	**1.0**	**1.0**
19–30 yr	**700**	**75**	5	**15**	90	**1.1**	**1.1**
31–50 yr	**700**	**75**	5	**15**	90	**1.1**	**1.1**
51–70 yr	**700**	**75**	10	**15**	90	**1.1**	**1.1**
>70 yr	**700**	**75**	15	**15**	90	**1.1**	**1.1**
PREGNANCY							
≤18 yr	**750**	**80**	5	**15**	75	**1.4**	**1.4**
19–30 yr	**770**	**85**	5	**15**	90	**1.4**	**1.4**
31–50 yr	**770**	**85**	5	**15**	90	**1.4**	**1.4**
LACTATION							
≤18 yr	**1,200**	**115**	5	**19**	75	**1.4**	**1.6**
19–30 yr	**1,300**	**120**	5	**19**	90	**1.4**	**1.6**
31–50 yr	**1,300**	**120**	5	**19**	90	**1.4**	**1.6**

[1] This table presents Recommended Dietary Allowances (RDAs) in **bold type** and Adequate Intakes (AIs) in unbolded type. Both RDAs and AIs may be used as goals for individual intake. RDAs are set to meet the needs of almost all (97 to 98%) individuals within a life stage group. For healthy breastfed infants, the AI is the mean intake. The AI for other life stages is believed to cover the needs of all individuals within the group, but lack of data or uncertainty in the data prevent confidence in the percent of individuals covered by this intake.

[2] As retinol activity equivalents (RAEs). 1 RAE = 1 mcg retinol, 12 mcg beta-carotene, 24 mcg alpha-carotene, or 24 mcg beta-cryptoxanthin. The RAE for dietary provitamin A carotenoids is two-fold greater than retinol equivalents (RE), whereas the RAE for preformed vitamin A is the same as RE.

[3] Calciferol (vitamin D2 and vitamin D3; 1 mcg calciferol = 40 IU vitamin D; RDI assumes the absence of adequate exposure to sunlight).

[4] As alpha-tocopherol. Alpha-tocopherol includes RRR-alpha-tocopherol, the only form of alpha-tocopherol that occurs naturally in foods, and the 2R-stereoisomeric forms of alpha-tocopherol (RRR-, RSR-, RRS-, and RSS-alpha tocopherol) that occur in fortified foods and supplements. It does not include the 2S-stereoisomeric forms of alpha-tocopherol (SRR-, SSR-, and SSS-alpha-tocopherol), also found in fortified foods and supplements.

Dietary Reference Intakes (DRIs)—Recommended Intakes for Vitamins[1] (continued)

Life Stage Group	Niacin[5] (mg/day)	Vit B6 (mg/day)	Folate[6] (mcg/day)	Vit B12[7] (mcg/day)	Pantothenic Acid (mg/day)	Biotin (mcg/day)	Choline[8] (mg/day)
INFANTS							
0–6 mo	2	0.1	65	0.4	1.7	5	125
7–12 mo	4	0.3	80	0.5	1.8	6	150
CHILDREN							
1–3 yr	6	0.5	150	0.9	2	8	200
4–8 yr	8	0.6	200	1.2	3	12	250
MALES							
9–13 yr	12	1.0	300	1.8	4	20	375
14–18 yr	16	1.3	400	2.4	5	25	550
19–30 yr	16	1.3	400	2.4	5	30	550
31–50 yr	16	1.3	400	2.4	5	30	550
51–70 yr	16	1.7	400	2.4	5	30	550
>70 yr	16	1.7	400	2.4	5	30	550
FEMALES							
9–13 yr	12	1.0	300	1.8	4	20	375
14–18 yr	14	1.2	400	2.4	5	25	400
19–30 yr	14	1.3	400	2.4	5	30	425
31–50 yr	14	1.3	400	2.4	5	30	425
51–70 yr	14	1.5	400	2.4	5	30	425
>70 yr	14	1.5	400	2.4	5	30	425
PREGNANCY							
≤18 yr	18	1.9	600	2.6	6	30	450
19–30 yr	18	1.9	600	2.6	6	30	450
31–50 yr	18	1.9	600	2.6	6	30	450
LACTATION							
≤18 yr	17	2.0	500	2.8	7	35	550
19–30	17	2.0	500	2.8	7	35	550
31–50	17	2.0	500	2.8	7	35	550

[5] As niacin equivalents (NE) except for 0–6 months where the value is for preformed niacin (not NE); 1 mg of niacin = 60 mg of tryptophan.

[6] As dietary folate equivalents (DFE). 1 DFE = 1 mcg food folate = 0.6 mcg of folic acid from fortified food or as a supplement consumed with food = 0.5 mcg of a supplement taken on an empty stomach. In view of evidence linking folate intake with neural tube defects in the fetus, it is recommended that all women capable of becoming pregnant consume 400 mcg from supplements or fortified foods in addition to intake of food folate from a varied diet. It is assumed that women will continue consuming 400 mcg from supplements or fortified foods until their pregnancy is confirmed and they enter prenatal care, which ordinarily occurs after the end of the periconceptional period—the critical time for formation of the neural tube.

[7] Because 10 to 30 percent of older people may malabsorb food-bound vitamin B12, it is advisable for those older than 50 years to meet their RDA mainly by consuming foods fortified with vitamin B12 or a supplement containing vitamin B12.

[8] Although AIs have been set for choline, there are few data to assess whether a dietary supply of choline is needed at all stages of the life cycle, and it may be that the choline requirement can be met by endogenous synthesis at some of these stages.

Sources:

National Academy of Sciences. *Dietary Reference Intakes for Calcium, Phosphorus, Magnesium, Vitamin D, and Fluoride* (1997); *Dietary Reference Intakes for Thiamin, Riboflavin, Niacin, Vitamin B6, Folate, Vitamin B12, Pantothenic Acid, Biotin, and Choline* (1998); *Dietary Reference Intakes for Vitamin C, Vitamin E, Selenium, and Carotenoids* (2000); and *Dietary Reference Intakes for Vitamin A, Vitamin K, Arsenic, Boron, Chromium, Copper, Iodine, Iron, Manganese, Molybdenum, Nickel, Silicon, Vanadium, and Zinc* (2001). National Academy Press, Washington DC. Available at www.nap.edu.

Dietary Reference Intakes (DRIs)—Recommended Intakes for Elements[1]

Life Stage Group	Ca mg/day	Cr mcg/day	Cu mcg/day	F mg/day	I mcg/day	Fe mg/day	Mg mg/day	Mn mg/day	Mo mcg/day	P mg/day	Se mcg/day	Zn mg/day
INFANTS												
0–6 mo	210	0.2	200	0.01	110	0.27	30	0.003	2	100	15	2
7–12 mo	270	5.5	220	0.5	130	**11**	75	0.6	3	275	20	**3**
CHILDREN												
1–3 yr	500	11	**340**	0.7	**90**	**7**	80	1.2	**17**	**460**	20	**3**
4–8 yr	800	15	**440**	1	**90**	**10**	130	1.5	**22**	**500**	30	**5**
MALES												
9–13 yr	1,300	25	**700**	2	**120**	**8**	240	1.9	**34**	**1,250**	40	**8**
14–18 yr	1,300	35	**890**	3	**150**	**11**	410	2.2	**43**	**1,250**	55	**11**
19–30 yr	1,000	35	**900**	4	**150**	**8**	400	2.3	**45**	**700**	55	**11**
31–50 yr	1,000	35	**900**	4	**150**	**8**	420	2.3	**45**	**700**	55	**11**
51–70 yr	1,200	30	**900**	4	**150**	**8**	420	2.3	**45**	**700**	55	**11**
>70 yr	1,200	30	**900**	4	**150**	**8**	420	2.3	**45**	**700**	55	**11**
FEMALES												
9–13 yr	1,300	21	**700**	2	**120**	**8**	240	1.6	**34**	**1,250**	40	**8**
14–18 yr	1,300	24	**890**	3	**150**	**15**	360	1.6	**43**	**1,250**	55	**9**
19–30 yr	1,000	25	**900**	3	**150**	**18**	310	1.8	**45**	**700**	55	**8**
31–50 yr	1,000	25	**900**	3	**150**	**18**	320	1.8	**45**	**700**	55	**8**
51–70 yr	1,200	20	**900**	3	**150**	**8**	320	1.8	**45**	**700**	55	**8**
>70 yr	1,200	20	**900**	3	**150**	**8**	320	1.8	**45**	**700**	55	**8**
PREGNANCY												
≤18 yr	1,300	29	**1,000**	3	**220**	**27**	400	2.0	**50**	**1,250**	60	**12**
19–30 yr	1,000	30	**1,000**	3	**220**	**27**	350	2.0	**50**	**700**	60	**11**
31–50 yr	1,000	30	**1,000**	3	**220**	**27**	360	2.0	**50**	**700**	60	**11**
LACTATION												
≤18 yr	1,300	44	**1,300**	3	**290**	**10**	360	2.6	**50**	**1,250**	70	**13**
19–30 yr	1,000	45	**1,300**	3	**290**	**9**	310	2.6	**50**	**700**	70	**12**
31–50 yr	1,000	45	**1,300**	3	**290**	**9**	320	2.6	**50**	**700**	70	**12**

[1] This table presents Recommended Dietary Allowances (RDAs) in **bold type** and Adequate Intakes (AIs) in unbolded type. Both RDAs and AIs may be used as goals for individual intake. RDAs are set to meet the needs of almost all (97 to 98%) individuals within a life stage group. For healthy breastfed infants, the AI is the mean intake. The AI for other life stages is believed to cover the needs of all individuals within the group, but lack of data or uncertainty in the data prevent confidence in the percent of individuals covered by this intake.

Sources:

National Academy of Sciences. *Dietary Reference Intakes for Calcium, Phosphorus, Magnesium, Vitamin D, and Fluoride* (1997); *Dietary Reference Intakes for Vitamin C, Vitamin E, Selenium, and Carotenoids* (2000); and *Dietary Reference Intakes for Vitamin A, Vitamin K, Arsenic, Boron, Chromium, Copper, Iodine, Iron, Manganese, Molybdenum, Nickel, Silicon, Vanadium, and Zinc* (2001). National Academy Press, Washington DC. Available at www.nap.edu.

Dietary Reference Intakes (DRIs)—Tolerable Upper Intakes for Vitamins[1]

Life Stage Group	Vit A[2] (mcg/day)	Vit C (mg/day)	Vit D (mcg/day)	Vit E[3,4] (mg/day)	Niacin[4] (mg/day)	Vit B6 (mg/day)	Folate[4] (mcg/day)	Choline (g/day)
INFANTS								
0–6 mo	600	ND	25	ND	ND	ND	ND	ND
7–12 mo	600	ND	25	ND	ND	ND	ND	ND
CHILDREN								
1–3 yr	600	400	50	200	10	30	300	1.0
4–8 yr	900	650	50	300	15	40	400	1.0
ADULTS								
9–13 yr	1,700	1,200	50	600	20	60	600	2.0
14–18 yr	2,800	1,800	50	800	30	80	800	3.0
19–70 yr	3,000	2,000	50	1,000	35	100	1,000	3.5
>70 yr	3,000	2,000	50	1,000	35	100	1,000	3.5
PREGNANCY								
≤18 yr	2,800	1,800	50	800	30	80	800	3.0
19–50 yr	3,000	2,000	50	1,000	35	100	1,000	3.5
LACTATION								
≤18 yr	2,800	1,800	50	800	30	80	800	3.0
19–50 yr	3,000	2,000	50	1,000	35	100	1,000	3.5

[1] UL = The maximum level of daily nutrient intake that is likely to pose no risk of adverse effects. Unless otherwise specified, the UL represents total intake from food, water, and supplements. Due to lack of suitable data, ULs could not be established for vitamin K, thiamin, riboflavin, vitamin B12, pantothenic acid, biotin, or the carotenoids. ND = Not determinable due to lack of data of adverse effects and concern with regard to lack of ability to handle excess amounts. In the absence of ULs, extra caution may be warranted in consuming levels above recommended intakes. Source of intake should be from food only to prevent high levels of intake. Carotene supplements are advised only to serve as a provitamin A source for individuals at risk of vitamin A deficiency.

[2] As preformed vitamin A only.

[3] As alpha-tocopherol; applies to any form of supplemental alpha-tocopherol.

[4] The ULs for vitamin E, niacin, and folate apply to synthetic forms obtained from supplements, fortified foods, or a combination of the two.

Sources:

National Academy of Sciences. *Dietary Reference Intakes for Calcium, Phosphorus, Magnesium, Vitamin D, and Fluoride* (1997); *Dietary Reference Intakes for Thiamin, Riboflavin, Niacin, Vitamin B6, Folate, Vitamin B12, Pantothenic Acid, Biotin, and Choline* (1998); *Dietary Reference Intakes for Vitamin C, Vitamin E, Selenium, and Carotenoids* (2000); and *Dietary Reference Intakes for Vitamin A, Vitamin K, Arsenic, Boron, Chromium, Copper, Iodine, Iron, Manganese, Molybdenum, Nickel, Silicon, Vanadium, and Zinc* (2001). National Academy Press, Washington DC. Available at www.nap.edu.

Dietary Reference Intakes (DRIs)—Tolerable Upper Intakes (ULs) for Elements[1]

Life Stage Group	B (mg/day)	Ca (mg/day)	Cu (mg/day)	F (mg/day)	I (mcg/day)	Fe (mg/day)	Mg[2] (mg/day)
INFANTS							
0–6 mo	ND[3]	ND	ND	0.7	ND	40	ND
7–12 mo	ND	ND	ND	0.9	ND	40	ND
CHILDREN							
1–3 yr	3	2,500	1	1.3	200	40	65
4–8 yr	6	2,500	3	2.2	300	40	110
ADULTS							
9–13 yr	11	2,500	5	10	600	40	350
14–18 yr	17	2,500	8	10	900	45	350
19–70 yr	20	2,500	10	10	1,100	45	350
>70 yr	20	2,500	10	10	1,100	45	350
PREGNANCY							
≤18 yr	17	2,500	8	10	900	45	350
19–50 yr	20	2,500	10	10	1,100	45	350
LACTATION							
≤18 yr	17	2,500	8	10	900	45	350
19–50 yr	20	2,500	10	10	1,100	45	350

[1] UL = The maximum level of daily nutrient intake that is likely to pose no risk of adverse effects. Unless otherwise specified, the UL represents total intake from food, water, and supplements. Due to lack of suitable data, ULs could not be established for arsenic, chromium, and silicon. In the absence of ULs, extra caution may be warranted in consuming levels above recommended intakes. Although the UL was not determined for arsenic, there is no justification for adding arsenic to food or supplements. Although silicon has not been shown to cause adverse effects in humans, there is no justification for adding silicon to supplements.

[2] The ULs for magnesium represent intake from a pharmacological agent only and do not include intake from food and water.

[3] ND = Not determinable due to lack of data of adverse effects and concern with regard to lack of ability to handle excess amounts. Source of intake should be only from food to prevent high levels of intake.

Dietary Reference Intakes (DRIs)—Tolerable Upper Intakes for Elements (continued)

Life Stage Group	Mn (mg/day)	Mo (mcg/day)	Ni (mg/day)	P (g/day)	Se (mcg/day)	V[4] (mg/day)	Zn (mg/day)
INFANTS							
0–6 mo	ND	ND	ND	ND	45	ND	4
7–12 mo	ND	ND	ND	ND	60	ND	5
CHILDREN							
1–3 yr	2	300	0.2	3	90	ND	7
4–8 yr	3	600	0.3	3	150	ND	12
ADULTS							
9–13 yr	6	1,100	0.6	4	280	ND	23
14–18 yr	9	1,700	1.0	4	400	ND	34
19–70 yr	11	2,000	1.0	4	400	1.8	40
>70 yr	11	2,000	1.0	3	400	1.8	40
PREGNANCY							
≤18 yr	9	1,700	1.0	3.5	400	ND	34
19–50 yr	11	2,000	1.0	3.5	400	ND	40
LACTATION							
≤18 yr	9	1,700	1.0	4	400	ND	34
19–50 yr	11	2,000	1.0	4	400	ND	40

[4] Although vanadium in food has not been shown to cause adverse effects in humans, there is no justification for adding vanadium to food, and vanadium supplements should be used with caution. The UL is based on adverse effects in laboratory animals; this data could be used to set a UL for adults, but not for children or adolescents.

Sources: National Academy of Sciences. *Dietary Reference Intakes for Calcium, Phosphorus, Magnesium, Vitamin C, and Fluoride* (1997); *Dietary Reference Intakes for Thiamin, Riboflavin, Niacin, Vitamin B6, Folate, Vitamin B12, Pantothenic Acid, Biotin, and Choline* (1998); *Dietary Reference Intakes for Vitamin C, Vitamin E, Selenium and Carotenoids* (2000); and *Dietary Reference Intakes for Vitamin A, Vitamin K, Arsenic, Boron, Chromium Copper, Iodine, Iron, Manganese, Molydenum, Nickel, Silicon, Vanadium, and Zinc* (2001). National Academy Press, Washington DC. Available at www.nap.edu.

Estimated Energy Requirements (EERs) for Men and Women 30 Years of Age[1]

Height M (in)	Physical activity level (PAL)	Weight; BMI = 18.5 Kg (lb)	Weight; BMI = 24.99 Kg (lb)	EER for Men; BMI = 18.5 Kcal/day	EER for Men; BMI = 24.99 Kcal/day	EER for Women; BMI = 18.5 Kcal/day	EER for Women; BMI = 24.99 Kcal/day
1.50	Sedentary	41.6	56.2	1,848	2,080	1,625	1,762
(59)	Low Active	(92)	(124)	2,009	2,267	1,803	1,956
	Active			2,215	2,506	2,025	2,198
	Very Active			2,554	2,898	2,291	2,489
1.65	Sedentary	50.4	68.0	2,068	2,349	1,816	1,982
(65)	Low Active	(111)	(150)	2,254	2,566	2,016	2,202
	Active			2,490	2,842	2,267	2,477
	Very Active			2,880	3,296	2,567	2,807
1.80	Sedentary	59.9	81.0	2,301	2,635	2,015	2,211
(71)	Low Active	(132)	(178)	2,513	2,884	2,239	2,459
	Active			2,782	3,200	2,519	2,769
	Very Active			3,225	3,720	2,855	3,141

[1] For each year below 30, add 7 kcal/day for women and 10 kcal/day for men. For each year above 30, subtract 7 kcal/day for women and 10 kcal/day for men. EERs are derived from the following regression equations based on doubly labeled water data:

adult man: EER = $662 - 9.53 \times$ age (yr) + PA $\times$ ($15.91 \times$ Wt [kg] + $539.6 \times$ Ht[m])

adult woman: EER = $354 - 6.91 \times$ age (yr) + PA $\times$ ($9.36 \times$ Wt[kg] + $726 \times$ Ht[m])

where PA refers to the coefficient for Physical Activity Levels (PAL).

PAL = total energy expenditure÷basal energy expenditure.

PA = 1.0 if PAL ≥ 1.0 < 1.4 (sedentary).

PA = 1.11 if PAL ≥ 1.4 < 1.6 (low active).

PA = 1.25 if PAL ≥ 1.6 < 1.9 (active).

PA = 1.48 if PAL ≥ 1.9 < 2.5 (very active).

BMI = Body Mass Index

Source:

National Academy of Sciences. *Dietary Reference Intakes for Energy, Carbohydrate, Fiber, Fat, Fatty Acids, Cholesterol, Protein, and Amino Acids.* National Academy Press, Washington DC. 2002. Available at www.nap.edu.

Acceptable Macronutrient Distribution Ranges

Macronutrient	Children, 1–3 yr (% energy)	Children, 4–18 yr (% energy)	Adults[3] (% energy)
Fat	30–40	25–35	20–35
n-6 PUFA[1]	5–10	5–10	5–10
n-3 PUFA[2]	0.6–1.2	0.6–1.2	0.6–1.2
Carbohydrate	45–65	45–65	45–65
Protein	5–20	10–30	10–35

[1] Primarily linoleic acid; however, approximately 10% of the total n-6 polyunsaturated fatty acids (PUFA) may come from longer-chain n-6 fatty acids.

[2] Primarily alpha-linolenic acid; however, approximately 10% of the total n-3 polyunsaturated fatty acids (PUFA) may come from longer-chain n-3 fatty acids.

[3] The adult category includes pregnant or lactating females regardless of age.

Source:

National Academy of Sciences. *Dietary Reference Intakes for Energy, Carbohydrate, Fiber, Fat, Fatty Acids, Cholesterol, Protein, and Amino Acids.* National Academy Press, Washington DC. 2002. Available at www.nap.edu.

Daily Values (DV) for Nutrition Labeling[1]

Mandatory Label Component	Daily Value (DV)	Voluntary Label Component	Daily Value (DV)
Total Fat	65 g	Vitamin D	400 IU[2]
Saturated Fat	20 g	Vitamin E	30 IU[2]
Cholesterol	300 mg	Vitamin K	80 mcg
Sodium	2,400 mg	Thiamin	1.5 mg
Total Carbohydrate	300 g	Riboflavin	1.7 mg
Dietary Fiber	25 g	Niacin	20 mg
Protein	50 g	Vitamin B6	2.0 mg
Vitamin A	5,000 IU[2]	Folic Acid	400 mcg
Vitamin C	60 mg	Vitamin B12	6.0 mcg
Calcium	1,000 mg	Biotin	300 mcg
Iron	18 mg	Pantothenic Acid	10 mg
		Phosphorus	1,000 mg
		Iodine	150 mcg
		Magnesium	400 mg
		Zinc	15 mg
		Selenium	70 mcg
		Copper	2.0 mg
		Manganese	2.0 mg
		Chromium	120 mcg
		Molybdenum	75 mcg
		Chloride	3,400 mg
		Potassium	3,500 mg

[1] Daily Values are based on a caloric intake of 2,000 kcal per day. This listing is for foods for adults and children four or more years of age.
[2] IU = International Units.
Source:
Code of Federal Regulations, Food and Drugs, Title 21, Part 101.9, Nutrition labeling of food. The Office of the Federal Register, National Archives and Records Administration. Washington DC. US Government Printing Office. 2003. Available at http://www.cfsan.fda.gov/~dms/flg-7a.html.

Food Component Definitions

MACRO COMPONENTS IN THE MAIN TABLE

KCAL: Kilocalories; measure of the energy value of a food when consumed; in nutrition, the term *kilocalories* is used synonymously with *calories* and *Calories.*

H_2O: Water (hydrogen oxide); molecular weight 18.016; 11.19% hydrogen, 88.81% oxygen; measured in grams.

PRO: Total protein; sum of the weight of proteins and free amino acids in a food; amino acids are the building blocks of protein molecules and are composed of carbon, hydrogen, oxygen, and nitrogen; each amino acid has an amino (nitrogen) group and an acid group; measured in grams.

CHO: Total carbohydrate; sum of mono- and di-saccharides (sugars) and polysaccharides (starch); usually includes the weight of dietary fiber; composed of carbon, hydrogen, and oxygen; measured in grams.

SUGR: Total sugars; sum of mono- and di-saccharides; measured in grams.

DFIB: Dietary fiber; includes cellulose, hemicellulose, lignin, pectin, and other nondigestible plant components; measured in grams. The main component of dietary fiber is cellulose ($C_6H_{10}O_6$), a nondigestible polysaccharide composed of glucose units.

WT: Weight; the mass of the serving of food measured in grams; food weights less than 5 grams were carried to the first decimal point; weights greater than or equal to 5 grams were rounded to the nearest whole number.

FAT: Total fat; sum of all fat-soluble components including fatty acids, phospholipids, and sterols; composed of carbon, hydrogen, and oxygen; measured in grams.

SFA: Saturated fat/fatty acids; sum of the fatty acids that contain no double carbon bonds; measured in grams.

MUFA: Monounsaturated fat/fatty acids; sum of the fatty acids with one double carbon bond; measured in grams.

PUFA: Polyunsaturated fat/fatty acids; sum of the fatty acids that contain two or more double carbon bonds; measured in grams.

CHOL: Cholesterol; $C_{27}H_{46}O$; molecular weight 386.64; 83.87% carbon, 11.99% hydrogen, 4.14% oxygen; principal sterol of animal fats and oils; measured in milligrams.

ESSENTIAL MINERALS/ELECTROLYTES IN THE MAIN TABLE

Na: Sodium (natrium); atomic weight 22.991; atomic number 11, valence 1; part of salt (sodium chloride); measured in milligrams.

K: Potassium; atomic weight 39.100; atomic number 19, valence 1; measured in milligrams.

Ca: Calcium; atomic weight 40.08; atomic number 20; valence 2; measured in milligrams.

P: Phosphorus; atomic weight 30.975; atomic number 15, valences 3, 5; measured in milligrams.

Mg: Magnesium; atomic weight 24.32; atomic number 12, valence 2; measured in milligrams.

Fe: Iron; atomic weight 55.85; atomic number 26, valences 2, 3; measured in milligrams.

Zn: Zinc; atomic weight 65.38; atomic number 30, valence 2; measured in milligrams.

Cu: Copper; atomic weight 63.54; atomic number 29, valences 1, 2; measured in milligrams.

Mn: Manganese; atomic weight 54.94; atomic number 25, valences 2, 4, 7; measured in milligrams.

Se: Selenium; atomic weight 78.96; atomic number 34, valences 2, 4, 6; measured in micrograms.

Cr: Chromium; atomic weight 52.01; atomic number 24, valences 2, 3, 6; measured in micrograms; in Section 32 only.

VITAMINS IN THE MAIN TABLE

A (RAE): Retinol measured in micrograms of Retinol Activity Equivalents (RAE); $C_{20}H_{30}O$; molecular weight 286.44; 83.86% carbon, 10.56% hydrogen, 5.59% oxygen.

A (IU): Retinol measured in International Units (IU); $C_{20}H_{30}O$; molecular weight 286.44; 83.86% carbon, 10.56% hydrogen, 5.59% oxygen.

C: L-Ascorbic acid; $C_6H_8O_6$; molecular weight 176.12; 40.91% carbon, 4.58% hydrogen, 54.51% oxygen; measured in milligrams.

E (tocopherol): Alpha-tocopherol, the most active form of vitamin E is $C_{28}H_{48}O_2$; molecular weight 416.66; 80.71% carbon, 11.61% hydrogen, 7.68% oxygen; measured as milligrams of alpha-tocopherol (ATE) equivalents. Beta-tocopherol, which is less biologically active than alpha-tocopherol as vitamin E, is $C_{28}H_{48}O_2$; molecular weight 416.66; 80.71% carbon, 11.61% hydrogen, 7.68% oxygen.

B-1: Thiamin(e); usually present as thiamin hydrochloride, $C_{12}H_{18}Cl_2N_4OS$; molecular weight 337.28; 42.73% carbon, 5.38% hydrogen, 21.03% chloride, 16.61% nitrogen, 4.74% nitrogen, 9.51% sulfur; measured in milligrams.

B-2: Riboflavin, $C_{17}H_{20}N_4O_6$; molecular weight 376.36; 54.25% carbon, 5.36% hydrogen, 14.89% nitrogen, 25.51% oxygen; measured in milligrams.

NIA: Niacin, nicotinic acid, nicotinamide; $C_6H_6N_2O$; molecular weight 122.12; 59.01% carbon, 4.95% hydrogen, 22.94% nitrogen, 13.10% oxygen; measured in milligrams.

B-6: Pyridoxal, $C_8H_9NO_3$; molecular weight 167.16; 57.48% carbon, 5.43% hydrogen, 8.38% nitrogen, 28.72% oxygen; Pyridoxamine dihydrochloride, $C_8H_{14}Cl_2N_2O_2$; molecular weight 241.12; 39.85 carbon, 5.85% hydrogen, 29.41% chloride, 11.62% nitrogen, 13.27% oxygen; and Pyridoxine hydrochloride, $C_8H_{12}ClNO_3$; molecular weight 205.64; 46.72% carbon, 5.88% hydrogen, 17.24% chloride, 6.81% nitrogen, 23.34% oxygen; measured in milligrams.

B-12: Cyanocobalamin; cobalt-containing B vitamin; $C_{63}H_{88}CoN_{14}P$; molecular weight 1355.38; 55.83% carbon, 6.54% hydrogen, 4.35% cobalt, 14.47% nitrogen, 16.53% oxygen, 2.28% phosporus; measured in micrograms.

FOL: Folacin; Folic acid, $C_{19}H_{19}N_7O_6$; molecular weight 441.40; 51.70% carbon, 4.34% hydrogen, 22.22% nitrogen, 21.75% oxygen; Pteroylhexaglutamylglutamic acid, $C_{49}H_{61}N_{13}O_{24}$; molecular weight 1216.13; 48.39% carbon, 5.06% hydrogen, 14.97% nitrogen, 31.58% oxygen; measured as micrograms of dietary folate equivalents (DFE).

PANT: Pantothenic acid; $C_9H_{17}NO_5$; molecular weight 219.23; 49.30% carbon, 7.82% hydrogen, 6.39% nitrogen, 36.49% oxygen; measured in milligrams.

FOOD COMPONENTS IN THE SUPPLEMENTARY TABLES

Alcohol, ethyl (ethanol): C_2H_5OH; molecular weight 46.07; 52.14% carbon, 13.13% hydrogen, 34.73% oxygen; alcohol in alcoholic beverages; made from starch, sugar, and other carbohydrates by fermentation with yeast; measured in percent volume and grams.

Amines

Histamine: $C_5H_9N_3$; molecular weight 111.15; 54.03% carbon, 8.16% hydrogen, 37.81% nitrogen; measured in milligrams.

Theobromine: $C_7H_8N_4O_2$; molecular weight 180.17; 46.66% carbon, 4.48% hydrogen, 31.10% nitrogen, 17.76% oxygen; principal alkaloid (methylxanthine) of the cacao bean which contains 1.5 to 3% of this compound; also present in coffee and tea; measured in milligrams.

Tryptamine: $C_{10}H_{12}N_2$; molecular weight 160.21; 74.96% carbon, 7.55% hydrogen, 17.49% nitrogen; measured in milligrams.

Tyramine: $C_8N_{11}NO$; molecular weight 137.18; 70.04% carbon, 8.08% hydrogen, 10.21% nitrogen, 11.66% oxygen; measured in milligrams.

Amino Acids

HIS: L-Histidine; $C_6H_9N_3O_2$; molecular weight 155.16; 46.44% carbon, 5.85% hydrogen, 27.08% nitrogen, 20.62% oxygen; measured in milligrams.

ISO: L-Isoleucine; $C_6H_{13}NO_2$; molecular weight 131.17; 54.94% carbon, 9.99% hydrogen, 10.68% nitrogen, 24.39% oxygen; measured in milligrams.

LEU: L-Leucine; $C_6H_{13}NO_2$; molecular weight 131.17; 54.94% carbon, 9.99% hydrogen, 10.67% nitrogen, 24.40% oxygen; measured in milligrams.

LYS: L-Lysine; $C_6H_{14}N_2O_2$; molecular weight 146.19; 49.29% carbon, 9.65% hydrogen, 19.16% nitrogen, 21.89% oxygen; measured in milligrams.

MET: L-Methionine; $C_5H_{11}NO_2S$; molecular weight 149.21; 40.25% carbon, 7.43% hydrogen, 9.39% nitrogen, 21.45% oxygen, 21.49% sulfur; measured in milligrams.

CYS: L-Cystine; $C_6H_{12}N_2O_4S_2$; molecular weight 240.30; 29.99% carbon, 5.03% hydrogen, 11.66% nitrogen, 26.63% oxygen, 26.69% sulfur; measured in milligrams.

PHE: L-Phenylalanine; $C_9H_{11}NO_2$; molecular weight 165.19; 65.43% carbon, 6.71% hydrogen, 8.48% nitrogen, 19.37% oxygen; measured in milligrams.

TYR: L-Tyrosine; $C_9H_{11}NO_3$; molecular weight 181.19; 59.66% carbon, 6.12% hydrogen, 7.73% nitrogen, 26.49% oxygen; measured in milligrams.

THR: L-Threonine; $C_4H_9NO_3$; molecular weight 119.12; 40.33% carbon, 7.62% hydrogen, 11.76% nitrogen, 40.29% oxygen; measured in milligrams.

TRY: L-Tryptophan; $C_{11}H_{12}N_2O_2$; molecular weight 204.22; 64.69% carbon, 5.92% hydrogen, 13.72% nitrogen, 15.67% oxygen; measured in milligrams.

VAL: L-Valine; $C_5H_{11}NO_2$; molecular weight 117.15; 51.26% carbon, 9.46% hydrogen, 11.96% nitrogen, 27.32% oxygen; measured in milligrams.

ARG: L-Arginine; $C_6H_{14}N_4O_2$; molecular weight 174.20; 41.36% carbon, 8.1% hydrogen, 32.16% nitrogen, 18.37% oxygen; measured in milligrams.

TAU: Taurine; $C_2H_7NO_3S$; molecular weight 125.14; 19.19% carbon, 5.64% hydrogen, 11.19% nitrogen, 38.35% oxygen, 25.63% oxygen, 25.62% sulphur; measured in milligrams; listed only in Section 32 of the main table.

CAR: L-Carnitine; $C_7H_{15}NO_3$; molecular weight 161.20; 52.15% carbon, 9.38% hydrogen, 8.69% nitrogen, 29.78% oxygen; measured in milligrams; listed only in Section 32 of the main table.

Caffeine: $C_6H_{10}N_4O_2$; molecular weight 194.19; 49.48% carbon, 5.19% hydrogen, 28.85% nitrogen, 16.48% oxygen; methylxanthine found in coffee, tea, chocolate, cocoa, and cola beverages; acts as central nervous system stimulant; measured in milligrams.

Carotenoids: Orange-yellow-red pigments, some of which have provitamin A activity; includes alpha-carotene, beta-carotene, beta-cryptoxanthin, lutein+zeaxanthin, and lycopene; measured in micrograms.

Alpha-Carotene: $C_{40}H_{56}$; molecular weight 536.85; 89.49% carbon, 10.51% hydrogen; provitamin A; about half as active as beta-carotene as provitamin A.

Beta-Carotene: $C_{40}H_{56}$; molecular weight 536.85; 89.49% carbon, 10.51% hydrogen; most active/important of the provitamins A.

Beta-Cryptoxanthin: $C_{40}H_{56}O$; molecular weight 552.85; 86.90% carbon, 10.21% hydrogen, 2.89% oxygen; some vitamin A activity.

Lutein: $C_{40}H_{56}O_2$; molecular weight 568.85; 84.45% carbon, 9.92% hydrogen, 5.63% oxygen; carotenoid alcohol (xanthophyll); not a vitamin A precursor.

Lycopene: $C_{40}H_{56}$; molecular weight 536.85; 89.48% carbon, 10.51% hydrogen; not a vitamin A precursor; major source is tomatoes.

Zeaxanthin: $C_{40}H_{56}O_2$; molecular weight 568.85; 84.45% carbon, 9.92% hydrogen, 5.63% oxygen; carotenoid alcohol (xanthophylls); not a vitamin A precursor.

Dietary Fiber Components

Lignin: Coniferyl, para-coumaryl and sinapyl alcohols such as matairesinol and secoisolariciresinol found in various plants (e.g., whole grains, beans, peas); most abundant natural aromatic organic polymer in vascular plants; measured in grams

Pectin: Polysaccharide in cell walls of plants; consists primarily of partially methoxylated polygalacturonase acids; molecular weight from 20,000 to 400,000; measured in grams.

Fatty Acids

Omega-3 Fatty Acids: Polyunsaturated fatty acids with the endmost double bond three carbons back from the end of the carbon chain; sum of available data for alpha-linolenic acid (ALA; 18:3 n-3), eicosapentaenoic acid (EPA; 20:5 n-3), docosapentaenoic acid (DPA; 22:5 n-3), and docosahexaenoic acid (DHA; 22:6 n-3); measured in grams.

Trans Fatty Acids: Sum of available data for trans palmitoleic acid (16:1), trans oleic acid (18:1), and trans linoleic acid (18:2); measured in grams.

Flavonoids:

Anthocyanidins: Sum of available data for cyanidin, delphinidin, malvidin, pelargonidin, peonidin, and petunidin; measured in milligrams.

Flavan-3-ols: $C_{15}H_{114}O_7$; molecular weight 306.26: 58.82% carbon, 4.61% hydrogen, 36.57% oxygen; sum of available data for (+) catechin, (+) gallocatechin, (−) epicatechin, (−) epigallocatechin, (−) epicatechin 3-gallate, (−) epigallocatechin 3-gallate, theaflavin, theaflavin 3-gallate, theaflavin 3'-gallate, theaflavin 3,3'digallate, and thearubigins; measured in milligrams.

Flavonols: Sum of available data for quercetin, kaempferol, myricetin, and isorhamnetin; measured in milligrams.

Flavanones: Sum of available data for hesperetin, narigenin, and eriodictyol; measured in milligrams.

Flavones: $C_{15}H_{10}O_2$; molecular weight 222.23; 81.06% carbon, 4.54% hydrogen, 14.40% oxygen; sum of available data for luteolin and apigenin; measured in milligrams.

Isoflavones: Includes the most prominent isoflavones, diadzein, genistein, and glycitein as well as total isoflavones; $C_{15}H_{10}O_2$; molecular weight 222.23; 81.06% carbon, 4.54% hydrogen, 14.40% oxygen; measured in milligrams.

Coumesterol, Formononetin, & Biochanin A: Compounds that share the estrogenic/antiestrogenic, antioxidant, and antiproliferative activities of the prominent isoflavones (daidzein, genistein, and glycitein).

Coumesterol: The most common coumestan; has a structure similar and competes with estradiol for cytoplasmic receptors in mammary tumor cells; $C_{15}H_8O_5$; molecular weight 268.21; 67.17% carbon, 3.01% hydrogen, 29.83% oxygen; measured in milligrams.

Formononetin: 4-methyl ether derivative of daidzein; reduced to daidzein by intestinal bacteria; $C_{16}H_{12}O4$; molecular weight 268.26; 71.63% carbon, 4.51% hydrogen, 23.86% oxygen; measured in milligrams.

Biochanin A: 4-methyl ether derivative of genistein; reduced to genistein by intestinal bacteria; $C_{16}H_{12}O_5$; measured in milligrams.

Glutathione: Tripeptide; $C_{10}H_{17}N_3O_6S$; molecular weight 307.33; 39.08% carbon, 5.58% hydrogen, 13.67% nitrogen, 31.24% oxygen, 10.43% sulfur; a bioactive component; measured in milligrams.

Gluten: A mixture of plant proteins occurring in cereal grains, especially wheat, and composed chiefly of gliadin and glutenin; allergy to these proteins results in celiac disease and requires a gluten-free or low-gluten diet.

Minerals:

Iodine (I): atomic weight 126.91; atomic number 53, valences 1, 3, 5, 7; measured in micrograms.

Molybdenum (Mo): atomic weight 95.95; atomic number 42, valences 2, 3, 4, 6; measured in micrograms.

Plant Acids:

Oxalic acid: $C_2H_2O_4$; molecular weight 126.07; 26.68% carbon, 2.24% hydrogen, 71.08% oxygen; may bind with minerals and prevent complete mineral absorption; measured in milligrams.

Phytic acid: $C_{18}H_{24}O_6$; molecular weight 660.08; 10.92% carbon, 2.75% hydrogen, 28.16% phosphorus, 58.18% oxygen; measured in milligrams.

Salicylic acid: $C_7H_6O_3$; molecular weight 138.12; 60.87% carbon, 4.38% hydrogen, 34.75% oxygen; measured in micrograms.

Plant Sterols:

Phytosterol: Generic name for sterols from plants; includes stigmasterol, sitosterol, fucosterol, Brassica sterol, and campesterol; measured in milligrams.

Campesterol: $C_{28}H_{48}O$; molecular weight 400.66; 83.93% carbon, 12.08% hydrogen, 3.99% oxygen; found in rapeseed oil, soybean oil, wheat germ oil; measured in milligrams.

Beta-sitosterol: $C_{29}H_{50}O$; molecular weight 414.69; 83.99% carbon, 12.15% hydrogen, 3.86% oxygen; measured in milligrams.

Stigmasterol: $C_{29}H_{48}O$; molecular weight 412.67; 84.40% carbon, 11.72% hydrogen, 3.88% oxygen; measured in milligrams.

Purines: Sum of adenine, guanine, and other purines; constituents of nucleic acids; $C_5H_4N_4$; molecular weight 120.11; 50.00% carbon, 3.36% hydrogen, 46.65% nitrogen; measured in milligrams.

Sugar Alcohols:

Mannitol: $C_{14}H_{14}O_6$; molecular weight 182.17; 39.56% C, 7.74% H, 52.70% O; measured in grams.

Sorbitol: $C_6H_{14}O_6$; molecular weight 182.17; 39.56% C, 7.75% H, 52.70% O; measured in grams.

Sugars:

Galactose: $C_6H_{12}O_6$; molecular weight 180.16; 40.00% carbon, 6.72% hydrogen, 53.29% oxygen; monosaccharide; measured in grams.

Glucose (dextrose): $C_6H_{12}O_6$; molecular weight 180.16; 40.00% carbon, 6.72% hydrogen, 53.29% oxygen; monosaccharide; measured in grams.

Fructose: $C_6H_{12}O_6$; molecular weight 180.16; 40.00% carbon, 6.72% hydrogen, 53.29% oxygen; monosaccharide; measured in grams.

Lactose: $C_{12}H_{22}O_{11}$; molecular weight 342.30; 42.10% carbon, 6.48% hydrogen, 51.42% oxygen; disaccharide composed of glucose and galactose; major sources are mammal milks; measured in grams.

Sucrose: $C_{12}H_{22}O_{11}$; molecular weight 342.30; 42.10% carbon, 6.48% hydrogen, 51.42% oxygen; disaccharide composed of glucose and fructose; major sources are sugar cane and sugar beets; measured in grams.

Maltose: $C_{12}H_{22}O_{11}$; molecular weight 342.30; 42.10% carbon, 6.48% hydrogen, 51.42% oxygen; disaccharide composed of 2 glucose molecules; measured in grams.

Raffinose: $C_{18}H_{32}O_{16}$; molecular weight 504.46; 42.86% carbon, 6.39% hydrogen, 50.75% oxygen; trisaccharide composed of galactose, glucose, and fructose; measured in grams.

Stachyose: $C_{24}H_{42}O_{21}$; molecular weight 666; 43.24% carbon, 6.31% hydrogen, 50.45% oxygen; tetrasaccharide; measured in grams.

Vitamins/Vitamin-Like Components:

Biotin: $C_{10}H_{16}N_2O_3S$; molecular weight 244.31; 49.16% carbon, 6.6% hydrogen, 11.47% nitrogen, 19.65% oxygen, 13.12% sulfur; richest sources are liver, kidney, pancreas, yeast, milk, egg yolk; combines with the proteinaceous substance, avidin, in raw egg white and becomes inactive; older names are vitamin H and coenzyme R; measured in micrograms.

Choline: $C_5H_{15}NO_2$; molecular weight 121.18; 49.55% carbon, 12.46% hydrogen, 11.56% nitrogen, 26.41% oxygen; measured in milligrams.

Betaine: $C_5H_{11}NO_2$; molecular weight 117.15; 51.26% carbon, 9.46% hydrogen, 11.96% oxygen, 27.32% oxygen; measured in milligrams

Myo-Inositol: $C_6H_{12}O_6$; molecular weight 180.16; 40.00% carbon, 6.71% hydrogen, 53.29% oxygen; measured in milligrams.

Vitamin D$_3$ (Cholecalciferol, 7-dehydrocholesterol): $C_{27}H_{44}O$; molecular weight 384.62; 84.31% carbon, 11.53% hydrogen, 4.16% oxygen; measured in International Units (IU) and in micrograms.

Vitamin K (Phylloquinone): $C_{31}H_{46}O_2$; molecular weight 450.68; 82.61% carbon, 10.29% hydrogen, 7.10% oxygen; measured in micrograms.

Sources:

Shils ME, JA Olson, M Shike, AC Ross. *Modern Nutrition in Health and Disease.* Ninth Edition. Williams & Wilkins. Baltimore. 1999.

The Merck Index. An Encyclopedia of Chemicals, Drugs, and Biologicals. Eleventh Edition. Merck & Co., Inc. Rahway NJ. 1989.

Amino Acids and Pathways of Utilization

Indispensable	Conditionally Indispensable	Dispensable
Histidine	Arginine	Alanine
Isoleucine	Cysteine	Aspartic acid
Leucine	Glutamine	Glutamic acid
Lysine	Glycine	Serine
Methionine	Proline	Taurine
Phenylalanine	Tyrosine	
Threonine		
Tryptophan		
Valine		

Some amino acids are metabolized into other important compounds. Nonprotein pathways of some amino acids are listed below:

Amino Acid(s)	Metabolic Product(s)
Tryptophan	Serotonin, nicotinic acid
Tyrosine	Catecholamines, thyroid hormones, melanin
Lysine	Carnitine
Cysteine	Taurine
Arginine	Nitric oxide
Glycine	Heme
Glycine, arginine, methionine	Creatine
Methionine, glycine, serine	Methyl group metabolism
Glycine, taurine	Bile acids
Glutamic acid, cysteine, glycine	Glutathione
Glutamic acid, aspartic acid, glycine	Nucleic acid bases

Source:
National Academy of Sciences. *Dietary Reference Intakes for Energy, Carbohydrate, Fiber, Fat, Fatty Acids, Cholesterol, Protein, and Amino Acids.* National Academy Press, Washington DC. 2002. Available at www.nap.edu.

Abbreviations and Symbols[1]

AIs	Adequate Intakes	Delx	Deluxe
Al	aluminum	DFE	dietary folate equivalents
am	American	DFIB	dietary fiber
amt	amount	dia	diameter
ap	as purchased	dmplngs	dumplings
apl	apple	DRIs	Dietary Reference Intakes
ARG	arginine	drmstk	drumstick
ATE	alpha-tocopherol equivalents	drnd	drained
Avg	average	drnk	drink
B	boron	drsng	dressing
ban	banana	DV	Daily Value
bbq	barbecue	Ed	Edition
Bch-Nut	Beech-Nut	EER	estimated energy requirement
bcn	bacon	enr	enriched
Beg	Beginner	F	fluoride/fluorine
BIO	biotin	Fe	iron
bkd	baked	Fds	Foods
BMI	body mass index	FL	Florida/Floridian
brded	breaded	fl oz	fluid ounce(s)
Brkfst/brkfst	Breakfast/brkfst	flvrd	flavored
brld	broiled	flvrs	flavors
brly	barley	FOL	folacin/folic acid
broc	broccoli	fr	French
brwn	brown	frmla	formula
brwnie	brownie	frstd	frosted
bsct	biscuit	frt	fruit
Bty Crckr	Betty Crocker	fru	fructose
C	carbon	frzn	frozen (commercially)
CA	California/Californian	g	gram(s)
Ca	calcium	Gal	galactose
cal	calorie(s)	Gen	General
CAR	carnitine	Gerber Grad	Gerber Graduates
cc	cubic centimeter(s)	Gldn	Golden
ched	cheddar	Glu	glucose
chkn	chicken	Grbr	Gerber
CHLN	choline	grld	grilled
cho	carbohydrate	Grmt	Gourmet
choc	chocolate	grn	green
CHOL	cholesterol	grn bns	green beans
chpd	chopped	grnd	ground
chrbrld	charbroiled	Grn Gnt Sklt Mls	Green Giant Skillet Meals
chs	cheese	grvy	gravy
cinn	cinnamon	H	hydrogen
ckd	cooked	H_2O	water
Cl	chloride	hckry	hickory
Cmplt Sklt Mls	Complete Skillet Meals	HIS	histidine
cmprt	compartment	Hlthy	Healthy
cnd	canned (commercially)	Hlthy Chc	Healthy Choice
conc	concentrate	hmstyl	homestyle
cond	condensed	hny	honey
Cr	chromium	hp	heaping
crm	cream	hydg	hydrogenated
crmd	creamed	I	iodine/iodide
crnbrs	cranberries	ingrdnts	ingredients
Crnch	Crunch	INOS	inositol/myo-inositol
crspbrd	crispbread	inst	instant
Crt A Ml	Create A Meal	ISO	isoleucine
crts	carrots	IU	international units
Cu	copper	jce	juice
CYS	cystine	Jhnsn	Johnson

jr/Jr	junior/Junior	pcs	pieces
K	potassium	peprni	pepperoni
KCAL	calorie(s)	PHE	phenylalanine
Kg	kilogram(s)	pinaple	pineapple
L	liter	pkg	package
Lac	lactose	pkt	packet
lb	pound	pnt	peanut
LEU	leucine	porterhse stk	porterhouse steak
Lght	Light	pot	potatoes
Lmtd	Limited	prep	prepared
lqd	liquid	PRO/pro	protein
lt	light	pt hlvs	point halves
LYS	lysine	PUFA	polyunsaturated fatty acids
mac	macaroni	pwdr	powder
Mal	maltose	RAE	retinol activity equivalents
Mar Clndrs	Marie Callender's	rd	round
marg	margarine	RDAs	Recommended Dietary Allowances
mayo	mayonnaise	Rd Brn	Red Baron
mcg	micrograms	RE	retinol equivalents
mcrwv	microwave	recon	reconstituted
mct	medium-chain triglycerides	red cal	reduced cal
Md Jhnsn	Mead Johnson	REF	reference code[1]
mdlons	medallions	refrig	refrigerated
mdly	medley	reg	regular
mech	mechanically	rnd	round
med	medium	rstd	roasted
MET	methionine	rstrnt	restaurant
mex	Mexican	RTB	Ready-To-Bake
mg	milligrams	rtd	ready-to-drink
Mg	magnesium	rte	ready-to-eat
MgCl	magnesium chloride	rtf	ready-to-feed
min	minute(s)	rts	ready-to-serve
Min Maid	Minute Maid	S	sulfur/sulphur
Mn	manganese	sauge	sausage
micro ckd	microwave cooked	sce	sauce
ml	milliliter	scrmbld	scrambled
mlk	milk	Se	selenium
Mo	molybdenum	sec	second
mo	month(s)	SFA	saturated fatty acids
mont	Monterey	Sfwy Slct	Safeway Select
Mrngstr Frms	Morningstar Farms	sgr	sugar
mshd	mashed	shldr	shoulder
mshrm/mshrms	mushroom/mushrooms	shrd	shredded
mtbls	meatballs	slcs	slices
MUFA	monounsaturated fatty acids	smkd	smoked
mxd	mixed	spag	spaghetti
N	nitrogen	Spec	Special
n-3	omega three (fatty acids)	spp	species
n-6	omega six (fatty acids)	sq	square
Na	sodium	srvng	serving
ndls	noodles	Stfrs Hmstl	Stouffer's Homestyle
NE	niacin equivalents	Stfrs Ln Csn	Stouffer's Lean Cuisine
nfdm	nonfat dry milk solids	Stfrs Lch Exprs	Stouffer's Lunch Express
Ni	nickel	Stg	Stage
NIA	niacin	str/Str	strained/Strained
nutr	nutritional	strawbrs	strawberries
Nutr	Nutrition	strawbry	strawberry
O	oxygen	strog	stroganoff
orig	original	sub	submarine sandwich
oz	ounce	Suc	sucrose
P	phosphorus	SUGR/sugr	sugar(s)
PAL	physical activity level	supp	supplement
PANT	pantothenic acid	Suprm	Supreme
pckt(s)	pocket(s)	swt & sr	sweet & sour

syrp	syrup	vit E	vitamin E (tocopherol)
t	teaspoon	vit K	vitamin K
T	tablespoon	vol	volume
TAU	taurine	whl	whole
THR	threonine	whl mlk	whole milk
Tndr Hrvst	Tender Harvest	whpd	whipped
tndrlns	tenderloins	whsky	whiskey
tom	tomato(es)	wht	wheat
tr	trace	wng	wing
Trop	Tropicana	WT	weight
TRY	tryptophan	wtr	water
TYR	tyrosine	Wt Wtchrs	Weight Watchers
ULs	upper levels/tolerable upper intake levels	w/	with
		w/o	without
unckd	uncooked	ygrt	yogurt
unenr	unenriched	yr	year(s)
US	United States	Zn	zinc
V	vanadium	&	and
VAL	valine	~	approximately
van	vanilla	"	inch(es)
var	variety	#	number
veg	vegetable(s)	<	less than
vit A	vitamin A	≤	less than or equal to
vit B-1	vitamin B-1 (thiamine)	>	greater than
vit B-2	vitamin B-2 (riboflavin)	≥	greater than or equal to
vit B-6	vitamin B-6 (pyridoxine)	/	per/or
vit B-12	vitamin B-12 (cyanocobalamin)	%	percent
vit C	vitamin C (ascorbic acid)	0	zero/none
vit D	vitamin D	blank space	lack of information

[1] The acronymns and code numbers used for reference codes are explained in the section on *Reference Codes*.

Reference Codes

The reference code is provided in the lower right-hand position for each food in the main table and indicates the source of the data. The reference codes that are 7-digit numbers represent food names and data from the USDA Database for Standard Reference, Release 15 (2002). The alpha reference codes refer to the food companies and restaurants listed below. Data were obtained from these food companies and restaurants, their promotional materials, their websites, and/or the nutrition labels on the products.

Code	Data Source and Location
AMNS	American Natural Snacks, St Augustine FL
AMUN	AmmunoMed LLC, Toledo OH
ANBU	Anheuser-Busch, St Louis MO
ARBY	Arby's, Chicago IL
ARNO	Arnold Foods Company, Inc, Totowa NJ
ATCO	Ateeco, Inc, Shenandoah PA
AUBN	Au Bon Pain, Boston MA
BARB	Barbara's Bakery, Inc, Petaluma CA
BLDM	Blue Diamond Growers, Sacramento CA
BOCA	Boca Foods Company, Madison WI
BRCH	Brach's Confections, Inc, Chicago IL
BRGR	Burger King Corporation, Miami FL
BRYS	Breyers, Green Bay WI
BTTR	Better Than Milk, American Natural & Specialty Brands, St Augustine FL
BUMO	B&M, Burnham & Morrill, Portland ME
BUSH	Bush Brothers & Company, Knoxville TN
CHAT	Chatfield's, distributed by American Natural & Specialty Brands, St Augustine FL
CHCK	Chicken of the Sea International, Inc, San Diego CA
CKFL	Chick-Fil-A, Atlanta GA
CKOT	Chicken Out, Gaithersburg, MD
CLAX	Claxton Bakery, Inc, Claxton GA
CLIF	Clif Bar, Inc, Berkeley CA
CNAG	ConAgra Foods, Omaha NE
COLA	The Coca-Cola Company, Atlanta GA
CORS	Coors Brewing Company, Golden CO
DANN	Dannon Company, Tarrytown NY
DIGI	DiGiorno Pizza, Digiorno Foods Company, Glenview IL
DIHL	Diehl Specialties International, Defiance OH
DOLE	Dole Food Company, Thousand Oaks CA
DRPP	Dr. Pepper/Seven-Up Companies, Inc, Plano TX
DRSY	DrSoy Nutrition, LLC, Irving CA
DSGN	Designer Cookies, Nashville TN
DUNK	Dunkin Donuts, Randolf MA
EDEN	Eden Foods, Clinton MI
EDYS	Edy's/Dreyer's Grand Ice Cream, Oakland CA
EGBT	Egg Beaters, ConAgra Foods, Omaha NE
EGLD	Eggland's Best, Inc, King of Prussia PA
ETHM	Ethel M Chocolates, Inc, Las Vegas NV
FRTO	Frito-Lay, Inc, Plano TX
GBAF	Great Foods of America Brands (GFA)/Smart Balance, Cresskill NJ
GENI	GeniSoy, Fairfield CA
GENM	General Mills, Inc, Minneapolis MN
GERB	Gerber Products Company, Parsippany NJ
GOTZ	Goetze's, Baltimore MD
GTRD	Gatorade Company, Chicago IL
HADA	Harry and David, Meadford OR
HGND	Haagen-Dazs, San Ramon CA
HLCH	Healthy Choice, ConAgra Brands, Inc, Omaha NE
HRSH	Hershey Foods Corporation, Hershey PA
IMAG	Imagine Foods, Inc, San Carlos CA

JACK	Jack-in-the Box/Foodmaker, Inc, San Diego CA
KBLR	Keebler Company, Elmhurst IL
KELL	Kellogg's Company, Battle Creek MI
KFCN	Kentucky Fried Chicken, Louisville KY
KNSE	Knouse Foods, Inc, Peach Glen PA
KOZY	Kozy Shack, Inc, Hicksville NY
LAND	Land O Lakes, Inc, Arden Hills MN
LIBO	Liberty Orchards, Cashmere WA
MALT	Malt-O-Meal, Northfield MN
MCDS	McDonald's Nutrition, Oak Brook IL
MDJN	Mead Johnson Nutritionals, Evansville IN
MICH	Michelina's, Luigino's, Inc, Duluth MN
MILE	Milena's Pizza, Cousins Foods, Chicago IL
MNTM	The Minute Maid Company, Houston TX
MORT	Morton Salt, Elgin IL
MSDA	Mrs. Dash Seasoning Products, Melrose Park IL
MSSM	Mrs. Smith's Frozen Foods Company, Swanee GA
NBSC	Nabisco, East Hanover NJ
NEST	Nestle Clinical Nutrition, Deerfield IL
NRCH	Nature's Choice, Barbara's Bakery, Petaluma CA
NRPT	Nature's Path, Inc, Blaine WA
NSTL	Nestle, Glendale CA
NTRC	NutriCare Products, Burlingame CA
NUWL	Nu-World Amaranth Inc, Naperville IL
NVAR	Novartis Nutrition Corporation, St Louis Park MN
PEPP	Pepperidge Farm, Inc, Norwalk CT
PIZA	Pizza Hut, Dallas TX
PNTA	Pinata, distributed by Don Miguel Mexican Foods, Inc, Anaheim CA
PPTT	Papetti Foods, Gaylord MN
PULS	Pulse, Baxter International Inc, Deerfield IL
PWRB	PowerBar, Berkeley CA
QUAK	Quaker Oats Company, Chicago IL
RDBN	Red Baron, Marshall MN
RSSM	Ross Products Division, Abbott Labs, Medical Foods, Columbus OH
RSSP	Ross Products Division, Abbott Labs, Pediatric Formulas, Columbus OH
SAFE	Safeway/Safeway Select, Pleasanton CA
SARA	Sara Lee Bakery, Chicago IL
SHNA	SHS North America, Gaithersburg MD
SHST	Shasta Sales Inc, Columbia SC
SLIM	Slim-Fast Foods Company, West Palm Beach FL
SMPL	Simple Snacks, distributed by Wessanen, St Augustine FL and Tree of Life, Inc, St Augustine FL
SMRT	Smart Ones, Weight Watchers, Heinz Frozen Food, Allentown PA
STOF	Stouffer's Food Corporation, Nestle USA, Inc, Solon OH
STOR	Storck USA, Chicago IL
SUBW	Subway Restaurants, Milford CT
SYNT	SoyNut Butter Company, Glenview IL
TACO	Taco Bell Corporation, Irvine CA
TRAD	Trader Joe's, South Pasadena CA
TROP	Tropicana Products, Inc, Bradenton FL
TUMO	Tumaro's, Inc, Los Angeles CA
UNLV	Unilever Bestfoods North America, Somerset NH
USAM	Uncle Sam Cereal, US Mills, Inc, Needham MA
VYFN	Veryfine Products, Littleton MA
WASA	WASA Crispbread, Saddle Brook NJ
WLCH	Welch Foods Inc, Billerica MA
WLDW	Wildwood Natural Foods, Santa Cruz CA
WHWA	White Wave Inc, Boulder CO
WNDR	Wonder, Wessanen, St Augustine FL
WNDY	Wendy's International, Inc, Dublin OH
WRTH	Worthington (Kellogg/Worthington) Foods Inc, Worthington OH

Heat, Weight, & Volume Conversions

Heat Measures

kilojoules	kilocalories
1	.239
4.182	1

Weight Measures

mcg	mg	g	kg	oz	lb
1,000	1	.001	.000001	.000035	.000002
1,000,000	1,000	1	.001	.035	.002
1,000,000,000	1,000,000	1,000	1	35.36	2.2
28,350,000	28,350	28.35[1]	.028	1	.0625
453,590,000	453,590	453.59[2]	.454	16	1

[1] Often rounded to 28 g. [2] Often rounded to 454 g.

Volume Measures

t	T	fl oz	cups	pints	quarts	ml/cc	liters
.21	.07	.034	.004	.002	.001	1	.001
1	.33	.17	.021	.011	.005	4.9	.005
3	1	.5	.063	.031	.016	14.8	.015
6	2	1	.125	.063	.03	20.6	.021
12	4	2	.25	.125	.06	59.1	.059
16	5.33	2.6	.33	.167	.08	78.9	.079
24	8	4	.5	.25	.13	118.3	.118
32	10.67	5.3	.67	.34	.17	157.7	.158
36	12	6	.75	.38	.19	177.4	.177
42	14	7	.875	.44	.22	207.0	.207
48	16	8	1	.5	.25	236.6	.237
96	32	16	2	1	.5	473	.473
100.8	33.6	17	2.1	1.06	.53	500	.500
192	64	32	4	2	1	946	.946
201.6	67.2	34	4.2	2.11	1.06	1,000	**1.000**
768	256	128	16	8	4	3,785	3.785

Volume-Weight Relationships

The relationship between volume and weight measures is variable and depends on the density of the food. The weights of 1 level cup of various foods are provided below as examples:

Food	Weight/cup (g)
puffed wheat cereal	12
shredded wheat cereal	49
green beans (snap beans), boiled	125
strawberries, raw whole	144
green peas, canned	170
cottage cheese	210
mayonnaise	224
water	237
pickle relish	240
chicken noodle soup	241
orange juice	249
whole milk	244
macaroni & cheese, cnd	252
peanut butter	256
chili con carne w/ meat, cnd	256

The serving sizes for beverages and some other foods (soups, salad dressings, yogurt, infant formula, medical formulas) are usually provided in fluid ounces, which is a volume measure. The gram weight of one fluid ounce of these beverages and foods varies according to the density of the food. Some examples are provided below in the left-hand box. The volume weight of water is a commonly used reference point for the weight of other fluids. The box below on the right provides the weight of various volumes of water.

Food	Weight/fl oz (g)	Volume of Water	Weight of Water (g)
yogurt	28.4	1 ml/cc	1
coffee	29.5	1 T (15 ml/cc)	15g
water	29.6[1]	1 fl oz	29.6[1]
tea	29.7	1 cup	240
whole milk	30.5	1 quart	960
soy milk	30.6	1 liter	1,000 (1 kg)
cola	30.8		
fruit punch	31.0		
orange juice	31.1		
cranberry juice	31.6		

[1] Often rounded to 30 grams.

Gram-Ounce Equivalents (g-oz)[1]

g-oz	g-oz	g-oz	g-oz	g-oz	g-oz	g-oz	g-oz	g-oz	g-oz	g-oz
001–0.04	044–1.6	087–3.1	130–4.6	173–6.1	216–7.6	259–9.1	302–10.7	345–12.2	388–13.7	431–15.2
002–0.07	045–1.6	088–3.1	131–4.6	174–6.1	217–7.7	260–9.2	303–10.7	346–12.2	389–13.7	432–15.2
003–0.11	046–1.6	089–3.1	132–4.7	175–6.2	218–7.7	261–9.2	304–10.7	347–12.2	390–13.8	433–15.3
004–0.14	047–1.7	090–3.2	133–4.7	176–6.2	219–7.7	262–9.3	305–10.8	348–12.3	391–13.8	434–15.3
005–0.18	048–1.7	091–3.2	134–4.7	177–6.2	220–7.8	263–9.3	306–10.8	349–12.3	392–13.8	435–15.3
006–0.21	049–1.7	092–3.3	135–4.8	178–6.3	221–7.8	264–9.3	307–10.8	350–12.4	393–13.9	436–15.4
007–0.25	050–1.8	093–3.3	136–4.8	179–6.3	222–7.8	265–9.4	308–10.9	351–12.4	394–13.9	437–15.4
008–0.28	051–1.8	094–3.3	137–4.8	180–6.3	223–7.9	266–9.4	309–10.9	352–12.4	395–13.9	438–15.4
009–0.32	052–1.8	095–3.4	138–4.9	181–6.4	224–7.9	267–9.4	310–10.9	353–12.5	396–14.0	439–15.5
010–0.35	053–1.9	096–3.4	139–4.9	182–6.4	225–7.9	268–9.5	311–11.0	354–12.5	397–14.0	440–15.5
011–0.39	054–1.9	097–3.4	140–4.9	183–6.5	226–8.0	269–9.5	312–11.0	355–12.5	398–14.0	441–15.6
012–0.42	055–1.9	098–3.5	141–5.0	184–6.5	227–8.0	270–9.5	313–11.0	356–12.6	399–14.1	442–15.6
013–0.46	056–2.0	099–3.5	142–5.0	185–6.5	228–8.0	271–9.6	314–11.1	357–12.6	400–14.1	443–15.6
014–0.49	057–2.0	100–3.5	143–5.0	186–6.6	229–8.1	272–9.6	315–11.1	358–12.6	401–14.2	444–15.7
015–0.53	058–2.0	101–3.6	144–5.1	187–6.6	230–8.1	273–9.6	316–11.2	359–12.7	402–14.2	445–15.7
016–0.56	059–2.1	102–3.6	145–5.1	188–6.6	231–8.2	274–9.7	317–11.2	360–12.7	403–14.2	446–15.7
017–0.56	060–2.1	103–3.6	146–5.2	189–6.7	232–8.2	275–9.7	318–11.2	361–12.7	404–14.3	447–15.8
018–0.63	061–2.2	104–3.7	147–5.2	190–6.7	233–8.2	276–9.7	319–11.3	362–12.8	405–14.3	448–15.8
019–0.67	062–2.2	105–3.7	148–5.2	191–6.7	234–8.3	277–9.8	320–11.3	363–12.8	406–14.3	449–15.8
020–0.71	063–2.2	106–3.7	149–5.3	192–6.8	235–8.3	278–9.8	321–11.3	364–12.8	407–14.4	450–15.9
021–0.71	064–2.3	107–3.8	150–5.3	193–6.8	236–8.3	279–9.8	322–11.4	365–12.9	408–14.4	451–15.9
022–0.78	065–2.3	108–3.8	151–5.3	194–6.8	237–8.4	280–9.9	323–11.4	366–12.9	409–14.4	452–15.9
023–0.81	066–2.3	109–3.8	152–5.4	195–6.9	238–8.4	281–9.9	324–11.4	367–13.0	410–14.5	453–16.0
024–0.85	067–2.4	110–3.9	153–5.4	196–6.9	239–8.4	282–10.0	325–11.5	368–13.0	411–14.5	454–16.0
025–0.88	068–2.4	111–3.9	154–5.4	197–7.0	240–8.5	283–10.0	326–11.5	369–13.0	412–14.5	455–16.0
026–0.92	069–2.4	112–4.0	155–5.5	198–7.0	241–8.5	284–10.0	327–11.5	370–13.1	413–14.6	456–16.1
027–0.95	070–2.5	113–4.0	156–5.5	199–7.0	242–8.5	285–10.1	328–11.6	371–13.1	414–14.6	457–16.1
028–0.99	071–2.5	114–4.0	157–5.5	200–7.1	243–8.6	286–10.1	329–11.6	372–13.1	415–14.6	458–16.2
029–1.0	072–2.5	115–4.1	158–5.6	201–7.1	244–8.6	287–10.1	330–11.6	373–13.2	416–14.7	459–16.2
030–1.1	073–2.6	116–4.1	159–5.6	202–7.1	245–8.6	288–10.2	331–11.7	374–13.2	417–14.7	460–16.2
031–1.1	074–2.6	117–4.1	160–5.6	203–7.2	246–8.7	289–10.2	332–11.7	375–13.2	418–14.7	461–16.3
032–1.1	075–2.7	118–4.2	161–5.7	204–7.2	247–8.7	290–10.2	333–11.8	376–13.3	419–14.8	462–16.3
033–1.2	076–2.7	119–4.2	162–5.7	205–7.2	248–8.7	291–10.3	334–11.8	377–13.3	420–14.8	463–16.3
034–1.2	077–2.7	120–4.2	163–5.8	206–7.3	249–8.8	292–10.3	335–11.8	378–13.3	421–14.9	464–16.4
035–1.2	078–2.8	121–4.3	164–5.8	207–7.3	250–8.8	293–10.3	336–11.9	379–13.4	422–14.9	465–16.4
036–1.3	079–2.8	122–4.3	165–5.8	208–7.3	251–8.9	294–10.4	337–11.9	380–13.4	423–14.9	466–16.4
037–1.3	080–2.8	123–4.3	166–5.9	209–7.4	252–8.9	295–10.4	338–11.9	381–13.4	424–15.0	467–16.5
038–1.3	081–2.9	124–4.4	167–5.9	210–7.4	253–8.9	296–10.4	339–12.0	382–13.5	425–15.0	468–16.5
039–1.4	082–2.9	125–4.4	168–5.9	211–7.4	254–8.9	297–10.5	340–12.0	383–13.5	426–15.0	469–16.5
040–1.4	083–2.9	126–4.4	169–6.0	212–7.5	255–9.0	298–10.5	341–12.0	384–13.5	427–15.1	470–16.6
041–1.4	084–3.0	127–4.5	170–6.0	213–7.5	256–9.0	299–10.6	342–12.1	385–13.6	428–15.1	471–16.6
042–1.5	085–3.0	128–4.5	171–6.0	214–7.6	257–9.1	300–10.6	343–12.1	386–13.6	429–15.1	472–16.6
043–1.5	086–3.0	129–4.6	172–6.1	215–7.6	258–9.1	301–10.6	344–12.1	387–13.7	430–15.2	473–16.7

[1] Gram-ounce equivalents were calculated on the basis of 1 ounce weighing 28.35 grams.

Main Table for the
Nutrient Content of
Foods

1. BEVERAGES
1.1 CARBONATED, LOW CALORIE

	KCAL / WT (g)	H₂0 (g) / FAT (g)	PRO (g) / SFA (g)	CHO (g) / MUFA (g)	SUGR (g) / PUFA (g)	DFIB (g) / CHOL (mg)	Na (mg) / K (mg)	Ca (mg) / P (mg)	Mg (mg) / Fe (mg)	Zn (mg) / Cu (mg)	Mn (mg) / Se (mcg)	A (mcg RAE) / A (IU)	C (mg) / E (mg ATE)	B-1 (mg) / B-2 (mg)	NIA (mg) / B-6 (mg)	B-12 (mcg) / FOL (mcg DFE)	PANT (mg) / REF
club soda	0	354.6	0.0	0.0		0.0	75	18	4	0.36	0.004	0	0	0.00	0.0	0.00	0.00
12 fl oz	355	0.0	0.0	0.0	0.0	0	7	0	0.04	0.021	0.0	0	0.0	0.00	0.00	0.0	14121
crème soda, french van, Diet Barq's	1			<0.1			44										
12 fl oz	355						<1	0									COLA1
red, Diet Barq's	4			0.0			43										
12 fl oz	355						0	0									COLA2
Diet Cherry Coke	<1			0.1			28										
12 fl oz	355						19	23									COLA4
Diet Coke	1			0.1			28										
12 fl oz	355						12	18									COLA5
caffeine free	1			0.1			28										
12 fl oz	355						12	18									COLA7
w/lemon	2			0.1			28										
12 fl oz	355						12	18									COLA6
diet cola w/aspartame	4	354.3	0.4	0.4		0.0	21	14	4	0.28	0.124	0	0	0.02	0.0	0.00	0.00
12 fl oz	355	0.0	0.0	0.0	0.0	0	0	32	0.11	0.039	0.4	0	0.0	0.08	0.00	0.0	14416
w/aspartame, decaffeinated	4	354.3	0.4	0.4		0.0	21	14	4	0.28	0.124	0	0	0.02	0.0	0.00	0.00
12 fl oz	355	0.0	0.0	0.0	0.0	0	0	32	0.11	0.039	0.4	0	0.0	0.08	0.00	0.0	14146
w/Na saccharin	0	354.3	0.0	0.4		0.0	57	14	4	0.18	0.060	0	0	0.00	0.0	0.00	0.00
12 fl oz	355	0.0	0.0	0.0	0.0	0	7	39	0.14	0.089	0.4	0	0.0	0.00	0.00	0.0	14166
Diet Dr. Pepper	0		0.0	0.0			52										
12 fl oz	355																DRPP1
Diet Inca Kola	1			<0.1			34										
12 fl oz	355						7	0									COLA8
Diet Mello Yello	3			0.2			25										
12 fl oz	355						51	<1									COLA9
Diet Minute Maid Orange	2			0.0			24										
12 fl oz	355						44	0									COLA10
Diet Mr. Pibb	1			0.3			26										
12 fl oz	355						20	29									COLA11
diet soda other than cola/pepper	0	354.3	0.4	0.0		0.0	21	14	4	0.00	0.060	0	0	0.00	0.0	0.00	0.00
w/aspartame - *12 fl oz*	355	0.0	0.0	0.0	0.0	0	7	0	0.14	0.089	0.0	0	0.0	0.00	0.00	0.0	14143
	0	354.3	0.0	0.4		0.0	57	14	4	0.18	0.060	0	0	0.00	0.0	0.00	0.00
w/Na saccharin - *12 fl oz*	355	0.0	0.0	0.0	0.0	0	7	0	0.14	0.089	0.0	0		0.00	0.00	0.0	14537
Diet Sprite	2			0.0			24										
12 fl oz	355						73	0									COLA12
Fresca	2			0.1			24										
12 fl oz	355						59	<1									COLA13
root beer, Diet Barq's	1			0.1			48										
12 fl oz	355						9	0									COLA3
Shasta diet w/aspartame, avg for 14 flvrs[1] - *12 fl oz*	0		0.0	0.0	0.0	0.0	45	<1					<1				
	355	0.0				0			<0.01			<1					SHST6
w/saccharin & aspartame, avg for 12 flvrs[2] - *12 fl oz*	0		0.0	0.0	0.0	0.0	55	<1					<1				
	355	0.0				0			<0.01			<1					SHST8
Tab	1			0.1			28										
12 fl oz	355						12	30									COLA18

[1] Values are averages for black cherry, caffeine-free cola, cherry cola, cola, crème, Doc Shasta, ginger ale, grape, grapefruit, kiwi-strawberry, lime-lemon twist, orange, raspberry crème, and root beer.

[2] Values are averages for black cherry, cherry cola, crème, ginger ale, grape, grapefruit, lime-lemon twist, orange, pineapple-orange, root beer, strawberry, and strawberry-peach.

	KCAL	H2O (g)	PRO (g)	CHO (g)	SUGR (g)	DFIB (g)	Na (mg)	Ca (mg)	Mg (mg)	Zn (mg)	Mn (mg)	A (mcg RAE)	C (mg)	B-1 (mg)	NIA (mg)	B-12 (mcg)	PANT (mg)
	WT (g)	FAT (g)	SFA (g)	MUFA (g)	PUFA (g)	CHOL (mg)	K (mg)	P (mg)	Fe (mg)	Cu (mg)	Se (mcg)	A (IU)	E (mg ATE)	B-2 (mg)	B-6 (mg)	FOL (mcg DFE)	REF

1.2 CARBONATED, SUGAR-SWEETENED

	KCAL	H2O	PRO	CHO	SUGR	DFIB	Na	Ca	Mg	Zn	Mn	A	C	B-1	NIA	B-12	PANT
Cherry Coke	104			28.0			28										
12 fl oz	370						0	37									COLA33
choc flavored	155	329.1	0.0	39.5	39.5	0.0	325	15	4	0.59	0.133	0	0	0.00	0.0	0.00	0.00
12 fl oz	369	0.0	0.0	0.0	0.0	0	185	4	0.37	0.048	0.4	0	0.0	0.00	0.00	0.00	14552
Citra	91			25.0			40										
12 fl oz	370						2	<1									COLA34
Coca-Cola Classic	97			27.0			33										
12 fl oz	370						0	41									COLA35
caffeine free	97			27.0			33										
12 fl oz	370						0	41									COLA36
cola	152	330.8	0.0	38.5		0.0	15	11	4	0.04	0.130	0	0	0.00	0.0	0.00	0.00
12 fl oz	370	0.0	0.0	0.0	0.0	0	4	44	0.11	0.041	0.4	0	0.0	0.00	0.00	0.0	14400
w/higher caffeine	152	330.8	0.0	38.5		0.0	15	11	4	0.04	0.130	0	0	0.00	0.0	0.00	0.00
12 fl oz	370	0.0	0.0	0.0	0.0	0	4	44	0.11	0.041	0.4	0	0.0	0.00	0.00	0.0	14148
w/o caffeine	152	330.8	0.0	38.5		0.0	15	11	4	0.04	0.130	0	0	0.00	0.0	0.00	0.00
12 fl oz	370	0.0	0.0	0.0	0.0	0	4	44	0.11	0.041	0.4	0	0.0	0.00	0.00	0.0	14147
cream soda	189	321.7	0.0	49.3		0.0	45	19	4	0.26	0.048	0	0	0.00	0.00	0.00	0.00
12 fl oz	371	0.0	0.0	0.0	0.0	0	4	0	0.19	0.030	0.0	0	0.0	0.00	0.00	0.0	14130
french van, Barq's	112			30.0			44										
12 fl oz	370						0	0									COLA30
red, Barq's	115			31.0			43										
12 fl oz	370						0	0									COLA31
Dr. Pepper	162			40.5	40.5		52										
12 fl oz	370																DRPP2
Fanta, avg for 7 flvrs[1]	117			32.4			33										
12 fl oz	370						0	1									COLA37
ginger ale	124	333.8	0.0	31.8		0.0	26	11	4	0.18	0.048	0	0	0.00	0.0	0.00	0.00
12 fl oz	366	0.0	0.0	0.0	0.0	0	4	0	0.66	0.066	0.4	0	0.0	0.00	0.00	0.0	14136
grape	160	330.3	0.0	41.7		0.0	56	11	4	0.26	0.048	0	0	0.00	0.0	0.00	0.00
12 fl oz	372	0.0	0.0	0.0	0.0	0	4	0	0.30	0.082	0.0	0	0.0	0.00	0.00	0.0	14142
Inca Kola	96			26.0			31										
12 fl oz	370						0	0									COLA38
lemon-lime	147	329.4	0.0	38.3		0.0	40	7	4	0.18	0.048	0	0	0.00	0.1	0.00	0.00
12 fl oz	368	0.0	0.0	0.0	0.0	0	4	0	0.26	0.044	0.0	0	0.0	0.00	0.00	0.0	14145
w/caffeine	147	329.4	0.0	38.3		0.0	40	7	4	0.18	0.048	0	0	0.00	0.1	0.00	0.00
12 fl oz	368	0.0	0.0	0.0	0.0	0	4	0	0.26	0.044	0.0	0	0.0	0.00	0.00	0.0	14144
Manzana Mia	99			27.0			47										
12 fl oz	370						3	<1									COLA39
Mello Yello[2]	118			32.0			33										
12 fl oz	370						20	<1									COLA40
Minute Maid, avg for 7 flvrs[3]	115			31.1			35										
12 fl oz	370						11	0									COLA42
Orange	118			32.0			24										
12 fl oz	370						14	0									COLA41
Mr. Pibb	97			26.0			31										
12 fl oz	370						14	29									COLA43
orange	179	325.9	0.0	45.8		0.0	45	19	4	0.37	0.048	0	0	0.00	0.0	0.00	0.00
12 fl oz	372	0.0	0.0	0.0	0.0	0	7	4	0.22	0.056	0.0	0	0.0	0.00	0.00	0.0	14150
pepper type	151	329.0	0.0	38.3		0.0	37	11	0	0.15	0.129	0	0	0.00	0.0	0.00	0.00
12 fl oz	368	0.4	0.3	0.0	0.0	0	4	40	0.15	0.022	0.4	0		0.00	0.00	0.0	14153
Pibb Xtra	97			26.0			28										
12 fl oz	370						14	29									COLA44
Red Flash	105			28.0			21										
12 fl oz	370						12	0									COLA45
root beer	152	330.4	0.0	39.2		0.0	48	19	4	0.26	0.048	0	0	0.00	0.0	0.00	0.00
12 fl oz	370	0.0	0.0	0.0	0.0	0	4	0	0.19	0.026	0.4	0	0.0	0.00	0.00	0.0	14157
Barq's	111			30.0			48										
12 fl oz	370						<1	0									COLA32
Shasta, avg for 22 flvrs[4]	175		0.0	43.7	43.7	0.0	45	<1					<1				
12 fl oz	370	0.0				0		<0.01				<1					SHST9

	KCAL	H₂O (g)	PRO (g)	CHO (g)	SUGR (g)	DFIB (g)	Na (mg)	Ca (mg)	Mg (mg)	Zn (mg)	Mn (mg)	A (mcg RAE)	C (mg)	B-1 (mg)	NIA (mg)	B-12 (mcg)	PANT (mg)
	WT (g)	FAT (g)	SFA (g)	MUFA (g)	PUFA (g)	CHOL (mg)	K (mg)	P (mg)	Fe (mg)	Cu (mg)	Se (mcg)	A (IU)	E (mg ATE)	B-2 (mg)	B-6 (mg)	FOL (mcg DFE)	REF
Sprite	96			26.0			47										
12 fl oz	370						0	0									COLA46
Surge	116			31.0			27										
12 fl oz	370						35	<1									COLA47
tonic water	124	333.4	0.0	32.2		0.0	15	4	0	0.37	0.004	0	0	0.00	0.0	0.00	0.00
12 fl oz	366	0.0	0.0	0.0	0.0	0	0	0	0.04	0.022	0.0	0	0.0	0.00	0.00	0.0	14155

[1] Values are averages for apple, grape, lemon, orange, pineapple, pink grapefruit, and strawberry.

[2] Values are averages for original Mello Yello, Mello Yello cherry, and Mello Yello melon.

[3] Values are averages for black cherry, blueberry, fruit punch, grape, peach, pineapple, and strawberry.

[4] Values are averages for black cherry, caffeine-free cola, cherry cola, cola, crème, doc Shasta, fruit punch, ginger ale, grape, kiwi-strawberry, lime-lemon twist, moon mist, orange, peach, pineapple, pineapple-orange, quinine/tonic, raspberry crème, red pop, root beer, strawberry, and strawberry-peach.

1.3 COCKTAILS (MIXED DRINKS)

	KCAL	H₂O	PRO	CHO	SUGR	DFIB	Na	Ca	Mg	Zn	Mn	A(RAE)	C	B-1	NIA	B-12	PANT
bloody mary mix/mild tomato	42	168.0	1.6	8.9	4.7		883										
cocktail, Tabasco - *6 fl oz*	182	0.0							1.31			546					14133
daiquiri (rum, lime jce, & sgr)	259	154.4	0.0	32.5		0.0	83	0	2	0.06	0.010	0	3	<0.01	<0.1	0.00	0.01
6.8 fl oz can	207	0.0	0.0			0	23	4	0.02	0.033	0.2	4		<0.01	0.01	2.1	14009
	112	41.9	0.1	4.1		0.0	3	2	1	0.04	0.008	0	1	0.01	<0.1	0.00	0.01
2 fl oz cocktail	60	0.1	<0.1	<0.1	<0.1	0	13	4	0.09	0.026	0.1	2	0.0	<0.01	<0.01	1.2	14010
pina colada (pineapple jce, rum,	526	121.9	1.3	61.3		0.2	158	2	13	0.44	0.708	2	3	0.04	0.2	0.00	0.12
sgr, coconut crm) - *6.8 fl oz can*	222	16.9	14.6	1.0	0.3	0	184	80	0.07	0.193	1.6	53		0.01	0.04	13.3	14015
	252	91.6	0.6	31.9		0.4	8	11	11	0.20	0.746	0	7	0.04	0.2	0.00	0.09
4.5 fl oz cocktail	141	2.7	2.3	0.1	<0.1	0	100	11	0.30	0.121	1.0	3	0.1	0.02	0.06	16.9	14017
tequila sunrise	232	166.3	0.6	23.8		0.0	120	0	15	1.27	0.030	11	41	0.08	0.4	0.00	0.19
6.8 fl oz can	211	0.2	<0.1			0	21	21	0.04	0.089	0.0	205		0.03	0.11	23.2	14019
whiskey sour	249	160.7	0.0	28.0		0.2	92	0	2	0.13	0.013	2	3	0.02	<0.1	0.00	0.02
6.8 fl oz can	209	0.0	0.0			0	23	13	0.02	0.019	0.2	27		0.01	0.00	0.0	14027
prep from liquid mix	158	77.0	0.0	13.9		0.0	66	1	1	0.06	0.006	1	2	0.01	<0.1	0.00	0.01
2 fl oz mix in 1.5 fl oz whiskey	106	0.0	<0.1	<0.1	<0.1	0	19	6	0.08	0.010	0.1	14		0.01	0.00	0.0	14029
prep from powdered mix - *.6 oz*	169	71.2	0.1	16.4		0.0	47	46	4	0.05	0.006	0	<1	<0.01	<0.1	0.00	0.01
pkt, 1.5 fl oz whsky, 1.5 fl oz wtr	103	0.0	<0.1	<0.1	<0.1	0	4	4	0.08	0.034	0.1	5		0.00	0.00	0.0	14025
whiskey sour mix	55	50.8	0.1	13.9		0.0	66	1	1	0.05	0.000	1	2	0.01	0.0	0.00	0.01
liquid - *2 fl oz*	65	0.1	<0.1	<0.1	<0.1	0	18	4	0.07	0.000	0.1	14	0.0	0.01	0.0	0.0	14028
	65	0.1	0.1	16.5		0.0	47	46	3	0.02	0.000	<1	<1	<0.01	0.0	<0.01	0.01
powder - *.6 oz pkt*	17	<0.1	<0.1	<0.1	<0.1	0	3	2	0.07	0.022	0.1	5		0.00	0.00	0.0	14024

1.4 COFFEE & COFFEE BEVERAGES

	KCAL	H₂O	PRO	CHO	SUGR	DFIB	Na	Ca	Mg	Zn	Mn	A(RAE)	C	B-1	NIA	B-12	PANT
Caramocha, Planet Java	189		4.0	37.0	33.0	2.0	168	160						0.01	0.0	0.00	0.02
9.5 fl oz (281 ml)	285	3.0	2.0			16	385	180									COLA48
cereal coffee (grain beverage)	8	0.1	0.1	1.9		0.2	2	1	6	0.01	0.025	0	0	0.01	0.4	0.00	0.02
powder - *1 t*	2.3	0.1	<0.1	<0.1	<0.1	0	42	13	0.11	0.005	0.3	0	<0.1	<0.01	0.02	0.6	14236
prep from powder w/water	9	177.7	0.2	1.8		0.0	7	5	7	0.05	0.027	0	0	0.01	0.4	0.00	0.02
1 t powder in 6 fl oz water	180	0.0	<0.1	<0.1	<0.1	0	43	13	0.11	0.016	0.4	0	0.0	<0.01	0.02	0.0	14237
prep from powder w/whl mlk	120	161.0	6.1	10.4		0.2	91	220	30	0.70	0.030	52	2	0.07	0.5	0.65	0.57
1 t powder in 6 fl oz milk	185	6.1	3.8	1.8	0.3	24	318	183	0.20	0.022	10.2	229		0.30	0.08	9.3	14421
coffee, brewed	5	235.3	0.2	0.9		0.0	5	5	12	0.05	0.064	0	0	0.00	0.5	0.00	<0.01
8 fl oz	237	0.0	<0.1	0.0	<0.1	0	128	2	0.12	0.017	0.2	0	0.0	0.00	0.00	0.0	14209
decaffeinated	5	235.3	0.2	0.9		0.0	5	5	12	0.05	0.064	0	0	0.00	0.5	0.00	<0.01
8 fl oz	237	0.0	<0.1	0.0	<0.1	0	128	2	0.12	0.017	0.2	0	0.0	0.00	0.00	0.0	14201
coffee, inst powder	4	<0.1	0.2	0.6		0.0	1	2	5	0.01	0.026	0	0	<0.01	0.4	0.00	<0.01
1 rd t	1.5	<0.1	<0.1	<0.1	<0.1	0	53	5	0.07	0.002	0.2	0	0.0	<0.01	<0.01	0.0	14214
café francais, General Foods	62	0.3	0.5	7.2	3.9	0.4	93	3					0				
amt for 1 serving	13	3.5	0.8			<1	129	39	0.09			0					14230
cappuccino flvr w/sugar	62	0.2	0.4	10.7	4.3	0.0	98	4	7	0.04	0.028	0	0	0.02	0.3	0.00	0.01
2 rd t	14	2.1	0.4	1.7	<0.1	0	118	26	0.14	0.016	0.8	0	0.0	0.01	0.00	0.0	14228
decaffeinated	4	0.1	0.2	0.8		0.0	0	3	6	<0.01	0.022	0	0	<0.01	0.5	0.00	<0.01
1 rd t	1.8	<0.1	<0.1	<0.1	<0.1	0	63	5	0.07	0.001	0.2	0	0.0	0.02	<0.01	0.0	14218
french flvr w/sugar	57	0.3	0.5	6.6	3.5	0.0	82	4	5	0.01	0.027	0	0	<0.01	0.7	0.00	<0.01
2 rd t	12	3.4	0.7	2.7	<0.1	0	136	41	0.08	0.003	0.6	0	0.6	<0.01	<0.01	0.0	14229
french van, General Foods	65	0.2	0.4	10.0	7.6	0.2	56	2					0				
amt for 1 serving	14	2.7	0.6			0	76	28	0.05			0					14231

	KCAL / WT (g)	H2O (g) / FAT (g)	PRO (g) / SFA (g)	CHO (g) / MUFA (g)	SUGR (g) / PUFA (g)	DFIB (g) / CHOL (mg)	Na (mg) / K (mg)	Ca (mg) / P (mg)	Mg (mg) / Fe (mg)	Zn (mg) / Cu (mg)	Mn (mg) / Se (mcg)	A (mcg RAE) / A (IU)	C (mg) / E (mg ATE)	B-1 (mg) / B-2 (mg)	NIA (mg) / B-6 (mg)	B-12 (mcg) / FOL (mcg DFE)	PANT (mg) / REF
french van, sugar & fat free,	25	0.2	0.2	5.3	0.4	0.3	65	4					0				
Gen Foods - amt for 1 srvng	7	0.3	0.1			0	72	16	0.06			0					14232
mocha flvr w/sugar	51	0.2	0.5	8.4	6.2	0.4	31	4	8	0.11	0.051	0	0	<0.01	0.3	0.00	0.01
2 rd t	12	1.9	0.4	1.3	<0.1	0	119	29	0.23	0.050	0.4	0	0.0	<0.01	0.00	0.0	14224
suisse mocha, General Foods	57	0.2	0.5	9.4	7.1	0.4	33	2					0				
amt for 1 serving	13	2.2	0.6			0	117	29	0.27			0					14225
suisse mocha, sugar & fat free,	24	0.2	0.4	5.1	0.4	0.6	36	5					0				
Gen Foods - amt for 1 srvng	7	0.4	0.1			0	112	20	0.33			0					14205
w/chicory	6	0.1	0.2	1.3		0.0	5	2	4	0.01	0.022	0	0	0.00	0.4	0.00	<0.01
1 rd t	1.8	<0.1	<0.1	<0.1	<0.1	0	61	5	0.09	0.001	0.2	0		0.01	<0.01	0.0	14222
w/cocoa, whitener, & low cal	34	0.2	0.7	3.2		0.1	20	6	8	0.11		0	0	<0.01	0.3	0.00	
sweetener, decaffeinated - 1 t	6	2.0	1.7	0.1	0.1	0	119	29	0.22	0.050	0.1	0	<0.1	0.07	0.00		14204
coffee, prep from inst powder	4	177.2	0.2	0.7		0.0	5	5	7	0.05	0.032	0	0	0.00	0.5	0.00	<0.01
1 rd t in 6 fl oz water	179	0.0	<0.1	0.0	<0.1	0	64	5	0.09	0.013	0.2	0	0.0	<0.01	0.00	0.0	14215
decaffeinated	4	177.2	0.2	0.7		0.0	5	5	7	0.05	0.023	0	0	0.00	0.5	0.00	<0.01
1 rd t in 6 fl oz water	179	0.0	<0.1	0.0	<0.1	0	63	5	0.07	0.013	0.2	·0		0.03	0.00	0.0	14219
w/chicory	7	177.2	0.2	1.3		0.0	11	5	5	0.05	0.023	0	0	0.00	0.4	0.00	<0.01
1 rd t in 6 fl oz water	179	0.0	<0.1	0.0	<0.1	0	61	5	0.09	0.013	0.2	0		0.01	0.00	0.0	14223
espresso, from restaurant	16	174.1	0.0	2.7		0.0	25	4	142	0.09	0.089	0	<1	<0.01	9.3	0.00	0.05
6 fl oz	178	0.3	0.2	0.0	0.2	0	205	12	0.23	0.089	0.0	0	0.0	0.32	<0.01	1.8	14210
Javadelic, Planet Java	178		4.0	34.0	31.0	1.0	167	160									
9.5 fl oz (281 ml)	285	3.0	2.0			16	385	180									COLA49
Kaffree Roma, Natural Touch	8	0.1	0.1	1.7	0.1	0.1	2	1		0.01			0	0.00			
amt for 1 cup	2	<0.1				0	18	7	0.07			0		0.00			WRTH66
Tremble, Planet Java	178		4.0	34.0	31.0	1.0	167	160									
9.5 fl oz (281 ml)	285	3.0	2.0			16	385	180									COLA50

1.5 DISTILLED SPIRITS

	KCAL / WT (g)	H2O (g) / FAT (g)	PRO (g) / SFA (g)	CHO (g) / MUFA (g)	SUGR (g) / PUFA (g)	DFIB (g) / CHOL (mg)	Na (mg) / K (mg)	Ca (mg) / P (mg)	Mg (mg) / Fe (mg)	Zn (mg) / Cu (mg)	Mn (mg) / Se (mcg)	A (mcg RAE) / A (IU)	C (mg) / E (mg ATE)	B-1 (mg) / B-2 (mg)	NIA (mg) / B-6 (mg)	B-12 (mcg) / FOL (mcg DFE)	PANT (mg) / REF
all types, 80 proof	97	28.0	0.0	0.0		0.0	0	0	0	0.02	0.008	0	0	<0.01	<0.1	0.00	0.00
1.5 fl oz jigger	42	0.0	0.0	0.0	0.0	0	1	2	0.02	0.009	0.0	0	0.0	<0.01	<0.01	0.0	14037
gin, 90 proof	110	26.1	0.0	0.0		0.0	1	0	0	0.00	0.000	0	0	0.00	0.00	0.00	0.00
1.5 fl oz jigger	42	0.0	0.0	0.0	0.0	0	0	0	0.00	0.002	0.0	0	0.0	0.00	0.00	0.0	14049
rum, 80 proof	97	28.0	0.0	0.0		0.0	0	0	0	0.03	0.008	0	0	<0.01	0.00	0.00	0.00
1.5 fl oz jigger	42	0.0	0.0	0.0	0.0	0	1	2	0.05	0.021	0.0	0	0.0	0.00	0.00	0.0	14050
vodka, 80 proof	97	28.0	0.0	0.0		0.0	0	0	0	0.00	0.000	0	0	<0.01	0.00	0.00	0.00
1.5 fl oz jigger	42	0.0	0.0	0.0	0.0	0	<1	2	<0.01	0.004	0.0	0		<0.01	0.00	0.0	14051
whiskey, 86 proof	105	26.8	0.0	0.0		0.0	0	0	0	0.02	0.006	0	0	<0.01	<0.1	0.00	0.00
1.5 fl oz jigger	42	0.0	0.0	0.0	0.0	0	1	2	0.01	0.009	0.0	0	0.0	<0.01	0.00	0.0	14052

1.6 FRUIT DRINKS & FRUIT-FLAVORED BEVERAGES

	KCAL / WT (g)	H2O (g) / FAT (g)	PRO (g) / SFA (g)	CHO (g) / MUFA (g)	SUGR (g) / PUFA (g)	DFIB (g) / CHOL (mg)	Na (mg) / K (mg)	Ca (mg) / P (mg)	Mg (mg) / Fe (mg)	Zn (mg) / Cu (mg)	Mn (mg) / Se (mcg)	A (mcg RAE) / A (IU)	C (mg) / E (mg ATE)	B-1 (mg) / B-2 (mg)	NIA (mg) / B-6 (mg)	B-12 (mcg) / FOL (mcg DFE)	PANT (mg) / REF
berry punch, Tropicana	130		0.0	32.0	30.0		15										
8 fl oz	250	0.0															TROP2
citrus punch, Tropicana	140		0.0	36.0	32.0		15										
8 fl oz	250	0.0															TROP3
concord punch, Minute Maid Juice To	120			32.0	31.0		20	0					0	0.00			
Go - 8 fl oz (240 ml)	250						0										COLA51
cranberry grape, Minute Maid Juice	150			39.0	38.0		20	0					0	0.00			
To Go - 8 fl oz (240 ml)	250						0										COLA53
fruit punch drink, cnd	117	218.2	0.0	29.5	28.5	0.2	55	20	5	0.30	0.496	2	73	0.05	0.1	0.00	0.03
8 fl oz	248	0.0	<0.1	<0.1	<0.1	0	62	2	0.52	0.126	0.0	35	0.0	0.06	0.00	2.5	14267
fruit punch drink, from frzn conc	114	217.9	0.0	28.9		0.2	10	10	5	0.10	0.252	2	108	0.02	0.1	0.00	0.02
8 fl oz	247	0.0	<0.1	<0.1	<0.1	0	32	2	0.22	0.074	0.0	27		0.03	0.01	2.5	14269
fruit punch drink, from powder	97	236.8	0.0	24.9		0.0	37	42	3	0.08	0.008	0	31	0.00	<0.1	0.00	0.00
2 rd t in 8 fl oz water	262	0.0	<0.1	<0.1	<0.1	0	3	52	0.13	0.047	0.3	0		0.01	0.00	0.0	14266
fruit punch, Tropicana	130		0.0	32.0	32.0		15										
8 fl oz	250	0.0															TROP7
Fruitopia, avg for 9 flavors[1]	111			29.3	29.1		79						60				
8 fl oz (240 ml)	250							51									COLA56
gelatin drink powder, orange	41	0.7	7.4	2.7			18	7	2	0.01			30	<0.01	<0.1		
w/aspartame, Knox - 1 pkt	11	0.1	<0.1	<0.1	<0.1	0	1	5	0.10	0.171		0		0.02			14118
grape berry punch, Kool-Aid Splash	116	220.2	0.0	30.7	29.7	0.0	35	0					0				
8 fl oz	252	0.0	0.0			0	13	0	0.05			0					14178
grape drink, cnd	113	221.0	0.0	28.8		0.0	15	8	5	0.28	0.090	0	85	0.01	0.1	0.00	0.01
8 fl oz	250	0.0	<0.1	<0.1	<0.1	0	13	3	0.43	0.030	0.0	3	0.0	0.01	0.02	0.0	14277

	KCAL / WT (g)	H₂O (g) / FAT (g)	PRO (g) / SFA (g)	CHO (g) / MUFA (g)	SUGR (g) / PUFA (g)	DFIB (g) / CHOL (mg)	Na (mg) / K (mg)	Ca (mg) / P (mg)	Mg (mg) / Fe (mg)	Zn (mg) / Cu (mg)	Mn (mg) / Se (mcg)	A (mcg RAE) / A (IU)	C (mg) / E (mg ATE)	B-1 (mg) / B-2 (mg)	NIA (mg) / B-6 (mg)	B-12 (mcg) / FOL (mcg DFE)	PANT (mg) / REF
Kool-Aid powder, cherry w/aspartame	3	<0.1	0.1	1.0	0.0		5						7				
& vit C - .125 pkt (amt for 1 serving)	1.2	<0.1															14127
tropical punch, unsweetened	1	<0.1	0.0	0.1	0.0	0.0	15	7					6				
amt for 1 serving	0.6	0.0	0.0			0	0	3	<0.01			0					14274
tropical punch w/sugar	64	<0.1	0.0	16.3	16.2	0.0	2	28					6				
amt for 1 serving	17	0.0	0.0			0	<1	13	0.01			0					14275
lemonade, from frzn conc	99	221.5	0.2	26.0		0.2	7	7	5	0.10	0.012	2	10	0.01	<0.1	0.00	0.03
8 fl oz	248	0.0	<0.1	<0.1	<0.1	0	37	5	0.40	0.045	0.2	52		0.05	0.01	5.0	14293
lemonade, from mix	103	236.8	0.0	26.9		0.0	13	71	3	0.11	0.000	0	8	0.01	<0.1	0.00	0.02
8 fl oz	264	0.0	0.0	0.0	<0.1	0	34	34	0.16	0.021	0.3	0		0.00	0.01	2.6	14288
lemonade, from mix w/aspartame	5	235.3	0.0	1.2		0.0	7	50	2	0.07	0.002	0	6	0.00	0.0	0.00	0.00
8 fl oz	237	0.0	0.0	0.0	0.0	0	0	24	0.09	0.017	0.2	0	0.0	0.00	0.00	0.0	14290
lemonade, Minute Maid Juice To Go	100			28.0	27.0		80	0					0	0.00			
8 fl oz (240 ml)	250						0										COLA57
lemonade mix w/vit C, Country Time	64	<0.1	0.0	17.7	15.4		13						7				
amt for 1 serving	18	0.2															14128
lemonade, mix w/vit C, pink, sugar free, Country Time - amt for 1 serving	5	<0.1	0.1	1.7	0.0		0						7				
	1.9	<0.1															14129
lemonade, pink, from frzn conc	99	220.6	0.2	25.9		0.0	7	7	5	0.10	0.012	0	10	0.01	<0.1	0.00	0.03
8 fl oz	247	0.0	<0.1	<0.1	<0.1	0	37	5	0.40	0.044	0.0	5		0.05	0.01	4.9	14543
lemonade, Tropicana	110		<1.0	28.0	26.0		20										
8 fl oz	250	0.0															TROP9
lemonade-flavored drink, from powder - 8 fl oz	112	237.0	0.0	28.7		0.0	19	29	3	0.08	0.000	0	34	0.00	0.0	0.00	0.00
	266	0.0	<0.1	<0.1	<0.1	0	3	3	0.05	0.027	0.3	0	<0.01	0.00	0.0	0.0	14297
limeade, from frzn conc, prep w/water - 8 fl oz	101	219.6	0.0	27.2		0.2	5	7	2	0.05	0.000	0	7	<0.01	0.1	0.00	0.05
	247	0.0	<0.1	<0.1	<0.1	0	32	2	0.07	0.012	0.0	0	<0.01	0.00	0.00	2.5	14303
mountain berry, Mad River	103			25.0	25.0		22						0				
8 fl oz (240 ml)	250						28					0					COLA58
orange breakfast drink, from frzn conc-8 fl oz	113	220.3	0.3	28.3		0.0	25	293	28	0.13	0.035	0	138	0.27	0.6	0.00	0.47
	250	0.0	<0.1	<0.1	<0.1	0	338	83	0.20	0.243	0.0	15		2.61	0.18	80.0	14427
orange breakfast drink, from powder - 8 fl oz	127	236.2	0.0	31.7		0.0	11	133	3	0.08	0.019	209	83	0.00	2.8	0.00	0.00
	271	0.0	0.0	0.0	0.0	0	65	60	0.05	0.019	0.3	694	2.8	0.24	0.28	0.0	14408
orange carrot medley, Mad River	88			22.0	21.0		25						1				
8 fl oz (240 ml)	250						82					4500					COLA59
orange drink, cnd	126	215.5	0.0	32.0		0.2	40	15	5	0.22	0.037	2	85	0.01	0.1	0.00	0.04
8 fl oz	248	0.0	<0.1	<0.1	<0.1	0	45	2	0.69	0.007	0.0	45	0.0	0.01	0.02	5.0	14323
orange flavor drink, breakfast type, low cal, powder - amt to make 8 fl oz	5	<0.1	0.1	2.1	0.1	0.1	2	34	7	0.00		150	60	0.00	2.0	0.00	0.00
	2.5	0.0	0.0	0.0	0.0	0	78	16	<0.01	<0.001	0.0	500	2.0	0.17	0.20	0.0	14409
orange gelatin drink, from powder	67	119.0	6.1	10.5		0.0	33	3	1	0.03	0.000	0	50	0.00	0.0	0.00	<0.01
1 pkt in 4 fl oz water	136	0.3	<0.1	<0.1	0.1	0	3	1	0.00	0.007	0.4	0		0.00	0.00	0.0	14397
passion fruit drink, Welch's Orchard Tropicals - 8 fl oz	491	124.0	0.7	122.3	95.2		109						36				
	248	0.0															14141
Smoothies, avg for 4 flavors, Tropicana[2] - 11.5 fl oz	260		4.0	62.0	48.0	5.0	58	250	95	2.25	0.575		60	0.23			0.90
	345	0.0					375		5.16			1750	30.0	0.26	0.30	80.0	TROP19
Squeezit 100, all flavors, Betty Crocker - 6.7 fl oz (200 ml)	90		0.0	22.0	18.0	0.0	15	0					0				
	~209	0.0	0.0			0			0.72			0					GENM2
Squeezit, all flavors, Betty Crocker 6.7 fl oz (200 ml)	108		0.0	26.3	24.3	0.0	0	0					0				
	~209	0.0	0.0			0			0.00			0					GENM1
Tang drink mix, orange	92	0.1	0.0	24.6	22.6	0.1	2	92	0	0.01			60	0.00	2.0	0.00	0.00
2 T (amt to make 8 fl oz)	25	0.0	0.0	0.0	0.0	0	48	42	0.02	0.004		500	2.0	0.17	0.20	0.0	14403
Tang drink mix, orange, sugar free	5	<0.1	0.1	2.1	0.1	0.1	2	34	7	0.00			60	0.00	2.0	0.00	0.00
amt to make 8 fl oz	2.5	0.0	0.0	0.0	0.0	0	78	16	<0.01	<0.001		500	2.0	0.17	0.20	0.0	14404
Tropical Harvest, Tropicana	120		<1.0	29.0	29.0		10						60				
8 fl oz	250	0.0					85					5000					TROP20
tropical punch, Kool-Aid Bursts	90	185.0	0.0	24.4	23.5	0.0	29	0					0				
6.8 fl oz	210	0.0	0.0			0	8	0	0.04			0					14276
Twister, avg for 12 flavors, Tropicana[3] - 8 fl oz	132		<0.8	31.8	29.5		18						49		2.0		1.00
	250	0.0										1750					TROP21
wild citrus, Mad River	111			28.0	27.0		21						2				
8 fl oz (240 ml)	250						46					200					COLA60

[1] Values are averages for beachside blast, berry lemonade, citrus excursion, fruit integration, kiwiberry ruckus, peachberry quencher, strawberry passion awareness, the grape beyond, and tremendously tangerine.

[2] Values are averages for mixed berry, peach, strawberry, and tropical orange.

[3] Values are averages for apple berry blackout, blue raspberry rush, cherry raspberry rampage, kinetic kiwi strawberry, kiwi grape combustion, mango tangerine mambo, orange cranberry clash, orange strawberry banana burst, passion fruit eruption, ruby red tangerine extreme, tropical fruit fury, and wild strawberry dragonfruit.

| | KCAL | H₂0 (g) | PRO (g) | CHO (g) | SUGR (g) | DFIB (g) | Na (mg) | Ca (mg) | Mg (mg) | Zn (mg) | Mn (mg) | A (mcg RAE) | C (mg) | B-1 (mg) | NIA (mg) | B-12 (mcg) | PANT (mg) |
	WT (g)	FAT (g)	SFA (g)	MUFA (g)	PUFA (g)	CHOL (mg)	K (mg)	P (mg)	Fe (mg)	Cu (mg)	Se (mcg)	A (IU)	E (mg ATE)	B-2 (mg)	B-6 (mg)	FOL (mcg DFE)	REF

1.7 LIQUEURS

coffee, 53 proof	175	16.1	0.1	24.3		0.0	4	1	2	0.02	0.009	0	0	<0.01	0.1	0.00	0.00
1.5 fl oz	52	0.2	0.1	<0.1	0.1	0	16	3	0.03	0.021	0.2	0	0.0	0.01	0.00	0.0	14414
coffee, 63 proof	160	21.5	0.1	16.7		0.0	4	1	2	0.02	0.009	0	0	<0.01	0.1	0.00	0.00
1.5 fl oz	52	0.2	0.1	<0.1	0.1	0	16	3	0.03	0.021	0.2	0		0.01	0.00	0.0	14534
coffee w/cream, 34 proof	154	21.9	1.3	9.8		0.0	43	8	1	0.08	0.016	21	0	0.00	<0.1	0.06	0.04
1.5 fl oz	47	7.4	4.5	2.1	0.3	7	15	24	0.06	0.019	0.1	82	0.1	0.03	0.01	0.0	14415
crème de menthe, 72 proof	186	14.2	0.0	20.8		0.0	3	0	0	0.02	0.020	0	0	0.00	<0.1	0.00	0.00
1.5 fl oz	50	0.2	<0.1	<0.1	0.1	0	0	0	0.04	0.040	0.2	0	0.0	0.00	0.00	0.0	14034

1.8 MALT BEVERAGES

Bacardi Silver, Anheuser-Busch	220		0.0	34.7													
12 fl oz	~356	0.0				0											ANBU1
beer	146	328.6	1.1	13.2		0.7	18	18	21	0.07	0.043	0	0	0.02	1.6	0.07	0.21
12 fl oz	356	0.0	0.0	0.0	0.0	0	89	43	0.11	0.032	4.3	0	0.0	0.09	0.18	21.4	14003
beer, light	99	337.0	0.7	4.6		0.0	11	18	18	0.11	0.057	0	0	0.03	1.4	0.04	0.13
12 fl oz	354	0.0	0.0	0.0	0.0	0	64	42	0.14	0.085	4.2	0	0.0	0.11	0.12	14.2	14006
Blue Moon Belgian White Ale, Coors - *12 fl oz*	171		2.3	12.9			6	17						<0.01	2.5		
	356						167							0.18			CORS10
Bud Dry, Anheuser-Busch	130		1.1	7.8													
12 fl oz	~356	0.0				0											ANBU2
Bud Ice, Anheuser-Busch	148		1.3	8.9													
12 fl oz	~356	0.0				0											ANBU3
Bud, Ice Light, Anheuser-Busch	110		1.0	6.5													
12 fl oz	~354	0.0				0											ANBU4
Bud Light, Anheuser-Busch	110		0.9	6.6													
12 fl oz	~354	0.0				0											ANBU5
Budweiser, Anheuser-Busch	143		1.2	10.8													
12 fl oz	~356	0.0				0											ANBU6
Busch, Anheuser-Busch	133		0.9	10.2													
12 fl oz	~356	0.0				0											ANBU7
Busch Ice, Anheuser-Busch	172		1.2	13.0													
12 fl oz	~356	0.0				0											ANBU8
Busch Light, Anheuser-Busch	110		0.8	6.7													
12 fl oz	~354	0.0				0											ANBU9
Busch NA (no alcohol), Anheuser-Busch - *12 fl oz*	60		0.6	12.9													
	~350	0.0				0											ANBU10
Coors Extra Gold	147		1.4	10.7			13	11						<0.01	2.1		
12 fl oz	356						103							0.07			CORS1
Coors Light	105		0.7	5.0			12	12						<0.01	1.4		
12 fl oz	354						61							<0.01			CORS2
Coors non-alcoholic	73		0.8	14.2			10	13						<0.01	1.4		
12 fl oz	350						57							0.07			CORS3
Coors Original	148		1.2	11.3			12	10						<0.01	1.8		
12 fl oz	356						110							<0.01			CORS4
Docs, Anheuser-Busch	165		0.3	16.5													
12 fl oz	~356	0.0				0											ANBU11
George Killian's Irish Red, Coors - *12 fl oz*	163		1.7	13.8			14	13						<0.01	2.5		
	356						114							0.21			CORS6
Hurricane, Anheuser-Busch	158		1.3	10.3													
12 fl oz	~356	0.0				0											ANBU12
Keystone, Coors	122		1.0	5.6			13	12						<0.01	1.4		
12 fl oz	356						83							0.07			CORS7
Keystone Ice, Coors	129		1.1	5.1			13	12						<0.01	1.4		
12 fl oz	356						78							0.04			CORS8
Keystone Light, Coors	100		0.7	5.0			13	13						<0.01	1.4		
12 fl oz	354						71							0.11			CORS9
King Cobra, Anheuser-Busch	166		1.1	12.2													
12 fl oz	~356	0.0				0											ANBU13

	KCAL WT (g)	H₂O (g) FAT (g)	PRO (g) SFA (g)	CHO (g) MUFA (g)	SUGR (g) PUFA (g)	DFIB (g) CHOL (mg)	Na (mg) K (mg)	Ca (mg) P (mg)	Mg (mg) Fe (mg)	Zn (mg) Cu (mg)	Mn (mg) Se (mcg)	A (mcg RAE) A (IU)	C (mg) E (mg ATE)	B-1 (mg) B-2 (mg)	NIA (mg) B-6 (mg)	B-12 (mcg) FOL (mcg DFE)	PANT (mg) REF
malt beverage, nonalcoholic	214	306.2	1.0	47.8		0.0	46	18	25	0.07	0.046	0	2	0.06	4.0	0.07	0.13
12 fl oz	356	0.4	0.1	0.1	0.2	0	28	78	0.14	0.039	4.3	7	0.0	0.17	0.10	49.8	14305
Michelob Amber Bock,	166		1.4	15.0													
Anheuser-Busch - 12 fl oz	~356	0.0				0											ANBU14
Michelob, Anheuser-Busch	155		1.3	13.3													
12 fl oz	~356	0.0				0											ANBU15
Michelob Black & Tan,	168		2.0	15.8													
Anheuser-Busch - 12 fl oz	~356	0.0				0											ANBU16
Michelob Golden Draft,	152		1.2	14.1													
Anheuser-Busch - 12 fl oz	~356	0.0				0											ANBU17
Michelob Golden Draft Light,	110		1.0	7.0													
Anheuser-Busch - 12 fl oz	~356	0.0				0											ANBU18
Michelob Hefeweizen,	176		2.5	16.9													
Anheuser-Busch - 12 fl oz	~356	0.0				0											ANBU19
Michelob Honey Lager,	175		2.0	17.9													
Anheuser-Busch - 12 fl oz	~356	0.0				0											ANBU20
Michelob Light, Anheuser-Busch	134		1.1	11.7													
12 fl oz	~354	0.0				0											ANBU21
Michelob Ultra, Anheuser-Busch	92		0.7	2.4													
12 fl oz	~356	0.0				0											ANBU22
Natural Ice, Anheuser-Busch	157		1.2	8.9													
12 fl oz	~356	0.0				0											ANBU23
Natural Light, Anheuser-Busch	110		0.8	6.6													
12 fl oz	~356	0.0				0											ANBU24
O'Doul's Amber (non-alcoholic),	90		1.9	18.0													
Anheuser-Busch - 12 fl oz	~356	0.0				0											ANBU25
O'Doul's (non-alcoholic),	70		1.2	13.3													
Anheuser-Busch - 12 fl oz	~356	0.0				0											ANBU26
Tequiza, Anheuser-Busch	127		0.9	9.0													
12 fl oz	~356	0.0				0											ANBU27
Zima, Coors	185		0.0	21.4			22	30						<0.01	<0.1		
12 fl oz	356						58							<0.01			CORS11
Zima Citrus, Coors	185		0.1	21.0			23	34						<0.01	<0.1		
12 fl oz	356						60							<0.01			CORS12

1.9 SPORT & ENERGY BEVERAGES

	KCAL WT (g)	H₂O (g) FAT (g)	PRO (g) SFA (g)	CHO (g) MUFA (g)	SUGR (g) PUFA (g)	DFIB (g) CHOL (mg)	Na (mg) K (mg)	Ca (mg) P (mg)	Mg (mg) Fe (mg)	Zn (mg) Cu (mg)	Mn (mg) Se (mcg)	A (mcg RAE) A (IU)	C (mg) E (mg ATE)	B-1 (mg) B-2 (mg)	NIA (mg) B-6 (mg)	B-12 (mcg) FOL (mcg DFE)	PANT (mg) REF
Gatorade mix, lemon lime	58	0.4	0.0	15.2	14.4		96										
3/4 scoop (amt for 1 serving)	16	0.0					32										14131
KMX	118			31.0			74								4.0	0.60	0.00
blue - 8.4 fl oz (250 ml)	252														0.40		COLA14
orange	120			31.0			74								20.0	4.80	5.00
8.4 fl oz (250ml)	252														2.00		COLA15
PowerAde, avg of 7 flavors[1]	72			19.0	15.0		53								2.0	0.60	
8 fl oz (240 ml)	240						33								0.20		COLA17
Light, Aleutian stream/Andean	26			7.0	7.0		49								2.0	0.60	
chill - 8 fl oz (240 ml)	240						34								0.20		COLA16
Propel Fitness Water, berry	20		0.0	6.0	4.0		70						12	10	0.48	5.00	
16.9 fl oz	507	0.0					80						6.0	1.00			GTRD2
Pulse Heart Health Formula	15					6.3	0	0	0				60		0.00		
16.9 fl oz bottle	~507										17.5		0.0		0.00	0.0	PULS1
Men's Health Formula	15					0	0	0	0				60		0.00		
16.9 fl oz bottle	~507										37.8		24.0		0.00		PULS2
Women's Health Formula	19					0	0	380	52				0		1.02		
16.9 fl oz bottle	~507										0.0		0.0		5.00	124.0	PULS3
Thirst quencher beverage	60	225.3	0.0	15.2		0.0	96	0	2	0.05	0.000	0	0	0.01	0.00	0.00	0.00
bottled - 8 fl oz	241	0.0	0.0	0.0	0.0	0	27	22	0.12	0.048	0.7	0	0.0	0.00	0.00	0.0	14382
fruit flavor, low cal	26	232.3	0.0	7.2		0.0	84	0	2	0.05	0.000	0	15	0.00	0.00	0.00	0.00
8 fl oz	240	0.0	0.0	0.0	0.0	0	24	22	0.12	0.048	0.2	0	0.0	0.00	0.00	0.0	14383

[1] Values are averages for arctic shatter, fruit punch, green squall, jagged ice, lemon lime, mountain blast, and infrared freeze.

	KCAL	H₂0 (g)	PRO (g)	CHO (g)	SUGR (g)	DFIB (g)	Minerals — Na (mg)	Ca (mg)	Mg (mg)	Zn (mg)	Mn (mg)	Vitamins — A (mcg RAE)	C (mg)	B-1 (mg)	NIA (mg)	B-12 (mcg)	PANT (mg)
	WT (g)	FAT (g)	SFA (g)	MUFA (g)	PUFA (g)	CHOL (mg)	K (mg)	P (mg)	Fe (mg)	Cu (mg)	Se (mcg)	A (IU)	E (mg ATE)	B-2 (mg)	B-6 (mg)	FOL (mcg DFE)	REF

1.10 TEA

Food / Serving	KCAL / WT	H₂0 / FAT	PRO / SFA	CHO / MUFA	SUGR / PUFA	DFIB / CHOL	Na / K	Ca / P	Mg / Fe	Zn / Cu	Mn / Se	A(RAE) / A(IU)	C / E	B-1 / B-2	NIA / B-6	B-12 / FOL	PANT / REF
brewed, black, 3 min	2	236.3	0.0	0.7		0.0	7	0	7	0.05	0.519	0	0	0.00	0.0	0.00	0.03
8 fl oz	237	0.0	<0.1	<0.1	<0.1	0	88	2	0.05	0.024	0.0	0	0.0	0.03	0.00	11.9	14355
brewed, black, 3 min, decaffeinated	2	236.3	0.0	0.7		0.0	7	0	7	0.05	0.519	0	0	0.00	0.0	0.00	0.03
8 fl oz	237	0.0	<0.1	<0.1	<0.1	0	88	2	0.05	0.024	0.0	0	0.0	0.03	0.00	11.9	14352
brewed, chamomile	2	236.3	0.0	0.5		0.0	2	5	2	0.09	0.104	2	0	0.02	0.0	0.00	0.03
8 fl oz	237	0.0	<0.1	<0.1	<0.1	0	21	0	0.19	0.036	0.0	47	0.2	0.01	0.00	2.4	14545
brewed, herbal, other than	2	236.3	0.0	0.5		0.0	2	5	2	0.09	0.104	0	0	0.02	0.0	0.00	0.03
chamomile - 8 fl oz	237	0.0	<0.1	<0.1	<0.1	0	21	0	0.19	0.036	0.0	0	0.0	0.01	0.00	2.4	14381
iced inst powder	2	<0.1	0.1	0.4		0.0	1	0	3	0.02	0.518	0	0	<0.01	0.1	0.00	0.03
1 t	0.7	<0.1	<0.1	<0.1	<0.1	0	46	3	0.03	0.006	<0.1	0	0.0	<0.01	<0.01	0.7	14366
avg for 4 flavors w/sugar,	80		0.0	19.0	19.0	0.0	0	0					6				
Lipton[1] - *1 1/3 T*	19	0.0	0.0			0			0.00			0					UNLV12
decaffeinated	2	<0.1	0.1	0.4		0.0	1	0	3	0.02	0.518	0	0	<0.01	0.1	0.00	0.03
1 t	0.7	<0.1	<0.1	<0.1	<0.1	0	46	3	0.03	0.006	<0.1	0	0.0	<0.01	<0.01	0.7	14353
decaffeinated, lemon, Lipton	5		0.0	1.0	0.0		0										
2 T	0.7	0.0															UNLV130
lemon	34	0.5	0.8	8.5		0.0	58	3	16	0.14	3.466	0	0	0.00	0.7	0.00	0.22
2 rd T	11	<0.1	<0.1	<0.1	<0.1	0	390	12	0.08	0.038	0.4	0	0.0	0.14	0.04	6.1	14368
lemon w/aspartame, Lipton	5		0.0	1.0	0.0		0										
1 T	2	0.0															UNLV131
lemon w/Na saccharin	48	0.5	0.5	11.7		0.0	151	3	18	0.13	4.373	0	0	0.00	0.6	0.00	0.17
4 T (1/4 cup)	14	0.1	<0.1	<0.1	<0.1	0	367	20	1.28	0.017	0.5	0	0.12	0.03		41.5	14375
lemon w/sugar	89	0.1	0.1	22.4		0.0	1	1	3	0.02	0.682	0	0	0.00	0.1	0.00	0.03
3 hp t	23	0.1	<0.1	<0.1	<0.1	0	50	3	0.04	0.006	0.2	0	0.0	0.05	<0.01	9.9	14370
lemon w/sugar, Lipton	70		0.0	18.0	18.0		0										
1 1/3 T	19	0.0															UNLV135
lemon w/saccharin, Lipton	0		0.0	0.0	0.0		5										
1 T	1.8	0.0															UNLV13
Lipton	0		0.0	0.0			0										
2 T	0.7	0.0															UNLV14
peach w/aspartame, Lipton	5		0.0	1.0	0.0		0										
1 1/3 T	2	0.0															UNLV132
raspberry w/aspartame, Lipton	5		0.0	0.0	0.0		0										
1 T	2	0.0															UNLV133
w/saccharin, Lipton	0		0.0	0.0	0.0		5										
1 T	1.8	0.0															UNLV134
iced, from inst powder	2	236.3	0.0	0.5		0.0	7	5	5	0.07	0.519	0	0	0.00	0.1	0.00	0.03
8 fl oz	237	0.0	0.0	0.0	0.0	0	47	2	0.05	0.019	0.0	0	0.0	<0.01	<0.01	0.0	14367
lemon	5	236.6	0.0	1.0		0.0	14	5	5	0.07	0.431	0	0	0.00	0.1	0.00	0.03
8 fl oz	238	0.0	0.0	0.0	<0.1	0	50	2	0.02	0.019	0.0	0	0.0	0.02	<0.01	0.0	14369
lemon w/Na Saccharin	5	235.3	0.0	1.2		0.0	24	5	5	0.07	0.486	0	0	0.00	0.1	0.00	0.02
8 fl oz	237	0.0	0.0	0.0	<0.1	0	40	2	0.14	0.017	0.0	0	0.0	0.01	<0.01	4.7	14376
lemon w/sugar	88	236.2	0.3	22.0		0.0	8	5	5	0.08	0.673	0	0	0.00	0.1	0.00	0.03
8 fl oz	259	0.0	<0.1	<0.1	<0.1	0	49	3	0.05	0.021	0.3	0	0.0	0.05	0.01	10.4	14371
iced, rtd, Cool from Nestea	82			22.0			68										
8 fl oz (240 ml)	237							89									COLA19
diet, Cool from Nestea	1			0.1			71										
8 fl oz (240 ml)	240							106									COLA21
diet lemon, Nestea	2			0.1			25										
8 fl oz (240 ml)	238							0									COLA20
earl grey, Nestea	65			17.0			26										
8 fl oz (240 ml)	240							34									COLA22
lemon green, Mad River	80			20.0	20.0		23						0				
8 fl oz (240 ml)	240						<1	0									COLA23
lemon/peach/raspberry, Nestea	78			21.0			24										
8 fl oz (240 ml)	240							0									COLA24
oolong w/honey, Mad River	80			20.0	20.0		23						0				
8 fl oz (240 ml)	240						<1	0									COLA25
Peach Frrreezer/Raspbrry Cooler,	87			23.0			68										
Cool from Nestea - *8 fl oz (240 ml)*	240							89									COLA26

	KCAL / WT (g)	H₂0 (g) / FAT (g)	PRO (g) / SFA (g)	CHO (g) / MUFA (g)	SUGR (g) / PUFA (g)	DFIB (g) / CHOL (mg)	Na (mg) / K (mg)	Ca (mg) / P (mg)	Mg (mg) / Fe (mg)	Zn (mg) / Cu (mg)	Mn (mg) / Se (mcg)	A (mcg RAE) / A (IU)	C (mg) / E (mg ATE)	B-1 (mg) / B-2 (mg)	NIA (mg) / B-6 (mg)	B-12 (mcg) / FOL (mcg DFE)	PANT (mg) / REF
red, Mad River	86			22.0	21.0		23						0				
8 fl oz (240 ml)	240						<1					0					COLA27
unsweetened, Nestea	2				0.2		25										
8 fl oz (240 ml)	240							21									COLA28
w/lemon, Nestea	89	218.9	0.0	20.4	18.0	0.0	0										
- 8 fl oz	240	0.7	0.1														14137
inst powder, decaffeinated, Lipton	0		0.0	0.0	0.0		0										
1.5 T	1	0.0															UNLV136

¹ Values are averages for lemonade, peach, raspberry, and strawberry kiwi.

1.11 WATER

	KCAL / WT (g)	H₂0 (g) / FAT (g)	PRO (g) / SFA (g)	CHO (g) / MUFA (g)	SUGR (g) / PUFA (g)	DFIB (g) / CHOL (mg)	Na (mg) / K (mg)	Ca (mg) / P (mg)	Mg (mg) / Fe (mg)	Zn (mg) / Cu (mg)	Mn (mg) / Se (mcg)	A (mcg RAE) / A (IU)	C (mg) / E (mg ATE)	B-1 (mg) / B-2 (mg)	NIA (mg) / B-6 (mg)	B-12 (mcg) / FOL (mcg DFE)	PANT (mg) / REF
Dasani	0			0.0	0.0		1										
8 fl oz (240 ml)	237						1										COLA29
Fruit₂0, raspberry, Veryfine	0		0.0	0.0	0.0	0.0	5	0					0				
8 fl oz	236	0.0	0.0			0				0.00		0					VYFN1
La Croix Spring Water	0		0.0	0.0	0.0	0.0	<1	<1					<1				
12 fl oz	356	0.0				0	<1			<0.01		<1					SHST4
Mt Shasta Natural Spring Water	0		0.0	0.0	0.0	0.0	<1	<1					<1				
20 fl oz	593	0.0				0	<1			<0.01		<1					SHST5
municipal tap	0	236.8	0.0	0.0		0.0	7	5	2	0.07	0.002	0	0	0.00	0.0	0.00	0.00
8 fl oz	237	0.0	0.0	0.0	0		0	0	0.02	0.014	0.0	0	0.0	0.00	0.00	0.0	14429
Perrier	0	236.8	0.0			0.0	2	33	0	0.00	0.000	0	0	0.00	0.00	0.00	0.00
8 fl oz	237	0.0	0.0	0.0	0		0	0	0.00	0.000	0.000	0		0.00	0.00	0.0	14384
Poland Spring	0	237.0	0.0	0.0		0.0	2	2	2	0.00	0.000	0	0	0.00	0.00	0.00	0.00
8 fl oz	237	0.0	0.0	0.0	0.0	0	0	0	0.02	0.000	0.0	0		0.00	0.00	0.0	14385

1.12 WINE

	KCAL / WT (g)	H₂0 (g) / FAT (g)	PRO (g) / SFA (g)	CHO (g) / MUFA (g)	SUGR (g) / PUFA (g)	DFIB (g) / CHOL (mg)	Na (mg) / K (mg)	Ca (mg) / P (mg)	Mg (mg) / Fe (mg)	Zn (mg) / Cu (mg)	Mn (mg) / Se (mcg)	A (mcg RAE) / A (IU)	C (mg) / E (mg ATE)	B-1 (mg) / B-2 (mg)	NIA (mg) / B-6 (mg)	B-12 (mcg) / FOL (mcg DFE)	PANT (mg) / REF
dessert, dry	130	82.5	0.2	4.2		0.0	9	8	9	0.07	0.123	0	0	0.02	0.2	0.00	0.03
3.5 fl oz	103	0.0	0.0	0.0	0.0	0	95	9	0.25	0.046	0.4	0		0.02	0.00	0.0	14536
dessert, sweet	158	74.7	0.2	12.2		0.0	9	8	9	0.07	0.123	0	0	0.02	0.2	0.00	0.03
3.5 fl oz	103	0.0	0.0	0.0	0.0	0	95	9	0.25	0.046	0.5	0	0.0	0.02	0.00	0.0	14057
nonalcoholic	6	100.2	0.5	1.1		0.0	7	9	10	0.08		0	0	0.00	0.1	0.00	
3.5 fl oz	102	0.0	0.0	0.0	0.0	0	90	15	0.41	0.011	0.2	0	0.0	0.01	0.02	1.0	14553
table, all types	72	91.6	0.2	1.4		0.0	8	8	10	0.07	0.149	0	0	<0.01	0.1	0.01	0.03
3.5 fl oz	103	0.0	0.0	0.0	0.0	0	92	14	0.42	0.014	0.2	0	0.0	0.02	0.02	1.0	14084
table, red	74	91.2	0.2	1.8		0.0	5	8	13	0.09	0.615	0	0	0.01	0.1	0.01	0.04
3.5 fl oz	103	0.0	0.0	0.0	0.0	0	115	14	0.44	0.021	0.2	0		0.03	0.04	2.1	14096
table, rose	73	91.6	0.2	1.4		0.0	5	8	10	0.06	0.108	0	0	<0.01	0.1	0.01	0.03
3.5 fl oz	103	0.0	0.0	0.0	0.0	0	102	15	0.39	0.054	0.2	0		0.02	0.02	1.0	14104
table, white	70	92.3	0.1	0.8		0.0	5	9	10	0.07	0.473	0	0	<0.01	0.1	0.00	0.02
3.5 fl oz	103	0.0	0.0	0.0	0.0	0	82	14	0.33	0.022	0.2	0		0.01	0.01	0.0	14106

2. CANDY

	KCAL / WT (g)	H₂0 (g) / FAT (g)	PRO (g) / SFA (g)	CHO (g) / MUFA (g)	SUGR (g) / PUFA (g)	DFIB (g) / CHOL (mg)	Na (mg) / K (mg)	Ca (mg) / P (mg)	Mg (mg) / Fe (mg)	Zn (mg) / Cu (mg)	Mn (mg) / Se (mcg)	A (mcg RAE) / A (IU)	C (mg) / E (mg ATE)	B-1 (mg) / B-2 (mg)	NIA (mg) / B-6 (mg)	B-12 (mcg) / FOL (mcg DFE)	PANT (mg) / REF
After Eight Mints, Nestle	147	2.6	0.9	31.5		0.9	5	9	18	0.24	0.089	<1	0	0.02	0.1	0.00	0.01
5 mints	41	5.6	3.4	1.8	0.2	0	69	23	0.63	0.101		8		0.02	0.01	0.4	19153
Almond Joy Bites, Hershey	218	0.5	2.2	23.0	20.7	1.7	16	44	15	0.32	0.000		<1	0.02	0.1		0.10
18 pieces	40	13.8	8.2	3.5	0.6	4	122	52	0.53	0.072	0.0	47	<0.1	0.06	0.02		19248
Almond Joy, Hershey	91	1.6	0.8	11.3	9.2	1.0	27	12					<1				
.7 oz snack bar	19	5.1	3.3	1.0	0.2	1	48	21	0.24			8	<0.1				19065b
	235	4.0	2.0	29.2	23.7	2.5	70	31					<1				
1.76 oz bar	49	13.2	8.6	2.6	0.6	2	124	55	0.62			21	<0.1				19065a
Almond Roca, Liberty Orchards	70		<1.0	6.0	6.0	0	40	0					0				
.42 oz piece	12	5.0	2.0			<5			0.00			0					LIBO1
apricots, choc glaceed, Liberty	95		0.0	21.0	21.0	0	0						1				
Orchards - 1.2 oz piece	33	1.5	1.0						0.00			300					LIBO2
Baby Ruth, Nestle	101	1.0	1.6	13.7	10.9	0.6	47	9	17	0.27	0.158	0	0	0.02	0.6	0.01	0.07
.7 oz fun size bar	21	4.4	2.6	1.4	0.7	1	83	32	0.04	0.104	0.7	0	0.4	0.02*	0.01	6.5	19111b
	289	2.9	4.5	39.1	31.2	1.7	136	25	48	0.78	0.451	0	0	0.06	1.7	0.03	0.20
2.1 oz bar	60	12.7	7.4	3.9	2.0	2	238	91	0.13	0.297	2.0	0	1.1	0.06	0.04	18.6	19111a
Berry Delights, Liberty Orchards	180		<1.0	37.0	29.0	0.0	60	0					0				
3 pieces	50	4.0	0.0			0			0.00			0					LIBO12

	KCAL / WT (g)	H₂0 (g) / FAT (g)	PRO (g) / SFA (g)	CHO (g) / MUFA (g)	SUGR (g) / PUFA (g)	DFIB (g) / CHOL (mg)	Na (mg) / K (mg)	Ca (mg) / P (mg)	Mg (mg) / Fe (mg)	Zn (mg) / Cu (mg)	Mn (mg) / Se (mcg)	A (mcg RAE) / A (IU)	C (mg) / E (mg ATE)	B-1 (mg) / B-2 (mg)	NIA (mg) / B-6 (mg)	B-12 (mcg) / FOL (mcg DFE)	PANT (mg) / REF
Butterfinger, Nestle	101	0.5	2.6	13.8	10.4	0.5	42	6	17	0.25	0.153	0	0	0.02	0.5	<0.01	0.06
.7 oz fun size bar	21	3.9	2.2	1.2	0.6	<1	80	28	0.16	0.101	0.7	0	0.3	0.01	0.01	5.7	19069a
	293	1.3	7.6	40.0	30.3	1.5	121	16	48	0.71	0.444	0	0	0.05	1.5	0.01	0.17
2.16 oz bar	61	11.4	6.3	3.4	1.7	1	232	80	0.45	0.292	2.0	0	1.0	0.04	0.04	16.5	19069b
butterscotch	111	1.5	0.0	25.6		0.0	111	1	0	0.01	0.007	8	0	<0.01	<0.1	<0.01	<0.01
1 oz (5 pieces)	28	0.9	0.6	0.3	<0.1	3	1	1	0.02	0.010	0.2	35	<0.1	0.01	<0.01	0.0	19070
butterscotch chips	916	1.3	3.7	114.1	115.8	0.0	151	58	9	0.20	0.010	0	<1	0.14	0.1	0.17	0.25
1 cup	170	49.4	41.0	3.9	0.7	0	318	54	0.14	0.053	2.2	0	3.8	0.00	0.03	1.7	19085
Hershey	80		<1.0	10.0			10										
1 T	15	4.0	4.0			0											HRSH1
caramel pecan clusters, Liberty	160		2.0	14.0	12.0	<1.0	35	20					0				
Orchards - 1 oz piece	28	11.0	3.0			10		0.00				100					LIBO3
Caramello, Hershey	208	3.1	2.8	28.7	25.6	0.5	55	96					1				
1.6 oz bar	45	9.5	5.7	2.4	0.3	12	153	68	0.49			136	0.1				19075
caramels	271	6.0	3.3	54.7	46.5	0.9	174	98	12	0.31	0.008	5	<1	0.01	0.2	0.00	0.42
2.5 oz (~10 pieces)	71	5.8	4.7	0.6	0.1	5	152	81	0.10	0.013	1.3	23	0.3	0.13	0.02	3.6	19074
choc coated, Riesen	170		2.0	25.0	15.0	0.0	35	30					0				
4 pieces (1.3 oz)	36	7.0	3.0			0		1.26				0					STOR1
choc crème filled, Hershey	80		<1.0	13.0			30										
Classic - 3 pieces (.74 oz)	21	3.0	2.0			<5											HRSH2
soft & chewy, Hershey Classic	80		<1.0	13.0			45										
Classic - 3 pieces (.74 oz)	21	2.3	1.5			<5											HRSH3
carob	470	1.3	7.1	49.0		3.3	93	264	31	3.07	0.122	6	<1	0.09	0.9	0.87	0.65
3 oz bar	87	27.3	25.2	0.4	0.3	3	551	110	1.12	0.159	4.5	21	1.4	0.15	0.11	24.4	19071
chewing gum	10	0.1	0.0	2.9		0.0	0	0	0	0.00	0.000	0	0	0.00	0.00	0.00	<0.01
1 stick	3	<0.1	<0.1	<0.1	<0.1	0	<1	0	0.00	0.000	<0.1	0	0	0.00	0.00	0.0	19163c
	27	0.2	0.0	7.7		0.0	0	0	0	0.00	0.000	0	0	0.00	0.00	0.0	<0.01
1 block	8	<0.1	<0.1	<0.1	<0.1	0	<1	0	0.00	0.000	<0.1	0	0	0.00	0.00	0.0	19163b
Chiclets	55	0.4	0.0	15.5		0.0	1	0	0	0.00	0.000	0	0	0.00	0.0	0.0	<0.01
10 Chiclets	16	<0.1	<0.1	<0.1	<0.1	0	1	0	0.00	0.000	0.1	0	0.0	0.00	0.00	0.0	19163a
Choc Dreamlets, Liberty Orchards	180		1.0	27.0	24.0	1.0	45	40					0				
3 pieces (1.6 oz)	45	10.0	6.0			15		0.36				200					LIBO4
choc truffles, Liberty Orchards	150		1.0	21.0	18.0	<1.0	15	40					0				
2 pieces (1.2 oz)	34	8.0	4.5			5		0.00				0					LIBO5
choc-coated almonds, Hershey	234		4.9	19.2	15.2	1.8	21	83					0				
Gldn Collection - 13 pcs (1.4 oz)	41	15.2	6.2			5		1.03				0					19084
choc-coated fondant	157	3.3	0.9	34.5		0.6	11	7	27	0.19	0.172	<1	0	0.01	0.2	0.00	0.01
1 large patty (1.5 oz)	43	4.0	2.3	1.3	0.1	0	72	41	0.67	0.185	0.6	9	0.1	0.02	<0.01	0.9	19083
choc-coated peanuts	208	0.8	5.2	19.8		1.9	16	42	38	0.78	0.332	0	0	0.05	1.7	0.11	0.23
10 pieces	40	13.4	5.8	5.2	1.7	4	201	85	0.52	0.188	2.0	0	1.0	0.07	0.08	3.2	19126
Goobers	200	0.7	5.3	19.0		2.4	16	50	46	0.85	0.324	0	0	0.05	2.0	0.11	0.22
1.38 oz pkg	39	13.1	4.8	5.7	2.0	4	196	115	0.52	0.316		0		0.08	0.08	3.1	19105
choc-coated raisins	176	5.0	1.8	30.7	28.0	1.9	16	39	20	0.36	0.127	3	<1	0.04	0.2	0.08	0.10
1/4 cup	45	6.7	4.0	2.1	0.2	1	231	64	0.77	0.153	1.0	17	0.4	0.07	0.04	2.3	19127
Raisinets	185	2.9	2.1	32.0			16	49	20				<1	0.04	0.2		
1.58 oz pkg	45	7.2	3.3	2.7	0.9	2	231	65	0.54			17	0.10				19149
choc flavor roll	259	3.5	2.0	53.8	48.0	1.0	60	56	23	0.40	0.134	0	<1	0.02	0.1	0.16	0.19
2.25 oz bar	64	4.0	0.8	1.0	2.0	1	176	70	0.77	0.147	2.0	3	0.4	0.10	0.02	3.2	19076
Chocolate N'Fruit, Harry and David	190		2.0	27.0	25.0	2.0	30	60					5				
~8 pieces	41	9.0	7.0			0		0.72				500					HADA1
Chunky, Nestle	198	1.2	3.6	22.8		1.9	21	57	29				<1	0.03	0.8		
1.4 oz piece	40	11.7	9.3	0.1	1.8	4	214	83	0.50			25	0.16				19119
Cookies'n Mint, Hershey	90		1.0	11.0			30										
.6 oz bar	17	4.5	2.0			<5											HRSH4
Cow Tales (caramel w/crème center),	110		1.0	20.0	11.0	<1.0	40	20					0				
Goetze's - 1 oz bar	28	3.0	1.0			<1		0.00				100					GOTZ1
Crispy Rice w/peanut butter, Hershey	60		<1.0	9.0			55										
.6 oz bar	16	2.0	0.5			0											HRSH5
Crunch, Nestle	200		2.0	26.0	21.0	<1.0	60	60					0				
4 fun size bars (1.4 oz)	40	10.0	7.0			10		0.00				0					NSTL1
	230	0.5	2.6	28.7	24.6	1.1	59	74					<1				
1.55 oz bar	44	11.6	6.7			6	151		0.22			30					19145

Minerals columns: Na, Ca, Mg, Zn, Mn (top) / K, P, Fe, Cu, Se (bottom). Vitamins columns: A, C, B-1, NIA, B-12, PANT (top) / A, E, B-2, B-6, FOL, REF (bottom).

	KCAL	H₂0 (g)	PRO (g)	CHO (g)	SUGR (g)	DFIB (g)	Na (mg)	Ca (mg)	Mg (mg)	Zn (mg)	Mn (mg)	A (mcg RAE)	C (mg)	B-1 (mg)	NIA (mg)	B-12 (mcg)	PANT (mg)
	WT (g)	FAT (g)	SFA (g)	MUFA (g)	PUFA (g)	CHOL (mg)	K (mg)	P (mg)	Fe (mg)	Cu (mg)	Se (mcg)	A (IU)	E (mg ATE)	B-2 (mg)	B-6 (mg)	FOL (mcg DFE)	REF
dark choc (bittersweet) w/almonds,	200		4.0	21.0	16.0	3.0	0	40				0	0				
Trader Joe's - 3 squares (1.35 oz)	38	14.0	6.0			0			1.44			0					TRAD1
dark choc (semi-sweet)	207	0.2	1.6	24.4		2.3	7	10	46	0.62	0.203	<1	0	0.01	0.3	0.00	0.03
1.45 oz bar	41	14.0	8.2	4.6	0.4	0	119	60	1.13	0.235	1.1	8	0.5	0.10	0.02	1.2	19081
Ethel M	210		2.0	24.0	20.0	2.0	0	0				0	0				
1.38 oz bar	39	13.0	8.0			5			0.72			0	0.03				ETHM1
Special Dark, Hershey	388	0.7	4.0	43.4	34.7	4.7	4	22	23	0.01	0.000		0	0.00	0.0	0.00	0.00
2.6 oz bar	73	23.7	14.0	3.8	0.3	4	366	37	1.55	0.015	0.2	44	0.1	0.01	0.00	0.0	19164
dark choc (semi-sweet) chips	805	1.2	7.1	106.0	95.6	9.9	18	54	193	2.72	1.344	2	0	0.09	0.7	0.00	0.18
1 cup (6 oz bag)	168	50.4	29.8	16.7	1.6	0	613	222	5.26	1.176	5.2	35	2.0	0.15	0.06	5.0	19080
Demet's Turtles, Nestle	825	10.4	10.9	98.6			160	269	88					0.26	0.6		
6 oz pkg	170	47.3	18.4	18.8	7.9	37	524		2.31			277		0.41			19158
Drops, Hershey	100		0.0	24.0			15										
9 pieces	26	0.0	0.0			0											HRSH6
Fifth Avenue, Hershey	270	1.3	4.9	35.1	26.4	1.7	126	41	35	0.63	0.028	6	<1	0.08	2.2	0.06	0.30
2 oz bar	56	13.4	3.7	5.9	2.8	3	194	79	0.67	0.118	0.3	31	<0.1	0.05	0.06	24.1	19098
fondant, homemade	60	1.1	0.0	14.9		0.0	3	0	0	0.01	0.002	0	0	<0.01	<0.1	0.00	<0.01
.56 oz piece	16	0.0	0.0	0.0	0.0	0	1	<1	0.01	0.006	0.1	0	0.0	<0.01	<0.01	0.0	19099
fruit chocolates, classic, Liberty	170		1.0	32.0	26.0	<1.0	45						0				
Orchards - *3 pieces*	45	6.0	2.5						0.00			0					LIBO7
fruit chocolates, tropical, Liberty	180		1.0	31.0	25.0	<1.0	45	0					0				
Orchards - *3 pieces*	45	7.0	3.0			0			0.00			0					LIBO6
Fruit Parfaits, Liberty Orchards	140		0.0	36.0	37.0	0.0	65	0					0				
3 pieces	42	0.0	0.0	0.0	0.0	0			0.00			0					LIBO8
fudge, homemade	70	1.6	0.4	13.0		0.3	10	8	6	0.09	0.034	8	<1	<0.01	<0.1	0.01	0.02
choc - *.6 oz piece*	17	1.8	1.1	0.6	0.1	3	23	13	0.12	0.043	0.3	32	<0.1	0.01	<0.01	0.3	19100
choc marshmallow	104	1.6	0.7	14.8		0.5	21	11	10	0.17	0.104	17	<1	0.01	0.1	0.01	0.03
w/nuts - *.78 oz piece*	22	4.6	2.2	1.2	0.9	5	37	19	0.25	0.074	0.4	73	0.2	0.02	0.01	1.8	19301
choc w/nuts	89	1.3	0.8	13.0		0.5	10	11	10	0.18	0.133	7	<1	0.01	0.1	0.01	0.04
.67 oz piece	19	3.7	1.2	0.8	1.4	2	36	22	0.20	0.088	0.4	32	0.1	0.02	0.02	3.2	19101
van	62	1.6	0.2	13.2		0.0	11	6	1	0.02	0.002	8	<1	<0.01	<0.1	0.01	0.02
.56 oz piece	16	0.9	0.5	0.2	<0.1	3	8	5	0.01	0.006	0.2	32	<0.1	0.01	<0.01	0.2	19103
van w/nuts	66	1.1	0.5	11.2		0.1	9	7	4	0.08	0.072	5	<1	0.01	<0.1	0.01	0.03
.53 oz piece	15	2.1	0.6	0.4	1.0	2	16	11	0.07	0.038	0.3	23	0.1	0.01	0.01	1.8	19104
Good & Plenty, Hershey	60		0.0	14.0			40										
snack size box	17	0.0	0.0			0											HRSH7
Good 'n Fruity, Hershey	60		0.0	15.0			10										
snack size box	17	0.0	0.0			0											HRSH8
gum drops	139	0.4	0.0	35.6		0.0	16	1	<1	0.00	0.004	0	0	0.00	<0.1	0.00	<0.01
10 gum drops	36	0.0	0.0	0.0	0.0	0	2	<1	0.14	0.004	0.2	0	0.0	<0.01	0.00	0.0	19106b
gummy bears	85	0.2	0.0	21.8		CHOL	10	1	<1	0.00	0.002	0	0	0.00	<0.1	0.00	<0.01
10 pieces	22	0.0	0.0	0.0	0.0	0	1	<1	0.09	0.003	0.1	0	0.0	0.00	0.00	0.0	19106a
halvah	230	1.8	6.1	29.6		2.2	96	16	107	2.12	0.428	0	<1	0.21	1.4	0.02	0.09
1.75 oz bar	49	10.5	2.0	4.0	4.2	0	92	297	2.22	0.589	5.6	1	1.4	0.04	0.17	31.9	19117
hard candy	112	0.4	0.0	27.8	17.8	0.0	11	1	1	<0.01	0.003	0	0	<0.01	<0.1	0.00	<0.01
1 oz (5 pieces)	28	0.1	0.0	0.0	0.0	0	1	1	0.09	0.008	0.2	0	0.0	<0.01	<0.01	0.0	19107
Heath Bar, Hershey	50		0.0	6.0			35										
.33 oz snack bar	9	3.0	1.0			<5											HRSH9
Heath Bites, Hershey	207	0.3	1.5	24.7	23.4	0.8	96	34	2	0.04	0.000		<1	0.01	<0.1		<0.01
15 pieces	39	11.8	6.1	3.4	1.0	7	82	28	0.30	0.012	0.0	90	<0.1	0.04	0.00		19243
Hi-C orange slices w/vit C, Brach	150		0.0	38.0	30.0	0.0	10	0					60				
3 pieces (1.6 oz)	45	0.0	0.0			0			0.00			0					BRAC1
Hugs, Hershey	25		0.0	3.0			0										
.16 oz piece	4.6	1.5	1.0			0											HRSH11
Hundred Grand, Nestle	200	2.2	2.1	30.4		0.6	89	49	10	0.33	0.107	10	<1	0.15	1.6	0.17	0.14
1.5 oz bar	43	7.8	4.8	2.5	0.3	8	83	51	0.13	0.050	2.0	35	0.2	0.20	0.17	56.3	19144
jelly beans	103	1.8	0.0	26.1		0.0	7	1	1	0.01	0.010	0	0	0.00	0.0	0.00	0.00
1 oz (10 large or 25 small)	28	0.1	<0.1	0.1	<0.1	0	10	1	0.31	0.008	0.2	0	0.0	0.00	0.00	0.0	19108
jelly candy, Chuckles	70		0.0	18.0			15										
2 pieces (.78 oz)	22	0.0	0.0			0											HRSH12
Jolly Rancher hard candy	70		0.0	17.0			10										
2 pieces (.6 oz)	17	0.0	0.0			0											HRSH13

	KCAL	H2O (g)	PRO (g)	CHO (g)	SUGR (g)	DFIB (g)	Na (mg)	Ca (mg)	Mg (mg)	Zn (mg)	Mn (mg)	A (mcg RAE)	C (mg)	B-1 (mg)	NIA (mg)	B-12 (mcg)	PANT (mg)
	WT (g)	FAT (g)	SFA (g)	MUFA (g)	PUFA (g)	CHOL (mg)	K (mg)	P (mg)	Fe (mg)	Cu (mg)	Se (mcg)	A (IU)	E (mg ATE)	B-2 (mg)	B-6 (mg)	FOL (mcg DFE)	REF
lollipop	60		0.0	16.0			10										
.6 oz lollipop	17	0.0	0.0			0											HRSH14
Jujubes, Chuckles	80		0.0	21.0			20										
7 pieces (.88 oz)	25	0.0	0.0			0											HRSH15
Heide	100		0.0	24.0			95										
45 pieces (1.1 oz)	31	0.0	0.0			0											HRSH16
Jujyfruits, Hershey	80		0.0	20.0			20										
.84 oz	24	0.0	0.0			0											HRSH17
Kisses, Hershey	25		0.0	3.0			0										
.16 oz piece	4.5	1.5	1.0			0											HRSH19
mini, Hershey	80		1.0	9.0			15										
11 pieces (.53 oz)	15	4.5	3.0			<5											HRSH20
w/almonds, Hershey	25		0.0	3.0			0										
.16 oz piece	4.5	1.5	1.0			0											HRSH18
Kit Kat Bites, Hershey	199	0.4	2.5	25.2	19.3	0.9	26	51	0	0.00	0.000		<1	0.01	<0.1		0.00
15 pieces	39	10.3	6.7	1.8	0.2	3	116	37	0.34	0.000	0.0	33	<0.1	0.06	0.00		19237
Kit Kat Wafer, Hershey	403	0.9	5.0	50.1	40.9	1.5	51	105	2	0.07	0.000	14	1	0.04	0.2	0.16	0.04
2.8 oz bar	78	21.1	13.6	3.7	0.4	7	226	88	0.66	0.016	3.7	70	0.1	0.13	0.01	2.3	19109
Krackel, Hershey	287	0.7	3.7	35.8	29.4	1.2	110	88	7	0.27	0.000		<1	0.03	0.1		0.24
2 oz bar	56	14.9	8.9	3.5	0.3	6	182	69	0.59	0.011	2.0	57	<0.1	0.11	0.02		19110
M&M's Peanut, M&M/Mars	253	0.9	4.6	29.6	24.9	1.7	24	49	37	1.18	0.342	13	<1	0.05	2.0	0.08	0.27
1.74 oz pkg (~25 pieces)	49	12.9	5.1	5.4	2.1	4	170	114	0.56	0.261	1.9	46	1.3	0.08	0.04	18.6	19140
M&M's Plain, M&M/Mars	236	0.8	2.1	34.2	30.6	1.2	29	50	12	0.29	0.070	10	<1	0.02	0.1	0.08	0.09
1.69 oz pkg (~69 pieces)	48	10.1	6.3	3.2	0.3	7	80	46	0.53	0.091	1.1	34	0.3	0.07	0.01	1.4	19141
milk choc mini baking bits,	71	0.3	0.7	9.6	8.7	0.4	10	16					<1				
M&M/Mars - .5 oz	14	3.3	2.1			2			0.17			32					19146
mini, M&M/Mars	209	1.0	2.0	28.2		1.1	29	49					<1				
1.5 oz	42	9.8	6.1			6			0.52			94				2.1	19157
semi-sweet choc mini baking	73	0.2	0.6	9.2	7.4	0.9	0	5	15	0.21	0.103	1	0	0.01	0.1	0.00	0.01
bits, M&M/Mars - 1 T	14	3.7	2.2	1.2	0.1	<1	47	17	0.41	0.090		10	0.1	0.01	0.01	3.9	19139
Mars Almond	234	2.3	4.1	31.4	26.1	1.0	85	84	36	0.56	0.184	24	<1	0.02	0.5	0.18	0.20
1.76 oz bar	50	11.5	3.6	5.3	2.0	9	163	117	0.55	0.125	0.8	94	2.3	0.16	0.03	9.5	19115
Marshmallow	23	1.2	0.1	5.8	4.0	0.0	3	0	<1	<0.01	0.001	0	0	<0.01	<0.1	0.00	<0.01
miniature - 10 pieces	7	<0.1	<0.1	<0.1	<0.1	0	<1	1	0.02	0.007	0.1	<1	0.0	<0.01	0.00	0.1	19116b
reg	23	1.2	0.1	5.8	4.0	0.0	3	0	<1	<0.01	0.001	0	0	<0.01	<0.1	0.00	<0.01
1 marshmallow	7	<0.1	<0.1	<0.1	<0.1	0	<1	1	0.02	0.007	0.1	<1	0.0	<0.01	0.00	0.1	19116c
Mexican Hats, Hershey	100		0.0	24.0			170										
9 pieces (1 oz)	29	0.0	0.0			0											HRSH21
milk choc	226	0.6	3.0	26.0		1.5	36	84	26	0.61	0.132	20	<1	0.03	0.1	0.17	0.19
1.55 oz bar	44	13.5	8.1	4.4	0.5	10	169	95	0.61	0.169	1.7	73	0.5	0.13	0.02	3.5	19120a
milk choc chips	862	2.2	11.6	99.5		5.7	138	321	101	2.32	0.502	77	1	0.13	0.5	0.66	0.71
1 cup	168	51.6	31.0	16.7	1.8	37	647	363	2.34	0.647	6.6	277	2.1	0.51	0.07	13.4	19120b
milk choc eggs, candy-coated,	90		1.0	12.0			10										
Hershey - 4 pieces (.63 oz)	18	4.0	2.5			<5											HRSH22
milk choc w/almond bites, Hershey	215	0.5	3.8	19.9	17.4	1.4	29	86	23	0.52	0.004		1	0.03	0.2		0.18
17 pieces	39	13.9	6.8	5.6	0.9	7	184	89	0.59	0.078	1.3	69	0.2	0.15	0.03		19236
milk choc w/almonds	231	0.7	4.0	23.4	19.3	2.7	33	99	40	0.59	0.275	5	<1	0.03	0.3	0.15	0.19
1.55 oz bar	44	15.1	7.5	5.9	1.0	8	195	116	0.72	0.186	1.8	33	0.8	0.19	0.02	5.3	19132
Golden Collection, Hershey	450		10.0	36.0	30.0	3.0	50	150					0				
2.8 oz pkg	78	30.0	13.0			10		1.44									19130
milk choc w/rice cereal	218	0.8	2.8	27.9	24.2	1.4	64	75	22	0.49	0.140	7	<1	0.03	0.2	0.15	0.26
1.55 oz bar	44	11.7	7.0	3.8	0.3	8	151	85	0.33	0.137	2.4	25	0.5	0.13	0.03	4.0	19134
Milk Duds, Hershey	90		<1.0	15.0			40										
7 pieces (.74 oz)	21	3.5	1.0			0											HRSH23
Milky Way, M&M/Mars	76	1.1	0.8	12.9	10.9	0.3	43	23	6	0.13	0.042	6	<1	0.01	0.1	0.06	0.05
.6 oz snack bar	18	2.9	1.4	1.1	0.1	3	43	26	0.14	0.027	1.0	19	0.1	0.04	0.01	1.8	19135b
	254	3.8	2.7	43.0	36.4	1.0	144	78	20	0.43	0.141	19	1	0.02	0.1	0.19	0.18
2.1 oz bar	60	9.7	4.7	3.6	0.4	8	145	86	0.46	0.090	3.4	65	0.4	0.13	0.03	6.0	19135a
Mounds, Hershey	258	4.8	2.4	31.1	24.5	2.0	77	11	0	0.00	0.000	1	<1	0.00	0.0	0.00	0.00
1.9 oz bar	53	14.1	10.9	0.2	0.1	1	170	0	1.11	0.000	0.0	10	<0.1	0.00	0.00		19142
Mr. Goodbar, Hershey	264	0.2	5.0	26.6	23.1	1.9	20	54	23	0.46	0.000	14	<1	0.07	1.7	0.12	0.21
1.75 oz bar	49	16.3	6.9	5.3	2.2	5	193	80	0.68	0.083	0.0	61	<0.1	0.07	0.03		19143

	KCAL / WT (g)	H₂O (g) / FAT (g)	PRO (g) / SFA (g)	CHO (g) / MUFA (g)	SUGR (g) / PUFA (g)	DFIB (g) / CHOL (mg)	Na (mg) / K (mg)	Ca (mg) / P (mg)	Mg (mg) / Fe (mg)	Zn (mg) / Cu (mg)	Mn (mg) / Se (mcg)	A (mcg RAE) / A (IU)	C (mg) / E (mg ATE)	B-1 (mg) / B-2 (mg)	NIA (mg) / B-6 (mg)	B-12 (mcg) / FOL (mcg DFE)	PANT (mg) / REF
Nibs, cherry, Hershey	139	6.0	0.9	31.7	20.5	0.2	78	3				0					
27 pieces	40	1.1	0.2	0.8	0.1	0	15	10	0.11			0	<0.1				19092
licorice	35		0.0	9.0			60										
8 pieces (.49 oz pkg)	14	0.0	0.0			0											HRSH25
Nuggets, cookies 'n crème, Hershey	45		<1.0	5.0			20										
.35 oz piece	10	2.5	1.5			0											HRSH31
cookies 'n mint, Hershey	50		<1.0	6.0			15										
.35 oz piece	10	2.5	1.0			0											HRSH32
dark choc w/almonds, Hershey	50		<1.0	5.0			0										
.35 oz piece	10	3.5	1.5			0											HRSH26
milk choc, Hershey	50		<1.0	6.0			10										
.35 oz piece	10	3.0	2.0			0											HRSH30
milk choc w/almonds & toffee, Hershey - *.35 oz piece*	50		<1.0	5.0			10										
	10	3.5	1.5			<5											HRSH27
milk choc w/almonds, Hershey	60		<1.0	5.0			5										
.35 oz piece	10	3.5	1.5			0											HRSH28
milk choc w/raisins & almonds, Hershey - *.35 oz piece*	50		<1.0	6.0			10										
	10	2.5	1.5			0											HRSH29
Oh Henry!, Nestle	246	3.4	6.2	36.9		2.0	135	62	35	0.69	0.283	5	<1	0.01	1.6	0.12	0.27
2 oz bar	57	9.6	3.8	3.8	1.6	5	185	94	0.32	0.164	2.0	27	1.1	0.09	0.04	17.1	19118
Payday, Hershey	90		2.0	10.0			65										
.7 oz bar	20	5.0	0.5			0											HRSH33
peanut bar	235	0.7	7.0	21.3	19.0	2.6	70	35	52	1.86	0.581	0	0	0.05	3.6	0.00	0.39
1.6 oz bar	45	15.2	2.1	7.5	4.8	0	183	145	0.44	0.369	2.2	0	2.1	0.06	0.07	35.1	19147
peanut brittle	134	0.4	2.1	19.5		0.7	129	8	12	0.25	0.167	11	0	0.04	0.7	0.00	0.15
1 oz	28	5.3	1.3	2.3	1.3	3	47	30	0.35	0.076	0.7	48	0.8	0.01	0.02	12.9	19148
peanut butter chips	835	9.6	30.7	75.4		14.1	420	185	185	3.36	2.352	2	<1	0.08	13.8	0.10	1.92
1 cup	168	50.1	22.0	16.1	9.0	0	848	521	2.86	0.672	4.5	34	5.0	0.34	0.37	161.3	19086
Rainblo bubble gum balls, Hershey	10		0.0	2.0			0										
1 piece (.07 oz)	2	0.0	0.0			0											HRSH34
raspberry chips, Hershey	80		<1.0	10.0			0										
1 T	15	4.0	2.5			0											HRSH35
Red Hot Dollars, Hershey	100		0.0	24.0			0										
7 pieces (1 oz)	28	0.0	0.0			0											HRSH36
Reese's Bites, Hershey	203	0.6	4.4	21.5	18.7	1.2	70	44	25	0.41	0.254		<1	0.06	1.7		0.22
16 pieces	39	11.6	7.0	2.8	0.7	3	149	76	0.33	0.117	0.6	23	0.2	0.08	0.04		19238
Reese's Crunchy Cookie Cups, Hershey - *5 miniature pieces*	198	0.4	3.3	23.2	19.0	1.2	102	31	16	0.27	0.000		<1	0.05	1.2		0.12
	39	11.0	4.5	3.8	1.6	3	132	51	0.48	0.062	0.1	28	0.1	0.05	0.02		19242b
	203	0.4	3.4	23.8	19.5	1.3	105	32	16	0.28	0.000		<1	0.06	1.2		0.12
1.44 oz pkg (2 cups)	40	11.3	4.6	3.9	1.6	3	136	53	0.49	0.064	0.1	28	0.1	0.05	0.02		19242a
Reese's Nutrageous, Hershey	176	0.5	3.8	18.0	13.7	1.3	48	23	23	0.44	0.000		<1	0.06	1.8		0.18
2 bars (1.2 oz)	34	10.9	3.0	4.3	2.8	1	124	60	0.42	0.092	0.1	12	0.4	0.03	0.03		19239a
	279	0.8	6.1	28.5	21.7	2.1	76	37	37	0.70	0.000		<1	0.10	2.8		0.29
1.92 oz bar	54	17.3	4.8	6.8	4.4	2	197	95	0.66	0.146	0.1	19	0.6	0.05	0.05		19239b
Reese's peanut butter chips, Hershey	80		3.0	7.0			35										
1 T	15	4.0	4.0			0											HRSH38
Reese's Peanut Butter Cups, Hershey	232	0.6	4.6	24.9	21.2	1.6	141	35	28	0.58	0.000	7	<1	0.07	2.0	0.12	0.28
2 pieces (1.6 oz)	45	13.7	4.8	5.2	2.5	3	154	72	0.54	0.108	0.6	25	0.1	0.05	0.05		19150
Reese's peanut butter eggs, Hershey	90		2.0	9.0			60										
.6 oz piece	17	5.0	1.5			0											HRSH39
Reese's Pieces, Hershey	229	0.5	5.7	27.5	24.5	1.4	89	32	40	0.53	0.506	0	0	0.08	2.8	0.06	0.28
1.6 oz pkg (58 pieces)	46	11.4	7.6	2.1	0.9	0	165	95	0.23	0.189	0.4	0	0.5	0.10	0.05	25.3	19151
Robin Eggs, large, Hershey	70		0.0	14.0			40										
2 pieces (.56 oz)	16	2.0	1.5			0											HRSH40
med, Hershey	90		0.0	16.0			45										
4 pieces (.67 oz)	19	2.5	2.0			0											HRSH41
mini, Hershey	70		0.0	13.0			40										
10 pieces (.56 oz)	16	2.5	2.0			0											HRSH42
Rolo caramels w/milk choc, Hershey	256	2.5	2.7	36.7	34.5	0.5	102	78	0	0.00	0.000	4	<1	0.01	<0.1	0.11	0.00
1.9 oz pkg (9 pieces)	54	11.3	7.8	2.0	0.2	6	102	38	0.23	0.000	0.0	65	<0.1	0.06	0.00	0.0	19152
sesame crunch	181	0.8	4.1	17.6		2.8	58	229	88	1.32	0.581	0	<1	0.19	1.3	0.00	0.01
20 pieces	35	11.7	1.6	4.4	5.1	0	113	148	1.49	0.333	1.4	<1	0.5	0.06	0.19	22.8	19154

	KCAL / WT (g)	H₂0 (g) / FAT (g)	PRO (g) / SFA (g)	CHO (g) / MUFA (g)	SUGR (g) / PUFA (g)	DFIB (g) / CHOL (mg)	Na (mg) / K (mg)	Ca (mg) / P (mg)	Mg (mg) / Fe (mg)	Zn (mg) / Cu (mg)	Mn (mg) / Se (mcg)	A (mcg RAE) / A (IU)	C (mg) / E (mg ATE)	B-1 (mg) / B-2 (mg)	NIA (mg) / B-6 (mg)	B-12 (mcg) / FOL (mcg DFE)	PANT (mg) / REF
Sixlets, Hershey	90		0.0	14.0			50										
24 pieces (3 tubes)	20	3.5	2.5			0											HRSH43
Skittles Candies, M&M/Mars	231	2.2	0.1	51.7	43.3	0.0	9	0	1	0.02	0.022	0	38	<0.01	<0.1	0.00	<0.01
2 oz pkg (54 pieces)	57	2.5	0.5	1.7	0.1	0	3	1	0.01	0.025	0.4	0	0.2	0.01	<0.01		19370
Skor Toffee Baking Bits, Hershey	70		0.0	7.0			60										
1 T	13	4.5	2.5			10											HRSH44
Skor Toffee Bar, Hershey	209	0.6	1.2	24.1	23.4	0.5	124	T	4	0.07	0.000		<1	0.01	<0.1		0.02
1.4 oz bar	39	12.6	7.3	3.6	0.5	21	60	24	0.22	0.016	0.0	280	<0.1	0.04			19136
Snickers, M&M/Mars	273	3.1	4.6	33.7	28.1	1.4	152	54	28	0.62	0.285	21	<1	0.06	0.9	0.09	0.29
2 oz bar	57	14.0	5.1	4.2	1.7	7	148	86	0.43	0.181	2.6	87	0.8	0.09	0.03	16.0	19155
Soft Drops, Hershey	100		0.0	24.0			15										
9 pieces (.92 oz)	26	0.0	0.0			0											HRSH45
Soft Hot Dollars, Hershey	90		0.0	23.0			15										
11 pieces (.85 oz)	24	0.0	0.0			0											HRSH46
Star Brites peppermints, Brach	59	0.3	0.0	14.7	9.4		6										
3 pieces	15	<0.1															19179
Starburst Fruit Chews, M&M/Mars	234	4.0	0.2	49.9	39.3	0.0	33	2	1	0.00	0.009	0	31	<0.01	<0.1	0.00	0.02
2.07 oz pkg (6 pieces)	59	4.9	0.7	2.1	1.8	0	1	4	0.08	0.007	0.5	0	0.9	<0.01	0.00	0.0	19156
Super Bubble Gum, Hershey	15		0.0	4.0			0										
.21 oz piece	6	0.0	0.0			0											HRSH51
Sweet Escapes, caramel & peanut	80		1.0	13.0			70										
butter crispy, Hershey - .7 oz bar	20	2.5	1.0			0											HRSH52
choc toffee crisp, Hershey	80		1.0	12.0			40										
.66 oz bar	19	3.5	2.0			<5											HRSH53
crispy caramel fudge, Hershey	70		<1.0	13.0			50										
.7 oz bar	20	2.0	1.0			0											HRSH54
crunchy peanut butter, Hershey	90		2.0	13.0			40										
.7 oz bar	20	3.0	1.0			0											HRSH55
triple choc wafer, Hershey	80		<1.0	13.0			30										
.7 oz bar	20	2.5	1.5			0											HRSH56
Symphony, Hershey	223	0.4	3.6	24.4	22.7	0.7	42	105					1				
1.5 oz bar	42	12.8	7.7	3.3	0.3	10	184	87	0.38			96	0.1				19093
Tastetations, butterscotch, Hershey	60		0.0	12.0			85										
3 pieces (.49 oz)	14	1.5	1.0			<5											HRSH60
caramel, Hershey	60		0.0	12.0			85										
3 pieces (.49 oz)	14	1.5	1.0			<5											HRSH61
choc, Hershey	60		0.0	12.0			30										
3 pieces (.49 oz)	14	1.5	1.0			<5											HRSH62
choc mint, Hershey	60		0.0	12.0			30										
3 pieces (.49 oz)	14	1.5	1.0			<5											HRSH63
peppermint, Hershey	60		0.0	15.0			15										
3 pieces (.56 oz)	16	0.0	0.0			0											HRSH64
Three Musketeers, M&M/Mars	250	3.5	1.9	46.1	39.7	1.0	116	50	17	0.33	0.096	14	<1	0.02	0.1	0.10	0.14
2.13 oz bar	60	7.7	3.9	2.6	0.3	7	80	55	0.44	0.093	1.5	48	0.4	0.08	0.01	0.0	19159
Twix Cookie Bar, caramel, M&M/Mars	289	2.5	2.7	38.0	27.9	0.6	112	52	14	0.38	0.140	6	<1	0.10	0.8	0.13	0.18
2.06 oz pkg (2 bars)	58	14.1	5.2	3.1	5.1	3	103	64	0.47	0.082	1.2	23	2.0	0.14	0.02	33.6	19160
peanut butter, M&M/Mars	307	1.1	5.9	30.5	20.5	2.0	158	45	43	0.81	0.504	10	<1	0.06	2.3	0.08	0.28
2.06 oz pkg (2 bars)	58	18.7	6.6	8.6	2.4	3	206	110	0.53	0.183	6.0	42	0.6	0.09	0.08	14.5	19161
Twizzlers, Cherry Bits, Hershey	135	6.0	1.2	31.8		0.0	104	5					0				
1.4 oz (8 pieces)	40	0.7	0.1	0.2	<0.1	0	6	19	0.22			0	0.0				19067
Cherry Pull 'n' Peel, Hershey	100		1.0	25.0			85										
1 oz piece	28	0.0	0.0			0											HRSH69
choc, Hershey	25		0.0	6.0			20										
.28 oz piece	8	0.0	0.0			0											HRSH70
licorice, Hershey	30		0.0	7.0			45										
.32 oz piece	9	0.0	0.0			0											HRSH71
Strawberry Twists, Hershey	249		1.8	56.6	28.1	0.0	204	0					0				
2.5 oz pkg	71	1.6	0.0			0				0.36		0					19112
Whatchamacallit, Hershey	237	1.5	3.9	30.4	23.5	0.9	144	57	13	0.21	0.158	18	<1	0.05	1.2	0.12	0.12
1.7 oz bar	48	11.4	8.2	1.8	0.4	6	145	66	0.54	0.058	0.3	64	0.1	0.10	0.02	8.6	19162
white candy chips	916	2.2	10.0	102.0	102.0	0	153	338	20	1.26	0.044	2	1	0.11	1.3	1.04	1.03
1 cup	170	54.6	33.0	15.5	1.7	36	486	299	0.41	0.102	9.0	10	3.8	0.48	0.10	28.9	19087

	KCAL / WT (g)	H2O (g) / FAT (g)	PRO (g) / SFA (g)	CHO (g) / MUFA (g)	SUGR (g) / PUFA (g)	DFIB (g) / CHOL (mg)	Na (mg) / K (mg)	Ca (mg) / P (mg)	Mg (mg) / Fe (mg)	Zn (mg) / Cu (mg)	Mn (mg) / Se (mcg)	A (mcg RAE) / A (IU)	C (mg) / E (mg ATE)	B-1 (mg) / B-2 (mg)	NIA (mg) / B-6 (mg)	B-12 (mcg) / FOL (mcg DFE)	PANT (mg) / REF
white choc chips, Hershey Premier	80		1.0	9.0			30										
1 T	15	4.0	3.0			0											HRSH72
Whoppers malted milk balls,	90		<1.0	15.0			65										
Hershey - 10 pieces (.7oz)	18	3.5	3.0			0											HRSH73
Willy Wonka's Everlasting	59	1.2	0.0	14.8			1										
Gobstoppers, Sunmark - 6 pieces	16	0.0															19180
Wunderbeans gourmet jelly beans,	100		0.0	24.0			5										
Hershey - 33 pieces (.95 oz)	27	0.0	0.0			0											HRSH74
yogurt chips	522	1.9	5.9	63.9		0.0	87	205	18	0.71	0.007	1	1	0.06	0.2	0.61	0.59
3.5 oz	100	27.0	24.1	0.5	0.5	1	289	159	0.09	0.031	4.7	6	1.0	0.26	0.06	8.0	19079
York Bites, Hershey	154	3.5	0.7	31.8	29.3	0.8	18	4	<1	<0.01	0.000	0		0.00	0.0		0.00
15 pieces	39	2.9	1.7	0.2	<0.1	<1	42	1	0.37	0.000	0.0	3	<0.1	0.00	0.00		19181
York Peppermint Pattie, Hershey	165	3.9	0.9	34.8	27.4	0.9	12	5				0					
1.5 oz patty	43	3.1	1.9	0.2	<0.1	<1	48	0	0.40			3	<0.1				19091
Zagnut, Hershey	70		<1.0	9.0			25										
.5 oz snack size bar	14	3.0	1.5			0											HRSH75
Zero, Hershey	70		<1.0	12.0			35										
.6 oz bar	17	2.5	1.5			0											HRSH76

3. CEREALS & GRAINS, COOKED

	KCAL / WT (g)	H2O (g) / FAT (g)	PRO (g) / SFA (g)	CHO (g) / MUFA (g)	SUGR (g) / PUFA (g)	DFIB (g) / CHOL (mg)	Na (mg) / K (mg)	Ca (mg) / P (mg)	Mg (mg) / Fe (mg)	Zn (mg) / Cu (mg)	Mn (mg) / Se (mcg)	A (mcg RAE) / A (IU)	C (mg) / E (mg ATE)	B-1 (mg) / B-2 (mg)	NIA (mg) / B-6 (mg)	B-12 (mcg) / FOL (mcg DFE)	PANT (mg) / REF
barley, pearled, ckd	193	108.0	3.5	44.3		6.0	5	17	35	1.29	0.407	0	0	0.13	3.2	0.00	0.21
1 cup	157	0.7	0.1	0.1	0.3	0	146	85	2.09	0.165	13.5	11	0.1	0.10	0.18	25.1	20006
scotch, reg/quick dry, Quaker	97	2.7	3.0	21.4		2.9	2	8	17	0.41	0.353	<1	0	0.07	1.3	0.00	0.08
1 oz	28	0.6	0.1	0.1	0.3	0	73	62	0.56	0.106		6	0.1	0.03	0.07	6.4	08232
buckwheat groats, roasted, ckd	155	127.1	5.7	33.5		4.5	7	12	86	1.02	0.677	0	0	0.07	1.6	0.00	0.60
1 cup	168	1.0	0.2	0.3	0.3	0	148	118	1.34	0.245	3.7	0	0.4	0.07	0.13	23.5	20010
bulgur, ckd	151	141.5	5.6	33.8		8.2	9	18	58	1.04	1.108	0	0	0.10	1.8	0.00	0.63
1 cup	182	0.4	0.1	0.1	0.2	0	124	73	1.75	0.137	1.1	0	0.1	0.05	0.15	32.8	20013
corn grits, inst dry, Quaker	96	2.4	2.4	22.1	0.1	1.3	305	6	10	0.19	0.087	0	0	0.18	2.5	0.00	0.12
1 oz pkt	28	0.3	<0.1	<0.1	0.1	0	41	31	8.51	0.028	4.8	0	<0.1	0.21	0.06	83.2	08092
butter flavor, Quaker	101	2.5	2.3	20.8	0.2	1.3	323	2	8	0.11	0.025	16	0	0.18	2.4	0.00	0.11
1 oz pkt	28	1.4	0.3	0.3	0.3	0	54	25	8.10	0.020	4.5	54	0.2	0.20	0.03	79.0	08221
cheddar cheese flavor, Quaker	102	2.1	2.3	20.5	0.6	1.2	522	13	10	0.21	0.076	1	0	0.17	2.2	0.06	0.11
1 oz pkt	28	1.6	0.5	0.4	0.2	1	48	39	8.10	0.031	4.5	4	<0.1	0.18	0.04	71.4	08094
w/imit bacon bits, Quaker	98	2.0	2.8	21.7	0.1	1.5	341	11	10	0.26	0.028	0	0	0.18	2.3	0.00	0.11
1 oz pkt	28	0.5	0.1	0.1	0.2	0	71	39	8.10	0.020	4.5	0	<0.1	0.20	0.06	78.4	08096
w/imit ham bits, Quaker	95	2.1	2.8	21.1	0.1	1.4	493	15	14	0.24	0.123	0	0	0.17	2.3	0.06	0.11
1 oz pkt	28	0.5	0.1	0.1	0.1	0	50	37	8.10	0.050	4.5	0	<0.1	0.20	0.06	73.6	08098
corn grits, inst, prep, Quaker	159	201.9	3.9	36.9		2.2	517	15	20	0.37	0.147	0	0	0.27	2.5	0.00	0.89
1 cup	245	0.5	<0.1	0.1	0.1	0	69	51	14.65	0.059	7.6	0	<0.1	0.15	0.10	139.7	08093
cheddar cheese flavor, Quaker	99	116.8	2.3	19.9		1.1	510	14	38	0.24	0.074	1	0	0.14	1.3	0.06	0.11
1 pkt prep	142	1.6	0.5	0.4	0.2	0	45	24	7.87	0.037	4.3	3	<0.1	0.08	0.04	69.6	08095
w/imit bacon bits, Quaker	94	115.9	2.7	20.8		1.4	331	13	10	0.28	0.028	0	0	0.15	1.4	0.00	0.11
1 pkt prep	141	0.5	0.1	0.1	0.2	0	68	38	8.01	0.025		0	<0.1	0.09	0.06	76.1	08097
w/imit ham bits, Quaker	92	116.0	2.7	20.1		1.3	510	17	14	0.25		0	0	0.16	0.1	0.06	0.11
1 pkt prep	141	0.5	0.1	0.1	0.1	0	58	31	7.91	0.055		0	<0.1	0.08	0.06	71.9	08099
corn grits, white, reg/quick, enr, ckd	145	206.4	3.4	31.5		0.5	0	0	10	0.17	0.041	0	0	0.24	2.0	0.00	0.15
1 cup	242	0.5	0.1	0.1	0.2	0	53	29	1.55	0.029	7.5	0	0.1	0.15	0.06	125.8	08091
unenr, ckd	145	206.4	3.4	31.5		0.5	0	0	10	0.17	0.041	0	0	0.05	0.5	0.00	0.15
1 cup	242	0.5	0.1	0.1	0.2	0	53	29	0.48	0.029		0	<0.1	0.02	0.06	2.4	08162
corn grits, yellow, reg/quick, enr, ckd	145	206.4	3.4	31.5		0.5	0	0	10	0.17	0.041	7	0	0.24	2.0	0.00	0.15
1 cup	242	0.5	0.1	0.1	0.2	0	53	29	1.55	0.029		145	<0.1	0.15	0.06	125.8	08164
unenr, ckd	145	206.4	3.4	31.5		0.5	0	0	10	0.17	0.041	7	0	0.05	0.5	0.00	0.15
1 cup	242	0.5	0.1	0.1	0.2	0	53	29	0.48	0.029		145	<0.1	0.02	0.06	2.4	08166
couscous, ckd	176	113.9	6.0	36.5		2.2	8	13	13	0.41	0.132	0	0	0.10	1.5	0.00	0.58
1 cup	157	0.3	<0.1	<0.1	0.1	0	91	35	0.60	0.064	43.2	0	<0.1	0.04	0.08	23.6	20029
Cream of Rice, ckd	127	213.5	2.2	27.8		0.2	2	7	7	0.39	0.351	0	0	0.00	1.0	0.00	0.19
1 cup	244	0.2	0.1	0.1	0.1	0	49	41	0.49	0.083	7.3	0	<0.1	0.00	0.07	7.3	08101
Cream of Wheat, inst, prep	154	203.4	4.3	31.6		2.9	7	60	14	0.41		0	0	0.24	1.7	0.00	0.17
1 cup	241	0.5	0.1	0.1	0.3	0	48	43	12.05	0.092	27.5	0	<0.1	0.00	0.03	248.2	08107

	KCAL	H₂0 (g)	PRO (g)	CHO (g)	SUGR (g)	DFIB (g)	Na (mg)	Ca (mg)	Mg (mg)	Zn (mg)	Mn (mg)	A (mcg RAE)	C (mg)	B-1 (mg)	NIA (mg)	B-12 (mcg)	PANT (mg)
	WT (g)	FAT (g)	SFA (g)	MUFA (g)	PUFA (g)	CHOL (mg)	K (mg)	P (mg)	Fe (mg)	Cu (mg)	Se (mcg)	A (IU)	E (mg ATE)	B-2 (mg)	B-6 (mg)	FOL (mcg DFE)	REF
quick, ckd	129	207.0	3.6	26.8		1.2	139	50	12	0.33		0	0	0.24	1.4	0.00	0.17
1 cup	239	0.5	0.1	0.1	0.3	0	45	100	10.28	0.067	30.6	0	<0.1	0.00	0.03	176.9	08105
reg, ckd	133	218.6	3.8	27.6		1.8	3	50	10	0.33		0	0	0.25	1.5	0.00	0.19
1 cup	251	0.5	0.1	0.1	0.3	0	43	43	10.29	0.075		0	<0.1	0.00	0.04	70.3	08103
Cream of Wheat Mix & Eat	102	116.6	2.7	21.4		0.4	241	20	7	0.24		376	0	0.43	5.0	0.00	0.13
inst, prep - *1 pkt prep*	142	0.3	<0.1	<0.1	0.2	0	38	20	8.09	0.041		1252	<0.1	0.28	0.57	164.7	08109
apple, banana, maple, inst, prep	132	117.5	2.4	29.0		0.5	242	41	9	0.23		375	0	0.45	5.0	0.00	0.12
1 pkt prep	150	0.5	0.1			0	56	20	8.10	0.057		1251		0.30	0.45	165.0	08111
Creamy Wheat (farina), dry, cinn,	152	5.3	5.3	32.8	0.1	1.6	1	15	6	0.24	0.119		<1	0.19	1.5	0.00	0.16
Quaker - *1/4 cup (amt for 1 serving)*	44	0.3	0.1	<0.1	0.3	0	46	39	13.20	0.031		2	0.1	0.11	0.02	110.4	08317
dry, Quaker	154	5.1	4.8	33.5	0.1	1.3	1	5	7	0.27	0.123		0	0.19	1.5	0.00	0.19
1/4 cup (amt for 1 serving)	44	0.4	0.1	<0.1	0.2	0	43	37	13.20	0.053		0	0.1	0.11	0.02	108.2	08230
prep, Quaker	119	202.7	3.6	26.2		0.9	7	9	7	0.23	0.096		0	0.16	1.8	0.00	0.12
1 cup	233	0.2	<0.1	0.1	0.1	0	33	30	11.02	0.035		0	<0.1	0.11	0.02	86.2	08237
farina, dry, Malt-O-Meal	120		4.0	26.0	0.0	1.0	0	100					0	0.37	5.0		
3 T	35	0.0	0.0			0	35		10.80			0		0.25	0.40	80.0	MALT8
enr, ckd	117	204.8	3.3	24.7		3.3	0	5	5	0.16	0.219		0	0.19	1.3	0.00	0.13
1 cup	233	0.2	<0.1	<0.1	0.1	0	30	28	1.17	0.026	21.2	0	<0.1	0.12	0.02	88.5	08113
unenr, ckd	117	204.8	3.3	24.7		3.3	0	5	5	0.16	0.219		0	0.02	0.2	0.00	0.13
1 cup	233	0.2	<0.1	<0.1	0.1	0	30	28	0.05	0.026		0	<0.1	0.02	0.02	4.7	08174
hominy grits, white, quick dry,	97	2.9	2.4	22.2	0.3	1.3	1	1	14	0.26	0.062		0	0.16	1.3	0.00	0.09
Quaker - *1 oz*	28	0.4	0.1	0.1	0.2	0	41	46	0.99	0.031				0.09	0.08	72.5	08314
white, reg dry, Quaker	97	2.9	2.4	22.2	0.3	1.3	1	1	14	0.26	0.062		0	0.16	1.3	0.00	0.09
1 oz	28	0.4	0.1	0.1	0.2	0	41	46	0.99	0.031		0		0.09	0.08	72.5	08316
yellow, quick dry, Quaker	94	3.3	2.3	21.8	0.3	1.6	1	1	11	0.20	0.028		0	0.14	1.2	0.00	0.09
1 oz	28	0.5	0.1	0.2	0.2	0	47	35	1.15	0.020		159	0.1	0.07	0.07	72.5	08315
Maltex, ckd	179	201.7	5.7	39.6		3.0	10	17	57	1.87			0	0.25	2.4	0.00	0.23
1 cup	249	1.0	0.2	0.1	0.4	0	266	179	1.79	0.336	36.1	0	0.9	0.10	0.08	22.4	08115
Malt-O-Meal, plain/choc, ckd	122	210.2	3.6	25.7		1.0	2	5	5	0.17			0	0.48	5.8	0.00	0.14
1 cup	240	0.2	0.1	0.1	<0.1	0	31	24	9.60	0.026		0	<0.1	0.24	0.02	4.8	08117
Maypo, ckd	170	198.5	5.8	31.9		5.8	10	125	50	1.49		701	29	0.72	9.4	2.88	0.34
1 cup	240	2.4	0.4	0.7	0.9	0	211	247	8.40	0.158	18.5	2338	1.7	0.72	0.96	9.6	08119
millet, ckd	207	124.3	6.1	41.2		2.3	3	5	77	1.58	0.473		0	0.18	2.3	0.00	0.30
1 cup	174	1.7	0.3	0.3	0.9	0	108	174	1.10	0.280	1.6	0	0.1	0.14	0.19	33.1	20032
MultiGrain Oatmeal, dry, Quaker	133	4.4	4.5	29.4		4.8	1	14	46	1.28	1.048		0	0.12	1.4	0.00	0.20
1/2 cup (amt for 1 serving)	40	1.0	0.2	0.2	0.5	0	164	138	1.19	0.176	16.7	3	0.2	0.05	0.10	10.4	08200
prep w/water, Quaker	143	195.6	4.9	31.6		5.1	7	19	51	1.43	1.128		0	0.12	1.5	0.00	0.22
1 cup	234	1.1	0.2	0.2	0.5	0	176	150	1.31	0.201		2	0.3	0.06	0.10	18.7	08249
Nutr for Women, Gldn brwn sugr,	170		5.0	33.0	13.0	3.0	330	350	40				0	0.30	4.0	1.20	
inst dry, Quaker - *1.6 oz pkt*	46	2.0	0.5	1.0	0.5	0	150	150	6.30			1000	10.5	0.34	0.70	140.0	QUAK1
Oat Bran, dry, Quakers/Mother's	146	3.6	6.8	25.2		5.7	2	32	96	1.68	2.280		2	0.39	0.3	0.00	0.34
1/2 cup (amt for 1 serving)	40	3.2	0.6	1.0	1.2	0	232	278	3.23	0.120		40	0.2	0.12	0.04	15.2	08231
prep w/water, Quakers/Mother's	101	208.4	4.8	17.5		4.0	7	26	70	1.24	1.589		2	0.27	0.2	0.00	0.24
1 cup	234	2.2	0.4	0.7	0.8	0	161	194	2.27	0.096		28	0.1	0.08	0.03	11.7	08236
oatmeal, inst dry, apples & cinn,	190		4.0	41.0	17.0	5.0	260	150					0	0.45	6.0		
Malt-O-Meal - *1.8 oz pkt*	53	2.0	0.5			0	135	100	5.40			1500		0.51	0.60	120.0	MALT16
baked apple, Quaker Express	200		4.0	42.0	19.0	4.0	320	100	40				0	0.30	4.0		
1.9 oz container	54	2.5	0.5			0		150	3.60			1000		0.34	0.40	80.0	QUAK2
cinn spice, Malt-O-Meal	250		6.0	54.0	24.0	5.0	360	150					0	0.45	6.0		
2.4 oz pkt	69	3.0	0.5			0	142	150	5.40			1500		0.51	0.60	120.0	MALT17
fruit & cream, Quaker	135	2.2	2.9	26.3		2.2	169	106	28	0.61	0.833		<1	0.31	4.2	0.01	0.13
1.2 oz pkt	35	2.5	0.5	0.8	0.6	0	97	105	4.00	0.067		1050	0.1	0.36	0.42	136.2	08225
Malt-O-Meal	150		5.0	28.0	0.0	4.0	120	150					0	0.45	6.0		
1.5 oz pkt	42	3.0	0.5			0	140	150	10.80			1500		0.51	0.60	120.0	MALT19
maple & brown sugar, Malt-O-	230		6.0	49.0	20.0	5.0	360	150					0	0.45	6.0		
Meal - *2.3 oz pkt*	65	3.0	0.5			0	148	150	5.40			1500		0.51	0.60	120.0	MALT18
oatmeal, inst, prep	138	200.1	5.9	23.9		4.0	377	215	56	1.15	1.369	599	0	0.70	7.2	0.00	0.47
1 cup prep	234	2.3	0.4	0.7	0.9	0	131	176	8.33	0.129	19.0	1996	0.3	0.37	0.98	208.3	08123
apples & cinn, Quaker	125	117.1	3.2	26.1		2.5	121	104	30	0.70	0.915	305	<1	0.30	4.1	0.00	0.15
1 pkt prep	149	1.4	0.3	0.5	0.6	0	106	113	3.89	0.085	7.6	1019	0.1	0.35	0.41	152.0	08125
bran & raisins	158	156.0	4.9	30.4		5.5	248	174	57	1.35	1.589	480	0	0.57	8.1	0.00	0.45
1 pkt prep	195	2.0	0.4			0	236	207	7.62	0.285		1599		0.64	0.76	253.5	08127

	KCAL / WT (g)	H₂O / FAT (g)	PRO / SFA (g)	CHO / MUFA (g)	SUGR / PUFA (g)	DFIB (g) / CHOL (mg)	Na / K (mg)	Ca / P (mg)	Mg / Fe (mg)	Zn / Cu (mg)	Mn (mg) / Se (mcg)	A (mcg RAE) / A (IU)	C / E (mg ATE)	B-1 / B-2 (mg)	NIA / B-6 (mg)	B-12 / FOL (mcg/DFE)	PANT (mg) / REF
cinn spice	177	117.9	4.8	35.1		2.6	280	172	52	0.97	1.473	473	0	0.56	5.7	0.00	0.38
1 pkt prep	161	1.9	0.4	0.6	0.7	0	105	145	6.63	0.119	10.0	1578	0.4	0.34	0.77	247.9	08129
fruit & cream, Quaker	183	110.3	3.9	35.7		2.9	233	146	39	0.87	1.133	429	<1	0.42	5.7	0.02	0.18
1 pkt prep	155	3.4	0.7	1.0	0.8	0	132	143	5.44	0.096		1428	0.2	0.49	0.57	186.0	08227
maple & brown sugar, Quaker - *1 pkt prep*	153	116.1	4.2	31.4		2.6	234	105	39	0.90	1.203	302	0	0.30	4.0	0.00	0.34
	155	1.8	0.4	0.6	0.7	0	112	132	3.86	0.098		1008	0.2	0.34	0.40	130.2	08131
raisins & spice	161	118.5	4.3	31.9		2.2	226	166	36	0.71		441	0	0.51	5.5	0.00	0.37
1 pkt prep	158	1.7	0.3	0.6	0.6	0	150	133	6.59	0.100	9.0	1468	0.2	0.36	0.75	243.3	08133
raisins, dates, & walnuts, Quaker - *1 pkt prep*	187	113.7	4.6	37.8		3.4	333	150	47	1.03	1.367	438	<1	0.43	5.8	0.00	0.23
	161	2.8	0.5	0.9	1.1	0	180	151	5.57	0.140		1457	0.2	0.49	0.59	188.4	08235
oatmeal, microwave, dry, Quick & Hearty - *1 oz pkt*	106	2.8	3.8	19.1	0.3	2.4	153	108	39	0.86	1.204	315	0	0.31	4.2	0.00	0.20
	29	2.1	0.4	0.7	0.7	0	110	136	8.53	0.087		1050		0.36	0.42	138.3	08304
apple spice, Quick & Hearty *1.6 oz pkt*	166	2.9	3.7	34.8	15.2	3.0	306	108	36	0.83	1.139	315	<1	0.31	4.2	0.00	0.20
	45	2.0	0.4	0.7	0.6	0	138	132	3.97	0.099		1050	0.3	0.36	0.42	135.9	08300
brown sugar cinn, Quick & Hearty - *1.5 oz pkt*	155	3.0	3.9	31.4	11.6	2.6	255	108	40	0.90		315	<1	0.31	4.2	0.00	0.20
	42	2.2	0.4	0.8	0.7	0	125	140	3.97	0.092		1050		0.36	0.42	136.1	08301
cinn double raisin, Quick & Hearty - *1.7 oz pkt*	169	4.2	3.9	35.0	15.5	2.9	275	108	39	0.84		315	<1	0.31	4.2		0.19
	47	2.2	0.4	0.7	0.7	0	188	139	3.97	0.118		1050		0.36	0.42	135.4	08302
honey bran, Quick & Hearty *1.4 oz pkt*	151	2.9	3.9	30.6	11.4	2.7	253	108	41	0.90		315	0	0.31	4.2	0.00	0.21
	41	2.1	0.4	0.7	0.7	0	118	142	3.97	0.094		1050		0.36	0.42	136.1	08303
oatmeal, quick/reg, ckd *1 cup*	145	199.6	6.1	25.3		4.0	2	19	56	1.15	1.369	0	0	0.26	0.3	0.00	0.47
	234	2.3	0.4	0.7	0.9	0	131	178	1.59	0.129	19.0	0	0.2	0.05	0.05	9.4	08121
dry *1/3 cup (.95 oz)*	104	2.4	4.3	18.1		2.9	1	14	40	0.83	0.980	0	0	0.20	0.2	0.00	0.34
	27	1.7	0.3	0.5	0.6	0	95	128	1.13	0.093	9.2	0	0.2	0.04	0.03	8.6	08120
dry, Quaker *1/2 cup*	150		5.0	27.0	1.0	4.0	0	0				0					
	40	3.0	0.5	1.0	1.0	0			1.80			0					QUAK3
Ralston, ckd *1 cup*	134	217.8	5.6	28.3		6.1	5	13	58	1.42		0	0	0.20	2.0	0.10	0.33
	253	0.8	0.1	0.1	0.4	0	154	147	1.64	0.200		0	0.3	0.18	0.11	17.7	08135
rice, brown, long grain, ckd *1 cup*	216	142.5	5.0	44.8		3.5	10	20	84	1.23	1.765	0	0	0.19	3.0	0.00	0.56
	195	1.8	0.4	0.6	0.6	0	84	162	0.82	0.195	19.1	0	0.4	0.05	0.28	7.8	20037
med grain, ckd *1 cup*	218	142.3	4.5	45.8		3.5	2	20	86	1.21	2.139	0	0	0.20	2.6	0.00	0.76
	195	1.6	0.3	0.6	0.6	0	154	150	1.03	0.158		0		0.02	0.29	7.8	20041
Rice Medley, frzn, Green Giant *10 oz pkg*	280		8.0	52.0	4.0	4.0	970	40					6				
	283	4.0	0.5			0			3.60			200					GENM3
rice, oriental, frzn, Green Giant *10 oz pkg*	340		7.0	52.0	7.0	4.0	1240	40					6				
	283	12.0	2.0			0			3.60			2500					GENM4
rice pilaf, frzn, Green Giant *10 oz pkg*	230		6.0	44.0	5.0	3.0	1250	40					4				
	283	3.5	2.0			5			4.50			2250					GENM5
rice, white & wild, frzn, Green Giant *10 oz pkg*	280		6.0	51.0	3.0	3.0	1350	60					4				
	283	6.0	1.0			0			4.50			100					GENM6
rice, white, glutinous, enr, ckd *1 cup*	169	133.3	3.5	36.7		1.7	9	3	9	0.71	0.456	0	0	0.03	0.5	0.00	0.37
	174	0.3	0.1	0.1	0.1	0	17	14	0.24	0.085	9.7	0	0.1	0.02	0.05	1.7	20055
long grain, enr, ckd[1] *1 cup*	205	108.1	4.3	44.5		0.6	2	16	19	0.77	0.746	0	0	0.26	2.3	0.00	0.62
	158	0.4	0.1	0.1	0.1	0	55	68	1.90	0.109	11.9	0	0.1	0.02	0.15	153.3	20045
long grain, enr, inst, ckd *1 cup*	162	126.1	3.4	35.1		1.0	5	13	8	0.40	0.388	0	0	0.12	1.5	0.00	0.29
	165	0.3	0.1	0.1	0.1	0	7	23	1.04	0.107	6.9	0	0.1	0.02	0.02	194.7	20049
long grain, enr, parboiled, ckd *1 cup*	200	126.9	4.0	43.3		0.7	5	33	21	0.54	0.455	0	0	0.44	2.5	0.00	0.57
	175	0.5	0.1	0.1	0.1	0	65	74	1.98	0.165	14.4	0	0.1	0.03	0.03	222.3	20047
med grain, enr, ckd[2] *1 cup*	242	127.6	4.4	53.2		0.6	0	6	24	0.78	0.701	0	0	0.31	3.4	0.00	0.76
	186	0.4	0.1	0.1	0.1	0	54	69	2.77	0.071	14.0	0		0.03	0.09	180.4	20051
short grain, enr, ckd[2] *1 cup*	242	127.5	4.4	53.4		0.6	0	2	15	0.74	0.664	0	0	0.31	2.8	0.00	0.74
	186	0.4	0.1	0.1	0.1	0	48	61	2.72	0.134	14.0	0		0.03	0.11	184.1	20053
rice, wild, ckd *1 cup*	166	121.2	6.5	35.0		3.0	5	5	52	2.20	0.462	0	0	0.09	2.1	0.00	0.25
	164	0.6	0.1	0.1	0.3	0	166	134	0.98	0.198	1.3	0	0.4	0.14	0.22	42.6	20089
Roman Meal, prep *1 cup*	147	199.3	6.5	33.0		8.2	2	29	108	1.78		0	0	0.24	3.1	0.00	0.37
	241	1.0	0.1			0	301	214	2.12	0.321		0		0.12	0.11	24.1	08137
w/oats, prep *1 cup*	170	195.6	7.2	34.1		7.0	10	26	74	1.94		0	0	0.31	3.3	0.00	0.25
	240	1.9	0.2			0	257	235	1.39	0.149		22		0.22	0.38	24.0	08155
wheat cereal, dry, Malt-O-Meal *3 T (1.2 oz)*	120		5.0	26.0	0.0	1.0	0	100					0	0.37	5.0		
	35	0.5	0.0			0	40	40	10.80			0		0.25	0.40	80.0	MALT29
choc flavor, Malt-O-Meal *3 T (1.2 oz)*	120		4.0	27.0	7.0	1.0	0	100					0	0.37	5.0		
	35	0.5	0.0			0	85	40	10.80			0		0.25	0.40	80.0	MALT27

	KCAL / WT (g)	H₂0 (g) / FAT (g)	PRO (g) / SFA (g)	CHO (g) / MUFA (g)	SUGR (g) / PUFA (g)	DFIB (g) / CHOL (mg)	Na (mg) / K (mg)	Ca (mg) / P (mg)	Mg (mg) / Fe (mg)	Zn (mg) / Cu (mg)	Mn (mg) / Se (mcg)	A (mcg RAE) / A (IU)	C (mg) / E (mg ATE)	B-1 (mg) / B-2 (mg)	NIA (mg) / B-6 (mg)	B-12 (mcg) / FOL (mcg DFE)	PANT (mg) / REF
maple brown sugar, Malt-O-Meal - 3 T (1.2 oz)	120		3.0	28.0	11.0	1.0	0	100					0	0.37	5.0		
	35	0.0	0.0			0	50	40	10.80			0		0.25	0.40	80.0	MALT28
Wheatena, ckd	136	207.5	4.9	28.7		6.6	5	10	49	1.68	1.997	0	0	0.02	1.3	0.00	0.10
1 cup	243	1.2	0.2	0.2	0.6	0	187	146	1.36	0.126		0	0.9	0.05	0.05	17.0	08143
Whole Wheat Hot Natural Cereal, ckd - 1 cup	150	202.3	4.8	33.2		3.9	0	17	53	1.16	1.411	0	0	0.17	2.2	0.00	0.40
	242	1.0	0.1	0.1	0.5	0	172	167	1.50	0.201		0	0.5	0.12	0.18	26.6	08145

¹ Unenriched rice contains 0.32 mg iron, 0.03 mg thiamin, and 0.6 mg niacin.   ² Unenriched rice contains 0.37 mg iron, 0.04 mg thiamin, and 0.7 mg niacin.

4. CEREALS, READY-TO-EAT

	KCAL / WT (g)	H₂0 (g) / FAT (g)	PRO (g) / SFA (g)	CHO (g) / MUFA (g)	SUGR (g) / PUFA (g)	DFIB (g) / CHOL (mg)	Na (mg) / K (mg)	Ca (mg) / P (mg)	Mg (mg) / Fe (mg)	Zn (mg) / Cu (mg)	Mn (mg) / Se (mcg)	A (mcg RAE) / A (IU)	C (mg) / E (mg ATE)	B-1 (mg) / B-2 (mg)	NIA (mg) / B-6 (mg)	B-12 (mcg) / FOL (mcg DFE)	PANT (mg) / REF
Alpha-Bits, frosted, Post	130	0.4	2.7	26.7	12.5	1.3	212	10	25	1.50			0	0.37	5.0	1.50	
1 cup (1.1 oz)	32	1.3	0.3			0	62	67	2.70	0.099		750		0.43	0.50	165.4	08325
marshmallow, Post	115	0.4	1.7	25.1	12.6	0.5	206	4	12	1.50			0	0.37	5.0	1.50	
1 cup (1 oz)	29	1.0	0.2			0	29	38	2.70	0.029		750		0.43	0.50	166.2	08326
Amaranth Cereal Snaps	183		7.5	33.0	0.0	5.0	3	60					1				
1 cup (1.6 oz)	45	2.7	0.0			0			7.02			0					NUWL1
Apple Cinn Squares, Kellogg's	182	5.2	4.0	44.1	11.7	4.7	20	21	48	1.49	1.701		0	0.39	5.0	1.49	0.35
3/4 cup (1.9 oz)	55	1.0	0.2	0.3	0.5	0	166	154	16.23	0.110	2.3	0	0.6	0.44	0.50	179.9	08254
Apple Jacks, Kellogg's	117	0.9	0.9	27.3	14.7	1.0	143	8	17	1.50	0.089	47	14	0.51	4.6	1.38	0.08
1 cup (1.1 oz)	30	0.6	0.1	0.2	0.3	0	36	38	4.17	0.042	2.2	156	<0.1	0.39	0.45	154.2	08003
Apple Zaps, Quaker	118	0.8	1.1	26.6	14.1	0.7	135	3	15	4.12	0.105	165	7	0.41	5.5	0.00	0.11
3/4 cup (1.1 oz)	30	1.0	0.3	0.2	0.2	0	53	45	4.95	0.042	0.0	550	0.2	0.47	0.55	710.1	08293
Apple Zings, Malt-O-Meal	130		1.0	30.0	16.0	1.0	150	100	8	3.70			15	0.37	5.0	1.50	
1 cup (1.1 oz)	33	1.0	0.0			0	35	20	4.50	0.040		750		0.42	0.50	100.0	MALT1
Banana Nut Crunch, Post	249	2.7	5.0	43.7	12.0	4.0	253	21	48	1.50			<1	0.38	5.0	1.50	
1 cup (2.1 oz)	59	6.1	0.8			0	171	183	16.20	0.226		750		0.42	0.50	161.7	08320
Basic 4, General Mills	202	3.6	4.4	42.4	13.8	3.2	316	196	40	2.97	0.912	118	0	0.30	3.9	1.16	0.29
1 cup (1.9 oz)	55	2.8	0.4	1.0	1.1	0	155	232	3.52	0.165	9.4	393	0.7	0.34	0.39	126.5	08262
Berry Colossal Crunch, Malt-O-Meal	120		1.0	26.0	13.0	1.0	210	0		3.70			0	0.37	5.0		
3/4 cup (1 oz)	30	1.5	0.0			0	35		4.50			0		0.42	0.50	100.0	MALT2
Blueberry Morning, Post	211	4.0	3.6	43.4	11.4	2.1	266	15	24	0.90			0	0.37	5.0	1.50	
1 1/4 cups (1.9 oz)	55	2.5	0.3			0	91	70	1.80	0.074		750		0.42	0.50	162.8	08321
Boo Berry, General Mills	118	0.7	0.9	27.0	14.1	0.3	211	20	3	3.75	0.015	0	6	0.38	5.0	1.50	0.03
1 cup (1.1 oz)	30	0.8	0.1	0.5	0.1	0	14	20	4.50	0.012	2.0	0	<0.1	0.43	0.50	165.9	08273
bran, 100%, Post	83	0.8	3.7	22.7	7.1	8.3	121	22	81	3.75			0	0.37	5.0	0.00	
1/3 cup (1 oz)	29	0.6	0.1			0	275	236	8.10	0.266		750		0.43	0.50	166.2	08343
All-Bran Buds	75	0.9	2.1	24.0	8.1	12.9	203	19	62	1.50	2.461	153	6	0.36	5.1	6.00	0.45
1/3 cup (1.1 oz)	30	0.6	0.1	0.2	0.4	0	300	150	4.50	0.144	8.7	510	0.5	0.42	2.01	677.4	08005
All-Bran, Kellogg's	81	0.9	3.9	22.9	5.9	9.9	80	102	118	1.86	2.834	163	6	0.37	5.0	6.20	0.54
1/2 cup (1.1 oz)	31	1.0	0.2	0.2	0.6	0	350	350	4.96	0.248	2.9	542	0.6	0.43	1.86	681.4	08001
All-Bran w/extra fiber	50	0.8	2.9	20.0	0.1	13.0	124	108	88	1.56	1.887	160	7	0.39	5.2	6.24	0.41
1/2 cup (.92 oz)	26	0.9	0.2	0.2	0.6	0	273	234	4.68	0.156	2.4	532	0.6	0.44	2.08	178.1	08253
bran flakes, Balance, Malt-O-Meal	90		3.0	23.0	5.0	5.0	230	0	60	3.70			15	0.37	5.0	1.50	
3/4 cup (1 oz)	29	0.5	0.0			0	170	150	8.10	0.120		1250		0.42	0.50	100.0	MALT3
Post	96	1.1	2.8	24.1	5.7	5.3	220	17	64	1.50			0	0.38	5.0	1.50	
3/4 cup (1.1 oz)	30	0.7	0.1			0	185	152	8.10	0.193		750		0.43	0.50	165.9	08322
Brown Sugar Bliss Oatmeal, Quaker	188	1.2	4.3	39.0		3.6	249	146	51	5.88	1.387	235	2	0.59	7.8	0.00	0.30
1 cup (1.7 oz)	49	2.7	0.6	0.8	0.7	0	160	155	4.95	0.167	1.1	784	2.9	0.67	0.78	734.0	08360
Cap'n Crunch, Quaker	108	0.7	1.2	22.9	11.8	0.7	202	4	15	4.28	0.181	2	0	0.43	5.7	0.00	0.09
3/4 cup (.95 oz)	27	1.6	0.4	0.3	0.2	0	54	45	5.16	0.043	1.8	40	0.2	0.48	0.57	710.4	08010
Crunchberries, Quaker	104	0.7	0.7	22.1	11.6	0.7	182	5	15	4.11	0.169	2	<1	0.41	5.5	0.01	0.10
3/4 cup (.92 oz)	26	1.5	0.4	0.3	0.2	0	54	44	4.94	0.042	1.7	37	0.2	0.47	0.55	684.1	08011
Peanut Butter Crunch, Quaker	112	0.7	1.9	21.3	9.0	0.8	200	3	19	18.80	0.194	2	0	0.41	5.6	0.00	0.13
3/4 cup (.95 oz)	27	2.5	0.6	0.8	0.6	0	64	52	4.95	0.068	1.8	41	0.2	0.47	0.55	710.1	08012
Cheerios, General Mills	111	1.0	3.3	22.2	1.2	2.7	273	100	40	3.75	0.090	150	6	0.38	5.0	1.50	0.02
1 cup (1.1 oz)	30	1.8	0.4	0.6	0.2	0	96	100	8.10	0.040	11.3	500	0.2	0.43	0.50	336.3	08013
apple cinn, General Mills	118	0.6	1.8	25.2	12.6	1.3	120	100	20	3.75	0.424	150	6	0.38	5.0	1.50	0.15
3/4 cup (1.1 oz)	30	1.5	0.3	0.7	0.4	0	58	65	4.50	0.060	11.3	500	0.3	0.43	0.50	336.3	08263
frosted, General Mills	115	0.8	1.5	25.8	13.2	0.9	210	100	16	3.75	0.415	150	6	0.38	5.0	1.50	0.15
1 cup (1.1 oz)	30	0.9	0.2	0.3	0.3	0	42	40	4.50	0.057	11.3	500	0.2	0.43	0.50	336.3	08267
honey nut, General Mills	112	0.7	2.7	24.0	10.5	1.8	269	100	32	3.75	0.753	150	6	0.38	5.0	1.50	0.15
1 cup (1.1 oz)	30	1.2	0.2	0.4	0.5	0	92	100	4.50	0.040	7.1	500	0.3	0.43	0.50	336.3	08045

	KCAL / WT (g)	H₂0 (g) / FAT (g)	PRO (g) / SFA (g)	CHO (g) / MUFA (g)	SUGR (g) / PUFA (g)	DFIB (g) / CHOL (mg)	Na (mg) / K (mg)	Ca (mg) / P (mg)	Mg (mg) / Fe (mg)	Zn (mg) / Cu (mg)	Mn (mg) / Se (mcg)	A (mcg RAE) / A (IU)	C (mg) / E (mg ATE)	B-1 (mg) / B-2 (mg)	NIA (mg) / B-6 (mg)	B-12 (mcg) / FOL (mcg DFE)	PANT (mg) / REF
multi-grain, General Mills	108	0.8	2.4	24.3	6.0	2.7	201	95	28	14.22	0.531	142	14	1.42	19.0	5.67	9.48
1 cup (1.1 oz)	30	1.2	0.3	0.5	0.3	0	88	98	17.04	0.052	5.0	474	19.1	1.61	1.90	640.2	08087
Chex, corn, General Mills	112	0.7	2.1	25.8	3.3	0.6	288	100	8	3.75	0.191	150	6	0.38	5.0	1.50	0.00
1 cup (1.1 oz)	30	0.3	0.1	0.1	0.1	0	25	22	9.00	0.232	2.9	500	0.1	0.43	0.50	336.3	08019
frosted mini, General Mills	110		1.0	27.0	10.0	0.0	200	100					6				
3/4 cup (1.1 oz)	30	0.0	0.0	0.0	0.0	0	25		9.00			500					GENM7
honey nut, General Mills	114	0.6	1.5	26.1	9.6	0.3	224	100	5	0.18	0.189	0	6	0.38	5.0	1.50	0.19
3/4 cup (1.1 oz)	30	0.6	0.1	0.3	0.2	0	30	20	9.00	0.036	0.5	0	0.3	0.00	0.50	165.9	08057
multi-bran, General Mills	166	1.0	3.4	41.2	10.8	6.4	322	89	53	3.33	0.759	134	5	0.33	4.5	1.32	0.00
1 cup (1.7 oz)	49	1.2	0.2	0.3	0.5	0	190	178	14.46	0.071	3.9	445	0.2	0.38	0.45	591.4	08345
rice, General Mills	117	0.9	1.9	26.7	2.5	0.3	292	103	9	3.88	0.307	155	6	0.39	5.2	1.55	
1 1/4 cups (1.1 oz)	31	0.3	0.1	0.1	0.1	0	30	35	9.30	0.000	1.2	517	0	0.44	0.52	350.6	08064
wheat, General Mills	104	0.7	3.0	24.3	3.0	3.3	267	60	24	2.40	1.100	90	4	0.23	3.0	0.90	0.00
1 cup (1.1 oz)	30	0.6	0.1	0.1	0.2	0	113	90	8.70	0.096	1.5	300	0.4	0.26	0.30	404.1	08082
Chex Morning Mix, banana nut,	130		2.0	24.0	9.0	1.0	170	100					0				
General Mills - *1.1 oz pouch*	32	3.5	0.5			0	70		5.40			400					GENM8
cinn, General Mills	130		2.0	24.0	8.0	1.0	180	100					0				
1.1 oz pouch	32	3.5	0.5			0	75		5.40			500					GENM9
fruit 'n nut, General Mills	130		2.0	24.0	8.0	1.0	190	100					0				
1.1 oz pouch	32	3.5	0.5	1.5	1.0	0	75		5.40			400					GENM10
honey nut, General Mills	130		2.0	24.0	8.0	1.0	190	100					0				
1.1 oz pouch	32	3.5	0.5			0	80		6.30			500					GENM11
Cinn Grahams, General Mills	113	0.8	1.5	25.8	11.4	1.0	237	100	8	3.75	0.000	150	6	0.38	5.0	1.50	0.00
3/4 cup (1.1 oz)	30	0.8	0.2	0.3	0.3	0	44	20	4.50	0.026	1.3	500	0.2	0.43	0.50	165.9	08139
Cinn Oatmeal Squares, Quaker	227	1.5	6.1	47.9	14.2	4.6	263	116	65	4.13	1.764	165	7	0.41	5.5	0.00	0.37
1 cup (2.1 oz)	60	2.6	0.5	0.9	1.0	0	250	202	16.86	0.180	3.8	550	2.2	0.46	0.55	706.2	08215
Cinn Toast Crunch, General Mills	127	0.8	1.5	23.7	10.2	1.2	206	100	8	3.75	0.821	150	6	0.38	5.0	1.50	0.23
3/4 cup (1.1 oz)	30	3.3	0.5	1.5	1.0	0	43	80	4.50	0.060	1.3	500	0.3	0.43	0.50	165.9	08272
Cocoa Blasts, Quaker	130	0.8	1.2	29.3	15.9	0.8	135	2	17	4.13	0.125	165	7	0.41	5.5	0.00	0.10
1 cup (1.2 oz)	33	1.2	0.3	0.2	0.2	0	62	50	4.95	0.059	2.1	550	0.2	0.47	0.55	709.5	08294
Cocoa Dyno-Bites, Malt-O-Meal	120		1.0	26.0	13.0	0.0	160	0	8	1.50			0	0.37	5.0	1.50	
3/4 cup (1.1 oz)	29	1.0	0.5			0	40	20	1.80	0.040		750		0.42	0.50	100.0	MALT4
Cocoa Krispies, Kellogg's	118	0.9	1.1	27.0	14.0	1.0	190	5	12	1.49	0.724	153	15	0.37	5.0	1.52	0.28
3/4 cup (1.1 oz)	31	1.0	0.5	0.3	0.2	0	50	30	4.65	0.062	4.3	508	0.1	0.43	0.50	172.7	08014
Cocoa Pebbles, Post	115	0.8	1.0	25.5	12.8	0.5	157	3	11	1.50			0	0.37	5.0	1.50	
3/4 cup (1 oz)	29	1.2	1.1			0	42	23	1.80	0.062		750		0.43	0.50	166.2	08323
Cocoa Puffs, General Mills	117	0.8	1.2	26.4	14.1	0.7	171	100	8	3.75	0.033	0	6	0.38	5.0	1.50	0.03
1 cup (1.1 oz)	30	1.0	0.2	0.5	0.2	0	50	20	4.50	0.042	2.0	0	0.1	0.43	0.50	165.9	08271
Coco-Roos, Malt-O-Meal	120		1.0	27.0	14.0		190	100		3.70			6	0.37	5.0	1.50	
3/4 cup (1.1 oz)	30	1.0	0.0			0	45		4.50			500		0.42	0.50	100.0	MALT5
Colossal Crunch, Malt-O-Meal	120	0.8	1.1	25.7	13.0	0.8	230	3	15	3.75	0.070	0	0	0.38	5.0	0.00	0.09
3/4 cup (1.1 oz)	30	1.7	0.4	0.6	0.1	0	40	43	4.50	0.047	2.7	0	0.4	0.43	0.50	165.9	08346
berry, Malt-O-Meal	120	0.8	1.2	25.7	13.0	0.8	220	2	6	3.75	0.015	0	0	0.38	5.0	0.00	0.01
3/4 cup (1.1 oz)	30	1.7	0.4	0.6	0.1	0	40	17	4.50	0.041	2.0	0	0.5	0.43	0.50	165.9	08347
Cookie Crisp, choc chip/van,	117	0.7	1.2	26.4	12.6	0.5	178	100	8	3.75	0.236	150	6	0.38	5.0	1.50	0.07
General Mills - *1 cup (1.1 oz)*	30	0.9	0.2	0.4	0.2	0	27	40	4.50	0.090	2.2	500	0.1	0.43	0.50	165.9	08017
Corn Bursts, Malt-O-Meal	118	0.7	1.0	28.7	14.0	0.4	122	11	1	1.50	0.132	225	15	0.75	10.0	1.50	0.08
1 cup (1.1 oz)	31	0.1	0.1	<0.1	<0.1	0	16	6	1.80	0.028	2.5	750	0.1	0.85	1.00	165.5	08083
Corn Flakes, Country, General Mills	111	0.5	1.8	25.5	2.4	0.5	263	250	7	3.75	0.031	150	6	0.38	5.0	1.50	0.07
1 cup (1.1 oz)	30	0.4	0.1	0.1	0.1	0	32	20	8.10	0.030	1.5	500	0.1	0.43	0.50	336.3	08269
Kellogg's	101	0.8	2.0	24.1	2.0	1.0	203	2	3	0.08	0.067	150	6	0.36	5.0	1.51	0.09
1 cup (1 oz)	28	0.2	0.1	0.1	0.1	0	25	14	8.40	0.020	1.4	501	<0.1	0.43	0.50	170.0	08020
Malt-O-Meal	110		2.0	26.0	2.0	1.0	320	0					15	0.37	5.0		
1 cup (1.1 oz)	30	0.0	0.0			0	25		8.10			750		0.42	0.50	100.0	MALT6
Post Toasties	101	1.0	1.9	24.3	1.8	1.3	266	1	4	0.13			0	0.38	5.0	1.50	
1 cup (1 oz)	28	<0.1	0.0			0	33	15	5.40	0.009		750		0.43	0.50	166.3	08338
Corn Pops, Kellogg's	118	0.9	1.1	27.9	14.0	0.2	120	5	2	1.52	0.076	150	6	0.37	5.0	1.52	0.09
1 cup (1.1 oz)	31	0.2	0.1	0.1	0.1	0	26	10	1.92	0.012	2.0	501	<0.1	0.43	0.50	169.3	08068
Count Chocula, General Mills	119	0.5	1.2	26.4	14.1	0.5	175	20	9	3.75	0.036	0	6	0.38	5.0	1.50	0.03
1 cup (1.1 oz)	30	1.1	0.2	0.6	0.2	0	41	20	4.50	0.040	2.0	0	0.1	0.43	0.50	165.9	08270
Cracklin' Oat Bran, Kellogg's	225	1.7	4.6	39.3	17.1	6.4	157	23	68	1.71	1.657	252	17	0.42	5.7	1.71	0.41
3/4 cup (1.9 oz)	55	8.0	2.3	4.6	1.2	0	248	179	2.04	0.182	12.1	842	0.4	0.48	0.56	184.3	08023

	KCAL	H₂0 (g)	PRO (g)	CHO (g)	SUGR (g)	DFIB (g)	Na (mg)	Ca (mg)	Mg (mg)	Zn (mg)	Mn (mg)	A (mcg RAE)	C (mg)	B-1 (mg)	NIA (mg)	B-12 (mcg)	PANT (mg)
	WT (g)	FAT (g)	SFA (g)	MUFA (g)	PUFA (g)	CHOL (mg)	K (mg)	P (mg)	Fe (mg)	Cu (mg)	Se (mcg)	A (IU)	E (mg ATE)	B-2 (mg)	B-6 (mg)	FOL (mcg DFE)	REF
Cranberry Macadamia Nut, Quaker	245	2.6	4.0	46.2	17.2	3.6	251	76	39	2.99	1.002	232	11	0.46	6.5	0.00	0.25
1 cup (2.1 oz)	60	5.9	1.0	3.9	0.5		134	107	10.29	0.168	0.8	773	1.2	0.56	0.67	533.4	08400
crisped rice	111	0.7	1.8	24.8		0.3	206	5	12	0.46	0.363	371	15	0.52	6.9	0.08	0.11
1 cup (1 oz)	28	0.1	<0.1	<0.1	<0.1	0	27	31	0.70	0.061	4.3	1235	<0.1	0.59	0.69	234.4	08025
Crispix, Kellogg's	109	0.9	2.0	24.9	3.0	0.1	210	6	7	1.45	0.528	150	6	0.38	5.2	1.51	0.27
1 cup (1 oz)	29	0.2	0.1	0.1	0.1	0	38	26	8.12	0.035	3.2	500	0.1	0.44	0.49	336.4	08259
Crispy Rice, Malt-O-Meal	125	1.0	2.0	28.7	3.2	0.2	320	0	8	0.60	0.313	225	15	0.45	6.0	1.80	0.29
1 cup (1.2 oz)	33	0.4	0.1	0.1	0.1	0	46	20	1.80	0.040	4.4	750	<0.1	0.51	0.50	203.3	08348
Crispy Wheaties 'n Raisins, General Mills - 1 cup (1.9 oz)	183	3.9	3.9	44.6	18.2	5.0	251	0	42	7.48	1.443	150	0	0.75	10.0	3.03	0.36
	55	0.9	0.2	0.1	0.4	0	227	140	7.48	0.176	3.9	500	0.6	0.85	1.00	324.5	08026
Crunchy Bran, Quaker	90	0.5	1.5	23.3	5.5	4.7	232	19	14	4.13	0.213	2	0	0.14	5.5	0.00	0.11
3/4 cup (.95 oz)	27	1.0	0.2	0.2	0.3	0	56	36	8.32	0.041	3.2	42	0.2	0.47	0.55	676.4	08018
Fiber One, General Mills	59	1.1	2.4	24.3	0.0	14.4	129	100	60	3.75	1.673	0	6	0.38	5.0	1.50	0.33
1/2 cup (1.1 oz)	30	0.8	0.1	0.1	0.4	0	232	150	4.50	0.160	2.7	0	0.1	0.43	0.50	165.9	08244
Frankenberry, General Mills	118	0.7	0.9	27.0	14.1	0.3	213	20	3	3.75	0.040	0	6	0.38	5.0	1.50	0.04
1 cup (1.1 oz)	30	0.8	0.1	0.4	0.2	0	14	20	4.50	0.024	5.9	0	0.1	0.43	0.50	165.9	08268
French Toast Crunch, General Mills	117	0.7	1.2	26.4	12.0	0.3	178	80	3	3.75	0.020	150	6	0.38	5.0	1.50	0.00
3/4 cup (1.1 oz)	30	1.0	0.2	0.5	0.1	0	22	60	4.50	0.000	1.2	500	0.3	0.43	0.50	165.9	08086
Froot Loops, Kellogg's	118	0.9	1.0	26.3	14.1	0.9	141	23	9	1.41	0.085	145	14	0.36	4.7	1.41	0.08
1 cup (1.1 oz)	30	1.2	0.6	0.3	0.4	0	33	19	4.23	0.030	2.2	483	0.1	0.39	0.48	155.7	08030
Frosted Flakes, Kellogg's	114	0.9	1.0	28.0	11.8	1.0	148	2	2	0.06	0.076	160	6	0.37	5.0	1.55	0.11
3/4 cup (1.1 oz)	31	0.2	<0.1	0.1	0.1	0	23	11	4.50	0.012	1.4	533	<0.1	0.47	0.50	172.1	08069
Malt-O-Meal	120		1.0	28.0	14.0	1.0	200	0					15	0.75	10.0	1.50	
3/4 cup (1.1 oz)	31	0.0	0.0			0	20		4.50			750		0.85	1.00	100.0	MALT9
Frosted Krispies, Kellogg's	114	0.9	1.0	27.0	12.0	0.1	218	3	8	0.27	0.225	151	6	0.39	5.1	1.53	0.21
3/4 cup (1.1 oz)	30	0.2	0.1	0.1	0.1	0	28	28	1.80	0.030	4.6	501	<0.1	0.42	0.51	340.8	08032
Frosted Mini-Spooners, Malt-O-Meal	190		5.0	45.0	11.0	6.0	0	0	60	1.50		0		0.37	5.0	1.50	
1 cup (1.9 oz)	55	1.0	0.0			0	160	150	16.20	0.200		0		0.42	0.50	100.0	MALT10
Frosted Mini-Wheats, bite size, Kellogg's - 1 cup (1.9 oz)	189	3.3	5.6	44.6	11.1	5.5	4	18	65	1.76	1.533	0		0.41	5.4	1.62	0.00
	55	0.9	0.2	0.1	0.6	0	190	162	15.40	0.176	2.3	0	0.0	0.46	0.54	176.0	08319
regular, Kellogg's - 1 cup (1.8 oz)	173	3.1	5.0	41.0	10.0	5.1	5	16	60	1.63	1.422	0		0.38	5.0	1.50	0.38
	51	0.8	0.2	0.1	0.5	0	173	150	14.79	0.163	2.1	0	0.5	0.42	0.50	163.2	08031
Fruit & Fibre (dates, raisins, walnuts), Post - 1 cup (1.9 oz)	212	4.7	3.9	41.9	16.4	5.3	280	24	66	1.50				0.37	5.0	1.50	
	55	3.1	0.4			0	244	162	5.40	0.260		750		0.42	0.50	162.8	08327
Fruity Dyno-Bites, Malt-O-Meal	100	<1.0		24.0	12.0	0.0	160	0		1.50				0.37	5.0	1.50	
3/4 cups (.95 oz)	27	0.5	0.0			0	20		1.80			750		0.42	0.50	100.0	MALT11
Fruity Pebbles, Post	108	0.8	1.0	23.7	11.9	0.2	158	1	5	1.50				0.38	5.0	1.50	
3/4 cup (.95 oz)	27	1.1	0.2			0	30	16	1.80	0.032		750		0.42	0.50	166.3	08324
Golden Crisp, Post	107	0.8	1.5	24.5	14.6	0.0	41	4	16	1.50				0.38	5.0	1.50	
3/4 cup (.95 oz)	27	0.4	0.1			0	34	37	1.80	0.059		750		0.42	0.50	166.3	08328
Golden Grahams, General Mills	112	0.8	1.5	24.9	10.5	0.9	269	350	8	3.75	0.213	150	6	0.38	5.0	1.50	0.09
3/4 cup (1.1 oz)	30	1.1	0.2	0.4	0.4	0	50	200	4.50	0.048	1.7	500	0.2	0.43	0.50	165.9	08035
Golden Puffs, Malt-O-Meal	100		2.0	25.0	15.0	<1.0	40	0	16	1.50				0.37	5.0	1.50	
3/4 cup (.95 oz)	27	0.0	0.0			0	35	40	1.80	0.040		750		0.42	0.50	100.0	MALT12
Granola, fruit, low fat, Nature Valley - 3/5 cup (1.9 oz)	212	3.7	4.4	44.0	18.7	2.8	207	20	24	0.61	1.104	0	0	0.09		0.00	
	55	2.5	0.5	1.2	0.6	0	153	150	1.10	0.120	9.5	0	0.8	0.03	0.06	7.2	08277
homemade - 1 cup (4.3 oz)	570	6.5	17.9	64.7		12.8	29	99	217	4.95		0	2	0.90	2.5	0.00	0.74
	122	30.0	5.8	9.6	12.9	0	656	564	5.12	0.747	24.8	11	15.7	0.34	0.39	104.9	08037
low fat, Kellogg's - 1/2 cup (1.7 oz)	186	1.7	4.0	39.0	14.0	3.0	120	20	40	3.77	1.350	234	2	0.39	5.3	5.98	0.00
	49	2.5	0.5	1.3	0.7	0	123	117	1.81	0.098	8.5	779	0.7	0.43	2.06	673.3	08189
low fat w/raisins, Kellogg's - 3/5 cup (2.1 oz)	230	2.1	4.8	48.0	17.0	3.0	148	25	45	3.78	1.385	225	4	0.38	5.0	6.00	0.00
	60	3.0	0.9	1.5	0.6	0	180	140	1.80	0.120	10.4	750	5.0	0.42	1.98	677.4	08284
w/almonds, Quaker Sun Country - 1/2 cup (2 oz)	266	0.8	6.7	38.3	11.6	3.0	19	49	52	1.14	1.528	0	<1	0.18	0.5	0.04	0.32
	57	10.3	1.3	3.3	1.8	0	221	168	2.48	0.165	9.9	0	1.2	0.10	0.07	19.4	08212
Grape-Nuts Flakes, Post	106	0.9	2.9	23.6	5.1	2.6	140	11	30	1.20				0.37	5.0	1.50	
3/4 cup (1 oz)	29	0.8	0.2			0	99	88	8.10	0.145		750		0.43	0.50	166.2	08330
Grape-Nuts, Post	208	2.0	6.3	47.2	7.0	5.0	354	20	58	1.20				0.38	5.0	1.50	
1/2 cup (2 oz)	58	1.1	0.2			0	178	139	16.20	0.212		750		0.42	0.50	161.8	08329
Great Grains, crunchy pecan, Post	216	3.1	4.9	37.8	8.1	3.7	214	15	46	1.20			<1	0.38	5.0	1.50	
3/5 cup (1.9 oz)	53	6.3	0.7			0	170	118	2.70	0.179		750		0.45	0.50	163.2	08331
raisin, date, & pecan, Post	204	4.7	4.3	39.5	13.3	4.0	156	17	45	1.20			<1	0.38	5.0	1.50	
3/5 cup (1.9 oz)	54	4.5	0.6			0	176	106	3.60	0.166		750		0.43	0.50	162.5	08332

Food / Serving	KCAL / WT (g)	H₂0 (g) / FAT (g)	PRO (g) / SFA (g)	CHO (g) / MUFA (g)	SUGR (g) / PUFA (g)	DFIB (g) / CHOL (mg)	Na (mg) / K (mg)	Ca (mg) / P (mg)	Mg (mg) / Fe (mg)	Zn (mg) / Cu (mg)	Mn (mg) / Se (mcg)	A (mcg RAE) / A (IU)	C (mg) / E (mg ATE)	B-1 (mg) / B-2 (mg)	NIA (mg) / B-6 (mg)	B-12 (mcg) / FOL (mcg DFE)	PANT (mg) / REF
Harmony, General Mills	200		5.0	44.0	13.0	2.0	350	600					30				
1 1/4 cups (1.9 oz)	55	1.0	0.0	0.0	0.0	0	90		9.00			500					GENM13
Heartland Natural, Heartland Co	499	4.7	11.6	78.5		7.0	293	75	147	3.04		3	1	0.36	1.6	0.00	0.96
1 cup (4.1 oz)	115	17.7	4.5	4.8	7.1	0	385	416	4.34	0.297	19.9	64	0.8	0.16	0.19	64.4	08040
w/coconut, Heartland Co	463	3.5	10.9	71.3		7.5	213	66	138	2.74		3	1	0.35	1.8	0.00	0.84
1 cup (3.7 oz)	105	17.1	6.2	4.0	5.7	0	384	380	5.39	0.532	18.2	57	0.7	0.15	0.16	56.7	08041
w/raisins, Heartland Co	468	5.5	10.7	75.9		6.1	226	66	141	2.83		3	1	0.32	1.5	0.00	0.91
1 cup (3.9 oz)	110	15.6	4.0	4.2	6.2	0	415	376	4.02	0.462	19.0	63	0.8	0.14	0.20	44.0	08042
Honey Bunches of Oats, honey	118	0.9	2.1	24.6	6.5	1.5	193	6	17	0.30			0	0.38	5.0	1.50	
roasted, Post - 3/4 cup (1.1 oz)	30	1.7	0.2			0	52	48	8.10	0.081		750		0.43	0.50	165.9	08333
w/almonds, Post	126	0.9	2.4	24.2	6.5	1.4	187	11	21	0.30			<1	0.38	5.0	1.50	
3/4 cup (1.1 oz)	31	2.6	0.3			0	70	60	8.10	0.069		750		0.42	0.50	166.2	08334
Honey Buzzers, Malt-O-Meal	110		1.0	26.0	11.0	<1.0	220	0	8	1.50			0	0.37	5.0	1.50	
1 oz	28	0.5	0.0			0	35	20	2.70			750		0.42	0.50	100.0	MALT13
Honey Crunch Corn Flakes,	117	0.8	2.0	26.1	9.9	1.0	210	7	7	0.09	0.045		6	0.38	5.0	1.50	0.07
Kellogg's - 3/4 cup (1.1 oz)	30	1.0	0.2	0.5	0.3	0	31	18	1.86	0.030	1.5	500	0.6	0.45	0.51	165.9	08309
Honey Graham Oh!s, Quaker	111	0.7	1.1	22.6	12.2	0.6	162	3	0	4.42	0.143	177	7	0.44	5.9	0.00	0.08
3/4 cup (.95 oz)	27	2.0	0.5	0.4	0.2	0	42	38	5.31	0.032	1.3	590	0.1	0.50	0.59	710.4	08211
Honey Graham Squares,	120		1.0	25.0	10.0	1.0	270	350	8	3.70			6	0.37	5.0	1.50	
Malt-O-Meal - 3/4 cup (1.1 oz)	30	1.0	0.0			0	50	200	4.50			500		0.42	0.50	100.0	MALT14
Honey Nut Clusters, General Mills	214	1.4	4.4	45.7		2.8	249	20	32	3.74	2.704	0	0	0.37	5.0	1.49	0.63
1 cup (1.9 oz)	55	2.7	0.3	1.4	0.7	0	135	100	4.51	0.080	5.9	0	3.0	0.42	0.50	162.8	08243
Honeycomb, Post	115	0.4	1.5	25.8	11.1	0.7	215	5	11	1.50			0	0.37	5.0	1.50	
1 1/3 cups (1 oz)	29	0.6	0.2			0	35	27	2.70	0.020		750		0.43	0.50	166.2	08335
Just Right, fruit & nut, Kellogg's	220	3.5	4.2	49.0	15.0	3.1	280	21	31	0.78	1.013	149	0	0.36	5.0	6.00	0.00
1 cup (2.1 oz)	60	2.0	0.3	0.9	0.8	0	170	107	16.20	0.120	3.1	497	2.0	0.42	1.98	673.2	08283
Kaboom, General Mills	115	0.7	2.7	24.3	6.0	1.8	285	100	16	3.75	0.490	150	6	0.38	5.0	1.50	0.18
1 1/4 cups (1.1 oz)	30	1.1	0.3	0.3	0.4	0	63	80	8.10	0.057	2.0	500	0.1	0.43	0.50	336.3	08278
King Vitaman, Quaker	120	0.6	2.0	26.3	6.3	1.2	260	4	26	3.88	0.282	310	12	0.39	5.2	1.55	0.17
1 1/2 cups (1.1 oz)	31	1.1	0.2	0.2	0.3	0	86	79	8.99	0.074	2.0	1033	2.1	0.44	0.51	698.4	08047
Kix, General Mills	113	0.6	1.8	25.8	3.3	0.9	267	150	8	3.75	0.289	159	6	0.38	5.0	1.50	0.12
1 1/3 cups (1.1 oz)	30	0.6	0.2	0.2	0.2	0	35	40	8.10	0.030	2.0	529	0.1	0.43	0.50	336.3	08048
berry berry, General Mills	118	0.7	1.2	26.1	9.3	0.8	178	50	6	3.75	0.156	150	6	0.38	5.0	1.50	0.08
3/4 cup (1.1 oz)	30	1.3	0.2	0.7	0.3	0	25	37	4.50	0.024	2.0	500	0.2	0.43	0.50	165.9	08274
Life, oat cinn, Quaker	120	1.3	2.9	25.5	8.5	2.0	153	105	28	4.07	0.806	1	<1	0.41	5.4	0.00	0.14
3/4 cup (1.1 oz)	32	1.3	0.2	0.4	0.4	0	82	120	6.61	0.070	0.8	10	0.2	0.46	0.54	703.0	08210
oat, Quaker	120	1.3	3.2	25.0	6.2	2.1	164	112	31	4.13	0.874	1	<1	0.40	5.5	0.00	0.18
3/4 cup (1.1 oz)	32	1.4	0.3	0.5	0.5	0	91	133	8.95	0.083	7.6	13	0.2	0.47	0.55	703.0	08049
Lucky Charms, General Mills	114	0.7	2.1	24.9	12.9	1.5	203	100	16	3.75	0.639	150	6	0.38	5.0	1.50	0.21
1 cup (1.1 oz)	30	1.1	0.2	0.3	0.3	0	57	60	4.50	0.040	5.9	500	0.1	0.43	0.50	336.3	08050
Marshmallow Mateys, Malt-O-Meal	115	0.8	2.3	25.1	12.8	1.4	211	100	18	4.22	0.003	150	6	0.38	5.0	1.50	<0.01
1 cup (1.1 oz)	30	1.0	0.2	0.4	0.3	0	62	75	5.71	0.075	5.2	500	0.1	0.43	0.50	335.7	08138
Mueslix, raisin almond crnch w/dates,	196	4.8	5.0	40.2	17.1	4.0	170	32	49	3.74	1.197	90	<1	0.44	5.5	6.05	2.53
Kellogg's - 3/5 cup (1.9 oz)	55	3.0	0.4	1.6	1.0	0	240	100	4.51	0.110	9.5	300	5.9	0.44	2.04	682.6	08286
Natural Cereal, 100% w/oats &	232	1.1	5.4	33.9	13.3	3.7	24	61	57	1.20	1.250	1	<1	0.16	1.0	0.13	0.42
honey, Quaker - 1/2 cup (1.8 oz)	51	9.6	4.2	2.3	1.0	1	252	175	1.32	0.352	0.9	6	1.8	0.14	0.09	18.4	08054
w/oats, honey, & Raisins, Quaker	225	1.8	4.9	34.9	15.4	3.5	27	56	51	1.07	1.107	1	<1	0.15	0.9	0.11	0.37
1/2 cup (1.8 oz)	51	8.4	3.7	2.0	0.9	1	262	158	1.26	0.326	0.8	6	1.5	0.13	0.09	16.3	08218
Nestle Nesquick, choc, General	120		1.0	25.0	12.0		190	100					6				
Mills - 3/4 cup (1.1 oz)	30	2.0	0.0	0.5	0.5	0	65		4.50			500					GENM14
Oat Bran Flakes, Common Sense,	105	0.9	3.3	23.1	6.0	3.9	210	16	45	3.75	1.195	235	6	0.38	5.1	6.03	0.32
Kellogg's - 3/4 cup (1.1 oz)	30	1.1	0.2	0.5	0.3	0	120	105	8.40	0.090	5.1	781	0.4	0.44	2.10	681.9	08258
Oat Bran, Quaker	212	2.3	7.1	42.7	9.3	5.6	207	109	96	3.96	2.195	165	7	0.41	5.5	0.00	0.48
1 1/4 cups (2 oz)	57	2.9	0.5	0.9	1.2	0	250	295	17.07	0.180	4.0	550	2.1	0.47	0.55	706.2	08216
Oatmeal Crisp, almond, General Mills	218	1.3	5.5	41.8	15.4	4.4	237	20	60	3.74	1.108	0	6	0.37	5.0	1.49	0.35
1 cup (1.9 oz)	55	4.6	0.6	2.4	1.2	0	184	150	4.51	0.120	9.5	0	3.1	0.42	0.50	162.8	08202
apple, General Mills	207	1.6	5.0	45.1	18.7	3.9	253	20	40	3.75	1.127	0	6	0.37	5.0	1.49	0.42
1 cup (1.9 oz)	55	2.1	0.4	0.8	0.7	0	171	100	4.51	0.080	9.5	0	0.4	0.42	0.50	162.8	08190
raisin, General Mills	204	3.2	5.0	44.6	17.6	3.9	216	20	40	3.75	1.058	0	6	0.37	5.0	1.49	0.34
1 cup (1.9 oz)	55	2.0	0.4	0.7	0.6	0	200		4.51	0.080	9.5	0	1.4	0.42	0.50	162.8	08245
Oatmeal Squares, Quaker	212	1.5	6.2	43.9		4.0	269	113	66	4.24	1.814	167	6	0.39	5.6	0.00	0.34
1 cup (2 oz)	56	2.4	0.5	0.8	1.0	0	205	206	17.07	0.179	3.9	555	1.5	0.48	0.55	739.8	08214

Header groups: columns A (mcg RAE)–PANT and A (IU)–FOL fall under **Vitamins**; columns Na–Mn and K–Se fall under **Minerals**.

	KCAL / WT (g)	H₂0 (g) / FAT (g)	PRO (g) / SFA (g)	CHO (g) / MUFA (g)	SUGR (g) / PUFA (g)	DFIB (g) / CHOL (mg)	Na (mg) / K (mg)	Ca (mg) / P (mg)	Mg (mg) / Fe (mg)	Zn (mg) / Cu (mg)	Mn (mg) / Se (mcg)	A (mcg RAE) / A (IU)	C (mg) / E (mg ATE)	B-1 (mg) / B-2 (mg)	NIA (mg) / B-6 (mg)	B-12 (mcg) / FOL (mcg DFE)	PANT (mg) / REF
Optimum, Nature's Path	190		8.0	41.0	16.0	10.0	230	250					1				
1 cup (1.9 oz)	55	2.5	0.0			0			2.70			0					NRPT1
Optimum Slim, Nature's Path	100		5.0	21.0	5.0	6.0	140	250					0				
1/2 cup	30	1.0	0.0			0			1.44			0					NRPT2
Oreo O's, Post	112	0.7	1.3	21.5	11.4	1.5	128	5	15	1.50			0	0.38	5.0	1.50	
3/4 cup (.95 oz)	27	2.4	0.4			0	49	32	1.80	0.081		750		0.42	0.50	166.3	08336
Para su Familia, frutis, General	120		1.0	26.0	6.0	0.0	210	100					6				
Mills - *1 cup (1.1 oz)*	30	1.0	0.0	0.0	0.0	0	20		8.10			500					GENM16
cinn stars, General Mills	120		1.0	26.0	6.0	0.0	240	100					6				
1 cup (1.1 oz)	30	1.0	0.0	0.0	0.0	0	25		8.10			500					GENM15
Product 19, Kellogg's	109	0.9	2.3	24.9	4.0	1.0	169	5	16	15.30	0.512	225	61	1.50	20.0	6.00	10.08
1 cup (1.1 oz)	30	0.4	0.1	0.1	0.2	0	50	40	18.09	0.036	3.6	750	20.1	1.71	2.07	675.9	08058
Puffed Amaranth	122		6.0	15.0	0.0	3.0	1	90					1				
1 cup (.8 oz)	23	1.0	0.0			0			7.92			0					NUWL2
puffed rice	56	0.4	0.9	12.6		0.2	0	1	4	0.14	0.210	0		0.36	4.9	0.00	0.04
1 cup (.49 oz)	14	0.1	<0.1			0	16	14	4.44	0.024	1.5	0		0.25	0.01	2.7	08156
Malt-O-Meal	60		1.0	13.0	0.0		0	0				0		0.37	5.0		
1 cup (.53 oz)	15	0.0	0.0			0	20	20	4.50			0		0.25			MALT20
Quaker	54	0.5	1.0	12.3		0.2	1	1	4	0.15	0.132	0		0.04	0.0	0.00	0.05
1 cup (.49 oz)	14	0.1	<0.1	<0.1	<0.1	0	16	17	0.49	0.132	1.5	0	<0.1	0.49	0.00	36.3	08066
puffed wheat	44	0.4	1.8	9.6		0.5	0	3	17	0.28	0.211	0		0.31	4.2	0.00	0.06
1 cup (.42 oz)	12	0.1	<0.1			0	42	43	3.80	0.049	14.8	0		0.22	0.02	3.8	08157
Malt-O-Meal	50		2.0	11.0	0.0	1.0	0	0				0		0.37	5.0		
1 cup (.5 oz)	15	0.0	0.0			0	60	40	4.50			0		0.25			MALT21
Quaker	55	0.6	2.4	11.5	0.2	1.4	1	4	20	0.46	0.300	0		0.09	0.8	0.06	0.07
1 1/4 cups (.53 oz)	15	0.3	0.1	<0.1	0.2	0	55	50	0.66	0.092	18.5	0	0.0	0.06	0.02	38.9	08146
Puffins, Barbara's Bakery	100		2.0	26.0	6.0	6.0	150	0					9				
3/4 cup (1.1 oz)	30	1.0	0.0			0	45		0.18			0					BARB2
Raisin Bran Crunch, Kellogg	188	2.8	3.2	45.0	20.0	4.0	209	19	47	1.59			1	0.37	5.3	1.54	
1 cup (1.9 oz)	53	1.0	0.2	0.4	0.4	0	213	137	4.51	0.159		541		0.42	0.48		08380
Raisin Bran, Gold Medal	170		5.0	41.0	12.0	6.0	320	700					0				
1 1/3 cups (1.9 oz)	55	1.5	0.0	0.0	0.0	0	330		18.00			500					GENM17
Kellogg's	188	4.9	5.0	45.0	18.9	7.0	350	28	80	1.50	1.823	150	<1	0.38	5.0	1.50	0.39
1 cup (2.1 oz)	59	1.5	0.3	0.3	0.9	0	360	250	4.48	0.201	4.1	500	0.5	0.42	0.50	162.8	08060
Malt-O-Meal	190		6.0	45.0	17.0	8.0	350	40	80	3.70			0	0.37	5.0	1.50	
1 cup (2.1 oz)	59	1.5	0.0			0	360	200	4.50	0.300		750		0.42	0.50	100.0	MALT22
Post	187	5.3	4.7	46.1	19.7	7.7	360	27	89	2.25			0	0.38	5.0	1.50	
1 cup (2.1 oz)	59	1.1	0.2			0	357	208	10.80	0.251		750		0.42	0.50	161.7	08337
Raisin Nut Bran, General Mills	209	2.5	5.2	41.5	16.0	5.1	250	20	40	3.74	1.305	0	0	0.37	5.0	1.49	0.34
1 cup (1.9 oz)	55	4.4	0.8	2.4	0.9	0	238	150	4.51	0.160	3.9	0	2.0	0.42	0.50	162.8	08261
Raisin Squares Mini-Wheats,	185	5.2	5.2	43.6	11.6	5.2	3	21	43	1.54	1.273	0	0	0.39	5.2	1.60	0.00
Kellogg's - *3/4 cup (1.9 oz)*	55	0.9	0.2	0.2	0.5	0	265	156	15.40	0.138	2.3	0	0.3	0.44	0.52	169.4	08287
Reese's Peanut Butter Puffs,	128	0.9	1.8	23.4	12.0	0.0	167	100	16	3.75	0.293	150		0.38	5.0	1.50	
General Mills - *3/4 cup (1.1 oz)*	30	2.9	0.6	1.2	0.9	0	42	20	4.50	0.063	2.0	500	0.6	0.43	0.50	165.9	08194
Rice Krispies, Kellogg's	128	1.0	2.0	29.0	3.0	0.1	319	5	13	0.46	0.347	153	6	0.38	5.0	1.49	0.32
1 1/4 cups (1.2 oz)	33	0.4	0.1	0.1	0.2	0	44	46	1.82	0.066	5.1	510	<0.1	0.46	0.50	175.9	08065
Rice Krispies Treats, Kellogg's	122	0.9	1.2	26.1	9.0	0.1	189	3	7	0.24	0.176	152	6	0.39	5.1	1.50	0.10
3/4 cup (1.1 oz)	30	1.5	0.4	0.9	0.2	0	24	24	1.86	0.030	3.6	504	<0.1	0.42	0.51	345.9	08288
Shredded Spoonfuls, Barbara's Bakery	120		4.0	24.0	5.0	4.0	200	<1					5				
3/4 cup (1.1 oz)	32	1.5	0.0			0	125		0.72			0	1.2				BARB1
Shredded Wheat, Post	82	1.0	2.6	19.8	0.0	2.6	0	10	31	0.63	0.875	0		0.06	1.0	0.00	0.22
1 rectangular biscuit (.85 oz)	24	0.3	<0.1	<0.1	0.1	0	104	103	0.75	0.084	1.4	0	0.2	0.00	0.08	8.4	08147a
	129	1.5	4.2	31.3	0.0	4.1	0	16	49	0.99	1.386	0		0.10	1.7	0.00	0.35
2 round biscuits (1.3 oz)	38	0.4	0.1	<0.1	0.2	0	165	163	1.19	0.132	2.2	0	0.4	0.00	0.13	13.3	08147b
	156	1.8	4.8	38.1	0.4	5.3	3	20	54	1.26			0	0.12	2.6	0.00	
2 biscuits (1.6 oz)	46	0.6	0.1			0	196	168	1.44	0.143		0		0.05	0.18		08340
frosted, bite size, Post	183	3.1	4.1	43.6	11.6	5.0	10	7	48	1.50			0	0.37	5.0	1.50	
1 cup (1.8 oz)	52	1.0	0.2			0	170	144	1.80	0.090		0		0.43	0.50	162.8	08339

	KCAL	H2O (g)	PRO (g)	CHO (g)	SUGR (g)	DFIB (g)	Na (mg)	Ca (mg)	Mg (mg)	Zn (mg)	Mn (mg)	A (mcg RAE)	C (mg)	B-1 (mg)	NIA (mg)	B-12 (mcg)	PANT (mg)
	WT (g)	FAT (g)	SFA (g)	MUFA (g)	PUFA (g)	CHOL (mg)	K (mg)	P (mg)	Fe (mg)	Cu (mg)	Se (mcg)	A (IU)	E (mg ATE)	B-2 (mg)	B-6 (mg)	FOL (mcg DFE)	REF
n' bran, Post	197	2.7	7.4	47.1	0.6	7.9	3	27	81	1.93			0	0.15	3.7	0.00	
1 1/4 cups (2.1 oz)	59	0.8	0.1			0	248	235	2.47	0.236		0		0.07	0.19	38.4	08341
spoon size, Post	167	2.0	5.0	40.7	0.4	5.6	3	21	57	1.31			0	0.13	2.7	0.00	
1 cup (1.7 oz)	49	0.5	0.1			0	203	175	1.56	0.162		0		0.06	0.20	28.4	08342
Smacks, Kellogg's	104	0.7	1.7	24.0	15.1	1.0	50	6	16	0.35	0.378	153	6	0.38	5.0	1.51	0.10
3/4 cup (.95 oz)	27	0.5	0.1	0.2	0.2	0	41	46	0.35	0.054	13.1	509	0.1	0.43	0.51	168.5	08071
Smart Start, Kellogg's	182	1.5	3.1	43.0	15.5	2.3	281	17	32	15.10	1.096	231	16	1.55	20.0	6.00	10.00
1 cup (1.8 oz)	50	0.6	0.2	0.2	0.3	0	102	101	18.00	0.090	10.7	770	20.1	1.70	2.00	677.5	08318
Special K, Kellogg's	117	0.9	7.0	22.0	4.0	0.7	224	9	19	0.90	0.853	230	21	0.53	7.1	6.05	0.49
1 cup (1.1 oz)	31	0.5	0.1	0.1	0.2	0	61	68	8.37	0.062	17.0	767	7.1	0.59	1.98	675.8	08067
Red Berries, Kellogg	114	0.9	3.8	25.0	10.0	1.0	220	19	12	0.50			21	0.52	7.0	2.11	
1 cup (1.1 oz)	31	0.3	0.1	0.1	0.2	0	75	50	8.12	0.053	4.0	750	7.1	0.62	0.70		08383
Strawberry Squares Mini-Wheats,	168	4.8	4.0	40.0	9.3	4.9	15	23	60	1.55	1.158	0	0	0.38	5.0	1.50	0.00
Kellogg's - 3/4 cup (1.8 oz)	50	1.0	0.2	0.2	0.7	0	172	150	16.20	0.135	2.1	0	0.3	0.43	0.50	148.0	08289
Sunrise, organic, General Mills	110		2.0	26.0	10.0	1.0	190	0					6				
3/4 cup (1.1 oz)	30	0.5	0.0	0.0	0.0	0	50		4.50			0					GENM18
Sweet Crunch/Quisp, Quaker	109	0.5	1.2	23.0		0.7	200	3	15	4.13	0.178	11	3	0.41	5.5	0.00	0.09
1 cup (.95 oz)	27	1.6	0.4	0.3	0.2	0	51	45	4.96	0.054	1.8	36	0.2	0.47	0.55	710.4	08059
Sweet Puffs, Quaker	133	0.8	2.3	29.9	16.1	1.2	80	3	19	0.42	0.303	0	0	0.05	1.5	0.05	0.11
1 cup (1.2 oz)	34	0.7	0.1	0.1	0.3	0	50	48	0.65	0.078	2.2	1	0.4	0.04	0.02	6.5	08299
Toasted Cinn Twists, Malt-O-Meal	130		1.0	24.0	10.0	1.0	210	100	8	3.70			6	0.37	5.0	1.50	
3/4 cup (1.1 oz)	30	3.5	0.5			0	45	60	4.50	0.040		500		0.42	0.50	100.0	MALT23
Toasted Oatmeal, honey nut, Quaker	192	1.3	4.5	37.9	13.0	3.5	216	133	60	5.39	1.343	216	1	0.59	7.2	0.00	0.30
1 cup (1.7 oz)	49	3.7	0.5	1.7	1.0	0	181	166	6.81	0.191	1.1	718	2.7	0.67	0.72	735.5	08219
Toasty Os, Malt-O-Meal	112	1.2	3.3	22.4	1.0	2.7	284	40	32	3.75	0.090	375	15	0.38	5.0	0.00	0.02
1 cup (1.1 oz)	30	1.8	0.4	0.7	0.6	0	94	100	8.10	0.039	11.3	1250	0.2	0.43	0.50	165.9	08350
apple cinn, Malt-O-Meal	120		2.0	25.0	13.0	1.0	160	100	16	3.70			6	0.37	5.0	1.50	
3/4 cup (1.1 oz)	30	1.5	0.0			0	55	60	4.50			500		0.42	0.50	200.0	MALT24
honey & nut, Malt-O-Meal	110		3.0	24.0	11.0	2.0	270	100	32	3.70			6	0.37	5.0	1.50	
1 cup (1.1 oz)	30	1.0	0.0			0	95	100	4.50	0.080		500		0.42	0.50	200.0	MALT25
Tootie Fruities, Malt-O-Meal	125	1.0	1.6	28.1	14.0	0.7	149	100	8	3.75	0.039	225	15	0.37	5.0	1.50	0.02
1 cup (1.1 oz)	32	1.0	0.3	0.3	0.2	0	39	20	4.50	0.032	3.2	750	0.3	0.43	0.50	165.4	08349
Total, General Mills	97	0.9	2.4	22.5	5.1	2.4	192	1000	24	15.00	0.999	150	60	1.50	20.0	6.00	9.90
3/4 cup (1.1 oz)	30	0.8	0.2	0.2	0.3	0	89	80	18.00	0.080	1.4	500	20.1	1.70	2.00	675.9	08077
brown sugar & oat, General	110		2.0	23.0	9.0	1.0	200	1000					60				
Mills - 3/4 cup (1.1 oz)	30	0.5	0.0	0.0	0.0	0	80		18.00			500					GENM19
corn, General Mills	112	0.8	1.8	25.7	3.3	0.8	209	1000	8	15.00	0.029	129	60	1.50	20.0	6.00	9.90
1 1/3 cups (1.1 oz)	30	0.5	0.1	0.1	0.1	0	28	110	18.00	0.000	1.5	429	20.1	1.70	2.00	675.9	08246
raisin bran, General Mills	171	4.5	3.9	41.3	19.8	5.0	239	1000	40	15.02	2.550	150	0	1.50	20.0	6.00	9.90
1 cup (1.9 oz)	55	1.1	0.2	0.1	0.5	0	354	100	17.99	0.160	3.9	500	20.3	1.70	2.00	672.7	08247
whole grain, General Mills	110		2.0	23.0	5.0	3.0	190	1000					60				
3/4 cup (1.1 oz)	30	1.0	0.0	0.0	0.0	0	90		18.00			500					GENM20
Trix, General Mills	117	0.6	0.9	26.7	13.2	0.9	194	100	4	3.75	0.018	150	6	0.38	5.0	1.50	
1 cup (1.1 oz)	30	1.1	0.2	0.6	0.3	0	17	20	4.50	0.087	1.5	500	0.6	0.43	0.50	165.9	08078
Uncle Sam	190		7.0	38.0	<1.0	10.0	135	40					1	0.75	10.0		
1 cup (1.9 oz)	55	5.0	0.5			0			1.80			0		0.85			USAM1
Waffelos	122	0.8	1.7	25.9			125	8	6	0.24		397	16	0.39	5.3	1.59	0.05
1 cup (1.1 oz)	30	1.3				0	26	245	4.77	0.034		1323		0.45	0.54	3.3	08079
Waffle Crisp, Post	129	0.8	1.8	23.7	9.5	0.5	130	6	12	1.50	0.425		0	0.38	5.0	1.50	0.14
1 cup (1.1 oz)	30	2.9	0.4	1.2	1.1	0	34	34	1.80	0.035	1.6	750	<0.1	0.43	0.50	165.9	08344
Wheat Bran Flakes, Kellogg's	92	0.9	2.9	22.9	4.9	5.1	207	15	41	3.77	1.224	375	16	0.38	5.0	6.00	0.27
Complete - 3/4 cup (1 oz)	29	0.6	0.1	0.1	0.3	0	171	157	8.12	0.145	3.0	1250	5.2	0.44	2.03	403.1	08028
Wheaties Energy Crunch, General	210		6.0	42.0	13.0	4.0	310	350					12				
Mills - 1 cup (1.9 oz)	55	3.0	0.0	1.0	0.5	0	135		18.00			500					GENM21
Wheaties, General Mills	107	0.9	3.0	24.3	4.2	3.0	218	0	32	7.50		150	6	0.75	10.0	3.00	0.24
1 cup (1.1 oz)	30	1.0	0.2	0.3	0.4	0	111	100	8.10	0.080	1.4	500	0.4	0.85	1.00	336.3	08089
honey frosted, General Mills	112	0.8	1.5	26.7	11.7	0.6	204	100	11	7.50	0.305	150	6	0.75	10.0	3.00	0.11
3/4 cup (1.1 oz)	30	0.3	0.1	0.1	0.1	0	33	20	8.10	0.030	1.4	500	0.0	0.85	1.00	675.9	08266

	KCAL	H₂O (g)	PRO (g)	CHO (g)	SUGR (g)	DFIB (g)	Na (mg)	Ca (mg)	Mg (mg)	Zn (mg)	Mn (mg)	A (mcg RAE)	C (mg)	B-1 (mg)	NIA (mg)	B-12 (mcg)	PANT (mg)
	WT (g)	FAT (g)	SFA (g)	MUFA (g)	PUFA (g)	CHOL (mg)	K (mg)	P (mg)	Fe (mg)	Cu (mg)	Se (mcg)	A (IU)	E (mg ATE)	B-2 (mg)	B-6 (mg)	FOL (mcg DFE)	REF

5. CHEESE & CHEESE PRODUCTS
5.1 CHEESE

Food																	
american processed	106	11.1	6.3	0.5		0.0	405	175	6	0.85	0.004	77	0	0.01	<0.1	0.20	0.14
1 oz	28	8.9	5.6	2.5	0.3	27	46	211	0.11	0.009	4.1	343	0.1	0.10	0.02	2.3	01042
nonfat, Kraft Free Singles	31	12.2	4.8	2.5	1.4	0.0	273	150		0.53			<1					
1 slice	21	0.2	0.1			3	50	194	0.01			455		0.06			01190
blue	100	12.0	6.1	0.7		0.0	395	150	7	0.75	0.003	56	0	0.01	0.3	0.35	0.49
1 oz	28	8.1	5.3	2.2	0.2	21	73	110	0.09	0.011	4.1	204	0.2	0.11	0.05	10.2	01004
brick	105	11.7	6.6	0.8		0.0	159	191	7	0.74	0.003	83	0	<0.01	<0.1	0.36	0.08
1 oz	28	8.4	5.3	2.4	0.2	27	39	128	0.12	0.007	4.1	307	0.1	0.10	0.02	5.7	01005
brie	95	13.7	5.9	0.1		0.0	178	52	6	0.67	0.010	50	0	0.02	0.1	0.47	0.20
1 oz	28	7.8	4.9	2.3	0.2	28	43	53	0.14	0.005	4.1	189	0.2	0.15	0.07	18.4	01006
camembert	85	14.7	5.6	0.1		0.0	239	110	6	0.67	0.011	70	0	0.01	0.2	0.37	0.39
1 oz	28	6.9	4.3	2.0	0.2	20	53	98	0.09	0.006	4.1	262	0.2	0.14	0.06	17.6	01007
caraway	107	11.1	7.1	0.9		0.0	196	191	6	0.83	0.006	77	0	0.01	0.1	0.08	0.05
1 oz	28	8.3	5.3	2.3	0.2	26	26	139	0.18	0.007	4.1	299		0.13	0.02	5.1	01008
cheddar	114	10.4	7.1	0.4		0.0	176	204	8	0.88	0.003	76	0	0.01	<0.1	0.24	0.12
1 oz	28	9.4	6.0	2.7	0.3	30	28	145	0.19	0.009	3.9	300	0.1	0.11	0.02	5.1	01009a
low fat	49	17.9	6.9	0.5		0.0	174	118	5	0.52	0.002	18	0	<0.01	<0.1	0.14	0.05
1 oz	28	2.0	1.2	0.6	0.1	6	19	137	0.12	0.006	4.1	66	<0.1	0.06	0.01	3.1	01168
low Na	113	11.1	6.9	0.5		0.0	6	199	8	0.88	0.003	76	0	0.01	<0.1	0.24	0.09
1 oz	28	9.2	5.9	2.6	0.3	28	32	137	0.20	0.010	4.1	297	0.1	0.11	0.02	5.1	01169
shredded	455	41.5	28.1	1.4		0.0	702	815	32	3.51	0.011	303	0	0.03	0.1	0.94	0.47
1 cup	113	37.4	23.8	10.6	1.1	119	111	579	0.77	0.035	15.7	1197	0.4	0.42	0.08	20.3	01009b
cheshire	110	10.7	6.6	1.4		0.0	198	182	6	0.79	0.003	66	0	0.01	<0.1	0.24	0.12
1 oz	28	8.7	5.5	2.5	0.2	29	27	132	0.06	0.012	4.1	279		0.08	0.02	5.1	01010
colby	112	10.8	6.7	0.7		0.0	171	194	7	0.87	0.003	75	0	<0.01	<0.1	0.24	0.06
1 oz	28	9.1	5.7	2.6	0.3	27	36	130	0.22	0.012	4.1	293	0.1	0.11	0.02	5.1	01011
cottage cheese, 1% fat	163	186.4	28.0	6.1		0.0	918	138	11	0.86	0.007	25	0	0.05	0.3	1.42	0.49
1 cup	226	2.3	1.5	0.7	0.1	9	194	303	0.32	0.063	20.3	84	0.2	0.37	0.15	27.1	01016
2% fat	203	179.2	31.1	8.2		0.0	918	156	14	0.95	0.007	47	0	0.05	0.3	1.60	0.55
1 cup	226	4.4	2.8	1.2	0.1	18	217	341	0.36	0.063	23.1	158	0.1	0.42	0.17	29.4	01015
creamed, large curd	216	165.8	26.2	5.6		0.0	851	126	11	0.78	0.006	92	0	0.04	0.3	1.30	0.45
1 cup	210	9.5	6.0	2.7	0.3	32	176	277	0.29	0.059	18.9	342	0.3	0.34	0.14	25.2	01012a
creamed, small curd	232	177.7	28.1	6.0		0.0	911	135	11	0.83	0.007	99	0	0.05	0.3	1.40	0.48
1 cup	225	10.1	6.4	2.9	0.3	34	189	297	0.32	0.063	20.3	367	0.3	0.37	0.15	27.0	01012b
creamed w/fruit	280	162.9	22.4	30.1		0.0	915	108	9	0.66	0.007	81	0	0.04	0.2	1.11	0.38
1 cup	226	7.7	4.9	2.2	0.2	25	151	237	0.25	0.063	16.0	278	0.2	0.29	0.12	22.6	01013
cream cheese	51	7.8	1.1	0.4		0.0	43	12	1	0.08	0.001	54	0	<0.01	<0.1	0.06	0.04
1 T	15	5.1	3.2	1.4	0.2	16	17	15	0.17	0.002	0.3	207	0.1	0.03	0.01	1.9	01017
edam	101	11.8	7.1	0.4		0.0	274	207	9	1.06	0.003	70	0	0.01	<0.1	0.44	0.08
1 oz	28	7.9	5.0	2.3	0.2	25	53	152	0.12	0.010	4.1	260	0.2	0.11	0.02	4.5	01018
feta	75	15.7	4.0	1.2		0.0	316	140	5	0.82	0.008	36	0	0.04	0.3	0.48	0.27
1 oz	28	6.0	4.2	1.3	0.2	25	18	96	0.18	0.009	4.3	127	<0.1	0.24	0.12	9.1	01019
fontina	110	10.8	7.3	0.4		0.0	227	156	4	0.99	0.004	78	0	0.01	<0.1	0.48	0.12
1 oz	28	8.8	5.4	2.5	0.5	33	18	98	0.07	0.007	4.1	333	0.1	0.06	0.02	1.7	01020
gjetost	132	3.8	2.7	12.1		0.0	170	113	20	0.32	0.011	95	0	0.09	0.2	0.69	0.95
1 oz	28	8.4	5.4	2.2	0.3	27	399	126	0.15	0.023	4.1	316		0.39	0.08	1.4	01021
goat, hard	128	8.2	8.7	0.6		0.0	98	254	15	0.45	0.071	136	0	0.04	0.7	0.03	0.12
1 oz	28	10.1	7.0	2.3	0.2	30	14	207	0.53	0.178	1.6	451	0.2	0.34	0.02	1.1	01156
semi-soft	103	12.9	6.1	0.7		0.0	146	84	8	0.19	0.026	114	0	0.02	0.3	0.06	0.05
1 oz	28	8.5	5.9	1.9	0.2	22	45	106	0.46	0.160	1.1	378	0.2	0.19	0.02	0.6	01157
soft	76	17.2	5.3	0.3		0.0	104	40	5	0.26	0.028	80	0	0.02	0.1	0.05	0.19
1 oz	28	6.0	4.1	1.4	0.1	13	7	73	0.54	0.208	0.8	267	0.1	0.11	0.07	3.4	01159
gouda	101	11.8	7.1	0.6		0.0	232	198	8	1.11	0.003	48	0	0.01	<0.1	0.44	0.08
1 oz	28	7.8	5.0	2.2	0.2	32	34	155	0.07	0.010	4.1	183	0.1	0.09	0.02	6.0	01022
gruyere	117	9.4	8.5	0.1		0.0	95	287	10	1.11	0.005	81	0	0.02	<0.1	0.45	0.16
1 oz	28	9.2	5.4	2.8	0.5	31	23	172	0.05	0.009	4.1	346	0.1	0.08	0.02	2.8	01023
limburger	93	13.7	5.7	0.1		0.0	227	141	6	0.60	0.011	98	0	0.02	<0.1	0.29	0.33
1 oz	28	7.7	4.7	2.4	0.1	26	36	111	0.04	0.006	4.1	363	0.2	0.14	0.02	16.4	01024
mexican, queso asadero	101	12.0	6.4	0.8		0.0	186	187	7	0.86	0.010	16	0	0.01	0.1	0.28	0.07
1 oz	28	8.0	5.1	2.3	0.2	30	24	126	0.14	0.007	4.1	63	<0.1	0.06	0.02	2.3	01166

	KCAL	H₂0 (g)	PRO (g)	CHO (g)	SUGR (g)	DFIB (g)	Na (mg)	Ca (mg)	Mg (mg)	Zn (mg)	Mn (mg)	A (mcg RAE)	C (mg)	B-1 (mg)	NIA (mg)	B-12 (mcg)	PANT (mg)
	WT (g)	FAT (g)	SFA (g)	MUFA (g)	PUFA (g)	CHOL (mg)	K (mg)	P (mg)	Fe (mg)	Cu (mg)	Se (mcg)	A (IU)	E (mg ATE)	B-2 (mg)	B-6 (mg)	FOL (mcg DFE)	REF
queso anejo	106	10.8	6.1	1.3		0.0	321	193	8	0.83	0.010	16	0	0.01	<0.1	0.39	0.07
1 oz	28	8.5	5.4	2.4	0.3	30	25	126	0.13	0.002	4.1	63	<0.1	0.06	0.01	0.3	01165
queso chihuahua	106	11.1	6.1	1.6		0.0	175	185	7	0.99	0.020	16	0	0.01	<0.1	0.29	0.08
1 oz	28	8.4	5.3	2.4	0.3	30	15	125	0.13	0.007	4.1	64	0.1	0.06	0.02	0.6	01167
monterey	106	11.6	6.9	0.2		0.0	152	211	8	0.85	0.003	59	0	<0.01	<0.1	0.24	0.06
1 oz	28	8.6	5.4	2.5	0.3	25	23	126	0.20	0.009	4.1	269	0.1	0.11	0.02	5.1	01025
mozzarella nuggets, frzn, Banquet	280		9.0	19.0	3.0	1.0	1060	150					0				
6 pieces (3 oz)	85	18.0	6.0			40		0.36				0					CNAG43
mozzarella, part nonfat	72	15.2	6.9	0.8		0.0	132	183	7	0.78	0.003	43	0	0.01	<0.1	0.23	0.02
1 oz	28	4.5	2.9	1.3	0.1	16	24	131	0.06	0.007	4.1	166	0.1	0.09	0.02	2.6	01028
part nonfat, low moisture	79	13.8	7.8	0.9		0.0	150	207	7	0.89	0.003	53	0	0.01	<0.1	0.26	0.03
1 oz	28	4.9	3.1	1.4	0.1	15	27	149	0.07	0.008	4.6	199	0.1	0.10	0.02	2.8	01029
whole milk	80	15.3	5.5	0.6		0.0	106	147	5	0.63	0.002	58	0	<0.01	<0.1	0.18	0.02
1 oz	28	6.1	3.7	1.9	0.2	22	19	105	0.05	0.006	4.1	225	0.1	0.07	0.02	2.0	01026
whole milk, low moisture	90	13.7	6.1	0.7		0.0	118	163	6	0.70	0.003	67	0	<0.01	<0.1	0.21	0.02
1 oz	28	7.0	4.4	2.0	0.2	25	21	117	0.06	0.006	4.6	256	0.2	0.08	0.02	2.3	01027
muenster	104	11.8	6.6	0.3		0.0	178	203	8	0.80	0.002	86	0	<0.01	<0.1	0.42	0.05
1 oz	28	8.5	5.4	2.5	0.2	27	38	133	0.12	0.009	4.1	318	0.1	0.09	0.02	3.4	01030
neufchatel	74	17.6	2.8	0.8		0.0	113	21	2	0.15	0.001	84	0	<0.01	<0.1	0.07	0.16
1 oz	28	6.6	4.2	1.9	0.2	22	32	39				321		0.06	0.01	3.1	01031
parmesan, grated	23	0.9	2.1	0.2		0.0	93	69	3	0.16	0.001	7	0	<0.01	<0.1	0.07	0.03
1 T	5	1.5	1.0	0.4	<0.1	4	5	40	0.05	0.002	1.3	35	<0.1	0.02	0.01	0.4	01032
hard	111	8.3	10.1	0.9		0.0	454	336	12	0.78	0.006	33	0	0.01	0.1	0.34	0.13
1 oz	28	7.3	4.7	2.1	0.2	19	26	197	0.23	0.009	6.4	171	0.2	0.09	0.03	2.0	01033
pimento, processed	106	11.1	6.3	0.5		0.0	405	174	6	0.84	0.005	71	1	0.01	<0.1	0.20	0.14
1 oz	28	8.8	5.6	2.5	0.3	27	46	211	0.12	0.009	4.1	358	0.1	0.10	0.02	2.3	01043
port du salut	100	12.9	6.7	0.2		0.0	151	184	7	0.74	0.003	93	0	<0.01	<0.1	0.43	0.06
1 oz	28	8.0	4.7	2.6	0.2	35	39	102	0.12	0.006	4.1	378	0.1	0.07		5.1	01034
provolone	100	11.6	7.3	0.6		0.0	248	214	8	0.92	0.003	66	0	0.01	<0.1	0.41	0.13
1 oz	28	7.5	4.8	2.1	0.2	20	39	141	0.15	0.007	4.1	231	0.1	0.09	0.02	2.8	01035
ricotta, part nonfat	171	92.3	14.1	6.4		0.0	155	337	19	1.66	0.012	135	0	0.03	0.1	0.36	0.30
1/2 cup	124	9.8	6.1	2.9	0.3	38	155	227	0.55	0.042	20.7	536	0.3	0.23	0.02	16.1	01037
whole milk	216	88.9	14.0	3.8		0.0	104	257	14	1.44	0.007	151	0	0.02	0.1	0.42	0.26
1/2 cup	124	16.1	10.3	4.5	0.5	63	130	196	0.47	0.026	18.0	608	0.4	0.24	0.05	14.9	01036
romano	110	8.8	9.0	1.0		0.0	340	302	12	0.73	0.006	29	0	0.01	<0.1	0.32	0.12
1 oz	28	7.6	4.9	2.2	0.2	29	24	215	0.22	0.009	4.1	162	0.2	0.10	0.02	2.0	01038
roquefort (sheep's milk)	105	11.2	6.1	0.6		0.0	513	188	9	0.59	0.009	83	0	0.01	0.2	0.18	0.49
1 oz	28	8.7	5.5	2.4	0.4	26	26	111	0.16	0.010	4.1	297		0.17	0.04	13.9	01039
swiss	107	10.5	8.1	1.0		0.0	74	272	10	1.11	0.005	66	0	0.01	<0.1	0.48	0.12
1 oz	28	7.8	5.0	2.1	0.3	26	31	172	0.05	0.009	3.6	240	0.1	0.10	0.02	1.7	01040
processed	95	12.0	7.0	0.6		0.0	388	219	8	1.02	0.004	64	0	<0.01	<0.1	0.35	0.07
1 oz	28	7.1	4.5	2.0	0.2	24	61	216	0.17	0.008	4.5	229	0.2	0.08	0.01	1.7	01044
tilsit, whole milk	96	12.2	6.9	0.5		0.0	213	198	4	0.99	0.004	71	0	0.02	0.1	0.60	0.10
1 oz	28	7.4	4.8	2.0	0.2	29	18	142	0.07	0.007	4.1	296	0.2	0.10	0.02	5.7	01041

5.2 CHEESE PRODUCTS

	KCAL	H₂0	PRO	CHO	SUGR	DFIB	Na	Ca	Mg	Zn	Mn	A	C	B-1	NIA	B-12	PANT
	WT	FAT	SFA	MUFA	PUFA	CHOL	K	P	Fe	Cu	Se	A	E	B-2	B-6	FOL	REF
cheese 'n salsa dip, low fat,	30		<1.0	3.0	0.0	0.0	240	20					0				
med, Old El Paso - 2 T (1 oz)	29	1.5	1.0			<5		0.00				0					GENM22
mild/medium, Old El Paso	40		<1.0	3.0	0.0	0.0	300	20					0				
2 T (1 oz)	29	3.0	1.0			<5		0.00				0					GENM23
cheese fondue[1]	247	66.5	15.4	4.1		0.0	143	514	25	2.12	0.107	118	0	0.03	0.2	0.90	0.25
1/2 cup	108	14.5	9.4	3.8	0.5	49	113	330	0.42	0.028	9.7	447		0.21	0.06	11.9	01163
cheese food, american cold pack	94	12.2	5.6	2.4		0.0	274	141	9	0.85	0.003	45	0	0.01	<0.1	0.36	0.28
1 oz	28	6.9	4.4	2.0	0.2	18	103	113	0.24	0.009	4.6	200		0.13	0.04	1.4	01045
american	93	12.2	5.6	2.1		0.0	337	163	9	0.85	0.003	58	0	0.01	<0.1	0.32	0.16
1 oz	28	7.0	4.4	2.0	0.2	18	79	130	0.24	0.009	4.6	259	0.2	0.13	0.04	2.4	01046
swiss	92	12.4	6.2	1.3		0.0	440	205	8	1.01	0.003	67	0	<0.01	<0.1	0.65	0.14
1 oz	28	6.8	4.4	1.9	0.2	23	81	149	0.17	0.009	4.6	243		0.11	0.01	1.7	01047
cheese sauce, homemade[2]	59	20.1	3.1	1.6		0.0	148	93	6	0.38	0.012	50	<1	0.01	0.1	0.11	0.07
2 T	30	4.5	2.4	1.4	0.4	11	43	69	0.11	0.006	2.0	182		0.07	0.01	3.3	01164
cheese sauce mix, four cheese,	60		2.0	7.0	1.0	0.0	740	20					0				
Knorr - 2 T (1/2 cup prep)	14	3.0	1.0			<5		0.00				0					UNLV69

	KCAL	H₂0 (g)	PRO (g)	CHO (g)	SUGR (g)	DFIB (g)	Na (mg)	Ca (mg)	Mg (mg)	Zn (mg)	Mn (mg)	A (mcg RAE)	C (mg)	B-1 (mg)	NIA (mg)	B-12 (mcg)	PANT (mg)
	WT (g)	FAT (g)	SFA (g)	MUFA (g)	PUFA (g)	CHOL (mg)	K (mg)	P (mg)	Fe (mg)	Cu (mg)	Se (mcg)	A (IU)	E (mg ATE)	B-2 (mg)	B-6 (mg)	FOL (mcg DFE)	REF
cheese sauce, rts	110	44.4	4.2	4.3	0.3	0.3	522	116	6	0.62	0.006	50	<1	<0.01	<0.1	0.09	0.08
1/4 cup	63	8.4	3.8	2.4	1.6	18	19	99	0.13	0.011	2.0	199	0.2	0.07	0.01	2.5	06930
basic cheddar, Chef-Mate	82	46.0	1.8	8.0	0.1	0.0	471	46	4	0.33	0.004		1	<0.01	<0.1	0.06	0.09
1/4 cup	62	4.7	1.6			6	16	51	0.18	0.008		39	1.2	0.04	0.01		06921
golden, Chef-Mate	139	40.8	6.7	2.3	0.4	0.7	501	161	6	0.65	0.005		0	<0.01	<0.1	0.09	0.08
1/4 cup	63	11.4	5.6	3.1	2.1	29	20	105	0.14	0.010		200	0.3	0.08	0.01		06908
jalapeno, Que Bueno	81	46.8	2.0	7.7	0.1	0.0	571	54	4	0.34	0.004		<1	<0.01	<0.1	0.06	0.09
1/4 cup	63	4.7	1.8	1.7	0.8	6	16	52	0.12	0.008		71	0.3	0.04	0.01		06922
nacho mild, Que Bueno	119	44.4	4.5	2.5	0.0	0.5	492	118	6	0.65	0.005		<1	<0.01	<0.1	0.09	0.08
1/4 cup	63	10.1	4.2	3.1	2.1	20	20	105	0.20	0.010		128	0.3	0.08	0.01		06909
nacho, Que Bueno	128	41.9	5.2	4.0	0.5	0.4	580	181	6	0.65	0.005		<1	<0.01	<0.1	0.09	0.08
1/4 cup	63	10.1	5.8			29	20	105	0.15	0.010		481	0.3	0.08	0.01		06910
nacho w/jalapeno peppers, La Victoria - *1/4 cup*	122	51.8	1.3	7.4	1.9	0.2	551	64					1				
	72	9.7	2.7	4.6	1.8	4		0.86				39					06278
sharp cheddar, Chef-Mate	133	42.6	5.5	1.8	0.3	0.6	473	136	6	0.65	0.005		<1	<0.01	<0.1	0.09	0.08
1/4 cup	63	11.5	4.6	3.1	2.1	23	20	105	0.13	0.010		302	0.3	0.08	0.01		06907
cheese spread, American	82	13.5	4.7	2.5		0.0	381	159	8	0.73	0.006	50	0	0.01	<0.1	0.11	0.19
1 oz	28	6.0	3.8	1.8	0.2	16	69	202	0.09	0.009	3.2	223	0.2	0.12	0.03	2.0	01048
Cheez Whiz, Kraft	91	17.0	4.0	3.0	2.2	0.1	541	118		0.54			<1				
2 T	33	6.9	4.3			25	79	266	0.06			214		0.08			01188
Cheez Whiz Light, Kraft	75	18.0	5.7	5.7	2.9	0.1	597	146		0.83			<1				
2 T	35	3.3	2.2			12	104	330	0.06			220		0.12			01189
Velveeta, Kraft	85	12.8	4.6	2.7	2.3	0.0	420	130		0.52			<1				
1 oz	28	6.2	4.0			22	94	242	0.05			310		0.10			01191
Velveeta Light, red fat, Kraft	62	14.4	5.5	3.3	2.4	0.0	444	161		0.70			<1				
1 oz	28	3.0	2.0			12	97	287	0.04			275		0.18			01192
creamy cheddar slices, Smart Balance	40		4.0	2.0	1.0		290	150									
.67 oz slice	19	2.0	0.5	0.5	0.5	<5	60	95				200	0.0				GBAF2
mozzarella cheese substitute	70	13.4	3.3	6.7		0.0	194	173	12	0.54	0.008	124	<1	0.01	0.1	0.23	0.02
1 oz	28	3.5	1.1	1.8	0.5	0	129	165	0.11	0.031	5.4	413	0.6	0.13	0.01	3.1	01161
Slices, Smart Beat	25		4.0	3.0	2.0		180	150									
1 oz	28	0.0	0.0	0.0	0.0	0						200	0.0				GBAF7

[1] Contains table wine, Swiss cheese, and all-purpose enriched flour. [2] Thin white sauce made with cheddar cheese and salt.

6. CREAMS & CREAM SUBSTITUTES

	KCAL	H₂0	PRO	CHO	SUGR	DFIB	Na	Ca	Mg	Zn	Mn	A	C	B-1	NIA	B-12	PANT
creamer, liquid/frzn w/hydg veg oils[1]	20	11.6	0.2	1.7		0.0	12	1	0	<0.01	0.000	1	0	0.00	0.0	0.00	0.00
1 T (1/2 fl oz container)	15	1.5	0.3	1.1	<0.1	0	29	10	<0.01	0.000	0.2	13	0.2	0.00	0.00	0.0	01067
w/lauric acid oils[2]	20	11.6	0.2	1.7		0.0	12	1	0	<0.01	0.006	1	0	0.00	0.0	0.00	0.00
1 T (1/2 fl oz container)	15	1.5	1.4	<0.1	<0.1	0	29	10	<0.01	0.004	0.2	13		0.00	0.00	0.0	01068
creamer, powdered	11	<0.1	0.1	1.1		0.0	4	0	<1	0.01	0.004	<1	0	0.00	0.00	0.00	0.00
1 t	2	0.7	0.7	<0.1	<0.1	0	16	8	0.02	0.002	<0.1	4	<0.1	<0.01	0.00	0.0	01069
creamer, soy milk, Silk	15		0.0	1.0	0.0	0.0	5	0					0				
1 T (1/2 fl oz)	~15	1.0	0.0			0				0.00		0					WHWA3
french van, Silk	20		0.0	3.0	3.0	0.0	5	0					0				
1 T (1/2 fl oz)	~15	1.0	0.0			0				0.00		0					WHWA1
hazelnut, Silk	15		0.0	1.0	0.0	0.0	5	0					0				
1 T (1/2 fl oz)	~15	1.0	0.0			0				0.00		0					WHWA2
half & half (milk & cream)	20	12.1	0.4	0.6		0.0	6	16	2	0.08	<0.001	15	<1	0.01	<0.1	0.05	0.04
1 T (1/2 fl oz container)	15	1.7	1.1	0.5	0.1	6	20	14	0.01	0.002	0.3	65	<0.1	0.02	0.01	0.5	01049
light (coffee/table) cream	29	11.1	0.4	0.5		0.0	6	14	1	0.04	<0.001	27	<1	<0.01	<0.1	0.03	0.04
1 T	15	2.9	1.8	0.8	0.1	10	18	12	0.01	0.001	0.1	95	<0.1	0.02	<0.01	0.3	01050
sour cream, cultured	26	8.5	0.4	0.5		0.0	6	14	1	0.03	<0.001	22	<1	<0.01	<0.1	0.04	0.04
1 T	12	2.5	1.6	0.7	0.1	5	17	10	0.01	0.002	0.3	95	0.1	0.02	<0.01	1.3	01056
fat free, Breakstone's Free	29	24.9	1.5	4.8	2.3	0.0	23	45					<1				
2 T	32	0.4	0.3			3	70	37	0.02			217					01194
imitation	59	20.2	0.7	1.9		0.0	29	1	2	0.33	0.031	0	0	0.00	0.0	0.00	0.00
1 oz	28	5.5	5.0	0.2	<0.1	0	46	13	0.11	0.016	0.7	0	<0.1	0.00	0.00	0.0	01074
red fat	20	12.0	0.4	0.6		0.0	6	16	2	0.08	<0.001	16	<1	0.01	<0.1	0.05	0.05
1 T	15	1.8	1.1	0.5	0.1	6	19	14	0.01	0.002	0.3	68	<0.1	0.02	<0.01	1.7	01055
red fat, Breakstone's	47	23.6	1.4	2.0	2.0	0.0	18	50					<1				
2 T	31	3.7	2.4			16	65	34	0.02			326					01193

Food	KCAL / WT (g)	H_2O / FAT (g)	PRO / SFA (g)	CHO / MUFA (g)	SUGR / PUFA (g)	DFIB (g) / CHOL (mg)	Na / K (mg)	Ca / P (mg)	Mg / Fe (mg)	Zn / Cu (mg)	Mn (mg) / Se (mcg)	A (mcg RAE) / A (IU)	C (mg) / E (mg ATE)	B-1 / B-2 (mg)	NIA / B-6 (mg)	B-12 (mcg) / FOL (mcg DFE)	PANT (mg) / REF
whipped topping, from mix, prep	8	2.7	0.1	0.7			3	4	<1	0.01	<0.001	1	<1	<0.01	<0.1	0.01	0.01
w/whole milk - *1 T*	4	0.5	0.4	<0.1	<0.1	<1	6	3	<0.01	<0.001	0.2	14	<0.1	<0.01	<0.01	0.2	01071
frzn	13	2.0	0.1	0.9		0.0	1	0	<1	<0.01	0.002	2	0	0.00	0.0	0.00	0.00
1 T	4	1.0	0.9	0.1	<0.1	0	1	<1	<0.01	0.001	0.1	34	<0.1	0.00	0.00	0.0	01073
pressurized	11	2.4	0.0	0.6		0.0	2	0	<1	<0.01	0.002	1	0	0.00	0.0	0.00	0.00
1 T	4	0.9	0.8	0.1	<0.1	0	1	1	<0.01	0.001	0.1	19	<0.1	0.00	0.00	0.0	01072
whipping cream, heavy fluid	52	8.7	0.3	0.4		0.0	6	10	1	0.03	<0.001	62	<1	<0.01	<0.1	0.03	0.04
1 T	15	5.6	3.5	1.6	0.2	21	11	9	<0.01	0.001	0.1	221	0.1	0.02	<0.01	0.6	01053
light fluid	44	9.5	0.3	0.4		0.0	5	10	1	0.04	<0.001	43	<1	<0.01	<0.1	0.03	0.04
1 T	15	4.6	2.9	1.4	0.1	17	15	9	<0.01	0.001	0.1	169	0.1	0.02	<0.01	0.6	01052
pressurized	8	1.8	0.1	0.4		0.0	4	3	<1	0.01	<0.001	6	0	<0.01	<0.1	0.01	0.01
1 T	3	0.7	0.4	0.2	<0.1	2	4	3	<0.01	<0.001	<0.1	25	<0.1	<0.01	<0.01	0.1	01054

[1] Contains hydrogenated vegetable oil and soy protein; vegetable oils are usually soybean, cottonseed, safflower, or blends thereof.

[2] Contains lauric acid oils and sodium caseinate; lauric oils include modified coconut oil, hydrogenated coconut oil, and/or palm kernel oil.

7. DESSERTS
7.1 BROWNIES & BARS

Food	KCAL / WT (g)	H_2O / FAT (g)	PRO / SFA (g)	CHO / MUFA (g)	SUGR / PUFA (g)	DFIB (g) / CHOL (mg)	Na / K (mg)	Ca / P (mg)	Mg / Fe (mg)	Zn / Cu (mg)	Mn (mg) / Se (mcg)	A (mcg RAE) / A (IU)	C (mg) / E (mg ATE)	B-1 / B-2 (mg)	NIA / B-6 (mg)	B-12 (mcg) / FOL (mcg DFE)	PANT (mg) / REF
brownie	227	7.6	2.7	35.8		1.2	175	16	17	0.40	0.072	12	0	0.14	1.0	0.04	0.31
1 brownie (2 3/4" × 7/8")	56	9.1	2.4	5.0	1.3	10	83	57	1.26	0.125	3.5	39	1.2	0.12	0.02	15.1	18151a
Little Debbie	247	8.3	2.9	39.0		1.3	190	18	19	0.44	0.078	13	0	0.16	1.0	0.04	0.33
1 twin wrapped pkg (2 pieces)	61	9.9	2.6	5.5	1.4	10	91	62	1.37	0.137	3.8	42	1.3	0.13	0.02	16.5	18151b
brownie, from mix, choc chunk, Betty Crocker Supreme - *1 brownie*	180		2.0	25.0	18.0	0.0	95	20				0		0.03	0.4		
	~40	9.0	2.5			20	95		1.08			0		0.07		8.0	GENM24
dark choc fudge, Betty Crocker Supreme - *1 brownie*	170		2.0	24.0	17.0	0.0	110	20				0		0.03	0.4		
	~38	7.0	1.5	2.5	2.0	20	90		0.72			0		0.07		8.0	GENM25
dark choc w/Hershey syrp, Betty Crocker Supreme - *1 brownie*	170		2.0	25.0	18.0	0.0	110	20				0		0.03	0.4		
	~42	7.0	1.5			20	100		1.08			0		0.07		8.0	GENM26
frosted, Betty Crocker Supreme *1 brownie*	210		2.0	30.0	22.0	1.0	135	20				0		0.03	0.4		
	~48	9.0	1.5			20	105		1.08			0		0.07		8.0	GENM27
fudge, Betty Crocker *1 brownie*	190		2.0	27.0	19.0	1.0	125	20				0		0.03	0.4		
	~47	8.0	1.5			25	100		1.08			0		0.07		8.0	GENM28
fudge, Betty Crocker Supreme *1 brownie*	170		2.0	24.0	17.0	0.0	105	20				0		0.03	0.4		
	~42	7.0	1.5			20	85		1.08			0		0.03		8.0	GENM29
fudge, red fat, Sweet Rewards *1 brownie*	140		2.0	27.0	19.0	0.0	110	0				0		0.03	0.4		
	~40	3.5	1.0			20	90		1.08			0		0.07		8.0	GENM31
german choc, Betty Crocker Supreme - *1 brownie*	200		2.0	29.0	21.0	1.0	130	20				0		0.03	0.4		
	~49	8.0	2.0	2.5	1.5	20	115		0.72			0		0.07		8.0	GENM32
original fudge, Betty Crocker Supreme - *1 brownie*	160		2.0	27.0	19.0	0.0	110	20				0		0.03	0.4		
	~42	6.0	1.0	2.0	1.5	20	105		0.72			0		0.07		8.0	
peanut butter w/Reese's Pieces, Bty Crckr Suprm - *1 brownie*	180		3.0	23.0	17.0	0.0	105	20				0		0.03	0.4		
	~40	9.0	2.5	2.5	2.0	20	120		0.72			0		0.03		8.0	GENM35
turtle, Betty Crocker Supreme *1 brownie*	170		2.0	23.0	16.0	0.0	100	20				0		0.03	0.0		
	~40	8.0	1.5	3.0	2.0	20	95		0.72			0		0.03		8.0	GENM36
walnut, Betty Crocker Supreme *1 brownie*	180		2.0	22.0	15.0	0.0	95	20				0		0.03	0.4		
	~39	9.0	1.5	3.0	3.0	20	105		0.72			0		0.03		8.0	GENM37
brownie, from refrig dough, fudge, Pillsbury RTB - *1/12 pkg (1.6 oz)*	180		2.0	25.0	15.0	<1.0	105	0				0					
	44	8.0	2.0			0			1.08			0					GENM38
brownie, homemade	112	3.0	1.5	12.0			82	14	13	0.23	0.141	42	<1	0.03	0.2	0.04	
1 brownie (2" sq)	24	7.0	1.8	2.6	2.3	18	42	32	0.44	0.093	2.8	198		0.05	0.02	9.4	GENM30
brownie mix, fudge, low fat, Sweet Rewards[1] - *1/18 pkg (1.1 oz)*	130		2.0	27.0	18.0	1.0	115					0		0.03	0.4		0.08
	32	2.5	1.0	1.0	0.0	0	95		1.08			0		0.03		8.0	18154
w/mini Kisses, Betty Crocker Stir 'n Bake[1] - *1/6 pkg (1.7 oz)*	220		2.0	36.0	27.0	1.0	160	0				0		0.06	0.4		
	48	7.0	2.5			0	140		1.44			0		0.03		8.0	GENM34
date bar mix, Betty Crocker Classic[2]	150		1.0	23.0	14.0	1.0	90	0				0		0.06	0.0		
1/12 pkg (1.2 oz)	33	6.0	2.0			0	95		0.72			0		0.03		8.0	GENM41
Sunkist Lemon bar, from mix, Betty Crocker - *1 bar*	140		2.0	24.0	17.0	0.0	90	0				0		0.03	0.0		
	~40	4.5	1.0			40	20		0.00			0		0.07		8.0	GENM43

[1] Water is the only ingredient added to the dry mix to prepare the brownies.

[2] Water is the only ingredient added to the dry mix to prepare the date bars.

	KCAL	H₂O (g)	PRO (g)	CHO (g)	SUGR (g)	DFIB (g)	Na (mg)	Ca (mg)	Mg (mg)	Zn (mg)	Mn (mg)	A (mcg RAE)	C (mg)	B-1 (mg)	NIA (mg)	B-12 (mcg)	PANT (mg)
	WT (g)	FAT (g)	SFA (g)	MUFA (g)	PUFA (g)	CHOL (mg)	K (mg)	P (mg)	Fe (mg)	Cu (mg)	Se (mcg)	A (IU)	E (mg ATE)	B-2 (mg)	B-6 (mg)	FOL (mcg DFE)	REF

7.2 CAKES & SNACK CAKES

	KCAL/WT	H₂O/FAT	PRO/SFA	CHO/MUFA	SUGR/PUFA	DFIB/CHOL	Na/K	Ca/P	Mg/Fe	Zn/Cu	Mn/Se	A RAE/IU	C/E	B-1/B-2	NIA/B-6	B-12/FOL	PANT/REF
angel food	72	9.3	1.7	16.2		0.4	210	39	3	0.02	0.024	0	0	0.03	0.2	0.02	0.06
1/12 cake (1 oz)	28	0.2	<0.1	<0.1	0.1	0	26	9	0.15	0.022	2.0	0		0.14	0.01	16.0	18086
from mix	129	16.5	3.1	29.4		0.1	255	42	4	0.07	0.032	0	0	0.05	0.1	0.02	0.06
1/12 cake of 10″ dia cake	50	0.2	<0.1	<0.1	0.1	0	68	116	0.12	0.034	7.7	0	<0.1	0.10	<0.01	24.0	18088
angel food mix, one-step white,	140		3.0	32.0	24.0	0.0	320	60					0	0.00	0.0		
SuperMoist¹ - *1/12 pkg (1.4 oz)*	40	0.0	0.0	0.0	0.0	0	40		0.00			0		0.07		0.0	GENM44
boston cream pie (cake), frzn	232	41.8	2.2	39.5		1.3	132	21	6	0.15	0.046	21	<1	0.38	0.2	0.15	0.28
1/6 of 19.5 oz cake	92	7.8	2.2	4.2	0.9	34	36	45	0.35	0.039	3.8	74	1.0	0.25	0.02	18.4	18090
butter pecan, from mix, SuperMoist	240		3.0	35.0	20.0	0.0	280	80					0	0.09	0.8		
1/12 cake	~77	10.0	2.0	3.5	2.0	55	30		0.72			0		0.10		32.0	GENM45
carrot bites w/crm cheese icing &	80		<1.0	7.0	5.0	0.0	35	<1					<1				
nuts, frzn, Sara Lee - *.56 oz piece*	16	5.0	3.5			<5			<0.01			200					SARA1
from mix, SuperMoist	320		4.0	42.0	24.0		360	100					0	0.12	0.8		
1/10 cake	~83	15.0	3.0			65	75		0.72			0		0.14		32.0	GENM46
w/crm cheese icing, frzn, Mrs.	300		3.0	37.0	28.0	1.0	360	0					0				
Smith's - *1/6 cake (2.9 oz)*	83	16.0	3.5			30			0.72			2000					MSSM1
carrot mix w/crm cheese icing, Bty	250		2.0	46.0	29.0	0.0	300	40					0	0.09	0.8		
Crckr Stir 'n Bake¹ - *1/6 pkg (2.2 oz)*	61	7.0	2.0			0	45		0.72			0		0.07		24.0	GENM47
cheesecake, from mix	257	36.5	4.4	20.4		0.3	166	41	9	0.41	0.112	114	<1	0.02	0.2	0.14	0.46
1/6 of 17 oz cake	80	18.0	7.9	6.9	1.3	44	72	74	0.50	0.016	4.2	438	1.3	0.15	0.04	16.0	18147
no-bake type	271	43.8	5.4	35.1		1.9	376	170	19	0.46	0.119	95	<1	0.12	0.5	0.31	0.61
1/8 of 9″ cake	99	12.6	6.6	4.5	0.8	29	209	232	0.47	0.029	4.7	362		0.26	0.05	37.6	18148
cherry chip, from mix, SuperMoist	300		4.0	41.0	23.0	0.0	340	60					0	0.12	0.8		
1/10 cake	~83	13.0	3.0	4.5	2.5	65	45		1.08			0		0.14		32.0	GENM51
cherry fudge w/choc icing	187	32.7	1.7	27.0		0.9	160	34	13	0.20	0.048	28	10	0.02	0.5	0.15	0.33
1/8 of 20 oz cake	71	8.9	3.6	3.1	1.7	30	118	75	0.78	0.040	2.4	158	0.8	0.13	0.04	7.8	18095
choc, butter recipe, from mix,	250		4.0	35.0	21.0	1.0	420	40					0	0.09	0.4		
SuperMoist - *1/12 cake*	~76	11.0	6.0			75	170		1.80			300		0.14		16.0	GENM52
homemade	340	23.2	5.0	50.7		1.5	299	57	30	0.66	0.266	38	<1	0.13	1.1	0.15	0.29
1/12 of 9″ dia cake	95	14.3	5.2	5.7	2.6	55	133	101	1.53	0.197	11.3	133	1.5	0.20	0.04	37.1	18101
w/choc icing	235	14.7	2.6	34.9		1.8	214	28	22	0.44	0.205	17	<1	0.02	0.4	0.09	0.13
1/8 of 18 oz cake	64	10.5	3.1	5.6	1.2	27	128	78	1.41	0.155	2.1	54		0.09	0.03	14.7	18096
choc chip, from mix, SuperMoist	250		3.0	35.0	20.0	0.0	270	80					0	0.12	0.8		
1/12 cake	~77	11.0	2.5	3.5	2.5	55	55		1.08			0		0.14		32.0	GENM53
choc cupcake w/icing, low-fat	131	9.8	1.8	28.9		1.8	178	15	11	0.24	0.096	0	0	0.02	0.3	0.00	0.10
1.5 oz cupcake	43	1.6	0.5	0.8	0.2	0	96	79	0.66	0.076	2.4	0		0.06	<0.01	9.5	18452
choc fudge, from mix, SuperMoist	270		3.0	35.0	21.0	1.0	340	40					0	0.09	0.8		
1/12 cake	~80	12.0	2.5			55	125		1.44			0		0.14		24.0	GENM54
choc snack cake, crème-filled	188	9.9	1.7	30.2		0.4	213	37	21	0.26	0.165	3	0	0.11	1.2	0.03	0.11
w/icing - *1.8 oz snack cake*	50	7.3	1.4	2.8	2.6	9	61	47	1.68	0.104	1.4	9	1.7	0.15	0.01	22.0	18127
crème-filled w/icing, Ding Dongs,	368	10.0	3.1	45.4	32.4	1.8	241	3									
Hostess - *2.8 oz snack cake*	80	19.4	11.0	4.0	1.2	14			1.84								18606
choc w/fudge swirls, from mix,	210		3.0	32.0	19.0	1.0	250	40					0	0.06	0.4		
SuperMoist - *1/9 cake*	~65	8.0	2.5	2.5	1.5	50	140		1.80			300		0.14		24.0	GENM55
coffeecake, cinn w/crumb topping	263	13.8	4.3	29.4		1.3	221	34	14	0.51	0.284	21	<1	0.13	1.1	0.11	0.41
1/9 of 20 oz cake	63	14.7	3.7	8.2	2.0	20	77	68	1.20	0.079	10.8	70	2.1	0.14	0.02	51.0	18104
cinn w/crumb topping, from	178	17.1	3.1	29.6		0.7	236	76	10	0.25	0.174	22	<1	0.09	0.9	0.08	0.15
mix - *1/8 of 8″× 5 3/4″ cake*	56	5.4	1.0	2.2	1.8	27	63	120	0.80	0.083	9.4	78	0.9	0.10	0.03	40.9	18108
cream/neufchatel cheese	258	24.5	5.3	33.7		0.8	258	45	11	0.45	0.131	65	<1	0.08	0.5	0.26	0.30
1/6 of 16 oz cake	76	11.6	4.1	5.4	1.3	65	220	77	0.49	0.040	10.1	218	1.2	0.10	0.04	40.3	18103
crème filled w/choc icing	298	26.2	4.5	48.4		1.8	291	34	14	0.40	0.171	33	<1	0.07	0.4	0.18	0.35
1/6 of 19 oz cake	90	9.7	2.5	5.1	1.3	62	70	68	0.46	0.063	13.0	111		0.07	0.04	52.2	18105
w/fruit	156	15.9	2.6	25.8		1.3	193	23	9	0.33	0.120	4	<1	0.02	1.3	0.01	0.33
1/8 of 14 oz cake	50	5.1	1.2	2.8	0.7	4	45	59	1.22	0.015	8.3	70	0.4	0.10	0.02	33.5	18106
coffeecake mix, cinn streusel, Bty	200		2.0	36.0	20.0	0.0	220	60					0	0.12	0.8		
Crckr Stir 'n Bake¹ - *1/6 pkg (1.7 oz)*	47	6.0	1.5			10	45		1.08			0		0.07		24.0	GENM56
devil's food, from mix, red fat,	200		4.0	36.0	20.0	1.0	380	40					0	0.09	0.8		
Sweet Rewards - *1/12 cake*	~76	5.0	1.5			55	150		1.80			0		0.14		32.0	GENM58
SuperMoist	270		3.0	35.0	21.0	1.0	340	40					0	0.09	0.4		
1/12 cake	~80	13.0	2.5	4.5	3.0	55	150		1.44			0		0.14		24.0	GENM57

	KCAL	H₂O (g)	PRO (g)	CHO (g)	SUGR (g)	DFIB (g)	Na (mg)	Ca (mg)	Mg (mg)	Zn (mg)	Mn (mg)	A (mcg RAE)	C (mg)	B-1 (mg)	NIA (mg)	B-12 (mcg)	PANT (mg)
	WT (g)	FAT (g)	SFA (g)	MUFA (g)	PUFA (g)	CHOL (mg)	K (mg)	P (mg)	Fe (mg)	Cu (mg)	Se (mcg)	A (IU)	E (mg ATE)	B-2 (mg)	B-6 (mg)	FOL (mcg DFE)	REF
devils' food mix w/choc icing, Bty	240		2.0	43.0	27.0	1.0	270	40					0	0.09	0.8		
Crckr Stir 'n Bake[1] - 1/6 pkg (2 oz)	58	7.0	2.0			0	130		1.44			0		0.03		16.0	GENM59
double choc swirl, from mix,	270		4.0	35.0	21.0	1.0	330	40					0	0.09	0.8		
SuperMoist - 1/12 cake	~80	13.0	2.5	4.5	3.0	55	160		1.44			0		0.14		24.0	GENM60
french van, from mix, SuperMoist	240		3.0	35.0	20.0	0.0	290	80					0	0.09	0.8		
1/12 cake	~77	10.0	2.5	3.5	2.0	55	30		0.72			0		0.10		32.0	GENM61
fruitcake	139	10.9	1.2	26.5		1.6	116	14	7	0.12	0.095	2	<1	0.02	0.3	<0.01	0.10
1 piece (1.5 oz)	43	3.9	0.5	1.8	1.4	2	66	22	0.89	0.022	0.9	9	0.7	0.04	0.02	12.9	18110
dark, Claxton	210		3.0	36.0	18.0	4.0	50	220					0				
1/8 cake (1″ × 2″ × 1 1/2″)	57	6.0	1.0			18			1.26			0					CLAX1
supreme, Safeway	280		3.0	48.0	24.0	1.0	180	20					0	0.06	0.4		
2.6 oz slice	74	8.0	1.0			20			1.80			0		0.07			SAFE40
fudge marble, from mix, SuperMoist	290		4.0	43.0	25.0	0.0	330	80					0	0.12	0.8		
1/10 cake	~87	12.0	2.5	4.0	2.5	65	75		1.08			0		0.14		32.0	GENM62
german choc, from mix, SuperMoist	270		3.0	36.0	21.0	0.0	330	40					0	0.09	0.8		
1/12 cake	~80	13.0	2.5	4.5	3.0	55	80		1.08			0		0.14		24.0	GENM63
gingerbread, from mix, Betty	230		3.0	39.0	18.0	0.0	350	0					0	0.12	0.8		
Crocker Classic - 1/8 cake	~82	6.0	1.5	2.0	0.5	25	150		1.08			0		0.10		32.0	GENM64
homemade	263	20.7	2.9	36.4			242	53	52	0.29	0.505	10	<1	0.14	1.3	0.04	0.28
1/9 of 8″ sq cake	74	12.1	3.1	5.3	3.1	24	325	40	2.13	0.144	12.1	36		0.12	0.14	37.7	18116
golden van, from mix, SuperMoist	240		3.0	35.0	20.0	0.0	290	80					0	0.09	0.8		
1/12 cake	~77	10.0	2.5	3.5	2.0	55	30		0.72			0		0.10		32.0	GENM65
lemon, from mix, SuperMoist	240		3.0	36.0	20.0	0.0	290	80					0	0.09	0.8		
1/12 cake	~75	10.0	2.5	3.5	2.0	55	30		0.72			0		0.10		32.0	GENM66
milk choc, from mix, SuperMoist	240		4.0	34.0	20.0	1.0	300	100					0	0.09	0.4		
1/12 cake	~77	10.0	2.5	3.5	2.0	55	130		1.08			0		0.14		24.0	GENM67
party swirl, from mix, SuperMoist	250		3.0	35.0	19.0	0.0	280	40					0	0.12	0.8		
1/12 cake	~75	11.0	2.5	3.5	2.5	55	40		0.72			0		0.14		32.0	GENM68
pineapple, from mix, SuperMoist	250		3.0	35.0	20.0	0.0	290	80					0	0.09	0.8		
1/12 cake	~77	10.0	2.5	3.5	2.0	55	30		0.72			0		0.10		32.0	GENM69
pineapple upside down, from mix,	400		3.0	64.0	43.0	0.0	330	60					0	0.12	0.8		
Betty Crocker Classic - 1/6 cake	~127	14.0	3.5	5.0	2.5	35	80		0.72			200		0.10		32.0	GENM70
homemade	367	37.1	4.0	58.1		0.9	367	138	15	0.36	0.403	71	1	0.18	1.4	0.09	0.23
1/9 of 8″ sq cake	115	13.9	3.4	6.0	3.8	25	129	94	1.70	0.100	10.8	291	1.5	0.18	0.04	44.9	18119
pound, fat free	80	8.8	1.5	17.3		0.3	97	12	3	0.09	0.039	8	0	0.04	0.2	0.00	0.10
1 oz	28	0.3	0.1	<0.1	0.1	0	31	41	0.58	0.016	1.5	27	<0.1	0.09	<0.01	16.4	18451
from mix, Betty Crocker Classic	260		4.0	45.0	26.0	0.0	210	40					0	0.12	1.2		
1/8 cake	~82	8.0	3.0	2.5	1.0	55	35		1.08			0		0.14		40.0	GENM71
made w/butter	116	7.4	1.7	14.6		0.2	119	11	3	0.14	0.027	45	0	0.04	0.4	0.08	0.13
1/10 of 10.6 oz cake	30	6.0	3.5	1.8	0.3	66	36	41	0.41	0.011	2.6	182		0.07	0.01	18.6	18120
made w/veg shortening	117	6.9	1.6	15.8		0.3	120	19	4	0.12	0.026	11	<1	0.04	0.4	0.04	0.09
1/10 of 10.6 oz cake	30	5.4	1.4	3.0	0.7	17	32	40	0.49	0.016	2.0	35	0.7	0.08	0.01	16.5	18121b
pound snack cake	276	16.4	3.7	37.3		0.7	284	45	9	0.28	0.062	25	<1	0.10	1.0	0.10	0.20
2.5 oz snack cake	71	12.7	3.3	7.1	1.6	41	75	95	1.15	0.038	4.8	84	1.7	0.18	0.02	39.1	18121a
rainbow chip, from mix, SuperMoist	300		4.0	41.0	23.0	0.0	340	60					0	0.12	0.8		
1/10 cake	~83	13.0	3.0	4.5	3.0	65	45		1.08			0		0.14		32.0	GENM72
shortcake, biscuit-type, homemade	98	8.1	1.7	13.7			143	58	5	0.14	0.094	5	<1	0.09	0.7	0.02	0.07
1 oz shortcake	28	4.0	1.1	1.7	1.0	1	30	41	0.72	0.022	4.8	20		0.08	0.01	23.5	18126
sour cream white, from mix,	280		3.0	41.0	22.0	0.0	370	60					0	0.12	0.8		
SuperMoist - 1/10 cake	~82	12.0	2.5	4.0	2.5	0	45		0.72			0		0.14		32.0	GENM73
spice, from mix, SuperMoist	240		3.0	35.0	20.0	0.0	290	80					0	0.09	0.8		
1/12 cake	~77	10.0	2.0	3.5	2.0	55	40		1.08			0		0.14		32.0	GENM74
sponge	110	11.3	2.1	23.2		0.2	93	27	4	0.19	0.080	17	0	0.09	0.7	0.09	0.18
1/12 of 16 oz cake	38	1.0	0.3	0.4	0.2	39	38	52	1.03	0.024	3.5	59	0.1	0.10	0.02	21.7	18133
homemade	113	11.2	2.8	21.9			87	16	3	0.22	0.063	29	0	0.06	0.5	0.14	0.21
1/12 of 16 oz cake	38	1.6	0.5	0.6	0.2	65	54	38	0.60	0.021	7.0	98		0.11	0.02	20.1	18134
sponge snack cake, crème-filled	157	8.7	1.3	27.5		0.2	157	19	3	0.12	0.072	2	<1	0.07	0.5	0.05	0.12
1.5 oz snack cake	43	4.9	1.1	1.8	1.4	7	37	80	0.55	0.024	1.3	7	0.9	0.06	0.01	19.8	18128
strawberry, from mix, SuperMoist	250		3.0	35.0	21.0	0.0	280	80					0	0.09	0.8		
1/12 cake	~77	10.0	2.0	3.5	2.0	55	30		0.72			0		0.10		32.0	GENM75
white, from mix, SuperMoist	230		3.0	34.0	18.0	0.0	300	40					0	0.09	0.8		
1/12 cake	~72	10.0	2.0	3.0	2.0	0	35		0.72			0		0.10		24.0	GENM76

	KCAL / WT (g)	H₂O (g) / FAT (g)	PRO (g) / SFA (g)	CHO (g) / MUFA (g)	SUGR (g) / PUFA (g)	DFIB (g) / CHOL (mg)	Na (mg) / K (mg)	Ca (mg) / P (mg)	Mg (mg) / Fe (mg)	Zn (mg) / Cu (mg)	Mn (mg) / Se (mcg)	A (mcg RAE) / A (IU)	C (mg) / E (mg ATE)	B-1 (mg) / B-2 (mg)	NIA (mg) / B-6 (mg)	B-12 (mcg) / FOL (mcg DFE)	PANT (mg) / REF
white, homemade	264	17.2	4.0	42.3		0.6	242	96	9	0.24	0.146	12	<1	0.14	1.1	0.06	0.14
1/12 of 9" cake	74	9.2	2.4	3.9	2.3	1	70	69	1.12	0.044	9.6	41	0.7	0.18	0.02	37.0	18139
w/coconut icing	399	23.2	4.9	70.8		1.1	318	101	13	0.37	0.310	12	<1	0.14	1.2	0.07	0.19
1/12 of 9" cake	112	11.5	4.4	4.1	2.4	1	111	78	1.30	0.075	12.0	43	0.8	0.21	0.03	38.1	18102
yellow, from mix, butter recipe	260		3.0	36.0	20.0	0.0	370	80					0	0.12	0.8		
SuperMoist - 1/12 cake	~77	11.0	6.0			75	35		0.72			300		0.14		32.0	GENM78
SuperMoist	250		3.0	35.0	20.0	0	290	80					0	0.09	0.8		
1/12 cake	~77	10.0	2.5	3.0	4.0	55	30		0.72			0		0.10		32.0	GENM79
yellow, homemade	245	17.1	3.6	36.0		0.5	233	99	8	0.31	0.129	27	<1	0.12	1.0	0.11	0.21
1/12 of 8" cake	68	9.9	2.7	4.2	2.4	37	62	80	1.12	0.038	9.3	95	0.8	0.16	0.02	34.7	18146
yellow mix w/choc icing, Bty Crckr	240		2.0	43.0	26.0	<1.0	240	60					0	0.09	0.8		
Stir 'n Bake[1] - 1/6 pkg (2 oz)	58	7.0	2.0			10	60		1.08			0		0.07		24.0	GENM81
yellow w/choc icing	243	14.0	2.4	35.5		1.2	216	24	19	0.40	0.166	21	0	0.08	0.8	0.11	0.18
1/8 of 18 oz cake	64	11.1	3.0	6.1	1.4	35	114	103	1.33	0.120	2.2	70	1.5	0.10	0.02	20.5	18140
yellow w/van icing	239	14.1	2.2	37.6		0.2	220	40	4	0.16	0.061	12	0	0.06	0.3	0.10	0.22
1/8 of 18 oz cake	64	9.3	1.5	3.9	3.3	35	34	92	0.68	0.022	3.5	40		0.04	0.02	25.6	18141

[1] Water is the only ingredient added to the dry mix to prepare the cake.

7.3 COOKIES

	KCAL / WT (g)	H₂O (g) / FAT (g)	PRO (g) / SFA (g)	CHO (g) / MUFA (g)	SUGR (g) / PUFA (g)	DFIB (g) / CHOL (mg)	Na (mg) / K (mg)	Ca (mg) / P (mg)	Mg (mg) / Fe (mg)	Zn (mg) / Cu (mg)	Mn (mg) / Se (mcg)	A (mcg RAE) / A (IU)	C (mg) / E (mg ATE)	B-1 (mg) / B-2 (mg)	NIA (mg) / B-6 (mg)	B-12 (mcg) / FOL (mcg DFE)	PANT (mg) / REF
animal	254	2.2	3.9	42.2		0.6	224	25	10	0.36	0.241	0	0	0.20	2.0	0.03	0.21
2 oz box (23 pieces)	57	7.9	2.0	4.4	1.1	0	57	65	1.57	0.089	4.0	0	1.1	0.19	0.01	77.0	18150b
anisette sponge	47	2.5	1.4	7.8		0.1	19	6	2	0.15	0.031	22	0	0.04	0.3	0.10	0.15
1 piece	13	1.2	0.5	0.6	0.2	47	15	22	0.47	0.012		72	0.2	0.06	0.02	13.7	18423b
apple 'n raisin, Archway Gourmet	111	2.8	1.4	17.1	9.2	0.7	121	7					0	0.07	0.4		
1 cookie	26	4.2	0.9	1.7	0.4	5	57		0.58			8		0.04			18549
apricot filled, Archway Home Style	100	3.7	1.3	16.2	8.1	0.4	80	5					0	0.06	0.5		
1 cookie	25	3.5	1.4	1.1	0.2	7	32		0.51			14		0.05			18517
arrowroot	22	0.2	0.3	3.6		0.1	19	2	1	0.03	0.021	0	0	0.02	0.2	<0.01	0.02
1 cookie	5	0.7	0.2	0.4	0.1	0	5	6	0.13	0.008	0.3	0	0.1	0.02	<0.01	6.6	18150a
biscotti dipped in dark choc,	130		2.0	19.0	11.0	1.0	65	20					0				
Safeway Select - 1.2 oz biscotti	33	5.0	2.5			5			0.72			100					SAFE1
black walnut ice box, Archway Home	119	1.4	1.3	14.9	6.7	0.3	77	5					0	0.07	0.5		
Style - 1 cookie	24	6.2	1.4	2.2	0.6	10	20		0.66			15		0.06			18519
breakfast treat	88	4.7	2.5	14.3		0.2	35	11	3	0.27	0.058	40	0	0.07	0.5	0.18	0.27
1 piece	24	2.2	0.8	1.0	0.4	88	27	42	0.86	0.023		133	0.3	0.10	0.03	25.2	18423c
butter	132	1.3	1.7	19.5		0.2	100	8	3	0.11	0.048	45	0	0.10	0.9	0.10	0.14
1 oz (5 cookies)	28	5.3	3.1	1.6	0.3	33	31	29	0.63	0.057	2.4	191	0.1	0.09	0.01	17.6	18155
caramel delights, Snackwell's	69	2.4	0.8	12.6	8.3	0.3	33	8	5	0.10			<1	<0.01	0.1	0.02	
1 cookie	18	2.0	0.5	0.6	0.1	0	22	17	0.16	0.031		1		0.02	<0.01		18650
carrot cake, Archway Gourmet	120	3.1	1.1	18.0	10.6	0.5	176	11					0	0.06	0.4		
1 cookie	28	5.0	1.5	1.6	0.6	4	11		0.72			251		0.04			18550
cherry filled, Archway Home Style	100	3.7	1.3	16.2	7.9	0.4	83	6					0	0.07	0.5		
1 cookie	25	3.5	1.4	1.1	0.2	7	30		0.53			22		0.05			18520
choc chip, 12–17% fat	45	0.4	0.6	7.3		0.4	38	2	3	0.07	0.045	0	0	0.03	0.3	0.00	0.03
1 cookie (2 1/4" dia)	10	1.5	0.4	0.6	0.5	0	12	8	0.31	0.025	0.6	<1		0.03	0.03	11.5	18158
18–28% fat	48	0.4	0.5	6.7		0.3	32	3	3	0.06	0.045	0	0	0.02	0.3	<0.01	0.02
1 cookie (2 1/4" dia)	10	2.3	0.7	0.7	0.2	0	14	11	0.28	0.021	0.6	<1	0.3	0.03	0.01	6.5	18159a
drop, Archway Home Style	101	4.0	1.4	15.5	7.9	0.3	78	10					0	0.06	0.5		
.9 oz	25	3.7	1.1	1.4	0.3	14	27		0.57			21		0.06			18521
ice box, Archway Home	117	1.5	1.1	15.4	8.4	0.2	59	5					0	0.06	0.5		
Style - 1 cookie	24	5.7	1.7	2.1	0.3	8	27		0.63			12		0.05			18522
n' toffee, Archway Gourmet	131	2.2	1.2	17.9	9.1	0.5	124	4					0	0.07	0.6		
1 cookie	28	6.1	1.8	2.3	0.5	6	21		0.61			20		0.05			18551
red fat, Chips Ahoy	140		2.0	22.0	10.0	<1.0	150	0					0				
3 cookies (1.1 oz)	31	5.0	2.5			0			1.08			0					NBSC1
soft type	69	1.7	0.5	8.9		0.5	49	2	5	0.07	0.056	0	0	0.02	0.2	0.00	0.04
1 cookie	15	3.6	1.1	2.0	0.5	0	14	8	0.36	0.024		<1		0.03	0.02	9.5	18160
sugar free, Archway Home	108	1.1	1.1	16.0	0.2	0.2	64	62					0	0.06	0.4		
Style - 1 cookie	24	5.3	1.5	2.0	0.3	<1	19		0.48			5		0.05			18565
choc chip, from mix, Betty	160		2.0	22.0	14.0	0.0	105	0					0	0.06	0.4		
Crocker - 2 cookies	~32	8.0	2.5			10	55		0.36			200		0.03		8.0	GENM84

	KCAL	H₂0 (g)	PRO (g)	CHO (g)	SUGR (g)	DFIB (g)	Na (mg)	Ca (mg)	Mg (mg)	Zn (mg)	Mn (mg)	A (mcg RAE)	C (mg)	B-1 (mg)	NIA (mg)	B-12 (mcg)	PANT (mg)
	WT (g)	FAT (g)	SFA (g)	MUFA (g)	PUFA (g)	CHOL (mg)	K (mg)	P (mg)	Fe (mg)	Cu (mg)	Se (mcg)	A (IU)	E (mg ATE)	B-2 (mg)	B-6 (mg)	FOL (mcg DFE)	REF
choc chip, from refrig dough	59	0.4	0.6	8.2		0.2	28	3	3	0.07	0.057	2	0	0.02	0.2	0.01	0.02
1 cookie	12	2.7	0.9	1.4	0.3	3	24	9	0.30	0.024	0.7	7		0.02	<0.01	8.4	18164
Pillsbury	140		1.0	17.0	10.0	<1.0	90	0					0				
1 oz cookie	28	7.0	2.0			<5			0.72			0					GENM85
w/walnuts, Pillsbury	130		1.0	16.0	9.0	<1.0	90	0					0				
1 oz cookie	28	7.0	2.0			5			0.72			0					GENM86
choc chip, homemade w/butter	78	0.9	0.9	9.3			55	6	9	0.15	0.106	22	<1	0.03	0.2	0.01	0.04
1 cookie (2 1/4″ dia)	16	4.5	2.3	1.3	0.7	11	35	16	0.40	0.062	1.8	95		0.03	0.01	7.5	18378
w/marg	78	0.9	0.9	9.3		0.4	58	6	9	0.15	0.106	23	<1	0.03	0.2	0.01	0.04
1 cookie (2 1/4″ dia)	16	4.5	1.3	1.7	1.3	5	36	16	0.39	0.061	1.8	109	0.5	0.03	0.01	7.5	18165
choc chip refrig dough, Pillsbury	127	2.9	1.2	17.9	10.4	0.7	88										
1 cookie	28	5.7	1.8	2.5	0.5												18630
choc chunk & chip, from refrig dough, Pillsbury RTB - *.9 oz cookie*	120		1.0	15.0	9.0	<1.0	70	0					0				
	26	6.0	2.0			<5			0.72			0					GENM83
choc chunk, from refrig dough, Pillsbury - *1 oz cookie*	140		1.0	17.0	10.0	<1.0	85	0					0				
	28	7.0	2.0			5			0.72			0					GENM87
choc chunk pecan, Pepperidge Farm	58	0.5	0.6	8.0		0.3	38	3	4	0.08	0.054	0	0	0.03	0.3	<0.01	0.03
1 cookie	12	2.7	0.9	1.4	0.3	0	16	13	0.34	0.025	0.7	<1	0.3	0.03	0.01	7.8	18159b
choc peanut butter, from mix, Betty Crocker - *2 cookies*	150		3.0	20.0	12.0	0.0	120	0					0	0	0.03	0.4	
	~33	7.0	2.5			10	80		0.72			0		0.03		8.0	GENM88
choc sandwich w/crème filling	82	0.3	0.6	11.2		0.9	55	6	7	0.10	0.063	0	0	0.02	0.2	0.01	0.03
1 cookie	17	4.5	1.3	2.5	0.5	0	41	15	0.53	0.054	0.5	1	0.6	0.03	0.01	4.4	18167
w/crème filling, choc coated	47	0.2	0.5	7.0		0.3	60	3	5	0.08	0.053	0	0	0.01	0.2	<0.01	0.02
1 cookie	10	2.1	0.4	0.9	0.7	0	18	10	0.39	0.035	0.5	<1	0.3	0.02	<0.01	7.0	18166
w/extra crème filling	65	0.2	0.5	8.9		0.3	64	3	4	0.08	0.050	0	0	0.01	0.2	<0.01	0.03
1 cookie	13	3.3	0.5	1.4	1.2	0	16	12	0.37	0.045	0.3	0	0.6	0.02	<0.01	9.1	18168
choc wafers[1]	123	1.3	1.9	20.5		1.0	164	9	15	0.31	0.197	1	0	0.06	0.8	0.03	0.11
5 wafers (1 oz)	28	4.0	1.2	1.4	1.2	1	60	37	1.14	0.131	1.6	4	0.4	0.08	0.01	21.8	18157
cinn apple, Archway Home Style	106	3.3	1.3	17.2	8.0	0.4	132	8					0	0.07	0.6		
1 cookie	26	3.7	0.9	1.4	0.2	0	23		0.63			<1		0.05			18523
cinn honey hearts, fat free, Archway Home Style - *1 cookie*	106	3.2	1.4	24.7	12.8	0.4	123	6					0	0.10	0.8		
	30	0.2	0.1	0.1	0.1	0	20		0.81			0		0.06			18552
coconut macaroon, Archway Home Style - *1 cookie*	106	2.4	0.9	12.4	9.5	0.5	38	3					0	0.01	0.1		
	22	6.1	5.4	0.4	0.1	0	57		0.35			0		0.01			18524
Homemade	97	2.5	0.9	17.3		0.4	59	2	5	0.17	0.227	0	0	<0.01	<0.1	0.01	0.06
1 cookie (2″ dia)	24	3.0	2.7	0.1	<0.1	0	37	10	0.18	0.034	2.5	0	0.1	0.03	0.02	1.0	18169
Crazy for Cats, Designer Cookies	120		2.0	16.0	6.0		75	20					0				
2 cookies	26	5.0	2.5			20			0.72			200					DSGN1
devil's food, fat free, Archway Home Style - *1 cookie*	68	2.6	1.0	15.9	8.2	0.6	79	2					0	0.06	0.4		
	20	0.2	0.1	0.1	0.1	0	54		0.53			0		0.04			18553
Snackwell's	49	2.8	0.8	11.9	6.9	0.3	28	5	4	0.07			<1	0.01	0.2	0.01	0.01
1 cookie	16	0.2	0.1	<0.1	<0.1	0	18	11	0.44	0.027	0.3	<1	<0.1	0.03	<0.01		18651
double choc chunk, from mix, Betty Crocker - *2 cookies*	150		2.0	21.0	14.0	0.0	100	0					0	0.03	0.4		
	~30	6.0	2.0			10	65		0.72			0		0.03		8.0	GENM89
double choc, from refrig dough, Pillsbury - *1 oz cookie*	140		1.0	17.0	10.0	<1.0	85	0					0				
	28	7.0	2.5			5			0.72			0					GENM90
Dunkaroos, Betty Crocker[2]	123		1.0	20.3	13.7	<0.3	98	0					0				
1 oz tray	28	4.5	1.2			0			0.24			0					GENM91
dutch cocoa, Archway Home Style - *1 cookie*	98	2.7	1.1	16.5	8.2	0.6	87	3					0	0.06	0.5		
	24	3.3	0.8	1.2	0.2	3	46		0.64			5		0.04			18528
fig bar	56	2.6	0.6	11.3		0.7	56	10	4	0.06	0.055	<1	<1	0.03	0.3	0.01	0.06
1 bar	16	1.2	0.2	0.5	0.4	0	33	10	0.46	0.024	0.5	5	0.2	0.03	0.01	6.2	18170b
	198	9.4	2.1	40.4		2.6	200	36	15	0.22	0.196	2	<1	0.09	1.1	0.05	0.21
2 oz pkg (two 3″bars)	57	4.2	0.6	1.7	1.6	0	118	35	1.65	0.084	1.9	19	0.7	0.12	0.04	22.2	18170a
Fig Newtons, Nabisco	110		1.0	22.0	14.0	1.0	115	20					0				
2 cookies	31	2.5	0.0			0			0.72			0					NBSC21
	200		2.0	39.0	22.0	2.0	200	20					0				
2 cookies (2 oz pkg)	57	4.0	0.5			0			1.08			0					NBSC20
Fortune	30	0.6	0.3	6.7		0.1	22	1	1	0.01	0.015	<1	0	0.01	0.1	<0.01	0.02
1 cookie	8	0.2	0.1	0.1	<0.1	<1	3	3	0.12	0.005	0.2	<1	<0.1	0.01	<0.01	7.0	18171
frosty lemon, Archway Home Style - *1 cookie*	112	3.1	1.1	16.8	8.7	0.2	95	11					0	0.06	0.5		
	26	4.4	1.5	1.5	0.2	0	24		0.42			0		0.05			18529

	KCAL	H₂0 (g)	PRO (g)	CHO (g)	SUGR (g)	DFIB (g)	Na (mg)	Ca (mg)	Mg (mg)	Zn (mg)	Mn (mg)	A (mcg RAE)	C (mg)	B-1 (mg)	NIA (mg)	B-12 (mcg)	PANT (mg)
	WT (g)	FAT (g)	SFA (g)	MUFA (g)	PUFA (g)	CHOL (mg)	K (mg)	P (mg)	Fe (mg)	Cu (mg)	Se (mcg)	A (IU)	E (mg ATE)	B-2 (mg)	B-6 (mg)	FOL (mcg DFE)	REF
frosty orange, Archway Home	113	2.9	1.2	16.9	8.8	0.2	94	11					0	0.06	0.5		
Style - *1 cookie*	26	4.6	1.4	1.5	0.5	0	24		0.42			0		0.05			18530
fruit & honey bar, Archway	103	3.5	1.2	17.5	9.3	0.5	107	6					0	0.07	0.6		
Home Style - *1 cookie*	26	3.3	0.8	1.2	0.3	6	44		0.65			11		0.05			18531
fudge, cake type	73	2.5	1.1	16.4		0.6	40	7	7	0.12	0.068	0	<1	0.05	0.3	0.02	0.05
1 cookie	21	0.8	0.2	0.4	0.1	0	29	17	0.52	0.061	0.8	<1		0.04	0.01	14.1	18156
Fudge Marshmallow, Safeway	90		<1.0	13.0	8.0	0.0	30	0					0	0.30	4.0	1.20	
.63 oz cookie	18	3.0	3.0			0			0.36			0		0.34	0.40	80.0	SAFE5
Fudge Mint, Safeway	170		1.0	23.0	10.0	<1.0	120	0					0				
2 cookies (1.16 oz)	33	8.0	6.0			0			1.08			0					SAFE4
Fudge Sticks, Keebler	150		1.0	19.0	15.0	0.0	55	0					0				
3 cookies (1 oz)	29	8.0	4.0			0			0.36			0					KBLR2
gingerbread, from refrig dough,	140		1.0	18.0	9.0	0.0	105	0					0				
Pillsbury - *1 oz cookie*	28	7.0	2.0			15			0.72			0					GENM92
gingersnaps	29	0.4	0.4	5.4		0.2	46	5	3	0.04	0.109	0	0	0.01	0.2	0.00	0.03
1 small cookie	7	0.7	0.2	0.4	0.1	0	24	6	0.45	0.021	0.4	<1	0.1	0.02	0.01	8.3	18172a
1 large (3 1/2"–4" dia)	133	1.7	1.8	24.6		0.7	209	25	16	0.18	0.498	0	0	0.06	1.0	0.00	0.12
	32	3.1	0.8	1.7	0.4	0	111	27	2.05	0.098	1.6	1	0.4	0.09	0.03	37.8	18172b
iced, Archway Home Style	172	1.7	1.4	26.2	14.1	0.4	132	8					0	0.10	0.9		
5 cookies	37	7.0	2.1	2.2	0.8	0	25		1.26			0		0.07			18558
red fat, Archway Home Style	136	1.6	1.4	24.6	12.0	0.4	141	9					0	0.11	0.9		
5 cookies	32	3.6	0.9	1.4	0.3	0	47		1.35			0		0.07			18562
Golden Grahams Treats, all flvrs,	90		1.0	16.3	8.0	0.0	105	7					0				
Betty Crocker - *.78 oz bar*	22	2.7	0.5			0	28		0.84			0					GENM93
graham crackers, choc coated	68	0.4	1.0	9.3		0.4	41	8	8	0.14	0.102	<1	0	0.02	0.3	0.00	0.03
1 cracker (2 1/2" sq)	14	3.2	1.9	1.1	0.1	0	29	19	0.50	0.060	2.0	2	0.2	0.03	0.01	3.1	18174
Fudge Graham, Safeway	120		1.0	15.0	8.0	1.0	100	0					0				
.85 oz cookie	24	6.0	4.0			0			0.36			0					SAFE2
Keebler	126	0.8	1.9	19.4	7.2		96										
3 cookies	27	4.5	0.8														18608
graham crackers, plain/honey³	59	0.6	1.0	10.8	2.6	0.4	85	3	4	0.11	0.113	0	0	0.03	0.6	0.00	0.08
2 crackers (2 1/2" sq)	14	1.4	0.2	0.6	0.5	0	19	15	0.52	0.028	1.4	0	0.3	0.04	0.01	12.6	18173
Nabisco	159	1.0	1.1	19.6	10.0	0.3	69	13	2	0.09				0.05	0.8	0.03	
8 small sections	31	8.4	1.6	5.8	0.4	3	21	26	0.55	0.016		3		0.06	0.01		18618b
hermits, Archway Home Style	95	3.7	1.3	16.6	8.2	0.5	147	13					0	0.07	0.6		
1 cookie	25	2.7	0.7	1.0	0.3	5	37		0.72			9		0.06			18525
holiday shapes, from refrig	130		1.0	16.0	7.0	0.0	100	0					0				
dough, Pillsbury⁴ - *1 oz cookie*	28	7.0	2.0			<5			0.72			0					GENM94
ice cream cone, cake/wafer	17	0.2	0.3	3.2		0.1	6	1	1	0.03	0.023	0	0	0.01	0.2	0.00	0.02
1 cone	4	0.3	<0.1	0.1	0.1	0	4	4	0.14	0.008	0.2	0	0.1	0.01	<0.01	6.8	18271b
sugar, rolled	40	0.3	0.8	8.4		0.2	32	4	3	0.08	0.073	0	0	0.05	0.5	0.00	0.04
1 cone	10	0.4	0.1	0.1	0.1	0	15	10	0.44	0.027	0.5	0	<0.1	0.04	0.01	13.8	18272
Waffle	121	1.5	2.3	22.9		0.9	41	7	8	0.19	0.166	0	0	0.07	1.3	0.00	0.14
large waffle cone	29	2.0	0.4	0.5	0.9	0	32	28	1.04	0.059	1.4	0	0.5	0.10	0.01	49.3	18271a
ladyfinger	40	2.1	1.2	6.6		0.1	16	5	1	0.13	0.026	18	0	0.03	0.2	0.08	0.12
1 ladyfinger	11	1.0	0.4	0.5	0.2	40	12	19	0.39	0.010		61	0.1	0.05	0.01	11.6	18423a
w/lemon jce & rind	40	2.1	1.2	6.6		0.1	16	5	1	0.13	0.026	18	<1	0.03	0.2	0.08	0.12
1 ladyfinger	11	1.0	0.4	0.5	0.2	40	12	19	0.39	0.010	2.3	61	0.1	0.05	0.01	11.6	18175
lemon drops, Archway Home	93	4.2	1.2	14.8	6.6	0.3	95	9					0	0.07	0.5		
Style - *.85 oz cookie*	24	3.3	0.8	1.2	0.3	9	20		0.53			14		0.06			18534
lemon nuggets, fat free, Archway	115	3.0	1.4	26.9	14.8	0.4	117	4					0	0.10	0.8		
Home Style - *1.13 oz cookie*	32	0.2	0.1	0.1	0.1	0	20		0.68			0		0.06			18554
lemon snaps, Archway Home	152	1.6	1.6	20.1	8.8	0.3	117	9					0	0.10	0.7		
Style - *1.1 oz cookie*	31	7.3	1.7	2.7	0.4	7	24		0.66			11		0.07			18559
M&M cookies, from refrig dough,	130		1.0	18.0	11.0	<1.0	75	0					0				
Pillsbury - *1 oz cookie*	28	6.0	2.0			<5			0.72			0					GENM95
marshmallow, choc coated	55	1.3	0.5	8.8		0.3	22	6	5	0.08	0.037	0	<1	0.01	0.1	0.02	0.06
1 small cookie (1 3/4" × 3/4")	13	2.2	0.6	1.2	0.3	0	24	13	0.33	0.034	0.6	1	0.3	0.03	0.01	3.9	18176b
marshmallow pie	164	3.9	1.6	26.4		0.8	66	18	14	0.25	0.111	0	<1	0.04	0.3	0.07	0.19
1 cookie (3" dia × 3/4")	39	6.6	1.8	3.6	0.8	0	71	38	0.99	0.102	1.7	2	0.8	0.08	0.02	11.7	18176a
mint crème, Snackwell's	108	1.1	1.0	19.0	13.3	0.7	72	5	10	0.16	<0.001		0	0.02	0.3	<0.01	0.01
1 cookie	25	3.6	0.9	0.8	0.2	0	37	21	0.60	0.070		<1	<0.1	0.03	0.01		18649

	KCAL / WT (g)	H₂O (g) / FAT (g)	PRO (g) / SFA (g)	CHO (g) / MUFA (g)	SUGR (g) / PUFA (g)	DFIB (g) / CHOL (mg)	Na (mg) / K (mg)	Ca (mg) / P (mg)	Mg (mg) / Fe (mg)	Zn (mg) / Cu (mg)	Mn (mg) / Se (mcg)	A (mcg RAE) / A (IU)	C (mg) / E (mg ATE)	B-1 (mg) / B-2 (mg)	NIA (mg) / B-6 (mg)	B-12 (mcg) / FOL (mcg DFE)	PANT (mg) / REF
molasses	138	1.9	1.8	23.6		0.3	147	24	17	0.14	0.402	0		0.11	1.0		0.13
1 large cookie (3 1/2–4″ dia)	32	4.1	1.0	2.3	0.6	0	111	30	2.06	0.119	1.8	0	0.5	0.08	0.03	38.7	18177b
Archway Home Style	103	2.9	1.2	18.2		0.3	144	9				0		0.07	0.7		
1 cookie	26	3.0	0.7	1.1	0.2	8	29		1.14			12		0.06			18535
dark, Archway Home Style	115	2.2	1.2	20.1	10.2	0.3	154	13				0		0.08	0.8		
1 cookie	28	3.4	0.8	1.3	0.2	0	95		1.23			0		0.06			18526
iced, Archway Home Style	114	3.1	1.0	19.6	10.0	0.3	130	7				0		0.08	0.7		
1 cookie	28	3.6	1.1	1.1	0.5	0	21		1.17			0		0.06			18532
Little Debbie	86	1.2	1.1	14.8		0.2	92	15	10	0.09	0.251	0	0	0.07	0.6	0.00	0.08
1 cookie	20	2.6	0.6	1.4	0.3	0	69	19	1.29	0.075	1.1	0	0.3	0.05	0.02	24.2	18177a
old fashioned, Archway Home Style - *1 cookie*	105	2.7	1.2	18.4	9.8	0.3	138	9				0		0.08	0.7		
	26	3.0	0.7	0.7	0.2	8	29		1.24			12		0.06			18539
mud pie, Archway Home Style	107	3.3	1.3	14.9	7.6	0.7	103	7				0		0.05	0.5		
1 cookie	25	4.9	2.2	1.5	0.2	5	67		0.72			8		0.05			18536
Nutty Bars, Little Debbie	312	1.7	4.6	31.5	19.4		127						1				
1 bar	57	18.7	3.6														18612
oatmeal	81	1.0	1.1	12.4		0.5	69	7	6	0.14	0.151	<1	<1	0.05	0.4	0.00	0.07
1 cookie	18	3.3	0.8	1.8	0.5	0	26	25	0.46	0.024	1.8	3	0.5	0.04	0.01	13.0	18178
Archway Home Style	106	2.5	1.5	16.7	8.0	0.7	87	8				0		0.07	0.5		
1 cookie	25	3.8	0.9	1.4	0.3	3	46		0.60			7		0.04			18537
fat-free	92	3.5	1.7	22.3		2.1	84	11	10	0.18	0.225	0	0	0.04	0.3	0.00	0.10
2 cookies (1 oz)	28	0.4	0.1	0.1	0.2	0	60	30	0.62	0.061	2.3	0	0.1	0.07	0.02	16.2	18456
from mix, Betty Crocker	150		2.0	22.0	12.0	<1.0	105	0				0		0.06	0.4		
2 cookies	~32	6.0	1.0			10	45		0.72			0		0.03		8.0	GENM98
from refrig dough	57	0.7	0.7	7.9		0.3	39	4	4	0.09	0.114	<1	<1	0.02	0.2	<0.01	0.03
1 cookie	12	2.5	0.6	1.4	0.4	3	20	14	0.29	0.015	1.2	8		0.02	0.01	4.9	18183
homemade	67	0.9	1.0	10.0			90	16	6	0.14	0.159	24	<1	0.04	0.2	0.01	0.05
1 cookie (2 5/8″ dia)	15	2.7	0.5	1.2	0.8	5	27	25	0.41	0.025	2.6	114		0.03	0.01	7.2	18377
iced, Archway Home Style	123	2.7	1.5	18.5	9.8	0.6	92	8				0		0.07	0.4		
1 cookie	28	4.9	1.5	1.5	0.7	3	45		0.55			5		0.04			18533
Ruth's, Archway Home Style	111	2.6	1.5	17.2	8.9	0.7	114	8				0		0.07	0.4		
1 cookie	26	4.1	0.9	1.5	0.6	4	48		0.72			9		0.04			18545
soft type	61	1.7	0.9	9.9		0.4	52	14	5	0.07	0.063	1	<1	0.03	0.3	<0.01	0.07
1 cookie	15	2.2	0.5	1.2	0.3	1	20	31	0.42	0.083	1.6	5		0.03	0.01	7.8	18179
sugar free, Archway Home Style	106	1.2	1.3	16.1	0.3	0.5	74	5				0		0.06	0.4		
1 cookie	24	5.0	1.2	1.9	0.3	0	21		0.47			<1		0.04			18513
oatmeal, apple filled, Archway Home Style - *1 cookie*	99	3.7	1.2	16.4	8.0	0.5	103	7				0		0.07	0.4		
	25	3.2	0.7	1.2	0.2	2	46		0.77			3		0.04			18516
oatmeal choc chip, from mix, Betty Crocker - *2 cookies*	150		2.0	21.0	13.0	0.0	135	0				0		0.06	0.0		
	~35	7.0	2.0			10	60		0.36			0		0.03		8.0	GENM96
from refrig dough, Pillsbury	120		1.0	16.0	10.0	<1.0		0				0					
1 oz cookie	28	6.0	2.0			<5			0.72			0					GENM97
oatmeal, date filled, Archway Home Style - *1 cookie*	99	3.5	1.3	16.6	8.7	0.7	98	9				0		0.07	0.5		
	25	3.1	0.7	1.2	0.2	3	52		0.51			6		0.04			18527
oatmeal pecan, Archway Gourmet	134	2.6	1.7	16.1	7.3	0.8	103	6				0		0.07	0.4		
1 cookie	28	6.8	2.4	2.5	0.6	5	43		0.83			9		0.04			18560
oatmeal raisin, Archway Home Style	107	3.0	1.5	17.5	9.3	0.8	98	8				0		0.07	0.4		
1 cookie	26	3.5	0.8	1.3	0.3	3	60		0.59			7		0.04			18538
fat free, Archway Home Style	106	3.9	1.4	24.4	13.8	0.9	165	11				0		0.08	0.5		
1 cookie	31	0.5	0.1	0.2	0.2	0	87		0.98			1		0.04			18555
homemade	65	1.0	1.0	10.3			81	15	6	0.13	0.148	21	<1	0.04	0.2	0.01	0.05
1 cookie (2 5/8″ dia)	15	2.4	0.5	1.0	0.8	5	36	24	0.40	0.027	2.3	102		0.02	0.01	6.5	18184
oatmeal raspberry, fat free, Archway Home Style - *1 cookie*	109	3.3	1.4	24.9	14.3	0.9	166	12				0		0.08	0.5		
	31	0.5	0.1	0.2	0.2	0	89		1.00			1		0.04			18556
peanut butter	72	0.9	1.4	8.8		0.3	62	5	7	0.08	0.042	<1	0	0.03	0.6	0.01	0.09
1 cookie	15	3.5	0.7	1.9	0.8	<1	25	13	0.38	0.030	0.9	1	0.5	0.03	0.01	12.5	18185
Archway Home Style	101	1.3	1.9	12.3	6.8	0.6	85	7				0		0.05	0.9		
1 cookie	21	5.1	1.1	2.1	0.9	8	44		0.57			13		0.04			18541
old fashioned, Archway Gourmet - *1 cookie*	117	2.0	2.3	14.3	8.1	0.8	118	6				0		0.06	1.2		
	25	5.9	1.3	2.5	1.1	9	52		0.67			15		0.05			18561
Ruth's Golden, Archway Gourmet - *1 cookie*	122	3.1	1.6	17.7	9.2	0.8	107	8				0		0.08	0.5		
	28	5.0	1.0	2.2	0.7	4	59		0.57			8		0.05			18564

	KCAL	H_2O (g)	PRO (g)	CHO (g)	SUGR (g)	DFIB (g)	Na (mg)	Ca (mg)	Mg (mg)	Zn (mg)	Mn (mg)	A (mcg RAE)	C (mg)	B-1 (mg)	NIA (mg)	B-12 (mcg)	PANT (mg)
	WT (g)	FAT (g)	SFA (g)	MUFA (g)	PUFA (g)	CHOL (mg)	K (mg)	P (mg)	Fe (mg)	Cu (mg)	Se (mcg)	A (IU)	E (mg ATE)	B-2 (mg)	B-6 (mg)	FOL (mcg DFE)	REF
soft type	69	1.7	0.8	8.7		0.3	50	2	5	0.08	0.065	0		0.04	0.3	0.00	0.05
1 cookie	15	3.7	0.9	2.1	0.5	0	16	13	0.13	0.012	0.7	0		0.02	<0.01	16.5	18186
peanut butter, from mix, Betty	160		3.0	20.0	12.0	0.0	135	0					0	0.06	0.8		
Crocker - 2 cookies	~32	8.0	1.5			10	55		0.36			0		0.03		8.0	GENM99
peanut butter, from refrig dough	60	0.5	1.1	6.9		0.1	52	13	5	0.09	0.055	2	0	0.02	0.5	0.01	0.04
1 cookie	12	3.3	0.7	1.7	0.6	4	41	32	0.22	0.020	0.6	6		0.02	0.01	8.3	18188
Pillsbury	130		2.0	16.0	9.0	0.0	130	0					0				
1 oz cookie	28	6.0	1.5			5			0.36			0					GENM100
peanut butter, homemade	95	1.2	1.8	11.8			104	8	8	0.16	0.114	27	<1	0.04	0.7	0.02	0.07
1 cookie (3" dia)	20	4.8	0.9	2.2	1.4	6	46	23	0.45	0.037	3.0	129		0.04	0.02	16.2	18189
peanut butter sandwich	67	0.4	1.2	9.2		0.3	52	7	7	0.15	0.128	<1	<1	0.05	0.5	0.03	0.13
1 cookie	14	3.0	0.7	1.6	0.5	0	27	26	0.36	0.033	1.1	1	0.5	0.04	0.02	9.0	18190
Peanut Jumble, Archway Home Style	116	1.8	2.2	13.3	6.6	0.7	77	7					0	0.06	1.1		
1 cookie	24	6.2	1.6	2.4	1.1	4	59		0.98			8		0.04			18542
pecan ice box, Archway Home Style	120	1.4	1.1	14.9	6.9	0.3	75	4					0	0.07	0.6		
1 cookie	24	6.3	1.4	2.6	0.5	6	17		0.49			9		0.05			18543
pecan shortbread	76	0.5	0.7	8.2		0.3	39	4	3	0.08	0.086	<1	0	0.04	0.3	<0.01	0.05
1 cookie (2" dia)	14	4.6	1.1	2.6	0.6	5	10	12	0.34	0.021	0.4	<1		0.03	<0.01	14.3	18193
Pinwheels (choc & marshmallow),	130		1.0	21.0	15.0	<1.0	35	0					0				
Nabisco - 1.1 oz cookie	30	5.0	2.5			0			0.36			0					NBSC3
pound cake, Aunt Bea's,	105	4.4	1.3	15.8	8.4	0.3	83	10					0	0.07	0.5		
Archway - 1 cookie	26	4.1	1.0	1.5	0.3	15	21		0.54			22		0.06			18518
raisin, soft type	60	2.0	0.6	10.2		0.2	51	7	3	0.05	0.046	0	<1	0.03	0.3	<0.01	0.04
1 cookie	15	2.0	0.5	1.1	0.3	<1	21	12	0.34	0.062	0.4	1	0.3	0.03	0.01	10.4	18191
raspberry filled, Archway Home Style	101	3.6	1.3	16.3	8.2	0.4	84	6					0	0.08	0.5		
1 cookie	25	3.5	1.4	1.1	0.2	7	31		0.54			11		0.05			18544
rocky road, Archway Gourmet	127	2.5	1.6	17.5	9.3	0.7	71	5					0	0.06	0.5		
1 cookie	28	5.9	1.5	2.0	1.2	11	54		0.75			22		0.06			18563
sugar free, Archway Home Style	101	1.8	1.4	15.5	0.2	0.6	66	40					0	0.06	0.4		
1 cookie	24	4.9	1.2	2.1	0.5	<1	58		0.67			3		0.05			18514
shortbread	40	0.3	0.5	5.2		0.1	36	3	1	0.04	0.034	1	0	0.03	0.3	0.01	0.02
1 cookie (1 5/8" sq)	8	1.9	0.5	1.1	0.3	2	8	9	0.22	0.012	0.6	7	0.3	0.03	0.01	7.5	18192
strawberry filled, Archway	100	3.7	1.3	16.2	7.9	0.4	84	6					0	0.07	0.5		
Home Style - 1 cookie	25	3.5	1.4	1.1	0.2	7	34		0.56			11		0.05			18547
sugar free, Archway Home Style	107		1.1	15.8	0.3	0.2	47	2					0	0.06	0.5		
1 cookie	24	5.4	1.3	2.0	0.3	0	14		0.43			1		0.05			18515
sugar	72	0.7	0.8	10.2		0.1	54	3	2	0.06	0.002	4	<1	0.03	0.4	0.03	0.04
1 cookie	15	3.2	0.8	1.8	0.4	8	9	12	0.32	0.011	0.3	14	0.4	0.03	0.01	10.4	18204
Archway Home Style	98	2.5	1.2	16.6	7.5	0.3	162	7					0	0.07	0.6		
1 cookie	24	3.1	0.8	1.1	0.2	5	20		0.53			8		0.06			18548
drop, soft, Archway Home Style	109	4.8	1.5	17.6	9.0	0.3	93	11					0	0.07	0.5		
1 oz	28	3.7	0.9	1.4	0.2	16	23		0.55			22		0.07			18546
fat free, Archway Home Style	71	2.1	0.9	16.6	8.0	0.2	80	3					0	0.04	0.5		
1 cookie	20	0.2	0.1	<0.1	0.1	0	12		0.44			0		0.04			18557
sugar, from mix, Betty Crocker	160		2.0	22.0	13.0	0.0	115	0					0	0.06	0.4		
2 cookies	~33	8.0	1.5			10	20		0.36			200		0.07		16.0	GENM101
sugar, from refrig dough	73	0.8	0.7	9.8		0.1	70	14	1	0.04	0.043	2	0	0.03	0.4	0.01	0.02
1 cookie	15	3.5	0.9	2.0	0.4	5	24	28	0.28	0.006	0.5	6	0.5	0.02	<0.01	12.9	18206
Pillsbury	130		1.0	19.0	10.0	0.0	115	0					0				
2 cookies	28	5.0	1.5			10			0.72			0					GENM102
sugar, homemade w/marg	66	1.2	0.8	8.4		0.2	69	10	2	0.06	0.044	30	<1	0.04	0.3	0.01	0.03
1 cookie (3" dia)	14	3.3	0.7	1.4	1.0	4	11	13	0.33	0.011	2.5	145	0.5	0.04	<0.01	11.3	18208
sugar wafers w/crème filling	145	0.3	1.2	19.9		0.2	42	5	3	0.10	0.078	0	0	0.03	0.7	0.00	0.06
8 small wafers (1 oz)	28	6.9	1.0	2.9	2.6	0	17	16	0.55	0.026	0.7	0	1.2	0.06	<0.01	19.3	18209
van sandwich w/crème filling	48	0.2	0.5	7.2		0.2	35	3	1	0.04	0.029	0	0	0.03	0.3	0.00	0.04
1 round cookie (1 3/4" dia)	10	2.0	0.3	0.8	0.8	0	9	8	0.22	0.011	0.3	0	0.4	0.02	<0.01	9.8	18210a
	72	0.3	0.7	10.8		0.2	52	4	2	0.06	0.044	0	0	0.04	0.4	0.00	0.06
1 oval cookie (3 1/8" long)	15	3.0	0.4	1.3	1.1	0	14	11	0.33	0.017	0.5	0	0.5	0.04	<0.01	14.7	18210b
van wafers, 12–17% fat	125	1.4	1.4	20.9		0.5	88	14	4	0.10	0.074	2	0	0.08	0.9	0.04	0.12
7 wafers (1 oz)	28	4.3	1.1	1.9	1.1	14	27	29	0.67	0.028	3.2	8	0.4	0.09	0.02	22.4	18212
18–21% fat	134	1.2	1.2	20.2		0.6	87	7	3	0.09	0.109	0	0	0.10	0.8	0.01	0.08
5 wafers (1 oz)	28	5.5	1.4	3.1	0.7	0	30	18	0.63	0.035	3.2	<1		0.06	0.01	19.3	18213

	KCAL	H₂0 (g)	PRO (g)	CHO (g)	SUGR (g)	DFIB (g)	Na (mg)	Ca (mg)	Mg (mg)	Zn (mg)	Mn (mg)	A (mcg RAE)	C (mg)	B-1 (mg)	NIA (mg)	B-12 (mcg)	PANT (mg)
								Minerals				Vitamins					
	WT (g)	FAT (g)	SFA (g)	MUFA (g)	PUFA (g)	CHOL (mg)	K (mg)	P (mg)	Fe (mg)	Cu (mg)	Se (mcg)	A (IU)	E (mg ATE)	B-2 (mg)	B-6 (mg)	FOL (mcg DFE)	REF
Keebler	147	1.3	1.6	21.6	8.5		120										
8 wafers	31	6.0	1.1														18609
white choc chunk, from refrig	130		1.0	17.0	11.0	0.0	100	0					0				
dough, Pillsbury - *1 oz cookie*	28	6.0	1.5			5			0.72			0					GENM103
white chunk, from mix, Betty Crocker	160		2.0	22.0	15.0	0.0	110	0					0	0.06	0.4		
2 cookies	~34	8.0	2.5			10	35		0.36			200		0.03		16.0	GENM104
Windmill, old fashioned, Archway	91	0.8	1.1	14.2	6.4	0.5	93	7					0	0.07	0.6		
Home Style - *1 cookie*	20	3.5	0.7	1.4	0.3	0	20		0.66			3		0.05			18540

[1] Twenty-eight wafers (168 g) are equivalent to 1 1/2 cups of wafer crumbs.
[2] Values are averages for chocolate chip cookies with chocolate icing, cookies 'n crème chocolate cookies with vanilla icing, and cinnamon graham cookies with vanilla icing.

[3] Nine graham crackers (126 g) are equivalent to 1 1/2 cups of graham cracker crumbs.
[4] Values are for bunny, birthday balloon, candy cane, doughboy, flag, holiday tree, pumpkin, rudolph, shamrock, tulip, and valentine.

7.4 DOUGHNUTS

	KCAL	H₂0 (g)	PRO (g)	CHO (g)	SUGR (g)	DFIB (g)	Na (mg)	Ca (mg)	Mg (mg)	Zn (mg)	Mn (mg)	A (mcg RAE)	C (mg)	B-1 (mg)	NIA (mg)	B-12 (mcg)	PANT (mg)
	WT (g)	FAT (g)	SFA (g)	MUFA (g)	PUFA (g)	CHOL (mg)	K (mg)	P (mg)	Fe (mg)	Cu (mg)	Se (mcg)	A (IU)	E (mg ATE)	B-2 (mg)	B-6 (mg)	FOL (mcg DFE)	REF
cake	198	9.8	2.4	23.4		0.7	257	21	9	0.26	0.160	8	<1	0.10	0.9	0.13	0.13
1 doughnut (3 1/4″ dia)	47	10.8	1.7	4.4	3.7	17	60	126	0.92	0.048	4.4	27	1.8	0.11	0.03	34.8	18248
choc coated/frosted	204	6.2	2.2	20.6		0.9	184	15	17	0.26	0.170	5	<1	0.05	0.6	0.10	0.18
1 doughnut (3″ dia)	43	13.3	3.5	7.5	1.6	26	84	87	1.06	0.092	2.5	15	1.8	0.05	0.02	15.9	18249
choc, sugared/glazed	175	6.8	1.9	24.1		0.9	143	89	14	0.24	0.155	5	<1	0.02	0.2	0.04	0.14
1 doughnut (3″ dia)	42	8.4	2.2	4.7	1.0	24	45	68	0.95	0.080	1.7	16	1.1	0.03	0.01	22.3	18251
sugared/glazed	192	8.8	2.3	22.9		0.7	181	27	8	0.20	0.150	1	<1	0.10	0.7	0.11	0.20
1 doughnut (3″ dia)	45	10.3	2.7	5.7	1.3	14	46	53	0.48	0.045	4.3	5		0.09	0.01	31.5	18250
wheat, sugared/glazed	162	13.4	2.8	19.2		1.0	160	22	10	0.31	0.389	7	<1	0.10	0.8	0.08	0.20
1 doughnut (3″ dia)	45	8.7	1.4	3.6	3.2	9	67	47	0.50	0.050	8.7	24	1.6	0.11	0.04	10.8	18252
cruller, glazed	169	7.3	1.3	24.4		0.5	141	11	5	0.11	0.088	2	0	0.07	0.9	0.02	0.09
1 cruller (3″ dia)	41	7.5	1.9	4.3	0.9	5	32	50	0.99	0.029	0.9	7	1.0	0.09	0.01	22.1	18253
yeast, glazed	242	15.2	3.8	26.6		0.7	205	26	13	0.46	0.158	2	<1	0.22	1.7	0.05	0.28
1 doughnut (3 3/4″ dia)	60	13.7	3.5	7.7	1.7	4	65	56	1.22	0.101	11.9	8	1.8	0.13	0.03	34.8	18255
w/crème filling	307	32.5	5.4	25.5		0.7	263	21	17	0.68	0.191	17	0	0.29	1.9	0.12	0.56
1 oval doughnut (3 1/2″×2 1/2″)	85	20.8	4.6	10.3	2.6	20	68	65	1.56	0.096	9.2	55	2.3	0.13	0.06	84.2	18254
w/jelly filling	289	30.3	5.0	33.3		0.8	249	21	17	0.64	0.174	14	0	0.27	1.8	0.19	0.74
1 oval doughnut (3 1/2″×2 1/2″)	85	15.9	4.1	8.7	2.0	22	67	72	1.50	0.116	10.6	46	2.1	0.12	0.09	79.9	18256

7.5 FROZEN DESSERTS

	KCAL	H₂0 (g)	PRO (g)	CHO (g)	SUGR (g)	DFIB (g)	Na (mg)	Ca (mg)	Mg (mg)	Zn (mg)	Mn (mg)	A (mcg RAE)	C (mg)	B-1 (mg)	NIA (mg)	B-12 (mcg)	PANT (mg)
	WT (g)	FAT (g)	SFA (g)	MUFA (g)	PUFA (g)	CHOL (mg)	K (mg)	P (mg)	Fe (mg)	Cu (mg)	Se (mcg)	A (IU)	E (mg ATE)	B-2 (mg)	B-6 (mg)	FOL (mcg DFE)	REF
Caramel Fudge Cosmo, Edys	140		2.0	23.0	18.0		50	300									
1/2 cup	~113	4.0	2.5			10											EDYS1
Caramel Swirl Sandwich, Healthy	140		2.0	27.0	17.0	<1.0	120	20					0				
Choice - *4 fl oz bar*	~80	3.0	1.0			5			1.80			100					HLCH4
Eskimo Pie (van ice cream w/dark	166	23.2	2.1	12.3	9.2		34	60									
choc coating) - *1 bar*	50	12.1	7.3			14											19264
frozen yogurt, choc decadence/cookies	120		2.0	19.5	14.0		45	300									
'n crm, Edys - *1/2 cup*	~69	3.5	1.5			10											EDYS2
heath toffee crunch, Edys	120		2.0	18.0	15.0		45	300									
1/2 cup	~69	4.0	2.0			10											EDYS4
raspberry/van, Edys	95		2.0	16.5	13.0		28	250									
1/2 cup	67	2.5	1.5			10											EDYS5
ultimate tin roof sundae, Edys	130		3.0	20.0	15.0		50	300									
1/2 cup	~77	4.0	2.0			5											EDYS6
van/choc/strawberry, Breyers	140		3.0	22.0	17.0	0.0	45	100					0				
1/2 cup	74	4.5	2.5			15		0.00				100					BRYS3
frozen yogurt, fat free, avg for 6	95		3.2	20.8	14.3		52	300									
flvrs, Edys[1] - *1/2 cup*	~92	0.0	0.0			0											EDYS3
w/low cal sweetener, choc	199	136.7	8.2	36.6		3.7	151	296	74	0.91		2	1	0.07	0.4	0.91	
1 cup	186	1.5	0.9	0.4	0.1	7	631	240	0.07	0.378	5.2	13	0.1	0.33	0.07	22.3	42185
frozen yogurt, soft serve, choc	115	45.9	2.9	17.9		1.6	71	106	19	0.35	0.087	32	<1	0.03	0.2	0.21	0.49
1/2 cup	72	4.3	2.6	1.3	0.2	4	188	100	0.90	0.094	1.7	115	0.1	0.15	0.05	7.9	19393
van	114	47.0	2.9	17.4		0.0	63	103	10	0.30	0.006	41	1	0.03	0.2	0.21	0.46
1/2 cup	72	4.0	2.5	1.1	0.2	1	152	93	0.22	0.029	1.8	153	<0.1	0.16	0.06	4.3	19293
fruit juice bar	75	72.0	1.1	18.6		0.0	4	5	4	0.05	0.152	1	9	0.01	0.1	0.00	0.04
3 fl oz bar	92	0.1	0.0	0.0	<0.1	0	49	6	0.17	0.00	0.2	27	0.0	0.02	0.02	5.5	19263

	KCAL / WT (g)	H₂0 / FAT (g)	PRO / SFA (g)	CHO / MUFA (g)	SUGR / PUFA (g)	DFIB / CHOL (mg)	Na / K (mg)	Ca / P (mg)	Mg / Fe (mg)	Zn / Cu (mg)	Mn / Se (mcg)	A (mcg RAE) / A (IU)	C / E (mg ATE)	B-1 / B-2 (mg)	NIA / B-6 (mg)	B-12 / FOL (mcg DFE)	PANT / REF (mg)
orange juice bar	68	56.3	0.4	17.1		0.1	6	7	6	0.01		1	19	0.01	0.1	0.00	
1 bar	74	0.0	0.0	0.0	0.0	0	74	10	0.35	0.016	0.1	24	<0.1	0.02	0.01	16.3	43346
w/aspartame	12	47.5	0.3	3.2		0.0	3	1	1	0.02	0.011	0	0	0.00	0.1	0.00	0.00
1 bar	51	0.1	0.0			0	13	0	0.07	0.009	0.1	1		0.00	0.00	0.0	19217
fudge bar, low fat, Healthy Choice	80		3.0	13.0	2.0	0.0	60	80					0				
2.26 oz bar	64	1.0	0.5	0.5	0.0	5			0.36			500					HLCH1
Fudge Swirl Sandwich, Healthy Choice - *4 fl oz bar*	140		2.0	27.0	16.0	<1.0	150	20					0				
	~80	3.0	1.0			5			1.80			100					HLCH5
Fudgsicle, fat free, Good Humor	90		3.0	18.0	15.0	<1.0	60	80					0				
1.75 fl oz bar	51	1.5	1.0			5			0.36			0					BRYS5
ice cream, avg for 11 flvrs, Edys Homemade[2] - *1/2 cup*	150		2.8	16.9	15.9		62	64									
	~69	7.8	4.8			30											EDYS9
avg for 12 flavors, Edys Limited Edition[3] - *1/2 cup*	157		2.4	18.3	14.6		48	63									
	~72	8.0	4.6			25											EDYS11
avg for 31 flavors, Edys Grand[4] *1/2 cup*	157		2.5	17.8	14.5		45	59									
	~71	8.2	4.8			26											EDYS8
choc *1/2 cup*	143	36.8	2.5	18.6		0.8	50	72	19	0.38	0.092	77	<1	0.03	0.1	0.19	0.37
	66	7.3	4.5	2.1	0.3	22	164	71	0.61	0.089	1.7	257	0.2	0.13	0.04	10.6	19270
choc, rich *1 cup*	349	87.2	4.1	32.0		0.0	115	151	47	1.21		231	1	0.04	0.1	0.53	
	148	23.7	14.6	6.9	0.9	87	354	195	0.10	0.028	2.7	966	0.6	0.28	0.06	3.0	43541
dulce de leche caramel, Haagen-Dazs - *1/2 cup*	290		5.0	28.0	28.0	0.0	95	150					0				
	106	17.0	10.0			100			0.00			500					HGND1
strawberry *1/2 cup*	127	39.6	2.1	18.2		0.6	40	79	9	0.22	0.051	63	5	0.03	0.1	0.20	0.48
	66	5.5	3.4			19	124	66	0.14	0.024	1.3	211		0.17	0.03	7.9	19271
van, reg (10% fat) *1/2 cup*	145	43.9	2.5	17.0	12.7	0.5	58	92	10	0.50	0.006	86	<1	0.03	0.1	0.28	0.42
	72	7.9	4.9	2.3	0.3	32	143	76	0.06	0.017	1.3	280	0.2	0.17	0.03	2.9	19095
van, rich (16% fat) *1/2 cup*	259	61.2	3.7	24.2	22.1	0.0	153	104	7	0.41	0.013	195	1	0.03	0.1	0.27	0.34
	107	17.3	10.7	5.0	0.6	98	398	75	0.16	0.080	2.5	689	0.4	0.12	0.04	7.5	19089
ice cream, fat free, van, Breyers *1/2 cup*	90		2.0	21.0	14.0	4.0	35	80					0				
	67	1.5	1.0			5			0.00			200					BRYS2
ice cream, light, avg for 15 flvrs, Edys Grand Light[5] - *1/2 cup*	121		2.9	17.8	12.9		51	57									
	80	4.1	2.3			18											EDYS7
avg for 4 flavors, Edys Lmtd Ed[6] Grand Light - *1/2 cup*	118		2.8	18.3	13.5		50	60									
	~80	3.8	2.0			19											EDYS10
blueberry hill, Healthy Choice *1/2 cup*	120		2.0	23.0	17.0	1.0	50	100					0				
	71	2.0	1.0			<5			0.00			200					CNAG45
butter pecan crunch, Healthy Choice - *1/2 cup*	120		3.0	22.0	21.0	<1.0	60	100					0				
	71	2.0	1.0			5			0.00			200					CNAG46
butterscotch blondie, Healthy Choice - *1/2 cup*	140		3.0	26.0	22.0	<1.0	75	100					0				
	71	2.0	1.0			10			1.80			100					CNAG44
cappuccino choc chunk, Healthy Choice - *1/2 cup*	120		3.0	22.0	19.0	<1.0	60	100					0				
	71	2.0	1.0			10	172	94	0.00			200					CNAG47
cappuccino mocha crunch, Healthy Choice - *1/2 cup*	120		3.0	22.0	19.0	<1.0	55	100					0				
	71	2.0	1.0			5			0.36			300					CNAG48
cherry choc chunk, Healthy Choice *1/2 cup*	110		3.0	19.0	19.0	<1.0	55	100					0				
	71	2.0	1.0			<5			0.00			200					CNAG49
cherry van, Healthy Choice *1/2 cup*	120		2.0	22.0	17.0	<1.0	50	100					0				
	71	2.0	1.0			5			0.00			0					CNAG50
choc choc chunk, Healthy Choice *1/2 cup*	120		3.0	21.0	18.0	2.0	45	100					0				
	71	2.0	1.0			<5	221	96	0.72			200					CNAG51
coconut cream pie, Healthy Choice *1/2 cup*	120		3.0	23.0	17.0	1.0	75	100					0				
	71	2.0	1.0			5			0.00			200					CNAG52
cookie crème de mint, Healthy Choice - *1/2 cup*	130		3.0	24.0	20.0	<1.0	60	100					0				
	71	2.0	1.0			5			0.00			200					CNAG53
cookies'n cream, Healthy Choice *1/2 cup*	130		3.0	24.0	20.0	1.0	60	100					0				
	71	2.0	1.0			5	167	98	0.00			200					CNAG54
fudge brownie, Healthy Choice *1/2 cup*	120		3.0	22.0	20.0	<1.0	55	100					0				
	71	2.0	1.0			5			0.00			200					CNAG55
mint choc chip, Healthy Choice *1/2 cup*	120		3.0	21.0	20.0	<1.0	50	100					0				
	71	2.0	1.0			5	178	97	0.00			200					CNAG56

	KCAL / WT (g)	H₂O (g) / FAT (g)	PRO (g) / SFA (g)	CHO (g) / MUFA (g)	SUGR (g) / PUFA (g)	DFIB (g) / CHOL (mg)	Na (mg) / K (mg)	Ca (mg) / P (mg)	Mg (mg) / Fe (mg)	Zn (mg) / Cu (mg)	Mn (mg) / Se (mcg)	A (mcg RAE) / A (IU)	C (mg) / E (mg ATE)	B-1 (mg) / B-2 (mg)	NIA (mg) / B-6 (mg)	B-12 (mcg) / FOL (mcg DFE)	PANT (mg) / REF
peanut butter cup, Healthy Choice	110		3.0	19.0	18.0	<1.0	65	100					0				
1/2 cup	71	2.0	1.0			5	182	97	0.00			200					CNAG57
praline caramel, Healthy Choice	129	40.6	2.7	25.0	24.0		70	99					0				
1/2 cup	71	2.0	0.5	1.0	0.5	4			0.08			199					19259
rocky road, Healthy Choice	130		3.0	25.0	23.0	2.0	60	100					0				
1/2 cup	71	2.0	1.0			5	175	85	0.72			200					CNAG60
strawberry, Healthy Choice	110		2.0	20.0	17.0	1.0	35	100					4				
1/2 cup	71	2.0	1.0			0			0.00			200					CNAG61
turtle fudge cake, Healthy Choice	130		2.0	23.0	21.0	<1.0	70	100					0				
1/2 cup	71	2.0	1.0			10			0.72			100					CNAG62
van bean, Healthy Choice	110		3.0	19.0	18.0	<1.0	45	100					0				
1/2 cup	71	2.0	1.0			5			0.00			300					CNAG63
van/choc/strawberry, Breyers - *1/2 cup*	110		3.0	18.0	14.0	0.0	50	100					1				
	67	3.0	2.0			10			0.00			300					BRYS1
van, Healthy Choice	100		4.0	18.0	1.0	0.0	50	60					2				
1/2 cup	71	2.0	1.0			5	153	88	0.00			850					CNAG64
wild raspberry truffle, Healthy Choice - *1/2 cup*	120		3.0	22.0	15.0	<0.1	55	100					0				
	71	2.0	1.0			5			0.00			200					CNAG65
ice cream, low/red cal, light van (1/2 the fat) - *1/2 cup*	92	45.0	2.5	15.0		0.0	56	92	10	0.29	0.005	45	1	0.04	0.1	0.44	0.33
	66	2.8	1.7	0.8	0.1	9	139	72	0.07	0.008	1.8	167	0.0	0.17	0.04	4.0	19088
w/aspartame	99	44.8	2.9	12.3	5.7		58	127									
1/2 cup	65	4.2	2.4	1.0	0.1	11											19260
ice cream, no sugar added	87		3.0	13.0	4.0		47	73									
neopolitan/straw/van, Edys - *1/2 cup*	71	3.0	1.5			10											EDYS15
All About PB, Edys	130		3.0	15.0	4.0		95	60									
1/2 cup	~71	6.0	2.0			10											EDYS13
avg for 5 flavors, Edys[7]	102		3.0	15.0	3.4		55	64									
1/2 cup	~71	3.9	2.2			10											EDYS14
ice cream, no sugar added, fat free, avg for 6 flvrs, Edys[8] - *1/2 cup*	98		3.4	20.8	4.0		56	76									
	71	0.0	0.0			1											EDYS12
ice cream, soft serve, french van	185	51.4	3.5	19.1		0.0	52	113	10	0.45	0.004	123	1	0.04	0.1	0.43	0.44
1/2 cup	86	11.2	6.4	3.0	0.4	78	152	100	0.18	0.026	2.6	439	0.3	0.16	0.04	7.7	19090
low/red cal, light van (1/2 the fat)	111	61.2	4.3	19.2		0.0	62	138	12	0.47	0.007	43	1	0.05	0.1	0.44	0.39
1/2 cup	88	2.3	1.4	0.7	0.1	11	194	106	0.05	0.024	3.2	158	0.0	0.17	0.04	5.3	19096
ices, italian, from restaurant	61	100.2	0.0	15.7		0.0	5	1	0	0.03	0.023	9	1	0.01	0.8	0.00	0.01
1/2 cup	116	<0.1	0.0	0.0	0.0	0	7	0	0.10	0.012	0.1	194	0.0	0.01	<0.01	5.8	19281
lime	127	66.2	0.4	32.3		0.0	22	2	1	0.02	0.020	0	1	<0.01	<0.1	0.00	<0.01
1/2 cup	99	0.0	0.0	0.0	0.0	0	3	1	0.16	0.013	0.1	0	0.0	0.00	<0.01	0.0	19280
pineapple coconut	112	72.6	0.0	23.7		0.7	35	0	5	0.11	0.159	0	13	0.01	<0.1	0.00	0.04
1/2 cup	99	2.6	2.3	0.1	<0.1	0	17	9	3.49	0.044	0.9	0	0.1	<0.01	0.02	1.0	19387
Klondike Bar (van ice cream w/choc coating) - *1 bar*	488	69.1	6.2	35.7	30.6		108	212									
	148	35.7	19.4			40						247					19262
popsicle, ice pop	42	47.2	0.0	11.2		0.0	7	0	1	0.01	0.004	0	0	0.00	0.0	0.00	<0.01
2 fl oz bar	59	0.0	0.0	0.0	0.0	0	2	0	0.00	0.005	0.0	0	0.0	0.00	0.0	0.0	19283
ice pop w/vit C	42	47.2	0.0	11.2		0.0	7	0	1	0.01	0.004	0	6	0.00	0.0	0.00	<0.01
2 fl oz bar	59	0.0	0.0			0	2	0	0.00	0.005	0.0	0	0.0	0.00	0.0	0.0	19717
sugar free, orange, cherry, grape, Good Humor - *1.75 fl oz bar*	15		0.0	3.0	0.0		0						6				
	55	0.0															BRYS4
sherbet, avg for 6 flavors, Edys[9]	132		1.2	27.8	22.7		37	37									
1/2 cup	~74	1.6	0.9			6											EDYS16
orange	102	48.9	0.8	22.5	18.0	0.0	34	40	6	0.36	0.008	9	2	0.02	<0.1	0.14	0.13
1/2 cup	74	1.5	0.9	0.4	0.1	4	71	30	0.10	0.021	1.0	56	0.1	0.06	0.02	3.7	19097
Sherbet Cyclone, Good Humor	50		1.0	11.0	10.0	0.0	10	20					30				
1.75 oz bar	53	0.5	0.0			0			0.00			0					BRYS6
sorbet, avg for 7 flavors, Edys[10]	131		0.0	33.1	26.4		14	0									
1/2 cup	~97	0.0	0.0			0											EDYS20
coconut, Edys	140		1.0	28.0	21.0		20	0									
1/2 cup	~94	3.0	2.5			5											EDYS19
sorbet bar, avg for 5 flavors, Edys[11]	80		0.0	20.5	19.5		0	0									
1 bar	~60	0.0	0.0			0											EDYS18

							Minerals					Vitamins					
	KCAL	H20 (g)	PRO (g)	CHO (g)	SUGR (g)	DFIB (g)	Na (mg)	Ca (mg)	Mg (mg)	Zn (mg)	Mn (mg)	A (mcg RAE)	C (mg)	B-1 (mg)	NIA (mg)	B-12 (mcg)	PANT (mg)
	WT (g)	FAT (g)	SFA (g)	MUFA (g)	PUFA (g)	CHOL (mg)	K (mg)	P (mg)	Fe (mg)	Cu (mg)	Se (mcg)	A (IU)	E (mg ATE)	B-2 (mg)	B-6 (mg)	FOL (mcg DFE)	REF
coconut, Edys	120		3.0	21.0	16.0		40	80									
1 bar	~79	3.0	2.5			0											EDYS17
strawberry & cream bar, Healthy	90		2.0	17.0	15.0	<1.0	45	60					0				
Choice - *2.5 fl oz bar*	~51	1.5	1.0			5			0.00			500					HLCH6
van sandwich, Healthy Choice	130		2.0	24.0	14.0	<1.0	150	20					0				
4 fl oz bar	~66	3.0	1.0			5			1.80			100					HLCH7

[1] Values are averages for black cherry vanilla swirl, caramel praline crunch, chocolate fudge, coffee fudge sundae, vanilla, and vanilla chocolate swirl.
[2] Values are averages for all natural vanilla, apple pie a la mode, brownies a la mode, chocolate chip cookie jar, chocolate chip mousse, double chocolate chunk, grovestand peach, mint chocolate chunk, old fashioned butter pecan, strawberries & cream, and vanilla custard.
[3] Values are averages for apple pie, candy bar blast, cracker jack peanut & toffee crunch, Girl Scout cookies samoas, Girl Scout cookies thin mints, Girl Scout cookies tagalongs, Jeff's mint chocolate sundae, NFL peanut butter blitz, orbit city swirl, peppermint, pumpkin, and Scooby snack.
[4] Values are averages for black cherry vanilla, blue ribbon chocolate cake, butter pecan, cherry chocolate chip, chocolate, chocolate caramel swirl, chocolate chips, chocolate fudge mousse, chocolate fudge sundae, coffee, cookie dough, cookies 'n cream, double fudge brownie, espresso chip, French vanilla, French vanilla fudge pie, fudge tracks, ice cream sandwich, mint chocolate chips, Neapolitan, real strawberry, rocky road, spumoni, strawberry cupcake, tin roof sundae, turtle sundae, ultimate caramel cup, vanilla, vanilla bean, vanillaberry, and vanilla chocolate.
[5] Values are averages for butter pecan, chocolate fudge mousse, chocolate raspberry escape, cookie dough, cookies 'n cream, crazy for caramel, espresso fudge chip, French silk, mint chocolate chips, mocha almond fudge, peanut butter cups, rocky road, s'mores & more, strawberry shortcake, and vanilla.
[6] Values are averages for 50/50 bar, gingerbread man, peppermint, and scooby doo dough.
[7] Values are averages for butter pecan, chips 'n swirls, double fudge brownie, mint chocolate chips, and triple chocolate.
[8] Values are averages for blueberry cobbler, chocolate fudge, raspberry vanilla swirl, vanilla, vanilla chocolate swirl, and vanilla 'n caramel.
[9] Values are averages for berry rainbow, lime, orange cream, raspberry, Swiss orange, and tropical rainbow.
[10] Values are averages for boysenberry, lemon, mandarin orange, mango, peach, raspberry, and strawberry.
[11] Values are averages for lemonade, lime, strawberry, tangerine, and wildberry.

7.6 GELATIN DESSERTS

	KCAL / WT	H20 / FAT	PRO / SFA	CHO / MUFA	SUGR / PUFA	DFIB / CHOL	Na / K	Ca / P	Mg / Fe	Zn / Cu	Mn / Se	A / A	C / E	B-1 / B-2	NIA / B-6	B-12 / FOL	PANT / REF
dry mix, all flvrs, unsweetened	94	3.6	24.0	0.0		0.0	55	15	6	0.04	0.029	0	0	0.01	<0.1	0.00	0.04
1 oz pkg	28	<0.1	<0.1	<0.1	<0.1	0	4	11	0.31	0.605	11.1	0	0.0	0.06	<0.01	8.4	19177b
all flvrs w/aspartame	35	0.7	5.5	3.3		0.0	16	0	<1	0.01	0.005	0	0	<0.01	<0.1	0.00	0.01
.35 oz pkg	10	0.0	0.0			0	1	129	<0.01	0.102	2.6	0		0.01	<0.01	1.4	19704
all flvrs w/sugar	324	0.9	6.6	76.9		0.0	216	3	2	0.01	0.014	0	0	<0.01	<0.1	0.00	0.01
3 oz pkg	85	0.0	0.0	0.0	0.0	0	6	121	0.13	0.100	5.7	0	0.0	0.02	0.01	2.6	19172
prep from mix, all flvrs	8	114.7	1.3	0.8		0.0	56	2	1	0.04	0.002	0	0	0.00	<0.1	0.00	<0.01
w/aspartame - *1/2 cup*	117	0.0	0.0	0.0	0.0	0	0	32	0.01	0.032	0.6	0	0.0	<0.01	<0.01	0.0	19176
all flvrs w/sugar	80	114.2	1.6	18.9		0.0	57	3	1	0.04	0.004	0	0	0.00	<0.1	0.00	<0.01
1/2 cup	135	0.0	0.0	0.0	0.0	0	1	30	0.04	0.032	0.4	0	0.0	<0.01	<0.01	0.0	19173
rte, mandarin orange in orange gel,	80		0.0	20.0	19.0	0.0	85	20					27				
Dole Fruit-n-Gel Bowl - *4 oz bowl*	113	0.0	0.0			0			0.00			0					DOLE4
papaya in peach gel, Dole Fruit-n-	50		0.0	13.0	12.0	0.0	70	0					27				
Gel Bowl - *4.3 oz bowl*	123	0.0	0.0			0			0.00			200					DOLE5
peaches in strawberry gel, Dole	80		0.0	20.0	19.0	0.0	85	20					21				
Fruit-n-Gel Bowl - *4 oz bowl*	113	0.0	0.0			0			0.00			100					DOLE6
pears in kiwi-berry gel, Dole Fruit-	50		0.0	13.0	11.0	0.0	70	0					24				
n-Gel Bowl - *4.3 oz bowl*	123	0.0	0.0			0			0.00			0					DOLE8
pineapple in lime gel, Dole Fruit-	80		0.0	20.0	19.0	0.0	80	20					21				
n-Gel Bowl - *4 oz bowl*	113	0.0	0.0			0			0.00			0					DOLE7
strawberry, sugar free, Jell-O	7	90.0	1.3	0.0	0.0	0.0	45	0					0				
Gelatin Snacks - *1 container*	92	0.0	0.0			0	3	0	0.03			0					19291

7.7 PASTRIES, SWEET ROLLS, COBBLERS, STRUDELS, & TURNOVERS

	KCAL / WT	H20 / FAT	PRO / SFA	CHO / MUFA	SUGR / PUFA	DFIB / CHOL	Na / K	Ca / P	Mg / Fe	Zn / Cu	Mn / Se	A / A	C / E	B-1 / B-2	NIA / B-6	B-12 / FOL	PANT / REF
cobbler, apple, frzn, Marie	370		2.0	45.0	31.0	2.0	170	0					30				
Callender - *1/4 cobbler (4.2 oz)*	120	20.0	9.0			0			0.72			0					CNAG66
berry, frzn, Marie Callender	370		3.0	41.0	29.0	1.0	220	20					4				
1/4 cobbler (4.2 oz)	120	21.0	5.0			<5			1.08				0				CNAG67
cherry, frzn, Marie Callender	380		3.0	50.0	32.0	0.0	240	0					1				
1/4 cobbler (4.2 oz)	120	19.0	8.0			5			0.72			0					CNAG68
peach, frzn, Marie Callender	360		3.0	47.0	24.0	0.0	240	0					4				
1/4 cobbler (4.2 oz)	120	18.0	6.0			0			1.08			0					CNAG69
cream puff shell, homemade	239	26.7	5.9	15.0		0.5	368	24	8	0.48	0.139	184	0	0.14	1.0	0.26	0.41
1 shell	66	17.1	3.7	7.3	4.9	129	64	79	1.33	0.034	15.8	812	2.5	0.24	0.05	43.6	18237
croissant	231	13.2	4.7	26.1		1.5	424	21	9	0.43	0.188	101	<1	0.22	1.2	0.09	0.49
1 med croissant	57	12.0	6.6	3.1	0.6	38	67	60	1.16	0.046	12.9	424	0.2	0.14	0.03	49.0	18239

							Minerals					Vitamins					
	KCAL	H_2O (g)	PRO (g)	CHO (g)	SUGR (g)	DFIB (g)	Na (mg)	Ca (mg)	Mg (mg)	Zn (mg)	Mn (mg)	A (mcg RAE)	C (mg)	B-1 (mg)	NIA (mg)	B-12 (mcg)	PANT (mg)
	WT (g)	FAT (g)	SFA (g)	MUFA (g)	PUFA (g)	CHOL (mg)	K (mg)	P (mg)	Fe (mg)	Cu (mg)	Se (mcg)	A (IU)	E (mg ATE)	B-2 (mg)	B-6 (mg)	FOL (mcg DFE)	REF
apple	145	26.0	4.2	21.1		1.4	156	17	7	0.59	0.120	54	<1	0.13	0.9	0.11	0.34
1 med croissant	57	5.0	2.8	1.4	0.4	18	51	33	0.63	0.023	10.8	217		0.09	0.02	50.2	18240
cheese	236	12.0	5.2	26.8		1.5	316	30	14	0.54	0.194	106	<1	0.30	1.2	0.18	0.48
1 med croissant	57	11.9	6.1	3.7	1.4	32	75	74	1.23	0.057	15.3	459	0.6	0.19	0.04	58.7	18241
danish pastry, cinn	262	15.8	4.6	29.0		0.8	241	46	12	0.47	0.235	3	<1	0.20	1.9	0.07	0.26
1 pastry (4 1/4″ dia)	65	14.6	3.7	8.1	1.9	14	81	70	1.27	0.065	11.1	8	1.9	0.17	0.02	53.3	18244
	349	18.4	4.8	46.9			326	37	14	0.48	0.370	5	3	0.26	2.2	0.22	0.55
3.1 oz pastry	88	16.7	3.5	10.6	1.6	27	96	74	1.80	0.075	15.0	18		0.19	0.05	82.7	21016
cream/neufchatel cheese	266	22.3	5.7	26.4		0.7	320	25	11	0.50	0.249	31	<1	0.13	1.4	0.12	0.22
1 pastry (4 1/4″ dia)	71	15.5	4.8	8.0	1.8	11	70	77	1.14	0.063	13.4	104	1.8	0.18	0.03	60.4	18245
fruit[1]	263	19.2	3.8	33.9		1.3	251	33	11	0.38	0.180	16	3	0.19	1.4	0.06	0.45
1 pastry (4 1/4″ dia)	71	13.1	3.5	7.1	1.7	81	59	63	1.26	0.046	10.5	53	1.7	0.16	0.03	32.0	18246
lemon	263	19.2	3.8	33.9		1.3	251	33	11	0.38	0.180	38	3	0.05	0.5	0.06	0.45
1 pastry (4 1/4″ dia)	71	13.1	2.0	4.2	1.1	28	59	63	0.53	0.046		124	1.0	0.07	0.03	11.4	18433
nut[2]	280	13.3	4.6	29.7		1.3	236	61	21	0.57	0.549	10	1	0.14	1.5	0.14	0.46
1 pastry (4 1/4″ dia)	65	16.4	3.8	8.9	2.8	30	62	72	1.17	0.127	9.2	34	2.4	0.16	0.07	79.3	18247
raspberry	263	19.2	3.8	33.9		1.3	251	33	11	0.38	0.180	43	3	0.05	0.5	0.06	0.45
1 pastry (4 1/4″ dia)	71	13.1	2.0	4.2	1.1	28	59	63	0.53	0.046		142	1.0	0.07	0.03	11.4	18435
eclair, choc, frzn, Weight Watchers	140	28.3	2.4	23.5	10.9	0.9	186										
1 éclair	59	4.1	0.7			30											18640
w/custard filling & choc glaze,	262	52.4	6.4	24.2		0.6	337	63	15	0.61	0.128	185	<1	0.12	0.8	0.34	0.49
homemade - *1 éclair (5″ long)*	100	15.7	4.1	6.5	3.9	127	117	107	1.18	0.058	15.6	718	2.1	0.27	0.06	38.0	18257
puff pastry, frzn	223	3.0	3.0	18.3		0.6	101	4	6	0.22	0.198	0	0	0.13	1.5	0.00	0.00
1 pastry	40	15.4	2.2	3.5	8.9	0	25	24	1.04	0.046	9.8	0	1.0	0.10	0.01	29.6	18211
strudel, apple	195	30.9	2.3	29.2		1.6	191	11	6	0.13	0.135	6	1	0.03	0.2	0.16	0.19
2.5 oz piece	71	8.0	1.5	2.3	3.8	4	106	23	0.30	0.021	4.3	21	2.2	0.02	0.03	14.2	18354
sweet roll, from refrig dough,	170		2.0	24.0	10.0	<1.0	330	0					0				
caramel, Pillsbury - *1.7 oz roll*	49	7.0	1.5			0			1.08			0					GENM107
cinn raisin w/icing, Pillsbury	170		2.0	26.0	11.0	<1.0	320	0					0				
1.7 oz roll	49	6.0	1.5			0			1.08			0					GENM108
cinn w/butter crm icing, Grands!	340		5.0	52.0	23.0	1.0	690	20					0				
3.5 oz roll	99	12.0	3.0			0			1.80			0					GENM109
cinn w/cream cheese icing,	330		5.0	52.0	23.0	1.0	660	20					0				
Grands! - *3.5 oz roll*	99	11.0	3.0			<5			1.80			0					GENM110
cinn w/cream cheese icing,	150		2.0	23.0	9.0	<1.0	350	0					0				
Pillsbury - *1.6 oz roll*	44	6.0	1.5			0			0.72			0					GENM111
cinn w/icing	109	6.8	1.6	16.8			250	10	4	0.10	0.125	0	<1	0.12	1.1	0.02	0.08
1 roll	30	4.0	1.0	2.2	0.5	0	19	104	0.80	0.021	5.3	1		0.07	0.01	26.7	18358
cinn w/icing, Grands!	330		5.0	52.0	23.0	1.0	670	20					0				
3.5 oz roll	99	11.0	3.0			0			1.80			0					GENM112
cinn w/icing, Pillsbury	150	11.7	2.4	23.9	8.4		334										
1 roll	44	5.0	1.2														18635
orange w/icing, Pillsbury	170		2.0	25.0	10.0	<1.0	340	0					0				
1.7 oz roll	49	7.0	1.5			0			1.08			0					GENM116
sweet roll, frzn, honey bun, Morton	270		3.0	35.0	16.0	1.0	160	0					0				
2.3 oz bun (4/pkg)	65	13.0	3.0			0			0.72			0					CNAG70
honey bun, mini, Morton	160		2.0	19.0	6.0	1.0	100	0					0				
1.3 oz bun (12/pkg)	38	8.0	2.0			0			0.72			0					CNAG71
sweet roll, red fat, from refrig	310		5.0	54.0	24.0	1.0	680	20					0				
dough, cinn w/icing, Grands! - *3.5 oz roll*	99	8.0	2.0			0			1.80			0					GENM114
cinn w/icing, Pillsbury	140		2.0	24.0	9.0	<1.0	340	0					0				
1.6 oz roll	44	3.5	1.0			0			0.72			0					GENM115
sweet roll, rte, cheese	238	19.4	4.7	28.8		0.8	236	78	13	0.42	0.139		<1	0.10	0.5	0.20	0.27
(cream/Neufchatel) - *1 roll*	66	12.1	4.0	6.0	1.3	50	90	65	0.50	0.063	7.9	168		0.09	0.05	33.7	18355
cinn raisin	223	14.9	3.7	30.5		1.4	230	43	10	0.35	0.180	39	1	0.19	1.4	0.08	0.24
1 roll	60	9.8	1.8	2.9	4.5	40	67	46	0.96	0.053	10.2	129	2.6	0.16	0.06	43.2	18356
toaster pastry, apple/blueberry/	204	6.4	2.4	37.0		1.1	218	14	9	0.34	0.154	149	<1	0.15	2.0	0.01	0.29
cherry/strawberry - *1 pastry*	52	5.3	0.8	2.2	2.0	0	58	58	1.81	0.098	2.3	501	1.2	0.19	0.20	51.5	18362
toaster pastry, apple cinn danish,	256	10.4	3.0	37.0	11.0	0.9	190	20					0				
Pop-Tarts Pastry Swirls - *1 pastry*	62	11.0	3.0	3.6	4.4	0			1.08			0					18508
frosted, low fat, Pop-Tarts	191	6.5	2.2	40.0	19.9	0.6	206	6	5	0.16			0	0.16	2.0	0.00	0.00
1 pastry	52	2.9	0.6	1.5	0.8	0	28	21	1.82	0.000		500	0.0	0.16	0.21		18491

	KCAL / WT (g)	H₂0 (g) / FAT (g)	PRO (g) / SFA (g)	CHO (g) / MUFA (g)	SUGR (g) / PUFA (g)	DFIB (g) / CHOL (mg)	Na (mg) / K (mg)	Ca (mg) / P (mg)	Mg (mg) / Fe (mg)	Zn (mg) / Cu (mg)	Mn (mg) / Se (mcg)	A (mcg RAE) / A (IU)	C (mg) / E (mg ATE)	B-1 (mg) / B-2 (mg)	NIA (mg) / B-6 (mg)	B-12 (mcg) / FOL (mcg DFE)	PANT (mg) / REF
Pop-Tarts	205	6.5	2.3	37.5	17.5	0.6	174	12	6	0.34			0	0.15	2.0	0.00	0.00
1 pastry	52	5.3	0.9	3.1	1.4	0	47	28	1.82	0.021		500	0.0	0.17	0.20		18475
toaster pastry, blueberry, frosted,	211	5.3	2.5	34.2	15.4	0.7	185	15	8	1.21			0	0.15	2.0	0.00	0.00
Pop-Tarts - 1 pastry	50	7.4	1.1	3.9	2.4	0	56	47	1.80	0.040		500	0.0	0.17	0.20		18479c
low fat, Pop-Tarts	192	6.5	2.3	39.8	18.7	0.6	222	6	5	0.16			0	0.16	2.0	0.00	0.00
1 pastry	52	2.9	0.6	1.6	0.7	0	30	23	1.82	0.000		500	0.0	0.16	0.21		18492
Pop-Tarts	212	6.5	2.4	35.6	16.1	0.6	207	12	8	0.66			0	0.15	2.0	0.00	0.00
1 pastry	52	6.9	1.1	3.4	2.5	0	49	46	1.82	0.078		500	0.0	0.17	0.20		18476
toaster pastry, brown sugar cinn	206	5.4	2.6	34.1		0.5	212	17	12	0.32	0.161	148	<1	0.19	2.3	0.11	0.13
1 pastry	50	7.1	1.8	4.0	0.9	0	57	67	2.02	0.066	6.3	493		0.29	0.21	21.0	18361
frosted, low fat, Pop-Tarts	188	5.3	2.4	39.2	18.1	0.6	210	7	5	0.15			0	0.15	2.0	0.00	0.00
1 pastry	50	2.8	0.6	1.5	0.7	0	31	23	1.80	0.050		500	0.0	0.15	0.20		18494
frosted, Pop-Tarts	211	5.3	2.5	34.2	15.4	0.7	185	15	8	1.21			0	0.15	2.0	0.00	0.00
1 pastry	50	7.4	1.1	3.9	2.4	0	56	47	1.80	0.040		500	0.0	0.17	0.20		18479b
Pop-Tarts	219	5.3	2.7	32.2	12.7	0.8	214	16	8	0.61			0	0.15	2.0	0.00	0.00
1 pastry	50	9.2	1.0	3.6	4.6	0	68	32	1.80	0.040		500	0.0	0.17	0.20		18478
toaster pastry, cheese danish,	252	10.4	3.0	36.6	12.0	0.3	180	40					0				
Pop-Tarts Pastry Swirls - 1 pastry	62	11.0	3.0	3.6	4.4	1			1.08			0					18510
toaster pastry, cherry, frosted,	204	6.5	2.2	37.4	18.7	0.5	220	13	7	0.76			0	0.15	2.0	0.00	0.00
Pop-Tarts - 1 pastry	52	5.3	1.0	3.5	0.8	0	49	42	1.82	0.099		500	0.0	0.17	0.20		18481
low fat, Pop-Tarts	192	6.5	2.3	39.8	18.6	0.6	222	6	5	0.16			0	0.16	2.0	0.00	0.00
1 pastry	52	2.9	0.6	1.6	0.7	0	30	22	1.82	0.000		500	0.0	0.16	0.21		18493
Pop-Tarts	204	6.5	2.4	37.0	16.5	0.6	220	15	8	0.64			0	0.15	2.0	0.00	0.00
1 pastry	52	5.4	0.9	3.0	1.6	0	59	44	1.82	0.078		500	0.0	0.17	0.20		18480
toaster pastry, choc fudge,	190	6.5	2.7	39.5	18.8	0.6	249	14	15	0.26			0	0.16	2.0	0.00	0.00
frstd, low fat, Pop-Tarts - 1 pastry	52	3.0	0.5	1.2	0.9	0	62	40	1.82	0.104		500	0.0	0.16	0.21		18495
frosted, Pop-Tarts	201	6.5	2.7	37.3	19.8	0.6	203	20	15	0.26			0	0.16	2.0	0.00	0.00
1 pastry	52	4.8	1.0	2.7	1.1	0	82	44	1.82	0.104		500	0.0	0.16	0.21		18482
toaster pastry, choc van crème,	203	6.5	2.6	36.8	19.4	0.5	229	16	11	0.62			0	0.15	2.0	0.00	0.00
frosted, Pop-Tarts - 1 pastry	52	5.3	1.0	3.2	1.0	0	62	36	1.82	0.052		500	0.0	0.17	0.21		18483
toaster pastry, grape, frosted,	203	6.5	2.3	37.6	18.4	0.5	198	12	11	0.68			0	0.15	2.0	0.00	0.00
Pop-Tarts - 1 pastry	52	5.1	0.9	3.1	1.1	0	60	46	1.82	0.052		500	0.0	0.17	0.21		18484
toaster pastry, milk choc, Pop-Tarts	205	6.4	3.4	35.6	18.0	0.8	227	20	12	0.21			0	0.16	2.0	0.00	0.00
1 pastry	52	5.8	1.5	3.2	1.1	0	82	45	1.82	0.052		500	0.0	0.16	0.21		18485
toaster pastry, raspberry, frosted,	205	6.5	2.2	37.2	18.4	0.5	211	11	8	0.63			0	0.15	2.0	0.00	0.00
Pop-Tarts - 1 pastry	52	5.5	1.0	3.2	1.3	0	44	46	1.82	0.042		500	0.0	0.17	0.21		18486
toaster pastry, s'mores, Pop-Tarts	204	6.5	3.2	36.2	19.0	0.7	199	15	11	0.21			0	0.16	2.0	0.00	0.00
1 pastry	52	5.5	1.5	3.1	0.9	0	65	39	1.82	0.052		500	0.0	0.16	0.21		18487
toaster pastry, strawberry danish,	254	10.1	3.0	37.2	16.0	1.1	170	20					0				
Pop-Tarts Pastry Swirls - 1 pastry	62	11.0	3.0	3.6	4.4	0			1.08			0					18509
frosted, low fat, Pop-Tarts	191	6.5	2.1	40.3	20.7	0.6	201	5	4	0.16			0	0.16	2.0	0.00	0.00
1 pastry	52	3.0	0.6	1.4	1.0	0	25	20	1.82	0.000		500	0.0	0.16	0.21		18497
frosted, Pop-Tarts	203	6.5	2.3	37.6	19.5	0.5	169	11	5	0.16			0	0.16	2.0	0.00	0.00
1 pastry	52	5.0	1.4	2.9	0.7	0	44	27	1.82	0.000		500	0.0	0.16	0.21		18489
low fat, Pop-Tarts	192	6.5	2.3	39.8	18.6	0.6	220	6	5	0.16		25	0	0.16	2.0	0.00	0.00
1 pastry	52	2.9	0.6	1.5	0.7	0	28	22	1.82	0.000		500	0.0	0.16	0.21		18496
Pop-Tarts	205	6.5	2.4	36.9	17.2	0.6	185	12	6	0.16			0	0.16	2.0	0.00	0.00
1 pastry	52	5.5	1.5	3.2	0.8	0	48	29	1.82	0.000		500	0.0	0.16	0.21		18488
toaster pastry, wild berry,	210	6.8	2.3	39.4	21.0	0.5	168	11	5	0.16			0	0.16	2.0	0.00	0.00
frosted, Pop-Tarts - 1 pastry	54	5.0	1.4	2.9	0.7	0	44	26	1.78	0.000		500	0.0	0.16	0.22		18490
toaster pastry, wild watermelon,	202	6.5	2.2	37.9	20.2	0.5	162	111	5	0.16			0	0.16	1.9	0.00	0.00
frosted, Pop-Tarts - 1 pastry	52	4.8	1.4	2.8	0.7	0	43	25	1.72	0.000		482	0.0	0.16	0.21		18498
Toaster Strudel Pastries, avg for	193		2.9	25.1	9.9	<0.7	204	0					0	0.15	3.8	0.90	
14 flvrs, Gen Mills - 1.9 oz strudel	54	8.9	2.1			7			0.78			0		0.32	0.30	31.4	GENM117
turnover, apple, from refrig dough,	170		2.0	23.0	11.0	<1.0	310	0					0				
Pillsbury - 2 oz turnover	57	8.0	2.0			0			0.72			0					GENM105
apple, frzn, Pepperidge Farm	284	37.3	3.7	31.2	10.8	1.6	176						0				
1 turnover	89	16.0	4.0						1.22								18628
cherry, from refrig dough,	170		2.0	23.0	12.0	0.0	310	0					0				
Pillsbury - 2 oz turnover	57	8.0	2.0			0			0.72			0					GENM106

[1] Includes apple, cinnamon, raisin, lemon, raspberry, and strawberry.

[2] Includes almond, raisin nut, and cinnamon nut.

	KCAL	H₂0 (g)	PRO (g)	CHO (g)	SUGR (g)	DFIB (g)	Na (mg)	Ca (mg)	Mg (mg)	Zn (mg)	Mn (mg)	A (mcg RAE)	C (mg)	B-1 (mg)	NIA (mg)	B-12 (mcg)	PANT (mg)
	WT (g)	FAT (g)	SFA (g)	MUFA (g)	PUFA (g)	CHOL (mg)	K (mg)	P (mg)	Fe (mg)	Cu (mg)	Se (mcg)	A (IU)	E (mg ATE)	B-2 (mg)	B-6 (mg)	FOL (mcg DFE)	REF

7.8 PIES, PIE CRUSTS, & PIE FILLINGS

	KCAL / WT	H₂0 / FAT	PRO / SFA	CHO / MUFA	SUGR / PUFA	DFIB / CHOL	Na / K	Ca / P	Mg / Fe	Zn / Cu	Mn / Se	A RAE / A IU	C / E	B-1 / B-2	NIA / B-6	B-12 / FOL	PANT / REF
apple	296	65.3	2.4	42.5		2.0	333	14	9	0.20	0.228	36	4	0.04	0.3	0.01	0.15
1/8 of 9" pie	125	13.8	4.7	5.5	2.7	0	81	30	0.56	0.058	1.3	155	0.1	0.03	0.05	43.8	18301
frzn, Banquet	292	54.3	2.9	41.4	25.8	1.0	361	10					0				
4 oz serving	112	13.2	5.7	6.1	1.4	9			0.34			0					18600
homemade	411	73.3	3.7	57.5			327	11	11	0.29	0.287	17	3	0.23	1.9	0.00	0.14
1/8 of 9" pie	155	19.4	4.7	8.4	5.2	0	122	43	1.74	0.082	12.1	90		0.17	0.05	58.9	18302
apple pie filling, cnd	75	54.3	0.1	19.4		0.7	33	3	1	0.03	0.020	1	1	0.01	<0.1	0.00	0.03
1/8 can	74	0.1	<0.1	0.0	<0.1	0	33	5	0.21	0.041	0.3	10	0.0	0.01	0.01	0.0	19312
banana cream, from mix	231	46.8	3.1	29.1		0.6	267	67	11	0.30	0.098	87	<1	0.09	0.7	0.19	0.24
1/8 of 9" pie	92	11.9	6.4	4.2	0.7	27	104	154	0.42	0.040	4.5	375		0.13	0.03	28.5	18303
homemade	387	69.0	6.3	47.4		1.0	346	108	23	0.69	0.219	98	2	0.20	1.5	0.36	0.56
1/8 of 9" pie	144	19.6	5.4	8.2	4.7	73	238	132	1.50	0.075	13.1	376	2.1	0.30	0.19	54.7	18304
blueberry	290	65.6	2.3	43.6		1.3	406	10	6	0.20	0.220	40	3	0.01	0.4	0.01	0.17
1/8 of 9" pie	125	12.5	2.1	5.3	4.4	0	63	29	0.38	0.058	1.8	175	2.5	0.04	0.05	43.8	18305
homemade	360	75.3	4.0	49.2			272	10	12	0.29	0.441	3	1	0.22	1.8	0.00	0.18
1/8 of 9" pie	147	17.5	4.3	7.5	4.5	0	74	44	1.81	0.098	10.9	62		0.19	0.05	52.9	18306
cherry	325	57.8	2.5	49.8		1.0	308	15	10	0.23	0.175	59	1	0.03	0.3	0.01	0.40
1/8 of 9" pie	125	13.8	3.2	7.3	2.6	0	101	36	0.60	0.050	1.5	351	1.9	0.04	0.05	40.0	18308
homemade	486	82.4	5.0	69.3			344	18	16	0.36	0.360	52	2	0.27	2.3	0.00	0.22
1/8 of 9" pie	180	22.0	5.4	9.6	5.8	0	139	54	3.33	0.139	14.0	736		0.23	0.06	73.8	18309
cherry pie filling, cnd	85	52.7	0.3	20.7		0.4	13	8	5	0.04	0.022	7	3	0.02	0.1	0.00	0.05
1/8 can	74	0.1	<0.1	<0.1	<0.1	0	78	11	0.18	0.059	0.3	152		0.01	0.03	3.0	19314
choc cream/crème	344	49.2	2.9	38.0		2.3	154	41	24	0.26	0.226	0	0	0.04	0.8	0.01	0.44
1/6 of 8" pie	113	21.9	5.6	12.6	2.7	6	144	77	1.21	0.057	8.5	0	3.1	0.12	0.02	19.2	18310
choc mousse, from mix	247	47.2	3.3	28.1			437	73	30	0.57	0.119	118	<1	0.05	0.6	0.20	0.19
1/8 of 9" pie	95	14.6	7.8	4.8	0.8	33	271	219	1.03	0.193	5.8	392		0.14	0.03	39.9	18312
coconut cream	191	27.6	1.3	23.8		0.8	163	19	13	0.30	0.280	17	0	0.03	0.1	0.08	0.15
1/6 of 7" pie	64	10.6	4.5	4.6	1.0	0	42	54	0.51	0.044	3.4	58	1.2	0.05	0.04	5.1	18313
from mix	259	46.7	2.6	26.8		0.5	309	68	16	0.36	0.179	89	1	0.03	0.1	0.20	0.24
1/8 of 9" pie	94	16.5	8.4	6.2	1.1	22	133	159	0.38	0.075	4.7	381		0.10	0.04	21.6	18314
coconut custard	270	51.2	6.1	31.4		1.9	348	84	19	0.71	0.218	27	1	0.09	0.4	0.09	0.25
1/6 of 8" pie	104	13.7	6.1	5.7	1.2	36	182	127	0.83	0.066	6.7	114		0.15	0.01	19.8	18316
custard, egg	221	63.9	5.8	21.8		1.7	252	84	12	0.55	0.063	69	1	0.04	0.3	0.45	0.70
1/6 of 8" pie	105	12.2	2.5	5.0	3.9	35	111	118	0.61	0.025	7.5	244	2.0	0.22	0.05	28.4	18317
lemon meringue	303	47.1	1.7	53.3		1.4	165	63	17	0.55	0.068	60	4	0.07	0.2	0.19	0.90
1/6 of 8" pie	113	9.8	2.0	3.0	4.1	51	101	119	0.69	0.001	3.4	198	2.5	0.24	0.03	19.2	18320
homemade	362	55.0	4.8	49.7			307	15	8	0.36	0.163	55	4	0.15	1.2	0.15	0.27
1/8 of 9" pie	127	16.4	4.0	7.1	4.2	67	83	53	1.27	0.053	14.7	203		0.20	0.03	45.7	18321
mince, homemade	477	61.7	4.3	79.2		4.3	419	36	23	0.36	0.434	2	10	0.25	2.0	0.00	0.17
1/8 of 9" pie	165	17.8	4.4	7.7	4.7	0	335	69	2.46	0.186	10.9	36	3.1	0.17	0.11	59.4	18322
peach	261	63.6	2.2	38.5		0.9	316	9	7	0.11	0.178	6	1	0.07	0.2	0.00	0.13
1/6 of 8" pie	117	11.7	1.8	5.0	4.4	0	146	26	0.59	0.062	1.5	123	2.4	0.04	0.03	44.5	18323
pecan	452	21.8	4.5	64.6		4.0	479	19	20	0.64	0.892	53	1	0.10	0.3	0.11	0.48
1/6 of 8" pie	113	20.9	4.0	12.1	3.6	36	84	87	1.18	0.220	5.7	198	2.1	0.14	0.02	47.5	18324
homemade	503	23.8	6.0	63.7			320	39	32	1.24	0.869	100	<1	0.23	1.0	0.21	0.58
1/8 of 9" pie	122	27.1	4.9	13.6	7.0	106	162	115	1.81	0.257	14.6	436		0.22	0.07	41.5	18325
pie crust, from mix	100	2.1	1.3	10.1		0.4	146	12	3	0.08	0.061	0	0	0.06	0.5	0.00	0.03
1/8 of 9" crust	20	6.1	1.5	3.5	0.8	0	12	17	0.43	0.015	4.4	0		0.04	0.01	22.2	18333
pie crust, frzn	82	1.8	0.7	7.9		0.2	104	3	3	0.05	0.098	0	0	0.04	0.4	<0.01	0.03
1/8 of 9" crust	16	5.2	1.7	2.5	0.6	0	18	9	0.36	0.012	0.5	0	0.8	0.06	0.01	9.8	18335
9" deep dish, Pet Ritz	90		1.0	10.0	0.0	0.0	85	0					0				
1/8 crust (.74 oz)	21	5.0	2.0			<5			0.72			0					GENM119
9", Pet Ritz	80		<1.0	9.0	0.0	0.0	75	0					0				
1/8 crust (.63 oz)	18	4.0	1.5			<5			0.36			0					GENM120
9 5/8" extra large, Pet	110		1.0	13.0	<1.0	0.0	110	0					0				
Ritz - *1/8 crust (.95 oz)*	27	6.0	2.5			5			0.72			0					GENM121
pie crust, homemade	121	2.3	1.5	10.9		0.4	125	2	3	0.10	0.099	0	0	0.09	0.8	0.00	0.04
1/8 of 9" crust	23	8.0	2.0	3.5	2.1	0	15	15	0.66	0.021	4.9	0		0.06	0.01	24.4	18336

	KCAL / WT (g)	H₂O / FAT (g)	PRO / SFA (g)	CHO / MUFA (g)	SUGR / PUFA (g)	DFIB / CHOL (g/mg)	Na / K (mg)	Ca / P (mg)	Mg / Fe (mg)	Zn / Cu (mg)	Mn / Se (mg/mcg)	A (mcg RAE) / A (IU)	C / E (mg)	B-1 / B-2 (mg)	NIA / B-6 (mg)	B-12 / FOL (mcg/DFE)	PANT / REF (mg)
choc wafer	142	2.0	1.4	15.2		0.4	188	8	11	0.23	0.145	52	0	0.04	0.6	0.01	0.08
1/8 of 9" crust	28	8.7	1.9	4.1	2.2	<1	47	29	0.84	0.097	1.2	256	1.4	0.06	<0.01	25.2	18398
graham	148	1.3	1.3	19.6		0.5	171	6	5	0.14	0.139	52	0	0.03	0.6	0.01	0.07
1/8 of 9" crust	30	7.5	1.6	3.4	2.1	0	26	20	0.65	0.014	1.8	220	1.2	0.05	0.01	10.8	18330
van wafer	117	1.9	0.8	11.0		0.0	113	9	2	0.05	0.039	54	<1	0.04	0.5	0.02	0.07
1/8 of 9" crust	22	8.0	1.6	3.4	2.4	9	17	17	0.36	0.015	1.7	262	1.1	0.05	0.01	17.4	18401
pie crust, ready-to-use, Nilla,	144	0.9	1.0	17.7	9.0	0.3	63	11	2	0.08					0.05	0.7	0.03
Nabisco - *1 oz serving*	28	7.6	1.4	5.2	0.4	3	19	23	0.50	0.014		3		0.05	0.01		18618a
pie crust, refrig, Pillsbury All	120	<1.0		13.0	<1.0	0.0	110	0								0	
Ready - *1/8 crust (.95 oz)*	27	7.0	3.0			5		0.00				0					GENM118
pumpkin	229	63.3	4.3	29.8		2.9	307	65	16	0.49	0.262	227	1	0.06	0.2	0.28	0.55
1/6 of 8" pie	109	10.4	1.9	4.4	3.4	22	168	77	0.86	0.052	2.8	3743	1.9	0.17	0.06	26.2	18326
homemade	316	90.7	7.0	40.9			349	146	29	0.71	0.307	660	3	0.14	1.2	0.14	0.69
1/8 of 9" pie	155	14.4	4.9	5.7	2.8	65	288	152	1.97	0.102	11.0	12431		0.31	0.07	43.4	18327
pumpkin pie mix, cnd	281	193.0	2.9	71.3		22.4	562	100	43	0.73	1.083	1121	9	0.04	1.0	0.00	3.07
1 cup	270	0.4	0.2	<0.1	<0.1	0	373	122	2.86	0.184	3.0	22405		0.32	0.43	94.5	11426
snack pie, fried, cherry	404	48.1	3.8	54.5		3.3	479	28	13	0.29	0.287	12	2	0.18	1.8	0.10	0.14
1 snack pie (5"×3 3/4")	128	20.6	3.1	9.5	6.9	0	83	55	1.56	0.060	3.1	220		0.14	0.04	37.1	18444
fruit[1]	404	48.1	3.8	54.5		3.3	479	28	13	0.29	0.287	1	2	0.18	1.8	0.10	0.14
1 snack pie (5"×3 3/4")	128	20.6	3.1	9.5	6.9	0	83	55	1.56	0.060	3.1	35	3.8	0.14	0.04	37.1	18319
lemon	404	48.1	3.8	54.5		3.3	479	28	13	0.29	0.287	3	2	0.18	1.8	0.10	0.14
1 snack pie (5"×3 3/4")	128	20.6	3.1	9.5	6.9	0	83	55	1.56	0.060	3.1	41		0.14	0.04	37.1	18445
van cream, homemade	350	59.2	6.0	41.1		0.8	328	113	16	0.67	0.161	106	1	0.18	1.2	0.38	0.52
1/8 of 9" pie	126	18.1	5.1	7.6	4.3	78	159	131	1.29	0.049	12.0	386	1.7	0.27	0.06	46.6	18328

[1] Includes apple, blueberry, cherry, lemon, peach, and strawberry.

7.9 PUDDINGS & CUSTARDS

	KCAL / WT (g)	H₂O / FAT (g)	PRO / SFA (g)	CHO / MUFA (g)	SUGR / PUFA (g)	DFIB / CHOL (g/mg)	Na / K (mg)	Ca / P (mg)	Mg / Fe (mg)	Zn / Cu (mg)	Mn / Se (mg/mcg)	A (mcg RAE) / A (IU)	C / E (mg)	B-1 / B-2 (mg)	NIA / B-6 (mg)	B-12 / FOL (mcg/DFE)	PANT / REF (mg)
banana, from inst mix w/2% milk	154	109.5	4.1	29.0		0.0	435	150	18	0.49	0.004	68	1	0.05	0.1	0.44	0.39
1/2 cup	147	2.5	1.4	0.7	0.2	9	193	318	0.09	0.015	2.9	250	0.1	0.20	0.05	5.9	19121
w/whole milk	169	108.1	4.0	28.9		0.0	435	147	16	0.47	0.007	35	1	0.05	0.1	0.44	0.39
1/2 cup	147	4.2	2.5	1.2	0.2	16	188	315	0.09	0.018	2.6	154		0.20	0.05	5.9	19319
banana, from reg mix w/2% milk	141	106.3	4.1	25.8		0.0	230	153	18	0.49	0.006	70	1	0.04	0.1	0.35	0.39
1/2 cup	140	2.4	1.4	0.6	0.1	10	192	116	0.07	0.014	2.9	249	0.1	0.20	0.05	5.6	19122
w/whole milk	155	104.8	4.0	25.6		0.0	230	150	18	0.48	0.007	36	1	0.04	0.1	0.35	0.38
1/2 cup	140	4.2	2.5	1.1	0.2	17	188	115	0.07	0.017	2.7	154	0.1	0.20	0.05	5.6	19321
banana, ready-to-eat	180	102.2	3.4	30.1		0.1	278	121	11	0.40	0.011	9	1	0.03	0.2	0.26	0.23
5 oz serving	142	5.1	0.8	2.2	1.9	0	156	98	0.18	0.040	2.0	30		0.21	0.03	2.8	19311
choc, from inst mix w/lowfat milk	154	109.6	4.6	27.8		0.6	417	153	28	0.63	0.091	68	1	0.05	0.2	0.46	0.40
1/2 cup	147	2.8	1.6	0.8	0.2	9	247	350	0.59	0.100	3.4	250	0.1	0.22	0.06	7.4	19123
w/whole milk	163	108.2	4.6	27.6		1.5	417	150	26	0.62	0.062	38	1	0.05	0.1	0.44	0.40
1/2 cup	147	4.6	2.7	1.4	0.3	16	244	351	0.43	0.094	2.5	176	0.1	0.21	0.06	5.9	19185
choc, from reg mix w/2% milk	155	105.3	4.7	27.8		0.4	148	159	30	0.65	0.061	67	1	0.05	0.1	0.36	0.40
1/2 cup	142	2.8	1.7	0.8	0.1	10	237	136	0.51	0.104	3.1	250	0.1	0.25	0.05	5.7	19190
w/whole milk	158	105.6	4.5	25.6		1.4	146	158	21	0.64	0.061	37	1	0.04	0.1	0.36	0.39
1/2 cup	142	4.8	3.0	1.4	0.2	17	231	132	0.51	0.107	2.4	156	0.1	0.25	0.05	5.7	19189
choc, ready-to-eat	189	98.4	3.8	32.4		1.4	183	128	30	0.60	0.098	16	3	0.04	0.5	0.00	0.20
5 oz serving	142	5.7	1.0	2.4	2.0	4	256	114	0.72	0.165	3.1	51	0.2	0.22	0.04	4.3	19183
Jell-O	102	85.5	2.8	22.7	17.3	0.9	192	89					<1				
1 snack container	113	0.5	0.3			2	235	86	0.60			174					19288
coconut cream, from inst mix	157	109.4	4.3	28.2		0.1	362	150	21	0.49	0.028	66	1	0.05	0.1	0.44	0.40
w/2% milk - *1/2 cup*	147	3.4	2.0	0.9	0.3	9	194	295	0.22	0.037	2.9	221		0.20	0.06	5.9	19191
w/whole milk	172	107.9	4.3	28.1		0.1	362	147	21	0.49	0.028	35	1	0.05	0.1	0.44	0.39
1/2 cup	147	5.1	3.1	1.4	0.4	16	190	294	0.22	0.038	2.9	154		0.20	0.05	5.9	19323
coconut cream, from reg mix	146	105.8	4.3	24.9		0.3	228	158	22	0.52	0.052	69	1	0.04	0.1	0.36	0.41
w/2% milk - *1/2 cup*	140	3.5	2.5	0.7	0.1	10	223	125	0.28	0.035	3.2	238	0.1	0.20	0.20	5.6	19219
w/whole milk	160	104.4	4.2	24.8		0.3	227	155	22	0.50	0.052	36	1	0.04	0.1	0.35	0.40
1/2 cup	140	5.3	3.6	1.2	0.2	17	220	123	0.28	0.038	3.2	154		0.20	0.20	5.6	19325
custard, egg, from mix	148	99.4	5.4	23.2		0.0	118	193	25	0.69	0.007	81	1	0.07	0.2	0.60	0.85
w/2% milk - *1/2 cup*	133	3.6	1.8	1.1	0.3	64	298	184	0.47	0.020	6.1	290		0.28	0.09	12.0	19205
w/whole milk	161	98.0	5.4	23.0		0.0	117	190	25	0.68	0.009	49	1	0.07	0.2	0.59	0.85
1/2 cup	133	5.3	2.8	1.6	0.3	70	294	181	0.47	0.021	5.9	196		0.28	0.09	12.0	19170

	KCAL	H₂0 (g)	PRO (g)	CHO (g)	SUGR (g)	DFIB (g)	Minerals Na (mg)	Ca (mg)	Mg (mg)	Zn (mg)	Mn (mg)	Vitamins A (mcg RAE)	C (mg)	B-1 (mg)	NIA (mg)	B-12 (mcg)	PANT (mg)
	WT (g)	FAT (g)	SFA (g)	MUFA (g)	PUFA (g)	CHOL (mg)	K (mg)	P (mg)	Fe (mg)	Cu (mg)	Se (mcg)	A (IU)	E (mg ATE)	B-2 (mg)	B-6 (mg)	FOL (DFE)	REF
flan/crème caramel from mix	137	100.7	4.0	25.0		0.0	150	150	16	0.48	0.004	69	1	0.04	0.1	0.35	0.38
w/2% milk - *1/2 cup*	133	2.3	1.4	0.6	0.1	9	217	114	0.08	0.013	7.0	239	0.1	0.20	0.05	5.3	19231
w/whole milk	150	99.3	3.9	24.8		0.0	149	148	16	0.47	0.007	39	1	0.04	0.1	0.35	0.38
1/2 cup	133	4.0	2.4	1.1	0.1	16	213	112	0.08	0.015	6.9	150	0.1	0.19	0.05	5.3	19232
flan/crème caramel, rte, refrig,	160		4.0	28.0	20.0	0.0	100	100					1					
Kozy Shack - *4 oz cup*	113	4.0	2.0			40			0.36			200						KOZY1
lemon, from inst mix	157	109.0	4.1	29.7		0.0	394	148	16	0.49	0.004	68	1	0.05	0.1	0.44	0.39
w/2% milk - *1/2 cup*	147	2.5	1.4	0.7	0.1	9	191	304	0.09	0.013	2.9	250	0.1	0.20	0.05	5.9	19204
w/whole milk	169	107.6	4.0	29.5		0.0	392	146	16	0.47	0.004	35	1	0.05	0.1	0.44	0.39
1/2 cup	147	4.3	2.6	1.2	0.2	16	187	301	0.09	0.016	2.6	154		0.20	0.05	5.9	19331
lemon, from reg mix w/sugar, egg	165	106.4	1.0	36.0		0.0	93	12	3	0.23	0.010	34	0	0.01	<0.1	0.15	0.23
yolk, & water - *1/2 cup*	146	1.9	0.6	0.7	0.3	76	7	31	0.26	0.020	3.1	115	0.2	0.04	0.02	5.8	19333
lemon, ready-to-eat	178	101.7	0.1	35.5		0.1	199	3	1	0.04	0.011	0	<1	0.00	<0.1	0.00	0.01
5 oz serving	142	4.3	0.6	1.8	1.6	0	1	7	0.10	0.021	2.6	0		0.01	0.00		19380
rennin dessert, choc, from mix	116	109.3	4.4	18.3		0.7	71	171	27	0.69	0.090	68	1	0.05	0.1	0.45	0.40
w/2% milk - *1/2 cup*	136	2.8	1.7	0.8	0.1	10	248	133	0.41	0.110	3.1	231	0.1	0.21	0.06	6.8	19213
w/whole milk	131	107.8	4.4	18.1		0.7	69	169	27	0.68	0.092	37	1	0.05	0.1	0.44	0.39
1/2 cup	136	4.5	2.7	1.3	0.2	16	243	132	0.41	0.113	2.9	150	0.1	0.21	0.06	6.8	19221
rennin dessert, van, from mix	102	109.2	4.1	16.4		0.0	61	161	17	0.48	0.004	68	1	0.05	0.1	0.44	0.39
w/2% milk - *1/2 cup*	133	2.4	1.4	0.6	0.1	9	189	126	0.07	0.016	2.8	226	1	0.20	0.05	6.7	19214
w/whole milk	118	107.7	4.0	16.2		0.0	61	158	17	0.47	0.005	36	1	0.05	0.1	0.44	0.39
1/2 cup	133	4.1	2.5	1.1	0.2	17	186	124	0.07	0.019	2.5	153	0.1	0.20	0.05	6.7	19223
rice, from reg mix	160	105.7	4.7	30.0		0.1	157	151	19	0.55	0.082	66	1	0.11	0.6	0.35	0.41
w/2% milk - *1/2 cup*	144	2.3	1.4	0.6	0.1	9	187	125	0.53	0.026	2.7	248	0.1	0.20	0.05	5.8	19208
w/whole milk	174	104.3	4.7	29.8		0.1	156	148	19	0.55	0.085	42	1	0.11	0.6	0.35	0.41
1/2 cup	144	4.1	2.4	1.1	0.1	16	184	122	0.53	0.029	2.6	166	0.1	0.20	0.05	5.8	19195
rice, ready-to-eat	231	96.4	2.8	31.2		0.1	121	74	11	0.70	0.179	36	1	0.03	0.2	0.30	0.33
5 oz serving	142	10.7	1.7	4.6	4.0	1	85	97	0.43	0.031	3.1	121	2.0	0.10	0.04	4.3	19193
tapioca, from reg mix	148	105.8	4.1	27.6		0.0	171	148	17	0.49	0.010	66	1	0.04	0.1	0.35	0.39
w/2% milk - *1/2 cup*	141	2.4	1.4	0.6	0.1	8	188	116	0.08	0.017	2.8	226	0.1	0.20	0.05	5.6	19209
w/whole milk	162	104.3	4.0	27.4		0.0	169	145	17	0.48	0.013	35	1	0.04	0.1	0.35	0.38
1/2 cup	141	4.1	2.4	1.1	0.2	17	185	114	0.08	0.018	2.7	152	0.1	0.20	0.05	5.6	19199
tapioca, ready-to-eat	169	105.4	2.8	27.5	25.1	0.1	226	119	11	0.38	0.013	0	1	0.03	0.4	0.31	0.28
5 oz serving	142	5.3	0.9	2.2	1.9	1	138	112	0.33	0.038	2.0	0	0.1	0.14	0.03	4.3	19218
van, from inst mix	141	106.2	4.1	25.9		0.0	223	151	17	0.48	0.006	67	1	0.04	0.1	0.35	0.39
w/2% milk - *1/2 cup*	140	2.4	1.4	0.6	0.1	10	192	116	0.08	0.018	2.9	224	0.1	0.20	0.05	5.6	19212
w/whole milk	162	104.4	3.8	28.0		0.0	406	143	17	0.47	0.010	36	1	0.05	0.1	0.43	0.37
1/2 cup	142	4.1	2.5	1.2	0.2	16	182	280	0.10	0.034	2.3	149	0.1	0.19	0.05	5.7	19203
van, from reg mix w/whole milk	155	104.4	4.1	25.9		0.0	224	150	18	0.49	0.006	36	1	0.04	0.1	0.35	0.39
1/2 cup	140	4.2	2.6	1.2	0.2	17	190	115	0.07	0.017	2.5	154	0.1	0.20	0.05	5.6	19207
van, ready-to-eat	147	80.5	2.6	24.7		0.1	153	99	9	0.28	0.009	7	0	0.02	0.3	0.11	0.20
4 oz serving	113	4.1	0.6	1.7	1.5	8	128	77	0.15	0.034	1.6	24	<1	0.16	0.01	0.0	19201
Jell-O	104	85.8	2.4	23.2	17.9	0.1	241	86					<1					
4 oz serving	113	0.2	0.2			2	123	115	0.05			174						19289

7.10 SAUCES, SYRUPS, & TOPPINGS FOR DESSERTS

	KCAL	H₂0 (g)	PRO (g)	CHO (g)	SUGR (g)	DFIB (g)	Na (mg)	Ca (mg)	Mg (mg)	Zn (mg)	Mn (mg)	A (mcg RAE)	C (mg)	B-1 (mg)	NIA (mg)	B-12 (mcg)	PANT (mg)
	WT (g)	FAT (g)	SFA (g)	MUFA (g)	PUFA (g)	CHOL (mg)	K (mg)	P (mg)	Fe (mg)	Cu (mg)	Se (mcg)	A (IU)	E (mg ATE)	B-2 (mg)	B-6 (mg)	FOL (DFE)	REF
glaze, homemade	97	4.8	0.2	19.8		0.0	25	6	1	0.02	0.002	23	<1	<0.01	<0.1	0.02	0.02
1/12 recipe yield	27	2.1	0.5	0.9	0.6	1	8	5	0.02	0.009	0.2	112	0.2	0.01	<0.01	0.3	19375
Holiday Baking Bits, candy-coated,	70		<1.0	11.0			0										
Hershey - *1 T (.53 oz)*	15	3.0	2.0			0											HRSH10
icing mix, fluffy white, Betty	100		<1.0	24.0	23.0	0.0	60	0					0				
Crocker - *3 T (6 T prep)*	26	0.0	0.0			0	30		0.00			0					GENM122
icing/frosting, rts, Betty Crocker	137		0.0	21.7	18.7	0.1	78	0					0				
Creamy Deluxe - *2 T (1.2 oz)*	33	5.3	1.7			0	37		0.22			0					GENM123
choc	163	7.0	0.5	25.9	23.7	0.4	75	3	9	0.12	0.098	0	0	0.01	<0.1	0.00	0.01
2 T	41	7.2	2.3	3.7	0.9	0	80	32	0.58	0.082	0.3	<1	1.0	0.01	<0.01	0.4	19226
coconut nut	157	8.0	0.6	20.1	15.2	0.5	74	5	7	0.16	0.320	0	<1	0.01	0.1	0.00	0.10
1/12 pkg	38	9.1	2.7	4.6	1.3	0	71	24	0.21	0.048	1.2	0	0.4	0.01	0.02	2.3	19227
cream cheese	137	5.0	0.0	22.2	21.0	0.0	63	1	1	0.01	0.004	0	0	0.00	<0.1	0.00	<0.01
1/12 tub	33	5.7	1.5	1.2	2.0	0	12	1	0.05	0.007	0.2	0	1.4	<0.01	0.00	0.0	19228
red fat, Sweet Rewards[1]	123		0.3	25.3	23.3	0.3	52	0					0				
2 T	33	2.0	0.7			0	53		0.36			0					GENM124

Food	KCAL / WT (g)	H$_2$O / FAT (g)	PRO / SFA (g)	CHO / MUFA (g)	SUGR / PUFA (g)	DFIB (g) / CHOL (mg)	Na / K (mg)	Ca / P (mg)	Mg / Fe (mg)	Zn / Cu (mg)	Mn (mg) / Se (mcg)	A (mcg RAE) / A (IU)	C (mg) / E (mg ATE)	B-1 / B-2 (mg)	NIA / B-6 (mg)	B-12 (mcg) / FOL (mcg DFE)	PANT (mg) / REF
soft whpd, Betty Crocker[2]	98		<0.2	14.9	13.5	0.2	37	0					0				
2 T	24	4.6	1.5			0	30		0.23			0					GENM125
van	159	5.0	0.0	26.4	24.2	0.0	67	1	<1	0.00	0.015	0	0	0.00	<0.1	0.0	0.00
2 T	38	6.4	1.9	3.3	0.9	0	14	15	0.04	0.003	0.2	0	1.8	<0.01	0.00	0.0	19230
icing/frosting, from mix	170	6.0	0.5	29.8		0.8	63	5	13	0.26	0.108	33	0	<0.01	<0.1	<0.01	0.01
choc made w/butter - 1/12 pkg prep	42	5.4	2.3	1.0	0.1	10	59	21	0.39	0.096	0.5	134	0.4	0.01	0.03	1.3	19241
choc made w/marg	170	5.9	0.5	29.8		0.8	68	5	13	0.26		34	0	<0.01	<0.1	<0.01	0.01
1/12 pkg prep	42	5.4	0.7	1.7	1.2	0	60	21	0.39	0.095	0.5	165	0.9	0.01	0.03	0.8	19372
van made w/marg	178	5.2	0.1	31.9		0.0	49	3	1	<0.01		34	0	<0.01	<0.1	<0.01	0.01
1/12 pkg prep	43	5.5	0.7	1.7	1.2	0	4	3	<0.01	0.012	0.3	169	0.8	<0.01	<0.01	0.0	19371
white fluffy made w/water	63	9.2	0.4	16.3		0.0	41	1	1	0.01	0.001	0	0	<0.01	0.2	<0.01	0.01
1/12 pkg prep	26	0.0	0.0			0	20	1	0.02	0.007	0.7	0	0.0	0.01	<0.01	0.5	19247
Oreo Crunchies (cookie crumb topping), Nabisco - .4 oz	52	0.2	0.5	7.7	4.0	0.4	58	3	5	0.14				0.01	0.2	<0.01	<0.01
	11	2.4	0.5	0.3	0.1		21	11	0.54	0.030		<1	<0.1	0.02	<0.01		18619
Sprinkles, milk choc, candy coated, Hershey - 1 T	70		<1.0	10.0			10										
	15	3.0	2.0			<5											HRSH47
peanut butter & milk choc, Hershey - 1 T	70		1.0	10.0			25										
	15	3.5	2.0			0											HRSH48
sundae syrup, caramel, Hershey	100		<1.0	25.0			95										
2 T	38	0.0	0.0			0											HRSH49
double choc, Hershey	50		0.0	13.0			15										
1 T	20	0.0	0.0			0											HRSH50
syrup, choc	109	12.1	0.8	25.4	19.4	1.0	28	5	25	0.28	0.149	0	<1	<0.01	0.1	0.00	<0.01
2 T (1 fl oz)	39	0.4	0.2	0.1	<0.1	0	87	50	0.82	0.200	0.5	12	<0.1	0.02	<0.01	1.6	14181
Hershey	100		1.0	24.0			25										
2 T	39	0.0	0.0			0											HRSH58
lite, Hershey	51	22.3	0.3	12.1	10.0	0.4	35	3	7	0.10	0.053	0	0	<0.01	<0.1	0.00	<0.01
2 T	35	0.2	0.0	0.0	0.0	0	35	10	0.22	0.056	0.2	0	<0.1	0.01	<0.01	0.4	19345
malt, Hershey	100		<1.0	25.0			55										
2 T	39	0.0	0.0			0											HRSH57
syrup, strawberry, Hershey	100		0.0	26.0			10										
2 T	40	0.0	0.0			0											HRSH59
topping, butterscotch/caramel	103	13.1	0.6	27.0		0.4	143	22	3	0.08	0.021	11	<1	<0.01	<0.1	0.04	0.06
2 T	41	<0.1	<0.1	<0.1	0.0	<1	34	19	0.08	0.010	0.0	37		0.04	0.01	0.8	19364
topping, choc fudge	133	8.3	1.7	23.9	15.9	1.1	131	31	19	0.26	0.128	2	<1	0.02	0.1	0.08	0.18
2 T	38	3.4	1.5	1.5	0.1	1	138	51	0.49	0.109	1.4	6	1.1	0.08	0.02	1.5	19348
Hershey	70		<1.0	10.0			25										
1 T	19	3.0	2.0			<5											HRSH65
topping, double choc, Hershey Choc Shoppe - 1 T	60		<1.0	12.0			30										
	18	1.0	0.5			0											HRSH66
topping, hot fudge, fat-free, Hershey Choc Shoppe - 2 T	100		1.0	23.0			135										
	39	0.0	0.0			0											HRSH67
Hershey Choc Shoppe	70		<1.0	10.0			80										
1 T	19	2.5	1.0			<5											HRSH68
topping, marshmallow cream	91	5.6	0.2	22.4	13.3	0.0	14	1	1	0.01	0.002	0	0	<0.01	<0.1	0.00	<0.01
1 oz	28	0.1	<0.1	<0.1	<0.1	0	1	2	0.06	0.027	0.5	<1	0.0	<0.01	<0.01	0.3	19365
topping, nuts in syrup	167	7.6	1.8	21.9		0.7	17	16	26	0.43	0.426	1	<1	0.07	0.2	0.00	0.09
2 T	41	9.0	0.8	2.0	5.6	0	86	46	0.43	0.195	0.6	17	0.4	0.05	0.08	8.6	19367
topping, pineapple	106	13.9	0.0	27.9		0.4	26	9	1	0.20	0.299	<1	25	0.01	<0.1	0.00	0.01
2 T	42	<0.1	<0.1	<0.1	<0.1	0	133	3	0.20	0.014	1.3	9	0.0	<0.01	0.01	1.3	19366
topping, strawberry	107	13.9	0.1	27.8		0.4	9	10	2	0.21	0.017	<1	10	<0.01	0.1	0.00	0.05
2 T	42	<0.1	<0.1	<0.1	<0.1	0	31	5	0.41	0.012	0.8	8	0.1	0.01	0.01	0.8	19137

[1] Values are averages for chocolate, milk chocolate, and vanilla.

[2] Values are averages for butter cream, chocolate, cream cheese, fluffy white, French vanilla, lemon, milk chocolate, strawberry, and vanilla.

	KCAL	H₂0 (g)	PRO (g)	CHO (g)	SUGR (g)	DFIB (g)	Na (mg)	Ca (mg)	Mg (mg)	Zn (mg)	Mn (mg)	A (mcg RAE)	C (mg)	B-1 (mg)	NIA (mg)	B-12 (mcg)	PANT (mg)
	WT (g)	FAT (g)	SFA (g)	MUFA (g)	PUFA (g)	CHOL (mg)	K (mg)	P (mg)	Fe (mg)	Cu (mg)	Se (mcg)	A (IU)	E (mg ATE)	B-2 (mg)	B-6 (mg)	FOL (mcg DFE)	REF

8. EGGS, EGG DISHES, & EGG SUBSTITUTES

Item	KCAL/WT	H₂0/FAT	PRO/SFA	CHO/MUFA	SUGR/PUFA	DFIB/CHOL	Na/K	Ca/P	Mg/Fe	Zn/Cu	Mn/Se	A-RAE/A-IU	C/E	B-1/B-2	NIA/B-6	B-12/FOL	PANT/REF
chicken egg, boiled, hard/soft	78	37.3	6.3	0.6		0.0	62	25	5	0.53	0.013	84	0	0.03	<0.1	0.56	0.70
1 large egg	50	5.3	1.6	2.0	0.7	212	63	86	0.60	0.007	15.4	280	0.5	0.26	0.06	22.0	01129
dried	31	0.1	2.4	0.1		0.0	27	11	2	0.29	0.008	31	0	0.02	<0.1	0.53	0.34
1 T	5	2.2	0.7	0.9	0.3	101	26	36	0.41	0.014	6.1	103		0.06	0.02	9.7	01134
fried	92	31.5	6.2	0.6		0.0	162	25	5	0.55	0.013	113	0	0.03	<0.1	0.42	0.56
1 large egg	46	6.9	1.9	2.7	1.3	211	61	89	0.72	0.007	12.4	394	0.8	0.24	0.07	17.5	01128
omelet, plain	93	46.3	6.3	0.6		0.0	165	26	5	0.56	0.013	113	0	0.03	<0.1	0.43	0.57
1 large egg	61	7.0	1.9	2.8	1.3	214	62	90	0.73	0.008	13.7	399	0.8	0.24	0.07	17.7	01130
poached	75	37.5	6.2	0.6		0.0	140	25	5	0.55	0.013	95	0	0.02	<0.1	0.40	0.56
1 large egg	50	5.0	1.5	1.9	0.7	212	60	89	0.72	0.007	15.4	316	0.5	0.22	0.06	17.5	01131
raw	75	37.7	6.2	0.6		0.0	63	25	5	0.55	0.012	96	0	0.03	<0.1	0.50	0.63
1 large egg	50	5.0	1.6	1.9	0.7	213	61	89	0.72	0.007	15.4	318	0.5	0.25	0.07	23.5	01123
raw, Eggland's Best	70	37.7	6.3	0.6			63	25	5	0.55	0.012			0.03	<0.1	0.50	0.63
1 large egg	50	4.0	1.2	1.9	0.7	180	60	89	0.72	0.007		317	5.0	0.25	0.07	23.0	EGLD1
scrambled w/milk	101	44.6	6.8	1.3		0.0	171	43	7	0.61	0.013	118	<1	0.03	<0.1	0.47	0.61
1 large egg	61	7.4	2.2	2.9	1.3	215	84	104	0.73	0.009	13.7	416	0.8	0.27	0.07	18.3	01132
soufflé, spinach, homemade[1] - *1 cup*	219	100.6	11.0	2.8			763	230	38	1.29	1.098	267	3	0.09	0.5	1.36	0.88
	136	18.4	7.1	6.8	3.1	184	201	231	1.35	0.120	12.9	2883		0.30	0.12	92.5	11658
chicken egg white, raw	17	29.0	3.5	0.3		0.0	54	2	4	<0.01	0.001	0	0	<0.01	<0.1	0.07	0.04
white of 1 large egg	33	0.0	0.0	0.0	0.0	0	47	4	0.01	0.002	5.8	0	0.0	0.15	<0.01	1.0	01124
chicken egg, yolk, raw	61	8.3	2.8	0.3		0.0	7	23	2	0.53	0.012	99	0	0.03	<0.1	0.53	0.65
yolk of 1 large egg	17	5.2	1.6	2.0	0.7	218	16	83	0.60	0.004	7.7	331	0.5	0.11	0.07	24.8	01125
duck egg, whole	130	49.6	9.0	1.0		0.0	102	45	12	0.99	0.027	279	0	0.11	0.1	3.78	1.30
1 egg	70	9.6	2.6	4.6	0.9	619	155	154	2.70	0.043	25.5	930	0.5	0.28	0.18	56.0	01138
egg substitutes, Better'n Eggs, Morningstar Farms - *2 oz*	26	50.4	5.4	0.3	0.3	0.0	98	24		0.60			0	0.04	0.0	0.38	0.80
	57	0.4	0.1	0.1	0.1	1	60	35	0.83			640		0.37	0.11		WRTH46
Better 'n Eggs, Papetti Foods	30		6.0	1.0	1.0	0.0	100	100		0.60			0	0.06		0.60	0.80
1/4 cup	56	0.0	0.0			0	55		0.72			300	1.2	0.34	0.08	32.0	PPTT1
Egg Beaters	30		6.0	1.0	0.0	0.0	115	20		0.60			0	0.06		0.60	0.80
1/4 cup	61	0.0	0.0			0			1.08			0	1.0	0.85	0.08	32.0	EGBT1
Egg Beaters Garden Vegetable	30		6.0	1.0	0.0	0.0	160	20		0.60			0	0.12		1.20	1.00
1/4 cup	61	0.0	0.0			0			1.08			750	1.2	0.68	0.08	40.0	EGBT2
Egg Beaters Southwestern	30		6.0	1.0	0.0	0.0	180	20		0.60			0	0.12		1.20	1.00
1/4 cup	61	0.0	0.0			0			1.08			750	1.0	0.68	0.08	40.0	EGBT3
frzn	96	43.9	6.8	1.9		0.0	119	44	9	0.59	0.004	41	<1	0.07	0.1	0.20	1.00
1/4 cup	60	6.7	1.2	1.5	3.7	1	128	43	1.19	0.013	24.8	810	1.3	0.23	0.08	9.6	01142
liquid	39	38.9	5.6	0.3		0.0	83	25	4	0.61	0.003	51	0	0.05	0.1	0.14	1.27
1.5 fl oz	47	1.6	0.3	0.4	0.8	<1	155	57	0.99	0.011	11.7	1015	0.2	0.14	<0.01	7.1	01143
powdered	44	0.4	5.5	2.2		0	79	32	6	0.18	0.008	37	<1	0.02	0.1	0.35	0.34
.35 oz	10	1.3	0.4	0.5	0.2	57	74	47	0.31	0.020	12.6	122	0.2	0.17	0.01	12.4	01144
Scramblers, Morningstar Farms - *2 oz*	39	47.1	6.6	2.3	1.4	0.0	122	19		0.71			0	0.17	0.0	1.77	1.85
	57	0.4				2	95	59	0.62			311		0.40	0.13		WRTH47
goose egg, whole	266	101.4	20.0	1.9		0.0	199	86	23	1.92	0.055	553	0	0.21	0.3	7.34	2.53
1 egg	144	19.1	5.2	8.3	2.4	1227	302	300	5.24	0.089	53.1	1843	1.1	0.55	0.34	109.4	01139
quail egg, whole	14	6.7	1.2	0.0		0.0	13	6	1	0.13	0.003	8	0	0.01	<0.1	0.14	0.16
1 egg	9	1.0	0.3	0.4	0.1	76	12	20	0.33	0.006	2.9	27	0.1	0.07	0.01	5.9	01140
turkey egg, whole	135	57.3	10.8	0.9		0.0	119	78	10	1.25	0.030	131	0	0.09	<0.1	1.34	1.49
1 egg	79	9.4	2.9	3.6	1.3	737	112	134	3.24	0.049	27.1	438		0.37	0.10	56.1	01141

[1] Contains whole milk, spinach, egg white, cheddar cheese, egg yolk, butter, flour, salt, and pepper.

	KCAL	H₂O (g)	PRO (g)	CHO (g)	SUGR (g)	DFIB (g)	Na (mg)	Ca (mg)	Mg (mg)	Zn (mg)	Mn (mg)	A (mcg RAE)	C (mg)	B-1 (mg)	NIA (mg)	B-12 (mcg)	PANT (mg)
	WT (g)	FAT (g)	SFA (g)	MUFA (g)	PUFA (g)	CHOL (mg)	K (mg)	P (mg)	Fe (mg)	Cu (mg)	Se (mcg)	A (IU)	E (mg ATE)	B-2 (mg)	B-6 (mg)	FOL (mcg DFE)	REF

9. ENTREES & MEALS
9.1 CANNED ENTREES

Food	KCAL/WT	H₂O/FAT	PRO/SFA	CHO/MUFA	SUGR/PUFA	DFIB/CHOL	Na/K	Ca/P	Mg/Fe	Zn/Cu	Mn/Se	A RAE/IU	C/E	B-1/B-2	NIA/B-6	B-12/FOL	PANT/REF
baked beans w/beef	322	189.7	17.0	45.0			1264	120	67	3.19	1.596	29	5	0.14	2.5	0.00	0.49
1 cup (9.4 oz)	266	9.2	4.5	3.7	0.5	59	851	215	4.26	0.798	25.5	567		0.12	0.24	114.4	16007
w/franks	368	179.6	17.5	39.9		17.9	1114	124	73	4.84	1.088	21	6	0.15	2.3	0.00	0.36
1 cup (9.1 oz)	259	17.0	6.1	7.3	2.2	16	609	269	4.48	0.552	16.8	399	1.2	0.15	0.12	77.7	16008
w/pork	268	180.8	13.1	50.5		13.9	1047	134	86	3.69	0.913	23	5	0.13	1.1	0.00	0.25
1 cup (8.9 oz)	253	3.9	1.5	1.7	0.5	18	782	273	4.30	0.544	11.9	450		0.10	0.16	91.1	16009
beef ravioli in tomato & meat sce,	229	188.2	8.4	36.9	5.2	3.7	1174	20					<1				
Chef Boyardee - *8.6 oz serving*	244	5.4	2.5	2.0	0.2	15	354		2.42			642					22515
mini in tomato & meat sce, Chef	239	194.2	8.8	40.6	4.8	3.3	1197	23					<1				
Boyardee - *8.9 oz serving*	252	4.7	1.8	2.0	0.2	18			2.42			610					22517
beef stew	218	189.1	11.5	15.7	2.2	3.5	947	28	32	1.90	0.332	193	10	0.17	2.9	0.86	0.50
8.2 oz serving	232	12.5	5.2	5.5	0.5	37	404	128	1.65	0.183	1.6	3860	0.2	0.14	0.30	25.5	22905
Castleberry	331	185.7	15.2	20.3		2.2	1002										
8.6 oz serving	245	21.1	7.9	9.6	0.6	56						938					22693
Dinty Moore	222	192.5	11.3	16.1	2.3	2.6	984	19	24	2.60			3				
1 cup (8.3 oz)	236	13.1	5.6	6.3	0.7	38	396		1.65	0.000		3988					22694
Beefaroni (mac, beef, tom sce),	184	167.0	8.2	31.1	4.8	3.0	799	17					<1				
Chef Boyardee - *7.5 oz serving*	212	2.9	1.2	1.3	0.3	17			1.51			259					22516
chicken & dumplings, Sweet Sue	218	191.8	15.1	22.8		2.6	946										
8.5 oz serving	240	7.4	1.8	3.0	1.6	36			2.57			0					22703
chili con carne (no beans)	255	164.8	20.2	24.5	4.4	8.2	1032	67	56	2.42	0.559	44	1	0.15	2.1	0.58	0.46
7.8 oz serving	222	8.1	2.1	2.2	1.4	24	608	193	3.31	0.244	5.3	884	0.3	0.15	0.19	57.7	22904
Chef-Mate	430	176.4	18.6	17.6	0.2	3.0	1588	68	45	4.50	0.408		2	0.14	4.8	1.83	0.78
1 cup (8.8 oz)	250	31.6	14.4	13.6	1.8	85	530	163	4.45	0.360		2900	1.6	0.27	0.34		22216
El Rio	305	205.9	15.1	16.2		3.7	812										
9.2 oz serving	261	20.1	7.5	8.8	0.8	50			4.41			478					22704
Hormel	194	191.6	17.0	17.9	3.4	3.1	970	50	38	2.60			0				
1 cup (8.3 oz)	236	6.6	2.2	2.2	0.8	35	349		2.60	0.236		2384					22705
chili con carne w/beans	287	193.3	14.6	30.5		11.3	1336	120	115	5.12	0.343	44	4	0.12	0.9	0.00	3.64
1 cup (9 oz)	256	14.1	6.0	6.0	0.9	44	934	394	8.78	0.300	3.3	863	1.9	0.27	0.34	58.9	16059
Chef-Mate	412	175.8	17.7	29.0	0.2	11.1	1171	89	46	3.87	0.407		1	0.11	3.5	1.44	0.66
1 cup (8.9 oz)	253	25.0	10.9	10.7	1.4	56	511	167	4.83	0.329		3013	1.2	0.20	0.23		22215
Hormel	240	187.8	16.6	33.7	4.6	8.4	1163	69	59	2.72			<1				
1 cup (8.7 oz)	247	4.4	1.8	1.7	0.9	25	662		3.21	0.247		968					22719
Nalley	281	192.5	40.2	11.9		12.9	1231										
9.1 oz serving	258	8.0	2.8	3.0	0.8	26			4.59			0					22513
Old El Paso	249	175.3	17.6	21.7		9.8	588										
8 oz serving	228	10.3	2.1	4.3	2.2	36			2.69			(0)					22514
Stagg Classic	324	180.5	17.2	29.2	7.1	7.4	825	91	64	2.72			2				
1 cup (8.7 oz)	247	16.3	6.7	6.9	1.1	42	785		3.95	0.247		1161					22716
Stagg Country	319	182.2	15.5	29.0	5.9	5.9	1131	57	52	2.47			2				
1 cup (8.7 oz)	247	15.8	6.8	7.5	0.7	40	558		3.46	0.247		514					22717
Stagg Dynamite	333	178.1	18.3	30.7	6.6	8.2	862	104	69	2.72			3				
1 cup (8.7 oz)	247	15.4	5.7	6.8	0.9	44	778		4.45	0.247		1252					22714
Stagg Ranchhouse	284	183.0	19.2	31.6	5.7	8.6	813	114	82	1.98			5				
1 cup (8.7 oz)	247	8.9	2.6	4.1	2.0	47	867		4.20	0.494		1082					22715
Stagg Silverado	227	189.1	18.0	33.1	7.2	8.2	865	89	72	2.72			5				
1 cup (8.7 oz)	247	2.8	1.0	0.9	0.9	40	815		3.71	0.494		1247					22718
Chili Magic, Louisiana, cnd,	220		8.0	42.0	6.0	10.0	2140	80					0				
Bush's[1] - *1 cup (7.8 oz)*	260	3.0	0.0			0			3.60			2500					BUSH14
Texas, cnd, Bush's[1]	240		10.0	40.0	6.0	10.0	2260	120					0				
1 cup (7.8 oz)	260	4.0	0.0			0			3.60			1500					BUSH15
Traditional, cnd, Bush's[1]	220		10.0	38.0	4.0	10.0	1780	80					0				
1 cup (7.8 oz)	260	2.0	0.0			0			2.88			2500					BUSH16

	KCAL	H₂0 (g)	PRO (g)	CHO (g)	SUGR (g)	DFIB (g)	Minerals Na (mg)	Ca (mg)	Mg (mg)	Zn (mg)	Mn (mg)	Vitamins A (mcg RAE)	C (mg)	B-1 (mg)	NIA (mg)	B-12 (mcg)	PANT (mg)
	WT (g)	FAT (g)	SFA (g)	MUFA (g)	PUFA (g)	CHOL (mg)	K (mg)	P (mg)	Fe (mg)	Cu (mg)	Se (mcg)	A (IU)	E (mg ATE)	B-2 (mg)	B-6 (mg)	FOL (mcg DFE)	REF
corned beef hash, Armour	498	157.6	23.8	12.0		1.9	854										
1 cup (8.3 oz)	236	39.4	15.6	17.4	0.8	97			2.19			0					22692
Chef-Mate	486	163.9	24.2	29.1	2.2	6.1	1594	46	38	7.51	0.111		2	0.22	6.3	2.45	1.23
1 cup (8.9 oz)	253	30.3	13.4	14.7	1.1	89	536	240	2.99	0.339		0	0.3	0.30	0.58		22217
Hormel	387	166.0	20.6	21.9	0.8	2.6	1003	45	31	3.30			2				
1 cup (8.3 oz)	236	24.2	10.2	12.4	0.7	76	406		2.36	0.000		0					22698
cowpeas w/pork	199	186.2	6.6	39.7		7.9	840	41	103	2.50	0.941	0	<1	0.15	1.0	0.00	0.46
1 cup (8.5 oz)	240	3.8	1.5	1.6	0.5	17	427	230	3.41	0.408	5.5	0		0.12	0.11	122.4	16065
macaroni & cheese	199	206.4	7.6	29.0	1.8	3.0	1058	113				53	0	0.28	2.5		
8.9 oz serving	252	5.8	3.0		1.3	8	123		2.02			209		0.25			22247
pasta w/franks in tom sce	262	197.1	9.3	30.0		2.3	1215										
1 cup (8.9 oz)	252	11.6	3.7	4.8	1.5	23			2.29			295					22522
pasta w/meatballs in tom sce	260	196.2	10.9	31.0		6.8	1053	28	35	1.84	0.393	48	8	0.19	3.3	0.58	0.52
1 cup (8.9 oz)	252	10.3	4.0	4.2	0.6	20	416	116	2.34	0.214	19.2	920	1.3	0.16	0.17	93.2	22907
Chef Ninja Turtles	227	160.9	8.2	33.6	7.2	2.8	840	21					<1				
7.5 oz serving	212	6.8	3.0	2.8	0.3	21			0.93			278					22520
roast beef hash, Hormel	385	165.5	21.3	22.9	0.6	3.5	793	42	33	3.30			2				
1 cup (8.3 oz)	236	23.6	9.9	11.3	0.6	73	432		2.36	0.236		0					22721
spag & meatballs in tom sce, Chef Boyardee - 8.5 oz	250	185.0	9.1	34.1	6.6	2.2	941	17					1				
	240	8.6	3.9	3.7	0.4	22			1.78			343					22518
spanish rice, Old El Paso	140		3.0	30.0	3.0	1.0	860	0					0				
1 cup (8.7 oz)	246	1.0	0.0			0			0.72			0					GENM126
sweet & sour veg w/chicken, Chun King - 8.9 oz serving	165	214.6	5.8	31.8			564						30				
	254	1.8				23						0					22674
turkey chili w/beans, Hormel	203	194.8	18.7	25.6	5.7	6.4	1198	116	69	2.72			1				
1 cup (8.7 oz)	247	2.8	0.7	0.4	1.2	35	682		3.46	0.247		1650					22706
vegetarian chili w/beans, Hormel - 1 cup (8.7 oz)	205	192.5	11.9	38.0	6.2	9.9	778	96	82	1.73			1				
	247	0.7	0.1	0.1	0.4	0	803		3.46	0.494		1941					22720

[1] Prepared according to recipe with extra lean ground beef.

9.2 FROZEN BREAKFASTS

	KCAL	H₂0 (g)	PRO (g)	CHO (g)	SUGR (g)	DFIB (g)	Na (mg)	Ca (mg)	Mg (mg)	Zn (mg)	Mn (mg)	A (mcg RAE)	C (mg)	B-1 (mg)	NIA (mg)	B-12 (mcg)	PANT (mg)
	WT (g)	FAT (g)	SFA (g)	MUFA (g)	PUFA (g)	CHOL (mg)	K (mg)	P (mg)	Fe (mg)	Cu (mg)	Se (mcg)	A (IU)	E (mg ATE)	B-2 (mg)	B-6 (mg)	FOL (mcg DFE)	REF
bagel french toast w/maple syrup, Sunny Fresh - 2.5 oz *serving*	190	29.2	14.0	21.0	5.7	0.0	283	40	4	0.35	0.006		0	0.03	0.1	0.36	0.39
	71	5.3	1.3	1.7	1.3	129	68	89	0.68	0.018		183	0.2	0.15	0.04		22362
biscuit, egg & cheese, Sunny Fresh *3.5 oz serving*	224	53.0	9.9	24.6	1.8	0.0	563	101	3	0.30	0.007		0	0.24	2.0	0.27	0.33
	99	8.9	2.4	1.1	3.7	111	40	50	2.25	0.006		205	2.0	0.30	0.04		22360
egg, ham, & cheese, Sunny Fresh - 4.2 oz *serving*	242	69.6	12.2	25.1	2.1	0.1	722	106	4	0.32	0.007		<1	0.24	2.0	0.29	0.35
	120	9.7	2.6	1.2	3.8	114	47	54	2.44	0.007		212	2.4	0.31	0.04		22361
sausage, Jimmy Dean *2 biscuits (3.4 oz)*	385	32.2	9.5	23.1		1.4	881	76									
	96	28.2	8.6			32			1.58								22364
breakfast burrito, ham & cheese *3.5 oz breakfast entrée*	212	53.3	9.6	27.8		1.4	405										
	99	6.9	2.0	2.1	1.8	192			3.17			0					22679
egg & cheese pckts, Brkfst Stuff-Its, Sunny Fresh - 2.3 oz pckt	147	34.4	6.8	14.7	1.1	1.0	233	63	3	0.23	0.005		0	0.12	1.5	0.21	0.26
	64	7.6	3.1	0.9	0.6	93	31	38	0.94	0.005		220	0.1	0.20	0.03		22363
french toast, cinn swirl w/sausage *5.5 oz breakfast entrée*	415	79.2	13.1	38.2		2.3	502										
	156	23.2	7.3	9.4	3.4	98			2.54			0					22592
scrmbld eggs, sausage, hashed brn potatoes - 6.2 oz brkfst entrée	361	117.4	12.6	17.2		1.4	772										
	177	26.9	7.3	12.7	3.6	283			1.66			0					22595
Toaster Scrambles Pastries, bacon & sausage, Gen Mills - 1.66 oz entrée	180		4.0	14.0	1.0	0.0	370	0					0				
	47	12.0	3.0			25			0.72			0					GENM127
cheese, egg, & bacon, Gen Mills *1.66 oz entrée*	180		4.0	14.0	1.0	0.0	380	0					0				
	47	12.0	3.5			25			0.72			0					GENM128
cheese, egg, & ham, Gen Mills *1.66 oz entrée*	180		4.0	14.0	1.0	0.0	370	0					0				
	47	12.0	3.5			25			0.72			0					GENM129
cheese, egg, & sausage, Gen Mills *1.66 oz entrée*	180		4.0	14.0	1.0	0.0	370	0					0				
	47	12.0	3.5			25			0.72			0					GENM130
western style, Gen Mills *1.66 oz entrée*	170		4.0	14.0	1.0	0.0	340	0					1				
	47	11.0	2.5			25			0.72			0					GENM131

	KCAL	H₂O (g)	PRO (g)	CHO (g)	SUGR (g)	DFIB (g)	Na (mg)	Ca (mg)	Mg (mg)	Zn (mg)	Mn (mg)	A (mcg RAE)	C (mg)	B-1 (mg)	NIA (mg)	B-12 (mcg)	PANT (mg)
	WT (g)	FAT (g)	SFA (g)	MUFA (g)	PUFA (g)	CHOL (mg)	K (mg)	P (mg)	Fe (mg)	Cu (mg)	Se (mcg)	A (IU)	E (mg ATE)	B-2 (mg)	B-6 (mg)	FOL (mcg DFE)	REF

9.3 FROZEN ENTREES & SANDWICHES

beef, chipped & creamed,	175	93.6	9.9	7.1			621	190									
Stouffer's - 4.4 oz serving	125	11.9	5.0	3.5	1.2	44			0.91				0				22579
Hot Sandwich Toppers	120		7.0	8.0	4.0	0.0	700	60									
4 oz pkg	113	6.0	2.5			25			0.36				0				CNAG133
beef macaroni, Healthy Choice	211	187.7	14.1	33.5	9.1	4.6	444	46	36	1.22	0.547		58	0.28	3.1	0.12	0.41
8.5 oz entrée	240	2.2	0.7	1.2	0.3	14	365	134	2.71	0.307	24.2	514	1.5	0.16	0.19	158.4	22402
beef patty, chrbrld w/mshrm grvy,	250		11.0	6.0	2.0	2.0	750	20									
Banquet - 1 patty w/gravy (5 oz)	142	20.0	9.0			35			1.08				0				CNAG72
beef pepper steak oriental, Healthy	260		19.0	34.0	5.0	2.0	520	20					9				
Choice - 9.5 oz entrée	269	5.0	2.5			35			1.08				200				CNAG73
beef portabello w/mshrms, grvy,	250		14.0	37.0	18.0	4.0	610	100					0				
whpd pot, Stfrs Ln Csn - 9 oz entrée	255	5.0	1.5	2.0	1.0	25	540		0.72				4500				STOF1
beef pot roast w/whpd potatoes,	207	206.8	17.3	22.4		3.6	495										
Sfrs Ln Csn - 9 oz entrée	255	5.4	1.3	2.3	0.8	38							977				22578
beef, sliced w/brwn grvy, Banquet	140		13.0	5.0	2.0	<1.0	850	0					0				
2 slices w/gravy (5.6 oz)	159	8.0	3.5			40			1.44				0				CNAG77
beef steak, fried, grvy, mshd pot,	640		18.0	47.0	7.0	4.0	1960	80					0				
Marie Callender's - 1/4 pkg (12 oz)	340	42.0	14.0			75			1.80				0				CNAG74
beef stew, hearty, Banquet	170		10.0	18.0	4.0	4.0	1120	20					4				
1 cup (8.7 oz)	246	7.0	3.0			30			1.44				500				CNAG75
beef stir-fry kit w/rice & veg,	433	297.9	25.8	70.8			1584						25				
Tyson - 14.3 oz srvng (1/2 pkg yield)	405	5.0											2762				22686
beef tips francais, Healthy Choice	300		20.0	40.0	6.0	4.0	520	20					0				
9.5 oz entrée	269	7.0	2.5			40			1.80				0				CNAG76
beef tips w/bbq sce & rstd pot,	260		20.0	32.0	7.0	4.0	690	100					6				
Stfrs Ln Csn - 8.75 oz entrée	248	6.0	1.0	2.0	2.5	30	570		1.80				500				STOF2
Bread Stuffs, chicken broccoli,	310		17.0	50.0	11.0	2.0	600	100					6				
Healthy Choice - 6.1 oz entrée	173	4.0	1.5			25			2.70				0				CNAG78
ham, cheese, broccoli, Healthy	320		21.0	48.0	10.0	1.0	590	250					9				
Choice - 6.1 oz entrée	173	5.0	1.5			20			2.70				0				CNAG79
italian style meatball, Healthy	330		18.0	52.0	12.0	4.0	600	200					0				
Choice - 6.1 oz entrée	173	5.0	1.5			20			3.60				0				CNAG80
philly beef steak, Healthy Choice	310		17.0	50.0	10.0	3.0	600	200					0				
6.1 oz entrée	173	5.0	1.5			20			2.70				0				CNAG81
burrito, bean & cheese, Patio	300		9.0	46.0	4.0	4.0	690	40					0				
5 oz burrito	142	9.0	4.5			15			0.72				200				CNAG82
burrito, beef & bean, hot, Patio	320		10.0	43.0	4.0	4.0	840	20					1				
5 oz burrito	142	12.0	4.5			25			1.08				200				CNAG83
Las Campanas	296	52.9	8.7	38.2		0.8	579										
4 oz serving	114	12.1	4.2	5.5	0.8	13			3.11				0				22613
medium, Patio	310		10.0	45.0	5.0	4.0	860	0					1				
5 oz burrito	142	10.0	5.0			20			0.00				300				CNAG84
mild, Patio	330		10.0	45.0	3.0	4.0	890	20					1				
5 oz burrito	142	12.0	4.0			20			0.72				0				CNAG85
red hot chili peppers, Patio	320		10.0	42.0	4.0	4.0	850	20					0				
5 oz burrito	142	12.0	4.5			20			1.08				400				CNAG86
w/green chili, mild, Patio	325	70.6	9.9	44.4	2.9	3.9	879	29					0				
4.9 oz entrée	140	11.9	4.0	4.6	3.4	20			0.99				0				22584
burrito, chicken breast con queso,	350		14.0	60.0	11.0	6.0	590	100					6				
Healthy Choice - 10.5 oz entrée	299	6.0	2.5			35			1.80				1500				CNAG87
burrito, chicken, Patio	290		11.0	44.0	6.0	2.0	740	60					0				
5 oz burrito	142	8.0	3.0			20			0.72				0				CNAG88
burrito, shrd beef, grn chili, jack	324	72.1	14.9	39.9			768	125					0				
chs, Marquez Primera - 5 oz entrée	142	11.6	3.8	3.4	2.7	27			2.85				0				22676
cabbage, stuffed, whpd potatoes,	199	223.5	11.6	25.8		6.5	412	105					53				
Stfs Ln Csn - 9.5 oz entrée	269	5.6	1.7	2.4	0.7	24							0				22585
cheese & chicken tortellini,	250		11.0	40.0	5.0	6.0	600	100					36				
Healthy Choice Bowl - 8.7 oz bowl	247	5.0	2.0			30			1.80				1500				CNAG123

	KCAL	H₂0 (g)	PRO (g)	CHO (g)	SUGR (g)	DFIB (g)	Na (mg)	Ca (mg)	Mg (mg)	Zn (mg)	Mn (mg)	A (mcg RAE)	C (mg)	B-1 (mg)	NIA (mg)	B-12 (mcg)	PANT (mg)
	WT (g)	FAT (g)	SFA (g)	MUFA (g)	PUFA (g)	CHOL (mg)	K (mg)	P (mg)	Fe (mg)	Cu (mg)	Se (mcg)	A (IU)	E (mg ATE)	B-2 (mg)	B-6 (mg)	FOL (mcg DFE)	REF
cheesy rice & broccoli, Green Giant	300		8.0	56.0	7.0	2.0	970	100					21				
10 oz pkg	283	5.0	1.5			5			3.60			4000					GENM132
chicken alfredo w/fettucini & veg,	373	199.1	19.0	32.6		3.8	588	147					24				
Stfrs Lch Exprs - *9.6 oz entrée*	272	18.5	7.0	6.3	2.4	57						2426					22610
chicken & broccoli alfredo, Banquet	270		11.0	28.0	3.0	3.0	540	100					6				
1 cup (6.8 oz)	194	12.0	7.0			40			0.72			0					CNAG89
chicken & pasta, homestyle, Healthy	270		21.0	32.0	6.0	5.0	570	60					4				
Choice - *9 oz entrée*	255	6.0	2.5			35			1.44			1500					CNAG90
southwestern, Healthy Choice Bowl	320		31.0	39.0	2.0	6.0	350	40					24				
9.5 oz bowl	269	4.0	2.0			40			1.80			400					CNAG131
chicken & veg marsala, Healthy	240		20.0	32.0	4.0	3.0	440	40					4				
Choice - *11.5 oz entrée*	326	4.0	2.0			30			0.72			500					CNAG91
chicken & veg w/vermicelli,	252	237.9	18.7	32.1		5.0	582	104					15				
Stfrs Ln Csn - *10.5 oz entrée*	297	5.6	1.0	2.1	1.4	24			1.34			199					22577
chicken aussie pie, Mrs Paterson's	434	75.0	14.7	39.8			799										
5.5 oz pie	156	24.0	7.2	8.3	4.3	48			3.01			363					22539
chicken bake, country, Healthy	230		18.0	22.0	9.0	4.0	600	100					2				
Choice Bowl - *9.5 oz bowl*	269	8.0	2.5			50			1.08			1000					CNAG127
chicken, bbq glazed, sce, & veg,	217	159.9	18.8	25.9			405						22				
Weight Watchers - *7.4 oz entrée*	209	4.4	1.0	1.6	1.1	48			1.09			0					22618
chicken breast, country glazed,	230		17.0	29.0	4.0	3.0	600	0					1				
Healthy Choice - *8.5 oz entrée*	241	5.0	2.0			40			0.36			0					CNAG93
chicken breast strips w/mac & chs,	270		22.0	34.0	9.0	1.0	600	150					1				
Healthy Choice - *8 oz entrée*	227	5.0	2.5			40			0.72			0					CNAG92
chicken cordon bleu, Barber	344	104.3	25.5	14.6			754	144									
5.9 oz serving (1/2 pkg)	168	20.5	5.7	8.2	3.2	81						215					22575
chicken, country style & dmplngs,	290		12.0	30.0	6.0	2.0	1270	40					0				
Banquet - *1 cup (7 oz)*	198	14.0	5.0			40			1.44			0					CNAG98
chicken, escalloped & noodles,	419	205.7	17.0	31.4			1211	116					0				
Stouffer's - *10 oz entrée*	283	25.2	6.6		13.6	76			1.13			0					22614
chicken fajita kit, Tyson	129	76.9	8.0	17.4			350						10				
3.8 oz serving (1/7 pkg yield)	107	3.3	0.8	1.3	0.6	13						55					22687
chicken fettuccine alfredo, Healthy	280		25.0	28.0	3.0	3.0	570	100					0				
Choice - *8.5 oz entrée*	241	7.0	2.5			55			1.08			0					CNAG94
chicken, fiesta, Healthy Choice Bowl	220		15.0	34.0	6.0	3.0	550	40					0				
9.5 oz bowl	269	2.0	1.0			30			2.70			100					CNAG128
chicken, fried, gravy, mshd pot,	550		20.0	48.0	12.0	3.0	2160	80					0				
Marie Callender's - *1/4 pkg (12 oz)*	340	30.0	9.0			70			0.36			0					CNAG99
chicken, garlic lemon w/rice,	300		18.0	48.0	6.0	4.0	400	20					15				
Healthy Choice Bowl - *9.5 oz bowl*	269	4.0	1.5			40			1.08			2000					CNAG129
chicken, grilled w/mshd potatoes,	180		16.0	18.0	3.0	3.0	600	0					1				
Healthy Choice - *8 oz entrée*	227	4.0	2.0			45			0.72			200					CNAG100
chicken, honey mustard, Healthy	290		21.0	38.0	7.0	1.0	520	0					0				
Choice - *9.5 oz entrée*	269	6.0	2.5			40			0.36			1000					CNAG101
chicken in peanut sce w/linguini &	270		16.0	37.0	10.0	4.0	690	40					4				
veg, Stfrs Ln Csn - *9 oz entree*	255	6.0	2.5	2.0	0.5	35	1080		1.80			200					STOF3
chicken, mandarin, Healthy Choice	280		20.0	43.0	9.0	4.0	520	20					9				
10 oz entrée	284	3.5	0.5			35	436	199	0.72			750					CNAG102
chicken milano w/garlic, Healthy	260		18.0	34.0	4.0	3.0	510	100					18				
Choice - *9.5 oz entrée*	269	6.0	2.5			35			1.08			500					CNAG95
chicken piccata, lemon herb w/rice	250		15.0	36.0	3.0	2.0	510	40					5				
& veg, Smart Ones - *9 oz entrée*	255	5.0	1.5	3.0	0.5	45			1.08			500					SMRT1
chicken pie, colonial, Healthy	310		22.0	40.0	15.0	5.0	570	100					4				
Choice Bowl - *9.5 oz bowl*	269	7.0	2.5			45			1.44			1500					CNAG126
chicken pie, hearty, Banquet	460		11.0	39.0	14.0	2.0	1010	40					0				
1 cup (8 oz)	227	29.0	11.0			35			1.44			750					CNAG96
chicken, sesame, Healthy Choice	260		13.0	35.0	9.0	4.0	600	20					21				
9.7 oz entrée	255	6.0	2.0			30			0.36			1500					CNAG103
chicken sonoma, grilled, Healthy	230		18.0	30.0	9.0	3.0	530	20					12				
Choice - *9 oz entrée*	255	4.0	1.0			45			1.80			2500					CNAG97
chicken tndrlns w/mshrm grvy,	380		26.0	31.0	7.0	2.0	1010	250					12				
broc rice, Stfrs Hmstl - *10 oz entrée*	283	17.0	6.0			55			1.44			500					STOF20

						Minerals					Vitamins					
KCAL	H₂0 (g)	PRO (g)	CHO (g)	SUGR (g)	DFIB (g)	Na (mg)	Ca (mg)	Mg (mg)	Zn (mg)	Mn (mg)	A (mcg RAE)	C (mg)	B-1 (mg)	NIA (mg)	B-12 (mcg)	PANT (mg)
WT (g)	FAT (g)	SFA (g)	MUFA (g)	PUFA (g)	CHOL (mg)	K (mg)	P (mg)	Fe (mg)	Cu (mg)	Se (mcg)	A (IU)	E (mg ATE)	B-2 (mg)	B-6 (mg)	FOL (mcg DFE)	REF
chicken teriyaki w/rice, Healthy	330		19.0	45.0	10.0	5.0	600	20					15				
Choice Bowl - *9.5 oz bowl*	298	6.0	2.0			40	428	223	0.72			500					CNAG124
chicken, teriyaki w/veg, Budget	317	233.9	18.7	52.2		4.0	675						44				
Grmt Lght & Hlthy - *11 oz entrée*	311	3.7	0.6	0.9	1.6	25						880					22683
chicken w/garlic sce, pasta, & veg,	214	207.5	16.9	21.5		3.6	467										
Tyson - *9 oz entrée*	255	6.7	1.3	2.3	2.1	28			1.56								22712
chili & cornbread, Healthy Choice	350		21.0	49.0	18.0	8.0	600	100					4				
Bowl - *9.5 oz bowl*	269	8.0	2.5			35			3.60			750					CNAG125
chimichanga, beef & bean, Fiesta	422	132.3	24.1	55.6		6.1	804						6				
Café - *8 oz entrée*	227	11.6	2.2	3.9	3.5	36			6.81			0					22682
creamy broc, chicken, cheese, &	280		14.0	25.0	6.0	2.0	980	150					0				
rice, Banquet - *1 cup (8 oz)*	227	14.0	7.0			45			0.36			0					CNAG104
egg rolls, chicken, mini, Chun King	210		6.0	25.0	3.0	2.0	650	20					0				
6 mini rolls (2.9 oz)	82	9.0	2.5			15			1.08			100					CNAG105
mini, LaChoy	210		6.0	25.0	3.0	2.0	650	20					0				
6 mini rolls (2.9 oz)	82	9.0	2.5			15			1.08			100					CNAG106
restaurant style, LaChoy	210		6.0	25.0	4.0	2.0	550	20					1				
3 oz egg roll	85	9.0	4.5			15			1.08			500					CNAG107
restaurant-style, Chun King	190		6.0	22.0	4.0	2.0	550	20					1				
3 oz egg roll	85	9.0	5.0			20			1.08			500					CNAG108
egg rolls, pork & shrimp, bite	210		6.0	25.0	3.0	2.0	540	20					0				
size, LaChoy - *12 rolls (3 oz)*	85	10.0	2.5			10			0.72			100					CNAG109
mini, Chun King	210		6.0	27.0	4.0	2.0	540	20					0				
6 mini rolls (2.9 oz)	82	9.0	2.5			15			1.08			100					CNAG110
mini, LaChoy	210		6.0	27.0	4.0	2.0	540	20					0				
6 mini rolls (2.9 oz)	82	9.0	2.5			15			1.08			100					CNAG111
egg rolls, pork, restaurant style,	220		5.0	24.0	6.0	2.0	390	20					0				
LaChoy - *3 oz egg roll*	85	11.0	2.5			10			1.08			300					CNAG112
egg rolls, shrimp, mini, Chun King	190		5.0	28.0	3.0	2.0	730	20					0				
6 mini rolls (3 oz)	82	6.0	1.5			10			1.08			500					CNAG113
mini, LaChoy	190		5.0	28.0	3.0	2.0	730	20					0				
6 mini rolls (2.9 oz)	82	6.0	1.5			10			1.08			500					CNAG114
restaurant style, LaChoy	180		5.0	25.0	6.0	2.0	490	40					0				
3 oz egg roll	85	7.0	1.5			15			1.08			100					CNAG115
restaurant-style, Chun King	180		5.0	24.0	6.0	2.0	490	40					0				
3 oz egg roll	85	7.0	3.0			15			1.08			100					CNAG116
egg rolls, swt & sr chicken, rstrnt	220		6.0	29.0	10.0	2.0	550	20					2				
style, LaChoy - *3 oz egg roll*	85	9.0	2.0			15			1.08			100					CNAG117
egg rolls, veg w/lobster, mini,	190		5.0	27.0	3.0	2.0	440	0					1				
LaChoy - *6 mini rolls (2.9 oz)*	82	7.0	1.5			5			0.72			0					CNAG118
enchiladas, beef w/sce, Patio	210		5.0	29.0	1.0	5.0	940	100					0				
2 enchiladas (5.7 oz)	161	8.0	3.0			20			1.08			300					CNAG119
enchiladas, cheese w/sce, Patio	210		6.0	30.0	4.0	2.0	880	100					0				
2 enchiladas (5.7 oz)	161	7.0	3.5			20			0.72			400					CNAG120
enchilada(s), chicken & rice w/jack	376	203.5	12.5	48.4		4.5	1002	255					15				
chs sce, Stouffer's - *10 oz entrée*	283	14.7	3.4	4.4	3.7	25						756					22615
suiza, Healthy Choice	280		14.0	43.0	4.0	5.0	440	150					2				
10 oz entrée	284	6.0	3.0			40			1.08			300					CNAG121
suiza w/sour crm sce & chs,	283	193.5	16.1	33.2		3.6	518	250									
Weight Watchers - *9 oz entrée*	255	9.7	3.7	3.0	1.3	64						0					22671
suiza w/sour crm sce & rice,	298	184.1	11.5	52.0		4.3	538	184									
Stfrs Ln Csn - *9 oz entrée*	255	4.8	1.5	1.5	1.1	20						0					22611
fettucine alfredo, Healthy Choice	240		10.0	36.0	3.0	4.0	600	100					0				
8 oz entrée	227	6.0	2.0			15			0.72			0					CNAG122
gravy & salisbury steak, Hot	210		9.0	8.0	5.0	2.0	790	20					1				
Sandwich Toppers - *5 oz pkg*	142	16.0	7.0			25			1.08			0					CNAG134
gravy & sliced beef, Hot Sandwich	70		8.0	5.0	1.0	0	440	0					0				
Toppers - *4 oz pkg*	113	2.0	1.0			25			1.08			0					CNAG135
gravy & sliced turkey, Hot Sandwich	160		8.0	6.0	1.0	0.0	670	20					0				
Toppers - *5 oz pkg*	142	11.0	4.0			30			0.36			0					CNAG136
lasagna, italian sausage, Budget	456	209.5	20.6	39.9		3.0	903	316									
Gourmet - *10.5 oz entrée*	298	23.8	8.2	9.8	2.0	48			2.68			2161					22673

	KCAL	H₂0 (g)	PRO (g)	CHO (g)	SUGR (g)	DFIB (g)	Na (mg)	Ca (mg)	Mg (mg)	Zn (mg)	Mn (mg)	A (mcg RAE)	C (mg)	B-1 (mg)	NIA (mg)	B-12 (mcg)	PANT (mg)
	WT (g)	FAT (g)	SFA (g)	MUFA (g)	PUFA (g)	CHOL (mg)	K (mg)	P (mg)	Fe (mg)	Cu (mg)	Se (mcg)	A (IU)	E (mg ATE)	B-2 (mg)	B-6 (mg)	FOL (mcg DFE)	REF
lasagna, roma, Healthy Choice	420		26.0	59.0	14.0	6.0	580	150					6				
13.5 oz entrée	383	9.0	3.0			35			3.60			500					CNAG139
lasagna w/meat & sce, Stouffer's	277	155.9	18.7	26.4		3.2	735	230									
7.6 oz serving (1/3 pkg)	215	10.8	4.7	3.5	0.6	41						0					22570
lasagna w/meat sce & 4 cheeses, Michelina's - *9 oz entrée*	290		16.0	39.0	7.0	3.0	810	150					12				
	255	8.0	3.5			35						1250					MICH1
Banquet	270		14.0	33.0	3.0	2.0	960	100					54				
1 cup (8 oz)	227	10.0	6.0			45			1.44			300					CNAG138
Marie Callender's	350		15.0	35.0	10.0	3.0	670	400					0				
1 cup (8.9 oz)	252	17.0	9.0			50			2.70			500					CNAG137
macaroni & beef in tom sce, Stfrs Ln Csn - *10 oz entrée*	249	224.7	13.9	36.5		3.4	563						157				
	283	5.4	1.6	2.1	0.7	23			2.18			991					22576
Weight Watchers	282	201.5	15.6	44.7		6.7	492						27				
9.5 oz entrée	269	4.6	1.6	1.8	0.6	13			5.68			987					22680
macaroni & cheese, Banquet	230		8.0	33.0	7.0	3.0	1290	100					0				
1 cup (7 oz)	198	7.0	3.0			10			0.36			100					CNAG140
Healthy Choice	270		13.0	40.0	8.0	3.0	600	200					0				
9 oz entrée	255	6.0	2.5			25	228	237	1.08			0					CNAG141
Marie Callender's	300		15.0	41.0	9.0	3.0	1190	250					0				
1 cup (8 oz)	227	9.0	6.0			25			1.08			500					CNAG142
manicotti w/3 cheeses, Healthy Choice - *11 oz entrée*	290		14.0	46.0	25.0	3.0	600	400					0				
	312	5.0	3.0			35	802	303	1.80			750					CNAG143
meatloaf, grvy, mshd pot, Marie Callender's - *1/6 pkg (7.3 oz)*	300		12.0	26.0	3.0	2.0	1100	60					0				
	208	16.0	6.0			70			1.44			200					CNAG145
meatloaf w/savory grvy, Banquet	190		10.0	7.0	2.0	1.0	750	0					0				
1 patty w/gravy (4.7 oz)	132	13.0	7.0			35			1.08			0					CNAG144
noodles, escalloped & chkn Marie Callender's - *6 oz srvng (1/2 pkg)*	292	115.1	9.6	28.3	4.4		742	77					0				
	171	15.6	5.4	4.7	5.6				1.45			905					22685
noodles w/beef & brown gravy, Banquet - *1 cup (7 oz)*	150		11.0	16.0	1.0	2.0	1120	0					0				
	198	5.0	2.5			35			1.44			0					CNAG146
pepper steak & rice, Michelinas' Authentico - *8 oz entrée*	270		11.0	43.0	5.0	2.0	850	40					18				
	227	5.0	1.5			20			2.70			500					MICH2
peppers stuffed w/beef & tom sce, Stouffer's - *7.8 oz srvng (1/2 pkg)*	189	180.8	7.9	20.9		5.3	579						87				
	220	8.1	2.7	3.8	0.5	22						0					22569
pierogies, am cheese, Mrs. T's	180		6.0	31.0	1.0	1.0	420	40					5				
3 pierogies (4.2 oz)	120	3.0	1.0			10			1.44			100					ATCO1
broccoli cheese, Mrs. T's	200		6.0	34.0	2.0	2.0	570	40					12				
3 pierogies (4.2 oz)	120	4.5	1.0			10			1.80			300					ATCO2
cheese bacon rogies, Mrs. T's	140		5.0	24.0	1.0	1.0	420	20					4	0.30	2.0		
7 pierogies (3 oz)	85	3.0	0.5			5			1.08			100		0.14			ATCO3
jalapeno cheddar, Mrs. T's	200		6.0	36.0	2.0	2.0	580	40					9	0.38			
3 pierogies (4.2 oz)	120	3.0	1.0			10			1.80			200		0.17			ATCO4
potato cheese, Mrs. T's	190		6.0	35.0	1.0	2.0	540	40					6	0.38	3.0		
3 pierogies (4.2 oz)	120	2.5	1.0			10			1.80			100		0.17			ATCO6
potato cheese rogies, Mrs. T's	130		4.0	24.0	1.0	1.0	350	20					5	0.30	2.0		
7 pierogies (3 oz)	85	1.5	0.5			5			1.08			100		0.14			ATCO5
potato onion, Mrs. T's	180		5.0	34.0	1.0	2.0	420	20					9				
3 pierogies (4.2 oz)	120	2.0	0.0			5			1.44			100					ATCO7
rstd garlic, Mrs. T's	240		6.0	36.0	1.0	2.0	530	20					9				
3 pierogies (4.2 oz)	120	8.0	1.5			25			1.80			400					ATCO8
pocket sandwich, beef & cheddar, Hot Pockets - *5 oz pocket*	403	62.5	16.3	39.2			906	337									
	142	20.2	8.8	6.7	1.2	53			2.93			0					22534
broccoli & cheddar, Weight Watchers - *5 oz pocket*	266	80.1	13.4	39.6			388	92									
	141	6.1	1.8	2.3	1.0	14						235					22541
chicken, broccoli, & cheddar, Croissant Pockets - *4.5 oz pckt*	301	64.0	11.4	38.9		1.4	652						6				
	128	11.0	3.4	4.4	1.7	37			3.80			339					22535
chicken, glazed supreme, Lean Pockets - *4.5 oz pocket*	233	75.4	9.9	34.2			562	122									
	128	6.3	1.9	2.5	1.0	23						768					22538
ham & cheese, Red Baron Premium Pckts - *4.7 oz pckt*	356	61.4	14.9	36.2			1052	190									
	133	16.9	6.2	6.1	1.8	41						0					22540
ham 'n cheese, Hot Pockets	340	57.5	14.8	38.4			666	251									
4.5 oz pocket	128	14.2	5.8	4.4	1.5	50			2.61			0					22537

								Minerals					Vitamins				
	KCAL	H₂O (g)	PRO (g)	CHO (g)	SUGR (g)	DFIB (g)	Na (mg)	Ca (mg)	Mg (mg)	Zn (mg)	Mn (mg)	A (mcg RAE)	C (mg)	B-1 (mg)	NIA (mg)	B-12 (mcg)	PANT (mg)
	WT (g)	FAT (g)	SFA (g)	MUFA (g)	PUFA (g)	CHOL (mg)	K (mg)	P (mg)	Fe (mg)	Cu (mg)	Se (mcg)	A (IU)	E (mg ATE)	B-2 (mg)	B-6 (mg)	FOL (mcg DFE)	REF
pepperoni, Hot Pockets	367	54.8	13.6	38.7			676	280									
4.5 oz pocket	128	17.7	6.6	6.3	2.0	41			3.16			449					22536
pork patty, herb breaded, Healthy	280		18.0	38.0	4.0	4.0	570	100					4				
Choice - 8 oz entrée	227	6.0	2.5			30			4.50			500					CNAG147
pot pie, beef	449	113.5	13.3	44.2		2.2	737										
7 oz individual pot pie	198	24.4	8.5	9.7	2.7	38						1024					22529
Banquet	400		9.0	38.0	8.0	1.0	1000	20					0				
7 oz pot pie	198	23.0	11.0			30			1.08			750					CNAG148
Marie Callender's	660		16.0	53.0	7.0	1.0	1430	40					0				
9.5 oz pot pie	269	42.0	21.0			20			2.70			1000					CNAG149
pot pie, cheesy potato, broc,	410		9.0	40.0	8.0	2.0	1220	80					0				
ham, Banquet - 7 oz pot pie	198	23.0	10.0			25			0.72			0					CNAG150
pot pie, chicken	484	130.0	13.0	42.7	7.8	1.7	857	33	24	1.02	0.681	256	2	0.25	4.1	0.15	0.38
7.7 oz individual pot pie	217	29.1	9.7	12.5	4.5	41	256	119	2.06	0.171	0.7	2285	3.8	0.36	0.20	58.6	22906
& broccoli, Banquet	350		10.0	32.0	9.0	2.0	830	20					0				
7 oz pot pie	198	20.0	9.0			35			0.72			1000					CNAG151
au gratin, Marie Callender's	690		19.0	50.0	3.0	4.0	1300	150					0				
9.5 oz pot pie	269	46.0	21.0			30			2.70			1000					CNAG152
Banquet	382	127.2	9.9	36.0	5.9	1.0	948	28					0				
7 oz individual pot pie	198	22.0	8.9	10.4	2.7	40			1.13			2806					22525
Marie Callender's	501	143.6	12.4	44.2	9.4		1041	37					0				
1 cup (8.3 oz)	234	30.6	12.6	12.3	5.6	14						1133					22526
Stouffer's	572	182.3	23.2	36.5		3.1	942	102					0				
10 oz individual pot pie	283	37.1	10.7	12.4	10.4	76			3.00			4670					22527
pot pie, mac & cheese, Banquet	210		7.0	34.0	10.0	1.0	750	80					0				
6.5 oz pot pie	184	5.0	2.5			10			1.08			0					CNAG153
Morton	210		7.0	34.0	10.0	1.0	750	80					0				
6.5 oz pot pie	184	5.0	2.5			10			1.08			0					CNAG154
pot pie, turkey	681	254.3	25.2	68.5		4.3	1355										
13.7 oz individual pot pie	387	34.1	11.1	13.4	5.3	62			3.87			6838					22528
Banquet	370		10.0	38.0	6.0	3.0	850	40					0				
7 oz pot pie	198	20.0	8.0			45			1.08			750					CNAG155
Marie Callender's	690		13.0	56.0	10.0	5.0	1100	40					0				
9.5 oz pot pie	269	46.0	19.0			15			2.70			1250					CNAG156
pot pie, veg cheese, Banquet	340		6.0	39.0	19.0	1.0	920	80					0				
7 oz pot pie	198	17.0	7.0			10			0.72			1250					CNAG157
pot pie, veg w/beef, Morton	340		5.0	33.0	8.0	2.0	1380	20					0				
7 oz pot pie	198	21.0	9.0			20			1.08			500					CNAG158
pot pie, veg w/chicken, Morton	320		8.0	32.0	7.0	2.0	1040	40					0				
7 oz pot pie	198	18.0	7.0			25			1.08			500					CNAG159
pot pie, veg w/turkey, Morton	310		8.0	29.0	8.0	2.0	1060	40					0				
7 oz pot pie	198	18.0	9.0			25			1.08			500					CNAG160
potato, ham, & broc au gratin,	210		7.0	16.0	6.0	2.0	970	80					18				
Banquet - 2/3 cup (5.2 oz)	147	13.0	5.0			30			0.72			200					CNAG161
potatoes, rstd w/ham, Healthy	210		17.0	26.0	10.0	6.0	600	100					24				
Choice Bowl - 8.5 oz bowl	241	4.0	2.0			30			1.08			100					CNAG130
quiche, swiss cheese, spinach,	470		17.0	32.0	5.0	1.0	580	150					0				
mshrms, Trader Joe's - 6 oz quiche	170	30.0	14.0			190			2.70			1750					TRAD5
ravioli, cheese parmigiana, Healthy	260		11.0	44.0	14.0	6.0	290	150					0				
Choice - 9 oz entrée	255	5.0	2.5			20			1.80			750					CNAG162
rice, chicken, veg stir-fry, Stfrs Ln	270	193.8	11.7	39.5		5.9	632						24				
Csn Lnch Exprss - 9 oz entrée	255	7.4	0.9	3.5	2.0	26						5271					22609
rigatoni w/broc, chkn, cheese sce,	220		18.0	20.0	2.0	2.0	660	40					4				
Smart Ones - 9 oz entrée	255	7.0	2.0	2.5	2.5	25			1.08			200					SMRT2
salisbury steak & gravy w/mshd	330		14.0	21.0	3.0	2.0	1360	80					6				
pot, Michelina's - 8 oz entrée	227	21.0	9.0			55			1.80			300					MICH3
w/brown gravy, Banquet	240		9.0	7.0	2.0	1.0	900	0					0				
1 patty w/gravy (5 oz)	142	20.0	10.0			40			1.08			0					CNAG163
w/gravy & mac & chs, Stfrs	386	198.0	22.6	26.4			1015	196					0				
Hmstyl - 9.6 oz entrée	272	21.2	8.0	7.9	1.8	63			2.28			0					22583
w/red skinned pot, Budget Grmt	261	249.7	18.3	33.9		7.2	494						51				
Light & Healthy - 11 oz entrée	311	5.9	2.0	1.8	0.9	44			3.05			1452					22616

	KCAL	H₂0 (g)	PRO (g)	CHO (g)	SUGR (g)	DFIB (g)	Na (mg)	Ca (mg)	Mg (mg)	Zn (mg)	Mn (mg)	A (mcg RAE)	C (mg)	B-1 (mg)	NIA (mg)	B-12 (mcg)	PANT (mg)
	WT (g)	FAT (g)	SFA (g)	MUFA (g)	PUFA (g)	CHOL (mg)	K (mg)	P (mg)	Fe (mg)	Cu (mg)	Se (mcg)	A (IU)	E (mg ATE)	B-2 (mg)	B-6 (mg)	FOL (mcg DFE)	REF
shepherd's pie, beef, Safeway Select[1]	360		28.0	17.0	0.0	4.0	890	100					0				
1 cup	227	20.0	9.0			75			2.16			100					SAFE7
spaghetti bolognese, Healthy Choice	255	220.2	14.3	43.1	7.4	5.1	473	51	42	1.44	0.603		15	0.35	0.5	0.17	0.20
10 oz entrée	283	2.9	1.0	0.9	0.9	17	408	139	3.54	0.354	33.7	492	0.3	3.77	0.20	203.8	22401
bolognese w/meat sce, Michelina's	280		12.0	47.0	6.0	3.0	770	20					9				
Authentico - *8.5 oz entrée*	241	4.0	1.0			10						750					MICH4
w/meat sce, Stouffer's Lean	313	252.3	14.3	50.5		5.5	610						35				
Cuisine - *11.5 oz entrée*	326	5.9	1.4	2.3	1.3	13			2.12			544					22580
w/meatballs & pomodoro sce, low	312	210.7	13.6	48.6		6.2	1011						9				
fat, Michelina's - *10 oz entrée*	284	7.1	2.2	2.6	1.1	14			2.93			520					22608
w/meatballs & sce, Stouffer's	299	201.5	18.0	39.5		4.6	465	94									
Lean Cuisine - *9.5 oz entrée*	269	7.5	2.1	2.7	1.3	5			2.37			0					22572
w/seasoned beef sce, Healthy	280		14.0	43.0	7.0	5.0	470	40					15				
Choice - *10 oz entrée*	284	6.0	2.0			30			3.60			500					CNAG164
Stuffed Nachos, Totino's[2]	215		6.5	26.8	2.0	1.5	580	50					0				
6 nachos	87	9.3	2.8			10			0.81			0					GENM133
swedish meatballs w/pasta,	276	195.6	21.7	31.2		2.6	562						0				
Stfrs Ln Csn - *9.1 oz entrée*	258	7.2	2.4	2.3	1.0	46			2.06			0					22573
swt & sr chkn w/rice, Michelina's	360		10.0	70.0	24.0	2.0	800	60					12				
Yu Sing - *8.5 oz entrée*	241	4.0	0.5			15			2.70			3000					MICH5
tamale bake (masa, pork, corn	400		16.0	32.0	3.0	2.0	770	200					4				
pudding), Safeway Select - *1 cup*	181	23.0	9.0			85			2.70			500					SAFE8
tuna casserole, Healthy Choice	250		16.0	30.0	5.0	5.0	600	100					0				
9 oz entrée	255	7.0	2.0			20			1.44			0					CNAG165
turkey & gravy	95	120.8	8.3	6.5		0.0	787	20	11	0.99	0.007	18		0.03	2.6	0.34	0.30
5 oz pkg	142	3.7	1.2	1.4	0.7	26	87	115	1.32	0.031	27.3	60		0.18	0.14	5.7	05286
turkey breast, rstd, Healthy Choice	220		18.0	26.0	0.0	5.0	600	20					1				
8.5 oz entrée	241	5.0	2.0			25			0.36			1250					CNAG166
w/gravy & garlic mshd pot, Smart	240		16.0	39.0	7.0	4.0	780	150					1				
Ones - *10 oz entrée*	283	3.5	1.0	1.0	1.0	25			1.80			300					SMRT3
turkey divan, Healthy Choice Bowl	250		19.0	25.0	8.0	5.0	600	100					24				
9.5 oz bowl	312	8.0	2.5			30	625	280	1.80			500					CNAG132
turkey, gravy, mshd potatoes, Marie	310		23.0	18.0	6.0	2.0	1100	60					0				
Callender's - *1/4 pkg (9.2 oz)*	262	16.0	6.0			70			0.36			0					CNAG167
turkey, sliced & hmstyl grvy,	140		7.0	5.0	1.0	1.0	600	0					0				
Banquet - *2 slcs w/grvy (4.3 oz)*	123	10.0	4.0			40			0.72			0					CNAG168
turkey tndrlns w/whpd sweet pot,	250		14.0	37.0	18.0	4.0	610	100					0				
drsng, Stfrs Ln Csn - *9 oz entrée*	255	5.0	1.5	2.0	1.0	25	540		0.72			4500					STOF8
turkey w/mshrms, brwn grvy, rice	223	187.2	19.0	27.8	0.0	3.1	437	22					0				
pilaf, Hlthy Chc - *8.5 oz entrée*	240	3.9	1.2	1.8	0.9	26			1.03			864					22619
white rice & veg w/soy sce, Hanover	130	102.8	4.5	27.0		2.5	636						16				
Stir Fry - *1 cup (4.8 oz)*	137	0.4															22601

[1] Ground beef, carrots, and onions topped with mashed potatoes and cheddar cheese.

[2] Values are averages for beef & cheese, grande, nacho cheese, and taco.

9.4 FROZEN MEALS

beef & broc stir fry, Green Giant	290		27.0	15.0	6.0	4.0	1150	40					54				
Crt A Ml - *1 1/3 cups prep (10 oz)*	283	13.0	3.0			60			3.60			750					GENM135
beef, mesquite, bbq sce, mshd pot,	320	238.8	21.4	38.3	16.5	5.0	491	37									
corn, Hlthy Chc - *11 oz meal*	311	9.0	2.9	3.3	2.8	3	911	271	1.09			1225					22707
beef, oriental w/veg & rice,	242	198.1	13.5	36.2			497						27				
Stfrs Ln Csn - *9 oz meal*	255	4.8	1.8	2.0	0.4	23						2550					22582
beef, oven rstd, Healthy Choice	280		18.0	35.0	10.0	4.0	600	0					12				
10.2 oz meal	288	8.0	2.5			50			1.80			0					CNAG184
beef patty, charbroiled, Healthy	310		16.0	40.0	8.0	4.0	550	20					0				
Choice - *11 oz meal*	312	9.0	3.0			45			1.80			1000					CNAG170
beef patty, western style, Banquet	360		14.0	28.0	4.0	3.0	1400	40					0				
9.5 oz meal	269	21.0	10.0			40			1.80			0					CNAG172
beef patty, w/country style veg,	310		11.0	22.0	5.0	2.0	1090	40					1				
Banquet - *9.5 oz meal*	269	20.0	8.0			40			1.80			300					CNAG171

	KCAL	H₂O (g)	PRO (g)	CHO (g)	SUGR (g)	DFIB (g)	Na (mg)	Ca (mg)	Mg (mg)	Zn (mg)	Mn (mg)	A (mcg RAE)	C (mg)	B-1 (mg)	NIA (mg)	B-12 (mcg)	PANT (mg)
	WT (g)	FAT (g)	SFA (g)	MUFA (g)	PUFA (g)	CHOL (mg)	K (mg)	P (mg)	Fe (mg)	Cu (mg)	Se (mcg)	A (IU)	E (mg ATE)	B-2 (mg)	B-6 (mg)	FOL (mcg DFE)	REF
beef pot roast & gravy, Marie	500		23.0	55.0	13.0	3.0	1460	40					0				
Callender's - *15 oz meal*	425	17.0	6.0			110			3.60			3500					CNAG173
beef pot roast, Healthy Choice	300		20.0	41.0	24.0	8.0	600	20					18				
11 oz meal	312	6.0	2.0			40			1.80			1250					CNAG174
beef pot roast, yankee, Banquet	230		14.0	20.0	8.0	4.0	1130	40					4				
9.4 oz meal	266	10.0	4.0			60			1.80			750					CNAG175
Banquet Extra Helping	410		25.0	33.0	25.0	3.0	1680	60					1				
14.5 oz meal	411	20.0	7.0			50			1.44			750					CNAG176
beef roast, Marie Callender's	390		24.0	30.0	7.0	11.0	1240	80					12				
14.5 oz meal	411	19.0	8.0			70			2.70			0					CNAG177
beef, sliced, gravy, mshd potatoes,	207	207.1	15.3	25.5		3.6	648										
carrots, Freezer Queen - *9 oz meal*	255	4.8	1.3	1.2	1.7	31						10583					22710
beef, sliced, gravy, mshd potatoes,	270	197.1	26.4	18.8	11.7	4.1	742	46					8				
peas, Banquet - *9 oz meal*	255	10.0	4.3	4.9	0.8	71			3.75			102					22691
beef steak, chicken fried & gravy,	650		20.0	50.0	9.0	7.0	2260	100					24				
Marie Callender's - *15 oz meal*	425	37.0	13.0			50			2.70			750					CNAG178
Banquet	420		15.0	39.0	9.0	4.0	1200	100					0				
10 oz meal	284	23.0	12.0			35			1.80			100					CNAG180
Banquet Extra Helping	820		29.0	63.0	13.0	6.0	2260	150					0				
16 oz meal	454	50.0	23.0			70			2.70			0					CNAG179
beef stew, Green Giant Complete	180		11.0	27.0	5.0	4.0	1110	40					12				
Skillet Meals - *1 1/4 cups (8 oz)*	227	3.5	1.0			25			1.80			3000					GENM136
beef strog w/ndls, carrots, peas,	600	247.9	30.4	58.7	8.1	4.4	1141	70					0				
Marie Callender's - *13 oz meal*	368	27.0	11.1	12.0	4.0	70			1.80			217					22677
Healthy Choice	320		22.0	40.0	14.0	7.0	600	60					12				
11 oz meal	312	8.0	3.0			60			1.80			200					CNAG181
beef tips, mshrm sce, pot, grn bns,	430		25.0	39.0	14.0	6.0	1620	60					9				
crnbrs, Mar Clndrs - *13.6 oz meal*	386	19.0	7.0			50			2.70			300					CNAG182
portabello, Healthy Choice	270		23.0	34.0	24.0	7.0	600	40					12				
11.3 oz meal	319	5.0	2.5			40			1.80			500					CNAG183
beefy noodle, Green Giant Create A	350		26.0	31.0	4.0	3.0	1130	20					4				
Meal - *1 1/4 cups prep (10 oz)*	283	14.0	5.0			70			3.60			2000					GENM137
cheesy rice w/chicken & broccoli,	390		24.0	44.0	8.0	6.0	1220	350					30				
Marie Callender's - *12 oz meal*	340	13.0	9.0			55			0.72			500					CNAG185
chicken a l'orange in sce, broc,	268	188.4	24.5	38.5			360						18				
rice, Stfrs Ln Csn - *9 oz meal*	255	1.8	0.4	0.5	0.4	46						1530					22581
chicken alfredo, Green Giant Create	400		35.0	36.0	8.0	3.0	1100	250					18				
A Meal - *1 1/4 cups prep (10 oz)*	283	13.0	5.0			75			2.70			1500					GENM134
chicken alfredo pasta, prep w/2%	290		20.0	37.0	7.0	2.0	920	200					15				
milk, Grn Gnt Sklt Mls - *1 1/2 cups*	~207	7.0	3.5			40			2.70			1250					GENM138
chicken & dumplings, Marie	390		17.0	34.0	14.0	4.0	1650	60					5				
Callender's - *14 oz meal*	397	20.0	10.0			130			1.80			2500					CNAG186
chicken & noodles, Marie	520		21.0	42.0	7.0	5.0	1320	100					9				
Callender's - *13 oz meal*	369	30.0	11.0			80			2.70			4000					CNAG187
chicken brst, grilled & rice pilaf,	360		20.0	38.0	14.0	4.0	1070	20					1				
Marie Callender's - *11.7 oz meal*	333	14.0	4.0			40			1.08			2250					CNAG188
chicken broccoli alfredo, Healthy	300		25.0	34.0	5.0	2.0	530	100					12				
Choice - *11.5 oz meal*	326	7.0	3.0			50			1.80			100					CNAG189
chicken cacciatore, pasta, veg,	266	288.8	22.0	35.9	9.9	5.0	552	53									
Healthy Choice - *12.5 oz meal*	354	4.0	1.0	2.4	0.6	32	750	255	2.23			266					22606
chicken Cantonese, Healthy Choice	280		22.0	34.0	15.0	2.0	480	40					6				
10.8 oz meal	305	6.0	3.0			50			1.80			3000					CNAG190
chicken cheesy pasta, prep w/2%	300		19.0	39.0	9.0	3.0	970	150					5				
mlk, Grn Gnt Sklt Mls - *1 1/4 cups*	~224	7.0	3.5			40			2.70			2000					GENM139
chicken cordon bleu, Marie	610		33.0	58.0	9.0	6.0	1920	200					18				
Callender's - *13 oz meal*	369	28.0	9.0			75			2.70			1750					CNAG191
chicken, country breaded,	350		16.0	51.0	20.0	5.0	480	60					0				
Healthy Choice - *10.3 oz meal*	291	9.0	2.0			45			0.72			500					CNAG202
chicken, country fried & gravy,	620		24.0	63.0	16.0	6.0	2300	40					4				
Marie Callender's - *16 oz meal*	454	30.0	9.0			75			0.36			0					CNAG203
chicken, country herb, Healthy	320		18.0	44.0	23.0	3.0	540	40					0				
Choice - *12.1 oz meal*	344	8.0	3.0			45			0.72			1250					CNAG204

Minerals columns: Na, Ca, Mg, Zn, Mn. Vitamins columns: A, C, B-1, NIA, B-12, PANT.

	KCAL	H₂O (g)	PRO (g)	CHO (g)	SUGR (g)	DFIB (g)	Na (mg)	Ca (mg)	Mg (mg)	Zn (mg)	Mn (mg)	A (mcg RAE)	C (mg)	B-1 (mg)	NIA (mg)	B-12 (mcg)	PANT (mg)
	WT (g)	FAT (g)	SFA (g)	MUFA (g)	PUFA (g)	CHOL (mg)	K (mg)	P (mg)	Fe (mg)	Cu (mg)	Se (mcg)	A (IU)	E (mg ATE)	B-2 (mg)	B-6 (mg)	FOL (mcg DFE)	REF
chicken Dijon, Healthy Choice	270		23.0	33.0	6.0	6.0	470	80					18				
11 oz meal	312	5.0	2.0			40			1.44			4500					CNAG192
chicken fingers, Banquet	740		22.0	67.0	24.0	6.0	1070	40					0				
7.1 oz meal	201	43.0	11.0			70			2.70			0					CNAG193
chicken, french recipe, veg, pot	179	213.9	23.0	9.2		6.1	864										
Budget Grmt Light - *9 oz meal*	255	5.6	1.4	2.7	0.5	26						2295					22617
chicken, fried, Banquet Extra	910		34.0	70.0	8.0	5.0	2400	80					1				
Helping - *14.7 oz meal*	417	55.0	13.0			160			1.80			0					CNAG205
boneless, Banquet	540		16.0	41.0	10.0	3.0	1180	40					6				
8.25 oz meal	234	34.0	9.0			60			1.08			0					CNAG206
Morton	470		20.0	30.0	4.0	3.0	1100	40					6				
9 oz meal	255	30.0	10.0			90			0.72			2250					CNAG207
mshd potatoes, corn, Banquet	470	140.8	21.5	35.1	3.0	2.1	1500	39					1				
8 oz meal	228	27.0	9.3	15.4	2.4	89			1.37			0					22571
original, Banquet	470		21.0	35.0	4.0	2.0	1500	40					1				
9 oz meal	255	27.0	9.0			90			1.08			0					CNAG208
white, Banquet Extra Helping	690		24.0	40.0	3.0	8.0	1900	60					6				
13 oz meal	369	48.0	12.0			70			1.44			0					CNAG209
chicken, garlic herb, oven rstd, Grn	350		31.0	35.0	8.0	5.0	760	60					18				
Gnt Crt A Ml - *1 3/4 cups prep (10 oz)*	283	9.0	1.5			70			1.80			3500					GENM144
stir fry, Green Giant Create A Meal	380		32.0	30.0	3.0	3.0	870	100					18				
1 1/4 cups prep (10 oz)	283	15.0	6.0			80			1.80			1500					GENM145
chicken, glazed, Marie Callender's	490		25.0	40.0	2.0	1.0	2130	40					2				
13 oz meal	369	25.0	11.0			90			2.70			1250					CNAG210
chicken, grilled & mshd potatoes,	340		24.0	20.0	2.0	1.0	1090	20					0				
Marie Callender's - *10 oz meal*	284	18.0	6.0			90			0.36			0					CNAG211
Banquet	330		16.0	37.0	18.0	2.0	1210	40					5				
10 oz meal	281	13.0	3.0			50			1.08			0					CNAG212
Southwestern style, Marie	410		34.0	43.0	9.0	6.0	2020	150					4				
Callender's - *14 oz meal*	397	11.0	6.0			80			1.80			0					CNAG213
w/mshrm sce, Marie Callender's	480		33.0	54.0	0.0	7.0	1030	80					54				
14 oz meal	397	15.0	6.0			65			2.70			500					CNAG214
chicken, herb rstd, mshd potatoes,	580		42.0	26.0	16.0	7.0	2100	80					36				
Marie Callender's - *14 oz meal*	397	34.0	16.0			205			1.80			750					CNAG215
chicken, honey glazed, Healthy	270		21.0	32.0	11.0	4.0	600	40					6				
Choice - *10 oz meal*	284	7.0	2.5			45			1.44			1000					CNAG216
chicken, honey rstd, Marie	440		45.0	27.0	7.0	7.0	1170	100					12				
Callender's - *14 oz meal*	397	17.0	7.0			140			1.80			0					CNAG217
chicken, lemon pepper, oven rstd, Grn	310		29.0	30.0	7.0	5.0	1400	40					30				
Gnt Crt A Ml - *1 2/3 cups prep (10 oz)*	283	8.0	1.5			65			1.80			2500					GENM146
chicken lo mein, Green Giant	200		15.0	30.0	7.0	3.0	760	40					24				
Cmplt Sklt Mls - *1 cup (8 oz)*	227	2.5	0.0			25			1.80			2000					GENM140
chicken, mesquite bbq, rice, veg,	310	224.8	18.1	48.1	12.8	6.0	483	42					9				
cobbler, Hlthy Chc - *10.5 oz meal*	298	5.0	2.0	2.0	1.0	54			1.49			1794					22713
bbq sce, corn, pot au gratin,	321	180.8	17.8	45.0		4.3	793						0				
Tyson - *9 oz meal*	255	7.8	2.6	2.7	0.5	26						474					22688
w/bbq sce, Healthy Choice	310		18.0	48.0	15.0	6.0	480	40					9				
10.5 oz meal	298	5.0	2.0			55			1.44			1750					CNAG218
chicken noodle, prep w/2% mlk,	320		21.0	45.0	11.0	3.0	1310	150					5				
Grn Gnt Sklt Mls - *1 1/4 cups*	~280	6.0	2.5			35			2.70			1750					GENM141
chicken nuggets, Banquet	430		14.0	42.0	11.0	4.0	650	20					6				
6.7 oz meal	191	23.0	8.0			50			1.44			0					CNAG194
Morton	340		12.0	31.0	12.0	2.0	470	40					2				
7 oz meal	198	19.0	4.5			30			1.44			2000					CNAG195
chicken, oriental style & veg stir	360		19.0	57.0	16.0	5.0	600	40					5				
fry, Healthy Choice - *11.9 oz meal*	337	6.0	2.0			25			2.70			1750					CNAG219
chicken parmigiana, Banquet	320		10.0	29.0	7.0	3.0	900	60					30				
9.5 oz meal	269	18.0	7.0			50			1.80			100					CNAG196
Healthy Choice	330		19.0	46.0	23.0	3.0	490	80					9				
11.5 oz meal	326	8.0	3.0			40			1.08			3000					CNAG197
Marie Callender's	660		30.0	63.0	18.0	5.0	920	20					4				
16 oz meal	454	32.0	8.0			50			2.70			1000					CNAG198

	KCAL	H₂O (g)	PRO (g)	CHO (g)	SUGR (g)	DFIB (g)	Na (mg)	Ca (mg)	Mg (mg)	Zn (mg)	Mn (mg)	A (mcg RAE)	C (mg)	B-1 (mg)	NIA (mg)	B-12 (mcg)	PANT (mg)
	WT (g)	FAT (g)	SFA (g)	MUFA (g)	PUFA (g)	CHOL (mg)	K (mg)	P (mg)	Fe (mg)	Cu (mg)	Se (mcg)	A (IU)	E (mg ATE)	B-2 (mg)	B-6 (mg)	FOL (mcg DFE)	REF
chicken pasta, garlic, Green Giant	260		17.0	31.0	5.0	2.0	990	100					15				
Skillet Meals - *1 cup (8 oz)*	227	7.0	3.5			35			1.80			2000					GENM143
primavera, Banquet	320		11.0	40.0	9.0	6.0	840	60					0				
9.5 oz meal	269	12.0	6.0			25			1.80			2500					CNAG199
chicken patty, breaded, Morton	290		10.0	24.0	12.0	4.0	840	20					0				
6.7 oz meal	191	17.0	3.5			35			1.08			3000					CNAG200
chicken, rstd, Healthy Choice	230		20.0	23.0	9.0	4.0	580	20					4				
11 oz meal	312	5.0	3.0			50			1.44			2500					CNAG220
chicken, sesame, Healthy Choice	360		19.0	54.0	17.0	4.0	600	60					6				
10.8 oz meal	306	7.0	2.0			20			2.70			3000					CNAG221
chicken teriyaki, Marie Callender's	510		24.0	71.0	22.0	2.0	1510	60					42				
13 oz meal	369	13.0	2.5			55			3.60			3500					CNAG201
rice mdly, mxd veg, apple cherry	268	249.6	17.1	37.1	10.9	2.8	602	37					12				
compote, Hlthy Chc - *11 oz meal*	312	5.6	3.0	2.2	0.5	44	424	225	1.09			1182					22587
chili & cornbread, Marie Callender's	560		27.0	67.0	25.0	7.0	2110	80					0				
16 oz meal	454	21.0	9.0			60			1.80			500					CNAG222
chimichanga, Banquet	500		13.0	56.0	9.0	9.0	1180	60					1				
9.5 oz meal	269	24.0	8.0			20			2.70			400					CNAG223
enchiladas, 2 beef, 2 chs chili'n	670		19.0	80.0	6.0	12.0	2400	250					0				
Beans, Patio - *15.5 oz meal*	439	30.0	14.0			60			3.60			1500					CNAG224
enchiladas, 4 beef chili'n beans,	540		12.0	73.0	6.0	12.0	2690	250					0				
Patio - *15.5 oz meal*	439	22.0	10.0			50			4.50			1500					CNAG225
enchiladas, beef & tamale combo,	450		10.0	56.0	7.0	9.0	1530	150					0				
Banquet - *11 oz meal*	312	20.0	8.0			30			1.80			750					CNAG226
enchiladas, beef, Banquet	370		10.0	54.0	7.0	8.0	1330	150					0				
11 oz meal	312	12.0	5.0			20			1.80			750					CNAG227
Patio	370		12.0	52.0	4.0	9.0	1700	150					4				
12 oz meal	340	12.0	5.0			25			1.80			500					CNAG228
tamale, chili gravy, Morton	270		7.0	40.0	3.0	7.0	1000	80					6				
10 oz meal	284	9.0	3.5			10			1.80			500					CNAG229
enchiladas, cheese, Banquet	360		12.0	56.0	7.0	8.0	1500	200					2				
11 oz meal	312	10.0	4.0			20			1.80			750					CNAG230
Patio	370		11.0	54.0	7.0	7.0	1570	150					0				
12 oz meal	340	12.0	5.0			25			1.80			500					CNAG231
enchiladas, chicken, Banquet	350		12.0	54.0	7.0	9.0	1580	150					0				
11 oz meal	312	10.0	3.0			25			2.70			750					CNAG232
green chili sce, rice, corn,	298	251.5	13.0	46.0	8.0	4.2	563	134					18				
Hlthy Chc - *11.3 oz meal*	320	6.7	3.1	2.6	1.0	38	384	237	0.77			768					22588
enchiladas, combo, mexican style,	360		10.0	55.0	7.0	9.0	1390	150					4				
Banquet - *11 oz meal*	312	11.0	5.0			20			1.80			750					CNAG233
enchiladas, fiesta, Patio	350		11.0	53.0	5.0	7.0	1760	150					0				
12 oz meal	340	11.0	5.0			25			1.80			400					CNAG234
enchiladas, mexican style, Patio	470		15.0	59.0	5.0	10.0	2210	100					2				
13.3 oz meal	376	19.0	8.0			30			2.70			500					CNAG235
enchiladas, ranchera, Patio	470		13.0	55.0	4.0	9.0	2670	100					1				
13 oz meal	369	22.0	10.0			35			2.70			500					CNAG236
fettuccine alfredo & garlic bread,	920		23.0	82.0	5.0	3.0	1270	250					0				
Marie Callender's - *14 oz meal*	397	55.0	23.0			90			2.70			200					CNAG237
Banquet	350		11.0	40.0	5.0	4.0	850	100					6				
9.5 oz meal	269	16.0	7.0			25			1.08			200					CNAG238
supreme, Marie Callender's	450		15.0	35.0	1.0	4.0	680	150					1				
13 oz meal	369	27.0	12.0			80			1.80			200					CNAG239
fettuccine primavera w/tortellini,	750		19.0	57.0	10.0	6.0	1130	200					6				
Marie Callender's - *14 oz meal*	397	49.0	21.0			65			1.80			1250					CNAG240
fettuccine w/broccoli & chicken,	710		26.0	53.0	7.0	6.0	910	150					9				
Marie Callender's - *13 oz meal*	369	43.0	17.0			85			2.70			500					CNAG241
fish, breaded, mac & cheese, broc,	550		22.0	53.0	12.0	3.0	1400	300					24				
Marie Callender's - *12 oz meal*	340	28.0	9.0			60			1.80			1500					CNAG243
fish, herb baked, Healthy Choice	340		16.0	54.0	11.0	5.0	480	40					0				
10.9 oz meal	309	7.0	1.5			35			0.72			3000					CNAG244
fish, lemon pepper, Healthy Choice	320		14.0	50.0	20.0	5.0	480	20					30				
10.7 oz meal	303	7.0	2.0			30			1.08			500					CNAG245

	KCAL / WT (g)	H₂O (g) / FAT (g)	PRO (g) / SFA (g)	CHO (g) / MUFA (g)	SUGR (g) / PUFA (g)	DFIB (g) / CHOL (mg)	Na (mg) / K (mg)	Ca (mg) / P (mg)	Mg (mg) / Fe (mg)	Zn (mg) / Cu (mg)	Mn (mg) / Se (mcg)	A (mcg RAE) / A (IU)	C (mg) / E (mg ATE)	B-1 (mg) / B-2 (mg)	NIA (mg) / B-6 (mg)	B-12 (mcg) / FOL (mcg DFE)	PANT (mg) / REF
fish sticks, Banquet	290		11.0	33.0	14.0	4.0	820	60					4				
6.6 oz meal	187	13.0	4.5			30			1.80			500					CNAG242
fried rice w/chicken & egg rolls,	330		12.0	51.0	3.0	5.0	1270	40					0				
Banquet - *8.5 oz meal*	241	9.0	3.0			60			1.08			1000					CNAG246
garlic & ginger stir fry, Grn Gnt	270		27.0	25.0	14.0	4.0	1130	60					42				
Crt A Ml - *1 1/2 cups prep (10 oz)*	283	7.0	1.0			55			1.44			3000					GENM142
gravy & charbroiled beef patty,	310		10.0	26.0	3.0	5.0	1210	40					2				
Morton - *9 oz meal*	255	18.0	9.0			30			1.44			0					CNAG247
gravy & salisbury steak, Morton	310		7.0	24.0	7.0	3.0	1100	40					1				
9 oz meal	255	20.0	8.0			30			1.44			1500					CNAG248
gravy & turkey w/dressing,	240		10.0	27.0	5.0	4.0	1200	40					0				
Morton - *9 oz meal*	255	10.0	4.0			40			1.44			2500					CNAG249
ham steak w/macaroni & cheese,	490		29.0	63.0	32.0	5.0	2310	40					12				
Marie Callender's - *14 oz meal*	397	13.0	7.0			80			0.72			2000					CNAG250
lasagna, extra cheese, Marie	590		27.0	61.0	19.0	7.0	1230	800					0				
Callender's - *15 oz meal*	425	27.0	13.0			50			2.70			1250					CNAG253
w/meat sce, Banquet	260		10.0	38.0	10.0	3.0	820	80					1				
9.5 oz meal	269	8.0	3.0			15			1.80			750					CNAG252
w/meat sce, Marie Callender's	630		29.0	59.0	24.0	3.0	1230	500					0				
15 oz meal	425	31.0	15.0			75			2.70			1000					CNAG251
lo mein stir fry, Grn Gnt Crt A	320		30.0	33.0	9.0	3.0	920	40					21				
Ml - *1 1/4 cups prep (10 oz)*	283	7.0	1.5			60			1.80			2000					GENM147
macaroni & cheese, Banquet	420		15.0	57.0	7.0	5.0	1330	150					0				
12 oz meal	340	14.0	8.0			20			1.44			0					CNAG254
Marie Callender's	540		25.0	55.0	12.0	5.0	1930	400					0				
12 oz meal	340	24.0	15.0			50			1.44			100					CNAG255
Morton	240		9.0	34.0	10.0	3.0	1190	100					0				
16 oz meal	227	8.0	4.0			20			0.72			200					CNAG256
meatloaf & gravy w/mshd potatoes,	540		23.0	42.0	30.0	5.0	1570	60					0				
Marie Callender's - *14 oz meal*	397	30.0	12.0			95			1.08			1250					CNAG257
Banquet	280		12.0	23.0	9.0	3.0	1020	40					0				
9.5 oz meal	269	16.0	6.0			60			1.80			200					CNAG258
Banquet Extra Helping	610		29.0	34.0	12.0	6.0	1940	60					6				
16 oz meal	454	40.0	15.0			110			3.60			2000					CNAG259
mshd potatoes, gravy, grn bns,	560		29.0	38.0	5.0	5.0	1420	100					9				
carrots, Stfrs Hmstyle - *17 oz meal*	481	32.0	12.0			95			3.60			750					STOF4
tom sce, mshd pot, carrots,	612	343.4	29.1	33.6	12.2	6.3	1943	77					8				
Banquet Extra Help - *16 oz meal*	453	40.0	15.5	17.3	7.2	113			3.94			2088					22675
tom sce, pot, veg w/sce, apple	316	264.6	15.3	52.4	17.0	6.1	459	48					55				
crisp, Healthy Choice - *12 oz meal*	340	5.0	2.5	1.9	0.6	37			2.24			745					22709
w/tomato sce, Morton	250		9.0	24.0	17.0	3.0	1200	40					0				
9 oz meal	255	13.0	4.5			20			1.08			2500					CNAG260
mex style, tamales, enchiladas, chili	508	267.0	13.9	68.4		8.3	1812	241					5				
sce, beans, rice, Patio - *13.3 oz meal*	376	19.9	6.8	7.7	2.7	26			2.86			628					22586
noodles & chicken, escalloped,	740		21.0	60.0	10.0	5.0	1600	150					0				
Marie Callender's - *13 oz meal*	369	46.0	16.0			90			2.70			750					CNAG262
homestyle, Banquet	390		12.0	44.0	5.0	7.0	1080	60					0				
12 oz meal	340	19.0	7.0			50			1.80			3500					CNAG261
parmesan herb chkn, oven rstd, Grn	340		31.0	29.0	3.0	5.0	1050	80					30				
Gnt Crt A Ml - *1 3/4 cups prep (10 oz)*	283	11.0	2.0			70			1.80			3000					GENM148
pork chop, country fried, Marie	540		23.0	50.0	23.0	8.0	2240	100					6				
Callender's - *15 oz meal*	425	28.0	9.0			65			2.70			5000					CNAG263
pork cutlet, Banquet	420		11.0	38.0	21.0	4.0	1060	60					0				
10.3 oz meal	291	25.0	7.0			35			1.80			100					CNAG264
pork rib, Banquet	400		17.0	40.0	22.0	4.0	1070	80					2				
10 oz meal	284	19.0	8.0			45			1.80			0					CNAG265
pork riblet, Banquet Extra Helping	720		27.0	62.0	18.0	7.0	1590	100					0				
15.2 oz meal	432	40.0	15.0			80			3.60			500					CNAG266
pork w/bbq sce, rstd pot, corn,	480		27.0	62.0	18.0	5.0	1460	40					6				
Stfrs Hmstyle - *15.3 oz meal*	435	14.0	5.0			65			2.70			500					STOF5
ravioli, cheese, sce, garlic bread,	750		25.0	96.0	18.0	11.0	1070	500					0				
Marie Callender's - *16 oz meal*	454	29.0	9.0			30			4.50			1000					CNAG267

	KCAL / WT (g)	H_2O (g) / FAT (g)	PRO (g) / SFA (g)	CHO (g) / MUFA (g)	SUGR (g) / PUFA (g)	DFIB (g) / CHOL (mg)	Na (mg) / K (mg)	Ca (mg) / P (mg)	Mg (mg) / Fe (mg)	Zn (mg) / Cu (mg)	Mn (mg) / Se (mcg)	A (mcg RAE) / A (IU)	C (mg) / E (mg ATE)	B-1 (mg) / B-2 (mg)	NIA (mg) / B-6 (mg)	B-12 (mcg) / FOL (mcg DFE)	PANT (mg) / REF
salisbury steak & gravy, Marie	550		30.0	51.0	14.0	6.0	1680	250					4				
Callender's - *14 oz meal*	397	25.0	11.0			85			3.60			400					CNAG268
mshd pot, corn, Banquet	398	196.6	15.3	27.7		3.5											
9.5 oz meal	269	25.0	8.5	11.8	1.3	51			2.07			0					22711
mshd pot, corn, Banquet Extra	782	332.3	27.1	47.1	7.0	7.0	2195	112					0				
Helping - *16.5 oz meal*	468	54.1	21.3	25.5	7.3	131			1.87								22689
mshrm gravy, mshd pot, corn,	326	250.3	18.0	48.0	23.8	6.2	466	42					12				
Hlthy Chc - *11.5 oz meal*	326	6.9	3.0	2.8	1.1	49			2.22			1014					22708
rstd pot, corn, grn bns, Stfrs	550		28.0	49.0	7.0	5.0	1360	60					12				
Hmstyle - *16 oz meal*	453	27.0	9.0			60			3.60			400					STOF6
shrimp & veg, Healthy Choice	270		15.0	39.0	6.0	6.0	580	150					30				
11.8 oz meal	335	6.0	3.0			50			1.80			1000					CNAG269
spaghetti & meat sce, Morton	200		5.0	30.0	13.0	4.0	750	20					0				
8 oz meal	242	6.0	2.5			5			1.44			2500					CNAG271
w/garlic bread, Marie	670		27.0	85.0	20.0	9.0	1160	150					0				
Callender's - *17 oz meal*	482	25.0	11.0			35			2.70			750					CNAG270
steak teriyaki, Grn Gnt Cmplt	300		15.0	53.0	13.0	3.0	1030	40					27				
Sklt Mls - *1 1/2 cups (8 oz)*	227	3.5	1.0			20			2.70			2250					GENM149
stuffed pasta shells, Healthy	370		18.0	60.0	12.0	5.0	570	250					5				
Choice - *10.3 oz meal*	293	6.0	3.0			20			5.40			500					CNAG272
stuffed pasta trio, Marie	380		15.0	40.0	26.0	5.0	950	500					1				
Callender's - *10.5 oz meal*	298	18.0	9.0			50			1.80			750					CNAG273
swedish mtbls, rice, broc, crts,	520		28.0	44.0	3.0	3.0	1020	40					0				
Mar Clndrs - *12.5 oz meal*	354	26.0	12.0			65			2.70			100					CNAG274
sweet & sour chicken, Healthy	360		20.0	53.0	25.0	5.0	360	40					15				
Choice - *11 oz meal*	312	7.0	3.0			45			1.08			2000					CNAG275
Marie Callender's	570		23.0	86.0	55.0	7.0	700	40					0				
14 oz meal	397	15.0	2.5			40			1.80			2500					CNAG276
stir fry, Green Giant Create A	340		25.0	43.0	31.0	3.0	620	60					18				
Meal - *1 1/4 cups prep (10 oz)*	283	7.0	1.0			60			1.80			3500					GENM150
szechuan stir fry, Grn Gnt Crt	310		26.0	20.0	12.0	4.0	1390	40					24				
A Meal - *1 1/4 cups prep (10 oz)*	283	14.0	3.0			60			3.60			3000					GENM151
teriyaki stir fry, Grn Gnt Crt A	230		27.0	18.0	10.0	4.0	920	60					42				
Meal - *1 1/4 cups prep (10 oz)*	283	6.0	1.0			55			1.80			750					GENM152
tuna & noodles, Marie	600		18.0	52.0	12.0	5.0	1570	100					0				
Callender's - *12 oz meal*	340	35.0	18.0			90			2.70			100					CNAG277
turkey & grvy w/drsng, Banquet	620		28.0	54.0	11.0	10.0	2250	60					0				
Extra Helping - *17 oz meal*	482	32.0	8.0			80			1.44			0					CNAG278
turkey brst, drsng, grvy, mshd pot,	460		24.0	55.0	6.0	7.0	1620	100					9				
grn bns, crts, Stfrs Hmstyl - *16 oz meal*	453	16.0	5.0			60			2.70			1750					STOF7
grilled & rice pilaf, Marie	310		22.0	34.0	8.0	4.0	940	60					0				
Callender's - *11.7 oz meal*	333	10.0	3.5			40			0.72			750					CNAG279
Healthy Choice	290		22.0	40.0	20.0	5.0	460	20					36				
10.5 oz meal	298	4.5	2.0			45			1.44			400					CNAG280
honey roast, Banquet	270		11.0	29.0	8.0	4.0	1310	60					0				
9 oz meal	255	12.0	2.5			30			1.80			1500					CNAG281
turkey, country inn roast,	250		20.0	28.0	16.0	4.0	530	40					0				
Healthy Choice - *10 oz meal*	284	6.0	2.0			40			1.80			500					CNAG282
turkey, grvy, drsng, broc,	504	288.1	31.0	51.8	11.1		2037	131					24				
Marie Callender's - *14 oz meal*	397	19.0	9.1	8.2	1.7	79			4.37			397					22599
turkey, grvy, drsng, mshd pot,	280	200.4	14.0	34.0	6.6	2.9	1061	47									
corn, Banquet - *9.2 oz meal*	262	9.9	2.5	3.7	3.7	52			1.39			84					22607
turkey mdlns, mshrms, sce,	214	186.7	15.1	34.6		3.1	504										
rice, veg, Wt Wtchrs - *8.5 oz meal*	240	1.7	0.4	0.4	0.5	24			1.42			319					22672
veal parmigiana, tom sce, mshd	362	184.9	12.6	34.8	15.0	6.6	964	66					28				
pot, peas, Banquet - *9 oz meal*	255	19.0	6.2	9.4	3.5	26			2.30			252					22605
w/tom sce, Morton	290		8.0	30.0	8.0	4.0	950	40					18				
8.7 oz meal	248	15.0	4.5			25			1.80			2250					CNAG283

	KCAL	H₂O (g)	PRO (g)	CHO (g)	SUGR (g)	DFIB (g)	Na (mg)	Ca (mg)	Mg (mg)	Zn (mg)	Mn (mg)	A (mcg RAE)	C (mg)	B-1 (mg)	NIA (mg)	B-12 (mcg)	PANT (mg)
	WT (g)	FAT (g)	SFA (g)	MUFA (g)	PUFA (g)	CHOL (mg)	K (mg)	P (mg)	Fe (mg)	Cu (mg)	Se (mcg)	A (IU)	E (mg ATE)	B-2 (mg)	B-6 (mg)	FOL (mcg DFE)	REF

9.5 FROZEN MEALS FOR CHILDREN

	KCAL/WT	H₂O/FAT	PRO/SFA	CHO/MUFA	SUGR/PUFA	DFIB/CHOL	Na/K	Ca/P	Mg/Fe	Zn/Cu	Mn/Se	A(RAE)/A(IU)	C/E	B-1/B-2	NIA/B-6	B-12/FOL	PANT/REF
beef patty sandwich w/cheese,	410		12.0	58.0	27.0	4.0	600	150					0				
Buckaroo Kid Cuisine - *8.5 oz meal*	241	15.0	7.0			30			1.80			100					CNAG284
chicken, fried, High Flying Kid	440		18.0	48.0	20.0	3.0	940	80					0				
Cuisine - *10 oz meal*	286	20.0	9.0			70			1.44			0					CNAG287
chicken nuggets, Dino Mite Kid	300		11.0	10.0	3.0	1.0	540	0					0				
Cuisine - *4 pieces (3 oz)*	85	23.0	6.0			40			0.72			0					CNAG285
chicken nuggets, mac & cheese,	524	155.7	17.7	52.9		3.1	974	206					0				
corn, Kid Cuisine - *9.1 oz meal*	257	26.7	6.6	10.7	6.0	49			2.85			0					22690
chicken nuggets w/chs, Radical	300		11.0	12.0	3.0	1.0	620	60					0				
Racin' Kid Csn - *4 nuggets (5.3 oz)*	74	23.0	7.0			35			0.36			0					CNAG286
corn dog, Circus Show Kid Cuisine	490		8.0	70.0	46.0	5.0	800	80					12				
8.8 oz meal	249	20.0	7.0			30			1.80			0					CNAG288
corn dog, Mystical Mini Kid Cuisine	230		6.0	18.0	7.0	0.0	600	0					0				
4 pieces (2.7 oz)	76	14.0	4.0			35			0.00			0					CNAG289
fish sticks, Funtastic Kid Cuisine	410		9.0	57.0	30.0	4.0	550	60					0				
8.3 oz meal	234	16.0	3.5			20			1.44			0					CNAG290
mac & cheese, Magical Kid Cuisine	440		10.0	72.0	25.0	4.0	870	100					0				
10.6 oz meal	301	13.0	5.0			15			1.80			400					CNAG291
pizza, cheese, Fire Chief Kid	340		19.0	44.0	7.0	2.0	780	200					0				
Cuisine - *5.2 oz meal*	147	10.0	5.0			20			5.40			500					CNAG293
cheese, Pirate Kid Cuisine	430		12.0	71.0	34.0	5.0	480	150					0				
8 oz meal	227	11.0	5.0			30			1.80			100					CNAG294
hamburger, Big League Kid	400		14.0	61.0	32.0	5.0	550	100					1				
Cuisine - *8.3 oz meal*	235	11.0	3.5			35			1.80			200					CNAG295
pepperoni, Poolside Kid	380		18.0	44.0	7.0	2.0	990	150					0				
Cuisine - *5.2 oz meal*	147	14.0	7.0			35			5.40			500					CNAG296
pizza snacks, Backpacking Kid	230		8.0	23.0	4.0	1.0	480	60					1				
Cuisine - *6 pieces (2.7 oz)*	76	11.0	5.0			20			1.08			100					CNAG292
pork ribettes, Parachuting Kid	390		16.0	39.0	16.0	3.0	760	60					0				
Cuisine - *7.5 oz meal*	214	19.0	8.0			50			1.08			0					CNAG297
taco roll up, Game Time Kid Cuisine	420		9.0	55.0	25.0	4.0	740	100					0				
7.3 oz meal	208	18.0	7.0			25			1.44			0					CNAG298
waffle sticks, Wave Rider Kid	390		3.0	75.0	38.0	3.0	580	20					0				
Cuisine - *6.6 oz meal*	187	8.0	2.0			30			0.72			0					CNAG299

9.6 FROZEN PIZZA & PIZZA ROLLS

	KCAL/WT	H₂O/FAT	PRO/SFA	CHO/MUFA	SUGR/PUFA	DFIB/CHOL	Na/K	Ca/P	Mg/Fe	Zn/Cu	Mn/Se	A(RAE)/A(IU)	C/E	B-1/B-2	NIA/B-6	B-12/FOL	PANT/REF
bacon burger, Totino's Party Pizza	390		14.0	35.0	4.0	2.0	810	150					0				
1/2 of 10.5 oz pizza	149	21.0	5.0			15			1.80			0					GENM153
canadian bacon, Jeno's Crisp 'N	440		16.0	51.0	6.0	2.0	1120	150					0				
Tasty - *6.9 oz pizza*	195	19.0	3.5			15			1.44			0					GENM154
cheese, Jeno's Crisp 'N Tasty	460		19.0	52.0	6.0	2.0	860	350					0				
6.9 oz pizza	195	19.0	6.0			20			1.44			0					GENM155
Totino's Family Size Pizza	370		17.0	39.0	4.0	2.0	740	300					0				
1/3 pizza	160	16.0	6.0			20			1.80			0					GENM156
Totino's Microwave Pizza	240		10.0	26.0	3.0	1.0	540	200					0				
For One - *3.7 oz pizza*	104	11.0	3.5			15			1.80			0					GENM157
combination, Jeno's Crisp 'N Tasty	500		17.0	50.0	5.0	8.0	1100	150					0				
7 oz pizza	198	26.0	6.0			20			1.44			0					GENM158
Totino's Family Size	310		11.0	29.0	3.0	1.0	700	150					0				
1/4 pizza	125	17.0	4.0			15			1.80			0					GENM160
Totino's Microwave Pizza	300		10.0	26.0	3.0	1.0	700	100					0				
For One - *4 oz pizza*	119	17.0	4.0			15			1.80			0					GENM159
french bread pizza, cheese,	360		20.0	57.0	10.0	5.0	600	350					12				
Healthy Choice - *6 oz pizza*	170	5.0	1.5			10			3.60			200					CNAG300

	KCAL / WT (g)	H₂O / FAT (g)	PRO / SFA (g)	CHO / MUFA (g)	SUGR / PUFA (g)	DFIB (g) / CHOL (mg)	Na / K (mg)	Ca / P (mg)	Mg / Fe (mg)	Zn (mg) / Cu (mg)	Mn (mg) / Se (mcg)	A (mcg RAE) / A (IU)	C (mg) / E (mg ATE)	B-1 / B-2 (mg)	NIA / B-6 (mg)	B-12 (mcg) / FOL (mcg DFE)	PANT (mg) / REF
Marie Callender's	530		28.0	50.0	5.0	4.0	980	500					0				
7.2 oz pizza	204	24.0	14.0			60			3.60			300					CNAG301
french bread pizza, pepperoni,	360		21.0	56.0	10.0	6.0	600	250					12				
Healthy Choice - 6 oz pizza	170	5.0	1.5			30			3.60			400					CNAG302
Marie Callender's	570		29.0	50.0	5.0	4.0	1160	450					0				
7.5 oz pizza	213	28.0	14.0			65			4.50			500					CNAG303
french bread pizza, sausage &	448	89.7	17.7	43.5		2.5	860	154									
pepperoni, Stfrs - 6.2 oz (1/2 pkg)	177	22.5	7.1	9.3	2.8	37			2.99			0					22553
french bread pizza, sausage,	350		20.0	55.0	10.0	5.0	600	200					15				
Healthy Choice - 6 oz pizza	170	5.0	1.5			20			3.60			200					CNAG304
french bread pizza, sauge, peprni,	429	90.5	16.1	44.5		3.5	840	231					30				
mshrm, Stfr - 6.2 oz (1/2 pizza)	175	20.7	6.4	8.7	2.5	33			2.71			431					22554
french bread pizza, supreme,	360		20.0	58.0	11.0	8.0	600	200					4				
Healthy Choice - 6.35 oz pizza	180	5.0	1.5			15			3.60			300					CNAG305
Marie Callender's	510		26.0	50.0	5.0	4.0	1200	400					0				
7.5 oz pizza	213	23.0	11.0			50			4.50			400					CNAG306
french bread pizza, veg, Healthy	320		18.0	50.0	8.0	4.0	600	300					0				
Choice - 6 oz pizza	170	5.0	1.5			10			3.60			400					CNAG307
Hamburger, Jeno's Crisp 'N Tasty	500		18.0	51.0	5.0	2.0	1040	150					0				
7.3 oz pizza	206	25.0	6.0			25			1.80			0					GENM161
pepperoni	400	68.8	16.2	36.2		2.3	879	25		1.78	0.356	45	2	0.37	3.6	0.06	0.73
5.1 oz serving	146	21.1	7.1	8.4	2.4	34	222	222	2.61	0.111	19.0	305	1.6	0.35	0.11	78.8	22903
12" dia, Tombstone Original	312	52.1	14.5	28.3			551	202									
4 oz (1/3 pizza)	113	15.7	6.0	5.3	2.0	32						375					22556
9" dia, Tombstone Original	413	71.0	17.8	38.6			869	272									
5.4 oz (1/4 pizza)	152	20.8	7.8	7.1	2.4	41						220					22555
Banquet	480		11.0	56.0	30.0	5.0	790	200					0				
6.7 oz pizza	191	23.0	7.0			35			1.80			0					CNAG308
deep dish, Pappalo's For	525	88.2	22.7	64.7		3.2	983	249									
One - 7 oz individual pizza	199	19.5	7.3	7.3	1.9	38			3.60			0					22548
deep dish, Red Baron	480	75.6	16.0	47.9			889	153									
Singles - 6 oz srvng (1/2 pizza)	168	25.0	8.2	10.8	2.8	29			3.46			0					22551
Jack's Original	323	58.4	15.0	29.5			612	221									
4.3 oz (1/4 pizza)	122	16.1	6.2	5.2	2.1	40						310					22544
Jeno's Crisp 'n Tasty	516	93.9	18.6	45.9		3.1	1221	204									
6.8 oz individual pizza	192	28.8	6.5	14.5	3.9	23						0					22546
Red Baron	442	70.8	18.0	36.0			1023	219									
5.4 oz (1/4 pizza)	154	25.1	9.0	10.2	2.6	37			3.03			437					22549
w/4 chs, rising crust, Verdi Sfwy	370		16.0	42.0	3.0	1.0	960	150					12				
Slct - 5.2 oz slice (1/6 pizza)	147	15.0	6.0			25			2.70			400					SAFE3
w/crisp crust, Totino's	364	74.7	12.8	34.5			973	235									
Party - 5.1 oz (1/2 pizza)	145	19.4	3.8	10.4	2.3	12			2.18			0					22568
w/italian style crust,	406	60.9	14.9	36.3			834	215									
Tony's - 4.9 oz (1/3 pizza)	138	22.4	7.6	9.1	2.6	32			2.79			0					22562
pepperoni & sausage, Tombstone	317	57.3	13.3	27.3		1.7	728	184									
Original - 4.2 oz (1/3 pizza)	118	17.2	6.3	5.8	2.4	32						414					22560
pizza rolls, hamburger,	210		8.0	24.0	3.0	1.0	490	40					0				
Totino's - 6 rolls	85	9.0	2.0			10			1.08			0					GENM163
hamburger, Totino's	231	37.7	9.4	26.4			417										
3 oz (2/5 pkg)	85	9.8										0					22531
pepperoni supreme, Totino's	220		8.0	24.0	3.0	1.0	450	40					0				
6 rolls	85	10.0	3.0			10			1.08			0					GENM164
pepperoni, Totino's	385	65.3	14.4	39.5		2.3	866	103									
5 oz (7/10 pkg)	141	18.9	5.0	9.2	2.2	31						0					22533
sausage, Totino's	230		8.0	24.0	3.0	1.0	370	40					0				
6 rolls	85	11.0	2.5			10			1.08			0					GENM165

	KCAL	H₂0 (g)	PRO (g)	CHO (g)	SUGR (g)	DFIB (g)	Na (mg)	Ca (mg)	Mg (mg)	Zn (mg)	Mn (mg)	A (mcg RAE)	C (mg)	B-1 (mg)	NIA (mg)	B-12 (mcg)	PANT (mg)
	WT (g)	FAT (g)	SFA (g)	MUFA (g)	PUFA (g)	CHOL (mg)	K (mg)	P (mg)	Fe (mg)	Cu (mg)	Se (mcg)	A (IU)	E (mg ATE)	B-2 (mg)	B-6 (mg)	FOL (mcg DFE)	REF
sausage, Totino's	351	69.2	14.1	40.2		2.8	632	102									
5 oz (3/5 pizza)	141	14.9	3.5	7.2	2.2	24						0					22532
pizza snack, chs, frzn, Banquet	200		9.0	24.0	4.0	2.0	360	100					5				
Munchers - 6 pieces (3 oz)	85	8.0	4.0			20			1.08			100					CNAG309
pepperoni & sausage, frzn,	230		8.0	23.0	4.0	2.0	430	60					1				
Banquet Munchers - 6 pcs (3 oz)	85	11.0	5.0			20			1.08			100					CNAG310
pepperoni, frzn, Banquet	210		8.0	24.0	4.0	2.0	440	80					5				
Munchers - 6 pieces (3 oz)	85	9.0	4.0			20			1.08			100					CNAG311
sausage, deep dish, Tony's d'Primo	391	64.9	12.4	40.6			830	142									
5 oz (1/4 pizza)	141	19.9	5.7	7.3	4.2	16			2.90			0					22565
Jeno's Crisp 'N Tasty	480		16.0	51.0	5.0	2.0	1050	150					0				
7 oz pizza	198	24.0	5.0			20			1.44			0					GENM168
Milena's	340		16.0	35.0	1.0	2.0	690	250					4				
4.9 oz slice (1/11 of pizza)	140	15.0	6.0			30			1.80			100					MILE1
Totino's Microwave Pizza	280		9.0	27.0	3.0	1.0	630	100					0				
For One - 4.2 oz pizza	116	15.0	3.5			10			1.80			0					GENM170
sausage & mshrm, Tombstone	306	69.7	14.4	31.2			718	201									
Original - 4.7 oz (1/5 pizza)	132	13.7	5.1	4.4	2.1	26						466					22557
Totino's Party Pizza	360		13.0	34.0	4.0	2.0	780	150					0				
1/2 of 10.8 oz pizza	153	19.0	4.5			15			1.80			0					GENM166
sausage & pepperoni	385	71.0	15.8	36.2		2.3	854	191	26	1.61	0.397	64	3	0.37	3.6	0.35	0.57
5.1 oz serving	146	19.7	6.3	7.8	2.6	31	256	207	2.77	0.127	18.1	425	1.4	0.33	0.10	75.9	22902
Jack's Great Combinations	348	68.8	17.4	30.1			708	225									
4.8 oz (1/4 pizza)	137	17.5	6.6	6.1	2.3	44						415					22543
Jeno's Crisp n' Tasty	491	101.0	16.8	51.7		2.8	1239	166									
7 oz individual pizza	198	24.2	5.7	11.9	3.1	26						0					22545
Tombstone Original	328	60.8	14.4	30.6		2.1	790	179									
4.4 oz (1/5 pizza)	125	16.4	6.1	5.6	2.3	31						359					22559
Totino's Party Pizza	380		13.0	35.0	4.0	2.0	850	150					0				
1/2 of 10.7 oz pizza	152	21.0	5.0			15			1.80			0					GENM167
w/crisp crust, Totino's	385	77.4	14.1	36.0			1041	210									
Party - 5.4 oz (1/2 pizza)	152	20.4	4.4	10.3	2.5	12			2.66			0					22566
w/italian style crust,	434	64.2	15.0	41.5			719	169									
Tony's - 5.2 oz (1/3 pizza)	147	23.1	6.9	9.3	3.0	24			3.15			0					22563
sausage, mshrms, pepperoni, Red	344	69.2	13.6	31.8			738	223									
Baron Supreme - 4.8 oz (1/5 pizza)	136	18.1	6.1	7.2	2.5	23			2.28			0					22598
sausage, peppers, mshrms,	386	92.7	16.7	33.2			765	281									
Celeste Deluxe - 5.9 oz (1/4 pizza)	167	20.7	8.1	7.6	2.4	37						721					22542
special deluxe, bake to rise, Red	360		16.0	40.0	5.0	2.0	1180	250					2				
Baron[1] - 5.4 oz slice (1/6 pizza)	152	15.0	5.0			25			2.70			300					RDBN1
supreme, Jeno's Crisp 'N Tasty	500		17.0	50.0	5.0	2.5	1090	150					0				
7.2 oz pizza	204	26.0	6.0			20			1.44			0					GENM169
rising crust, DiGiorno	370		17.0	40.0	8.0	3.0	1000	150					1				
5.5 oz slice (1/6 of pizza)	155	16.0	7.0			35			1.80			400					DIGI1
sausage, pepperoni, vegs,	400	76.6	15.8	39.1			772	212									
Tony's - 5.5 oz (1/3 pizza)	155	20.0	6.7	7.9	2.8	28			2.95			0					22561
taco style (mex sausage, taco sce,	437	70.4	14.3	42.8			756	188									
corn crust) - 5.4 oz (1/3 pizza)	154	23.3	7.7	8.9	3.5	28			2.54			501					22564
three meat, Jeno's Crisp 'N Tasty	490		17.0	49.0	5.0	2.0	1150	150					0				
7 oz pizza	198	25.0	6.0			25			1.44			0					GENM171
two chs, sausage, peprni, onions,	337	64.2	12.0	32.0			704	147									
Rd Brn Spec Delx - 4.6 oz (1/5 pizza)	129	17.8	6.3	6.9	2.3	25			2.54			0					22550
zesty italiano, Totino's Party Pizza	390		13.0	36.0	4.0	2.0	850	150					0				
1/2 of 10.7 oz pizza	152	21.0	5.0			15			1.80			0					GENM172

[1] Contains sausage, pepperoni, green and red peppers, onions, and black olives.

9.7 PACKAGED ENTREES

Each food has two data rows. Column pairs: top label / bottom label.

Food	KCAL / WT (g)	H2O / FAT (g)	PRO / SFA (g)	CHO / MUFA (g)	SUGR / PUFA (g)	DFIB (g) / CHOL (mg)	Na / K (mg)	Ca / P (mg)	Mg / Fe (mg)	Zn / Cu (mg)	Mn / Se (mg/mcg)	A RAE(mcg) / A (IU)	C (mg) / E (mg ATE)	B-1 / B-2 (mg)	NIA / B-6 (mg)	B-12(mcg) / FOL(mcg DFE)	PANT (mg) / REF
Asian Side Dish, avg for 2 flvrs, Lipton[1] - 1/2 cup (1 cup prep)	230		6.0	47.0	2.5	1.0	825	0					1	0.34	2.5		
	62	2.0	0.0			0			2.25			350		0.10		80.0	UNLV137
Bowl Appetit, cheesy broc mshd pot, dry, Bty Crckr - 2.3 oz bowl	260		5.0	43.0	4.0	3.0	930	40					0	0.00	2.0		
	65	9.0	2.5			0	730		1.08			0		0.10		0.0	GENM173
herb chicken veg rice, dry, Betty Crocker - 2.4 oz bowl	260		7.0	50.0	2.0	2.0	750	20					0	0.15	2.0		
	68	5.0	1.0			15	160		1.80			500		0.00		60.0	GENM174
tomato parmesan penne, dry, Betty Crocker - 3.1 oz bowl	350		12.0	59.0	8.0	2.0	870	100					0	0.45	3.0		
	88	8.0	2.5			5	540		1.80			200		0.34		80.0	GENM175
burrito, prep, Old El Paso Dinner Kit - 1 burrito	270		14.0	27.0	2.0	1.0	840	100					0				
	~147	12.0	4.5			40			2.70			100					GENM176
Chicken Helper, cheddar & broc, prep[2] - 1 cup	310		27.0	28.0	5.0	<1.0	760	100					0	0.30	7.0		
	~231	9.0	3.0			60	350		1.44			200		0.34		40.0	GENM177
chicken & mshd potatoes, prep[2] 1 cup	250		20.0	24.0	2.0	1.0	790	40					0	0.00	6.0		
	~232	9.0	2.0			50	460		1.08			300		0.10			GENM179
chicken & stuffing, prep[2] 1 cup	290		25.0	28.0	3.0	1.0	830	20					0	0.15	7.0		
	~213	9.0	1.5			60	220		1.80			200		0.17		40.0	GENM180
chicken fried rice, prep[2] 1 cup	260		23.0	22.0	1.0	1.0	660	60					0	0.12	6.0		
	~164	8.0	2.0			120	220		1.44			400		0.14		40.0	GENM178
fettuccini alfredo, prep[2] 1 cup	290		26.0	28.0	4.0	1.0	830	80					0	0.30	8.0		
	~243	8.0	2.5			60	310		1.44			200		0.34		40.0	GENM181
southwestern chicken, prep[2] 1 cup	240		23.0	27.0	2.0	1.0	810	60					0	0.15	7.0		
	~178	5.0	1.0			55	290		1.80			500		0.10		40.0	GENM187
Chicken Helper Oven Favorites, ched & mozzarella, prep[2] - 8.4 oz	320		23.0	34.0	4.0	<1.0	750	60					0	0.30	7.0		
	238	11.0	3.0			50	260		1.44			200		0.26		60.0	GENM182
chicken & biscuit bake, prep[2] 8.3 oz	290		22.0	35.0	6.0	2.0	830	100					0	0.15	6.0		
	235	7.0	2.5			50	430		1.44			500		0.26		24.0	GENM183
creamy chicken & rice, prep[2] 8 oz	290		20.0	30.0	1.0	0.0	680	40					0	0.15	5.0		
	227	10.0	2.5			45	200		1.08			300		0.10		40.0	GENM184
homestyle stuffing & gravy, prep[2] 7.8 oz	310		21.0	32.0	3.0	1.0	980	40					0	0.15	6.0		
	221	11.0	2.0			50	210		1.80			300		0.17		32.0	GENM185
potatoes au gratin, prep[2] 8.1 oz	270		20.0	29.0	2.0	2.0	910	40					0	0.06	6.0		
	230	9.0	2.5			45	440		1.08			200		0.14		0.0	GENM186
fajitas, prep, Old El Paso Dinner Kit - 2 fajitas	300		24.0	36.0	3.0	2.0	1070	100					15				
	~208	7.0	1.5			55			2.70			100					GENM188
fettuccine alfredo cup, dry, Knorr 2.1 oz container	260		8.0	48.0	3.0	2.0	990	80					0				
	59	5.0	1.0			10			1.44			0					UNLV53
gordita w/ranch sce, prep, Old El Paso Dinner Kit - 1 gordita	390		20.0	34.0	2.0	1.0	1070	100					0				
	~142	19.0	4.0			45			2.70			100					GENM189
Hamburger Helper, cheddar & broccoli, prep[3] - 1 cup	270		14.0	31.0	3.0	0.0	805	70					0	0.26	2.8		
	~212	10.5	3.8			30	275		1.26			50		0.26		50.0	GENM190
cheeseburger mac, prep[3] 1 cup	360		23.0	32.0	4.0	1.0	940	150					0	0.30	5.0		
	~229	16.0	6.0			65	480		1.80			100		0.43		60.0	GENM191
chili mac, prep[3] 1 cup	300		20.0	30.0	4.0	1.0	820	20					0	0.23	5.0		
	~239	12.0	4.5			55	460		2.70			500		0.26		40.0	GENM192
four cheese lasagna, prep[3] 1 cup	350		23.0	31.0	6.0	0.0	800	100					0	0.23	4.0		
	~220	15.0	6.0			60	440		1.80			200		0.34		60.0	GENM193
rice oriental, prep[3] 1 cup	280		18.0	32.0	2.0	0.0	990	0					0	0.15	3.0		
	~235	10.0	3.5			50	280		2.70			0		0.14		40.0	GENM194
stroganoff, prep[3] 1 cup	320		21.0	30.0	7.0	0.0	830	100					0	0.23	5.0		
	~210	13.0	5.0			55	370		2.70			100		0.34		60.0	GENM195
zesty italian, prep[3] 1 cup	300		20.0	32.0	8.0	2.0	850	20					0	0.30	5.0		
	~236	10.0	4.0			50	460		2.70			300		0.26		60.0	GENM196
Noodles & Sce, avg for 11 flvrs, Lipton[4] - 2/3 cup (1 cup prep)	307		5.7	41.7		1.7	873	71					4	0.61	4.1		
	62	12.4	4.7			71			2.37			500		0.35		100.0	UNLV151
Pasta & Sce, avg for 8 flvrs, Lipton[5] - 2/3 cup (1 cup prep)	311		5.6	45.0		1.3	915	116					1	0.53	3.5		
	62	10.3	3.6			12			1.76			450		0.30		102.5	UNLV139
red bean chili cup, Knorr 1.73 oz container	170		9.0	32.0	8.0	8.0	970	80					6				
	49	1.0	0.0			0			1.80			500					UNLV87
Rice & Sce, avg for 13 flvrs, Lipton[6] - 1/2 cup (1 cup prep)	265		3.8	45.5	2.0	1.6	886	20					2	0.35	2.8		
	64	6.8	1.8			3			1.98			412		0.11		84.6	UNLV128

	KCAL	H₂0 (g)	PRO (g)	CHO (g)	SUGR (g)	DFIB (g)	Na (mg)	Ca (mg)	Mg (mg)	Zn (mg)	Mn (mg)	A (mcg RAE)	C (mg)	B-1 (mg)	NIA (mg)	B-12 (mcg)	PANT (mg)
	WT (g)	FAT (g)	SFA (g)	MUFA (g)	PUFA (g)	CHOL (mg)	K (mg)	P (mg)	Fe (mg)	Cu (mg)	Se (mcg)	A (IU)	E (mg ATE)	B-2 (mg)	B-6 (mg)	FOL (mcg DFE)	REF
tacos, crispy w/grnd beef, prep,	300	17.0	19.0	2.0	2.0	840	100					1					
Old El Paso Dinner Kit - *2 tacos*	~114	17.0	6.0			55			1.80			300					GENM198
soft w/grnd beef, prep, Old El	390		22.0	33.0	2.0	2.0	1270	80					1				
Paso Dinner Kit - *2 tacos*	~176	19.0	7.0			65			3.60			300					GENM199
three cheese & mac cup, Knorr	250		8.0	44.0	5.0	1.0	990	80					0				
2.1 oz container	59	4.5	2.0			10			1.08			0					UNLV97
tomato pasta cup, Knorr	170		5.0	34.0	7.0	0.0	820	20					0				
1.48 oz container	42	2.0	0.5			0	360		0.36			200					UNLV98
Tuna Helper, cheesy broc, prep[7]	290		15.0	37.0	7.0	1.0	860	100					0	0.30	5.0		
1 cup	~247	9.0	3.0			20	360		1.44			300		0.34		60.0	GENM200
creamy pasta, prep[7]	290		12.0	32.0	5.0	2.0	880	60					0	0.23	5.0		
1 cup	~246	13.0	3.5			15	280		1.44			500		0.17		60.0	GENM201
garden cheddar, prep[7]	290		13.0	36.0	6.0	1.0	990	100					0	0.30	5.0		
1 cup	~253	11.0	3.0			20	280		1.44			400		0.26		60.0	GENM202
tetrazzini, prep[7]	300		14.0	34.0	3.0	1.0	970	60					0	0.38	5.0		
1 cup	~239	12.0	3.0			20	210		1.80			400		0.26		60.0	GENM203
tuna melt, prep[7]	300		12.0	34.0	6.0	0.0	920	100					0	0.23	4.0		
1 cup	~238	13.0	3.5			20	280		1.08			400		0.26		40.0	GENM204

[1] Values are averages for chicken fried rice and teriyaki rice.

[2] Values are for entrées prepared with boneless, skinless chicken breasts according to package instructions.

[3] Values are for entrées prepared with lean ground beef according to package instructions.

[4] Values are averages for alfredo, alfredo broccoli, beef, butter, butter and herb, chicken, chicken broccoli, cream and chives, creamy chicken flavor, parmesan, and stroganoff.

[5] Values are averages for cheddar broccoli, cheesy cheddar, creamy garlic, creamy tomato parmesan, Italian cheese, roasted garlic and olive oil with sundried tomatoes, roasted garlic chicken cavatelli pasta, and three cheese rotini.

[6] Values are averages for Cajun, Cajun with beans, cheddar broccoli, chicken broccoli, chicken parmesan risotto, creamy chicken, creamy garlic parmesan risotto, herb and butter, mushroom, original wild rice, pilaf, rice medley, and Spanish.

[7] Values are for entrees prepared with water pack canned tuna according to package instructions.

10. FAST FOODS & RESTAURANT FOODS
10.1 GENERIC FAST FOODS

	KCAL	H₂0 (g)	PRO (g)	CHO (g)	SUGR (g)	DFIB (g)	Na (mg)	Ca (mg)	Mg (mg)	Zn (mg)	Mn (mg)	A (mcg RAE)	C (mg)	B-1 (mg)	NIA (mg)	B-12 (mcg)	PANT (mg)
	WT (g)	FAT (g)	SFA (g)	MUFA (g)	PUFA (g)	CHOL (mg)	K (mg)	P (mg)	Fe (mg)	Cu (mg)	Se (mcg)	A (IU)	E (mg ATE)	B-2 (mg)	B-6 (mg)	FOL (mcg DFE)	REF
biscuit, egg	373	68.1	11.6	31.9		0.8	891	82	19	0.99	0.261	180	<1	0.30	2.2	0.63	0.89
1 biscuit	136	22.1	4.7	9.1	6.4	245	238	388	2.90	0.061	27.3	620	3.3	0.49	0.11	80.2	21002
egg & bacon	458	70.0	17.0	28.6		0.8	999	189	24	1.64	0.279	56	3	0.14	2.4	1.04	1.22
1 biscuit	150	31.1	8.0	13.4	7.5	353	251	239	3.74	0.113	30.9	191	2.1	0.23	0.14	81.0	21003
egg & cheese	340	82.2	15.6	25.9		0.8	804	225	22	1.65	0.219	201	1	0.26	2.1	1.14	0.88
1 biscuit	146	19.4	6.6	8.3	2.6	291	188	302	2.98	0.110	33.7	669		0.57	0.13	140.2	21104
egg & ham	442	104.9	20.4	30.3		0.8	1382	221	31	2.23	0.305	252	0	0.67	2.0	1.19	1.67
1 biscuit	192	27.0	5.9	11.0	7.7	300	319	317	4.55	0.138	36.9	874	2.2	0.60	0.27	88.3	21004
egg & sausage	581	77.2	19.2	41.1		0.9	1141	155	25	2.16	0.315	184	0	0.50	3.6	1.37	1.53
1 biscuit	180	38.7	15.0	16.4	4.4	302	320	490	3.96	0.104	34.2	635	2.8	0.45	0.20	82.8	21005
egg & steak	410	77.7	17.9	21.3			888	138	25	2.80	0.244	206	<1	0.36	3.1	1.41	1.08
1 biscuit	148	28.4	8.6	11.7	5.8	272	306	225	5.30	0.107	31.4	704		0.52	0.18	75.5	21006
egg, cheese, & bacon	477	59.3	16.3	33.4			1260	164	20	1.54	0.255	190	2	0.30	2.3	1.05	1.18
1 biscuit	144	31.4	11.4	14.2	3.5	261	230	459	2.55	0.075	35.6	648		0.43	0.10	64.8	21007
ham	386	32.1	13.4	43.8		0.8	1433	160	23	1.65	0.362	34	<1	0.51	3.5	0.03	0.41
1 biscuit	113	18.4	11.4	4.8	1.0	25	197	554	2.72	0.036	19.3	133	2.2	0.32	0.14	59.9	21008
sausage	485	36.3	12.1	40.0		1.4	1071	128	20	1.55	0.360	16	<1	0.40	3.3	0.51	0.36
1 biscuit	124	31.8	14.2	12.8	3.0	35	198	446	2.58	0.050	23.2	56	3.1	0.29	0.11	71.9	21009
brownie	243	7.6	2.7	39.0			153	25	16	0.55	0.109	3	3	0.07	0.6	0.16	0.33
2.1 oz brownie (2" sq)	60	10.1	3.1	3.8	2.6	10	83	88	1.29	0.000	3.8	11		0.13	0.02	26.4	21027
burrito, bean	447	114.0	14.1	71.4			985	113	87	1.52	0.868	17	2	0.63	4.1	1.09	2.00
2 burritos	217	13.5	6.9	4.7	1.2	4	653	98	4.51	0.378	21.9	332		0.61	0.30	134.5	21060
bean & cheese	378	100.3	15.1	55.0			1166	214	80	1.64	0.432	99	2	0.22	3.6	0.89	1.60
2 burritos	186	11.7	6.8	2.5	1.8	28	497	180	2.27	0.352	16.9	1250		0.71	0.24	104.2	21061
bean & chili pepper	412	110.9	16.4	58.1			1044	100	71	3.41	0.783	10	1	0.45	4.4	1.16	1.88
2 burritos	204	14.7	7.6	5.4	1.0	33	579	114	4.55	0.333	18.4	204		0.71	0.29	136.7	21062
bean & meat	508	119.9	22.5	66.0			1335	106	83	3.83	0.832	32	2	0.53	5.4	1.73	2.24
2 burritos	231	17.8	8.3	7.0	1.2	49	656	141	4.90	0.377	30.5	635		0.83	0.37	145.5	21063
bean, cheese, & beef	331	131.8	14.6	39.7			991	130	51	2.35	0.396	150	5	0.30	3.9	1.10	1.66
2 burritos	203	13.3	7.1	4.5	1.0	124	410	140	3.74	0.329	17.7	800		0.71	0.22	85.3	21064
bean, cheese, & chili	662	187.4	33.3	85.2			2060	289	97	6.08	0.813	185	7	0.54	7.7	1.98	2.89
pepper - *2 burritos*	336	23.0	11.2	8.5	1.3	158	810	286	7.69	0.588	44.4	1596		1.21	0.40	178.1	21065

	KCAL / WT (g)	H₂O (g) / FAT (g)	PRO (g) / SFA (g)	CHO (g) / MUFA (g)	SUGR (g) / PUFA (g)	DFIB (g) / CHOL (mg)	Na (mg) / K (mg)	Ca (mg) / P (mg)	Mg (mg) / Fe (mg)	Zn (mg) / Cu (mg)	Mn (mg) / Se (mcg)	A (mcg RAE) / A (IU)	C (mg) / E (mg ATE)	B-1 (mg) / B-2 (mg)	NIA (mg) / B-6 (mg)	B-12 (mcg) / FOL (mcg DFE)	PANT (mg) / REF
beef	524	109.1	26.6	58.5			1492	84	81	4.73	0.785	13	1	0.24	6.4	1.96	2.99
2 burritos	220	20.8	10.5	7.4	0.9	64	739	174	6.09	0.409	36.7	277		0.92	0.31	193.6	21066
beef & chili pepper	426	109.4	21.5	49.4			1116	86	60	4.32	0.746	24	2	0.40	5.1	1.29	1.87
2 burritos	201	16.5	8.0	6.1	1.0	54	498	141	4.44	0.316	23.9	462		0.80	0.30	138.7	21067
beef, cheese, & chili	632	167.8	40.9	63.7			2092	222	70	7.90	0.608	198	4	0.61	8.3	2.07	3.01
pepper - 2 burritos	304	24.8	10.4	9.9	2.2	170	666	316	7.81	0.362	33.4	973		1.25	0.36	197.6	21068
fruit (apple/cherry)	231	26.4	2.5	35.0			212	16	7	0.40	0.130	21	1	0.17	1.9	0.51	0.95
1 small	74	9.5	4.6	3.4	1.1	4	104	15	1.07	0.081	6.9	406		0.18	0.07	39.2	21069a
	484	55.2	5.2	73.3			443	33	16	0.84	0.271	43	2	0.36	3.9	1.07	1.98
1 large	155	19.9	9.6	7.2	2.2	8	219	31	2.25	0.171	14.4	849		0.37	0.16	82.2	21069b
cheeseburger, large, double meat	704	131.8	38.0	39.7			1148	240	52	6.68	0.317	62	1	0.36	7.2	3.41	0.85
w/lettuce, & tomato - 1 sandwich	258	43.7	17.7	17.4	4.7	142	596	395	5.91	0.206	28.9	348		0.49	0.41	92.9	21100
single meat w/ham, lettuce, &	744	127.1	39.5	37.7			1712	302	51	6.63	0.373	84	7	0.53	9.2	2.87	1.04
tomato - 1 sandwich	254	48.2	21.1	18.9	3.9	122	538	531	5.03	0.246	32.5	505		0.56	0.38	99.1	21099
single meat w/lettuce, &	563	115.0	28.2	38.4			1108	206	44	4.60	0.311	140	8	0.39	7.4	2.56	0.72
tomato - 1 sandwich	219	32.9	15.0	12.6	2.0	88	445	311	4.66	0.186	37.4	613	1.2	0.46	0.28	118.3	21098
triple meat	796	164.5	56.1	26.7			1213	283	61	10.88	0.353	106	3	0.61	11.5	5.90	1.16
1 sandwich	304	51.0	21.7	21.5	3.2	161	821	541	8.30	0.258	25.5	359		0.64	0.61	82.1	21101
cheeseburger, reg, double meat	457	65.7	27.7	22.1			636	233	33	4.96	0.234	99	0	0.25	6.0	2.31	0.62
1 sandwich	155	28.5	13.0	11.0	1.9	110	308	374	3.41	0.130	32.1	332	1.2	0.37	0.25	96.1	21092
double meat & double-decker	461	69.4	22.1	44.3			891	224	34	4.35	0.304	83	0	0.34	6.0	1.92	0.66
bun - 1 sandwich	160	21.6	9.5	8.3	1.8	80	285	338	3.70	0.141	34.1	277		0.38	0.22	94.4	21094
double meat, double-decker bun	650	106.2	29.7	53.1			921	169	36	4.13	0.274	78	3	0.57	8.3	2.07	0.64
w/lettuce & tom - 1 sandwich	228	35.3	12.8	12.6	6.4	93	390	349	4.72	0.162	39.4	372	2.0	0.43	0.27	132.2	21095
double meat w/lettuce, & tom	417	85.0	21.2	35.2			1051	171	30	3.49	0.299	71	2	0.35	8.1	1.93	0.43
1 sandwich	166	21.1	8.7	7.8	2.7	60	335	242	3.42	0.149	23.6	398		0.28	0.18	88.0	21093
single meat	295	53.9	16.0	26.5			616	111	20	2.09	0.176	86	2	0.25	3.7	0.94	0.32
1 sandwich	113	14.1	6.3	5.3	1.1	37	223	176	2.43	0.101	19.8	462	0.5	0.23	0.11	79.1	21090
single meat w/lettuce & tom	359	85.0	17.8	28.1			976	182	26	2.62	0.293	82	2	0.32	6.4	1.23	0.34
1 sandwich	154	19.8	9.2	7.2	1.5	52	229	216	2.65	0.123	20.5	431		0.23	0.15	95.5	21091
chicken, breaded & fried, boneless	319	50.1	18.0	15.3	0.0	0.0	513	14	24	1.00	0.118	0	0	0.12	7.5	0.31	0.85
6 pieces	106	20.6	4.7	10.5	4.6	61	305	289	0.94	0.063	17.3	0	1.4	0.16	0.31	44.5	21037
w/bbq sce	330	67.4	17.1	25.0			829	21	25	1.12	0.163	17	1	0.10	7.0	0.30	0.96
6 pieces	130	18.0	5.6	8.8	2.4	61	319	215	1.46	0.173	17.2	342		0.16	0.34	31.2	21038
w/honey sce	329	52.2	16.8	26.9			537	17	20	1.08	0.138	30	<1	0.09	6.8	0.30	0.91
6 pieces	115	17.5	5.5	8.6	2.2	61	255	202	1.32	0.173	16.6	101		0.15	0.31	42.6	21039
w/mustard sce	322	70.5	17.4	20.9			790	25	26	1.14	0.165	22	<1	0.12	6.9	0.31	0.92
6 pieces	130	18.9	5.7	9.0	2.9	61	280	218	1.48	0.168	26.5	109		0.16	0.31	42.9	21040
w/sweet & sour sce	346	64.0	17.0	29.0			677	21	23	1.09	0.151	61	1	0.10	6.9	0.36	0.92
6 pieces	130	18.0	5.5	8.6	2.2	61	277	211	1.48	0.170	16.9	242		0.20	0.33	42.9	21041
chicken, breaded & fried, dark meat	431	72.5	30.1	15.7			755	36	37	3.24	0.127	67	0	0.13	7.2	0.83	2.46
drumstick & thigh	148	26.7	7.0	10.9	6.3	166	445	240	1.60	0.118	35.1	222		0.43	0.33	37.0	21035
light meat	494	74.5	35.7	19.6			975	60	37	1.55	0.155	57	0	0.15	12.0	0.67	2.59
side breast & wing	163	29.5	7.8	12.2	6.8	148	566	306	1.48	0.101	35.4	192		0.29	0.57	44.0	21036
chicken fillet sandwich	515	86.1	24.1	38.7			957	60	35	1.87	0.473	31	9	0.33	6.8	0.38	0.60
1 sandwich	182	29.4	8.5	10.4	8.4	60	353	233	4.68	0.231	40.4	100		0.24	0.20	149.2	21102
w/cheese	632	104.9	29.4	41.6			1238	258	43	2.90	0.381	164	3	0.41	9.1	0.46	1.35
1 sandwich	228	38.8	12.4	13.7	9.9	78	333	406	3.63	0.171	48.1	620		0.46	0.41	155.0	21103
chili con carne	256	194.1	24.6	21.9			1007	68	46	3.57	0.397	83	2	0.13	2.5	1.14	3.59
1 cup	253	8.3	3.4	3.4	0.5	134	691	197	5.19	0.595	44.0	1662		1.14	0.33	55.7	21042
chimichanga, beef	425	88.2	19.6	42.8			910	63	63	4.96	0.557	7	5	0.49	5.8	1.51	2.05
1 chimichanga	174	19.7	8.5	8.1	1.1	9	586	124	4.54	0.423	23.7	146		0.64	0.28	120.1	21070
beef w/cheese	443	96.4	20.1	39.3			957	238	60	3.37	0.489	132	3	0.38	4.7	1.30	1.79
1 chimichanga	183	23.4	11.2	9.4	0.7	51	203	187	3.84	0.351	23.1	540		0.86	0.22	131.8	21071
beef w/cheese & red chili	364	106.5	14.7	38.3			895	218	41	4.63	0.391	50	2	0.23	3.5	1.28	1.48
peppers - 1 chimichanga	180	17.6	8.4	7.1	0.5	50	329	146	3.15	0.563	24.7	702		0.95	0.16	129.6	21073
beef w/red chili peppers	424	103.1	18.1	45.8			1169	70	65	3.02	0.616	13	<1	0.29	5.3	1.08	2.19
1 chimichanga	190	19.1	8.3	7.8	1.1	10	614	112	4.18	0.276	24.3	262		0.67	0.23	131.1	21072
clams, breaded & fried	451	33.6	12.8	38.8			834	21	31	1.63	0.308	37	0	0.21	2.9	1.10	0.30
3/4 cup	115	26.4	6.6	11.4	6.8	87	266	238	3.05	0.095	9.5	122		0.26	0.03	65.6	21043
coleslaw	147	73.3	1.5	12.8			267	34	9	0.20	0.124	36	8	0.04	0.1		0.15
3/4 cup	99	11.0	1.6	2.4	6.4	5	177	36	0.72	0.042	1.0	338		0.03	0.11	38.6	21127

	KCAL / WT (g)	H₂0 (g) / FAT (g)	PRO (g) / SFA (g)	CHO (g) / MUFA (g)	SUGR (g) / PUFA (g)	DFIB (g) / CHOL (mg)	Na (mg) / K (mg)	Ca (mg) / P (mg)	Mg (mg) / Fe (mg)	Zn (mg) / Cu (mg)	Mn (mg) / Se (mcg)	A (mcg RAE) / A (IU)	C (mg) / E (mg ATE)	B-1 (mg) / B-2 (mg)	NIA (mg) / B-6 (mg)	B-12 (mcg) / FOL (mcg DFE)	PANT (mg) / REF
cookies, animal crackers	299	2.5	4.1	50.5			273	11	11	0.30	0.326	7	1	0.25	2.5	0.05	0.21
1 box	67	9.0	3.5	3.8	1.0	11	56	64	1.47	0.051	4.7	27	0.3	0.24	0.02	122.6	21029
choc chip	233	2.9	2.9	36.2			188	20	17	0.34	0.237	11	1	0.09	1.4	0.10	0.14
1 box	55	12.1	5.3	5.1	1.0	12	82	52	1.47	0.184	3.3	52	0.4	0.19	0.03	45.1	21030
corn dog (frank w/corn flour	460	81.7	16.8	55.8			973	102	18	1.31	0.193	60	0	0.28	4.2	0.44	1.35
coating) - 1 corn dog	175	18.9	5.2	9.1	3.5	79	263	166	6.18	0.245	22.2	207		0.70	0.09	134.8	21120
corn-on-the-cob w/butter	155	105.2	4.5	31.9			29	4	41	0.91	0.000	34	7	0.25	2.2	0.00	0.37
1 ear	146	3.4	1.6	1.0	0.6	6	359	108	0.88	0.000	1.0	391		0.10	0.32	43.8	21128
crab cake	160	32.0	11.3	5.1		0.2	491	202	25	2.12	0.282	93	<1	0.06	1.2	4.40	0.27
2.1 oz cake	60	10.4	2.2	4.3	3.1	82	162	227	1.12	0.366	25.3	313		0.08	0.15	35.4	21046
croissant, egg & cheese	368	57.7	12.8	24.3			551	244	22	1.75	0.226	277	<1	0.19	1.5	0.77	1.05
1 croissant	127	24.7	14.1	7.5	1.4	216	174	348	2.20	0.091	24.5	1001		0.38	0.10	54.6	21011
egg, cheese, & bacon	413	56.7	16.2	23.6			889	151	23	1.90	0.222	142	2	0.35	2.2	0.86	1.07
1 croissant	129	28.4	15.4	9.2	1.8	215	201	276	2.19	0.099	24.5	472		0.34	0.12	52.9	21012
egg, cheese, & ham	474	77.7	18.9	24.2			1081	144	26	2.17	0.220	131	11	0.52	3.2	1.00	1.25
1 croissant	154	33.6	17.5	11.4	2.4	213	272	336	2.13	0.126	27.2	451		0.30	0.23	51.7	21013
egg, cheese, & sausage	523	73.4	20.3	24.7			1115	144	24	2.14	0.253	123	<1	0.99	4.0	0.90	1.31
1 croissant	160	38.2	18.2	14.3	3.0	216	283	290	3.04	0.109	20.6	422		0.32	0.11	46.4	21014
danish pastry, cheese	353	30.8	5.8	28.7			319	70	15	0.63	0.350	45	3	0.26	2.5	0.23	0.57
3.2 oz pastry	91	24.6	5.1	15.6	2.4	20	116	80	1.85	0.086	17.2	155		0.21	0.05	82.8	21015
fruit	335	27.3	4.8	45.1			333	22	14	0.48	0.193	25	2	0.29	1.8	0.24	0.59
3.3 oz pastry	94	15.9	3.3	10.1	1.6	19	110	69	1.40	0.055	13.9	86		0.21	0.06	42.3	21017
eggs, scrambled	199	62.7	13.0	2.0		0.0	211	54	13	1.56	0.040	251	3	0.08	0.2	0.95	0.88
2 eggs	94	15.2	5.8	5.5	1.9	400	138	227	2.43	0.063	21.2	836	1.6	0.49	0.18	52.6	21018
enchilada w/cheese & beef	323	128.4	11.9	30.5			1319	228	83	2.69	0.584	98	1	0.10	2.5	1.02	1.44
1 enchilada	192	17.6	9.0	6.1	1.4	40	574	167	3.07	0.518	9.8	1135		0.40	0.27	67.2	21075
w/cheese & sour cream	319	103.1	9.6	28.5			784	324	51	2.51	0.240	99	1	0.08	1.9	0.75	1.52
1 enchilada	163	18.8	10.6	6.3	0.8	44	240	134	1.32	0.259	10.1	1161		0.42	0.39	86.4	21074
enchirito w/cheese, beef, & beans	344	121.0	17.9	33.8			1251	218	71	2.76	0.384	89	5	0.17	3.0	1.62	1.83
1 enchirito	193	16.1	7.9	6.5	0.3	50	560	224	2.39	0.270	8.1	1015		0.69	0.21	119.7	21076
english muffin w/butter	189	20.6	4.9	30.4			386	103	13	0.42	0.209	32	1	0.25	2.6	0.02	0.14
1 muffin	63	5.8	2.4	1.5	1.3	13	69	85	1.59	0.064	11.7	136	0.1	0.32	0.04	84.4	21019
w/cheese & sausage	393	43.4	15.3	29.2		1.5	1036	168	24	1.68	0.220	93	1	0.70	4.1	0.68	0.53
1 muffin sandwich	115	24.3	9.9	10.1	2.7	59	215	186	2.25	0.076	21.3	380	0.5	0.25	0.15	100.1	21020
w/egg, cheese, & canadian	289	77.8	16.7	26.7	2.8	1.5	729	151	23	1.56	0.012	177	2	0.49	3.3	0.67	0.89
bacon - *1 muffin sandwich*	137	12.6	4.7	4.7	1.6	234	199	270	2.44	0.070	34.0	586	0.9	0.45	0.15	86.3	21021
w/egg, cheese, & sausage	487	78.2	21.7	31.0			1135	196	30	2.36	0.299	196	1	0.84	4.5	1.37	1.40
1 muffin sandwich	165	30.9	12.4	12.7	3.3	274	294	287	3.47	0.119	31.0	660		0.50	0.20	113.9	21022
fish fillet, battered/breaded &	211	48.7	13.3	15.4		0.5	484	16	22	0.40	0.168	10	0	0.10	1.9	1.01	0.18
fried - 3.2 oz fillet	91	11.2	2.6	2.3	5.7	31	291	156	1.92	0.041	8.3	35		0.10	0.09	18.2	21047
fish sandwich w/tartar sce	431	74.8	16.9	41.0			615	84	33	1.00	0.365	33	3	0.33	3.4	1.07	0.58
1 sandwich	158	22.8	5.2	7.7	8.2	55	340	212	2.61	0.191	79.9	109	0.9	0.22	0.11	113.8	21105
w/tartar sce & cheese	523	82.7	20.6	47.6			939	185	37	1.17	0.362	130	3	0.46	4.2	1.08	0.44
1 sandwich	183	28.6	8.1	8.9	9.4	68	353	311	3.50	0.119	88.6	432	1.8	0.42	0.11	133.6	21106
french toast sticks	513	42.2	8.3	57.9		2.7	499	78	27	0.93	0.219	14	0	0.23	3.0	0.07	0.56
5 sticks	141	29.0	4.7	12.6	9.9	75	127	123	2.96	0.271	23.5	45	4.0	0.25	0.25	101.5	21024
french toast w/butter	356	68.5	10.3	36.0			513	73	16	0.59	0.209	136	<1	0.58	3.9	0.36	0.54
2 slices	135	18.8	7.7	7.1	2.4	116	177	146	1.89	0.065	20.9	473		0.50	0.05	102.6	21023
fries, fried in veg oil	458	47.4	5.8	53.3	0.0	4.7	265	19	52	0.63	0.346	0	16	0.11	3.8	0.00	0.67
20–25 fries (reg size)	134	24.7	5.2	14.3	4.2	0	923	173	1.05	0.201	0.8	0	1.6	0.05	0.48	50.9	21138b
	578	59.7	7.3	67.3	0.0	5.9	335	24	66	0.79	0.436	0	20	0.14	4.8	0.00	0.85
30–40 fries (large size)	169	31.1	6.5	18.0	5.3	0	1164	218	1.32	0.254	1.0	0	2.1	0.07	0.61	64.2	21138a
frijoles w/cheese	225	115.4	11.4	28.7			882	189	85	1.74	0.503	35	2	0.13	1.5	0.68	1.10
1 cup	167	7.8	4.1	2.6	0.7	37	605	175	2.24	0.341	2.8	456		0.33	0.20	111.9	21077
ham & cheese sandwich	352	74.2	20.7	33.3			771	130	16	1.37	0.139	96	3	0.31	2.7	0.54	1.04
1 sandwich	146	15.5	6.4	6.7	1.4	58	291	152	3.24	0.183	23.1	320	0.3	0.48	0.20	78.8	21116
ham, egg, & cheese sandwich	347	73.1	19.2	30.9			1005	212	26	1.99	0.243	166	3	0.43	4.2	1.23	0.94
1 sandwich	143	16.3	7.4	5.7	1.7	246	210	346	3.10	0.122	32.5	562	0.6	0.56	0.16	98.7	21117
hamburger, large, double meat	540	121.5	34.3	40.3			791	102	50	5.67	0.249	5	1	0.36	7.6	4.07	0.54
w/lettuce, & tomato - *1 sandwich*	226	26.6	10.5	10.3	2.8	122	570	314	5.85	0.219	25.5	102		0.38	0.54	110.7	21114
single meat	427	89.0	23.1	36.8	8.3	2.1	731	134	34	4.76	0.344	5	3	0.34	6.6	2.58	0.52
1 sandwich	172	21.0	7.9	9.3	1.6	71	396	213	4.15	0.273		110	<0.1	0.28	0.25	87.7	21202

| | KCAL | H₂O (g) | PRO (g) | CHO (g) | SUGR (g) | DFIB (g) | Na (mg) | Ca (mg) | Mg (mg) | Zn (mg) | Mn (mg) | A (mcg RAE) | C (mg) | B-1 (mg) | NIA (mg) | B-12 (mcg) | PANT (mg) |
	WT (g)	FAT (g)	SFA (g)	MUFA (g)	PUFA (g)	CHOL (mg)	K (mg)	P (mg)	Fe (mg)	Cu (mg)	Se (mcg)	A (IU)	E (mg ATE)	B-2 (mg)	B-6 (mg)	FOL (mcg DFE)	REF
triple meat	692	135.6	50.0	28.6			712	65	54	10.75	0.233	8	1	0.31	11.0	4.92	0.67
1 sandwich	259	41.5	15.9	18.2	2.7	142	785	394	8.31	0.197	55.7	158		0.54	0.62	106.2	21115
hamburger, reg, double meat	544	72.3	29.9	42.9			554	86	37	5.72	0.282	0	0	0.33	8.3	2.92	0.67
1 sandwich	176	27.9	10.4	12.1	2.3	99	363	234	4.56	0.167	39.6	0	1.3	0.37	0.32	105.6	21110
single meat	275	33.8	12.3	30.5			387	63	19	2.00	0.213	0	0	0.33	3.7	0.89	0.37
1 sandwich	90	11.8	4.1	5.5	0.9	35	145	103	2.40	0.090	21.7	0	0.5	0.27	0.06	72.9	21107
single meat w/lettuce &	279	54.4	12.9	27.3			504	63	22	2.06	0.253	4	2	0.23	3.7	0.88	0.30
tomato - 1 sandwich	110	13.5	4.1	5.3	2.6	26	227	124	2.63	0.102	20.6	83		0.20	0.12	74.8	21109
hash brown potatoes	151	43.3	1.9	16.1			290	7	16	0.22	0.110	1	5	0.08	1.1	0.01	0.34
1/2 cup	72	9.2	4.3	3.9	0.5	9	267	69	0.48	0.070	0.2	18	0.1	0.01	0.17	7.9	21026
hot dog	242	52.9	10.4	18.0			670	24	13	1.98	0.091	0	<1	0.24	3.6	0.51	0.51
1 hot dog	98	14.5	5.1	6.9	1.7	44	143	97	2.31	0.076	26.0	0		0.27	0.05	60.8	21118
w/chili	296	54.5	13.5	31.3			480	19	10	0.78	0.114	3	3	0.22	3.7	0.30	0.55
1 hot dog	114	13.4	4.9	6.6	1.2	51	166	192	3.28	0.103	13.0	58		0.40	0.05	88.9	21119
hush puppies	257	25.2	4.9	34.9			965	69	16	0.43	0.267	9	0	0.00	2.0	0.17	0.22
5 pieces	78	11.6	2.7	7.8	0.4	135	188	190	1.43	0.204	8.0	94		0.02	0.10	83.5	21129
ice milk, van, soft serve w/cone	164	67.4	3.9	24.1		0.1	92	153	15	0.57	0.021	49	1	0.05	0.3	0.21	0.27
1 cone	103	6.1	3.5	1.8	0.4	28	169	139	0.15	0.019	3.8	211	0.4	0.26	0.06	17.5	21028
nachos w/cheese	346	45.7	9.1	36.3			816	272	55	1.79	0.224	149	1	0.19	1.5	0.82	1.31
6–8 nachos	113	19.0	7.8	8.0	2.2	18	172	276	1.28	0.140	15.7	559		0.37	0.20	10.2	21078
& jalapeno peppers	608	87.1	16.8	60.1			1736	620	108	2.90	0.439	573	1	0.12	2.8	1.02	2.45
6–8 nachos	204	34.1	14.0	14.4	4.0	84	294	394	2.45	0.173	14.1	4062		0.49	0.37	18.4	21079
beans, grnd beef, &	569	142.7	19.8	55.8			1800	385	97	3.65	0.423	436	5	0.23	3.3	1.02	2.52
peppers - 6–8 nachos	255	30.7	12.5	11.0	5.7	20	451	388	2.78	0.745	13.8	3402		0.69	0.41	38.3	21080
nachos w/cinn & sugar	592	1.1	7.2	63.4			439	85	20	0.59	0.493	5	8	0.19	3.9	1.72	1.90
6–8 nachos	109	36.0	18.2	11.8	4.1	39	78	33	2.89	0.156	6.6	108		0.45	0.17	7.6	21081
onion rings, breaded & fried	276	30.8	3.7	31.3			430	73	16	0.35	0.296	1	1	0.08	0.9	0.12	0.20
8–9 rings	83	15.5	7.0	6.7	0.7	14	129	86	0.85	0.069	2.9	8	0.3	0.10	0.06	84.7	21130
oysters, battered/breaded & fried	368	66.7	12.5	39.9			677	28	24	15.64	0.424	108	4	0.31	4.4	1.01	1.06
6 oysters	139	17.9	4.6	6.9	4.6	108	182	196	4.46	0.796	92.2	363		0.35	0.03	43.1	21048
pancakes w/butter & syrup	520	115.4	8.3	90.9			1104	128	49	1.02	0.322	81	3	0.39	3.4	0.23	0.67
2 pancakes	232	14.0	5.9	5.3	2.0	58	251	476	2.62	0.151	19.3	281	1.4	0.56	0.12	62.6	21025
pizza, cheese	140	30.1	7.7	20.5			336	117	16	0.81	0.232	74	·1	0.18	2.5	0.33	0.22
1/8 of 12" pizza	63	3.2	1.5	1.0	0.5	9	110	113	0.58	0.081	13.5	382		0.16	0.04	43.5	21049
w/meat & veg	184	37.7	13.0	21.3			382	101	18	1.11	0.119	58	2	0.21	2.0	0.36	0.83
1/8 of 12" pizza	79	5.4	1.5	2.5	0.9	21	179	131	1.53	0.119	10.9	524		0.17	0.09	36.3	21050
w/pepperoni	181	33.0	10.1	19.9			267	65	9	0.52	0.099	53	2	0.13	3.0	0.18	0.25
1/8 of 12" pizza	71	7.0	2.2	3.1	1.2	14	153	75	0.94	0.064	13.1	282		0.23	0.06	46.2	21051
potato, baked w/cheese sce	474	194.6	14.6	46.5			382	311	65	1.89	0.515	252	26	0.24	3.3	0.18	1.30
1 potato	296	28.7	10.6	10.7	6.0	18	1166	320	3.02	0.630	7.7	835		0.21	0.71	26.0	21131
w/cheese sce & bacon	451	194.4	18.4	44.4			972	308	69	2.15	0.505	188	29	0.27	4.0	0.33	1.29
1 potato	299	25.9	10.1	9.7	4.8	30	1178	347	3.14	0.646	9.6	628		0.24	0.75	29.9	21132
w/cheese sce & broc	403	237.4	13.7	46.6			485	336	78	2.03	0.803	268	48	0.27	3.6	0.34	1.42
1 potato	339	21.4	8.5	7.7	4.2	20	1441	346	3.32	0.647	5.8	1695		0.27	0.78	61.0	21133
w/cheese sce & chili	482	276.8	23.2	55.9			699	411	111	3.79	0.675	186	32	0.28	4.2	0.24	2.57
1 potato	395	21.8	13.0	6.8	0.9	32	1572	498	6.12	0.826	5.5	766		0.36	0.95	47.4	21134
w/sour cream & chives	393	209.7	6.7	50.0			181	106	69	0.91	0.580	266	34	0.27	3.7	0.21	1.48
1 potato	302	22.3	10.0	7.9	3.3	24	1383	184	3.11	0.686	3.3	1347		0.18	0.79	33.2	21135
potato salad	108	74.8	1.5	12.9			312	13	8	0.19	0.070	29	1	0.07	0.3		0.35
1/3 cup	95	5.7	1.0	1.6	2.9	57	257	53	0.69	0.075	0.9	95		0.10	0.14	23.8	21140
potatoes, mashed	66	63.4	1.8	12.9			182	17	14	0.26	0.094	9	<1	0.07	1.0	0.04	0.38
1/3 cup	80	1.0	0.4	0.3	0.2	2	235	44	0.38	0.078	0.4	33		0.04	0.18	6.4	21139
roast beef sandwich	346	67.6	21.5	33.4			792	54	31	3.39	0.125	11	2	0.38	5.9	1.22	0.83
1 sandwich	139	13.8	3.6	6.8	1.7	51	316	239	4.23	0.097	29.2	210		0.31	0.26	68.1	21121

	KCAL	H₂O (g)	PRO (g)	CHO (g)	SUGR (g)	DFIB (g)	Na (mg)	Ca (mg)	Mg (mg)	Zn (mg)	Mn (mg)	A (mcg RAE)	C (mg)	B-1 (mg)	NIA (mg)	B-12 (mcg)	PANT (mg)
	WT (g)	FAT (g)	SFA (g)	MUFA (g)	PUFA (g)	CHOL (mg)	K (mg)	P (mg)	Fe (mg)	Cu (mg)	Se (mcg)	A (IU)	E (mg ATE)	B-2 (mg)	B-6 (mg)	FOL (mcg DFE)	REF
w/cheese	473	76.6	32.2	45.4			1633	183	40	5.37	0.312	58	0	0.39	5.9	2.06	0.69
1 sandwich	176	18.0	9.0	3.7	3.5	77	345	401	5.05	0.199	34.3	194		0.46	0.33	79.2	21122
salad, vegetable	33	197.7	2.6	6.7			54	27	23	0.43	0.304	118	48	0.06	1.1	0.00	0.25
1 1/2 cups	207	0.1	<0.1	<0.1	0.1	0	356	81	1.30	0.104	0.8	2352		0.10	0.17	76.6	21052
w/cheese & egg	102	196.3	8.8	4.8			119	100	24	1.00	0.273	104	10	0.09	1.0	0.30	0.52
1 1/2 cups	217	5.8	3.0	1.8	0.5	98	371	132	0.67	0.089	7.4	822		0.17	0.11	84.6	21053
w/chicken	105	189.8	17.4	3.7			209	37	33	0.89	0.249	52	17	0.11	5.9	0.20	0.59
1 1/2 cups	218	2.2	0.6	0.7	0.6	72	447	170	1.09	0.094	15.5	935		0.13	0.44	67.6	21054
w/pasta & seafood	379	335.1	16.4	32.0			1572	71	50	1.67	0.667	317	38	0.29	3.5	1.71	0.38
1 1/2 cups	417	20.9	2.6	4.8	9.1	50	600	204	3.17	0.363	44.6	6247		0.21	0.33	250.2	21055
w/shrimp	106	210.3	14.5	6.6			489	59	38	1.27	0.142	40	9	0.12	1.2	3.78	0.50
1 1/2 cups	236	2.5	0.7	0.8	0.5	179	404	160	0.90	0.160	38.2	791		0.17	0.14	87.3	21056
w/turkey, ham, & cheese	267	268.8	26.0	4.7			743	235	49	3.13	0.359	147	16	0.39	6.0	0.85	0.91
1 1/2 cups	326	16.1	8.2	5.2	1.4	140	401	401	1.96	0.166	36.8	1053		0.39	0.42	101.1	21057
scallops, breaded & fried	386	69.1	15.8	38.5			919	19	32	1.08	0.298	42	0	0.20	0.0	0.43	0.50
6 scallops	144	19.4	4.9	12.6	0.6	108	294	292	2.04	0.216	38.9	138		0.85	0.07	61.9	21058
shake, choc	264	148.7	7.1	42.6		1.7	202	235	35	0.85	0.081	46	1	0.12	0.3	0.71	0.81
10 fl oz	208	7.7	4.8	2.2	0.3	27	416	212	0.64	0.135	3.5	193	0.1	0.51	0.10	8.3	14346c
strawberry	320	209.7	9.6	53.5		1.1	235	320	37	1.02	0.042	74	2	0.13	0.5	0.88	1.39
10 fl oz	283	7.9	4.9			31	515	283	0.31	0.062	5.9	340		0.55	0.12	8.5	14428
van	231	155.4	7.3	37.2		0.8	171	254	25	0.75	0.029	64	2	0.09	0.4	0.75	0.87
10 fl oz	208	6.2	3.9	1.8	0.2	23	362	212	0.19	0.106	4.4	270	0.1	0.38	0.11	6.2	14347d
shrimp, breaded & fried	454	78.4	18.9	40.0			1446	84	39	1.21	0.333	36	0	0.21	0.0	0.15	0.48
6–8 shrimp	164	24.9	5.4	17.4	0.6	200	184	344	2.95	0.144	68.4	120		0.90	0.07	136.1	21059
steak sandwich w/lettuce,	459	104.2	30.3	52.0			798	90	49	4.53	0.367	20	6	0.41	7.3	1.57	0.92
tom, & mayo - 1 sandwich	204	14.1	5.3	5.3	3.3	73	524	298	5.16	0.220	42.0	367		0.37	0.37	128.5	21123
submarine sandwich, cheese	456	131.8	21.8	51.0			1651	189	68	2.58	0.531	71	12	1.00	5.5	1.09	0.89
& deli meats - 8 oz sub	228	18.6	6.8	8.2	2.3	36	394	287	2.51	0.303	30.8	424		0.80	0.14	109.4	21124
roast beef	410	127.4	28.6	44.3			845	41	67	4.38	0.432	30	6	0.41	6.0	1.81	0.78
8 oz sub	216	13.0	7.1	1.8	2.6	73	330	192	2.81	0.361	25.7	413		0.41	0.32	88.6	21125
tuna salad	584	139.0	29.7	55.4			1293	74	79	1.87	0.512	46	4	0.46	11.3	1.61	1.87
9 oz sub	256	28.0	5.3	13.4	7.3	49	335	220	2.64	0.428	60.2	187		0.33	0.23	135.7	21126
sundae, caramel	304	87.6	7.3	49.3		0.0	195	189	28	0.82	0.093	70	3	0.06	0.9	0.60	0.37
1 sundae	155	9.3	4.5	3.0	1.0	25	318	217	0.22	0.082	5.0	264	0.9	0.29	0.05	12.4	21032
hot fudge	284	94.3	5.6	47.7		0.0	182	207	33	0.95	0.126	58	2	0.06	1.1	0.65	0.33
1 sundae	158	8.6	5.0	2.3	0.8	21	395	228	0.58	0.130	5.2	221	0.7	0.30	0.13	9.5	21033
strawberry	268	93.2	6.3	44.6		0.0	92	161	24	0.66	0.168	57	2	0.06	0.9	0.64	0.44
1 sundae	153	7.8	3.7	2.7	1.0	21	271	155	0.32	0.077	4.4	222	0.8	0.28	0.08	18.4	21034
taco, large	568	153.6	31.8	41.1			1233	339	108	6.05	0.676	166	3	0.24	4.9	1.60	2.60
9.3 oz	263	31.6	17.5	10.1	1.5	87	729	313	3.71	0.316	36.0	1315		0.68	0.37	152.5	21082a
small	369	99.9	20.7	26.7			802	221	70	3.93	0.439	108	2	0.15	3.2	1.04	1.69
6 oz	171	20.6	11.4	6.6	1.0	56	474	203	2.41	0.205	23.4	855		0.44	0.24	99.2	21082b
taco salad	279	143.3	13.2	23.6			762	192	51	2.69	0.331	71	4	0.10	2.5	0.63	1.35
1 1/2 cups	198	14.8	6.8	5.2	1.7	44	416	143	2.28	0.224	4.4	588		0.36	0.22	112.9	21083
w/chili con carne	290	200.4	17.4	26.6			885	245	52	3.29	0.337	258	3	0.16	2.5	0.73	1.44
1 1/2 cups	261	13.1	6.0	4.5	1.5	5	392	154	2.66	0.300	7.6	1574		0.50	0.52	112.2	21084
tostada, beans & cheese	223	95.4	9.6	26.5			543	210	59	1.90	0.367	45	1	0.10	1.3	0.69	1.14
1 tostada	144	9.9	5.4	3.1	0.7	30	403	117	1.89	0.206	3.5	622		0.33	0.16	43.2	21085
beans, beef, & cheese	333	158.5	16.1	29.7			871	189	68	3.17	0.360	101	4	0.09	2.9	1.13	1.87
1 tostada	225	16.9	11.5	3.5	0.6	74	491	173	2.45	0.315	20.9	1276		0.50	0.25	85.5	21086
beef & cheese	315	101.1	19.0	22.8			897	217	64	3.68	0.504	51	3	0.10	3.1	1.17	1.89
1 tostada	163	16.3	10.4	3.3	1.0	41	572	179	2.87	0.264	19.1	712		0.55	0.23	117.4	21087
w/guacamole	360	189.3	12.5	32.0			799	423	73	4.07	0.352	209	4	0.13	2.0	0.99	2.01
2 tostadas	261	23.3	9.9	8.5	3.1	39	650	232	1.62	0.253	7.0	1751		0.57	0.26	117.5	21088

	KCAL	H₂O (g)	PRO (g)	CHO (g)	SUGR (g)	DFIB (g)	Na (mg)	Ca (mg)	Mg (mg)	Zn (mg)	Mn (mg)	A (mcg RAE)	C (mg)	B-1 (mg)	NIA (mg)	B-12 (mcg)	PANT (mg)
	WT (g)	FAT (g)	SFA (g)	MUFA (g)	PUFA (g)	CHOL (mg)	K (mg)	P (mg)	Fe (mg)	Cu (mg)	Se (mcg)	A (IU)	E (mg ATE)	B-2 (mg)	B-6 (mg)	FOL (mcg DFE)	REF

10.2 ARBY'S

Food	KCAL/WT	H₂O/FAT	PRO/SFA	CHO/MUFA	SUGR/PUFA	DFIB/CHOL	Na/K	Ca/P	Mg/Fe	A-RAE/A-IU	C/E	REF
biscuit w/bacon	360		9.0	27.0		1.0	1000	40		0		
3.4 oz biscuit	96	24.0	7.0			10			0.36			ARBY1
w/butter	280		5.0	27.0		0.5	780	40		0		
2.9 oz biscuit	82	17.0	4.0			0			0.00			ARBY2
w/ham	330		12.0	28.0		1.0	1610	40		0		
4.4 oz biscuit	125	20.0	5.0			30			0.72			ARBY3
w/sausage	460		12.0	28.0		1.0	1080	0		0		
4.3 oz biscuit	122	33.0	9.0			25			0.72			ARBY4
chicken finger 4-pack	640		31.0	42.0		0.0	1590	20		0		
6.8 oz	192	38.0	8.0			70			2.70			ARBY9
snack	580		19.0	55.0		3.0	1450	0			9	
6.4 oz serving	181	32.0	7.0			35			2.70			ARBY10
croissant w/bacon	340		10.0	28.0		1.0	520	0		0		
2.7 oz croissant	76	23.0	13.0			30			3.78			ARBY11
w/ham	310		13.0	29.0		0.0	1130					
3.7 oz croissant	105	19.0	11.0			50			3.42			ARBY12
w/sausage	440		13.0	29.0		0.0	600			0		
3.6 oz croissant	102	32.0	15.0			45			0.72			ARBY13
croutons, cheese & garlic	100		2.5	10.0		0.0	138					
.63 oz	18	6.3										ARBY14
seasoned	30		1.0	5.0		1.0	70	0		0		
.25 oz	7	1.0	0.0			0			0.36			ARBY15
french toast syrup	130		0.0	32.0		0.0	45	0		0		
~ 2 T (1 fl oz)	43	0.0	0.0			0			0.00			ARBY17
French Toastix	370		7.0	48.0		4.0	440	70		0		
4.4 oz serving	124	17.0	4.0			0			1.80			ARBY18
fries, curly cheddar	460		6.0	54.0		4.0	1290	60			15	
6 oz serving	170	24.0	6.0			5			1.80			ARBY19
large	620		8.0	78.0		7.0	1540	0			21	
7 oz serving	198	30.0	7.0			0			2.70			ARBY20
medium	400		5.0	50.0		4.0	990	0			15	
4.5 oz serving	128	20.0	5.0			0			1.80			ARBY21
small	310		4.0	39.0		3.0	770	0			12	
3.5 oz serving	99	15.0	3.5			0			1.44			ARBY22
fries, homestyle, child-size	220		3.0	32.0		3.0	430	0			12	
3 oz serving	85	10.0	2.5			0			0.72			ARBY23
large	560		6.0	79.0		6.0	1070	0			30	
7.5 oz serving	213	24.0	6.0			0			1.80			ARBY24
medium	370		4.0	53.0		4.0	710	0			21	
5 oz serving	142	16.0	4.0			0			1.08			ARBY25
small	300		3.0	42.0		3.0	570	0			15	
4 oz serving	113	13.0	3.5			0			0.72			ARBY26
hot chocolate	110		2.0	23.0		0.0	120	50		0		
8.6 oz	244	1.0	0.5			0			0.00			ARBY29
Jalapeno Bites	330		7.0	30.0		2.0	670	40			1	
4 oz serving	111	21.0	9.0			40			0.72			ARBY33
mozzarella sticks	470		18.0	34.0		2.0	1330	400			1	
4.8 oz serving	137	29.0	14.0			60			0.72			ARBY40
onion petals	410		4.0	43.0		2.0	300	40		0		
4 oz serving	113	24.0	3.5			0			0.72			ARBY42
potato, baked deluxe	650		20.0	67.0		6.0	750	100			36	
12.7 oz serving	361	34.0	20.0			90			3.60			ARBY45
w/broccoli'n cheddar	540		12.0	71.0		7.0	680	250			72	
13.5 oz serving	384	24.0	12.0			50			3.60			ARBY46
w/butter & sour cream	500		8.0	65.0		6.0	170	100			30	
11.3 oz serving	320	24.0	15.0			55			3.60			ARBY47
potato cakes	250		2.0	26.0		3.0	490	0			6	
2 cakes (3.5 oz)	100	16.0	4.0			0			0.72			ARBY44
salad, caesar	90		7.0	8.0		3.0	170	200			42	
8 oz salad	223	4.0	2.5			10			1.80			ARBY73

	KCAL / WT (g)	H₂O (g) / FAT (g)	PRO (g) / SFA (g)	CHO (g) / MUFA (g)	SUGR (g) / PUFA (g)	DFIB (g) / CHOL (mg)	Na (mg) / K (mg)	Ca (mg) / P (mg)	Mg (mg) / Fe (mg)	Zn (mg) / Cu (mg)	Mn (mg) / Se (mcg)	A (mcg RAE) / A (IU)	C (mg) / E (mg ATE)	B-1 (mg) / B-2 (mg)	NIA (mg) / B-6 (mg)	B-12 (mcg) / FOL (mcg DFE)	PANT (mg) / REF
caesar side	45		4.0	4.0		2.0	95	40					27				
5 oz salad	137	2.0	1.0			5			1.08								ARBY74
chicken finger	570		30.0	39.0		3.0	1300	60					42				
13 oz salad	367	34.0	9.0			65			1.80								ARBY75
garden	70		4.0	14.0		6.0	45	80					42				
12.3 oz salad	349	1.0	0.0			0			1.44								ARBY76
grilled chicken	210		30.0	14.0		6.0	800	80					42				
16.4 oz salad	464	4.5	1.5			65			1.80								ARBY77
grilled chicken caesar	230		33.0	8.0		3.0	920	200					42				
12 oz salad	338	8.0	3.5			80			1.80								ARBY78
roast chicken	160		20.0	15.0		6.0	700	80					42				
14.8 oz salad	420	2.5	0.0			40			1.80								ARBY79
side	25		2.0	5.0		2.0	20	20					9				
5.7 oz salad	161	0.0	0.0			0			0.72								ARBY80
turkey club	350		33.0	9.0		3.0	920	350					42				
11.5 oz salad	325	21.0	10.0			90			1.80								ARBY81
salad dressing, bbq vinaigrette	140		0.0	9.0	0.0		660	0					0				
2 oz	57	11.0	1.5			0			0.36								ARBY64
bleu cheese	300		2.0	3.0	0.0		580	20					0				
2 oz	57	31.0	6.0			45			0.00								ARBY65
buttermilk ranch	360		1.0	2.0	0.0		490	20					0				
2 oz	57	39.0	6.0			5			0.00								ARBY66
buttermilk ranch, red cal	60		1.0	13.0	1.0		750	0					0				
2 oz	57	0.0	0.0			0			0.00								ARBY67
caesar	310		1.0	1.0	0.0		470	0					1				
2 oz	57	34.0	5.0			60			0.00								ARBY68
honey french	290		0.0	18.0	<1.0		410	0					0				
2 oz	57	24.0	4.0			0			0.00								ARBY69
italian parmesan	240		1.0	4.0	0.0		950	20					1				
2 oz	57	24.0	4.0			0			0.00								ARBY70
italian, red cal	25		0.0	3.0	<1.0		1030	0					0				
2 oz	57	1.0	1.0			0			0.00								ARBY71
thousand island	290		1.0	9.0	0.0		480	0					0				
2 oz	57	28.0	4.5			35			0.00								ARBY72
sandwich, BLT	820		24.0	72.0		5.0	1480	40					15				
10.5 oz sandwich	297	49.0	11.0			110			1.80								ARBY5
sandwich, chicken bacon'n swiss	610		31.0	49.0		2.0	1550	150					2				
7.5 oz sandwich	213	33.0	8.0			110			2.70								ARBY6
breast fillet	540		24.0	47.0		2.0	1160	80					4				
7.3 oz sandwich	208	30.0	5.0			90			1.80								ARBY7
cordon bleu	630		34.0	47.0		2.0	1820	150					2				
8.5 oz sandwich	242	35.0	8.0			120			2.70								ARBY8
grilled deluxe	450		29.0	37.0		2.0	1050	60					1				
8.9 oz sandwich	252	22.0	4.0			110			2.70								ARBY27
sandwich, hot ham'n swiss	340		23.0	35.0		1.0	1450	150					1				
6 oz sandwich	170	13.0	4.5			90			2.70								ARBY30
sandwich, light grilled chicken	280		29.0	30.0		3.0	1170	80					0				
6.1 oz sandwich	174	5.0	1.5			55			1.80								ARBY35
roast chicken	260		23.0	33.0		3.0	1010	100					2				
6.8 oz sandwich	194	5.0	1.0			40			2.70								ARBY36
roast turkey deluxe	260		23.0	33.0		3.0	980	80					1				
6.8 oz sandwich	194	5.0	0.5			40			1.80								ARBY37
sandwich, roast beef & swiss	810		37.0	73.0		5.0	1780	200					2				
12.7 oz sandwich	360	42.0	13.0			130			2.70								ARBY48
Arby-Q	360		16.0	40.0		2.0	1530	80					5				
6.6 oz sandwich	186	14.0	4.0			70			3.60								ARBY49
Beef'N Cheddar	480		23.0	43.0		2.0	1240	100					1				
7 oz sandwich	198	24.0	8.0			90			3.60								ARBY50
Big Montana	630		47.0	41.0		3.0	2080	80					0				
11 oz sandwich	313	32.0	15.0			155			7.20								ARBY51
giant	480		32.0	41.0		3.0	1440	60					0				
8 oz sandwich	228	23.0	10.0			110			5.40								ARBY52
junior	310		16.0	34.0		2.0	740	60					0				
4.6 oz sandwich	129	13.0	4.5			70			2.70								ARBY53

									Minerals				Vitamins				
	KCAL / WT (g)	H₂O (g) / FAT (g)	PRO (g) / SFA (g)	CHO (g) / MUFA (g)	SUGR (g) / PUFA (g)	DFIB (g) / CHOL (mg)	Na (mg) / K (mg)	Ca (mg) / P (mg)	Mg (mg) / Fe (mg)	Zn (mg) / Cu (mg)	Mn (mg) / Se (mcg)	A (mcg RAE) / A (IU ATE)	C (mg) / E (mg ATE)	B-1 (mg) / B-2 (mg)	NIA (mg) / B-6 (mg)	B-12 (mcg) / FOL (mcg DFE)	PANT (mg) / REF
regular	350		21.0	34.0		2.0	950	60					0				
5.5 oz sandwich	157	16.0	6.0			85			3.60								ARBY54
super	470		22.0	47.0		3.0	1130	80					1				
8.6 oz sandwich	245	23.0	7.0			85			3.60								ARBY55
w/cheddar cheese, Arby's	340		16.0	36.0		2.0	890	80					0				
Melt - 5.3 oz sandwich	150	15.0	5.0			70			2.70								ARBY57
sandwich, roast chicken caesar	820		43.0	75.0		5.0	2160	40					9				
12.8 oz sandwich	363	38.0	9.0			140			1.44								ARBY58
chicken club	520		29.0	38.0		2.0	1440	150					2				
9.8 oz sandwich	278	28.0	7.0			115			2.70								ARBY59
ham & swiss	730		36.0	74.0		5.0	2180	200					4				
12.7 oz sandwich	360	34.0	8.0			125			1.44								ARBY60
turkey & swiss	760		43.0	75.0		5.0	1920	350					2				
12.7 oz sandwich	360	33.0	6.0			130			4.50								ARBY61
turkey ranch & bacon	880		48.0	74.0		5.0	2320	900					2				
13.5 oz sandwich	383	44.0	10.0			155			3.60								ARBY62
sandwich, sourdough w/bacon	420		16.0	66.0		3.0	960	80					0				
5.1 oz sandwich	144	10.0	2.5			10			2.16								ARBY94
w/ham	390		19.0	67.0		2.0	1570	80					0				
6.1 oz sandwich	173	6.0	1.0			30			1.80								ARBY95
w/sausage	520		19.0	67.0		2.0	1040	80					0				
6 oz sandwich	170	19.0	5.0			25			2.52								ARBY96
sauce, Arby's	15		0.0	4.0		0.0	180	0					1				
.5 oz pkt	14	0.0	0.0			0			0.00								ARBY82
au jus	5		0.3	0.9		0.0	386	0					0				
3 oz	85	<0.1	<0.1			0			0.00								ARBY83
bbq dipping	40		0.0	10.0		0.0	350	0					2				
1 oz	28	0.0	0.0			0			0.36								ARBY84
Bronco Berry	90		0.0	23.0		0.0	35	0					2				
1.5 oz	43	0.0	0.0			0			0.00								ARBY85
honey mustard	130		0.0	5.0		0.0	160	0					0				
1 oz	28	12.0	1.5			10			0.00								ARBY86
Horsey	60		0.0	3.0		0.0	150	0					0				
.5 oz	14	5.0	0.5			5			0.36								ARBY87
marinara	35		1.0	4.0		0.0	260	0					6				
1.5 oz	43	1.0	0.0			0			0.72								ARBY88
Tangy Southwest	250		0.0	3.0		0.0	290	0					0				
1.5 oz	43	26.0	4.5			30			0.00								ARBY89
shake, choc	480		10.0	84.0		0.0	370	500					2				
14 oz	397	16.0	8.0			45			0.72								ARBY90
jamocha	470		10.0	82.0		0.0	390	500					2				
14 oz	397	15.0	7.0			45											ARBY91
strawberry	500		11.0	87.0		0.0	340	350					1				
14 oz	397	13.0	8.0			15			0.36								ARBY92
van	470		10.0	83.0		0.0	360	500					2				
14 oz	397	15.0	7.0			45			1.08								ARBY93
sub, french dip	440		28.0	42.0		2.0	1680	80					1				
10 oz sandwich	285	18.0	8.0			100			4.50								ARBY16
hot ham 'n swiss	530		29.0	45.0		3.0	1860	300					2				
9.8 oz sandwich	278	27.0	8.0			110			2.70								ARBY31
italian	780		29.0	49.0		3.0	2440	250					2				
11 oz sandwich	312	53.0	15.0			120			2.70								ARBY32
philly beef 'n swiss	700		36.0	46.0		4.0	1940	300					9				
11 oz sandwich	311	42.0	15.0			130			4.50								ARBY43
roast beef	760		35.0	47.0		3.0	2230	300					4				
11.8 oz sandwich	334	48.0	16.0			130			4.50								ARBY56
turkey	630		26.0	51.0		2.0	2170	200					2				
10.8 oz sandwich	306	37.0	9.0			100			0.36								ARBY97
turnover, apple w/icing	420		4.0	65.0		2.0	230	10					3				
4.5 oz turnover	128	16.0	4.5			0			1.80								ARBY98
cherry w/icing	410		4.0	63.0		1.0	250	10					7				
4.5 oz turnover	128	16.0	4.5			0			1.62								ARBY99

Columns are paired: the upper value in each cell group corresponds to the first header listed; the lower value corresponds to the second header. Minerals group spans Na, Ca, Mg, Zn, Mn. Vitamins group spans A, C, B-1, NIA, B-12, PANT.

Food / Serving	KCAL / WT (g)	H_2O (g) / FAT (g)	PRO (g) / SFA (g)	CHO (g) / MUFA (g)	SUGR (g) / PUFA (g)	DFIB (g) / CHOL (mg)	Na (mg) / K (mg)	Ca (mg) / P (mg)	Mg (mg) / Fe (mg)	Zn (mg) / Cu (mg)	Mn (mg) / Se (mcg)	A (mcg RAE) / A (IU)	C (mg) / E (mg ATE)	B-1 (mg) / B-2 (mg)	NIA (mg) / B-6 (mg)	B-12 (mcg) / FOL (mcg DFE)	PANT (mg) / REF
10.3 AU BON PAIN																	
apple cider	250		0.0	62.0	62.0	0.0	125	0					0				
16 fl oz	496	0.0	0.0			0			0.72			0					AUBN1
bagel	300		12.0	61.0	5.0	3.0	470	20					0				
4.1 oz bagel	116	1.0	0.0			0			0.72			0					AUBN2
cinn crisp	430		11.0	96.0	25.0	3.0	430	60					1				
4.8 oz bagel	136	6.0	1.0			0			1.80			0					AUBN7
cinn raisin	330		12.0	71.0	5.0	3.0	480	40					1				
4.6 oz bagel	129	1.0	0.0			0			1.08			0					AUBN8
dutch apple	470		13.0	99.0	28.0	5.0	540	40					1				
5 oz bagel	142	4.0	0.5			0			1.44			0					AUBN9
everything	330		13.0	63.0	5.0	3.0	750	60					0				
4.7 oz bagel	133	3.0	0.0			0			0.72			0					AUBN10
french toast	420		11.0	76.0	14.0	3.0	440	40					0				
4.8 oz bagel	136	7.0	1.5			0			1.08			0					AUBN12
honey 9 grain	360		14.0	75.0	5.0	6.0	550	20					0				
5 oz bagel	142	2.0	0.0			0			1.80			0					AUBN13
jalapeno cheddar	290		12.0	55.0	5.0	2.0	550	80					0				
4.1 oz bagel	116	2.0	1.0			5			0.72			200					AUBN14
sesame seed	340		13.0	62.0	5.0	3.0	470	80					0				
4.4 oz bagel	123	4.0	0.5			0			1.80			0					AUBN16
bagel sandwich w/egg	400		25.0	63.0	5.0	3.0	730	40					0				
7.1 oz sandwich	201	4.0	1.0			120			1.08			300					AUBN3
w/egg & bacon	480		30.0	63.0	5.0	3.0	960	40					0				
7.6 oz sandwich	215	12.0	3.5			130			1.44			300					AUBN4
w/egg & cheese	480		31.0	63.0	5.0	3.0	870	200					0				
7.9 oz sandwich	223	11.0	5.0			140			1.08			500					AUBN5
w/egg, cheese, & bacon	560		35.0	63.0	5.0	3.0	1100	200					0				
8.4 oz sandwich	237	18.0	7.0			155			1.44			500					AUBN6
baguette	120		5.0	25.0	0.0	1.0	330	20					4				
1.8 oz slice	50	0.0	0.0			0			0.36			0					AUBN17
bread, ficelle	500		18.0	103.0	3.0	0.0	1130	40					21				
6.3 oz piece	179	1.0	0.0			0			1.08			0					AUBN21
focaccia	740		26.0	137.0	4.0	7.0	1700	60					6				
10.3 oz piece	292	9.0	1.5			0			1.80			0					AUBN22
multigrain	130		6.0	24.0	0.0	1.0	360	40					12				
1.8 oz slice	50	1.0	0.0			0			0.36			0					AUBN23
parisienne	120		5.0	25.0	0.0	1.0	330	40					6				
1.8 oz slice	50	0.0	0.0			0			0.36			0					AUBN24
white	110		5.0	23.0	0.0	1.0	290	0					4				
1.8 oz slice	50	0.0	0.0			0			0.36			0					AUBN25
bread bowl	640		28.0	127.0	3.0	6.0	1830	150					36				
9.2 oz bowl	262	3.0	0.0			0			1.44			0					AUBN18
bread stick, rosemary garlic	200		6.0	33.0	2.0	2.0	1430	60					2				
2.3 oz bread stick	65	5.0	0.5			0			1.44			100					AUBN19
brownie, blonde w/nuts	570		6.0	57.0	31.0	2.0	460	60					0				
4 oz brownie	113	36.0	14.0			65			3.60			1250					AUBN26
cheesecake	470		5.0	55.0	42.0	1.0	260	20					0				
4 oz brownie	113	26.0	9.0			95			1.80			1500					AUBN27
choc chip	480		5.0	61.0	46.0	2.0	220	20					0				
4 oz brownie	113	25.0	7.0			85			2.70			1500					AUBN28
pecan	510		5.0	55.0	40.0	3.0	200	20					0				
4 oz brownie	113	31.0	7.0			80			1.80			1250					AUBN30
cake, apple spice loaf	860		12.0	128.0	65.0	3.0	950	300					1				
7.8 oz slice	221	36.0	8.0			90			1.44			200					AUBN31
butter crumb	790		9.0	96.0	48.0	2.0	560	80					0				
6 oz slice	170	42.0	17.0			50			3.60			1000					AUBN32
raspberry crumb	770		9.0	94.0	47.0	2.0	550	80					0				
6 oz slice	170	41.0	16.0			50			3.60			1000					AUBN34
cappuccino, iced	220		14.0	22.0	20.0	0.0	220	450					0				
16 fl oz (med)	~570	8.0	5.0			35			0.00			750					AUBN35

	KCAL	H₂O (g)	PRO (g)	CHO (g)	SUGR (g)	DFIB (g)	Na (mg)	Ca (mg)	Mg (mg)	Zn (mg)	Mn (mg)	A (mcg RAE)	C (mg)	B-1 (mg)	NIA (mg)	B-12 (mcg)	PANT (mg)
	WT (g)	FAT (g)	SFA (g)	MUFA (g)	PUFA (g)	CHOL (mg)	K (mg)	P (mg)	Fe (mg)	Cu (mg)	Se (mcg)	A (IU)	E (mg ATE)	B-2 (mg)	B-6 (mg)	FOL (mcg DFE)	REF
cheese, brie	150		8.0	0.0	0.0	0.0	180	150					0				
1.5 oz	43	14.0	6.0			30			1.80			400					AUBN36
cambozola	200		6.0	0.0	0.0	0.0	320	150					0				
1.5 oz	43	18.0	12.0			25			0.00			500					AUBN37
cheddar	170		11.0	1.0	1.0	0.0	260	300					0				
1.5 oz	43	14.0	9.0			45			0.36			500					AUBN38
provolone	140		10.0	1.0	0.0	0.0	330	350					0				
1.5 oz	43	10.0	7.0			35			0.00			300					AUBN39
swiss	160		12.0	0.0	0.0	0.0	105	350					0				
1.5 oz	43	12.0	9.0			30			0.00			300					AUBN40
chili, chicken	210		12.0	28.0	1.0	5.0	580	80					60				
8 oz	227	5.0	1.5			20			10.80			1500					AUBN42
chili w/beans, classic	190		11.0	22.0	2.0	6.0	600	150					4				
8 oz	227	6.0	2.0			10			1.44			1500					AUBN41
cookie, choc chip	260		3.0	41.0	24.0	1.0	270	20					0				
2.2 oz cookie	62	10.0	4.5			20			0.72			200					AUBN43
choc chunk macadamia	290		4.0	38.0	21.0	0.0	270	40					0				
2.2 oz cookie	62	14.0	4.0			25			0.72			200					AUBN44
cranberry almond macaroon,	320		4.0	42.0	33.0	3.0	190	40					0				
choc dipped - *2.8 oz cookie*	79	16.0	8.0			0			1.08			0					AUBN46
engish toffee	200		2.0	33.0	19.0	0.0	170	20					0				
1.6 oz cookie	45	6.0	3.5			30			0.36			100					AUBN47
gingerbread man	270		4.0	46.0	21.0	0.0	270	40					0				
2.3 oz cookie	65	8.0	1.5			10			1.08			300					AUBN48
oatmeal raisin	240		4.0	43.0	15.0	2.0	210	20					0				
2.2 oz cookie	61	6.0	1.5			20			1.08			200					AUBN50
peanut butter chunk	270		7.0	34.0	18.0	2.0	300	20					0				
2.2 oz cookie	62	13.0	3.5			25			0.72			200					AUBN51
shortbread	270		5.0	48.0	13.0	1.0	280	40					0				
2.5 oz cookie	71	7.0	4.5			20			1.08			300					AUBN53
shortbread, choc dipped	300		6.0	52.0	17.0	1.0	290	40					0				
2.5 oz cookie	71	10.0	4.5			20			1.08			300					AUBN54
walnut raisin	280		4.0	34.0	19.0	2.0	260	20					0				
2.2 oz cookie	61	15.0	4.0			20			1.08			200					AUBN56
white choc, choc dipped	380		4.9	46.0	26.0	2.0	135	60					0				
shortbread - *2.8 oz cookie*	78	21.0	15.0			40			0.36			500					AUBN57
croissant	250		8.0	44.0	6.0	2.0	340	60					5				
2.8 oz croissant	78	6.0	3.0			25			1.08			200					AUBN58
almond	510		13.0	63.0	18.0	3.0	440	100					5				
4.7 oz croissant	133	25.0	10.0			95			1.44			500					AUBN59
apple	220		6.0	45.0	17.0	2.0	220	40					36				
3.6 oz croissant	101	3.0	1.5			20			0.72			100					AUBN60
choc	380		8.0	61.0	26.0	3.0	300	60					4				
3.4 oz croissant	96	15.0	7.0			20			1.44			200					AUBN61
cinn raisin	340		9.0	69.0	15.0	3.0	350	80					9				
3.8 oz croissant	108	5.0	2.5			20			1.44			200					AUBN62
ham & cheese	330		18.0	46.0	6.0	2.0	750	200					5				
1 croissant	~151	10.0	6.0			50			1.08			300					AUBN63
raspberry	340		9.0	55.0	20.0	2.0	370	60					4				
1 croissant	~142	11.0	6.0			50			0.72			300					AUBN64
spinach & cheese	250		10.0	32.0	5.0	2.0	400	200					6				
1 croissant	~113	9.0	6.0			35			0.72			2250					AUBN65
sweet cheese	350		9.0	52.0	17.0	1.0	400	60					4				
1 croissant	~150	14.0	8.0			65			0.72			400					AUBN66
fruit cup	70		1.0	16.0	15.0	1.0	10	20					42				
6 oz	170	0.0	0.0			0			0.36			1750					AUBN67
	140		2.0	32.0	30.0	2.0	20	40					84				
12 oz	340	1.0	0.0			0			0.72			3500					AUBN68
Mocha Blast	351		13.0	56.0	53.0	0.0	195	600					3				
24 fl oz	~726	7.0	4.5			32			0.00			950					AUBN69
Mocha Blast, frzn	270		10.0	43.0	41.0	0.0	150	400					2				
12 fl oz	~311	6.0	3.5			25			0.00			750					AUBN70

	KCAL	H₂0 (g)	PRO (g)	CHO (g)	SUGR (g)	DFIB (g)	Na (mg)	Ca (mg)	Minerals Mg (mg)	Zn (mg)	Mn (mg)	Vitamins A (mcg RAE)	C (mg)	B-1 (mg)	NIA (mg)	B-12 (mcg)	PANT (mg)
	WT (g)	FAT (g)	SFA (g)	MUFA (g)	PUFA (g)	CHOL (mg)	K (mg)	P (mg)	Fe (mg)	Cu (mg)	Se (mcg)	A (IU)	E (mg ATE)	B-2 (mg)	B-6 (mg)	FOL (mcg DFE)	REF
muffin, apple spice	510		7.0	78.0	41.0	2.0	540	200					1				
5.8 oz muffin	163	21.0	5.0			50			1.08			100					AUBN71
banana walnut	560		12.0	67.0	31.0	3.0	510	200					4				
5.4 oz muffin	152	30.0	5.0			50			1.44			200					AUBN72
blueberry	480		7.0	71.0	31.0	3.0	580	200					1				
5.6 oz muffin	159	20.0	4.5			60			1.08			100					AUBN73
carrot walnut spice	550		9.0	71.0	40.0	4.0	860	150					6				
5.5 oz muffin	156	27.0	5.0			60			1.80			9500					AUBN74
choc cake, lowfat	320		4.0	74.0	48.0	4.0	590	20					0				
4.2 oz muffin	118	2.0	0.5			20			1.62			0					AUBN75
corn	440		8.0	64.0	30.0	2.0	640	150					2				
5.5 oz muffin	156	18.0	3.0			70			1.08			200					AUBN76
cranberry nut	540		9.0	62.0	29.0	4.0	560	200					4				
5.4 oz muffin	153	29.0	6.0			55			1.08			100					AUBN77
double choc	540		9.0	80.0	44.0	3.0	470	200					0				
5.3 oz muffin	150	23.0	9.0			65			1.08			100					AUBN78
pumpkin	540		9.0	79.0	40.0	3.0	380	80					2				
6 oz muffin	170	19.0	3.0			70			2.70			9500					AUBN79
raisin bran	520		12.0	97.0	38.0	10.0	1220	100					1				
6 oz muffin	170	15.0	6.0			55			2.70			200					AUBN80
triple berry, lowfat	290		5.0	61.0	31.0	2.0	310	60					4				
4.4 oz muffin	123	2.0	0.5			25			0.72			0					AUBN81
oatmeal, dry	150		5.0	27.0	1.0	4.0	0	0					0				
1.4 oz	40	3.0	0.5			0			1.80			0					AUBN82
pastry, cinn roll	320		8.0	66.0	27.0	2.0	310	60					6				
4 oz roll	113	4.0	2.0			20			1.44			100					AUBN83
cranberry danish	370		8.0	63.0	25.0	2.0	390	80					9				
4.5 oz pastry	128	10.0	3.5			45			0.72			400					AUBN84
crème de fleur	550		12.0	71.0	32.0	1.0	540	60					4				
5.6 oz pastry	157	26.0	15.0			110			0.72			750					AUBN85
lemon danish	390		10.0	69.0	26.0	6.0	380	100					21				
4.3 oz pastry	120	11.0	4.0			50			1.80			400					AUBN86
pecan roll	750		14.0	112.0	48.0	4.0	560	150					12				
6 oz pastry	170	29.0	7.0			15			2.70			400					AUBN87
sweet cheese danish	430		10.0	61.0	23.0	1.0	440	80					9				
4.3 oz pastry	120	18.0	8.0			80			0.72			500					AUBN88
roll, braided	420		13.0	63.0	8.0	3.0	730	80					9				
5.1 oz roll	145	14.0	3.0			40			1.80			0					AUBN90
four grain	310		14.0	58.0	2.0	2.0	740	40					9				
4.1 oz roll	117	3.0	1.0			0			1.44			0					AUBN91
hearth	240		11.0	44.0	1.0	2.0	570	20					6				
3.2 oz roll	89	2.0	0.5			0			1.08			0					AUBN93
petit pain	200		8.0	40.0	0.0	0.0	550	40					12				
2.9 oz roll	81	0.0	0.0			0			0.36			0					AUBN89
salad, caesar	240		13.0	19.0	2.0	4.0	370	350					42				
7.8 oz salad	221	12.0	6.0			330			2.70			4500					AUBN105
chrbrld salmon filet	210		24.0	9.0	5.0	2.0	135	20					42				
w/peppers - 9.7 oz salad	275	7.0	1.0			50			2.70			1500					AUBN106
chef's	290		27.0	11.0	7.0	3.0	1290	300					12				
10.3 oz salad	292	15.0	1.5			65			1.80			400					AUBN107
chicken caesar	600		33.0	63.0	3.0	5.0	930	300					15				
10.5 oz salad	298	25.0	8.0			80			1.44			1750					AUBN108
cobb	460		40.0	26.0	5.0	8.0	1530	300					498				
11 oz salad	369	22.0	10.0			220			4.50			16000					AUBN110
garden	90		3.0	14.0	3.0	3.0	160	40					9				
5.2 oz salad	146	2.0	0.5			0			1.80			100					AUBN111
garden	160		6.0	26.0	6.0	5.0	400	60					15				
9.3 oz salad	264	4.0	1.0			0			3.60			200					AUBN112
mediterranean chicken	230		18.0	12.0	2.0	3.0	1010	80					18				
9.7 oz salad	275	12.0	3.0			50			1.80			500					AUBN114
mozzarella & red pepper	360		23.0	10.0	6.0	2.0	380	700					66				
10.5 oz salad	298	25.0	16.0			90			1.80			5500					AUBN115

	KCAL / WT (g)	H₂O (g) / FAT (g)	PRO (g) / SFA (g)	CHO (g) / MUFA (g)	SUGR (g) / PUFA (g)	DFIB (g) / CHOL (mg)	Na (mg) / K (mg)	Ca (mg) / P (mg)	Mg (mg) / Fe (mg)	Zn (mg) / Cu (mg)	Mn (mg) / Se (mcg)	A (mcg RAE) / A (IU)	C (mg) / E (mg ATE)	B-1 (mg) / B-2 (mg)	NIA (mg) / B-6 (mg)	B-12 (mcg) / FOL (mcg DFE)	PANT (mg) / REF
nicoise	350		28.0	21.0	6.0	4.0	950	60					18				
13.2 oz salad	376	16.0	3.0			245			1.80			750					AUBN116
thai chicken	260		17.0	28.0	14.0	4.0	1380	20					18				
11.2 oz salad	311	8.0	0.5			45			10.80			500					AUBN118
tomato w/basil pesto	280		16.0	11.0	7.0	3.0	180	500					27				
9.2 oz salad	260	19.0	11.0			60			1.80			1250					AUBN119
tuna	430		27.0	28.0	7.0	6.0	880	80					15				
13.3 oz salad	377	25.0	4.0			10			2.70			5000					AUBN120
salad dressing, balsamic	190		1.0	1.0	4.0	0.0	170	0					0				
vinaigrette - 2 T (1.1 oz)	30	19.0	3.0			0			0.00			0					AUBN94
blue cheese	130		1.0	3.0	2.0	0.0	280	20					0				
2 T (1.1 oz)	30	12.0	2.5			10			0.00			100					AUBN95
caesar	160		1.0	3.0	2.0	0.0	220	20					0				
2 T (1.1 oz)	30	16.0	2.5			15			0.00			0					AUBN96
dijon vinaigrette, lite	80		0.0	3.0	3.0	0.0	260	0					1				
2 T (1.1 oz)	30	8.0	1.0			0			0.00			0					AUBN97
honey mustard, lite	100		0.0	11.0	8.0	0.0	240	0					0				
2 T 1.1 oz)	30	6.0	1.0			15			0.00			0					AUBN98
mediterranean	80		0.0	2.0	1.0	0.0	270	20					0				
2 T (1.1 oz)	30	9.0	1.5			5			0.00			0					AUBN99
olive oil vinaigrette, lite	60		0.0	3.0	2.0	0.0	230	0					0				
2 T (1.1 oz)	30	6.0	1.0			0			0.00			100					AUBN100
parmesan & peppercorn	170		1.0	2.0	1.0	0.0	300	20					0				
2 T (1.1 oz)	30	16.0	2.5			10			0.36			100					AUBN101
ranch, lite	110		1.0	1.0	1.0	0.0	270	20					0				
2 T (1.1 oz)	30	10.0	1.5			10			0.00			0					AUBN102
raspberry, fat free	35		0.0	8.0	7.0	0.0	80	0					1				
2 T (1.1 oz)	30	0.0	0.0			0			0.00			0					AUBN103
thai peanut	70		1.0	8.0	6.0	0.0	530	0					0				
2 T (1.1 oz)	30	3.0	0.0			0			0.36			0					AUBN104
sandwich filling, chicken tarragon	210		18.0	1.0	0.0	0.0	590	0					2				
4 oz	113	14.0	2.5			70			1.08			0					AUBN122
country ham	150		21.0	2.0	2.0	0.0	1140	0					0				
3.8 oz	108	3.0	1.0			60			0.72			0					AUBN123
hummus	100		4.0	8.0	0.0	2.0	210	0					0				
2 oz	57	6.0	0.0			0			0.72			0					AUBN125
roast beef	150		26.0	1.0	0.0	0.0	460	0					1				
3.8 oz	106	5.0	2.0			70			4.50			0					AUBN126
tuna salad	170		25.0	3.0	1.0	0.0	450	20					2				
4.5 oz	128	8.0	1.0			0			0.36			5500					AUBN127
turkey breast	120		22.0	4.0	2.0	0.0	950	0					0				
4 oz	113	2.0	0.0			50			0.00			0					AUBN128
scone, asiago cheese	430		14.0	38.0	5.0	1.0	500	350					0				
4.3 oz scone	123	27.0	16.0			155			0.72			750					AUBN129
cinn	480		11.0	68.5	23.0	2.0	320	100					0				
4.2 oz scone	118	18.0	8.0			125			1.80			500					AUBN130
orange w/icing	410		11.0	62.0	12.0	2.0	340	80					2				
4.2 oz scone	118	14.0	8.0			125			1.44			500					AUBN131
soup, autumn pumpkin	140		2.0	15.0	2.0	4.0	640	40					1				
8 oz	227	7.0	3.5			15			0.72			23000					AUBN133
baked stuffed potato	240		6.0	20.0	1.0	1.0	720	80					12				
8 oz	227	15.0	6.0			25			0.72			500					AUBN134
black bean	170		11.0	32.0	2.0	17.0	870	80					84				
8 oz	227	0.0	0.0			0			16.20			1000					AUBN135
broccoli cheddar	230		6.0	13.0	5.0	2.0	960	150					36				
8 oz	227	16.0	9.0			50			0.72			1000					AUBN136
chicken florentine	170		5.0	17.0	2.0	1.0	780	40					2				
8 oz	227	9.0	4.5			35			0.72			1250					AUBN137
chicken noodle	90		7.0	11.0	2.0	0.0	670	20					2				
8 oz	227	2.0	0.0			15			0.72			1500					AUBN138
clam chowder	220		8.0	16.0	1.0	1.0	800	100					6				
8 oz	227	15.0	6.0			35			1.44			500					AUBN139

	KCAL	H₂0 (g)	PRO (g)	CHO (g)	SUGR (g)	DFIB (g)	Na (mg)	Ca (mg)	Mg (mg)	Zn (mg)	Mn (mg)	A (mcg RAE)	C (mg)	B-1 (mg)	NIA (mg)	B-12 (mcg)	PANT (mg)
	WT (g)	FAT (g)	SFA (g)	MUFA (g)	PUFA (g)	CHOL (mg)	K (mg)	P (mg)	Fe (mg)	Cu (mg)	Se (mcg)	A (IU)	E (mg ATE)	B-2 (mg)	B-6 (mg)	FOL (mcg DFE)	REF
corn & green chili bisque	160		4.0	17.0	3.0	2.0	920	60					66				
8 oz	227	8.0	5.0			25			6.30			1750					AUBN140
corn chowder	240		5.0	25.0	4.0	2.0	520	80					9				
8 oz	227	13.0	8.0			35			0.72			1250					AUBN141
curried rice & lentil	100		5.0	18.0	1.0	4.0	900	20					60				
8 oz	227	1.0	0.0			0			10.80			2500					AUBN142
french moroccan tomato lentil	110		6.0	19.0	3.0	6.0	470	40					96				
8 oz	227	1.0	1.0			0			9.00			3500					AUBN143
french onion	80		3.0	11.0	3.0	2.0	1280	40					5				
8 oz	227	3.0	1.5			10			0.72			300					AUBN144
garden vegetable	40		2.0	7.0	3.0	2.0	610	40					18				
8 oz	227	1.0	0.0			0			0.72			2000					AUBN145
lobster bisque	250		6.0	16.0	5.0	1.0	1110	60					5				
8 oz	227	18.0	8.0			55			0.72			2000					AUBN146
mediterranean pepper	190		9.0	30.0	3.0	7.0	450	40					306				
8 oz	227	4.0	0.0			0			45.00			5500					AUBN147
pasta e fagioli	160		7.0	24.0	2.0	5.0	510	60					1				
8 oz	227	4.0	1.0			5			1.80			1000					AUBN148
tomato	130		4.0	17.0	10.0	2.0	990	80					9				
8 oz	227	5.0	2.0			10			1.08			6500					AUBN149
stew, beef	210		12.0	16.0	2.0	2.0	780	40					12				
8 oz	227	10.0	3.0			40			1.44			2500					AUBN150
chicken	230		12.0	17.0	2.0	2.0	630	40					9				
8 oz	227	12.0	3.5			40			1.44			2000					AUBN151
mediterranean seafood	170		14.0	18.0	3.0	2.0	920	40					174				
8 oz	227	5.0	1.0			50			25.20			4000					AUBN152
strudel, apple	410		6.0	56.0	19.0	1.0	140	20					0				
4.4 oz strudel	123	18.0	0.0			0			0.36			1250					AUBN153
cherry	390		6.0	49.0	5.0	1.0	135	20					0				
4.2 oz	118	19.0	0.0			0			0.72			1500					AUBN154
yogurt, blueberry w/granola & fruit - 7.5 oz	310		10.0	56.0	36.0	2.0	130	200					66				
	241	6.0	2.0			10			1.08			100					AUBN156
plain, lowfat	190		6.0	36.0	31.0	0	95	200					2				
7 oz	198	2.0	1.5			10			0.36			100					AUBN159
strawberry w/granola & fruit	310		10.0	56.0	36.0	2.0	130	200					12				
8.5 oz	241	6.0	2.0			10			1.08			100					AUBN162

10.4 BURGER KING

	KCAL	H₂0 (g)	PRO (g)	CHO (g)	SUGR (g)	DFIB (g)	Na (mg)	Ca (mg)	Mg (mg)	Zn (mg)	Mn (mg)	A (mcg RAE)	C (mg)	B-1 (mg)	NIA (mg)	B-12 (mcg)	PANT (mg)
	WT (g)	FAT (g)	SFA (g)	MUFA (g)	PUFA (g)	CHOL (mg)	K (mg)	P (mg)	Fe (mg)	Cu (mg)	Se (mcg)	A (IU)	E (mg ATE)	B-2 (mg)	B-6 (mg)	FOL (mcg DFE)	REF
apple pie	340		2.0	52.0	23.0	1.0	470	0					0				
4 oz fried pie	113	14.0	3.0			1			1.44			100					BRGR1
big fish sandwich	710		24.0	66.0	7.0	4.0	1160	80					0				
9.2 oz sandwich	262	39.0	15.0			50			3.60			100					BRGR2
cheeseburger	360		19.0	31.0	6.0	2.0	790	150					1				
4.7 oz sandwich	133	17.0	8.0			50			3.60			300					BRGR3
double	540		32.0	32.0	6.0	2.0	1050	250					1				
6.7 oz sandwich	189	31.0	15.0			100			4.50			500					BRGR4
double Whopper	1150		64.0	53.0	11.0	4.0	1530	300					9				
15 oz sandwich	426	76.0	30.0			210			9.00			1250					BRGR6
double w/bacon	580		35.0	32.0	6.0	2.0	1240	250					1				
6.8 oz sandwich	193	34.0	17.0			110			4.50			500					BRGR5
smokehouse cheddar	720		39.0	32.0	3.0	2.0	1240	200					4				
Griller - *8.5 oz sandwich*	241	48.0	19.0			125			4.50			300					BRGR7
Whopper	850		39.0	53.0	11.0	4.0	1430	250					9				
13.9 oz sandwich	395	53.0	20.0			120			7.20			1250					BRGR8
Whopper Jr	440		19.0	32.0	6.0	2.0	790	150					4				
5.6 oz sandwich	160	26.0	9.0			55			3.60			500					BRGR9
chicken sandwich, specialty	560		25.0	52.0	5.0	3.0	1270	60					0				
7.2 oz sandwich	204	28.0	6.0			60			2.70			400					BRGR10
Whopper	580		39.0	48.0	7.0	3.0	1370	80					6				
9.6 oz sandwich	272	26.0	5.0			75			8.10			750					BRGR13

	KCAL	H₂0 (g)	PRO (g)	CHO (g)	SUGR (g)	DFIB (g)	Na (mg)	Ca (mg)	Mg (mg)	Zn (mg)	Mn (mg)	A (mcg RAE)	C (mg)	B-1 (mg)	NIA (mg)	B-12 (mcg)	PANT (mg)
	WT (g)	FAT (g)	SFA (g)	MUFA (g)	PUFA (g)	CHOL (mg)	K (mg)	P (mg)	Fe (mg)	Cu (mg)	Se (mcg)	A (IU)	E (mg ATE)	B-2 (mg)	B-6 (mg)	FOL (mcg DFE)	REF
Whopper Jr	350		26.0	30.0	4.0	2.0	900	60					4				
5.8 oz sandwich	165	14.0	2.5			45			5.40			300					BRGR14
chicken tenders	210		14.0	13.0	0.0		530	20					0				
5 pieces (2.7 oz)	77	12.0	3.5			30			0.36			0					BRGR11
	340		22.0	20.0	0.0		840	20					0				
8 pieces (4.3 oz)	123	19.0	5.0			50			0.72			100					BRGR12
cini-mini rolls w/o icing	440		6.0	51.0	20.0	1.0	710	60					1				
4 rolls (3.8 oz)	108	23.0	6.0			25			2.70			1000					BRGR15
cini-minis van icing	110		0.0	20.0	19.0	0.0	40										
1 oz	28	3.0	0.5			0											BRGR16
cookies	440		4.0	57.0	32.0	2.0	390	20					0				
3.4 oz serving	96	21.0	7.0			15			1.80			400					BRGR17
Croissan'wich, egg & cheese	320		12.0	24.0	3.0		730	300					0				
4 oz sandwich	112	19.0	7.0			185			3.60			400					BRGR18
sausage & cheese	420		14.0	23.0	4.0		840	100					0				
3.8 oz sandwich	107	31.0	11.0			45			3.60			200					BRGR19
sausage, egg, & cheese	520		19.0	24.0	4.0	1.0	1090	300					0				
5.5 oz sandwich	157	39.0	14.0			210			4.50			500					BRGR20
dipping sauce, barbecue	35		0.0	9.0	7.0	0.0	390										
1 oz	28	0.0	0.0			0											BRGR21
honey flavored	90		0.0	23.0	22.0	0.0	0										
1 oz	28	0.0	0.0			0											BRGR22
honey mustard	90		0.0	9.0	4.0	0.0	150										
1 oz	28	6.0	1.0			10											BRGR23
ranch	140		1.0	1.0	1.0	0.0	95										
1 oz	28	15.0	2.5			5											BRGR24
sweet & sour	40		0.0	10.0	5.0	0.0	65										
1 oz	28	0.0	0.0			0											BRGR25
zesty onion ring	150		0.0	3.0	2.0	0.0	210										
1 oz	28	15.0	2.5			15											BRGR26
Egg'wich, canadian bacon &	380		15.0	35.0	3.0	3.0	680	150					0				
egg - 5 oz sandwich	142	19.0	4.0			125			3.60			200					BRGR27
canadian bacon, egg, &	420		18.0	36.0	3.0	3.0	900	250					0				
cheese - 5.5 oz sandwich	155	23.0	7.0			140			3.60			400					BRGR28
egg & cheese	410		15.0	36.0	3.0	3.0	760	250					0				
4.9 oz sandwich	140	23.0	7.0			130			3.60			400					BRGR29
french fries, king	600		7.0	76.0	1.0	6.0	1070	20					12				
6.8 oz	194	30.0	8.0			0			1.08			0					BRGR33
large	500		6.0	63.0	1.0	5.0	880	20					12				
5.6 oz	160	25.0	7.0			0			1.08			0					BRGR32
med	360		4.0	46.0	1.0	4.0	640	20					9				
4.1 oz	117	18.0	5.0			0			0.72			0					BRGR31
small	230		3.0	29.0	0.0	2.0	410	20					5				
2.6 oz	74	11.0	3.0			0			0.36			0					BRGR30
french toast sticks	390		6.0	46.0	11.0	2.0	440	60					0				
5 sticks (4 oz)	113	20.0	4.5			0			1.80			0					BRGR34
Frozen Coca Cola Classic, large	460		0.0	116.0	116.0	0.0	<1	<1					<1				
19 oz	539	0.0	0.0			0			<0.01			<1					BRGR36
med	370		0.0	92.0	92.0	0.0	<1	<1					<1				
15.5 oz	439	0.0	0.0			0			<0.01			<1					BRGR35
Frozen Minute Maid cherry, large	460		0.0	116.0	116.0	0.0	<1	<1					<1				
19 oz	539	0.0	0.0			0			<0.01			<1					BRGR38
med	370		0.0	92.0	92.0	0.0	<1	<1					<1				
15.5 oz	439	0.0	0.0			0			<0.01			<1					BRGR37
hamburger	310		17.0	31.0	6.0	2.0	580	80					1				
4.3 oz sandwich	121	13.0	5.0			40			3.60			100					BRGR39
1/4 lb	490		26.0	50.0	10.0	3.0	950	100					2				
7.4 oz sandwich	210	21.0	8.0			60			5.40			200					BRGR40

	KCAL	H₂0 (g)	PRO (g)	CHO (g)	SUGR (g)	DFIB (g)	Na (mg)	Ca (mg)	Mg (mg)	Zn (mg)	Mn (mg)	A (mcg RAE)	C (mg)	B-1 (mg)	NIA (mg)	B-12 (mcg)	PANT (mg)
	WT (g)	FAT (g)	SFA (g)	MUFA (g)	PUFA (g)	CHOL (mg)	K (mg)	P (mg)	Fe (mg)	Cu (mg)	Se (mcg)	A (IU ATE)	E (mg ATE)	B-2 (mg)	B-6 (mg)	FOL (mcg DFE)	REF
double	450		28.0	31.0	6.0	2.0	620	100					1				
5.8 oz sandwich	164	24.0	10.0			75			4.50			100					BRGR41
double Whopper	1060		59.0	52.0	11.0	4.0	1100	200					9				
14 oz sandwich	401	69.0	25.0			185			9.00			1000					BRGR42
homestyle Griller	480		26.0	35.0	5.0	2.0	760	60					6				
8.5 oz sandwich	242	27.0	11.0			75			4.50			500					BRGR43
King Supreme	550		30.0	32.0	6.0	2.0	790	150					1				
6.9 oz sandwich	196	34.0	14.0			100			4.50			200					BRGR44
Whopper	760		35.0	52.0	11.0	4.0	1000	150					9				
10.7 oz sandwich	304	46.0	14.0			100			7.20			1000					BRGR45
Whopper Jr	390		17.0	32.0	6.0	2.0	570	80					4				
5.6 oz sandwich	158	22.0	7.0			45			3.60			500					BRGR46
hash brown rounds, large	390		3.0	38.0	0.0	4.0	760	20					1				
4.5 oz	128	25.0	7.0			0			0.72			0					BRGR48
small	230		2.0	23.0	0.0	2.0	450	0					1				
2.6 oz)	75	15.0	4.0			0			0.36			0					BRGR47
Hershey's sundae pie	310		3.0	33.0	20.0		135	40					0				
2.8 oz pie	79	18.0	13.0			10			1.44			0					BRGR49
hot fudge brownie royale	440		6.0	62.0	46.0	6.0	250	40					0				
4 oz serving	113	19.0	6.0			50			9.00			400					BRGR50
onion rings, king	550		8.0	70.0	8.0	5.0	800	200					0				
5.6 oz	159	27.0	7.0			5			0.00			0					BRGR54
large	480		7.0	60.0	7.0	5.0	690	150					0				
4.8 oz	137	23.0	6.0			0			0.00			0					BRGR53
med	320		4.0	40.0	5.0	3.0	460	100					0				
3.2 oz	91	16.0	4.0			0			0.00			0					BRGR52
small	180		2.0	22.0	3.0	2.0	260	60					0				
1.8 oz	51	9.0	2.0			0			0.00			0					BRGR51
salad, chicken caesar	160		25.0	5.0	3.0	3.0	730	100					6				
9 oz salad	257	6.0	3.0			40			3.60			750					BRGR60
garden	180		1.0	5.0	3.0	2.0	15	20					30				
5 oz salad	142	0.0	0.0			0			0.72			2500					BRGR61
salad dressing, catalina	180		0.0	10.0	9.0	0.0	530										
1.5 oz pkt	43	16.0	2.5			0											BRGR55
creamy Caesar	140		1.0	4.0	2.0	0.0	340										
1.5 oz pkt	43	13.0	2.0			10											BRGR56
light italian	50		0.0	4.0	3.0	0.0	360										
1.5 oz pkt	43	4.5	0.5			0											BRGR57
ranch	220		0.0	2.0	2.0	0.0	410										
1.5 oz pkt	43	23.0	3.5			10											BRGR58
thousand island	110		1.0	7.0	7.0	0.0	410										
1.5 oz pkt	43	9.0	1.5			10											BRGR59
shake, choc	790		15.0	89.0	75.0	2.0	380	450					0				
med (15 oz)	425	42.0	27.0			125			1.08			1500					BRGR62
strawberry, syrup added	780		15.0	88.0	75.0	1.0	300	450					0				
med (15 oz)	425	41.0	27.0			125			0.36			1500					BRGR63
van	720		15.0	73.0	60.0	1.0	280	400					0				
med (14 oz)	397	41.0	27.0			125			0.36			1500					BRGR64
veggie burger	330		14.0	45.0	6.0	4.0	770	60					6				
6.1 oz sandwich	173	10.0	1.5			0			6.30			400					BRGR65

10.5 CHICKEN OUT

	KCAL	H₂0 (g)	PRO (g)	CHO (g)	SUGR (g)	DFIB (g)	Na (mg)	Ca (mg)	Mg (mg)	Zn (mg)	Mn (mg)	A (mcg RAE)	C (mg)	B-1 (mg)	NIA (mg)	B-12 (mcg)	PANT (mg)
applesauce, chunky cinn	60		0.0	25.0													
6 oz	170	0.0															CKOT49
baguette	80		6.0	28.0													
1 baguette	~52	0.9															CKOT57
broccoli & carrots, steamed	30		9.0	6.0													
6 oz	170	0.0															CKOT47

	KCAL	H₂0 (g)	PRO (g)	CHO (g)	SUGR (g)	DFIB (g)	Na (mg)	Ca (mg)	Mg (mg)	Zn (mg)	Mn (mg)	A (mcg RAE)	C (mg)	B-1 (mg)	NIA (mg)	B-12 (mcg)	PANT (mg)
	WT (g)	FAT (g)	SFA (g)	MUFA (g)	PUFA (g)	CHOL (mg)	K (mg)	P (mg)	Fe (mg)	Cu (mg)	Se (mcg)	A (IU)	E (mg ATE)	B-2 (mg)	B-6 (mg)	FOL (mcg DFE)	REF
cheese & macaroni	311		4.0	39.0													
6 oz	170	12.0															CKOT44
chicken breast w/o skin	210		35.0	0.0													
6 oz	170	3.9															CKOT7
chicken, dark rotisserie w/o skin	232		31.0	0.0													
leg & thigh (~6.5 oz)	~185	6.1															CKOT2
chicken, white rotisserie,	196		35.0	0.0													
breast w/o skin - ~6.5 oz	~185	3.5															CKOT1
pulled meat	180		25.0	0.0													
6 oz	170	3.9															CKOT8
coleslaw, farm fresh	55		2.0	10.0													
6 oz	170	0.0															CKOT51
cranberry relish, mandarin walnut	240		0.0	66.0													
6 oz	170	0.5															CKOT50
green beans, oriental	34		2.0	8.0													
6 oz	170	0.0															CKOT48
peas, corn, & carrots, rstd	120		8.0	22.0													
6 oz	170	0.2															CKOT46
potato wedges, baked	110		2.3	26.0													
6 oz	170	0.1															CKOT42
potatoes, red skin, mshd	181		3.0	26.0													
6 oz	170	6.3															CKOT39
rice pilaf	140		4.0	28.0													
6 oz	170	0.9															CKOT45
salad, apricot chicken	300		38.5	0.9													
6 oz	170	8.2															CKOT3
bbq pulled chicken	263		43.8	8.0													
6 oz	170	4.9															CKOT6
pesto chicken	285		36.3	1.3													
6 oz	170	7.9															CKOT5
signature chicken	230		37.2	0.5													
6 oz	170	4.5															CKOT4
salad dressing, balsamic	18		0.0	4.0													
vinaigrette - 1 oz	28	0.0															CKOT20
caesar	55		0.0	0.5													
1 oz	28	5.0															CKOT19
chinese	72		0.0	1.5													
1 oz	28	6.5															CKOT23
lowfat honey mustard	23		1.0	5.0													
1 oz	28	0.5															CKOT24
ranch	90		0.5	1.0													
1 oz	28	6.0															CKOT21
southwestern	85		0.5	3.0													
1 oz	28	7.0															CKOT22
soup, chicken noodle	130		11.0	8.0													
6 oz	170	2.5															CKOT59
vegetable minestrone	98		3.0	12.0													
6 oz	170	1.5															CKOT61
spinach, creamed w/artichokes	160		8.0	20.0													
6 oz	170	5.9															CKOT38
stuffing, apple cornbread	215		6.0	42.0													
6 oz	170	2.0															CKOT43
sweet potatoes, mshd	120		0.0	40.0													
6 oz	170	<0.1															CKOT40
vegetarian baked beans	150		7.0	26.0													
6 oz	170	0.9															CKOT41

Minerals / Vitamins (column group headers)

	KCAL / WT (g)	H_2O (g) / FAT (g)	PRO (g) / SFA (g)	CHO (g) / MUFA (g)	SUGR (g) / PUFA (g)	DFIB (g) / CHOL (mg)	Na (mg) / K (mg)	Ca (mg) / P (mg)	Mg (mg) / Fe (mg)	Zn (mg) / Cu (mg)	Mn (mg) / Se (mcg)	A (mcg RAE) / A (IU)	C (mg) / E (mg ATE)	B-1 (mg) / B-2 (mg)	NIA (mg) / B-6 (mg)	B-12 (mcg) / FOL (mcg DFE)	PANT (mg) / REF

10.6 CHICK-FIL-A

Food	KCAL/WT	H₂O/FAT	PRO/SFA	CHO/MUFA	SUGR/PUFA	DFIB/CHOL	Na/K	Ca/P	Mg/Fe	Zn/Cu	Mn/Se	A(RAE)/A(IU)	C/E	B-1/B-2	NIA/B-6	B-12/FOL	PANT/REF
biscuit	260		4.0	38.0	5.0	1.0											
2.8 oz biscuit	78	11.0	2.5			0											CKFL25
& gravy	320		5.0	44.0	5.0	1.0	940										
6.8 oz	192	15.0	4.0			5											CKFL37
chicken	400		16.0	43.0	5.0	2.0	1200										
4.8 oz	137	18.0	4.5			30											CKFL27
chicken w/cheese	400		16.0	43.0	5.0	2.0	1200										
5.3 oz	150	18.0	4.5			30											CKFL28
w/bacon	300		6.0	38.0	5.0	1.0	780										
3 oz	86	14.0	4.0			5											CKFL29
w/bacon & egg	390		13.0	38.0	5.0	1.0	860										
5 oz	142	20.0	6.0			250											CKFL30
w/bacon, egg, & cheese	430		16.0	38.0	5.0	1.0	1070										
5.5 oz	155	24.0	9.0			265											CKFL31
w/butter	270		4.0	38.0	5.0	1.0	680										
2.8 oz biscuit	79	12.0	3.0			0											CKFL26
w/egg	340		11.0	38.0	5.0	1.0	740										
4.8 oz	135	16.0	4.5			245											CKFL32
w/egg & cheese	390		13.0	38.0	5.0	1.0	960	150					0				
5.2 oz	148	21.0	7.0			260			2.70			500					CKFL33
w/sausage	410		9.0	42.0	5.0	1.0	740										
4.2 oz	119	23.0	9.0			20											CKFL34
w/sausage & egg	500		15.0	43.0	5.0	1.0	810										
6.2 oz	176	29.0	11.0			265											CKFL35
w/sausage, egg, & cheese	540		18.0	43.0	5.0	1.0	1030	150					0				
6.7 oz	189	33.0	13.0			280			3.60			500					CKFL36
brownie, fudge nut	330		4.0	45.0	29.0	2.0	210	20					0				
2.6 oz brownie	74	15.0	3.5			20			1.80			1250					CKFL52
cheesecake	340		6.0	30.0	25.0	2.0	270	60					0				
3.3 oz slice	93	21.0	12.0			90			0.00			500					CKFL50
chicken filet	230		23.0	10.0	2.0	0.0	990	40					0				
3.7 oz filet	105	11.0	2.5			60			1.08			200					CKFL4
chargrilled	100		20.0	1.0	1.0	0.0	690	0					0				
2.8 oz filet	79	1.5	0.0			60			0.36			0					CKFL8
Chick-fil-A Nuggets	260		26.0	12.0	3.0	<1.0	1090	40					0				
8 nuggets	113	12.0	2.5			70			1.08			0					CKFL12
Chick-n-Strips	250		25.0	12.0	2.0	0.0	570	40					0				
4 strips	108	11.0	2.5			70			1.08			0					CKFL11
coleslaw	210		1.0	14.0	9.0	2.0	180	40					27				
3.7 oz salad	105	17.0	2.5			20			0.36			300					CKFL23
Cool Wrap, chargrilled chicken	390		31.0	53.0	6.0	3.0	1120	200					5				
8.4 oz wrap	240	7.0	3.0			70			3.60			2250					CKFL15
chicken caesar	460		38.0	51.0	5.0	3.0	1540	400					0				
8 oz wrap	227	11.0	6.0			85			3.60			750					CKFL16
spicy chicken	390		31.0	51.0	5.0	3.0	1150	200					5				
7.9 oz wrap	225	7.0	3.5			70			3.60			200					CKFL14
croutons, garlic & butter	90		3.0	3.0	1.0	<1.0	0	0					0				
.6 oz pkt	17	4.0	0.0			0			0.36			0					CKFL65
danish	430		6.0	63.0	<1.0	2.0	160						0				
4.6 oz danish	132	17.0	4.5			25											CKFL39
hash browns	170		2.0	20.0	<1.0	2.0	350										
3 oz	84	9.0	4.5			10											CKFL38
honey mustard sce	45		0.0	10.0	10.0	0.0	150	0					0				
1 oz pkt	28	0.0	0.0			0			0.00			0					CKFL64
iced tea	0		0.0	0.0	0.0	0.0	0	0					0				
small (9 oz)	~270	0.0	0.0			0			0.36			0					CKFL43
sweetened	80		0.0	19.0	19.0	0.0	0	0					0				
small (9 oz)	~291	0.0	0.0			0			0.36			0					CKFL42
Icedream cone	160		4.0	28.0	24.0	0.0	80	100					0				
small (4.7 oz)	133	4.0	2.0			15			0.36			200					CKFL49

	KCAL	H₂0 (g)	PRO (g)	CHO (g)	SUGR (g)	DFIB (g)	Na (mg)	Ca (mg)	Mg (mg)	Zn (mg)	Mn (mg)	A (mcg RAE)	C (mg)	B-1 (mg)	NIA (mg)	B-12 (mcg)	PANT (mg)
	WT (g)	FAT (g)	SFA (g)	MUFA (g)	PUFA (g)	CHOL (mg)	K (mg)	P (mg)	Fe (mg)	Cu (mg)	Se (mcg)	A (IU)	E (mg ATE)	B-2 (mg)	B-6 (mg)	FOL (mcg DFE)	REF
cream cheese	190		4.0	4.0	2.0	0.0	190	40					0				
1 pkt	~54	17.0	13.0			55			0.00			500					DUNK31
lite	110		4.0	6.0	0.0		230	40					0				
1 pkt	~42	9.0	7.0			30			0.00			500					DUNK36
w/chives	170		4.0	4.0	2.0	2.0	230	80					0				
1 pkt	~54	17.0	11.0			45			0.00			500					DUNK32
w/garden vegetables	170		2.0	4.0	2.0	0.0	340	40					0				
1 pkt	~46	15.0	11.0			45			0.00			400					DUNK33
w/salmon	170		4.0	2.0	0.0	0.0	180	200					0				
1 pkt	~50	17.0	11.0			45			0.00			500					DUNK34
w/strawberry	190		4.0	9.0	9.0	0.0	150	40					2				
1 pkt	~65	17.0	9.0			45			0.00			500					DUNK35
croissant	330		5.0	37.0	3.0	0.0	270	0					0				
1 croissant	~78	18.0	4.5			5			0.00			0					DUNK37
cruller, french	150		2.0	17.0	8.0	1.0	105	0					0				
1 cruller	~33	8.0	2.0			20			0.00			0					DUNK38
danish, apple	250		4.0	36.0	15.0	0.0	220	0					0				
3 oz danish	85	10.0	2.5			5			0.00			0					DUNK43
cheese	270		4.0	32.0	11.0	0.0	210	0					0				
3 oz danish	85	14.0	4.5			15			0.00			0					DUNK44
strawberry cheese	250		4.0	33.0	12.0	0.0	200	0					0				
3 oz danish	85	12.0	3.5			10			0.00			0					DUNK45
donut, apple crumb	230		3.0	34.0	12.0	1.0	270	0					0				
1 donut	~67	10.0	3.0			0			0.72			0					DUNK51
donut, apple n'spice	200		3.0	29.0	7.0	1.0	270	0					0				
1 donut	~57	8.0	1.5			0			0.72			0					DUNK52
donut, bavarian kreme	210		3.0	30.0	9.0	1.0	270	0					0				
1 donut	~60	9.0	2.0			0			0.72			0					DUNK53
donut, bismark w/choc icing	340		3.0	50.0	31.0	1.0	290	0					0				
1 donut	~97	15.0	3.5			0			0.72			0					DUNK54
donut, black raspberry	210		3.0	32.0	10.0	1.0	280	0					0				
1 donut	~61	8.0	1.5			0			0.72			0					DUNK55
donut, blueberry crumb	240		3.0	36.0	15.0	1.0	260	0					0				
1 donut	~70	10.0	3.0			0			0.72			0					DUNK56
donut, boston kreme	240		3.0	36.0	14.0	1.0	280	0					0				
1 donut	~69	9.0	2.0			0			0.72			0					DUNK57
donut, bow tie	300		4.0	34.0	10.0	1.0	340	0					0				
1 donut	~72	17.0	3.5			0			0.72			0					DUNK58
donut, cake, blueberry	290		3.0	35.0	16.0	1.0	400	0					0				
1 donut	~68	16.0	3.5			10			1.08			0					DUNK61
choc coconut	300		4.0	31.0	12.0	1.0	370	0					0				
1 donut	~70	19.0	6.0			0			0.00			0					DUNK63
cinnamon	330		4.0	34.0	14.0	1.0	340	20					0				
1 donut	~73	20.0	5.0			25			1.80			0					DUNK64
double choc	310		3.0	37.0	18.0	2.0	370	40					0				
1 donut	~72	17.0	3.5			0			0.00			0					DUNK66
glazed	350		4.0	41.0	21.0	1.0	340	20					0				
1 donut	~85	19.0	5.0			25			1.44			0					DUNK67
old fashioned	300		4.0	28.0	9.0	1.0	330	20					0				
1 donut	~65	19.0	5.0			25			1.44			0					DUNK68
powdered	330		4.0	36.0	17.0	1.0	330	20					0				
1 donut	~75	19.0	5.0			25			1.44			0					DUNK69
whole wheat, glazed	310		4.0	32.0	14.0	2.0	380	0					0				
1 donut	~79	19.0	4.0			0			1.08			0					DUNK72
w/choc glaze	290		3.0	33.0	14.0	1.0	370	0					0				
1 donut	~66	16.0	3.5			0			0.00			0					DUNK59
w/choc icing	360		4.0	40.0	15.0	1.0	350	20					0				
1 donut	~81	20.0	5.0			25			1.44			0					DUNK60

Minerals columns: Na, Ca, Mg, Zn, Mn (row 1); K, P, Fe, Cu, Se (row 2). Vitamins columns: A, C, B-1, NIA, B-12, PANT (row 1); A (IU), E, B-2, B-6, FOL, REF (row 2).

	KCAL / WT (g)	H_2O (g) / FAT (g)	PRO (g) / SFA (g)	CHO (g) / MUFA (g)	SUGR (g) / PUFA (g)	DFIB (g) / CHOL (mg)	Na (mg) / K (mg)	Ca (mg) / P (mg)	Mg (mg) / Fe (mg)	Zn (mg) / Cu (mg)	Mn (mg) / Se (mcg)	A (mcg RAE) / A (IU)	C (mg) / E (mg ATE)	B-1 (mg) / B-2 (mg)	NIA (mg) / B-6 (mg)	B-12 (mcg) / FOL (mcg DFE)	PANT (mg) / REF
donut, choc kreme-filled	270		3.0	35.0	16.0	1.0	260	0					0				
1 donut	~73	13.0	3.0			0			0.72			0					DUNK73
donut, éclair	270		3.0	39.0	17.0	1.0	290	0					0				
1 donut	~86	11.0	2.5			0			0.72			0					DUNK82
donut, glazed	180		3.0	25.0	6.0	1.0	250	0					0				
1 donut	~48	8.0	1.5			0			0.72			0					DUNK75
donut, jelly-filled	210		3.0	32.0	14.0	1.0	280	0					0				
1 donut	~66	8.0	1.5			0			0.72			0					DUNK76
donut, lemon burst	300		3.0	35.0	25.0	3.0	300	0					0				
1 donut	~80	14.0	5.0			0			1.80			0					DUNK77
donut, strawberry	210		3.0	32.0	11.0	1.0	260	0					0				
1 donut	~66	8.0	1.5			0			0.72			0					DUNK78
donut, sugar, raised	170		3.0	22.0	4.0	1.0	250	0					0				
1 donut	~44	8.0	1.5			0			0.72			0					DUNK79
donut, van kreme-filled	270		3.0	36.0	17.0	1.0	250	0					0				
1 donut	~80	13.0	3.0			0			0.72			0					DUNK80
donut w/choc icing	200		3.0	29.0	10.0	1.0	260	0					0				
1 donut	~48	9.0	2.0			0			0.72			0					DUNK46
donut w/maple icing	210		3.0	30.0	12.0	1.0	260	0					0				
1 donut	~49	9.0	2.0			0			0.72			0					DUNK47
donut w/marble icing	200		3.0	29.0	11.0	1.0	260	0					0				
1 donut	~48	9.0	2.0			0			0.72			0					DUNK48
donut w/strawberry icing	210		3.0	30.0	12.0	1.0	260	0					0				
1 donut	~49	9.0	2.0			0			0.72			0					DUNK49
Dunkaccino	230		2.0	35.0	25.0	0.0	210	40					0				
10 fl oz	~362	10.0	3.0			5			0.00			0					DUNK81
english muffin w/ham, egg, & cheese	310		21.0	35.0	3.0	1.0	1300	150					0				
1 sandwich	~124	10.0	5.0			145			5.40			300					DUNK83
fritter, apple	300		4.0	41.0	12.0	1.0	360	0					0				
1 fritter	~74	14.0	3.0			0			1.08			0					DUNK84
glazed	260		4.0	31.0	7.0	1.0	330	0					0				
1 fritter	~61	14.0	0.0			0			1.08			0					DUNK85
hot chocolate	220		2.0	38.0	28.0	2.0	280	40					0				
10 fl oz	~310	8.0	2.0			0			0.36			0					DUNK86
iced coffee w/cream	60		1.0	2.0	0.0	0.0	20	40					0				
16 fl oz	~450	6.0	3.5			20			0.00			200					DUNK87
w/cream & sugar	110		1.0	14.0	12.0	0.0	20	40					0				
16 fl oz	~462	6.0	3.5			20			0.00			200					DUNK88
jelly stick	530		4.0	61.0	32.0	1.0	320	0					0				
1 stick	~146	29.0	7.0			35			6.30			0					DUNK89
muffin, banana nut	540		10.0	73.0	35.0	3.0	550	80					0				
1 muffin	~177	23.0	6.0			75			2.70			1750					DUNK90
blueberry	490		8.0	75.0	39.0	2.0	630	60					0				
1 muffin	~168	18.0	6.0			75			2.70			200					DUNK91
blueberry, red fat	450		9.0	74.0	35.0	2.0	650	80					0				
1 muffin	~160	13.0	3.5			70			2.70			0					DUNK92
choc chip	590		9.0	85.0	47.0	3.0	570	80					0				
1 muffin	~195	23.0	10.0			75			2.70			200					DUNK93
coffee cake	710		11.0	102.0	59.0	2.0	650	100					0				
6.5 oz muffin	184	29.0	9.0			85			3.60			200					DUNK94
corn	510		9.0	81.0	35.0	1.0	950	60					0				
1 muffin	~160	17.0	5.0			85			2.70			300					DUNK95
cranberry orange	460		8.0	71.0	35.0	3.0	530	800					5				
1 muffin	~158	16.0	5.0			70			2.70			200					DUNK96
honey bran raisin	490		10.0	81.0	45.0	5.0	510	100					0				
1 muffin	~175	14.0	3.5			60			3.60			0					DUNK97
Munchkins, cake	270		3.0	27.0	9.0	1.0	240	0					0				
4 munchkins	~58	16.0	4.0			25			5.40			0					DUNK99

	KCAL	H₂O (g)	PRO (g)	CHO (g)	SUGR (g)	DFIB (g)	Na (mg)	Ca (mg)	Mg (mg)	Zn (mg)	Mn (mg)	A (mcg RAE)	C (mg)	B-1 (mg)	NIA (mg)	B-12 (mcg)	PANT (mg)
	WT (g)	FAT (g)	SFA (g)	MUFA (g)	PUFA (g)	CHOL (mg)	K (mg)	P (mg)	Fe (mg)	Cu (mg)	Se (mcg)	A (IU)	E (mg ATE)	B-2 (mg)	B-6 (mg)	FOL (mcg DFE)	REF
cinnamon	270		3.0	31.0	14.0	1.0	210	20					0				
4 munchkins	~62	15.0	3.5			25			4.50			0					DUNK101
coco, glazed	200		2.0	26.0	13.0	1.0	250	0					0				
3 munchkins	~33	10.0	2.0			0			0.00			0					DUNK107
glazed	280		3.0	38.0	22.0	1.0	190	0					0				
3 munchkins	~46	13.0	3.0			20			4.50			0					DUNK103
powdered	270		3.0	31.0	15.0	1.0	210	0					0				
4 munchkins	~61	14.0	3.5			25			4.50			0					DUNK104
Munchkins, yeast, glazed	200		3.0	27.0	12.0	1.0	220	0					0				
5 munchkins	~52	9.0	2.0			0			0.36			0					DUNK108
jelly-filled	210		3.0	30.0	15.0	1.0	240	0					0				
5 munchkins	~65	9.0	2.0			0			0.72			0					DUNK109
lemon-filled	170		2.0	23.0	9.0	0.0	190	0					0				
4 munchkins	~42	8.0	1.5			0			0.00			0					DUNK110
sugar-raised	220		4.0	26.0	5.0	1.0	290	0					0				
7 munchkins	~53	12.0	2.5			0			0.72			0					DUNK111
scone, blueberry	410		5.0	55.0	24.0	1.0	320	40					1				
4 oz scone	113	19.0	5.0			40			1.44			0					DUNK112
maple walnut	470		6.0	62.0	25.0	1.0	320	60					0				
4 oz scone	113	22.0	5.0			40			1.80			0					DUNK113
raspberry white choc	450		6.0	59.0	27.0	1.0	330	60					1				
4 oz scone	~113	22.0	7.0			40			1.44			0					DUNK98
vanilla chai	230		1.0	40.0	32.0	0.0	50	20					0				
10 fl oz	~240	8.0	6.0			5			0.72			0					DUNK115

10.8 JACK-IN-THE-BOX

	KCAL		PRO	CHO	SUGR	DFIB	Na										
	WT	FAT	SFA			CHOL	K										REF
bacon cheddar potato wedges	770		21.0	52.0	2.0	3.0	1330										
9.3 oz serving	262	53.0	16.0			45	950										JACK25
biscuit, sausage	380		11.0	25.0	2.0	2.0	730										
3.6 oz biscuit	103	27.0	8.0			35	260										JACK48
sausage, egg & cheese	760		25.0	33.0	4.0	2.0	1390										
7.9 oz biscuit	223	60.0	20.0			280	240										JACK50
Breakfast Jack®	310		13.0	33.0	4.0	1.0	720										
4.7 oz sandwich	129	14.0	5.0			205	200										JACK44
cake, double fudge	310		3.0	49.0	37.0	4.0	270										
3 oz serving	85	11.0	3.0			25	220										JACK58
cheese sticks	240		11.0	21.0	1.0	1.0	420										
3 sticks (2.5 oz)	71	12.0	5.0			25	60										JACK26
	400		18.0	35.0	2.0	2.0	700										
5 sticks (4.2 oz)	118	21.0	8.0			40	100										JACK27
cheeseburger	360		19.0	31.0	6.0	1.0	740										
4.1 oz sandwich	127	18.0	8.0			60	130										JACK4
bacon bacon	910		38.0	58.0	10.0	3.0	1780										
11 oz sandwich	314	59.0	19.0			100	460										JACK7
bacon ultimate	1120		52.0	59.0	12.0	2.0	2260										
12.5 oz sandwich	353	75.0	28.0			160	600										JACK8
big	700		26.0	59.0	13.0	2.0	1340										
8.4 oz sandwich	239	40.0	16.0			70	330										JACK9
Big Texas	610		26.0	55.0	8.0	2.0	1280										
8 oz sandwich	228	32.0	15.0			65	280										JACK10
chili	440		20.0	45.0	7.0	2.0	880										
6 oz sandwich	173	20.0	9.0			45	230										JACK1
Jack's Western	660		24.0	59.0	12.0	2.0	1100										
8.8 oz sandwich	249	37.0	14.0			60	330										JACK11
jr bacon	540		22.0	31.0	6.0	1.0	940										
5.4 oz sandwich	153	36.0	10.0			75	160										JACK5
Ultimate	990		41.0	59.0	12.0	2.0	1620										
11.6 oz sandwich	328	66.0	28.0			130	480										JACK15

	KCAL / WT (g)	H₂0 (g) / FAT (g)	PRO (g) / SFA (g)	CHO (g) / MUFA (g)	SUGR (g) / PUFA (g)	DFIB (g) / CHOL (mg)	Na (mg) / K (mg)	Ca (mg) / P (mg)	Mg (mg) / Fe (mg)	Zn (mg) / Cu (mg)	Mn (mg) / Se (mcg)	A (mcg RAE) / A (IU)	C (mg) / E (mg ATE)	B-1 (mg) / B-2 (mg)	NIA (mg) / B-6 (mg)	B-12 (mcg) / FOL (mcg DFE)	PANT (mg) / REF
cheesecake	310		7.0	34.0	23.0	0.0	220										
3.6 oz serving	103	16.0	9.0			55	180										JACK56
chicken breast pieces	360		27.0	24.0	0.0	1.0	970										
5 pieces (5.3 oz)	150	17.0	3.0			80	430										JACK16
chicken fajita pita	330		24.0	35.0	4.0	3.0	910										
8.1 oz sandwich	230	11.0	4.5			55	430										JACK17
chicken sandwich	410		15.0	39.0	4.0	2.0	740										
5.8 oz sandwich	165	21.0	4.5			35	290										JACK18
grilled fillet	430		23.0	34.0	6.0	2.0	910										
7.6 oz sandwich	216	22.0	6.0			60	390										JACK22
supreme	830		31.0	70.0	5.0	3.0	1920										
10.6 oz sandwich	308	46.0	7.0			60	230										JACK19
chicken teriyaki bowl	550		26.0	103.0	27.0	3.0	1720										
16.3 oz bowl	461	3.0	0.5			35	420										JACK20
croissant, sausage	680		18.0	41.0	5.0	2.0	760										
6.6 oz croissant	188	50.0	15.0			250	230										JACK49
supreme	570		19.0	41.0	5.0	1.0	1040										
6 oz croissant	171	37.0	9.0			240	270										JACK52
croutons	60		2.0	10.0	0.0	0.0	130										
.49 oz	14	1.5	0.0			0	20										JACK86
Curly Fries, chili cheese	630		13.0	54.0	6.0	6.0	1640										
8.3 oz serving	236	40.0	11.0			30	800										JACK28
seasoned	400		6.0	45.0	1.0	5.0	890										
4.4 oz serving	125	23.0	5.0			0	580										JACK36
dipping sce, bbq	45		1.0	11.0	4.0	0.0	330										
1 oz	28	0.0	0.0			0	65										JACK62
buttermilk house	130		0.0	3.0	0.0	0.0	210										
.88 oz	25	13.0	2.0			10	15										JACK64
Frank's Red Hot Buffalo	10		0.0	2.0	0.0	0.0	840										
1 oz	28	0.0	0.0			0	15										JACK66
sweet & sour	45		0.0	11.0	6.0	0.0	160										
1 oz	28	0.0	0.0			0	5										JACK70
egg roll	130		5.0	15.0	1.0	2.0	310										
2 oz egg roll	57	6.0	2.0			5	140										JACK29
	400		14.0	44.0	4.0	6.0	920										
3 egg rolls (6 oz)	170	19.0	6.0			15	430										JACK30
Extreme Sausage Sandwich	720		26.0	35.0	5.0	2.0	1180										
7.7 oz sandwich	219	53.0	18.0			280	310										JACK45
fish & chips	610		18.0	66.0	0.0	5.0	1240										
8 oz serving	227	31.0	7.0			40	660										JACK21
french fries	330		3.0	44.0	0.0	3.0	550										
4 oz serving	113	16.0	3.5			0	440										JACK31
jumbo	410		4.0	55.0	0.0	4.0	690										
5 oz serving	142	20.0	4.5			0	550										JACK32
Super Scoop	580		6.0	77.0	0.0	6.0	960										
7 oz serving	198	28.0	6.0			0	770										JACK33
French Toast Sticks	430		8.0	57.0	11.0	2.0	460										
4 pieces (4.4 oz)	124	18.0	4.0			10	140										JACK46
guacamole	90		1.0	5.0	1.0	3.0	240										
1.6 oz	46	7.0	2.0			0	180										JACK88
hamburger	310		17.0	30.0	6.0	1.0	600										
4.2 oz sandwich	119	14.0	6.0			45	120										JACK3
hash browns	150		1.0	13.0	0.0	2.0	230										
2 oz serving	57	10.0	2.5			0	190										JACK47
ice cream shake, choc	660		11.0	89.0	79.0	1.0	270										
16 fl oz shake	315	29.0	18.0			110	720										JACK57
Oreo Cookie	670		11.0	81.0	62.0	1.0	350										
16 fl oz shake	301	33.0	19.0			110	660										JACK59
strawberry	640		10.0	84.0	71.0	0.0	220										
16 fl oz shake	313	28.0	18.0			110	610										JACK60

	KCAL	H₂0 (g)	PRO (g)	CHO (g)	SUGR (g)	DFIB (g)	Na (mg)	Ca (mg)	Mg (mg)	Zn (mg)	Mn (mg)	A (mcg RAE)	C (mg)	B-1 (mg)	NIA (mg)	B-12 (mcg)	PANT (mg)
	WT (g)	FAT (g)	SFA (g)	MUFA (g)	PUFA (g)	CHOL (mg)	K (mg)	P (mg)	Fe (mg)	Cu (mg)	Se (mcg)	A (IU)	E (mg ATE)	B-2 (mg)	B-6 (mg)	FOL (mcg DFE)	REF
van	570		12.0	65.0	54.0	0.0	220										
16 fl oz shake	285	29.0	18.0			115	630										JACK61
Jack's Spicy Chicken	650		26.0	67.0	9.0	4.0	1190										
10 oz sandwich	283	31.0	6.0			60	460										JACK23
jelly, grape	35		0.0	9.0	9.0		10										
.49 oz	14	0.0	0.0			0	0										JACK87
Jumbo Jack	600		22.0	58.0	12.0	3.0	980										
9.5 oz sandwich	269	31.0	11.0			45	390										JACK12
w/cheese	690		27.0	61.0	13.0	3.0	1360										
10.4 oz sandwich	314	38.0	16.0			70	470										JACK13
ketchup	10		0.0	2.0	2.0	0.0	105										
.32 oz	9	0.0	0.0			0	30										JACK89
marinara sce	15		0.0	3.0	3.0	0.0	210										
.88 oz	25	0.0	0.0			0	85										JACK68
onion rings	500		6.0	51.0	3.0	3.0	420										
4.2 oz serving	119	30.0	5.0			0	140										JACK35
philly cheesesteak	580		35.0	55.0	6.0	3.0	1660										
8.3 oz sandwich	264	22.0	11.0			90	390										JACK6
salad dressing, blue cheese	260		1.0	5.0	4.0	0.0	670										
2 oz	57	26.0	4.5			30	25										JACK63
buttermilk house	310		1.0	3.0	2.0	0.0	470										
2 oz	57	33.0	5.0			20	45										JACK65
Italian, low cal	15		0.0	4.0	2.0	0.0	510										
2 oz	57	0.0	0.0			0	25										JACK67
thousand island	160		1.0	12.0	10.0	0.0	490										
2 oz	57	12.0	2.0			15	45										JACK73
salad, side	50		3.0	4.0	2.0	2.0	65										
4.6 oz salad	130	3.0	1.5			10	280										JACK37
salsa	10		0.0	2.0	1.0	0.0	220										
1 oz	28	0.0	0.0			0	55										JACK91
sour cream	60		1.0	2.0	0.0	0.0	20										
1 oz	28	5.0	3.0			15	35										JACK92
Sourdough Breakfast Sandwich	440		17.0	36.0	3.0	2.0	880										
5.8 oz sandwich	159	26.0	8.0			215	210										JACK51
Sourdough Grilled Chicken Club	520		33.0	33.0	5.0	3.0	1330										
8.8 oz sandwich	249	28.0	6.0			85	540										JACK24
Sourdough Jack®	700		30.0	36.0	7.0	3.0	1220										
8.6 oz sandwich	244	49.0	16.0			80	450										JACK14
soy sce	5		0.0	1.0	0.0	0.0	480										
.32 oz	9	0.0	0.0			0	35										JACK69
stuffed jalapeños	230		7.0	22.0	2.0	2.0	690										
3 peppers (2.5 oz)	72	13.0	6.0			20	105										JACK38
	530		15.0	51.0	5.0	4.0	1600										
7 peppers (5.9 oz)	168	30.0	13.0			45	240										JACK39
taco	170		6.0	15.0	2.0	2.0	210										
2.7 oz taco	77	9.0	3.0			20	190										JACK40
Monster	260		9.0	21.0	4.0	3.0	340										
4.4 oz taco	119	15.0	5.0			30	130										JACK34
taco sce	0		0.0	0.0	0.0	0.0	80										
.32 oz	9	0.0	0.0			0	20										JACK71
taquitos	320		14.0	28.0	1.0	3.0	440										
3 pieces (4 oz)	114	17.0	7.0			40	200										JACK41
	480		19.0	47.0	2.0	5.0	650										
5 pieces (6.2 oz)	175	24.0	9.0			50	330										JACK42
tartar sce	210		0.0	2.0	1.0	0.0	370										
1.5 oz	43	22.0	3.5			20	30										JACK72
turnover, apple	170		6.0	15.0	2.0	2.0	210										
3.7 oz turnover	105	9.0	3.0			20	190										JACK40
Ultimate Breakfast Sandwich	730		30.0	66.0	9.0	2.0	1870										
10 oz sandwich	284	40.0	11.0			440	390										JACK53

	KCAL / WT (g)	H₂O / FAT (g)	PRO / SFA (g)	CHO / MUFA (g)	SUGR / PUFA (g)	DFIB (g) / CHOL (mg)	Na / K (mg)	Ca / P (mg)	Mg / Fe (mg)	Zn / Cu (mg)	Mn (mg) / Se (mcg)	A (mcg RAE) / A (IU)	C (mg) / E (mg ATE)	B-1 (mg) / B-2 (mg)	NIA (mg) / B-6 (mg)	B-12 (mcg) / FOL (mcg DFE)	PANT (mg) / REF

10.9 KENTUCKY FRIED CHICKEN

Item	KCAL / WT	H₂O / FAT	PRO / SFA	CHO / MUFA	SUGR / PUFA	DFIB / CHOL	Na / K	Ca / P	Mg / Fe	Zn / Cu	Mn / Se	A-RAE / A-IU	C / E	B-1 / B-2	NIA / B-6	B-12 / FOL	PANT / REF
baked beans, bbq	190		6.0	33.0	13.0	6.0	760	80									
5.5 oz serving	156	3.0	1.0			5			1.80			400					KFCN39
biscuit	180		4.0	20.0	2.0	<1.0	560	20					<1				
1 biscuit	56	10.0	2.5			0			1.08								KFCN44
cake, double choc chip	320		4.0	41.0	28.0	1.0	230	40				0					
2.7 oz piece	76	16.0	4.0			55			1.80			0					KFCN45
chicken breast, Extra Crispy	470		34.0	19.0	0.0	0.0	1230	20					<1				
5.7 oz piece	162	28.0	8.0			135			1.44								KFCN6
Hot & Spicy	450		33.0	20.0	0.0	0.0	1450						<1				
6.3 oz piece	179	27.0	8.0			130			1.08								KFCN10
Original Recipe	370		40.0	11.0	0.0	0.0	1145	20					<1				
5.7 oz piece	161	19.0	6.0			145			1.08								KFCN2
chicken drumstick, Extra Crispy	160		12.0	5.0	0.0	0.0	415						<1				
2.1 oz piece	60	10.0	2.5			70			0.72								KFCN7
Hot & Spicy	140		13.0	4.0	0.0	0.0	380	20					<1				
2.1 oz piece	60	9.0	2.5			65			0.72								KFCN11
Original Recipe	140		14.0	4.0	0.0	0.0	440						<1				
2.1 oz piece	59	8.0	2.0			75			0.72								KFCN3
chicken pieces, honey bbq	607		33.0	33.0	18.0	1.0	1145	40					5				
6 pieces (6.7 oz)	189	38.0	10.0			193			1.44			400					KFCN32
Hot Wing	471		27.0	18.0	0.0	2.0	1230	40					<1				
6 pieces (4.8 oz)	135	33.0	8.0			150			1.44								KFCN31
chicken pot pie	770		29.0	69.0	8.0	5.0	2160	100					1				
13 oz serving	368	42.0	13.0			70			1.80			4000					KFCN30
chicken thigh, Extra Crispy	370		21.0	12.0	0.0	0.0	710	20					<1				
4 oz piece	114	26.0	7.0			120			1.08								KFCN8
Hot & Spicy	390		22.0	14.0	0.0	0.0	1240	·					<1				
4.5 oz piece	128	28.0	8.0			125			1.44								KFCN12
Original Recipe	360		22.0	12.0	0.0	0.0	1060						<1				
4.4 oz piece	126	25.0	7.0			165			1.08								KFCN4
chicken wing, Extra Crispy	190		10.0	10.0	0.0	0.0	390						<1				
1.8 oz piece	52	12.0	3.5			55			0.36								KFCN5
Hot & Spicy	180		11.0	9.0	0.0	0.0	420						<1				
1.9 oz piece	55	11.0	3.0			60			0.72								KFCN9
Original Recipe	145		11.0	5.0	0.0	0.0	370						<1				
1.7 oz piece	47	9.0	2.5			60			0.36								KFCN1
coleslaw	190		1.0	22.0	13.0	3.0	300	40					24				
5 oz serving	142	11.0	2.0			5			0.00			1250					KFCN40
corn on the cob	150		5.0	26.0	10.0	7.0	10	60					6				
5.7 oz piece	162	3.0	1.0			0			1.08			0					KFCN38
Crunch Melt, honey bbq	556		33.0	48.0	7.0	2.0	1010	40					<1				
8.1 oz serving	231	26.0	5.0			60			1.80								KFCN24
green beans	50		5.0	5.0	2.0	2.0	460	0					1				
4.7 oz serving	132	1.5	0.5			5			0.72			750					KFCN42
macaroni & cheese	180		7.0	21.0	2.0	2.0	860	150					<1				
5.4 oz serving	153	8.0	3.0			10			<0.36			1000					KFCN37
mashed potatoes w/gravy	120		1.0	17.0	0.0	2.0	440						<1				
4.8 oz serving	136	6.0	1.0			<1			0.36								KFCN35
Mean Greens	70		4.0	11.0	1.0	5.0	650	200					6				
5.4 oz serving	152	3.0	1.0			10			1.80			3000					KFCN43
parfait, choc cream	290		3.0	37.0	25.0	2.0	330	40				0					
4 oz serving	113	15.0	11.0			15			1.08								KFCN48
fudge brownie	280		3.0	44.0	35.0	1.0	190	20				0					
3.5 oz serving	99	10.0	3.5			145			1.08			100					KFCN46
lemon crème	410		7.0	62.0	50.0	4.0	290	200					2				
4.5 oz serving	127	14.0	8.0			20			0.72			100					KFCN47
strawberry shortcake	200		1.0	33.0	26.0	1.0	220	20					5				
3.5 oz serving	99	7.0	6.0			10			0.72								KFCN49

	KCAL	H₂O (g)	PRO (g)	CHO (g)	SUGR (g)	DFIB (g)	Na (mg)	Ca (mg)	Mg (mg)	Zn (mg)	Mn (mg)	A (mcg RAE)	C (mg)	B-1 (mg)	NIA (mg)	B-12 (mcg)	PANT (mg)
	WT (g)	FAT (g)	SFA (g)	MUFA (g)	PUFA (g)	CHOL (mg)	K (mg)	P (mg)	Fe (mg)	Cu (mg)	Se (mcg)	A (IU)	E (mg ATE)	B-2 (mg)	B-6 (mg)	FOL (mcg DFE)	REF
pie, apple	310		2.0	44.0	23.0	0.0	280	0					0				
4 oz slice	113	14.0	3.0			0			1.08			0					KFCN51
pecan	490		5.0	66.0	31.0	2.0	510	20					0				
4 oz slice	113	23.0	5.0			65			1.44			200					KFCN50
strawberry creme	280		4.0	32.0	22.0	2.0	130	0					2				
2.8 oz slice	78	15.0	8.0			15			0.72			100					KFCN52
popcorn chicken, large	620		30.0	36.0	0.0	0.0	1046	20					0				
6 oz serving	170	40.0	10.0			73			0.72			0					KFCN29
small	362		17.0	21.0	0.0	0.2	610	0					0				
3.5 oz serving	99	23.0	6.0			43			0.36			0					KFCN28
potato salad	180		2.0	22.0	5.0	1.0	470	0					6				
5.6 oz serving	160	9.0	1.5			5			0.36			0					KFCN41
potato wedges	240		4.0	30.0	0.0	3.0	830	20					4				
5.5 oz serving	156	12.0	3.0			0			1.80			0					KFCN36
sandwich, honey bbq chicken	310		28.0	37.0	7.0	2.0	560	60					<1				
6.3 oz sandwich	178	6.0	2.0			125			1.80			300					KFCN21
sandwich, Original Recipe chicken	450		29.0	33.0	0.0	2.0	940	40					<1				
w/sce - 7 oz sandwich	200	22.0	5.0			70			1.80			100					KFCN13
w/o sce	360		29.0	21.0	<1.0	<1.0	890	40					<1				
6.6 oz sandwich	187	13.0	3.5			60			1.80			100					KFCN14
sandwich, Tender Roast chicken	350		32.0	26.0	1.0	1.0	880	40					<1				
w/sce - 7.4 oz sandwich	211	15.0	3.0			75			1.80			200					KFCN19
w/o sce	270		31.0	23.0	<1.0		690	40					<1				
6.2 oz sandwich	177	5.0	1.5			65			1.80								KFCN20
sandwich, Triple Crunch chicken	490		28.0	39.0	0.0	2.0	710	40					<1				
w/sce - 6.7 oz sandwich	189	29.0	6.0			70			1.80			100					KFCN15
w/o sce	390		25.0	29.0	0.0	2.0	650	40					<1				
6.2 oz sandwich	176	15.0	4.5			50			2.70								KFCN16
sandwich, Triple Crunch Zinger	550		28.0	39.0	3.0	2.0	830	40					<1				
chicken w/sce - 7.4 oz sandwich	210	32.0	7.0			85			1.80			300					KFCN17
w/o sce	390		25.0	36.0	0.0	2.0	650	40					<1				
6.2 oz sandwich	176	15.0	4.5			50			1.80								KFCN18
Strips, Blazin	315		26.0	21.0	1.0	1.0	1541						1				
3 strips (4.6 oz)	129	16.0	4.0			56			1.26			100					KFCN34
Strips, crispy Colonels	340		28.0	20.0	0.0	0.0	1140						<1				
3 strips (5.3 oz)	150	16.0	4.5			70			0.72								KFCN25
honey bbq	377		27.0	33.0	12.0	4.0	1709	40					<1				
3 strips (6.3 oz)	178	15.0	4.0			45			0.36			100					KFCN27
spicy crispy	335		25.0	23.0	<1.0	<1.0	1140	20					<1				
3 strips (4.1 oz)	115	15.0	4.0			70			0.90			100					KFCN26
Twister	600		22.0	52.0	4.0	4.0	1430	100					<1				
8.5 oz serving	240	34.0	7.0			50			1.80			100					KFCN22
Blazin	719		30.0	56.0	4.0	4.0	1986	360					2				
8.7 oz serving	246	43.0	12.0			70			1.98			250					KFCN33
Crispy Caesar	744		27.0	66.0	4.0	5.0	1616	170					<1				
9.5 oz serving	270	41.0	9.0			55			2.52			400					KFCN23

10.10 MCDONALD'S

	KCAL	H₂O (g)	PRO (g)	CHO (g)	SUGR (g)	DFIB (g)	Na (mg)	Ca (mg)	Mg (mg)	Zn (mg)	Mn (mg)	A (mcg RAE)	C (mg)	B-1 (mg)	NIA (mg)	B-12 (mcg)	PANT (mg)
bagel, ham, egg, & cheese	550		26.0	58.0	10.0	2.0	1500	200					<1				
7.7 oz bagel	218	23.0	8.0			255			4.50			750					MCDS1
spanish omelete	710		27.0	59.0	10.0	3.0	1520	250					15				
9.1 oz bagel	258	40.0	15.0			275			4.50			750					MCDS2
steak, egg, & cheese	640		31.0	57.0	9.0	2.0	1540	200					<1				
8.6 oz bagel	241	31.0	12.0			265			5.40			750					MCDS3
biscuit	240		4.0	30.0	1.0	1.0	640	40					<1				
2.4 oz biscuit	69	11.0	2.5			0			1.80								MCDS4
bacon, egg, & cheese	480		21.0	31.0	3.0	1.0	1360	150					<1				
5.4 oz biscuit	152	31.0	10.0			250			2.70			500					MCDS5

	KCAL	H₂0 (g)	PRO (g)	CHO (g)	SUGR (g)	DFIB (g)	Minerals					Vitamins					
							Na (mg)	Ca (mg)	Mg (mg)	Zn (mg)	Mn (mg)	A (mcg RAE)	C (mg)	B-1 (mg)	NIA (mg)	B-12 (mcg)	PANT (mg)
	WT (g)	FAT (g)	SFA (g)	MUFA (g)	PUFA (g)	CHOL (mg)	K (mg)	P (mg)	Fe (mg)	Cu (mg)	Se (mcg)	A (IU)	E (mg ATE)	B-2 (mg)	B-6 (mg)	FOL (mcg DFE)	REF
sausage	410		10.0	30.0	2.0	1.0	930	40					<1				
4 oz biscuit	112	28.0	8.0			35			2.70								MCDS6
sausage & egg	490		16.0	31.0	2.0	1.0	1010	80					<1				
5.7 oz biscuit	162	33.0	10.0			245			2.70			300					MCDS7
burrito, sausage	290		13.0	24.0	2.0	2.0	680	150					12				
4 oz burrito	113	16.0	6.0			170			2.70			500					MCDS8
cheeseburger	330		15.0	35.0	7.0	2.0	800	250					2				
4.3 oz sandwich	121	14.0	6.0			45			2.70			200					MCDS9
Big Mac	590		24.0	47.0	8.0	3.0	1070	300					4				
7.6 oz sandwich	215	34.0	11.0			85			4.50			300					MCDS10
Big N' Tasty	580		26.0	37.0	8.0	2.0	1030	300					9				
9.3 oz sandwich	247	37.0	12.0			95			4.50			500					MCDS11
Quarter Pounder	530		28.0	38.0	9.0	2.0	1250	350					2				
7.05 oz sandwich	199	30.0	13.0			95			4.50			500					MCDS12
Chicken McGrill sandwich	400		25.0	37.0	6.0	2.0	890	200					6				
7.5 oz sandwich	213	17.0	3.0			60			2.70			300					MCDS13
Chicken McNugget sce, barbeque	45		0.0	10.0	10.0	0.0	250						4				
1 oz pkt	28	0.0	0.0			0			<0.01								MCDS15
honey	45		0.0	12.0	11.0	0.0	0						<1				
.5 oz pkt	14	0.0	0.0			0			<0.01								MCDS16
honey mustard	50		0.0	3.0	3.0	0.0	95						<1				
.5 oz pkt	14	4.5	0.5			10			<0.01								MCDS17
hot mustard	60		<1.0	7.0	6.0	<1.0	240						<1				
1 oz pkt	28	3.5	0.0			5			0.72								MCDS18
lite mayonnaise	45		0.0	<1.0	0.0	0.0	100						<1				
.4 oz pkt	12	4.5	0.5			10			<0.01								MCDS19
sweet' n sour	50		0.0	11.0	10.0	0.0	140						<1				
1 oz pkt	28	0.0	0.0			0			<0.01			300					MCDS20
Chicken McNuggets	210		10.0	12.0	0.0	1.0	460						1				
4 pieces (2.5 oz)	72	13.0	2.5			35			0.72								MCDS21
	310		15.0	18.0	0.0	2.0	680	20					1				
6 pieces (3.8 oz)	108	20.0	4.0			50			0.72								MCDS22
	510		25.0	30.0	0.0	3.0	1140	20					2				
10 pieces (6.3 oz)	180	33.0	6.0			85			1.44								MCDS23
cinnamon roll	340		5.0	52.0	28.0	3.0	250	250					<1				
3.4 oz roll	99	15.0	5.0			35			1.08			100					MCDS24
cookies, choc chip	280		3.0	37.0	20.0	1.0	170	20					<1				
2 oz bag	57	14.0	8.0			40			1.44			400					MCDS25
McDonaldland	230		3.0	38.0	12.0	1.0	250						<1				
2 oz bag	57	8.0	2.0			0			1.80								MCDS26
Crispy Chicken sandwich	500		22.0	46.0	6.0	2.0	1100	200					6				
7.7 oz sandwich	219	26.0	4.5			50			2.70			300					MCDS27
danish, apple	340		5.0	47.0	21.0	2.0	340	60					15				
3.7 oz danish	105	15.0	3.0			20			1.44								MCDS28
cheese	400		7.0	45.0	16.0	2.0	400	80					<1				
3.7 oz danish	105	21.0	5.0			40			1.44			300					MCDS29
eggs, scrambled	160		13.0	1.0	1.0	0.0	170	60					<1				
2 eggs (3.6 oz)	101	11.0	3.5			425			1.08			500					MCDS30
english muffin	150		5.0	27.0	2.0	2.0	270	200					<1				
2 oz muffin	57	2.0	1.0			0			1.80								MCDS31
Filet-O-Fish sandwich	470		15.0	45.0	5.0	1.0	730	200					<1				
5.5 oz sandwich	156	26.0	5.0			50			1.80			200					MCDS32
french fries, large	540		8.0	68.0	0.0	6.0	350	20					21				
6.2 oz	176	26.0	4.5			0			1.44								MCDS36
med	450		6.0	57.0	0.0	5.0	290	20					18				
5.2 oz	147	22.0	4.0			0			1.08								MCDS35
small	210		3.0	26.0	0.0	2.0	135						9				
2.4 oz	68	10.0	1.5			0			0.36								MCDS34
super size	610		9.0	77.0	0.0	7.0	390	20					24				
7 oz	198	29.0	5.0			0			1.44								MCDS33

	KCAL / WT (g)	H₂O / FAT (g)	PRO / SFA (g)	CHO / MUFA (g)	SUGR / PUFA (g)	DFIB (g) / CHOL (mg)	Minerals Na / K (mg)	Ca / P (mg)	Mg / Fe (mg)	Zn / Cu (mg)	Mn (mg) / Se (mcg)	Vitamins A (mcg RAE) / A (IU)	C (mg) / E (mg ATE)	B-1 (mg) / B-2 (mg)	NIA (mg) / B-6 (mg)	B-12 (mcg) / FOL (mcg DFE)	PANT (mg) / REF
fruit & yogurt parfait	280		8.0	53.0	40.0	<1.0	115	250					24				
11 oz serving	310	4.0	2.0			15			1.08			100					MCDS37
w/granola	380		10.0	76.0	49.0	2.0	240	300					24				
12 oz serving	338	5.0	2.0			15			1.80			100					MCDS38
hamburger	280		12.0	35.0	7.0	2.0	560	200					2				
3.8 oz sandwich	105	10.0	4.0			30			2.70								MCDS39
Big N' Tasty	530		24.0	37.0	8.0	2.0	790	200					9				
8.85 oz sandwich	232	32.0	10.0			80			4.50			300					MCDS40
Quarter Pounder	420		23.0	36.0	8.0	2.0	780	200					2				
6.07 oz sandwich	171	21.0	8.0			70			4.50								MCDS41
hash browns	130		1.0	14.0	0.0	1.0	330						2				
1.9 oz serving	53	8.0	1.5			0			0.36								MCDS42
ice cream, van, red fat in cone	150		4.0	23.0	17.0	0.0	75	100					1				
3.2 oz cone	90	4.5	3.0			20			0.36			300					MCDS43
McFlurry, Butterfinger	620		16.0	90.0	76.0	<1.0	260	450					2				
12.3 oz serving	348	22.0	14.0			70			0.36			1250					MCDS44
M&M	630		16.0	90.0	81.0	1.0	210	500					2				
12.3 oz serving	348	23.0	15.0			75			0.36			1250					MCDS45
Nestle Crunch	630		16.0	89.0	78.0	<1.0	230	500					2				
12.3 oz serving	348	24.0	16.0			75			0.36			1250					MCDS46
Oreo	570		15.0	82.0	69.0	<1.0	280	450					2				
11.9 oz serving	337	20.0	12.0			70			1.08			1250					MCDS47
McMuffin, egg	300		18.0	29.0	3.0	2.0	840	300					1				
4.9 oz sandwich	138	12.0	5.0			235			2.70			500					MCDS48
sausage	370		14.0	28.0	2.0	2.0	790	250					<1				
4 oz sandwich	114	23.0	9.0			50			2.70			200					MCDS49
sausage & egg	450		20.0	29.0	3.0	2.0	930	300					<1				
5.8 oz sandwich	164	28.0	10.0			260			2.70			500					MCDS50
pancakes w/margarine & syrup	600		9.0	104.0	40.0	0.0	770	100					<1				
8 oz serving	228	17.0	3.0			20			4.50			400					MCDS52
pie, apple, baked	260		3.0	34.0	13.0	<1.0	200	20					24				
2.7 oz serving	77	13.0	3.5			0			1.08								MCDS54
salad, chef	150		17.0	5.0	2.0	2.0	740	150					15				
7.3 oz salad	206	8.0	4.0			95			1.44			1500					MCDS61
grilled chicken caesar	100		17.0	3.0	<1.0	2.0	240	100					12				
5.7 oz salad	163	2.5	1.5			40			1.08			1250					MCDS63
salad dressing, herb vinaigrette, fat free -1.5 fl oz (44 ml) pkt	35	0.0	0.0	8.0	6.0	0.0	260						5				
~23	~23	0.0	0.0			0			<0.01								MCDS56
honey mustard	160		1.0	13.0	10.0	<1.0	260						5				
1.5 fl oz (44 ml) pkt	~22	11.0	1.5			15			<0.01								MCDS57
ranch	170		0.0	3.0	1.0	0.0	460						5				
1.5 fl oz (44 ml) pkt	~22	18.0	2.5			15			<0.01								MCDS58
red french, red cal	130		0.0	18.0	11.0	0.0	360						5				
1.5 fl oz (44 ml) pkt	~23	6.0	1.0			0			<0.01			750					MCDS59
thousand island	130		0.0	11.0	6.0	<1.0	350						5				
1.5 fl oz (44 ml) pkt	~22	9.0	1.5			15			<0.01								MCDS60
sausage	170		6.0	0.0	0.0	0.0	290						<1				
1.5 oz serving	43	16.0	5.0			35			0.36								MCDS64
shake, choc, small	318	178.8	8.5	51.3		2.0	243	283	43	1.03	0.098	55	1	0.15	0.4	0.85	0.98
12 fl oz	250	9.3	5.8	2.7	0.4	33	500	255	0.78	0.163	4.3	233	0.2	0.61	0.13	10.0	14346d
med	423	238.1	11.3	68.3		2.7	323	376	57	1.37	0.130	73	1	0.19	0.5	1.13	1.30
16 fl oz	333	12.3	7.7	3.6	0.5	43	666	340	1.03	0.216	5.7	310	0.2	0.82	0.17	13.3	14346b
large	582	327.5	15.6	93.9		3.7	444	518	78	1.88	0.179	101	2	0.27	0.7	1.56	1.79
22 fl oz	458	16.9	10.6	4.9	0.6	60	916	467	1.42	0.298	7.8	426	0.3	1.12	0.23	18.3	14346a
shake, strawberry	560		14.0	89.0	79.0	<1.0	190	450					9				
16 fl oz	333	16.0	11.0			65			0.36			1250					MCDS66
shake, van, small	278	186.8	8.8	44.8		1.0	205	305	30	0.90	0.035	78	2	0.11	0.5	0.90	1.05
12 fl oz	250	7.5	4.6	2.2	0.3	28	435	255	0.23	0.128	5.3	325	0.1	0.46	0.13	7.5	14347c
med	370	248.8	11.7	59.6		1.3	273	406	40	1.20	0.047	103	3	0.15	0.6	1.20	1.39
16 fl oz	333	10.0	6.2	2.9	0.4	37	579	340	0.30	0.170	7.0	433	0.2	0.61	0.17	10.0	14347b
large	508	342.1	16.0	82.0		1.8	376	559	55	1.65	0.064	142	4	0.21	0.8	1.65	1.91
22 fl oz	458	13.7	8.5	3.9	0.5	50	797	467	0.41	0.234	9.6	595	0.3	0.83	0.24	13.7	14347a

	KCAL / WT (g)	H₂0 (g) / FAT (g)	PRO (g) / SFA (g)	CHO (g) / MUFA (g)	SUGR (g) / PUFA (g)	DFIB (g) / CHOL (mg)	Na (mg) / K (mg)	Ca (mg) / P (mg)	Mg (mg) / Fe (mg)	Zn (mg) / Cu (mg)	Mn (mg) / Se (mcg)	A (mcg RAE) / A (IU)	C (mg) / E (mg ATE)	B-1 (mg) / B-2 (mg)	NIA (mg) / B-6 (mg)	B-12 (mcg) / FOL (mcg DFE)	PANT (mg) / REF
soft drink, Coca-Cola, super size	410	0.0	0.0	113.0	113.0	0.0	40						<1				
42 fl oz	1294	0.0	0.0			0			<0.01								MCDS68
Hi-C orange, super size	460	0.0	0.0	124.0	124.0	0.0	75						252				
42 fl oz	1294	0.0	0.0			0			<0.01								MCDS69
Sprite, super size	410	0.0	0.0	109.0	109.0	0.0	150						<1				
42 fl oz	1294	0.0	0.0			0			<0.01								MCDS70
sundae, hot caramel	360	7.0	61.0	47.0	0.0		180	250					1				
6.4 oz sundae	182	10.0	6.0			35			<0.01			500					MCDS71
hot fudge	340	8.0	52.0	47.0	1.0		170	250					1				
6.3 oz sundae	179	12.0	9.0			30			0.72			500					MCDS72
strawberry	290	7.0	50.0	46.0	<1.0		95	200					1				
6.3 oz sundae	178	7.0	5.0			30			0.36			500					MCDS73

10.11 PIZZA HUT

	KCAL / WT (g)	H₂0 (g) / FAT (g)	PRO (g) / SFA (g)	CHO (g) / MUFA (g)	SUGR (g) / PUFA (g)	DFIB (g) / CHOL (mg)	Na (mg) / K (mg)	Ca (mg) / P (mg)	Mg (mg) / Fe (mg)	Zn (mg) / Cu (mg)	Mn (mg) / Se (mcg)	A (mcg RAE) / A (IU)	C (mg) / E (mg ATE)	B-1 (mg) / B-2 (mg)	NIA (mg) / B-6 (mg)	B-12 (mcg) / FOL (mcg DFE)	PANT (mg) / REF
bread stick	130		3.0	20.0	1.0	1.0	170										
1.3 oz serving	38	4.0	1.0			0			1.08								PIZA1
buffalo wing dip 'n dressing,	220		2.0	2.0	2.0	0.0	440	20					0				
blue cheese *-1.5 oz serving*	42	24.0	4.0			40			0.00			0					PIZA2
ranch	220		1.0	2.0	2.0	0.0	420	0					0				
1.5 oz serving	42	24.0	4.0			10			0.00			0					PIZA3
buffalo wings, hot	210		22.0	4.0	0.0	<1.0	900	20									
4 pieces (3.1 oz)	87	12.0	3.0			130			0.72			1000					PIZA4
mild	200		23.0	<1.0	0.0	0.0	510	20									
5 pieces (3 oz)	84	12.0	3.5			150			0.72			300					PIZA5
cavatina pasta	480		21.0	66.0	12.0	9.0	1170	150									
12.6 oz serving	357	14.0	6.0			8			3.60			1250					PIZA6
supreme	560		24.0	73.0	11.0	10.0	1400	150									
14 oz serving	396	19.0	8.0			10			4.50			1500					PIZA7
dessert pizza, apple	250		3.0	48.0	25.0	2.0	230										
2.9 oz slice	81	4.5	1.0			0			1.08								PIZA8
cherry	250		3.0	47.0	24.0	3.0	220										
2.9 oz slice	81	4.5	1.0			0			1.44			450					PIZA9
garlic bread	150		3.0	16.0	<1.0	1.0	240	40									
1.3 oz slice	37	8.0	1.5			0			1.44			500					PIZA10
ham & cheese sandwich	550		33.0	57.0	6.0	4.0	2150	300									
9.7 oz sandwich	276	21.0	7.0			22			4.50			500					PIZA11
pizza, hand tossed, beef	330		16.0	29.0	1.0	3.0	880	200					2				
4.7 oz slice	134	17.0	8.0			25			1.80			750					PIZA12
cheese	240		12.0	28.0	1.0	2.0	650	200					2				
3.7 oz slice	106	10.0	5.0			10			1.44			750					PIZA13
chicken supreme	230		13.0	29.0	2.0	2.0	650	100					6				
4.4 oz slice	124	7.0	3.5			15			1.80			500					PIZA14
ham	260		14.0	28.0	1.0	2.0	800	200					2				
4.2 oz slice	118	10.0	5.0			20			1.80			750					PIZA15
italian sausage	340		16.0	28.0	2.0	2.0	910	200					2				
4.7 oz slice	134	18.0	8.0			30			1.80			750					PIZA16
meat lover's	320		14.0	28.0	2.0	2.0	900	150					2				
4.6 oz slice	129	17.0	7.0			30			1.80			500					PIZA17
pepperoni	280		13.0	28.0	2.0	2.0	790	200					24				
4.1 oz slice	116	13.0	6.0			20			1.80			750					PIZA18
pepperoni lover's	250		11.0	27.0	2.0	2.0	730	100					2				
3.7 oz slice	106	11.0	4.5			15			1.80			500					PIZA19
pork	320		16.0	29.0	2.0	3.0	920	200					2				
4.7 oz slice	134	16.0	7.0			25			1.80			750					PIZA20
super supreme	290		13.0	29.0	2.0	2.0	850	150					6				
4.9 oz slice	139	14.0	6.0			25			1.80			500					PIZA21
supreme	270		13.0	29.0	2.0	3.0	730	150					6				
4.6 oz slice	129	12.0	5.0			20			1.80			500					PIZA22

	KCAL	H₂0 (g)	PRO (g)	CHO (g)	SUGR (g)	DFIB (g)	Na (mg)	Ca (mg)	Mg (mg)	Zn (mg)	Mn (mg)	A (mcg RAE)	C (mg)	B-1 (mg)	NIA (mg)	B-12 (mcg)	PANT (mg)
	WT (g)	FAT (g)	SFA (g)	MUFA (g)	PUFA (g)	CHOL (mg)	K (mg)	P (mg)	Fe (mg)	Cu (mg)	Se (mcg)	A (IU)	E (mg ATE)	B-2 (mg)	B-6 (mg)	FOL (mcg DFE)	REF
veggie lover's	220		9.0	29.0	2.0	2.0	580	100					9				
4.4 oz slice	126	8.0	3.0			5			1.80			500					PIZA23
pizza, pan pizza, beef	330		14.0	29.0	<1.0	3.0	690	150					2				
4.3 oz slice	123	18.0	7.0			20			2.70			500					PIZA24
cheese	290		12.0	28.0	<1.0	2.0	590	200					2				
3.9 oz slice	110	14.0	6.0			10			1.80			750					PIZA25
chicken supreme	270		13.0	29.0	2.0	2.0	580	100					6				
4.4 oz slice	128	12.0	4.0			15			1.80			500					PIZA26
ham	260		11.0	28.0	<1.0	2.0	610	100					2				
3.7 oz slice	107	12.0	4.0			15			1.80			500					PIZA27
italian sausage	340		13.0	29.0	<1.0	2.0	720	150					2				
4.3 oz slice	123	20.0	7.0			25			1.80			500					PIZA28
meat lover's	360		14.0	29.0	1.0	3.0	840	150					2				
4.6 oz slice	133	21.0	7.0			30			1.80			500					PIZA29
pepperoni	280		11.0	28.0	<1.0	2.0	610	100					2				
4.1 oz slice	106	14.0	5.0			15			1.80			500					PIZA30
pepperoni lover's	330		14.0	29.0	<1.0	2.0	760	200					2				
3.9 oz slice	122	18.0	7.0			20			1.80			750					PIZA31
pork	320		13.0	29.0	<1.0	3.0	730	150					2				
4.7 oz slice	123	17.0	6.0			20			1.80			500					PIZA32
super supreme	340		14.0	30.0	1.0	3.0	780	150					6				
4.8 oz slice	143	18.0	6.0			25			1.80			500					PIZA33
supreme	320		13.0	29.0	1.0	3.0	670	150					6				
4.6 oz slice	133	17.0	6.0			20			1.80			500					PIZA34
veggie lover's	270		10.0	30.0	2.0	3.0	510	100					12				
4.4 oz slice	130	12.0	4.0			5			1.80			500					PIZA35
pizza, sicilian, beef	260		11.0	31.0	3.0	2.0	640	150					6				
4.2 oz slice	111	11.0	4.5			15			1.80			400					PIZA36
cheese	290		12.0	31.0	3.0	2.0	630	200					6				
4.1 oz slice	115	13.0	6.0			10			1.80			750					PIZA37
chicken supreme	270		12.0	32.0	3.0	2.0	620	150					9				
4.5 oz slice	130	11.0	4.0			15			1.80			500					PIZA38
ham	257		11.0	30.0	3.0	2.6	745	130					0				
3.8 oz slice	108	10.0	4.9			14			1.80			350					PIZA39
italian sausage	333		13.0	31.0	3.0	2.8	855	140					1				
4.4 oz slice	124	18.0	7.4			24			1.98			450					PIZA40
meat lover's	350		14.0	31.0	3.0	2.0	830	150					6				
4.6 oz slice	133	19.0	7.0			25			2.70			500					PIZA41
pepperoni	280		10.0	31.0	3.0	2.0	630	150					6				
3.9 oz slice	110	13.0	5.0			15			1.80			400					PIZA42
pepperoni lover's	320		13.0	31.0	3.0	2.0	780	200					6				
4.4 oz slice	125	16.0	7.0			20			1.80			500					PIZA43
pork	320		13.0	31.0	3.0	2.0	750	150					6				
4.4 oz slice	125	16.0	6.0			20			2.70			500					PIZA44
super supreme	340		13.0	32.0	3.0	2.0	780	150					6				
4.5 oz slice	142	18.0	6.0			20			2.70			500					PIZA45
supreme	310		12.0	32.0	3.0	2.0	690	150					9				
4.6 oz slice	134	15.0	6.0			15			2.70			500					PIZA46
veggie lover's	270		12.0	32.0	3.0	2.0	620	150					15				
4.1 oz slice	132	11.0	4.0			15			1.80			500					PIZA47
pizza, stuffed crust, beef	390		19.0	40.0	2.0	3.0	1150	250					4				
5.7 oz slice	166	18.0	8.0			30			2.70			750					PIZA48
cheese	360		18.0	39.0	2.0	3.0	1090	300					4				
5.7 oz slice	157	16.0	8.0			25			1.80			1000					PIZA49
chicken supreme	350		21.0	41.0	3.0	3.0	1130	250					9				
6.6 oz slice	186	13.0	6.0			35			2.70			750					PIZA50
ham	330		18.0	39.0	2.0	3.0	1130	250					4				
5.7 oz slice	156	13.0	6.0			30			1.80			750					PIZA51

Food	KCAL / WT (g)	H₂0 (g) / FAT (g)	PRO (g) / SFA (g)	CHO (g) / MUFA (g)	SUGR (g) / PUFA (g)	DFIB (g) / CHOL (mg)	Na (mg) / K (mg)	Ca (mg) / P (mg)	Mg (mg) / Fe (mg)	Zn (mg) / Cu (mg)	Mn (mg) / Se (mcg)	A (mcg RAE) / A (IU)	C (mg) / E (mg ATE)	B-1 (mg) / B-2 (mg)	NIA (mg) / B-6 (mg)	B-12 (mcg) / FOL (mcg DFE)	PANT (mg) / REF
italian sausage	400		19.0	40.0	2.0	3.0	1180	250					4				
6.1 oz slice	166	20.0	8.0			35			2.70			750					PIZA52
meat lover's	470		22.0	40.0	2.0	3.0	1430	250					4				
6.9 oz slice	190	25.0	11.0			50			2.70			750					PIZA53
pepperoni lover's	420		21.0	40.0	2.0	3.0	1350	300					4				
6.8 oz slice	176	21.0	9.0			40			2.70			750					PIZA54
pork	380		19.0	40.0	2.0	3.0	1190	250					4				
6.1 oz slice	166	18.0	8.0			30			2.70			750					PIZA55
super supreme	430		21.0	41.0	3.0	3.0	1360	250					9				
7 oz slice	204	22.0	9.0			40			2.70			750					PIZA56
supreme	410		20.0	41.0	3.0	3.0	1220	250					9				
6.9 oz slice	191	20.0	9.0			35			2.70			750					PIZA57
veggie lover's	340		16.0	42.0	3.0	3.0	1030	250					15				
6.8 oz slice	188	14.0	6.0			20			2.70			750					PIZA58
pizza, the big new yorker,	380		19.0	41.0	<0.1	7.0	1140	350					0				
cheese - 5.9 oz slice	174	17.0	9.0			20			1.80			1000					PIZA59
pepperoni	370		17.0	41.0	<0.1	7.0	1150	250					0				
5.6 oz slice	167	16.0	7.0			20			1.80			750					PIZA60
supreme	450		22.0	43.0	<0.1	8.0	1350	250					9				
7.4 oz slice	224	23.0	10.0			35			2.70			750					PIZA61
pizza, the new edge, chicken	90		7.0	9.0	2.0	<1.0	290	60					9				
supreme - 2.5 oz slice	70	3.5	1.5			15			0.00			300					PIZA62
meat lover's	160		7.0	8.0	<1.0	<1.0	440	80					0				
2 oz slice	58	11.0	4.5			20			0.36			300					PIZA63
the works	110		5.0	9.0	2.0	<1.0	270	80					9				
2.2 oz slice	63	6.0	2.5			10			0.36			300					PIZA64
veggie lover's	70		4.0	9.0	2.0	<1.0	180	60					6				
1.9 oz slice	54	3.0	1.5			<5			0.00			300					PIZA65
pizza, thin n' crispy, beef	270		13.0	22.0	1.0	2.0	750	150					2				
3.5 oz slice	106	15.0	7.0			25			1.80			500					PIZA66
cheese	200		10.0	22.0	1.0	2.0	590	200					2				
2.8 oz slice	85	9.0	5.0			10			1.44			750					PIZA67
chicken supreme	200		12.0	23.0	2.0	2.0	620	100					9				
3.6 oz slice	113	7.0	3.5			20			1.44			500					PIZA68
ham	170		9.0	21.0	1.0	2.0	610	100					2				
2.6 oz slice	82	7.0	3.5			15			1.44			500					PIZA69
italian sausage	290		12.0	22.0	1.0	2.0	800	150					2				
3.4 oz slice	106	17.0	7.0			30			1.80			750					PIZA70
meat lover's	310		14.0	22.0	1.0	2.0	910	150					2				
3.8 oz slice	116	19.0	8.0			35			1.80			500					PIZA71
pepperoni lover's	250		12.0	22.0	1.0	2.0	760	200					2				
2.9 oz slice	97	13.0	6.0			20			1.44			750					PIZA72
pork	270		13.0	22.0	1.0	2.0	820	150					2				
3.4 oz slice	106	14.0	6.0			25			1.80			500					PIZA73
super supreme	280		13.0	23.0	2.0	2.0	840	150					9				
4.2 oz slice	130	15.0	6.0			25			1.80			500					PIZA74
supreme	250		12.0	23.0	2.0	2.0	710	150					9				
3.9 oz slice	117	13.0	6.0			20			1.80			500					PIZA75
veggie lover's	190		8.0	24.0	3.0	2.0	520	100					12				
3.8 oz slice	115	7.0	3.0			5			1.44			500					PIZA76
sandwich, supreme	640		34.0	62.0	7.0	4.0	2150	300									
10.3 oz sandwich	292	28.0	10.0			28			5.40			750					PIZA80
spaghetti w/marinara sce	490		18.0	91.0	10.0	8.0	730	150									
16.7 oz serving	473	6.0	1.0			0			3.60			1000					PIZA77
w/meat sce	600		23.0	98.0	10.0	9.0	910	100									
16.5 oz serving	467	13.0	5.0			8			3.60			1750					PIZA78
w/meatballs	850		37.0	120.0	12.0	10.0	1120	150									
18.9 oz serving	537	24.0	10.0			17			5.40			2000					PIZA79

KCAL	H₂O (g)	PRO (g)	CHO (g)	SUGR (g)	DFIB (g)	Na (mg)	Ca (mg)	Mg (mg)	Zn (mg)	Mn (mg)	A (mcg RAE)	C (mg)	B-1 (mg)	NIA (mg)	B-12 (mcg)	PANT (mg)
WT (g)	FAT (g)	SFA (g)	MUFA (g)	PUFA (g)	CHOL (mg)	K (mg)	P (mg)	Fe (mg)	Cu (mg)	Se (mcg)	A (IU)	E (mg ATE)	B-2 (mg)	B-6 (mg)	FOL (mcg DFE)	REF

10.12 SUBWAY

breakfast sandwich, bacon & egg - *4.5 oz sandwich*

KCAL	H₂O	PRO	CHO	SUGR	DFIB	Na	Ca	Mg	Zn	Mn	A-RAE	C	B-1	NIA	B-12	PANT
320		14.0	34.0	3.0	3.0	520	80					4				
127	16.0	4.5			185			3.60			300					SUBW1
320		14.0	34.0	3.0	3.0	550	150					4				
130	15.0	5.0			185			3.60			400					SUBW2
340		21.0	35.0	4.0	3.0	1100	80					4				
147	14.0	4.0			200			3.60			300					SUBW3
300		14.0	36.0	3.0	3.0	530	80					12				
167	12.0	3.5			180			3.60			400					SUBW4
280		16.0	11.0	1.0	3.0	1590	100					30				
312	19.0	8.0			55			1.08			1000					SUBW5
230		14.0	11.0	1.0	3.0	1370	150					30				
316	15.0	6.0			55			1.80			1000					SUBW6
320		17.0	17.0	2.0	4.0	1050	100					36				
346	20.0	9.0			55			1.80			1250					SUBW7
200		9.0	17.0	1.0	4.0	970	100					30				
314	11.0	3.5			25			1.08			1000					SUBW8
180		17.0	12.0	2.0	4.0	890	100					30				
315	8.0	3.5			35			3.60			1000					SUBW9
200		17.0	11.0	1.0	3.0	1410	100					30				
318	10.0	4.5			45			1.08			1000					SUBW10
240		13.0	10.0	0.0	3.0	880	100					30				
279	16.0	4.0			40			1.08			1000					SUBW11
480		23.0	46.0	6.0	4.0	1900	150					24				
250	24.0	9.0			55			3.60			500					SUBW12
440		21.0	47.0	6.0	4.0	1680	150					24				
254	21.0	7.0			55			5.40			500					SUBW13
530		24.0	53.0	7.0	6.0	1360	150					27				
284	26.0	10.0			55			5.40			750					SUBW14
410		16.0	52.0	6.0	5.0	1280	150					24				
252	16.0	4.5			25			3.60			500					SUBW15
390		24.0	48.0	7.0	5.0	1210	150					24				
253	14.0	5.0			35			8.10			500					SUBW16
410		24.0	47.0	6.0	4.0	1730	150					24				
256	16.0	6.0			45			3.60			500					SUBW17
450		20.0	46.0	5.0	4.0	1190	150					24				
252	22.0	6.0			40			3.60			500					SUBW18
220		2.0	30.0	18.0	1.0	160	0					0				
48	10.0	4.0			15			1.08			200					SUBW19
220		2.0	30.0	17.0	1.0	105	0					0				
48	10.0	4.0			10			1.08			0					SUBW20
220		2.0	30.0	17.0	1.0	105	0					0				
48	10.0	4.0			15			1.08			0					SUBW21
200			30.0	16.0	2.0	180	0					0				
48	8.0	2.5			15			1.08			0					SUBW22
220		4.0	26.0	16.0	1.0	200	0					0				
48	12.0	4.0			10			1.08			200					SUBW23
230		2.0	28.0	14.0	0.0	135	0					0				
48	12.0	4.0			15			1.08			0					SUBW24
220		2.0	28.0	17.0	1.0	160	0					0				
48	11.0	4.0			15			1.08			300					SUBW25
210		11.0	35.0	3.0	3.0	770	60					12				
147	4.0	1.5			10			3.60			200					SUBW26
220		13.0	35.0	3.0	3.0	660	60					12				
157	4.5	2.0			15			5.40			200					SUBW27
330		13.0	36.0	2.0	3.0	830	150					12				
173	16.0	4.5			25			3.60			400					SUBW28

Row labels, in order:
- **breakfast sandwich**, bacon & egg - *4.5 oz sandwich* (SUBW1)
- cheese & egg — *4.6 oz sandwich* (SUBW2)
- ham & egg — *5.2 oz sandwich* (SUBW3)
- western egg — *5.9 oz sandwich* (SUBW4)
- **classic salad**, BMT — *11 oz salad* (SUBW5)
- cold cut trio — *11.1 oz salad* (SUBW6)
- meatball — *12.2 oz salad* (SUBW7)
- seafood & crab — *11 oz salad* (SUBW8)
- steak & cheese — *11.1 oz salad* (SUBW9)
- subway melt — *11.2 oz salad* (SUBW10)
- tuna — *9.8 oz salad* (SUBW11)
- **classic sub**, BMT — *6" sub (8.8 oz)* (SUBW12)
- cold cut trio — *6" sub (9 oz)* (SUBW13)
- meatball — *6" sub (10 oz)* (SUBW14)
- seafood & crab — *6" sub (8.9 oz)* (SUBW15)
- steak & cheese — *6" sub (8.9 oz)* (SUBW16)
- subway melt — *6" sub (9 oz)* (SUBW17)
- tuna — *6" sub (8.9 oz)* (SUBW18)
- **cookie**, choc chip — *1.7 oz cookie* (SUBW19)
- choc chunk — *1.7 oz cookie* (SUBW20)
- M&M — *1.7 oz cookie* (SUBW21)
- oatmeal raisin — *1.7 oz cookie* (SUBW22)
- peanut butter — *1.7 oz cookie* (SUBW23)
- sugar — *1.7 oz cookie* (SUBW24)
- white macadamia nut — *1.7 oz cookie* (SUBW25)
- **deli sub**, ham — *5.2 oz sub* (SUBW26)
- roast beef — *5.5 oz sub* (SUBW27)
- tuna — *6.1 oz sub* (SUBW28)

	KCAL / WT (g)	H₂0 (g) / FAT (g)	PRO (g) / SFA (g)	CHO (g) / MUFA (g)	SUGR (g) / PUFA (g)	DFIB (g) / CHOL (mg)	Na (mg) / K (mg)	Ca (mg) / P (mg)	Mg (mg) / Fe (mg)	Zn (mg) / Cu (mg)	Mn (mg) / Se (mcg)	A (mcg RAE) / A (IU)	C (mg) / E (mg ATE)	B-1 (mg) / B-2 (mg)	NIA (mg) / B-6 (mg)	B-12 (mcg) / FOL (mcg DFE)	PANT (mg) / REF
turkey breast	220		13.0	36.0	3.0	3.0	730	60					12				
5.5 oz sub	157	3.5	1.5			15			3.60			200					SUBW29
Fruizle Express, berry lishus	110		1.0	28.0	27.0	1.0	30	0					66				
small (13 oz)	369	0.0	0.0			0			1.80			0					SUBW30
peach pizzazz	100		0.0	26.0	26.0	0.0	25	0					66				
small (12 oz)	341	0.0	0.0			0			0.00			100					SUBW31
pineapple delight	130		1.0	33.0	33.0	1.0	25	0					90				
small (13 oz)	369	0.0	0.0			0			0.00			0					SUBW32
sunrise refresher	120		1.0	29.0	28.0	1.0	20	20					126				
small (12 oz)	341	0.0	0.0			0			0.00			200					SUBW33
salad dressing, french, fat free	70		0.0	17.0	12.0		390	0					0				
2 oz	57	0.0	0.0			0			0.00			0					SUBW34
italian, fat free	20		0.0	4.0	3.0	0.0	610	0					0				
2 oz	57	0.0	0.0			0			0.00			0					SUBW35
ranch, fat free	60		0.0	14.0	6.0	0.0	530	0					0				
2 oz	57	0.0	0.0			0			0.00			0					SUBW36
select sub, southwest chicken	260		3.0	41.0	24.0	1.0	270	20					0				
6" sub (10.5 oz)	298	10.0	4.5			20			0.72			200					SUBW43
southwest steak & cheese	440		24.0	49.0	9.0	5.0	1160	150					24				
6" sub (9 oz)	255	19.0	6.0			45			8.10			500					SUBW44
seven under 6 salad, ham	110		11.0	11.0	1.0	3.0	1070	40					30				
10.2 oz salad	289	3.0	1.0			25			1.08			750					SUBW45
roast beef	120		12.0	10.0	1.0	3.0	720	40					30				
10.2 oz salad	290	3.0	1.5			20			1.80			750					SUBW46
rstd chicken breast	140		16.0	12.0	2.0	3.0	800	40					30				
10.7 oz salad	304	3.0	1.0			45			1.08			750					SUBW47
subway club	150		17.0	12.0	2.0	3.0	1110	40					30				
11.4 oz salad	323	3.5	1.5			35			1.80			750					SUBW48
turkey breast	110		11.0	11.0	1.0	3.0	820	40					30				
10.2 oz salad	290	2.0	0.0			20			1.08			750					SUBW49
turkey breast & ham	120		13.0	11.0	1.0	3.0	1030	40					30				
10.5 oz salad	299	3.0	0.5			25			1.08			750					SUBW50
veggie delite	50		2.0	9.0	0.0	3.0	310	40					30				
8.2 oz salad	233	1.0	0.0			0			1.08			750					SUBW51
seven under 6 sub, ham	290		18.0	46.0	6.0	4.0	1270	60					21				
6" sub (7.7 oz)	219	5.0	1.5			25			3.60			300					SUBW52
roast beef	290		19.0	45.0	6.0	4.0	910	60					21				
6" sub (7.8 oz)	220	5.0	2.0			20			6.30			300					SUBW53
rstd chicken breast	320		23.0	47.0	7.0	5.0	1000	60					21				
6" sub (8.3 oz)	234	5.0	2.0			45			5.40			300					SUBW54
subway club	320		24.0	46.0	6.0	4.0	1300	60					21				
6" sub (8.9 oz)	253	6.0	2.0			35			5.40			300					SUBW55
turkey breast	280		18.0	46.0	5.0	4.0	1010	60					21				
6" sub (7.8 oz)	220	4.5	1.5			20			3.60			300					SUBW56
turkey breast & ham	290		20.0	46.0	6.0	4.0	1220	60					21				
6" sub (8.1 oz)	229	5.0	1.5			25			3.60			300					SUBW57
veggie delite	230		9.0	44.0	5.0	4.0	510	60					21				
6" sub (5.7 oz)	163	3.0	1.0			0			3.60			300					SUBW58
soup, black bean	180		9.0	27.0	4.0	15.0	1160	60					4				
1 cup (8 fl oz)	240	4.5	2.0			10			1.80			500					SUBW59
brown & wild rice w/chicken	190		6.0	17.0	3.0	2.0	990	300					24				
1 cup (8 fl oz)	240	11.0	4.5			20			0.00			500					SUBW60
cheese w/ham & bacon	230		8.0	13.0	4.0	2.0	1270	200					0				
1 cup (8 fl oz)	240	16.0	6.0			20			0.00			100					SUBW61
chicken & dumpling	130		7.0	16.0	2.0	1.0	1030	20					0				
1 cup (8 fl oz)	240	4.5	2.5			30			0.00			1000					SUBW62
cream of broccoli	130		5.0	15.0	0.0	2.0	860	150					12				
1 cup (8 fl oz)	240	6.0	0.0			10			0.00			200					SUBW63
cream of potato w/bacon	210		5.0	20.0	3.0	4.0	970	100					6				
1 cup (8 fl oz)	240	12.0	4.0			20			1.80			750					SUBW64

	KCAL	H₂O (g)	PRO (g)	CHO (g)	SUGR (g)	DFIB (g)	Na (mg)	Ca (mg)	Minerals Mg (mg)	Zn (mg)	Mn (mg)	A (mcg RAE)	C (mg)	B-1 (mg)	NIA (mg)	B-12 (mcg)	PANT (mg)
	WT (g)	FAT (g)	SFA (g)	MUFA (g)	PUFA (g)	CHOL (mg)	K (mg)	P (mg)	Fe (mg)	Cu (mg)	Se (mcg)	A (IU)	E (mg ATE)	B-2 (mg)	B-6 (mg)	FOL (mcg DFE)	REF
golden broccoli cheese	180		6.0	12.0	4.0	9.0	910	150					9				
1 cup (8 fl oz)	240	12.0	4.0			10			1.80			100					SUBW65
minestrone	70		3.0	11.0	2.0	2.0	1030	40					6				
1 cup (8 fl oz)	240	1.0	0.0			10			0.00			2000					SUBW67
new england style clam chowder	140		5.0	19.0	2.0	7.0	900	60					0				
1 cup (8 fl oz)	240	4.5	1.0			15			1.80			750					SUBW68
potato cheese chowder	210		7.0	22.0	3.0	2.0	1010	200					0				
1 cup (8 fl oz)	240	10.0	7.0			25			0.00			1500					SUBW69
rstd chicken noodle	90		7.0	7.0	1.0	1.0	1180	20					4				
1 cup (8 fl oz)	240	4.0	1.0			20			0.00			2000					SUBW70
tomato bisque	90		1.0	15.0	7.0	3.0	750	20					4				
1 cup (8 fl oz)	240	2.5	0.5			0			0.00			750					SUBW71
vegetable beef	90		5.0	14.0	4.0	2.0	1340	20					4				
1 cup (8 fl oz)	240	1.5	0.5			10			0.00			2000					SUBW72

10.13 TACO BELL

	KCAL	H₂O (g)	PRO (g)	CHO (g)	SUGR (g)	DFIB (g)	Na (mg)	Ca (mg)	Mg (mg)	Zn (mg)	Mn (mg)	A (mcg RAE)	C (mg)	B-1 (mg)	NIA (mg)	B-12 (mcg)	PANT (mg) / REF
breakfast burrito	530		17.0	48.0	2.0	5.0	1540	300					0				
8.4 oz burrito	239	26.0	9.0			390			4.50			4500					TACO1
gordita	400		12.0	28.0	3.0	3.0	740	200					6				
5 oz gordita	142	25.0	7.0			210			1.80			1500					TACO2
quesadilla	420		15.0	38.0	2.0	1.0	1100	300					1				
5.5 oz quesadilla	155	21.0	8.0			210			2.70			2000					TACO3
steak burrito	530		22.0	40.0	3.0	<1.0	1450	250					0				
8.4 oz burrito	239	27.0	9.0			420			4.50			2500					TACO4
steak quesadilla w/green sce	470		22.0	39.0	2.0	1.0	1320	300					0				
6.9 oz quesadilla	197	23.0	9.0			235			3.60			1250					TACO5
burrito, 7 layer	520		16.0	65.0	4.0	13.0	1270	200					6				
10 oz burrito	284	22.0	7.0			25			3.60			1500					TACO12
bean	370		13.0	54.0	3.0	12.0	1080	150					0				
7 oz burrito	198	12.0	3.5			10			2.70			2250					TACO13
chili cheese	330		13.0	40.0	2.0	4.0	900	150					0				
5.5 oz burrito	156	13.0	5.0			25			1.08			1000					TACO14
burrito fiesta, beef	380		14.0	49.0	3.0	4.0	1100	100					0				
6.5 oz burrito	183	15.0	5.0			30			1.80			1500					TACO6
chicken	370		17.0	48.0	2.0	3.0	1000	100					1				
6.5 oz burrito	183	12.0	3.5			35			1.44			1500					TACO7
steak	370		18.0	47.0	2.0	3.0	1020	100					0				
6.5 oz burrito	183	12.0	4.0			25			1.80			1500					TACO8
burrito grilled stuft, beef	730		27.0	75.0	4.0	11.0	2090	350					9				
11.5 oz burrito	325	35.0	11.0			65			5.40			1500					TACO15
chicken	690		33.0	73.0	4.0	8.0	1900	300					9				
11.5 oz burrito	325	29.0	8.0			70			5.40			1250					TACO16
steak	690		30.0	72.0	4.0	8.0	1970	300					6				
11.5 oz burrito	325	30.0	8.0			60			6.30			1250					TACO17
burrito supreme, beef	430		17.0	50.0	4.0	9.0	1210	150					5				
8.7 oz burrito	247	18.0	7.0			40			2.70			2500					TACO9
chicken	410		20.0	49.0	4.0	8.0	1120	150					5				
8.7 oz burrito	247	16.0	6.0			45			1.80			2250					TACO10
steak	420		21.0	48.0	4.0	8.0	1140	150					4				
8.7 oz burrito	247	16.0	6.0			35			2.70			2250					TACO11
chalupa baja, beef	420		14.0	30.0	3.0	3.0	760	150					5				
5.4 oz chalupa	154	27.0	7.0			35			2.70			300					TACO18
chicken	400		17.0	28.0	3.0	2.0	660	100					5				
5.4 oz chalupa	154	24.0	5.0			40			1.80			200					TACO19
steak	400		17.0	27.0	3.0	2.0	680	100					4				
5.4 oz chalupa	154	24.0	6.0			30			2.70			100					TACO20
chalupa nacho cheese, beef	370		13.0	30.0	3.0	3.0	740	100					5				
5.4 oz chalupa	152	22.0	6.0			25			1.80			400					TACO21
chicken	350		16.0	29.0	3.0	2.0	640	80					5				
5.4 oz chalupa	152	19.0	4.5			25			1.80			300					TACO22

	KCAL / WT (g)	H₂O (g) / FAT (g)	PRO (g) / SFA (g)	CHO (g) / MUFA (g)	SUGR (g) / PUFA (g)	DFIB (g) / CHOL (mg)	Na (mg) / K (mg)	Ca (mg) / P (mg)	Mg (mg) / Fe (mg)	Zn (mg) / Cu (mg)	Mn (mg) / Se (mcg)	A (mcg RAE) / A (IU)	C (mg) / E (mg ATE)	B-1 (mg) / B-2 (mg)	NIA (mg) / B-6 (mg)	B-12 (mcg) / FOL (mcg DFE)	PANT (mg) / REF
steak	350		16.0	28.0	2.0	1.0	660	80					4				
5.4 oz chalupa	152	19.0	4.5			20			2.70			200					TACO23
chalupa supreme, beef	380		14.0	29.0	3.0	3.0	580	150					5				
5.4 oz chalupa	152	23.0	8.0			40			1.80			300					TACO24
chicken	360		17.0	28.0	3.0	2.0	490	100					5				
5.4 oz chalupa	152	20.0	7.0			45			1.80			200					TACO25
steak	360		17.0	27.0	3.0	2.0	500	150					4				
5.4 oz chalupa	152	20.0	7.0			35			2.70			100					TACO26
cheese, cheddar/3 cheese blend	25		2.0	0.0	0.0	0.0	53	50					0				
.25 oz	7	2.0	1.3			5			0.90			50					TACO27
cinnamon twist	150		1.0	27.0	13.0	<1.0	190	0					0				
1.2 oz twist	35	4.5	1.0			0			0.36			0					TACO28
enchirito, beef	370		18.0	33.0	2.0	9.0	1300	300					1				
7.4 oz enchirito	211	19.0	9.0			50			1.80			5000					TACO29
chicken	350		21.0	32.0	2.0	7.0	1210	250					1				
7.4 oz enchirito	211	16.0	8.0			55			1.80			5000					TACO30
steak	350		22.0	31.0	2.0	7.0	1220	250					0				
7.4 oz enchirito	211	16.0	8.0			45			2.70			4500					TACO31
gordita baja, beef	360		13.0	29.0	4.0	4.0	810	150					4				
5.4 oz gordita	153	21.0	5.0			35			1.80			300					TACO32
chicken	340		16.0	28.0	4.0	3.0	710	150					4				
5.4 oz gordita	153	18.0	4.0			40			1.80			200					TACO33
steak	340		15.0	28.0	3.0	3.0	760	150					6				
5.4 oz gordita	153	18.0	4.0			35			2.70			200					TACO34
gordita nacho cheese, beef	310		13.0	30.0	4.0	4.0	780	100					4				
5.4 oz gordita	152	15.0	4.0			25			1.80			400					TACO35
chicken	290		15.0	29.0	4.0	3.0	690	100					4				
5.4 oz gordita	152	13.0	2.5			25			1.44			300					TACO36
steak	290		16.0	28.0	3.0	2.0	700	100					4				
5.4 oz gordita	152	13.0	3.0			20			1.80			200					TACO37
gordita supreme, beef	300		17.0	27.0	4.0	3.0	550	150					4				
5.4 oz gordita	152	14.0	5.0			35			1.80			100					TACO38
chicken	300		16.0	28.0	4.0	3.0	530	150					4				
5.4 oz gordita	152	13.0	5.0			45			1.44			200					TACO39
steak	300		17.0	27.0	4.0	3.0	550	150					4				
5.4 oz gordita	152	14.0	5.0			35			1.80			100					TACO40
guacamole	35		0.0	2.0	<1.0	<1.0	100	0					0				
.74 oz	21	3.0	0.0			0			0.00			0					TACO41
mexican pizza	540		20.0	42.0	2.0	8.0	1040	250					6				
7.6 oz pizza	215	35.0	10.0			45			3.60			1750					TACO42
mexican rice	190		5.0	23.0	<1.0	<1.0	750	150					1				
4.6 oz serving	130	9.0	3.5			15			1.44			5000					TACO43
meximelt	290		15.0	22.0	2.0	4.0	830	200					0				
4.5 oz meximelt	127	15.0	7.0			45			1.08			400					TACO44
nachos	320		5.0	34.0	2.0	3.0	560	100					0				
3.2 oz serving	90	18.0	4.0			<5			0.72			300					TACO45
bellgrande	760		20.0	83.0	4.0	17.0	1300	200					5				
10.8 oz serving	307	39.0	11.0			35			3.60			500					TACO46
supreme	440		14.0	44.0	3.0	9.0	800	150					4				
6.8 oz serving	194	24.0	7.0			35			2.70			0					TACO47
pintos 'n cheese	180		9.0	18.0	1.0	10.0	640	150					0				
4.5 oz serving	127	8.0	4.0			15			1.80			2250					TACO48
quesadilla, cheese	490		19.0	39.0	3.0	4.0	1080	400					0				
5 oz serving	141	28.0	11.0			55			0.72			500					TACO49
chicken	540		28.0	40.0	3.0	4.0	1270	400					1				
6.5 oz serving	183	30.0	12.0			80			1.08			500					TACO50
salsa	5		0.0	1.0	<1.0	<1.0	60	0					2				
.74 oz	21	0.0	0.0			0			0.00			100					TACO52
sauce, border, fire	0		0.0	<1.0	0.0	0.0	95	0					0				
.3 oz pkt	8	0.0	2.5			0			0.00			300					TACO53
border, hot	0		0.0	0.0	0.0	0.0	80	0					0				
.3 oz pkt	8	0.0	0.0			0			0.00			300					TACO54

	KCAL	H₂0 (g)	PRO (g)	CHO (g)	SUGR (g)	DFIB (g)	Na (mg)	Ca (mg)	Mg (mg)	Zn (mg)	Mn (mg)	A (mcg RAE)	C (mg)	B-1 (mg)	NIA (mg)	B-12 (mcg)	PANT (mg)
	WT (g)	FAT (g)	SFA (g)	MUFA (g)	PUFA (g)	CHOL (mg)	K (mg)	P (mg)	Fe (mg)	Cu (mg)	Se (mcg)	A (IU)	E (mg ATE)	B-2 (mg)	B-6 (mg)	FOL (mcg DFE)	REF
border, mild	0		0.0	0.0	0.0	0.0	60	0					0				
.3 oz pkt	8	0.0	0.0			0			0.00			400					TACO55
green	10		0.0	2.0	0.0	0.0	85	0					0				
1 oz	28	0.0	0.0			10			0.00			0					TACO56
nacho cheese	110		2.0	4.0	2.0	0.0	460	40					0				
2 oz	56	10.0	2.0			<5			0.00			300					TACO57
pepper jack cheese	80		<1.0	1.0	<1.0	0.0	135	0					2				
.5 oz	16	8.0	1.5			10			0.00			0					TACO58
picante	0		0.0	<1.0	0.0	0.0	105	0					0				
.3 oz pkt	9	0.0	0.0			0			0.00			0					TACO59
red	10		0.0	2.0	0.0	0.0	220	0					0				
1 oz	28	0.0	0.0			0			0.00			2000					TACO60
sour cream	45		<1.0	<1.0	<1.0	0.0	15	0					0				
.74 oz	21	4.0	2.5			10			0.00			200					TACO61
taco	210		9.0	18.0	<1.0	3.0	330	80					0				
2.75 oz taco	78	12.0	4.0			30			1.08			400					TACO62
double decker	380		15.0	43.0	2.0	9.0	740	100					0				
5.5 oz taco	156	17.0	5.0			30			1.80			400					TACO70
taco salad express w/chips	620		27.0	60.0	9.0	13.0	1390	250					18				
16.8 oz salad	475	31.0	13.0			65			4.50			1500					TACO63
w/salsa & shell	850		30.0	69.0	12.0	16.0	2250	300					30				
18.7 oz salad	531	52.0	14.0			70			6.30			14500					TACO64
w/salsa, w/o shell	400		24.0	31.0	9.0	15.0	1510	250					21				
16.3 oz salad	461	22.0	10.0			70			4.50			7500					TACO65
taco supreme	260		10.0	20.0	2.0	4.0	350	100					4				
4 oz taco	113	16.0	6.0			40			1.08			400					TACO66
double decker	420		15.0	45.0	3.0	10.0	760	150					4				
6.7 oz taco	191	21.0	8.0			40			1.80			400					TACO67
soft, beef	260		11.0	22.0	3.0	3.0	630	150					5				
4.7 oz taco	134	14.0	7.0			40			1.80			500					TACO68
soft, chicken	230		15.0	21.0	3.0	1.0	570	150					5				
4.7 oz taco	134	10.0	5.0			45			1.08			400					TACO69
taco soft, beef	210		11.0	20.0	1.0	3.0	570	80					0				
3.5 oz taco	99	10.0	4.0			30			1.08			400					TACO71
chicken	190		13.0	19.0	1.0	2.0	480	80					1				
3.5 oz taco	99	7.0	2.5			35			0.72			200					TACO72
grilled steak	280		12.0	20.0	2.0	2.0	630	80					4				
4.5 oz taco	127	17.0	4.0			35			1.44			300					TACO73
tostada	250		10.0	27.0	2.0	11.0	640	150					1				
6 oz tostada	169	12.0	4.5			15			1.80			2500					TACO74

10.14 WENDY'S

	KCAL	H₂0 (g)	PRO (g)	CHO (g)	SUGR (g)	DFIB (g)	Na (mg)	Ca (mg)	Mg (mg)	Zn (mg)	Mn (mg)	A (mcg RAE)	C (mg)	B-1 (mg)	NIA (mg)	B-12 (mcg)	PANT (mg)
	WT (g)	FAT (g)	SFA (g)	MUFA (g)	PUFA (g)	CHOL (mg)	K (mg)	P (mg)	Fe (mg)	Cu (mg)	Se (mcg)	A (IU)	E (mg ATE)	B-2 (mg)	B-6 (mg)	FOL (mcg DFE)	REF
cheeseburger, jr	310		17.0	34.0	7.0	2.0	820	150					4				
4.6 oz cheeseburger	129	12.0	5.0			45	230		3.60			300					WNDY5
jr bacon	380		20.0	34.0	6.0	2.0	890	150					9				
5.8 oz cheeseburger	165	18.0	7.0			55	320		3.60			400					WNDY6
jr deluxe	350		17.0	37.0	8.0	2.0	890	150					9				
6.3 oz cheeseburger	179	16.0	6.0			45	320		3.60			500					WNDY7
kid's meal	310		17.0	34.0	6.0	2.0	820	150					4				
4.3 oz cheeseburger	122	12.0	5.0			45	220		3.60			300					WNDY8
chicken sandwich, breast fillet	430		27.0	46.0	6.0	2.0	750	100					12				
7.3 oz sandwich	207	16.0	3.0			55	470		2.70			200					WNDY9
club	470		30.0	47.0	6.0	2.0	920	100					15				
7.6 oz sandwich	215	19.0	4.0			65	500		2.70			200					WNDY10
grilled	300		24.0	36.0	8.0	2.0	740	80					9				
6.6 oz sandwich	188	7.0	1.5			55	430		2.70			200					WNDY16
spicy	430		27.0	47.0	6.0	3.0	1240	100					9				
7.65 oz sandwich	217	15.0	3.0			60	500		2.70			200					WNDY17
chicken nugget sauce, barbeque	40		1.0	10.0	7.0	0.0	160	0					0				
1 oz pkt	28	0.0	0.0			0	105		0.72			0					WNDY12

	KCAL / WT (g)	H₂O / FAT (g)	PRO / SFA (g)	CHO / MUFA (g)	SUGR / PUFA (g)	DFIB / CHOL (mg)	Na / K (mg)	Ca / P (mg)	Mg / Fe (mg)	Zn / Cu (mg)	Mn / Se (mcg)	A (mcg RAE) / A (IU)	C / E (mg ATE)	B-1 / B-2 (mg)	NIA / B-6 (mg)	B-12 / FOL (mcg)	PANT (mg) / REF
honey mustard	130		0.0	6.0	5.0	0.0	210	0					0				
1 oz pkt	28	12.0	2.0			10	15		0.00			0					WNDY11
sweet & sour	45		0.0	12.0	10.0	0.0	115	0					1				
1 oz pkt	28	0.0	0.0			0	15		0.00			0					WNDY13
chicken nuggets	180		9.0	10.0	0.0	0.0	380	20					1				
4 pieces (2.1 oz kid's meal)	60	11.0	2.5			25	150		0.36			0					WNDY14
	220		11.0	13.0	0.0	0.0	480	20					1				
5 pieces (2.6 oz)	75	14.0	3.0			35	190		0.72			0					WNDY15
chili, large	300		25.0	31.0	7.0	7.0	1310	150					4				
12 oz	340	9.0	3.5			50	700		3.60			1000					WNDY20
small	200		17.0	21.0	5.0	5.0	870	80					2				
8 oz	227	6.0	2.5			35	470		1.80			750					WNDY21
chili topping, cheddar cheese	70		4.0	1.0	0.0	0.0	110	100					0				
2 T	17	6.0	3.5			15	15		0.00			200					WNDY18
hot chili seasoning	5		0.0	2.0	1.0	0.0	280	0					0				
.25 oz pkt	7	0.0	0.0			0	0		0.00			0					WNDY19
french fries, biggie	440		5.0	63.0	0.0	7.0	380	20					4				
5.6 oz	159	19.0	3.5			0	860		1.44			0					WNDY23
great biggie	530		6.0	75.0	1.0	8.0	450	20					4				
6.7 oz	190	23.0	4.5			0	1030		1.80			0					WNDY24
kid's meal	250		3.0	36.0	0.0	4.0	220	20					2				
3.2 oz	91	11.0	2.0			0	490		0.72			0					WNDY25
medium	390		4.0	56.0	0.0	6.0	340	20					4				
5 oz	142	17.0	3.0			0	770		1.44			0					WNDY26
frosty dairy dessert, junior	170		4.0	28.0	21.0	0.0	100	150					0				
6 fl oz	113	4.0	2.5			20	290		0.72			400					WNDY28
medium	440		11.0	73.0	56.0	0.0	260	400					0				
16 fl oz	298	11.0	7.0			50	770		1.44			1000					WNDY27
small	330		8.0	56.0	43.0	0.0	200	300					0				
12 fl oz	227	8.0	5.0			35	590		1.08			750					WNDY29
hamburger, big bacon classic	570		34.0	46.0	11.0	3.0	1460	200					15				
9.9 oz hamburger	282	29.0	12.0			100	580		5.40			750					WNDY30
classic single w/everything	410		24.0	37.0	8.0	2.0	890	100					9				
7.7 oz hamburger	218	19.0	7.0			70	440		5.40			300					WNDY31
junior	270		14.0	34.0	6.0	2.0	600	100					4				
4.2 oz hamburger	117	9.0	3.0			30	220		3.60			100					WNDY32
kid's meal	270		14.0	33.0	6.0	2.0	600	100					4				
3.9 oz hamburger	110	9.0	3.0			30	210		3.60			100					WNDY33
potato, baked	310		7.0	72.0	5.0	7.0	25	20					36				
10 oz	284	0.0	0.0			0	1190		3.60			0					WNDY3
w/bacon & cheese	580		18.0	79.0	6.0	7.0	950	200					42				
13.4 oz	380	22.0	6.0			40	1410		3.60			500					WNDY1
w/broccoli & cheese	480		9.0	81.0	6.0	9.0	510	200					72				
14.5 oz	411	14.0	3.0			5	1400		4.50			1750					WNDY2
w/sour cream & chives	370		7.0	73.0	5.0	7.0	40	60					36				
11 oz	312	6.0	4.0			15	1230		3.60			400					WNDY4
salad additions, crispy rice noodles	60		1.0	10.0	1.0	0.0	180	0					0				
.5 oz pkt	14	2.0	0.5			0	15		0.36			0					WNDY34
garlic croutons	70		1.0	9.0	0.0	0.0	120	0					0				
.5 oz pkt	14	2.5	0.0			0	15		0.36			0					WNDY35
honey rstd pecans	130		2.0	5.0	3.0	2.0	65	20					0				
.7 oz pkt	20	13.0	1.0			0	65		0.36			0					WNDY36
rstd almonds	130		4.0	4.0	1.0	2.0	70	60					0				
.74 oz pkt	21	12.0	1.0			0	150		0.72			0					WNDY37
taco chips	220		3.0	25.0	0.0	2.0	150	60					0				
1.5 oz pkt	43	11.0	2.0			0	95		0.72			0					WNDY38
salad, caesar side	70		7.0	2.0	1.0	1.0	250	150					21				
3.5 oz salad	99	4.0	2.0			15	280		1.08			2250					WNDY48
chicken blt	310		33.0	10.0	4.0	4.0	1100	300					30				
13.3 oz salad	376	16.0	8.0			60	610		1.80			2500					WNDY49
mandarin chicken	150		20.0	17.0	11.0	3.0	650	60					30				
12.3 oz salad	348	1.5	0.0			10	420		1.80			1750					WNDY50

	KCAL / WT (g)	H₂0 (g) / FAT (g)	PRO (g) / SFA (g)	CHO (g) / MUFA (g)	SUGR (g) / PUFA (g)	DFIB (g) / CHOL (mg)	Na (mg) / K (mg)	Ca (mg) / P (mg)	Mg (mg) / Fe (mg)	Zn (mg) / Cu (mg)	Mn (mg) / Se (mcg)	A (mcg RAE) / A (IU)	C (mg) / E (mg ATE)	B-1 (mg) / B-2 (mg)	NIA (mg) / B-6 (mg)	B-12 (mcg) / FOL (mcg DFE)	PANT (mg) / REF
side	35		2.0	7.0	4.0	3.0	20	40					18				
5.9 oz salad	167	0.0	0.0			0	350		0.72			7000					WNDY51
spring mix	180		11.0	12.0	5.0	5.0	230	300					30				
11.1 oz salad	315	11.0	6.0			30	620		1.80			8500					WNDY52
taco supremo	360		27.0	29.0	8.0	8.0	1090	350					27				
17.5 oz salad	495	17.0	9.0			65	950		3.60			2500					WNDY53
salad dressing, blue cheese	260		2.0	2.0	1.0	0.0	460	40					0				
2.5 oz pkt	64	27.0	6.0			40	30		0.36			0					WNDY39
caesar	150		1.0	1.0	0.0	0.0	240	0					0				
.9 oz pkt	28	16.0	2.5			20	5		0.00			0					WNDY40
creamy ranch	250		1.0	5.0	3.0	0.0	640	60					0				
2.5 oz pkt	71	25.0	4.5			15	70		0.00			0					WNDY41
creamy ranch, red fat	110		1.0	7.0	3.0	1.0	610	60					0				
2.5 oz pkt	71	9.0	1.5			15	80		0.00			0					WNDY42
french, fat free	90		0.0	21.0	18.0	1.0	240	0					0				
2.5 oz pkt	71	0.0	0.0			0	10		0.72			0					WNDY43
honey mustard	310		1.0	12.0	11.0	0.0	410	0					0				
2.5 oz pkt	71	29.0	4.5			25	10		0.00			0					WNDY44
honey mustard, red fat	120		0.0	23.0	18.0	0.0	370	0					0				
2.5 oz pkt	71	3.5	0.0			0	15		0.00			0					WNDY45
house vinaigrette	220		0.0	9.0	8.0	0.0	830	0					1				
2.5 oz pkt	71	20.0	3.0			0	5		0.00			0					WNDY46
oriental sesame	280		2.0	21.0	19.0	0.0	620	20					1				
2.5 oz pkt	71	21.0	3.0			0	40		0.72			0					WNDY47

11. FATS, OILS, SHORTENINGS, AND SPREADS
11.1 ANIMAL FATS

	KCAL / WT (g)	H₂0 (g) / FAT (g)	PRO (g) / SFA (g)	CHO (g) / MUFA (g)	SUGR (g) / PUFA (g)	DFIB (g) / CHOL (mg)	Na (mg) / K (mg)	Ca (mg) / P (mg)	Mg (mg) / Fe (mg)	Zn (mg) / Cu (mg)	Mn (mg) / Se (mcg)	A (mcg RAE) / A (IU)	C (mg) / E (mg ATE)	B-1 (mg) / B-2 (mg)	NIA (mg) / B-6 (mg)	B-12 (mcg) / FOL (mcg DFE)	PANT (mg) / REF
beef fat, ckd	193	5.3	3.0	0.0	0.0	0.0	12	4	2	0.40	0.002	0	0	0.01	0.4	0.46	0.04
1 oz	28	19.9	8.1	8.6	0.8	27	34	22	0.30	0.013	4.9	0	0.1	0.03	0.04	0.9	13020
beef suet, raw	242	1.1	0.4	0.0		0.0	2	1	<1	0.06	<0.001	0	0	<0.01	0.1	0.08	0.01
1 oz	28	26.6	14.8	8.9	0.9	19	5	4	0.05	0.002	0.1	0	0.4	<0.01	0.01	0.3	13335
beef tallow, raw	115	0.0	0.0	0.0		0.0	0	0	0	0.00		0	0	0.00	0.00	0.00	0.00
1 T	13	12.8	6.4	5.4	0.5	14	0	0	0.00	0.000	<0.1	0	0.3	0.00	0.00	0.0	04001
chicken fat, raw	115	<0.1	0.0	0.0		0.0	0	0	0	0.00		0	0	0.00	0.0	0.00	0.00
1 T	13	12.8	3.8	5.7	2.7	11	0	0	0.00	0.000	<0.1	0	0.3	0.00	0.00	0.0	04542
duck fat, raw	115	<0.1	0.0	0.0		0.0	0	0	0	0.00		0	0	0.00	0.00	0.00	0.00
1 T	13	12.8	4.2	6.3	1.7	13	0	0	0.00	0.000	<0.1	0	0.3	0.00	0.00	0.0	04574
goose fat, raw	115	<0.1	0.0	0.0		0.0	0	0	0	0.00		0	0	0.00	0.00	0.00	0.00
1 T	13	12.8	3.5	7.3	1.4	13	0	0	0.00		<0.1	0	0.3	0.00	0.00	0.0	04576
lamb fat, ckd	166	7.4	3.4	0.0		0.0	16	7	4	0.49	0.001	0	0	0.02	2.2	0.67	0.16
1 oz	28	16.8	7.7	6.9	1.3	32	55	32	0.37	0.025	5.3	0		0.05	0.01	0.9	17006
lard (pork fat), raw	115	0.0	0.0	0.0		0.0	0	0	0	0.01	0.000	0	0	0.00	0.00	0.00	0.00
1 T	13	12.8	5.0	5.8	1.4	12	0	0	0.00	0.000	<0.1	0	0.2	0.00	0.00	0.0	04002
mutton tallow, raw	115	0.0	0.0	0.0		0.0	0	0	0	0.00		0	0	0.00	0.00	0.00	0.00
1 T	13	12.8	6.1	5.2	1.0	13	0	0	0.00	0.000	<0.1	0	0.4	0.00	0.00	0.0	04520
pork backfat, raw	230	2.2	0.8	0.0		0.0	3	1	1	0.10	0.001	1	<1	0.02	0.3	0.05	0.03
1 oz	28	25.1	9.1	11.9	2.9	16	18	11	0.05	0.005	2.3	4	0.2	0.01	0.01	0.3	10004
pork fat, ckd	178	6.6	3.5	0.0		0.0	10	15	2	0.36	0.001	1	0	0.09	0.7	0.13	0.09
1 oz	28	18.1	6.9	7.8	1.8	26	67	46	0.10	0.015	4.6	4	0.2	0.03	0.04	0.6	10007
raw	181	7.0	1.8	0.0		0.0	5	13	1	0.20	0.001	1	0	0.07	0.5	0.09	0.07
1 oz	28	19.2	6.7	8.5	2.0	26	34	26	0.08	0.008	2.3	3		0.03	0.01	0.6	10006
salt pork, raw	212	3.1	1.4	0.0		0.0	404	2	2	0.26	0.001	0	0	0.06	0.5	0.08	0.06
1 oz	28	22.8	8.3	10.8	2.7	24	19	15	0.12	0.014	1.6	0	0.1	0.02	0.02	0.3	10165
turkey fat, raw	115	<0.1	0.0	0.0		0.0	0	0	0	0.00		0	0	0.00	0.00	0.00	0.00
1 T	13	12.8	3.8	5.5	3.0	13	0	0	0.00	0.000	<0.1	0	0.4	0.00	0.00	0.0	04575

	KCAL / WT (g)	H₂O (g) / FAT (g)	PRO (g) / SFA (g)	CHO (g) / MUFA (g)	SUGR (g) / PUFA (g)	DFIB (g) / CHOL (mg)	Na (mg) / K (mg)	Ca (mg) / P (mg)	Mg (mg) / Fe (mg)	Zn (mg) / Cu (mg)	Mn (mg) / Se (mcg)	A (mcg RAE) / A (IU)	C (mg) / E (mg ATE)	B-1 (mg) / B-2 (mg)	NIA (mg) / B-6 (mg)	B-12 (mcg) / FOL (mcg DFE)	PANT (mg) / REF

11.2 FISH OILS

	KCAL/WT	H₂O/FAT	PRO/SFA	CHO/MUFA	SUGR/PUFA	DFIB/CHOL	Na/K	Ca/P	Mg/Fe	Zn/Cu	Mn/Se	A(RAE)/A(IU)	C/E	B-1/B-2	NIA/B-6	B-12/FOL	PANT/REF
cod liver oil	123	0.0	0.0	0.0		0.0	0	0	0	0.00	0.000	4080	0		0.0	0.00	0.00
1 T	14	13.6	3.1	6.4	3.1	78	0	0	0.00	0.000	0.0	13600		0.00	0.00	0.0	04589
herring oil	123	0.0	0.0	0.0		0.0	0	0	0	0.00	0.000	0	0		0.0	0.00	0.00
1 T	14	13.6	2.9	7.7	2.1	104	0	0	0.00	0.000	0.000	0		0.00	0.00	0.0	04590
menhaden oil	123	0.0	0.0	0.0		0.0	0	0	0	0.00	0.000	0	0		0.0	0.00	0.00
1 T	14	13.6	4.1	3.6	4.7	71	0	0	0.00	0.000	0.0	0		0.00	0.00	0.0	04591
fully hydg	113	0.0	0.0	0.0		0.0	0	0	0	0.00	0.000	0	0		0.0	0.00	0.00
1 T	13	12.5	12.0	0.0	0.0	63	0	0	0.00	0.000	0.0	0		0.00	0.00	0.0	04592
salmon oil	123	0.0	0.0	0.0		0.0	0	0	0	0.00	0.000	0	0		0.0	0.00	0.00
1 T	14	13.6	2.7	3.9	5.5	66	0	0	0.00	0.000	0.0	0		0.00	0.00	0.0	04593
sardine oil	123	0.0	0.0	0.0		0.0	0	0	0	0.00	0.000	0	0		0.0	0.00	0.00
1 T	14	13.6	4.1	4.6	4.3	97	0	0	0.00	0.000	0.0	0		0.00	0.00	0.0	04594

11.3 SHORTENINGS

	KCAL/WT	H₂O/FAT	PRO/SFA	CHO/MUFA	SUGR/PUFA	DFIB/CHOL	Na/K	Ca/P	Mg/Fe	Zn/Cu	Mn/Se	A(RAE)/A(IU)	C/E	B-1/B-2	NIA/B-6	B-12/FOL	PANT/REF
beef tallow & cottonseed,	115	0.0	0.0	0.0		0.0	0	0	0	0.00		0	0	0.00	0.00	0.0	0.00
for frying - 1 T	13	12.8	5.7	4.9	1.1	13	0	0	0.00		0.0	0	0.5	0.00	0.00	0.0	04550
coconut (hydg) & palm kernel,	113	0.0	0.0	0.0		0.0	0	0	0	0.00		0	0	0.00	0.00	0.0	0.00
for confectionery - 1 T	13	12.8	11.7	0.3	0.1	0	0	0	0.00	0.000	0.0	0	0.3	0.00	0.00	0.0	04551
lard & veg oil	115	0.0	0.0	0.0		0.0	0	0	0	0.00		0	0	0.00	0.00	0.0	0.00
1 T	13	12.8	5.2	5.7	1.4	7	0	0	0.00	0.000	0.0	0	0.2	0.00	0.00	0.0	04544
palm, for confectionery	120	0.0	0.0	0.0		0.0	0	0	0	0.00		0	0	0.00	0.00	0.0	0.00
1 T	14	13.6	8.9	4.0	0.1	0	0	0	0.00		0.0	0	2.6	0.00	0.00	0.0	04570

11.4 SPREADS

	KCAL/WT	H₂O/FAT	PRO/SFA	CHO/MUFA	SUGR/PUFA	DFIB/CHOL	Na/K	Ca/P	Mg/Fe	Zn/Cu	Mn/Se	A(RAE)/A(IU)	C/E	B-1/B-2	NIA/B-6	B-12/FOL	PANT/REF
Brummel & Brown 34% spread,	50		0.0	3.0	2.0	0.0	45	0				0					
avg for 3 flvrs, Lipton[1] - 1 T	12	4.0	1.0	1.0	2.0	0		0.00				400					UNLV143
yogurt-based 35% spread	45		0.0	0.0	0.0	0.0	90	0				0					
1 T	14	5.0	1.0	1.0	2.5	0		0.00				500					UNLV144
butter	102	2.3	0.1	0.0		0.0	117	3	<1	0.01	0.001	101	0	<0.01	<0.1	0.02	0.02
1 T	14	11.5	7.2	3.3	0.4	31	4	3	0.02	0.002	0.1	434	0.2	<0.01	<0.01	0.4	01001
sweet (unsalted)	102	2.5	0.1	0.0		0.0	2	3	<1	0.01	0.001	101	0	<0.01	<0.1	0.02	0.02
1 T	14	11.5	7.2	3.3	0.4	31	4	3	0.02	0.002	0.1	434	0.2	<0.01	<0.01	0.4	01145
whipped	67	1.5	0.1	0.0		0.0	78	2	<1	<0.01	<0.001	67	0	<0.01	<0.1	0.01	0.01
1 T	9	7.6	4.7	2.2	0.3	21	2	2	0.02	0.002	0.1	287	0.1	<0.01	<0.01	0.3	01002
Country Crock 39% soft	50		0.0	0.0			95	100				0					
w/Ca & vit E - 1 T	14	5.0	1.0	1.5	2.5	0		0.00				500	3.0				UNLV2
48% soft	60		0.0	0.0	0.0	0.0	110	0				0					
1 T	14	7.0	1.5	1.0	3.0	0		0.00				500					UNLV3
55% squeeze	70		0.0	0.0	0.0	0.0	95	0				0					
1 T	14	8.0	1.5	2.0	4.5	0		0.00				500					UNLV4
60% quarters	80		0.0	0.0	0.0	0.0	110	0				0					
1 T	14	8.0	1.5	2.5	2.5	0		0.00				500					UNLV5
light 39% soft spread	50		0.0	0.0	0.0	0.0	85	0				0					
1 T	14	5.0	1.0	1.5	2.5	0		0.00				500					UNLV8
Country Crock Churnstyle	60		0.0	0.0	0.0	0.0	85	0				0					
48% soft - 1 T	14	7.0	1.5	1.5	3.0	0		0.00				500					UNLV6
60% quarters	80		0.0	0.0	0.0	0.0	85	0				0					
1 T	14	8.0	1.5	2.5	2.5	0		0.00				500					UNLV7
Earth Balance Natural	100		0.0	0.0	0.0		120	0				0					
1 T	14	11.0	3.0	4.0	3.0	0						500	0				GBAF9
Filbert's 48% soft spread	60		0.0	0.0	0.0	0.0	120	0				0					
1 T	14	7.0	4.5	1.5	3.0	0		0.00				500					UNLV145
53% quarters	70		0.0	0.0	0.0	0.0	100	0				0					
1 T	14	7.0	1.5	2.0	2.0	0		0.00				500					UNLV146

	KCAL / WT (g)	H₂0 (g) / FAT (g)	PRO (g) / SFA (g)	CHO (g) / MUFA (g)	SUGR (g) / PUFA (g)	DFIB (g) / CHOL (mg)	Na (mg) / K (mg)	Ca (mg) / P (mg)	Mg (mg) / Fe (mg)	Zn (mg) / Cu (mg)	Mn (mg) / Se (mcg)	A (mcg RAE) / A (IU)	C (mg) / E (mg ATE)	B-1 (mg) / B-2 (mg)	NIA (mg) / B-6 (mg)	B-12 (mcg) / FOL (mcg DFE)	PANT (mg) / REF
garlic butter w/olive oil, Land	100		0.0	0.0	0.0	0.0	95	0					0				
O Lakes - *1 T*	14	11.0	5.0			20			0.00			400					LAND1
I Can't Believe It's Not Butter	50		0.0	0.0	0.0	0.0	85	0					0				
37% soft spread - *1 T*	14	5.0	1.0	1.5	2.5	0			0.00			500					UNLV147
40% quarters	50		0.0	0.0	0.0	0.0	85	0					0				
1 T	14	6.0	1.0	1.5	1.5	0			0.00			500					UNLV9
40% sweet cream & Ca	50		0.0	0.0	0.0	0.0	110	100									
soft spread - *1 T*	14	5.0	1.0	1.5	2.5	0						500					UNLV148
55% Squeeze	70		0.0	0.0	0.0	0.0	95	0					0				
1 T	14	8.0	1.5	2.0	4.5	0			0.00			500					UNLV149
70% quarters	90		0.0	0.0	0.0	0.0	90	0					0				
1 T	14	10.0	2.0	3.0	2.5	0			0.00			500					UNLV116
70% quarters, unsalted	90		0.0	0.0	0.0	0.0	0	0					0				
1 T	14	10.0	2.0	3.0	2.5	0			0.00			500					UNLV10
70% whipped	90		0.0	0.0	0.0	0.0	90	0					0				
1 T	14	10.0	2.0	3.0	2.5	0			0.00			500					UNLV11
fat free	5		0.0	0.0	0.0	0.0	90	0					0				
1 T	14	0.0	0.0	0.0	0.0	0			0.00			500					UNLV114
70% soft spread	90		0.0	0.0	0.0	0.0	90	0					0				
1 T	14	10.0	2.0	2.5	4.5	0			0.00			500					UNLV150
Imperial, 1/3 less fat, 52%	70		0.0	0.0	0.0	0.0	105	0					0				
quarters - *1 T*	14	7.0	1.5	1.5	2.0	0			0.00			500					UNLV138
48% soft spread	60		0.0	0.0	0.0	0.0	85						0				
1 T	14	7.0	4.5	1.5	3.0	0			0.00			500					UNLV106
65% quarters	80		0.0	0.0	0.0	0.0	105	0					0				
1 T	14	9.0	2.0	2.5	2.0	0			0.00			500					UNLV107
80% soft	100		0.0	0.0	0.0	0.0	105	0					0				
1 T	14	11.0	2.0	2.5	5.0	0			0.00			500					UNLV15
82% Butter Blend cubes	100		0.0	0.0	0.0	0.0	115	0					0				
1 T	14	11.0	2.5	3.5	2.5	0			0.00			500					UNLV16
margarine, corn & soy,	99	2.4	0.0	0.3		0.0	92	0	<1	0.02				<0.01	<0.1		0.00
80% fat, stick - *1 T*	14	11.0	2.1	5.2	3.2	0	3	1	0.02				0.9	0.00	0.00	0.1	04628
corn, soft	34	0.8	0.0	0.0		0.0	51	1	<1	0.00		34	<1	<0.01	<0.1	<0.01	<0.01
1 t	5	3.8	0.7	1.5	1.5	0	2	1	0.00		0.0	168	0.5	<0.01	<0.01	0.0	04092
corn, stick	34	0.7	0.0	0.0		0.0	44	1	<1	0.00		34	<1	<0.01	<0.1	<0.01	<0.01
1 t	5	3.8	0.7	1.8	1.1	0	2	1	0.00	0.000	0.0	168	0.7	<0.01	<0.01	0.0	04065
liquid	102	2.2	0.3	0.0		0.0	111	9	1	0.00		104	<1	<0.01	<0.1	0.03	0.03
1 T	14	11.4	1.9	4.0	5.1	0	13	7	0.00	0.000	0.0	507	0.7	0.01	<0.01	0.4	04105
soy, soft	34	0.8	0.0	0.0		0.0	1	1	<1	0.00		34	<1	<0.01	<0.1	<0.01	<0.01
1 t	5	3.8	0.6	1.7	1.3	0	2	1	0.00		0.0	168	0.2	<0.01	<0.01	0.0	04093
soy, stick	34	0.7	0.0	0.0		0.0	44	1	<1			34	<1	<0.01	<0.1	<0.01	<0.01
1 t	5	3.8	0.6	1.8	1.2	0	2	1	0.00		0.0	168	0.1	<0.01	<0.01	0.0	04080
margarine-butter blend, 60%	102	2.2	0.1	0.1		0	127	4	<1	<0.01	<0.001	104	<1	<0.01	<0.1	0.01	0.01
corn oil, 40% butter - *1 T*	14	11.5	4.0	4.7	2.3	12	5	3	0.01	0.001	0.1	507	1.1	<0.01	<0.01	0.3	04585
mayonnaise, extra heavy,	100		0.0	0.0	0.0	0.0	85	0					0				
Hellmann's - *1 T*	14	11.0	1.5			10			0.00			0					UNLV59
fat free, Kraft	11	13.1	0.0	2.0	1.1	0.3	120	1					0				
1 T	16	0.4	0.1			2	8	4	0.02			16	0.5				04013
Hellmann's/Best Foods	100		0.0	0.0	0.0	0.0	85	0					0				
1 T	14	11.0	1.5			5			0.00			0					UNLV62
imitation, soy	35	9.4	0.0	2.4		0.0	75	0	0	0.02		0	0	0.00	0.0	0.00	0.00
1 T	15	2.9	0.5	0.7	1.6	4	2	0	0.00	0.002	0.2	0	1.0	0.00	0.00	0.0	04027
light, Hellmann's/Best	50		0.0	1.0	0.0	0.0	120	0					0				
Foods - *1 T*	15	5.0	1.0			5			0.00			0	3.0				UNLV60
light, Kraft Mayo Light	50	8.3	0.1	1.3	0.6	0.0	120	1					<1				
1 T	15	4.9	0.8			5	8	9	0.03			28	0.6				04011
red fat, Hellmann's/Best	25		0.0	2.0	<1.0	0.0	130	0					0				
Foods Just 2 Good - *1 T*	15	2.0	0.5			0			0.00			0					UNLV61
safflower & soy	99	2.1	0.2	0.4		0.0	78	2	<1	0.02		12	0	0.00	<0.1	0.04	0.04
1 T	14	11.0	1.2	1.8	7.6	8	5	4	0.07		0.2	39	3.0	0.00	0.08	1.1	04026
soy	99	2.1	0.2	0.4		0.0	78	2	<1	0.02		12	0	0.00	<0.1	0.04	0.03
1 T	14	11.0	1.6	3.1	5.7	8	5	4	0.07	0.001	0.2	39	0.3	0.00	0.08	1.1	04025
Smart Balance Light Mayo	50		0.0	2.0	0.0		125	0									
1 T	15	5.0	0.0	2.5	1.5	5	125					0	2.0				GBAF5

	KCAL WT (g)	H₂O (g) FAT (g)	PRO (g) SFA (g)	CHO (g) MUFA (g)	SUGR (g) PUFA (g)	DFIB (g) CHOL (mg)	Na (mg) K (mg)	Ca (mg) P (mg)	Mg (mg) Fe (mg)	Zn (mg) Cu (mg)	Mn (mg) Se (mcg)	A (mcg RAE) A (IU)	C (mg) E (mg ATE)	B-1 (mg) B-2 (mg)	NIA (mg) B-6 (mg)	B-12 (mcg) FOL (mcg DFE)	PANT (mg) REF
Smart Beat	10		0.0	3.0	1.0		135	0									
1 T	16	0.0	0.0	0.0	0.0	0						0	0.0				GBAF6
Miracle Whip, light, Kraft	37	10.1	0.1	2.3	1.6	0.0	131	1					0				
1 T	16	3.0	0.5			4	4	2	0.03			5	0.1				04012
nonfat, Kraft	13	12.6	0.0	2.5	1.6	0.3	126	1					0				
1 T	16	0.4	0.1			1	8	1	0.02			11	<0.1				04014
Promise 60% whpd soft	80		0.0	0.0	0.0	0.0	70	0					0				
1 T	14	8.0	1.5	2.0	4.5	0			0.00			500					UNLV22
68% quarters	90		0.0	0.0	0.0	0.0	90	0					0				
1 T	14	10.0	2.5	2.5	4.0	0			0.00			500					UNLV108
Buttery Light Soft	45		0.0	0.0	0.0	0.0	55	0					0				
1 T	14	5.0	1.0	1.0	2.5	0			0.00			500					UNLV109
Ultra 26% soft spread	35		0.0	0.0	0.0	0.0	90	0					0				
1 T	14	3.5	1.0	1.0	1.5	0			0.00			500					UNLV111
Promise Take Control	40		0.0	0.0	0.0	0.0	110	0					0				
32% light - *1 T*	14	4.5	0.5	2.0	1.5	5			0.00			500					UNLV24
35% soft	45		0.0	0.0	0.0	0.0	85	0					0				
1 T	14	5.0	0.5	2.0	2.0	5			0.00			500	4.5				UNLV25
40% soft	50		0.0	0.0			110										
1 T	14	6.0	1.0	2.5	2.0	5			0.00			500	1.8				UNLV23
60% soft	80		0.0	0.0		0.0	85										
spread - *1 T*	14	8.0	1.0	4.5	2.0	<5						500					UNLV110
sandwich spread	58	6.1	0.1	3.4		0.1	150	2	<1	0.12		10	0	<0.01	<0.1	0.03	0.00
1 T	15	5.1	0.8	1.1	3.0	11	5	4	0.03	0.002	0.2	33	1.0	<0.01	<0.01	0.9	04030
Sandwich Spred, Hellmann's/Best	50		0.0	2.0	2.0	0.0	180	0					0				
Foods - *1 T*	15	5.0	0.5			<5			0.00			0					UNLV89
Shedd's 52% quarters	60		0.0	0.0	0.0	0.0	115	0					0				
1 T	14	7.0	1.5	2.0	1.5	0			0.00			500					UNLV26
60% garlic	80		0.0	0.0	0.0	0.0	90	0					0				
1 T	14	8.0	1.5	2.0	4.0	0			0.00			500					UNLV27
80% margarine	100		0.0	0.0	0.0	0.0	110	0					0				
1 T	14	11.0	2.0	3.5	2.5	0			0.00			500					UNLV28
80% soft margarine	100		0.0	0.0	0.0	0.0	110	0					0				
1 T	14	11.0	2.0	2.5	5.0	0			0.00			500					UNLV29
80% soft whpd margarine	100		0.0	0.0	0.0	0.0	110	0					0				
1 T	14	11.0	2.0	2.5	2.5	0			0.00			500					UNLV30
80% unsalted	100		0.0	0.0	0.0	0.0	0	0					0				
1 T	14	11.0	2.0	3.5	2.5	0			0.00			500					UNLV31
Smart Balance Buttery	80		0.0	0.0	0.0		90	0									
1 T	14	9.0	2.5	3.5	2.5	0	5	5				500	0.0				GBAF10
Light	45		0.0	0.0	0.0		90	0									
1 T	14	5.0	1.5	2.0	1.5	0	5	1				500	0.0				GBAF11
Smart Beat Squeeze	5		0.0	1.0	0.0		100	0									
margarine - *1 T*	14	0.0	0.0	0.0	0.0	0						500	0.0				GBAF3
Superlight margarine	20		0.0	0.0	0.0		105	0									
1 T	14	2.0	0.0	1.5	0.5	0						500	2.0				GBAF4
spread, corn, 40% fat, stick	17	2.8	0.0	0.0		0.0	46	1	<1	0.00		35	<1	<0.01	<0.1	<0.01	<0.01
1 t	5	1.9	0.3	0.7	0.8	0	1	1	0.00		0.0	171	0.2	<0.01	<0.01	0.0	04107
spread, fat-free, bottle	7	13.3	0.0	0.8		0.0	128	1	1	0.03	0.000	0		0.15	<0.1	0.00	
1 T	15	0.4	0.1	0.1	0.2	<1	32	6	0.03	0.000	0.0		0.1	0.01	<0.01	0.0	04632
tub	6	13.2	0.0	0.6		0.0	85	1	<1	0.01	0.000	0		0.15	0.1	0.00	0.04
1 T	15	0.4	0.3	0.1	0.1	0	5	<1	0.01	0.000	0.0		0.1	0.00	<0.01	0.0	04631
spread, soy, 40% fat, stick	17	2.8	0.0	0.0		0.0	46	1	<1	0.00		35	<1	<0.01	<0.1	<0.01	<0.01
1 t	5	1.9	0.3	0.9	0.5	0	1	1	0.00		0.0	171	0.4	<0.01	<0.01	0.0	04110
70% fat	87	3.8	0.0	0.2			98	1	<1	0.01	0.002			0.01			<0.01
1 T	14	9.7	1.8	5.1	2.3	0	6	1	0.02					<0.01	<0.01	0.1	04629
spread, soy & cottonseed,	26	1.8	0.0	0.0		0.0	48	1	<1	0.00		35	<1	<0.01	<0.1	<0.01	<0.01
60% fat, soft - *1 t*	5	2.9	0.6	1.9	0.3	0	1	1	0.00		0.0	171	0.2	<0.01	<0.1	<0.01	04106
spread, soy & palm, 60%	26	1.8	0.0	0.0		0.0	48	1	<1	0.00		35	<1	<0.01	<0.1	<0.01	<0.01
fat, stick - *1 t*	5	2.9	0.7	1.2	0.9	0	1	1	0.00		0.0	171	0.2	<0.01	<0.1	<0.01	04526
Wendy's soft whpd	100		0.0	0.0	0.0	0.0	110	0					0				
margarine - *1 T*	14	11.0	2.0	2.5	2.5	0			0.00			500					UNLV37

¹ Values are averages for apple and cinnamon, blueberry, and strawberry.

	KCAL	H₂O (g)	PRO (g)	CHO (g)	SUGR (g)	DFIB (g)	Na (mg)	Ca (mg)	Mg (mg)	Zn (mg)	Mn (mg)	A (mcg RAE)	C (mg)	B-1 (mg)	NIA (mg)	B-12 (mcg)	PANT (mg)
	WT (g)	FAT (g)	SFA (g)	MUFA (g)	PUFA (g)	CHOL (mg)	K (mg)	P (mg)	Fe (mg)	Cu (mg)	Se (mcg)	A (IU)	E (mg ATE)	B-2 (mg)	B-6 (mg)	FOL (mcg DFE)	REF

11.5 VEGETABLE OILS & VEGETABLE OIL SPRAYS

	KCAL/WT	H₂O/FAT	PRO/SFA	CHO/MUFA	SUGR/PUFA	DFIB/CHOL	Na/K	Ca/P	Mg/Fe	Zn/Cu	Mn/Se	A/A	C/E	B-1/B-2	NIA/B-6	B-12/FOL	PANT/REF
almond oil	120	0.0	0.0	0.0		0.0	0	0	0	0.00		0	0	0.00	0.0	0.00	0.00
1 T	14	13.6	1.1	9.5	2.4	0	0	0	0.00	0.000	0.0	0	5.3	0.00	0.00	0.0	04529
apricot kernel oil	120	0.0	0.0	0.0		0.0	0	0	0	0.00		0	0	0.00	0.0	0.00	0.00
1 T	14	13.6	0.9	8.2	4.0	0	0	0	0.00		0.0	0	1.2	0.00	0.00	0.0	04530
avocado oil	124	0.0	0.0	0.0		0.0	0	0	0	0.00	0.000	0	0	0.00	0.00	0.00	0.00
1 T	14	14.0	1.6	9.9	1.9	0	0	0	0.00	0.000	0.0	0		0.00	0.00	0.0	04581
babassu oil	120	0.0	0.0	0.0		0.0	0	0	0	0.00		0	0	0.00	0.00	0.00	0.00
1 T	14	13.6	11.0	1.6	0.2	0	0	0	0.00		0.0	0	2.6	0.00	0.00	0.0	04534
canola oil	124	0.0	0.0	0.0		0.0	0	0	0	0.00	0.000	0	0	0.00	0.00	0.00	0.00
1 T	14	14.0	1.0	8.2	4.1	0	0	0	0.00	0.000	0.0	0	2.9	0.00	0.00	0.0	04582
canola, Smart Balance	120		0.0	0.0		0.0	0						0				
1 T	14	14.0	1.0	7.0	5.0	0	0					0	2.0				GBAF1
cocoa (cacao) oil	120	0.0	0.0	0.0		0.0	0	0	0	0.00	0.000	0	0	0.00	0.00	0.00	0.00
1 T	14	13.6	8.1	4.5	0.4	0	0	0	0.00	0.000	0.0	0	0.2	0.00	0.00	0.0	04501
coconut oil	117	0.0	0.0	0.0		0.0	0	0	0	0.00	0.000	0	0	0.00	0.00	0.00	0.00
1 T	14	13.6	11.8	0.8	0.2	0	0	0	0.01	0.000		0	<0.1	0.00	0.00	0.0	04047
corn oil	120	0.0	0.0	0.0		0.0	0	0	0	0.00		0	0	0.00	0.00	0.00	0.00
1 T	14	13.6	1.7	3.3	8.0	0	0	0	0.00	0.000	0.0	0	2.9	0.00	0.00	0.0	04518
cottonseed oil	120	0.0	0.0	0.0		0.0	0	0	0	0.00		0	0	0.00	0.00	0.00	0.00
1 T	14	13.6	3.5	2.4	7.1	0	0	0	0.00	0.000	0.0	0	5.2	0.00	0.00	0.0	04502
hazelnut oil	120	0.0	0.0	0.0		0.0	0	0	0	0.00		0	0	0.00	0.00	0.00	0.00
1 T	14	13.6	1.0	10.6	1.4	0	0	0	0.00		0.0	0	6.4	0.00	0.00	0.0	04532
I Can't Believe It's Not Butter,	0		0.0	0.0	0.0	0.0	0	0					0				
40% spray - 1/3 sec spray	0	0.0	0.0	0.0	0.0	0			0.00			0					UNLV112
mustard oil	124	0.0	0.0	0.0		0.0	0	0	0	0.00	0.000	0	0	0.00	0.00	0.00	0.00
1 T	14	14.0	1.6	8.3	3.0		0	0	0.00	0.000	0.0	0		0.00	0.00	0.0	04583
No Stick Mazola spray	0	0.0	0.0	0.0	0.0	0.0	0	0					0	0			
1/4 sec spray	0.2	0.0	0.0	0.0	0.0	0			0.00			0					UNLV64
nutmeg oil	120	0.0	0.0	0.0		0.0	0	0	0	0.00		0	0	0.00	0.00	0.00	0.00
1 T	14	13.6	12.2	0.7	0.0	0	0	0	0.00		0.0	0	<0.1	0.00	0.00	0.0	04572
oat oil	120	0.0	0.0	0.0		0.0	0	0	0	0.00	0.000	0	0	0.00	0.00	0.00	0.00
1 T	14	13.6	2.7	4.8	5.6	0	0	0	0.00	0.000	0.0	0	2.0	0.00	0.00	0.0	04588
olive oil	119	0.0	0.0	0.0		0.0	0	0	0	0.01		0	0	0.00	0.00	0.00	0.00
1 T	14	13.5	1.8	9.9	1.1	0	0	<1	0.05	0.000	0.0	0	1.7	0.00	0.00	0.0	04053
palm kernel oil	117	0.0	0.0	0.0		0.0	0	0	0	0.00	0.000	0	0	0.00	0.00	0.00	0.00
1 T	14	13.6	11.1	1.6	0.2	0	0	0	0.00	0.000		0	0.5	0.00	0.00	0.0	04513
palm oil	120	0.0	0.0	0.0		0.0	0	0	0	0.00		0	0	0.00	0.00	0.00	0.00
1 T	14	13.6	6.7	5.0	1.3	0	0	0	<0.01	0.000	0.0	0	3.0	0.00	0.00	0.0	04055
peanut oil	119	0.0	0.0	0.0		0.0	0	0	0	<0.01		0	0	0.00	0.00	0.00	0.00
1 T	14	13.5	2.3	6.2	4.3	0	0	0	<0.01	0.000	0.0	0	1.7	0.00	0.00	0.0	04042
poppyseed oil	120	0.0	0.0	0.0		0.0	0	0	0	0.00		0	0	0.00	0.00	0.00	0.00
1 T	14	13.6	1.8	2.7	8.5	0	0	0	0.00		0.0	0	1.6	0.00	0.00	0.0	04514
Pro Chef spray, Mazola	0	0.0	0.0		0.0	0.0	0						0	0			
1/3 sec spray	0.3	0.0	0.0	0.0	0.0	0	0		0.00			0					UNLV86
rice bran oil	120	0.0	0.0	0.0		0.0	0	0	0	0.00		0	0	0.00	0.00	0.00	0.00
1 T	14	13.6	2.7	5.3	4.8	0	0	0	0.01		0.0	0	4.4	0.00	0.00	0.0	04037
Right Blend (canola &	120	0.0	0.0		0.0	0.0	0										
corn), Mazola - 1 T	14	14.0	1.0	7.0	4.5	0							2.0				UNLV88
safflower oil, >70%	120	0.0	0.0	0.0		0.0	0	0	0	0.00		0	0	0.00	0.0	0.00	0.00
linoleic acid - 1 T	14	13.6	0.8	2.0	10.1	0	0	0	0.00	0.000	0.0	0	5.9	0.00	0.00	0.0	04510
>70% oleic acid	120	0.0	0.0	0.0		0.0	0	0	0	0.00	0.000	0	0	0.00	0.0	0.00	0.00
1 T	14	13.6	0.8	10.2	2.0	0	0	0	0.00	0.000	0.0	0	4.7	0.00	0.00	0.0	04511
sesame oil	120	0.0	0.0	0.0		0.0	0	0	0	0.00		0	0	0.00	0.00	0.00	0.00
1 T	14	13.6	1.9	5.4	5.7	0	0	0	0.00	0.000	0.0	0	0.6	0.00	0.00	0.0	04058
sheanut oil	120	0.0	0.0	0.0		0.0	0	0	0	0.00		0	0	0.00	0.00	0.00	0.00
1 T	14	13.6	6.3	6.0	0.7	0	0	0	0.00		0.0	0	0.0	0.00	0.00	0.0	04536
Smart Balance spray	10		0.0	0.0													
1 sec spray	2	1.5	0.0	0.5	0.5	0											GBAF8

	KCAL	H₂0 (g)	PRO (g)	CHO (g)	SUGR (g)	DFIB (g)	Na (mg)	Ca (mg)	Mg (mg)	Zn (mg)	Mn (mg)	A (mcg RAE)	C (mg)	B-1 (mg)	NIA (mg)	B-12 (mcg)	PANT (mg)
	WT (g)	FAT (g)	SFA (g)	MUFA (g)	PUFA (g)	CHOL (mg)	K (mg)	P (mg)	Fe (mg)	Cu (mg)	Se (mcg)	A (IU)	E (mg ATE)	B-2 (mg)	B-6 (mg)	FOL (mcg DFE)	REF
soy (hydg) & cottonseed	120	0.0	0.0	0.0		0.0	0	0	0	0.00		0	0	0.00	0.0	0.00	0.00
oil - *1 T*	14	13.6	2.4	4.0	6.5	0	0	0	0.00	0.000	0.0	0	3.8	0.00	0.00	0.0	04543
soy lecithin[1]	104	0.0	0.0	0.0		0.0	0	0	0	0.00		0	0	0.00	0.0	0.00	0.00
1 T	14	13.6	2.0	1.5	6.2	0	0	0	0.00	0.000	0.0	0	0.7	0.00	0.00	0.0	04531
soy oil	120	0.0	0.0	0.0		0.0	0	0	0	0.00		0	0	0.00	0.00	0.00	0.00
1 T	14	13.6	2.0	3.2	7.9	0	0	0	<0.01	0.000	0.0	0	2.5	0.00	0.00	0.0	04044
hydg	120	0.0	0.0	0.0		0.0	0	0	0	0.00		0	0	0.00	0.0	0.00	0.00
1 T	14	13.6	2.0	5.8	5.1	0	0	0	0.00	0.000	0.0	0	2.5	0.00	0.00	0.0	04034
sunflower oil, hydg	124	0.0	0.0	0.0		0.0	0	0	0	0.00	0.000	0	0	0.00	0.00	0.00	0.00
1 T	14	14.0	1.4	11.7	0.5	0	0	0	0.00	0.000	0.0	0		0.00	0.00	0.0	04584b
<60% linoleic acid	120	0.0	0.0	0.0		0.0	0	0	0	0.00		0	0	0.00	0.00	0.00	0.00
1 T	14	13.6	1.4	6.2	5.5	0	0	0	<0.01		0.0	0	8.1	0.00	0.00	0.0	04060
>60% linoleic acid	120	0.0	0.0	0.0		0.0	0	0	0	0.00		0	0	0.00	0.00	0.00	0.00
1 T	14	13.6	1.4	2.7	8.9	0	0	0	0.00	0.000	0.0	0	6.9	0.00	0.00	0.0	04506
>70% oleic acid	124	0.0	0.0	0.0		0.0	0	0	0	0.00	0.000	0	0	0.00	0.00	0.00	0.00
1 T	14	14.0	1.4	11.7	0.5	0	0	0	0.00	0.000	0.0	0		0.00	0.00	0.0	04584c
walnut oil	120	0.0	0.0	0.0		0.0	0	0	0	0.00		0	0	0.00	0.00	0.00	0.00
1 T	14	13.6	1.2	3.1	8.6	0	0	0	0.00	0.000	0.0	0	0.4	0.00	0.00	0.0	04528
wheat germ oil	120	0.0	0.0	0.0		0.0	0	0	0	0.00		0	0	0.00	0.00	0.00	0.00
1 T	14	13.6	2.6	2.1	8.4	0	0	0	0.00	0.000	0.0	0	26.2	0.00	0.00	0.0	04038

[1] Seventy percent phosphatide in 30% oil.

12. FISH & SEAFOOD
12.1 CRUSTACEA

	KCAL	H₂0 (g)	PRO (g)	CHO (g)	SUGR (g)	DFIB (g)	Na (mg)	Ca (mg)	Mg (mg)	Zn (mg)	Mn (mg)	A (mcg RAE)	C (mg)	B-1 (mg)	NIA (mg)	B-12 (mcg)	PANT (mg)
	WT (g)	FAT (g)	SFA (g)	MUFA (g)	PUFA (g)	CHOL (mg)	K (mg)	P (mg)	Fe (mg)	Cu (mg)	Se (mcg)	A (IU)	E (mg ATE)	B-2 (mg)	B-6 (mg)	FOL (mcg DFE)	REF
crab, alaska king, ckd by	82	65.9	16.4	0.0		0.0	911	50	54	6.48	0.034	8	6	0.05	1.1	9.78	0.34
moist heat - *3 oz*	85	1.3	0.1	0.2	0.5	45	223	238	0.65	1.005	34.0	25		0.05	0.15	43.4	15137
imitation, made from	87	62.6	10.2	8.7		0.0	715	11	37	0.28	0.009	17	0	0.03	0.2	1.36	0.06
surimi - *3 oz*	85	1.1	0.2	0.2	0.6	17	77	240	0.33	0.027	19.0	56	0.1	0.02	0.03	1.7	15138
raw	71	67.6	15.5	0.0		0.0	711	39	42	5.06	0.030	6	6	0.04	0.9	7.65	0.30
3 oz	85	0.5	0.1	0.1	0.1	36	173	186	0.50	0.784	30.9	20		0.04	0.13	37.4	15136
crab, blue, ckd by moist	87	65.8	17.2	0.0		0.0	237	88	28	3.59	0.162	2	3	0.09	2.8	6.21	0.37
heat - *3 oz*	85	1.5	0.2	0.2	0.6	85	275	175	0.77	0.548	34.2	5	0.9	0.04	0.15	43.4	15140
cnd	84	64.7	17.4	0.0		0.0	283	86	33	3.42	0.162	2	2	0.07	1.2	0.39	0.31
3 oz	85	1.0	0.2	0.2	0.4	76	318	221	0.71	0.646	27.0	4	0.9	0.07	0.13	36.6	15141
raw	74	67.2	15.4	0.0		0.0	249	76	29	3.01	0.128	2	3	0.07	2.3	7.65	0.30
3 oz	85	0.9	0.2	0.2	0.3	66	280	195	0.63	0.569	31.8	4	0.9	0.03	0.13	37.4	15139
crab cake[1]	93	42.6	12.1	0.3		0.0	198	63	20	2.45	0.114	34	2	0.05	1.7	3.56	0.30
1 cake	60	4.5	0.9	1.7	1.4	90	194	128	0.65	0.366	24.4	151		0.05	0.10	36.6	15142
crab, dungeness, ckd by	94	62.3	19.0	0.8		0.0	321	50	49	4.65	0.082	26	3	0.05	3.1	8.82	0.34
moist heat - *3 oz*	85	1.1	0.1	0.2	0.3	65	347	149	0.37	0.624	40.5	88		0.17	0.15	35.7	15226
raw	73	67.3	14.8	0.6		0.0	251	39	38	3.63	0.068	23	3	0.04	2.7	7.65	0.30
3 oz	85	0.8	0.1	0.1	0.3	50	301	155	0.31	0.573	31.5	77		0.14	0.13	37.4	15143
crab, queen, ckd by moist	98	63.8	20.2	0.0		0.0	587	28	54	3.05	0.031	44	6	0.08	2.5	8.82	0.34
heat - *3 oz*	85	1.3	0.2	0.3	0.5	60	170	109	2.45	0.528	37.7	147		0.21	0.15	35.7	15227
raw	77	68.5	15.7	0.0		0.0	458	22	42	2.38	0.026	38	6	0.07	2.1	7.65	0.30
3 oz	85	1.0	0.1	0.2	0.4	47	147	113	2.13	0.485	29.4	128		0.17	0.13	37.4	15144
crayfish, farmed, ckd by	74	68.7	14.9	0.0		0.0	82	43	28	1.26	0.184	13	<1	0.04	1.4	2.64	0.44
moist heat - *3 oz*	85	1.1	0.2	0.2	0.4	116	202	205	0.94	0.493	29.1	43		0.07	0.11	9.4	15243
raw	61	71.4	12.6	0.0		0.0	53	21	26	0.86	0.124	13	<1	0.04	1.6	1.79	0.48
3 oz	85	0.8	0.2	0.2	0.3	91	222	185	0.47	0.201	24.1	43		0.03	0.06	25.5	15242
crayfish, wild, ckd by	70	67.5	14.3	0.0		0.0	80	51	28	1.50	0.444	13	1	0.04	1.9	1.83	0.49
moist heat - *3 oz*	85	1.0	0.2	0.2	0.3	113	252	230	0.71	0.582	31.2	43	1.3	0.07	0.06	37.4	15146
raw	65	69.9	13.6	0.0		0.0	49	23	23	1.11	0.192	14	1	0.06	1.9	1.70	0.46
3 oz	85	0.8	0.1	0.1	0.2	97	257	218	0.71	0.356	26.9	44	2.4	0.03	0.09	31.5	15145
lobster, northern, ckd by	83	64.6	17.4	1.1		0.0	323	52	30	2.48	0.052	22	0	0.01	0.9	2.64	0.24
moist heat - *3 oz*	85	0.5	0.1	0.1	0.1	61	299	157	0.33	1.649	36.3	74	0.9	0.06	0.07	9.4	15148
raw	77	65.2	16.0	0.4		0.0	252	41	23	2.57	0.047	18	0	0.01	1.2	0.79	1.39
3 oz	85	0.8	0.2	0.2	0.1	81	234	122	0.26	1.414	35.2	60	1.2	0.04	0.05	7.7	15147

	KCAL	H₂O (g)	PRO (g)	CHO (g)	SUGR (g)	DFIB (g)	Na (mg)	Ca (mg)	Mg (mg)	Zn (mg)	Mn (mg)	A (mcg RAE)	C (mg)	B-1 (mg)	NIA (mg)	B-12 (mcg)	PANT (mg)
	WT (g)	FAT (g)	SFA (g)	MUFA (g)	PUFA (g)	CHOL (mg)	K (mg)	P (mg)	Fe (mg)	Cu (mg)	Se (mcg)	A (IU)	E (mg ATE)	B-2 (mg)	B-6 (mg)	FOL (mcg DFE)	REF
shrimp, breaded & fried[2]	206	44.9	18.2	9.7		0.3	292	57	34	1.17	0.085	48	1	0.11	2.6	1.59	0.30
3 oz (11 large)	85	10.4	1.8	3.2	4.3	150	191	185	1.07	0.233	35.4	161		0.12	0.08	20.4	15150
ckd by moist heat	84	65.7	17.8	0.0		0.0	190	33	29	1.33	0.029	56	2	0.03	2.2	1.27	0.29
3 oz (15 1/2 large)	85	0.9	0.2	0.2	0.4	166	155	116	2.63	0.164	33.7	186	0.4	0.03	0.11	3.4	15151
cnd	102	61.7	19.6	0.9		0.0	144	50	35	1.07	0.051	15	2	0.02	2.3	0.95	0.19
3 oz	85	1.7	0.3	0.2	0.6	147	179	198	2.33	0.255	33.7	51	0.8	0.03	0.09	1.7	15152
raw	90	64.5	17.3	0.8		0.0	126	44	31	0.94	0.043	46	2	0.02	2.2	0.99	0.23
3 oz	85	1.5	0.3	0.2	0.6	129	157	174	2.05	0.224	32.3	153	0.7	0.03	0.09	2.6	15149
shrimp, imitation, made from surimi - *3 oz*	86	63.7	10.5	7.8		0.0	599	16	37	0.28	0.009	17	0	0.02	0.1	1.36	0.06
	85	1.2	0.2	0.2	0.6	31	76	240	0.51	0.027	19.5	56		0.03	0.03	1.7	15153
spiny lobster, ckd by dry heat - *3 oz*	122	56.7	22.4	2.7		0.0	193	54	43	6.18	0.015	5	2	0.01	4.2	3.43	0.34
	85	1.6	0.3	0.3	0.6	77	177	195	1.20	0.353	50.3	17		0.05	0.15	0.9	15228
raw	95	63.0	17.5	2.1		0.0	150	42	34	4.82	0.013	4	2	0.01	3.6	2.98	0.30
3 oz	85	1.3	0.2	0.2	0.5	60	153	202	1.04	0.324	39.3	14	1.2	0.04	0.13	0.9	15154

[1] Prepared with crab meat, egg, onion, and margarine.

[2] Breading consists of bread crumbs, egg, milk, and salt.

12.2 FINFISH

	KCAL	H₂O (g)	PRO (g)	CHO (g)	SUGR (g)	DFIB (g)	Na (mg)	Ca (mg)	Mg (mg)	Zn (mg)	Mn (mg)	A (mcg RAE)	C (mg)	B-1 (mg)	NIA (mg)	B-12 (mcg)	PANT (mg)
	WT (g)	FAT (g)	SFA (g)	MUFA (g)	PUFA (g)	CHOL (mg)	K (mg)	P (mg)	Fe (mg)	Cu (mg)	Se (mcg)	A (IU)	E (mg ATE)	B-2 (mg)	B-6 (mg)	FOL (mcg DFE)	REF
anchovies, cnd in olive oil	42	10.1	5.8	0.0		0.0	734	46	14	0.49	0.020	4	0	0.02	4.0	0.18	0.18
5 anchovies	20	1.9	0.4	0.8	0.5	17	109	50	0.93	0.068	13.6	14	1.0	0.07	0.04	2.6	15002
raw	111	62.4	17.3	0.0		0.0	88	125	35	1.46	0.060	13	0	0.05	11.9	0.53	0.55
3 oz	85	4.1	1.1	1.0	1.4	51	326	148	2.76	0.179	31.0	43	0.5	0.22	0.12	7.7	15001
bass, freshwater, ckd by dry heat - *3 oz*	124	58.5	20.6	0.0		0.0	77	88	32	0.71	0.969	30	2	0.07	1.3	1.96	0.74
	85	4.0	0.9	1.6	1.2	74	388	218	1.62	0.101	13.8	98		0.08	0.12	14.5	15187
raw	97	64.3	16.0	0.0		0.0	60	68	26	0.55	0.756	26	2	0.06	1.1	1.70	0.64
3 oz	85	3.1	0.7	1.2	0.9	58	303	170	1.27	0.079	10.7	85		0.06	0.10	12.8	15003
bass, striped, ckd by dry heat - *3 oz*	105	62.4	19.3	0.0		0.0	75	16	43	0.43	0.016	26	0	0.10	2.2	3.75	0.74
	85	2.5	0.6	0.7	0.9	88	279	216	0.92	0.034	39.8	88		0.03	0.29	8.5	15188
raw	82	67.3	15.1	0.0		0.0	59	13	34	0.34	0.013	23	0	0.09	1.8	3.25	0.64
3 oz	85	2.0	0.4	0.6	0.7	68	218	168	0.71	0.026	31.0	77	0.4	0.03	0.26	7.7	15004
bluefish, ckd by dry heat	135	53.2	21.8	0.0		0.0	65	8	36	0.88	0.023	117	0	0.06	6.2	5.29	0.81
3 oz	85	4.6	1.0	2.0	1.2	65	405	247	0.53	0.058	39.8	390		0.08	0.39	1.7	15189
raw	105	60.2	17.0	0.0		0.0	51	6	28	0.69	0.018	102	0	0.05	5.1	4.58	0.70
3 oz	85	3.6	0.8	1.5	0.9	50	316	193	0.41	0.045	31.0	338	0.4	0.07	0.34	1.7	15005
burbot, ckd by dry heat	98	62.4	21.0	0.0		0.0	105	54	35	0.82	0.762	4	0	0.36	1.7	0.78	0.13
3 oz	85	0.9	0.2	0.1	0.3	65	440	218	0.98	0.218	13.8	14	–	0.15	0.29	0.9	15190
raw	77	67.4	16.4	0.0		0.0	82	43	27	0.65	0.595	4	0	0.32	1.4	0.68	0.13
3 oz	85	0.7	0.1	0.1	0.3	51	343	170	0.77	0.170	10.7	13		0.12	0.26	0.9	15006
butterfish, ckd by dry heat - *3 oz*	159	56.8	18.8	0.0		0.0	97	24	27	0.84	0.016	28	0	0.12	4.9	1.56	0.74
	85	8.7				71	409	262	0.54	0.059	39.8	93		0.16	0.29	14.5	15191
raw	124	63.0	14.7	0.0		0.0	76	19	21	0.65	0.013	26	0	0.10	3.8	1.62	0.64
3 oz	85	6.8	2.9	2.9	0.5	55	319	204	0.43	0.046	31.0	85		0.13	0.26	12.8	15007
carp, ckd by dry heat	138	59.2	19.4	0.0		0.0	54	44	32	1.62	0.043	9	1	0.12	1.8	1.25	0.74
3 oz	85	6.1	1.2	2.5	1.6	71	363	451	1.35	0.062	13.8	27		0.06	0.19	14.5	15009
raw	108	64.9	15.2	0.0		0.0	42	35	25	1.26	0.036	8	1	0.10	1.4	1.30	0.64
3 oz	85	4.8	0.9	2.0	1.2	56	283	353	1.05	0.048	10.7	25	0.5	0.05	0.16	12.8	15008
catfish, channel, breaded[1] & fried - *3 oz*	195	50.0	15.4	6.8		0.6	238	37	23	0.73	0.034	7	0	0.06	1.9	1.62	0.62
	85	11.3	2.8	4.8	2.8	69	289	184	1.22	0.086	11.8	24		0.11	0.16	33.2	15011
catfish, channel, farmed, ckd by dry heat - *3 oz*	129	60.8	15.9	0.0		0.0	68	8	22	0.89	0.017	13	1	0.36	2.1	2.38	0.52
	85	6.8	1.5	3.5	1.2	54	273	208	0.70	0.104	12.3	43		0.06	0.14	6.0	15235
raw	115	64.1	13.2	0.0		0.0	45	8	20	0.63	0.015	13	1	0.31	2.0	2.10	0.51
3 oz	85	6.5	1.5	3.0	1.3	40	254	172	0.43	0.086	10.7	43	1.0	0.06	0.16	8.5	15234
catfish, channel, wild, ckd by dry heat - *3 oz*	89	66.0	15.7	0.0		0.0	43	9	24	0.52	0.023	13	1	0.19	2.0	2.47	0.77
	85	2.4	0.6	0.9	0.5	61	356	258	0.30	0.033	12.2	43		0.06	0.09	8.5	15233
raw	81	68.3	13.9	0.0		0.0	37	12	20	0.43	0.021	13	1	0.18	1.6	1.90	0.65
3 oz	85	2.4	0.6	0.7	0.7	49	304	178	0.26	0.029	10.7	43	0.5	0.06	0.10	8.5	15010
cisco, raw	83	67.1	16.1	0.0		0.0	47	10	14	0.31	0.057	26	0	0.07	2.1	0.85	
3 oz	85	1.6	0.4	0.4	0.5	43	301	129	0.34	0.061	10.7	85	0.1	0.09	0.26	12.8	15013
smoked	150	59.3	13.9	0.0		0.0	409	22	14	0.26	0.018	241	0	0.04	2.0	3.62	0.26
3 oz	85	10.1	1.5	4.7	1.9	27	249	128	0.42	0.183	15.4	802	0.2	0.14	0.23	1.7	15014
cod, atlantic, ckd by dry heat - *3 oz*	89	64.5	19.4	0.0		0.0	66	12	36	0.49	0.017	12	1	0.07	2.1	0.89	0.15
	85	0.7	0.1	0.1	0.2	47	207	117	0.42	0.031	32.0	39	0.3	0.07	0.24	6.8	15016

	KCAL	H₂0 (g)	PRO (g)	CHO (g)	SUGR (g)	DFIB (g)	Na (mg)	Ca (mg)	Mg (mg)	Zn (mg)	Mn (mg)	A (mcg RAE)	C (mg)	B-1 (mg)	NIA (mg)	B-12 (mcg)	PANT (mg)
	WT (g)	FAT (g)	SFA (g)	MUFA (g)	PUFA (g)	CHOL (mg)	K (mg)	P (mg)	Fe (mg)	Cu (mg)	Se (mcg)	A (IU)	E (mg ATE)	B-2 (mg)	B-6 (mg)	FOL (mcg DFE)	REF
cnd	89	64.3	19.3	0.0		0.0	185	18	35	0.49	0.017	12	1	0.07	2.1	0.89	0.14
3 oz	85	0.7	0.1	0.1	0.2	47	449	221	0.42	0.031	32.4	39	0.2	0.07	0.24	6.8	15017
dried & salted	247	13.7	53.4	0.0		0.0	5973	136	113	1.35	0.043	36	3	0.23	6.4	8.50	1.42
3 oz	85	2.0	0.4	0.3	0.7	129	1239	808	2.13	0.150	125.6	120	0.5	0.20	0.73	21.3	15018
raw	70	69.0	15.1	0.0		0.0	46	14	27	0.38	0.013	10	1	0.06	1.8	0.77	0.13
3 oz	85	0.6	0.1	0.1	0.2	37	351	173	0.32	0.024	28.1	34	0.2	0.06	0.21	6.0	15015
cod, pacific, ckd by dry	89	64.6	19.5	0.0		0.0	77	8	26	0.43	0.013	9	3	0.02	2.1	0.88	0.14
heat - *3 oz*	85	0.7	0.1	0.1	0.3	40	439	190	0.28	0.028	39.8	27		0.04	0.39	6.8	15192
raw	70	69.1	15.2	0.0		0.0	60	6	20	0.34	0.010	7	2	0.02	1.7	0.77	0.12
3 oz	85	0.5	0.1	0.1	0.2	31	343	148	0.22	0.022	31.0	24	0.2	0.04	0.34	6.0	15019
croaker, atlantic, breaded[2]	188	50.8	15.5	6.4		0.3	296	27	36	0.44	0.068	20	0	0.08	3.7	1.79	0.63
& fried - *3 oz*	85	10.8	3.0	4.5	2.5	71	289	184	0.73	0.055	33.0	64		0.11	0.22	38.3	15021
raw	88	66.3	15.1	0.0		0.0	48	13	34	0.36	0.021	15	0	0.06	3.6	2.13	0.64
3 oz	85	2.7	0.9	1.0	0.4	52	293	179	0.31	0.036	31.0	51	0.9	0.08	0.26	12.8	15020
cusk, ckd by dry heat	95	59.2	20.7	0.0		0.0	34	11	34	0.42	0.016	18	0	0.04	2.8	1.02	0.27
3 oz	85	0.7				45	428	223	0.90	0.020	39.8	59		0.14	0.38	1.7	15193
raw	74	64.9	16.1	0.0		0.0	26	9	26	0.32	0.013	15	0	0.04	2.3	0.88	0.24
3 oz	85	0.6	0.1	0.1	0.2	35	333	173	0.71	0.015	31.0	51		0.11	0.33	1.7	15022
dolphinfish, ckd by dry	93	60.5	20.2	0.0		0.0	96	16	32	0.50	0.016	53	0	0.02	6.3		0.74
heat - *3 oz*	85	0.8	0.2	0.1	0.2	80	453	156	1.23	0.045	39.8	177		0.07	0.39	5.1	15194
raw	72	65.9	15.7	0.0		0.0	75	13	26	0.39	0.013	46	0	0.02	5.2	0.51	0.64
3 oz	85	0.6	0.2	0.1	0.1	62	354	122	0.96	0.035	31.0	153	0.3	0.06	0.34	4.3	15023
drum, freshwater, ckd by	130	60.3	19.1	0.0		0.0	82	65	32	0.72	0.762	50	1	0.07	2.4	1.96	0.74
dry heat - *3 oz*	85	5.4	1.2	2.4	1.3	70	300	196	0.98	0.252	13.8	167		0.18	0.29	14.5	15195
raw	101	65.7	14.9	0.0		0.0	64	51	26	0.56	0.595	43	1	0.06	2.0	1.70	0.64
3 oz	85	4.2	1.0	1.9	1.0	54	234	153	0.77	0.197	10.7	145		0.14	0.26	12.8	15024
eel, ckd by dry heat	201	50.4	20.1	0.0		0.0	55	22	22	1.77	0.034	966	2	0.16	3.8	2.46	0.24
3 oz	85	12.7	2.6	7.8	1.0	137	297	235	0.54	0.025	7.1	3219	4.3	0.04	0.07	14.5	15026
raw	156	58.0	15.7	0.0		0.0	43	17	17	1.38	0.030	887	2	0.13	3.0	2.55	0.20
3 oz	85	9.9	2.0	6.1	0.8	107	231	184	0.43	0.020	5.5	2954	3.4	0.03	0.06	12.8	15025
fish pieces, frzn, reheated	155	26.4	8.9	13.5		0.0	332	11	14	0.38	0.135	18	0	0.07	1.2	1.03	0.19
1 piece (4″ × 2″ × 1/2″)	57	7.0	1.8	2.9	1.8	64	149	103	0.42	0.058	9.5	60	0.8	0.10	0.03	37.1	15027a
fish sticks, frzn, reheated	76	13.0	4.4	6.7		0.0	163	6	7	0.18	0.066	9	0	0.04	0.6	0.50	0.09
1 stick (4″ × 1″ × 1/2″)	28	3.4	0.9	1.4	0.9	31	73	51	0.21	0.028	4.6	30	0.4	0.05	0.02	18.2	15027b
flounder/sole (flatfish), ckd	99	62.2	20.5	0.0		0.0	89	15	49	0.54	0.017	9	0	0.07	1.9	2.13	0.49
by dry heat - *3 oz*	85	1.3	0.3	0.2	0.5	58	292	246	0.29	0.022	49.5	32	1.6	0.10	0.20	7.7	15029
raw	77	67.2	16.0	0.0		0.0	69	15	26	0.38	0.014	9	1	0.08	2.5	1.29	0.43
3 oz	85	1.0	0.2	0.2	0.3	41	307	156	0.31	0.027	27.8	28	1.6	0.06	0.18	6.8	15028
gefiltefish w/broth, sweet	35	33.7	3.8	3.1		0.0	220	10	4	0.34	0.031	11	<1	0.03	0.4	0.35	0.08
1 piece	42	0.7	0.2	0.3	0.1	13	38	31	1.04	0.082	4.4	37		0.02	0.03	1.3	15030
grouper, ckd by dry heat	100	62.4	21.1	0.0		0.0	45	18	31	0.43	0.010	43	0	0.07	0.3	0.59	0.74
3 oz	85	1.1	0.3	0.2	0.3	40	404	122	0.97	0.038	39.8	140		0.01	0.30	8.5	15032
raw	78	67.3	16.5	0.0		0.0	45	23	26	0.41	0.012	37	0	0.06	0.3	0.51	0.64
3 oz	85	0.9	0.2	0.2	0.3	31	411	138	0.76	0.017	31.0	122	0.4	<0.01	0.26	7.7	15031
haddock, ckd by dry heat	95	63.1	20.6	0.0		0.0	74	36	43	0.41	0.026	16	0	0.03	3.9	1.18	0.13
3 oz	85	0.8	0.1	0.1	0.3	63	339	205	1.15	0.028	34.4	54		0.04	0.29	11.1	15034
raw	74	67.9	16.1	0.0		0.0	58	28	33	0.31	0.021	14	0	0.03	3.2	1.02	0.11
3 oz	85	0.6	0.1	0.1	0.2	48	264	160	0.89	0.022	25.7	47	0.3	0.03	0.26	10.2	15033
smoked	99	60.8	21.4	0.0		0.0	649	42	46	0.43	0.026	19	0	0.04	4.3	1.36	0.14
3 oz	85	0.8	0.1	0.1	0.3	65	353	213	1.19	0.036	36.5	62	0.3	0.04	0.34	12.8	15035
halibut, atlantic & pacific,	119	60.9	22.7	0.0		0.0	59	51	91	0.45	0.017	46	0	0.06	6.1	1.16	0.32
ckd by dry heat - *3 oz*	85	2.5	0.4	0.8	0.8	35	490	242	0.91	0.030	39.8	152	0.9	0.08	0.34	11.9	15037
raw	94	66.2	17.7	0.0		0.0	46	40	71	0.36	0.013	40	0	0.05	5.0	1.00	0.28
3 oz	85	1.9	0.3	0.6	0.6	27	383	189	0.71	0.023	31.0	132	0.7	0.06	0.29	10.2	15036
halibut, greenland, ckd by	203	52.6	15.7	0.0		0.0	88	3	28	0.43	0.013	15	0	0.06	1.6	0.82	0.24
dry heat - *3 oz*	85	15.1	2.6	9.1	1.5	50	292	179	0.72	0.032	39.8	51		0.09	0.41	0.9	15196
raw	158	59.7	12.2	0.0		0.0	68	3	22	0.34	0.010	14	0	0.05	1.3	0.85	0.21
3 oz	85	11.8	2.1	7.1	1.2	39	228	139	0.56	0.026	31.0	47	0.7	0.07	0.36	0.9	15038
herring, atlantic, ckd by dry	173	54.5	19.6	0.0		0.0	98	63	35	1.08	0.034	26	1	0.10	3.5	11.17	0.63
heat - *3 oz*	85	9.9	2.2	4.1	2.3	65	356	258	1.20	0.100	39.8	87	1.1	0.25	0.30	10.2	15040
kippered	87	23.9	9.8	0.0		0.0	367	34	18	0.54	0.020	15	<1	0.05	1.8	7.48	0.35
1 piece (5″ × 1 3/4″ × 1/4″)	40	4.9	1.1	2.0	1.2	33	179	130	0.60	0.054	21.0	51	0.4	0.13	0.17	5.6	15042

	KCAL	H₂0 (g)	PRO (g)	CHO (g)	SUGR (g)	DFIB (g)	Na (mg)	Ca (mg)	Mg (mg)	Zn (mg)	Mn (mg)	A (mcg RAE)	C (mg)	B-1 (mg)	NIA (mg)	B-12 (mcg)	PANT (mg)
	WT (g)	FAT (g)	SFA (g)	MUFA (g)	PUFA (g)	CHOL (mg)	K (mg)	P (mg)	Fe (mg)	Cu (mg)	Se (mcg)	A (IU)	E (mg ATE)	B-2 (mg)	B-6 (mg)	FOL (mcg DFE)	REF
pickled	39	8.3	2.1	1.4		0.0	131	12	1	0.08	0.006	39	0	0.01	0.5	0.64	0.01
1 piece (1 3/4" × 7/8" × 1/2")	15	2.7	0.4	1.8	0.3	2	10	13	0.18	0.016	8.8	129	0.2	0.02	0.03	0.3	15041
raw	134	61.2	15.3	0.0		0.0	77	48	27	0.84	0.030	24	1	0.08	2.7	11.62	0.55
3 oz	85	7.7	1.7	3.2	1.8	51	278	201	0.94	0.078	31.0	80	0.9	0.20	0.26	8.5	15039
herring, pacific, ckd by	213	54.0	17.9	0.0		0.0	81	90	35	0.58	0.049	30	0	0.06	2.4	8.18	0.98
dry heat - *3 oz*	85	15.1	3.5	7.5	2.6	84	461	248	1.22	0.085	39.8	99		0.22	0.44	5.1	15197
raw	166	60.8	13.9	0.0		0.0	63	71	27	0.45	0.038	27	0	0.05	1.9	8.50	0.85
3 oz	85	11.8	2.8	5.8	2.1	65	360	194	0.95	0.066	31.0	90		0.17	0.38	4.3	15043
ling, ckd by dry heat	94	62.8	20.7	0.0		0.0	147	37	69	0.85	0.032	30	0	0.11	2.4	0.55	0.31
3 oz	85	0.7				43	413	216	0.71	0.120	39.8	98		0.20	0.30	6.8	15198
raw	74	67.7	16.1	0.0		0.0	115	29	54	0.66	0.026	26	0	0.09	2.0	0.48	0.27
3 oz	85	0.5	0.1	0.1	0.2	34	322	168	0.55	0.094	31.0	85		0.16	0.26	6.0	15044
lingcod, ckd by dry heat	93	64.3	19.2	0.0		0.0	65	15	28	0.49	0.022	14	0	0.03	2.0	3.53	0.74
3 oz	85	1.2	0.2	0.4	0.3	57	476	219	0.35	0.030	39.8	49		0.12	0.29	8.5	15199
raw	72	68.9	15.0	0.0		0.0	50	12	22	0.38	0.017	13	0	0.03	1.6	3.06	0.64
3 oz	85	0.9	0.2	0.3	0.3	44	371	171	0.27	0.023	31.0	43	0.2	0.10	0.26	7.7	15045
mackerel, atlantic, ckd by	223	45.3	20.3	-0.0		0.0	71	13	82	0.80	0.017	46	<1	0.14	5.8	16.15	0.84
dry heat - *3 oz*	85	15.1	3.5	6.0	3.7	64	341	236	1.33	0.080	43.9	153		0.35	0.39	1.7	15047
raw	174	54.0	15.8	0.0		0.0	77	10	65	0.54	0.013	43	<1	0.15	7.7	7.40	0.73
3 oz	85	11.8	2.8	4.6	2.8	60	267	184	1.39	0.062	37.5	140	1.3	0.27	0.34	0.9	15046
mackerel, jack, cnd	296	131.4	44.1	0.0		0.0	720	458	70	1.94	0.076	247	2	0.08	11.7	13.19	0.58
1 cup	190	12.0	3.5	4.2	3.1	150	369	572	3.88	0.279	71.6	825	2.7	0.40	0.40	9.5	15048
mackerel, king, ckd by	114	58.7	22.1	0.0		0.0	173	34	35	0.61	0.005	214	1	0.10	8.9	15.30	0.82
dry heat - *3 oz*	85	2.2	0.4	0.8	0.5	58	474	270	1.94	0.028	39.8	713		0.49	0.43	7.7	15200
raw	89	64.5	17.2	0.0		0.0	134	26	27	0.48	0.004	185	1	0.09	7.3	13.26	0.71
3 oz	85	1.7	0.3	0.6	0.4	45	370	211	1.51	0.022	31.0	618		0.40	0.38	6.8	15049
mackerel, pacific & jack,	171	52.5	21.9	0.0		0.0	94	25	31	0.73	0.016	12	2	0.11	9.1	3.60	0.31
ckd by dry heat - *3 oz*	85	8.6	2.4	2.9	2.1	51	443	136	1.27	0.101	39.8	40	1.1	0.46	0.32	1.7	15201
raw	134	59.6	17.1	0.0		0.0	73	20	24	0.57	0.013	11	2	0.09	7.1	3.74	0.27
3 oz	85	6.7	1.9	2.2	1.6	40	345	106	0.99	0.079	31.0	37	0.9	0.36	0.28	1.7	15050
mackerel, spanish, ckd by	134	58.2	20.1	0.0		0.0	56	11	32	0.53	0.010	28	1	0.11	4.3	5.95	0.74
dry heat - *3 oz*	85	5.4	1.5	1.8	1.5	62	471	230	0.63	0.055	34.5	93		0.18	0.39	0.9	15052
raw	118	60.9	16.4	0.0		0.0	50	9	28	0.42	0.012	26	1	0.11	2.0	2.04	0.64
3 oz	85	5.4	1.6	1.3	1.5	65	379	174	0.37	0.047	31.0	85	0.6	0.14	0.34	0.9	15051
milkfish, ckd by dry heat	162	53.2	22.4	0.0		0.0	78	55	32	0.89	0.022	28	0	0.01	7.0	2.78	0.74
3 oz	85	7.3				57	318	177	0.35	0.037	13.8	93		0.06	0.41	15.3	15202
raw	126	60.2	17.5	0.0		0.0	61	43	26	0.70	0.017	26	0	0.01	5.5	2.89	0.64
3 oz	85	5.7	1.4	2.2	1.6	44	248	138	0.27	0.029	10.7	85		0.05	0.36	13.6	15053
monkfish, ckd by dry heat	82	66.7	15.8	0.0		0.0	20	9	23	0.45	0.026	12	1	0.02	2.2	0.88	0.15
3 oz	85	1.7				27	436	218	0.35	0.031	39.8	39		0.06	0.24	6.8	15203
raw	65	70.8	12.3	0.0		0.0	15	7	18	0.35	0.020	10	1	0.02	1.8	0.77	0.13
3 oz	85	1.3	0.3	0.2	0.5	21	340	170	0.27	0.024	31.0	34		0.05	0.20	6.0	15054
mullet, striped, ckd by dry	128	59.9	21.1	0.0		0.0	60	26	28	0.75	0.019	36	1	0.09	5.4	0.21	0.75
heat - *3 oz*	85	4.1	1.2	1.2	0.8	54	389	207	1.20	0.120	39.8	120		0.09	0.42	8.5	15056
raw	99	65.5	16.4	0.0		0.0	55	35	25	0.44	0.014	31	1	0.08	4.4	0.19	0.65
3 oz	85	3.2	0.9	0.9	0.6	42	303	188	0.87	0.043	31.0	104	0.9	0.07	0.36	7.7	15055
ocean perch, atlantic, ckd	103	61.8	20.3	0.0		0.0	82	116	33	0.52	0.017	12	1	0.11	2.1	0.98	0.36
by dry heat - *3 oz*	85	1.8	0.3	0.7	0.5	46	298	235	1.00	0.028	47.2	39		0.11	0.23	8.5	15058
raw	80	66.9	15.8	0.0		0.0	64	91	26	0.41	0.013	10	1	0.09	1.7	0.85	0.31
3 oz	85	1.4	0.2	0.5	0.4	36	232	184	0.78	0.022	36.8	34	1.1	0.09	0.20	7.7	15057
orange roughy, ckd by dry	76	58.7	16.0	0.0		0.0	69	32	32	0.82	0.016	20	0	0.10	3.1	1.96	0.54
heat - *3 oz*	85	0.8	<0.1	0.5	<0.1	22	327	218	0.20	0.152	39.8	69		0.16	0.29	6.8	15232
raw	59	64.5	12.5	0.0		0.0	54	26	26	0.64	0.013	18	0	0.09	2.6	1.70	0.47
3 oz	85	0.6	<0.1	0.4	<0.1	17	255	170	0.15	0.119	31.0	60		0.13	0.26	6.0	15073
perch, ckd by dry heat	99	62.3	21.1	0.0		0.0	67	87	32	1.22	0.765	9	1	0.07	1.6	1.87	0.74
3 oz	85	1.0	0.2	0.2	0.4	98	292	218	0.99	0.163	13.7	27		0.10	0.12	5.1	15061
raw	77	67.3	16.5	0.0		0.0	53	68	26	0.94	0.595	7	1	0.06	1.3	1.62	0.64
3 oz	85	0.8	0.2	0.1	0.3	77	229	170	0.77	0.128	10.7	24	0.2	0.09	0.10	4.3	15060
pike, northern, ckd by	96	62.0	21.0	0.0		0.0	42	62	34	0.73	0.264	20	3	0.06	2.4	1.96	0.74
dry heat - *3 oz*	85	0.7	0.1	0.1	0.2	43	281	240	0.60	0.055	13.8	69		0.07	0.11	14.5	15063
raw	75	67.1	16.4	0.0		0.0	33	48	26	0.57	0.204	18	3	0.05	2.0	1.70	0.64
3 oz	85	0.6	0.1	0.1	0.2	33	220	187	0.47	0.043	10.7	60	0.2	0.05	0.10	12.8	15062

	KCAL	H₂O (g)	PRO (g)	CHO (g)	SUGR (g)	DFIB (g)	Na (mg)	Ca (mg)	Mg (mg)	Zn (mg)	Mn (mg)	A (mcg RAE)	C (mg)	B-1 (mg)	NIA (mg)	B-12 (mcg)	PANT (mg)
	WT (g)	FAT (g)	SFA (g)	MUFA (g)	PUFA (g)	CHOL (mg)	K (mg)	P (mg)	Fe (mg)	Cu (mg)	Se (mcg)	A (IU)	E (mg ATE)	B-2 (mg)	B-6 (mg)	FOL (mcg DFE)	REF
pike, walleye, ckd by	101	62.4	20.9	0.0		0.0	55	120	32	0.67	0.872	20	0	0.27	2.4	1.96	0.74
dry heat - 3 oz	85	1.3	0.3	0.3	0.5	94	424	229	1.42	0.194	13.8	69		0.17	0.12	14.5	15204
raw	79	67.4	16.3	0.0		0.0	43	94	26	0.53	0.680	18	0	0.23	2.0	1.70	0.64
3 oz	85	1.0	0.2	0.2	0.4	73	331	179	1.11	0.151	10.7	60	0.2	0.14	0.10	12.8	15064
pollock, atlantic, ckd	100	61.2	21.2	0.0		0.0	94	65	73	0.51	0.016	10	0	0.05	3.4	3.13	0.35
by dry heat - 3 oz	85	1.1	0.1	0.1	0.5	77	388	241	0.50	0.054	39.8	34		0.19	0.28	2.6	15205
raw	78	66.5	16.5	0.0		0.0	73	51	57	0.40	0.013	9	0	0.04	2.8	2.71	0.30
3 oz	85	0.8	0.1	0.1	0.4	60	303	188	0.39	0.043	31.0	30	0.2	0.16	0.24	2.6	15065
pollock, walleye, ckd by	96	63.0	20.0	0.0		0.0	99	5	62	0.51	0.017	20	0	0.06	1.4	3.57	0.14
dry heat -3 oz	85	1.0	0.2	0.1	0.4	82	329	410	0.24	0.047	36.9	65	0.2	0.06	0.06	3.4	15067
raw	69	69.3	14.6	0.0		0.0	84	4	48	0.37	0.013	17	0	0.06	1.1	2.64	0.12
3 oz	85	0.7	0.1	0.1	0.4	60	277	320	0.20	0.037	18.6	56	0.2	0.05	0.05	2.6	15066
pomano, florida, ckd by	179	53.5	20.1	0.0		0.0	65	37	26	0.59	0.021	31	0	0.58	3.2	1.02	0.74
dry heat - 3 oz	85	10.3	3.8	2.8	1.2	54	541	290	0.57	0.066	39.8	102		0.13	0.20	14.5	15069
raw	139	60.5	15.7	0.0		0.0	55	19	23	0.61	0.011	28	0	0.48	2.6	1.11	0.64
3 oz	85	8.0	3.0	2.2	1.0	43	324	166	0.51	0.032	31.0	94	0.2	0.10	0.17	12.8	15068
pout, ocean, ckd by dry	87	64.7	18.1	0.0		0.0	66	11	14	1.12	0.016	12	0	0.08	2.2	0.88	0.15
heat - 3 oz	85	1.0	0.3	0.4	<0.1	57	436	218	0.31	0.035	39.8	39		0.07	0.24	6.8	15206
raw	67	69.2	14.1	0.0		0.0	52	9	11	0.88	0.013	10	0	0.07	1.8	0.77	0.13
3 oz	85	0.8	0.3	0.3	<0.1	44	340	170	0.24	0.027	31.0	34		0.05	0.20	6.0	15059
rockfish, pacific, ckd by	103	62.4	20.4	0.0		0.0	65	10	29	0.45	0.017	56	0	0.04	3.3	1.02	0.74
dry heat - 3 oz	85	1.7	0.4	0.4	0.5	37	442	194	0.45	0.031	39.8	186	1.1	0.07	0.23	8.5	15071
raw	80	67.4	15.9	0.0		0.0	51	8	22	0.35	0.014	48	0	0.03	2.7	0.85	0.64
3 oz	85	1.3	0.3	0.3	0.4	30	344	151	0.35	0.025	31.0	162	1.1	0.06	0.20	7.7	15070
sablefish, ckd by dry heat	213	53.4	14.6	0.0		0.0	61	38	60	0.35	0.016	87	0	0.10	4.4	1.22	0.74
3 oz	85	16.7	3.5	8.8	2.2	54	390	183	1.39	0.024	39.8	287		0.10	0.29	14.5	15208
raw	166	60.4	11.4	0.0		0.0	48	30	47	0.27	0.013	79	0	0.09	3.4	1.28	0.64
3 oz	85	13.0	2.7	6.8	1.7	42	304	143	1.09	0.019	31.0	264	0.4	0.08	0.26	12.8	15074
smoked	218	51.1	15.0	0.0		0.0	626	43	63	0.37	0.017	105	0	0.11	4.5	1.70	0.84
3 oz	85	17.1	3.6	9.0	2.3	54	400	189	1.44	0.031	42.7	347		0.10	0.33	17.0	15075
salmon, atlantic, farmed,	175	55.0	18.8	0.0		0.0	52	13	26	0.37	0.014	13	3	0.29	6.8	2.38	1.25
ckd by dry heat - 3 oz	85	10.5	2.1	3.8	3.8	54	326	214	0.29	0.042	35.2	43		0.11	0.55	28.9	15237
raw	156	58.6	16.9	0.0		0.0	50	10	24	0.34	0.013	13	3	0.29	6.4	2.38	1.17
3 oz	85	9.2	1.9	3.3	3.3	50	308	198	0.31	0.042	31.0	43		0.10	0.54	22.1	15236
salmon, atlantic, wild, ckd	155	50.7	21.6	0.0		0.0	48	13	31	0.70	0.018	11	0	0.23	8.6	2.59	1.63
by dry heat - 3 oz	85	6.9	1.1	2.3	2.8	60	534	218	0.88	0.273	39.8	37		0.41	0.80	24.7	15209
raw	121	58.2	16.9	0.0		0.0	37	10	25	0.54	0.014	10	0	0.19	6.7	2.70	1.41
3 oz	85	5.4	0.8	1.8	2.2	47	417	170	0.68	0.213	31.0	34		0.32	0.70	21.3	15076
salmon, chinook, ckd by dry	196	55.8	21.9	0.0		0.0	51	24	104	0.48	0.016	127	3	0.04	8.5	2.44	0.74
heat - 3 oz	85	11.4	2.7	4.9	2.3	72	429	315	0.77	0.045	39.8	422		0.13	0.39	29.8	15210
raw	153	62.2	17.1	0.0		0.0	40	19	81	0.37	0.013	116	3	0.03	6.7	2.54	0.64
3 oz	85	8.9	2.1	3.8	1.8	56	335	246	0.60	0.035	31.0	387	1.0	0.10	0.34	25.5	15078
smoked (lox)	99	61.2	15.5	0.0		0.0	666	9	15	0.26	0.014	22	0	0.02	4.0	2.77	0.74
3 oz	85	3.7	0.8	1.7	0.8	20	149	139	0.72	0.196	27.5	75	1.1	0.09	0.24	1.7	15077
salmon, chum, ckd by dry heat	131	58.2	21.9	0.0		0.0	54	12	24	0.51	0.018	29	0	0.08	7.2	2.94	0.74
3 oz	85	4.1	0.9	1.7	1.0	81	468	309	0.60	0.060	39.8	97		0.19	0.39	4.3	15211
cnd w/bone	120	60.2	18.2	0.0		0.0	414	212	26	0.85	0.017	15	0	0.02	6.0	3.74	0.48
3 oz	85	4.7	1.3	1.6	1.3	33	255	301	0.60	0.085	36.8	52	1.4	0.14	0.32	17.0	15080
raw	102	64.1	17.1	0.0		0.0	43	9	19	0.40	0.013	26	0	0.07	6.0	2.55	0.64
3 oz	85	3.2	0.7	1.3	0.8	63	365	241	0.47	0.047	31.0	84	0.9	0.15	0.34	3.4	15079
salmon, coho, farmed, ckd by	151	57.0	20.7	0.0		0.0	44	10	29	0.40	0.018	50	1	0.09	6.3	2.69	1.08
dry heat - 3 oz	85	7.0	1.7	3.1	1.7	54	391	282	0.33	0.076	12.0	167		0.10	0.48	11.9	15239
raw	136	59.9	18.1	0.0		0.0	40	10	26	0.37	0.010	48	1	0.08	5.8	2.27	0.97
3 oz	85	6.5	1.5	2.8	1.6	43	383	248	0.29	0.041	10.7	160		0.09	0.56	11.1	15238
salmon, coho, wild, ckd by	118	60.8	19.9	0.0		0.0	49	38	28	0.48	0.016	33	1	0.06	6.8	4.25	0.69
dry heat - 3 oz	85	3.7	0.9	1.3	1.1	47	369	274	0.52	0.060	32.3	111	0.7	0.12	0.48	11.1	15247
ckd by moist heat	156	55.6	23.3	0.0		0.0	45	39	30	0.44	0.015	27	1	0.10	6.6	3.81	0.71
3 oz	85	6.4	1.4	2.3	2.1	48	387	253	0.60	0.055	39.3	92		0.14	0.47	7.7	15082
raw	124	61.8	18.4	0.0		0.0	39	31	26	0.35	0.012	26	1	0.10	6.1	3.54	0.70
3 oz	85	5.0	1.1	1.8	1.7	38	360	223	0.48	0.043	31.0	85	0.6	0.12	0.47	7.7	15081
salmon, pink, chunk, cnd w/o skin	60	45.0	10.0	0.0			280	6	12	0.24	0.000			0.02	2.9	0.90	0.29
or bone, Chicken of the Sea - 2 oz	57	2.0	0.5	0.4	0.3	20	116	94	0.21	0.000		5	0.0	0.09	0.13	7.0	CHCK1

	KCAL / WT (g)	H₂0 (g) / FAT (g)	PRO (g) / SFA (g)	CHO (g) / MUFA (g)	SUGR (g) / PUFA (g)	DFIB (g) / CHOL (mg)	Minerals Na (mg) / K (mg)	Ca (mg) / P (mg)	Mg (mg) / Fe (mg)	Zn (mg) / Cu (mg)	Mn (mg) / Se (mcg)	Vitamins A (mcg RAE) / A (IU)	C (mg) / E (mg ATE)	B-1 (mg) / B-2 (mg)	NIA (mg) / B-6 (mg)	B-12 (mcg) / FOL (mcg DFE)	PANT (mg) / REF
ckd by dry heat	127	59.2	21.7	0.0		0.0	73	14	28	0.60	0.016	35	0	0.17	7.2	2.94	0.74
3 oz	85	3.8	0.6	1.0	1.5	57	352	251	0.84	0.084	48.6	116		0.06	0.20	4.3	15212
cnd w/bone	118	58.5	16.8	0.0		0.0	471	181	29	0.78	0.017	14	0	0.02	5.6	3.74	0.47
3 oz	85	5.1	1.3	1.5	1.7	47	277	280	0.71	0.087	28.2	47	1.1	0.16	0.26	12.8	15084
raw	99	64.9	16.9	0.0		0.0	57	11	22	0.47	0.013	30	0	0.14	6.0	2.55	0.64
3 oz	85	2.9	0.5	0.8	1.2	44	275	196	0.65	0.065	37.9	100	0.9	0.05	0.17	3.4	15083
salmon, red, chunk, cnd w/o skin or	60	43.0	10.0	0.0		0.0	280	6	10	0.30	0.000			0.02	2.6	1.00	0.34
bone, Chicken of the Sea - 2 oz	57	2.0	0.5	0.4	1.0	20	100	82	0.21	0.000		30	0.2	0.09	0.06	13.0	CHCK2
salmon, sockeye, ckd by dry heat	184	52.6	23.2	0.0		0.0	56	6	26	0.43	0.017	54	0	0.18	5.7	4.93	0.60
3 oz	85	9.3	1.6	4.5	2.0	74	319	235	0.47	0.057	32.1	178		0.15	0.19	4.3	15086
cnd w/bone	130	58.4	17.4	0.0		0.0	457	203	25	0.87	0.026	45	0	0.01	4.7	0.26	0.47
3 oz	85	6.2	1.4	2.7	1.6	37	320	277	0.90	0.071	30.1	150	1.4	0.16	0.26	8.5	15087
raw	143	59.7	18.1	0.0		0.0	40	5	20	0.46	0.012	49	0	0.17	4.9	4.25	0.52
3 oz	85	7.3	1.3	3.5	1.6	53	332	183	0.40	0.044	28.6	163	0.9	0.13	0.16	3.4	15085
sardines, atlantic, cnd in soy oil	50	14.3	5.9	0.0		0.0	121	92	9	0.31	0.026	16	0	0.02	1.3	2.15	0.15
2 sardines	24	2.7	0.4	0.9	1.2	34	95	118	0.70	0.045	12.6	54	0.1	0.05	0.04	2.9	15088
sardines, pacific, cnd in tom sce	68	26.0	6.2	0.0		0.0	157	91	13	0.53	0.078	35	<1	0.02	1.6	3.42	0.28
1 sardine	38	4.6	1.2	2.1	0.9	23	130	139	0.87	0.103	15.4	139	1.4	0.09	0.05	9.1	15089
scup, ckd by dry heat	115	58.2	20.6	0.0		0.0	46	43	25	0.53	0.038	26	0	0.11	4.2	1.38	0.74
3 oz	85	3.0				57	313	201	0.58	0.055	39.8	88		0.10	0.29	14.5	15213
raw	89	64.1	16.0	0.0		0.0	36	34	20	0.41	0.030	23	0	0.09	3.5	1.19	0.64
3 oz	85	2.3	0.5	0.5	0.9	44	244	157	0.45	0.043	31.0	77	0.4	0.09	0.26	12.8	15090
sea bass, ckd by dry heat	105	61.3	20.1	0.0		0.0	74	11	45	0.44	0.017	54	0	0.11	1.6	0.26	0.74
3 oz	85	2.2	0.6	0.5	0.8	45	279	211	0.31	0.020	39.8	181		0.13	0.39	5.1	15092
raw	82	66.5	15.7	0.0		0.0	58	9	35	0.34	0.013	47	0	0.09	1.4	0.26	0.64
3 oz	85	1.7	0.4	0.4	0.6	35	218	165	0.25	0.016	31.0	156	0.4	0.10	0.34	4.3	15091
seatrout, ckd by dry heat	113	61.1	18.2	0.0		0.0	63	19	34	0.49	0.016	30	0	0.06	2.5	2.94	0.74
3 oz	85	3.9	1.1	1.0	0.8	90	371	273	0.30	0.032	39.8	98		0.18	0.39	5.1	15214
raw	88	66.4	14.2	0.0		0.0	49	14	26	0.38	0.013	26	0	0.05	2.0	2.55	0.64
3 oz	85	3.1	0.9	0.8	0.6	71	290	213	0.23	0.026	31.0	85	0.2	0.14	0.34	4.3	15093
shad, american, ckd by dry heat	214	50.3	18.5	0.0		0.0	55	51	32	0.40	0.046	31	0	0.16	9.2	0.12	0.74
3 oz	85	15.0				82	418	297	1.05	0.070	39.8	102		0.26	0.39	14.5	15215
raw	167	58.0	14.4	0.0		0.0	43	40	26	0.31	0.036	28	0	0.13	7.1	0.13	0.64
3 oz	85	11.7	2.7	4.9	2.8	64	326	231	0.82	0.054	31.0	94	0.9	0.20	0.34	12.8	15094
shark, batter-dipped & fried	194	51.1	15.8	5.4		0.0	104	43	37	0.41	0.043	46	0	0.06	2.4	1.03	0.53
3 oz	85	11.7	2.7	5.0	3.1	50	132	165	0.94	0.036	28.9	153		0.08	0.26	18.7	15096
raw	111	62.5	17.8	0.0		0.0	67	29	42	0.37	0.013	60	0	0.04	2.5	1.27	0.59
3 oz	85	3.8	0.8	1.5	1.0	43	136	179	0.71	0.028	31.0	198	0.9	0.05	0.34	2.6	15095
sheepshead, ckd by dry heat	107	58.7	22.1	0.0		0.0	62	31	30	0.54	0.018	30	0	0.01	1.5	1.96	0.74
3 oz	85	1.4	0.3	0.3	0.3	54	435	298	0.57	0.104	43.6	98		0.04	0.30	14.5	15098
raw	92	66.3	17.2	0.0		0.0	60	18	27	0.33	0.011	26	0	0.01	1.3	1.70	0.64
3 oz	85	2.0	0.5	0.6	0.4	43	343	266	0.39	0.026	31.0	85		0.03	0.26	12.8	15097
smelt, rainbow, ckd by dry heat	105	61.9	19.2	0.0		0.0	65	65	32	1.80	0.765	14	0	0.01	1.5	3.37	0.63
3 oz	85	2.6	0.5	0.7	1.0	77	316	251	0.98	0.151	39.8	49		0.12	0.14	4.3	15100
raw	82	67.0	15.0	0.0		0.0	51	51	26	1.40	0.595	13	0	0.01	1.2	2.92	0.54
3 oz	85	2.1	0.4	0.5	0.8	60	247	196	0.77	0.118	31.0	43	0.4	0.10	0.13	3.4	15099
snapper, ckd by dry heat	109	59.8	22.4	0.0		0.0	48	34	31	0.37	0.014	30	1	0.05	0.3	2.98	0.74
3 oz	85	1.5	0.3	0.3	0.5	40	444	171	0.20	0.039	41.7	98		<0.01	0.39	5.1	15102
raw	85	65.3	17.4	0.0		0.0	54	27	27	0.31	0.011	26	1	0.04	0.2	2.55	0.64
3 oz	85	1.1	0.2	0.2	0.4	31	354	168	0.15	0.024	32.5	85	0.4	<0.01	0.34	4.3	15101
spot, ckd by dry heat	134	58.8	20.2	0.0		0.0	31	15	46	0.55	0.038	30	0	0.16	7.2	2.94	0.74
3 oz	85	5.3	1.6	1.5	1.2	65	541	202	0.35	0.050	39.8	98		0.23	0.39	5.1	15216
raw	105	64.6	15.7	0.0		0.0	25	12	36	0.43	0.030	26	0	0.14	6.0	2.55	0.64
3 oz	85	4.2	1.2	1.1	0.9	51	422	158	0.27	0.039	31.0	85	1.3	0.19	0.34	4.3	15103
sturgeon, ckd by dry heat	115	59.4	17.6	0.0		0.0	59	14	38	0.46	0.026	207	0	0.07	8.6	2.13	0.74
3 oz	85	4.4	1.0	2.1	0.8	65	309	230	0.77	0.045	13.8	687	0.6	0.08	0.20	14.5	15105
raw	89	65.1	13.7	0.0		0.0	46	11	30	0.36	0.021	179	0	0.06	7.1	1.87	0.64
3 oz	85	3.4	0.8	1.6	0.6	51	241	179	0.60	0.035	10.7	595	0.4	0.06	0.17	12.8	15104
sturgeon, smoked	147	53.1	26.5	0.0		0.0	628	14	40	0.48	0.026	238	0	0.08	9.4	2.47	0.85
3 oz	85	3.7	0.9	2.0	0.4	68	322	239	0.79	0.043	17.1	793	0.4	0.08	0.23	17.0	15106
sucker, white, ckd by dry heat	101	62.9	18.3	0.0		0.0	43	77	32	0.82	0.654	50	0	0.01	1.2	1.96	0.74
3 oz	85	2.5	0.5	0.8	0.9	45	414	229	1.42	0.213	13.8	167		0.07	0.20	14.5	15217

	KCAL	H2O (g)	PRO (g)	CHO (g)	SUGR (g)	DFIB (g)	Na (mg)	Ca (mg)	Mg (mg)	Zn (mg)	Mn (mg)	A (mcg RAE)	C (mg)	B-1 (mg)	NIA (mg)	B-12 (mcg)	PANT (mg)
	WT (g)	FAT (g)	SFA (g)	MUFA (g)	PUFA (g)	CHOL (mg)	K (mg)	P (mg)	Fe (mg)	Cu (mg)	Se (mcg)	A (IU)	E (mg ATE)	B-2 (mg)	B-6 (mg)	FOL (mcg DFE)	REF
raw	78	67.8	14.2	0.0		0.0	34	60	26	0.64	0.510	43	0	0.01	1.0	1.70	0.64
3 oz	85	2.0	0.4	0.6	0.7	35	323	179	1.11	0.166	10.7	145		0.06	0.17	12.8	15107
sunfish, pumpkinseed, ckd by	97	62.7	21.1	0.0		0.0	88	88	32	1.69	0.762	14	1	0.08	1.2	1.96	0.74
dry heat - 3 oz	85	0.8	0.2	0.1	0.3	73	382	196	1.31	0.327	13.8	49		0.07	0.12	14.5	15218
raw	76	67.6	16.5	0.0		0.0	68	68	26	1.32	0.595	13	1	0.07	1.0	1.70	0.64
3 oz	85	0.6	0.1	0.1	0.2	57	298	153	1.02	0.255	10.7	43		0.06	0.10	12.8	15108
surimi	84	64.9	12.9	5.8		0.0	122	8	37	0.28	0.009	17	0	0.02	0.2	1.36	0.06
3 oz	85	0.8	0.2	0.1	0.4	26	95	240	0.22	0.027	23.9	56		0.02	0.03	1.7	15109
swordfish, ckd by dry heat	132	58.4	21.6	0.0		0.0	98	5	29	1.25	0.017	35	1	0.04	10.0	1.72	0.32
3 oz	85	4.4	1.2	1.7	1.0	43	314	286	0.88	0.138	52.4	116		0.10	0.32	1.7	15111
raw	103	64.3	16.8	0.0		0.0	77	3	23	0.98	0.016	31	1	0.03	8.2	1.49	0.35
3 oz	85	3.4	0.9	1.3	0.8	33	245	224	0.69	0.107	40.9	101	0.4	0.08	0.28	1.7	15110
tilefish, ckd by dry heat	125	59.7	20.8	0.0		0.0	50	22	28	0.45	0.013	18	0	0.12	3.0	2.13	0.74
3 oz	85	4.0	0.7	1.1	1.1	54	435	201	0.26	0.044	43.8	59		0.16	0.26	14.5	15113
raw	82	67.1	14.9	0.0		0.0	45	22	24	0.31	0.009	15	0	0.10	2.5	1.87	0.64
3 oz	85	2.0	0.4	0.5	0.5	43	368	159	0.21	0.035	31.0	51	0.3	0.14	0.22	12.8	15112
trout, mixed species, ckd by dry	162	53.9	22.6	0.0		0.0	57	47	24	0.72	0.927	16	<1	0.36	4.9	6.37	1.90
heat - 3 oz	85	7.2	1.3	3.5	1.6	63	394	267	1.63	0.205	13.8	54		0.36	0.20	12.8	15219
raw	126	60.7	17.7	0.0		0.0	44	37	19	0.56	0.723	14	<1	0.30	3.8	6.62	1.65
3 oz	85	5.6	1.0	2.8	1.3	49	307	208	1.28	0.160	10.7	49	0.2	0.28		11.1	15114
trout, rainbow, farmed, ckd by	144	57.4	20.6	0.0		0.0	36	73	27	0.42	0.017	73	3	0.20	7.5	4.22	1.11
dry heat - 3 oz	85	6.1	1.8	1.8	2.0	58	375	226	0.30	0.052	12.8	244		0.07	0.34	20.4	15241
raw	117	61.8	17.7	0.0		0.0	30	57	27	0.35	0.015	71	2	0.17	7.0	3.20	1.22
3 oz	85	4.6	1.3	1.3	1.5	50	383	240	0.23	0.039	10.7	236	<0.1	0.06	0.53	9.4	15240
trout, rainbow, wild, ckd by dry	128	59.9	19.5	0.0		0.0	48	73	26	0.43	0.018	13	2	0.13	4.9	5.36	0.91
heat - 3 oz	85	4.9	1.4	1.5	1.6	59	381	229	0.32	0.049	11.2	43		0.08	0.29	16.2	15116
raw	101	61.1	17.4	0.0		0.0	26	57	26	0.92	0.134	16	2	0.10	4.6	3.78	0.79
3 oz	85	2.9	0.6	1.0	1.1	50	409	230	0.60	0.093	10.7	53	0.2	0.09	0.35	10.2	15115
tuna, bluefin, ckd by dry heat	156	50.2	25.4	0.0		0.0	43	9	54	0.65	0.017	643	0	0.24	9.0	9.25	1.16
3 oz	85	5.3	1.4	1.7	1.6	42	275	277	1.11	0.094	39.8	2142		0.26	0.45	1.7	15118
raw	122	57.9	19.8	0.0		0.0	33	7	43	0.51	0.013	558	0	0.20	7.4	8.02	0.90
3 oz	85	4.2	1.1	1.4	1.2	32	214	216	0.87	0.073	31.0	1856	0.9	0.21	0.39	1.7	15117
tuna, chunk light, cnd in canola	110	37.0	13.0	0.0			250	5	15	0.40	0.000			0.03	6.3	1.10	0.10
oil, drnd, Chkn of the Sea - 2 oz	57	6.0	0.3	1.2	0.5	30	118	99	0.45	0.000		5	0.2	0.06	0.15	9.0	CHCK3
cnd in spring water, drnd, Chkn	60	42.0	13.0	0.0			250	5	11	0.49	0.000			0.03	6.4	1.50	0.10
of the Sea[3] - 2 oz	57	0.5	0.2	0.1	0.2	30	111	74	0.49	0.000		5	0.0	0.05	0.13	10.0	CHCK4
tuna, chunk white, cnd in spring	60	40.0	13.0	0.0			250	2	15	0.23	0.000			0.03	7.9	0.60	0.07
wtr, drnd, Chkn of the Sea[4] - 2 oz	57	1.0	0.1	0.1	0.2	25	124	97	0.18	0.000		5	0.0	0.00	0.13	9.0	CHCK5
tuna, light, cnd in oil, drained	168	50.9	24.8	0.0		0.0	301	11	26	0.77	0.013	20	0	0.03	10.5	1.87	0.31
3 oz	85	7.0	1.3	2.5	2.5	15	176	264	1.18	0.060	64.6	66	1.0	0.10	0.09	4.3	15119
cnd in water, drained	99	63.3	21.7	0.0		0.0	287	9	23	0.65	0.009	14	0	0.03	11.3	2.54	0.18
3 oz	85	0.7	0.2	0.1	0.3	26	201	139	1.30	0.043	68.3	48	0.5	0.06	0.30	3.4	15121
tuna salad, homemade[5]	159	53.7	13.6	8.0		0.0	342	14	16	0.48	0.034	20	2	0.03	5.7	1.02	0.22
3 oz	85	7.9	1.3	2.5	3.5	11	151	151	0.85	0.123	35.0	82		0.06	0.07	6.8	15128
tuna, skipjack, ckd by dry heat	112	52.9	24.0	0.0		0.0	40	31	37	0.89	0.016	15	1	0.03	15.9	1.86	0.41
3 oz	85	1.1	0.4	0.2	0.3	51	444	242	1.36	0.094	39.8	51		0.10	0.83	8.5	15220
raw	88	60.0	18.7	0.0		0.0	31	25	29	0.70	0.013	14	1	0.03	13.1	1.62	0.36
3 oz	85	0.9	0.3	0.2	0.3	40	346	189	1.06	0.073	31.0	44		0.09	0.72	7.7	15123
tuna, solid light, cnd in olive oil,	130	37.0	14.0	0.0			250	5	14	0.39	0.000			0.03	8.5	1.50	0.10
drnd, Chkn of the Sea - 2 oz	57	8.0	0.9	4.3	1.9	30	119	102	0.47	0.000		5	0.1	0.06	0.20	6.0	CHCK6
cnd in spring wtr, drnd, Chkn of	70	40.0	14.0	0.0			250	5	13	0.49	0.000			0.03	8.0	1.50	0.10
the Sea - 2 oz	57	1.0	0.2	0.1	0.2	30	120	100	0.49	0.000		5	0.0	0.05	0.15	10.0	CHCK7
tuna, solid white, cnd in canola	90	37.0	14.0	0.0			250	3	17	0.23	0.000			0.03	8.0	0.90	0.07
oil, drnd, Chkn of the Sea - 2 oz	57	3.0	0.4	1.1	0.5	25	155	146	0.19	0.000		5	0.3	0.00	0.21	3.0	CHCK8
cnd in spring wtr, drnd, Chkn of	70	40.0	15.0	0.0			250	3	15	0.24	0.000			0.03	6.5	0.80	0.07
the Sea - 2 oz	57	1.0	0.1	<0.1	0.1	25	130	109	0.19	0.000		5	0.2	0.00	0.19	3.0	CHCK9
tuna, white, cnd in oil, drained	158	54.4	22.6	0.0		0.0	337	3	29	0.40	0.014	20	0	0.01	9.9	1.87	0.31
3 oz	85	6.9	1.4	2.1	2.9	26	283	227	0.55	0.111	51.1	68		0.07	0.37	4.3	15124
cnd in water, drained	109	62.2	20.1	0.0		0.0	320	12	28	0.41	0.016	5	0	0.01	4.9	0.99	0.11
3 oz	85	2.5	0.7	0.7	0.9	36	201	184	0.82	0.033	55.8	16	1.4	0.04	0.18	1.7	15126
tuna, yellowfin, ckd by dry heat	118	53.4	25.5	0.0		0.0	40	18	54	0.57	0.016	17	1	0.43	10.1	0.51	0.74
3 oz	85	1.0	0.3	0.2	0.3	49	484	208	0.80	0.070	39.8	58		0.05	0.88	1.7	15221

	KCAL	H₂0 (g)	PRO (g)	CHO (g)	SUGR (g)	DFIB (g)	Na (mg)	Ca (mg)	Mg (mg)	Zn (mg)	Mn (mg)	A (mcg RAE)	C (mg)	B-1 (mg)	NIA (mg)	B-12 (mcg)	PANT (mg)
	WT (g)	FAT (g)	SFA (g)	MUFA (g)	PUFA (g)	CHOL (mg)	K (mg)	P (mg)	Fe (mg)	Cu (mg)	Se (mcg)	A (IU)	E (mg ATE)	B-2 (mg)	B-6 (mg)	FOL (mcg DFE)	REF
raw	92	60.3	19.9	0.0		0.0	31	14	43	0.44	0.013	15	1	0.37	8.3	0.44	0.64
3 oz	85	0.8	0.2	0.1	0.2	38	377	162	0.62	0.054	31.0	50	0.4	0.04	0.77	1.7	15127
turbot, european, ckd by dry heat	104	59.9	17.5	0.0		0.0	163	20	55	0.24	0.019	10	1	0.06	2.3	2.16	0.56
3 oz	85	3.2				53	259	140	0.39	0.040	39.8	34		0.08	0.21	7.7	15222
raw	81	65.4	13.6	0.0		0.0	128	15	43	0.19	0.014	9	1	0.06	1.9	1.87	0.48
3 oz	85	2.5	0.6	0.5	0.7	41	202	110	0.31	0.031	31.0	30		0.07	0.18	6.8	15129
whitefish, ckd by dry heat	146	55.3	20.8	0.0		0.0	55	28	36	1.08	0.073	33	0	0.15	3.3	0.82	0.74
3 oz	85	6.4	1.0	2.2	2.3	65	345	294	0.40	0.078	13.8	111		0.13	0.29	14.5	15223
raw	114	61.9	16.2	0.0		0.0	43	22	28	0.84	0.057	31	0	0.12	2.6	0.85	0.64
3 oz	85	5.0	0.8	1.7	1.8	51	269	230	0.31	0.061	10.7	102	0.2	0.10	0.26	12.8	15130
smoked	92	60.2	19.9	0.0		0.0	866	15	20	0.42	0.029	48	0	0.03	2.0	2.77	0.09
3 oz	85	0.8	0.2	0.2	0.2	28	360	112	0.43	0.268	11.5	162	0.2	0.09	0.33	6.0	15131
whiting, ckd by dry heat	99	63.5	20.0	0.0		0.0	112	53	23	0.45	0.111	29	0	0.06	1.4	2.21	0.21
3 oz	85	1.4	0.3	0.4	0.5	71	369	242	0.36	0.034	34.9	97	0.3	0.05	0.15	12.8	15133
raw	77	68.2	15.6	0.0		0.0	61	41	18	0.75	0.088	26	0	0.05	1.1	1.96	0.18
3 oz	85	1.1	0.2	0.2	0.4	57	212	189	0.29	0.026	27.3	84	0.3	0.04	0.13	11.1	15132
wolffish, atlantic, ckd by dry heat	105	63.1	19.1	0.0		0.0	93	7	32	0.85	0.016	111	0	0.18	2.2	2.00	0.56
3 oz	85	2.6	0.4	0.9	0.9	50	327	218	0.10	0.031	39.8	368		0.08	0.39	5.1	15224
raw	82	67.9	14.9	0.0		0.0	72	5	26	0.66	0.013	96	0	0.15	1.8	1.73	0.48
3 oz	85	2.0	0.3	0.7	0.7	39	255	170	0.08	0.025	31.0	319		0.07	0.34	4.3	15134
yellowtail, ckd by dry heat	159	57.2	25.2	0.0		0.0	43	25	32	0.57	0.016	26	2	0.15	7.4	1.06	0.58
3 oz	85	5.7				60	457	171	0.54	0.049	39.8	88		0.04	0.16	3.4	15225
raw	124	63.3	19.7	0.0		0.0	33	20	26	0.44	0.013	25	2	0.12	5.8	1.11	0.50
3 oz	85	4.5	1.1	1.7	1.2	47	357	133	0.42	0.038	31.0	81		0.03	0.14	3.4	15135

[1] Breading consists of cornmeal, egg, milk, and salt.
[2] Breading consists of bread crumbs, egg, milk, and salt.
[3] The low sodium product contains 90 mg sodium per 2 oz.

[4] The very low sodium product contains 35 mg sodium per 2 oz.
[5] Prepared with light tuna canned in oil, pickle relish, salad dressing, onion, and celery.

12.3 FISH EGGS

	KCAL	H₂0	PRO	CHO	SUGR	DFIB	Na	Ca	Mg	Zn	Mn	A	C	B-1	NIA	B-12	PANT
caviar, black & red, granular	40	7.6	3.9	0.6		0.0	240	44	48	0.15	0.008	90	0	0.03	<0.1	3.20	0.56
1 T	16	2.9	0.6	0.7	1.2	94	29	57	1.90	0.018	10.5	299	1.1	0.10	0.05	8.0	15012
roe, mixed species, ckd by dry heat	58	16.6	8.1	0.5		0.0	33	8	7	0.36	0.004	26	5	0.08	0.6	3.27	0.33
1 oz	28	2.3	0.5	0.6	1.0	136	80	146	0.22	0.036	14.7	86		0.27	0.05	26.1	15207
raw	40	19.2	6.3	0.4		0.0	26	6	6	0.28	0.003	22	5	0.07	0.5	2.84	0.28
1 oz	28	1.8	0.4	0.5	0.8	106	63	114	0.17	0.028	11.4	75	2.0	0.21	0.05	22.7	15072

12.4 MOLLUSKS

	KCAL	H₂0	PRO	CHO	SUGR	DFIB	Na	Ca	Mg	Zn	Mn	A	C	B-1	NIA	B-12	PANT
abalone, fried[1]	161	51.1	16.7	9.4		0.0	502	31	48	0.81	0.060	2	2	0.19	1.6	0.59	2.44
3 oz	85	5.8	1.4	2.3	1.4	80	241	184	3.23	0.194	44.0	4		0.11	0.13	17.0	15156
raw	89	63.4	14.5	5.1		0.0	256	26	41	0.70	0.034	2	2	0.16	1.3	0.62	2.55
3 oz	85	0.6	0.1	0.1	0.1	72	213	162	2.71	0.167	38.1	4	3.4	0.09	0.13	4.3	15155
clam liquid, cnd	5	234.5	1.0	0.2		0.0	516	31	26	0.24	0.178	22	2	0.02	0.4	12.00	0.10
1 cup	240	<0.1	<0.1	<0.1	<0.1	7	358	274	0.72	0.934	9.8	72	2.4	0.05	0.02	4.8	15162
clams, breaded & fried[2]	172	52.3	12.1	8.8			309	54	12	1.24	0.459	77	9	0.09	1.8	34.23	0.37
3 oz (9 small)	85	9.5	2.3	3.9	2.4	52	277	160	11.82	0.303	24.6	257		0.21	0.05	40.8	15158
ckd by moist heat[3]	126	54.1	21.7	4.4		0.0	95	78	15	2.32	0.850	145	19	0.13	2.9	84.06	0.58
3 oz (19 small)	85	1.7	0.2	0.1	0.5	57	534	287	23.77	0.585	54.4	485		0.36	0.09	24.7	15159
cnd, drained	126	54.1	21.7	4.4		0.0	95	78	15	2.32	0.850	145	19	0.13	2.9	84.06	0.58
3 oz	85	1.7	0.2	0.1	0.5	57	534	287	23.77	0.585	41.3	485	0.9	0.36	0.09	24.7	15160
minced, cnd, Progresso	25		4.0	2.0	0.0	0.0	250	0				0					
1/4 cup	60	0.0	0.0			10			0.72			0					GENM205
raw	63	69.5	10.9	2.2		0.0	48	39	8	1.16	0.425	77	11	0.07	1.5	42.02	0.31
3 oz (4 large or 9 small)	85	0.8	0.1	0.1	0.1	29	267	144	11.88	0.292	20.7	255	0.9	0.18	0.05	13.6	15157
cuttlefish, ckd by moist heat	134	52.0	27.6	1.4		0.0	632	153	51	2.94	0.178	173	7	0.01	1.9	4.59	0.77
3 oz	85	1.2	0.2	0.1	0.2	190	541	493	9.21	0.848	76.2	574		1.47	0.23	20.4	15229
raw	67	68.5	13.8	0.7		0.0	316	77	26	1.47	0.094	96	5	0.01	1.0	2.55	0.43
3 oz	85	0.6	0.1	0.1	0.1	95	301	329	5.12	0.499	38.1	319		0.77	0.13	13.6	15163
mussels, blue, ckd by moist heat	146	52.0	20.2	6.3		0.0	314	28	31	2.27	5.780	77	12	0.26	2.6	20.40	0.81
3 oz	85	3.8	0.7	0.9	1.0	48	228	242	5.71	0.127	76.2	258		0.36	0.09	64.6	15165
raw	73	68.5	10.1	3.1		0.0	243	22	29	1.36	2.890	41	7	0.14	1.4	10.20	0.43
3 oz	85	1.9	0.4	0.4	0.5	24	272	167	3.36	0.080	38.1	136	0.6	0.18	0.04	35.7	15164

	KCAL / WT (g)	H₂0 (g) / FAT (g)	PRO (g) / SFA (g)	CHO (g) / MUFA (g)	SUGR (g) / PUFA (g)	DFIB (g) / CHOL (mg)	Na (mg) / K (mg)	Ca (mg) / P (mg)	Mg (mg) / Fe (mg)	Zn (mg) / Cu (mg)	Mn (mg) / Se (mcg)	A (mcg RAE) / A (IU)	C (mg) / E (mg ATE)	B-1 (mg) / B-2 (mg)	NIA (mg) / B-6 (mg)	B-12 (mcg) / FOL (mcg DFE)	PANT (mg) / REF
octopus, ckd by moist heat	139	51.4	25.3	3.7		0.0	391	90	51	2.86	0.040	69	7	0.05	3.2	30.60	0.77
3 oz	85	1.8	0.4	0.3	0.4	82	536	237	8.11	0.628	76.2	230	1.0	0.06	0.55	20.4	15230
raw	70	68.2	12.7	1.9		0.0	196	45	26	1.43	0.021	38	4	0.03	1.8	17.00	0.43
3 oz	85	0.9	0.2	0.1	0.2	41	298	158	4.51	0.370	38.1	128	1.0	0.03	0.31	13.6	15166
oysters, eastern, breaded & fried[2]	173	57.0	7.7	10.2			367	55	51	76.67	0.431	80	3	0.13	1.5	13.75	0.24
6 med (3 oz)	88	11.1	2.8	4.1	2.9	71	215	140	6.12	3.779	58.5	266		0.18	0.06	37.8	15168
cnd	59	72.4	6.0	3.3		0.0	95	38	46	77.31	0.383	77	4	0.13	1.1	16.26	0.15
3 oz (~11 oysters)	85	2.1	0.5	0.2	0.6	47	195	118	5.70	3.792	30.4	255	0.7	0.14	0.08	7.7	15170
oysters, eastern, farmed, ckd by dry heat - 6 med	47	48.4	4.1	4.3		0.0	96	33	19	26.64	0.251	11	4	0.08	1.1	14.34	0.12
	59	1.3	0.4	0.1	0.4	22	90	68	4.58	0.846	45.7	37		0.03	0.04	14.2	15246
raw	50	72.4	4.4	4.6		0.0	150	37	28	31.85	0.331	7	4	0.09	1.1	13.61	0.13
6 med	84	1.3	0.4	0.1	0.5	21	104	78	4.86	0.620	53.5	21		0.05	0.05	15.1	15245
oysters, eastern, wild, ckd by dry heat - 6 med	42	49.1	4.9	2.8		0.0	144	27	27	43.42	0.170	0	2	0.05	1.0	16.40	0.13
	59	1.1	0.3	0.1	0.5	29	99	80	2.55	2.038	42.3	0		0.05	0.06	10.6	15244
ckd by moist heat	58	29.5	5.9	3.3		0.0	177	38	40	76.28	0.293	23	3	0.08	1.0	14.71	0.15
6 med	42	2.1	0.6	0.3	0.8	44	118	85	5.04	3.179	30.1	76		0.08	0.05	5.9	15169
raw	57	71.5	5.9	3.3		0.0	177	38	39	76.28	0.308	25	3	0.08	1.2	16.35	0.16
6 med	84	2.1	0.6	0.3	0.8	45	131	113	5.59	3.740	53.5	84	0.7	0.08	0.05	8.4	15167
oysters, pacific, ckd by moist heat	139	54.5	16.1	8.4		0.0	180	14	37	28.25	1.039	124	11	0.11	3.1	24.48	0.77
3 oz	85	3.9	0.9	0.6	1.5	85	257	207	7.82	2.277	130.9	413		0.38	0.08	12.8	15231
raw	69	69.8	8.0	4.2		0.0	90	7	19	14.13	0.547	69	7	0.06	1.7	13.60	0.43
3 oz	85	2.0	0.4	0.3	0.8	43	143	138	4.34	1.340	65.5	230	0.7	0.20	0.04	8.5	15171
scallops, breaded & fried[2]	67	18.1	5.6	3.1			144	13	18	0.33	0.043	7	1	0.01	0.5	0.41	0.06
2 large	31	3.4	0.8	1.4	0.9	19	103	73	0.25	0.024	8.3	23		0.03	0.04	15.5	15173
scallops, imitation, made from surimi - 3 oz	84	62.7	10.9	9.0		0.0	676	7	37	0.28	0.009	17	0	0.01	0.3	1.36	0.06
	85	0.3	0.1	0.1	0.2	19	88	240	0.26	0.027	20.1	56		0.01	0.03	1.7	15174
scallops, mixed species, raw	75	66.8	14.3	2.0		0.0	137	20	48	0.81	0.077	13	3	0.01	1.0	1.30	0.12
3 oz (6 large)	85	0.6	0.1	<0.1	0.2	28	274	186	0.25	0.045	18.9	43	0.9	0.06	0.13	13.6	15172
squid, fried[1]	149	54.9	15.2	6.6		0.0	260	33	32	1.48	0.060	9	4	0.05	2.2	1.05	0.43
3 oz	85	6.4	1.6	2.3	1.8	221	237	213	0.86	1.797	44.0	30		0.39	0.05	17.0	15176
raw	78	66.8	13.2	2.6		0.0	37	27	28	1.30	0.030	9	4	0.02	1.8	1.11	0.43
3 oz	85	1.2	0.3	0.1	0.4	198	209	188	0.58	1.607	38.1	28	1.0	0.35	0.05	4.3	15175
whelks (sea snails), ckd by moist heat - 3 oz	234	27.2	40.5	13.2		0.0	350	96	146	2.77	0.757	42	6	0.04	1.7	15.42	0.34
	85	0.7	0.1	<0.1	<0.1	111	590	240	8.55	1.751	76.2	138		0.18	0.55	9.4	15178
raw	116	56.1	20.3	6.6		0.0	175	48	73	1.39	0.380	22	3	0.02	0.9	7.71	0.18
3 oz	85	0.3	<0.1	<0.1	<0.1	55	295	120	4.28	0.876	38.1	72	0.1	0.09	0.29	5.1	15177

[1] Dipped in flour and salt before frying.
[2] Breading consists of bread crumbs, egg, milk, and salt.
[3] These values also apply to canned clams.

13. FLOUR & GRAIN FRACTIONS

	KCAL / WT (g)	H₂0 (g) / FAT (g)	PRO (g) / SFA (g)	CHO (g) / MUFA (g)	SUGR (g) / PUFA (g)	DFIB (g) / CHOL (mg)	Na (mg) / K (mg)	Ca (mg) / P (mg)	Mg (mg) / Fe (mg)	Zn (mg) / Cu (mg)	Mn (mg) / Se (mcg)	A (mcg RAE) / A (IU)	C (mg) / E (mg ATE)	B-1 (mg) / B-2 (mg)	NIA (mg) / B-6 (mg)	B-12 (mcg) / FOL (mcg DFE)	PANT (mg) / REF
amaranth flour	729	19.2	28.2	129.0		29.6	41	298	519	6.20	4.407	0	8	0.16	2.5	0.00	2.04
1 cup	195	12.7	3.2	2.8	5.6	0	714	887	14.80	1.515		0	2.0	0.41	0.43	95.6	20001
arrowroot flour	457	14.6	0.4	112.8		4.4	3	51	4	0.09	0.602	0	0	<0.01	0.0	0.00	0.17
1 cup	128	0.1	<0.1	<0.1	0.1	0	14	6	0.42	0.051		0		0.00	0.01	9.0	20003
barley flour/meal	511	17.9	15.5	110.3		14.9	6	47	142	2.96	1.530	0	0	0.55	9.3	0.00	0.21
1 cup	148	2.4	0.5	0.3	1.1	0	457	438	3.97	0.508		0		0.17	0.59	11.8	20130
barley malt flour	585	13.3	16.7	126.8		11.5	18	60	157	3.34	1.933	2	1	0.50	9.1	0.00	0.53
1 cup	162	3.0	0.6	0.4	1.5	0	363	491	7.63	0.437		31		0.50	1.06	61.6	20131
buckwheat flour, whole groat	402	13.4	15.1	84.7		12.0	13	49	301	3.74	2.436	0	0	0.50	7.4	0.00	0.53
1 cup	120	3.7	0.8	1.1	1.1	0	692	404	4.87	0.618	6.8	0	1.2	0.23	0.70	64.8	20011
carob (St John's bread) flour	229	3.7	4.8	91.5		41.0	36	358	56	0.95	0.523	1	<1	0.05	2.0	0.00	0.05
1 cup	103	0.7	0.1	0.2	0.2	0	852	81	3.03	0.588	5.5	14	0.6	0.47	0.38	29.9	16055
corn bran	170	3.6	6.4	65.1		65.0	5	32	49	1.19	0.106	3	0	0.01	2.1	0.00	0.48
1 cup	76	0.7	0.1	0.2	0.3	0	33	55	2.12	0.188	12.5	54	1.8	0.08	0.12	3.0	20015
corn flour, yellow, masa harina, enr	416	10.3	10.6	86.9		10.9	6	161	125	2.03	0.55	0	0	1.63	11.2	0.00	0.75
1 cup	114	4.3	0.6	1.1	2.0	0	340	254	8.22	0.193	17.1	0	0.3	0.86	0.42	343.1	20017
whole grain	422	12.8	8.1	89.9		15.7	6	8	109	2.02	0.538	27	0	0.29	2.2	0.00	0.77
1 cup	117	4.5	0.6	1.2	2.1	0	369	318	2.78	0.269	18.0	549	0.3	0.09	0.43	29.3	20016
cornmeal, white, bolted, enr, self-rising - *1 cup*	407	15.4	10.1	85.7		8.2	1521	440	105	2.44		0	0	0.81	6.5	0.00	0.52
	122	4.1	0.6	1.1	1.9	0	311	981	7.03	0.183		0		0.49	0.66	339.2	20323

	KCAL	H₂O (g)	PRO (g)	CHO (g)	SUGR (g)	DFIB (g)	Na (mg)	Ca (mg)	Mg (mg)	Zn (mg)	Mn (mg)	A (mcg RAE)	C (mg)	B-1 (mg)	NIA (mg)	B-12 (mcg)	PANT (mg)
	WT (g)	FAT (g)	SFA (g)	MUFA (g)	PUFA (g)	CHOL (mg)	K (mg)	P (mg)	Fe (mg)	Cu (mg)	Se (mcg)	A (IU)	E (mg ATE)	B-2 (mg)	B-6 (mg)	FOL (mcg DFE)	REF
bolted, enr, self-rising, wheat	592	17.6	14.3	124.8		10.7	2242	508	92	2.36		0	0	1.21	8.8	0.00	0.65
flour added - *1 cup*	170	4.8	0.7	1.3	2.2	0	352	1107	8.42	0.236		0		0.74	0.65	453.9	20324
degermed, enr, self-rising	490	14.0	11.6	103.2		9.8	1860	483	68	1.38		0	0	0.94	6.3	0.00	
1 cup	138	2.4	0.3	0.6	1.0	0	235	860	6.53	0.179		0		0.53	0.54	408.5	20325
whole grain	442	12.5	9.9	93.8		8.9	43	7	155	2.22	0.608	0	0	0.47	4.4	0.00	0.52
1 cup	122	4.4	0.6	1.2	2.0	0	350	294	4.21	0.235	18.9	0	0.4	0.25	0.37	30.5	20320
cornmeal, yellow, bolted, enr,	407	15.4	10.1	85.7		8.2	1521	440	105	2.44	0.608	28	0	0.81	6.5	0.00	0.52
self-rising - *1 cup*	122	4.1	0.6	1.1	1.9	0	311	981	7.03	0.183		572		0.49	0.66	339.2	20023
bolted, enr, self-rising, wheat	592	17.6	14.3	124.8		10.7	2242	508	92	2.36	0.877	24	0	1.21	8.8	0.00	0.65
flour added - *1 cup*	170	4.8	0.7	1.3	2.2	0	352	1107	8.42	0.236		488		0.74	0.65	453.9	20024
degermed, enr	505	16.0	11.7	107.2		10.2	4	7	55	0.99	0.145	29	0	0.99	6.9	0.00	0.43
1 cup	138	2.3	0.3	0.6	1.0	0	224	116	5.70	0.108	10.8	570	0.5	0.56	0.35	391.9	20022
degermed, enr, self-rising	490	14.0	11.6	103.2		9.8	1860	483	68	1.38	0.145	29	0	0.94	6.3	0.00	0.43
1 cup	138	2.4	0.3	0.6	1.0	0	235	860	6.53	0.179		570		0.53	0.54	408.5	20025
whole grain	442	12.5	9.9	93.8		8.9	43	7	155	2.22	0.608	28	0	0.47	4.4	0.00	0.52
1 cup	122	4.4	0.6	1.2	2.0	0	350	294	4.21	0.235	18.9	572	0.8	0.25	0.37	30.5	20020
cracker meal	440	8.7	10.7	93.0		3.0	32	26	28	0.79	1.086	0	0	0.80	6.6	0.00	0.54
1 cup	115	2.0	0.3	0.2	0.8	0	132	120	5.34	0.259	48.6	0	0.1	0.54	0.04	207.0	18236
oat bran, ckd	88	184.0	7.0	25.1		5.7	2	22	88	1.16	2.111	0	0	0.35	0.3	0.00	0.48
1 cup	219	1.9	0.4	0.6	0.7	0	201	261	1.93	0.145	16.9	0		0.07	0.05	13.1	20034
raw	231	6.2	16.3	62.2		14.5	4	55	221	2.92	5.292	0	0	1.10	0.9	0.00	1.40
1 cup	94	6.6	1.2	2.2	2.6	0	532	690	5.09	0.379	42.5	0	1.6	0.21	0.16	48.9	20033
potato flour	571	10.4	11.0	132.9		9.4	88	104	104	0.86	0.501	0	6	0.36	5.6	0.00	0.76
1 cup	160	0.5	0.1	<0.1	0.2	0	1602	269	2.21	0.315	1.8	0	0.4	0.08	1.23	40.0	11413
quinoa	636	15.8	22.3	117.1		10.0	36	102	357	5.61	3.842	0	0	0.34	5.0	0.00	1.78
1 cup	170	9.9	1.0	2.6	4.0	0	1258	697	15.73	1.394		0		0.67	0.38	83.3	20035
organic, andean, unckd, Eden	180		7.0	29.0	1.0	11.0	10	16	62	2.02			0	0.08	0.0		
Foods - *1/4 cup*	45	3.5	0.0			0	260	234	2.25	0.000		200	3.0	0.27	0.00	17.5	EDEN19
rice bran	373	7.2	15.8	58.6		24.8	6	67	922	7.13	16.768	0	0	3.25	40.1	0.00	8.72
1 cup	118	24.6	4.9	8.9	8.8	0	1752	1979	21.88	0.859	18.4	0	7.1	0.34	4.80	74.3	20060
rice flour, brown	574	18.9	11.4	120.8		7.3	13	17	177	3.87	6.341	0	0	0.70	10.0	0.00	2.51
1 cup	158	4.4	0.9	1.6	1.6	0	457	532	3.13	0.363		0	1.1	0.13	1.16	25.3	20090
rice flour, white	578	18.8	9.4	126.6		3.8	0	16	55	1.26	1.896	0	0	0.22	4.1	0.00	1.29
1 cup	158	2.2	0.6	0.7	0.6	0	120	155	0.55	0.205	23.9	0	0.2	0.03	0.69	6.3	20061
rye flour, dark	415	14.2	18.0	88.0		28.9	1	72	317	7.19	8.614	0	0	0.40	5.5	0.00	1.86
1 cup	128	3.4	0.4	0.4	1.5	0	934	809	8.26	0.960	45.7	0	3.3	0.32	0.57	76.8	20063
rye flour, light	374	9.0	8.6	81.8		14.9	2	21	71	1.79	2.009	0	0	0.34	0.8	0.00	0.68
1 cup	102	1.4	0.1	0.2	0.6	0	238	198	1.84	0.255	36.4	0	0.6	0.09	0.24	22.4	20065
rye flour, medium	361	10.0	9.6	79.0		14.9	3	24	77	2.03	5.569	0	0	0.29	1.8	0.00	0.50
1 cup	102	1.8	0.2	0.2	0.8	0	347	211	2.16	0.293	36.4	0	1.4	0.12	0.27	19.4	20064
semolina, enr	601	21.2	21.2	121.6		6.5	2	28	78	1.75	1.034	0	0	1.35	10.0	0.00	0.97
1 cup	167	1.8	0.3	0.2	0.7	0	311	227	7.28	0.316	149.3	0	0.4	0.95	0.17	352.4	20066
sorghum	651	17.7	21.7	143.3			12	54				0	0	0.46	5.6	0.00	
1 cup	192	6.3	0.9	1.9	2.6	0	672	551	8.45			0		0.27			20067
soy flour, defatted	329	7.3	47.0	38.4		17.5	20	241	290	2.46	3.018	2	0	0.70	2.6	0.00	2.00
1 cup	100	1.2	0.1	0.2	0.5	0	2384	674	9.24	4.065	1.7	40	0.2	0.25	0.57	305.0	16117
full fat	366	4.3	29.0	29.6		8.1	11	173	360	3.29	1.911	5	0	0.49	3.6	0.00	1.34
1 cup	84	17.3	2.5	3.8	9.8	0	2113	415	5.35	2.453	6.3	101	1.6	0.97	0.39	289.8	16115
full fat, roasted	375	3.2	29.6	28.6		8.2	10	160	314	3.04	1.765	5	0	0.35	2.8	0.00	1.03
1 cup	85	18.6	2.7	4.1	10.5	0	1735	405	4.95	1.888	6.4	94		0.80	0.30	193.0	16116
low fat	327	2.4	40.9	33.4		9.0	16	165	202	1.04	2.710	2	0	0.33	1.9	0.00	1.60
1 cup	88	5.9	0.9	1.3	3.3	0	2262	522	5.27	4.470	8.2	35	0.2	0.25	0.46	360.8	16118
soy meal, defatted, raw	414	8.5	54.8	49.0			4	298	373	6.17	4.636	2	0	0.84	3.2	0.00	2.41
1 cup	122	2.9	0.3	0.5	1.3	0	3038	855	16.71	2.440	4.0	49		0.31	0.69	369.7	16119
triticale flour, whole grain	439	13.0	17.1	95.1		19.0	3	46	199	3.46	5.441	0	0	0.49	3.7	0.00	2.82
1 cup	130	2.4	0.4	0.2	1.0	0	606	417	3.37	0.727		0	1.2	0.17	0.52	96.2	20070
wheat bran	125	5.7	9.0	37.4		24.8	1	42	354	4.22	6.670	0	0	0.30	7.9	0.00	1.26
1 cup	58	2.5	0.4	0.4	1.3	0	686	588	6.13	0.579	45.0	0	1.3	0.33	0.76	45.8	20077
wheat flour, white, all-purpose, enr	455	14.9	12.9	95.4		3.4	3	19	28	0.88	0.853	0	0	0.98	7.4	0.00	0.55
1 cup	125	1.2	0.2	0.1	0.5	0	134	135	5.80	0.180	42.4	0	0.2	0.62	0.06	386.3	20081
wheat flour, white, bread	495	18.3	16.4	99.4		3.3	3	21	34	1.16	1.085	0	0	1.11	10.3	0.00	0.60
1 cup	137	2.3	0.3	0.2	1.0	0	137	133	6.04	0.249	54.4	0	1.0	0.70	0.05	394.6	20083

	KCAL / WT (g)	H₂O (g) / FAT (g)	PRO (g) / SFA (g)	CHO (g) / MUFA (g)	SUGR (g) / PUFA (g)	DFIB (g) / CHOL (mg)	Na (mg) / K (mg)	Ca (mg) / P (mg)	Mg (mg) / Fe (mg)	Zn (mg) / Cu (mg)	Mn (mg) / Se (mcg)	A (mcg RAE) / A (IU)	C (mg) / E (mg ATE)	B-1 (mg) / B-2 (mg)	NIA (mg) / B-6 (mg)	B-12 (mcg) / FOL (mcg DFE)	PANT (mg) / REF
cake, enr	496	17.1	11.2	106.9		2.3	3	19	22	0.85	0.869	0		1.22	9.3	0.00	0.63
1 cup	137	1.2	0.2	0.1	0.5	0	144	116	10.03	0.190	6.7	0	<0.1	0.59	0.05	386.3	20084
self-rising, enr	443	13.2	12.4	92.8		3.4	1588	423	24	0.78	1.250	0	0	0.84	7.3	0.00	0.55
1 cup	125	1.2	0.2	0.1	0.5	0	155	744	5.84	0.140	43.0	0	0.1	0.52	0.06	383.8	20082
tortilla mix	450	11.2	10.7	74.5			751	228	23	0.71	0.682	0		0.82	6.5	0.00	0.44
1 cup	111	11.8	4.6	5.0	1.7	0	111	233	7.83	0.111		0		0.55	0.04	238.7	20086
wheat flour, whole wheat	407	12.3	16.4	87.1		14.6	6	41	166	3.52	4.559	0		0.54	7.6	0.00	1.21
1 cup	120	2.2	0.4	0.3	0.9	0	486	415	4.66	0.458	84.8	0	1.5	0.26	0.41	52.8	20080
wheat germ, crude	414	12.8	26.6	59.6		15.2	14	45	275	14.13	15.296	0		2.16	7.8	0.00	2.60
1 cup	115	11.2	1.9	1.6	6.9	0	1026	968	7.20	0.915	91.1	0		0.57	1.50	323.2	20078
honey crunch, Kretschmer	52	0.5	3.7	8.1	3.5	1.4	2	7	38	1.94	2.223	1	0	0.19	0.7	0.00	0.15
1.7 T	14	1.1	0.2	0.1	0.7	0	135	142	1.13	0.101	8.1	13	4.2	0.10	0.07	111.6	08085
toasted	432	6.3	32.9	56.0		14.6	5	51	362	18.84	22.550	0	7	1.89	6.3	0.00	1.57
1 cup	113	12.1	2.1	1.7	7.5	0	1070	1295	10.27	0.701	73.5	0	20.5	0.93	1.11	397.8	08084

14. FRUIT & VEGETABLE JUICES & JUICE DRINKS

	KCAL / WT (g)	H₂O (g) / FAT (g)	PRO (g) / SFA (g)	CHO (g) / MUFA (g)	SUGR (g) / PUFA (g)	DFIB (g) / CHOL (mg)	Na (mg) / K (mg)	Ca (mg) / P (mg)	Mg (mg) / Fe (mg)	Zn (mg) / Cu (mg)	Mn (mg) / Se (mcg)	A (mcg RAE) / A (IU)	C (mg) / E (mg ATE)	B-1 (mg) / B-2 (mg)	NIA (mg) / B-6 (mg)	B-12 (mcg) / FOL (mcg DFE)	PANT (mg) / REF
acerola jce, raw	56	228.2	1.0	11.6		0.7	7	24	29	0.24		61	3872	0.05	1.0	0.00	0.50
8 fl oz	242	0.7	0.2	0.2	0.2	0	235	22	1.21	0.208	0.2	1232	0.1	0.15	0.01	33.9	09002
apple jce, cnd/bottled	117	218.1	0.1	29.0		0.2	7	17	7	0.07	0.280	0	2	0.05	0.2	0.00	0.16
8 fl oz	248	0.3	<0.1	<0.1	0.1	0	295	17	0.92	0.055	0.2	2	<0.1	0.04	0.07	0.0	09016
from frzn conc	112	210.1	0.3	27.6		0.2	17	14	12	0.10	0.151	0	1	0.01	0.1	0.00	0.15
8 fl oz	239	0.2	<0.1	<0.1	0.1	0	301	17	0.62	0.033	0.2	0	<0.1	0.04	0.08	0.0	09018
from frzn conc, Minute Maid - 8 fl oz	110		2.0	27.0	24.0		25	20					72	0.15	0.4		
(8 fl oz)	239	0.0					480								0.08	60.0	MNTM1
jce box, Minute Maid	110		2.0	27.0	24.0		25	20					72	0.15	0.4		
6.8 fl oz	211	0.0					480								0.08	60.0	MNTM2
w/Ca & vit C, Tropicana	140		<1.0	35.0	32.0		30	100					60				
8 fl oz	248	0.0					310										TROP1
apple raspberry cherry jce cocktail, Veryfine - 8 fl oz	129	215.3	0.2	32.2	24.8		12						80				
(8 fl oz)	248	0.0															14122
apricot nectar, cnd	141	213.0	0.9	36.1		1.5	8	18	13	0.23	0.080	166	2	0.02	0.7	0.00	0.24
8 fl oz	251	0.2	<0.1	0.1	<0.1	0	286	23	0.95	0.183	0.5	3303	0.2	0.04	0.06	2.5	09036
beef broth & tomato jce, cnd	62	151.0	1.0	14.3		0.2	220	18	5	0.03	0.047	10	2	<0.01	0.3	0.08	0.06
5.5 fl oz	168	0.2	0.1	<0.1	<0.1	0	161	22	0.97	0.029	1.2	215		0.05	0.04	6.7	14114
carrot jce, cnd	94	209.7	2.2	21.9		1.9	68	57	33	0.42	0.307	1291	20	0.22	0.9	0.00	0.54
8 fl oz	236	0.4	0.1	<0.1	0.2	0	689	99	1.09	0.109	1.4	25833	<0.1	0.13	0.51	9.4	11655
cherry jce, jce box, Minute Maid	110		2.0	27.0	24.0		25	20					72	0.15	0.4		
6.8 fl oz	215	0.0					480								0.08	60.0	MNTM3
Eden Foods	140		1.0	33.0	25.0	0.0	30	20					0				
8 fl oz	235	1.0	0.0			0	370		1.44			200					EDEN3
citrus fruit jce drink, from frzn conc - 8 fl oz	114	217.7	0.7	28.5		0.0	7	22	15	0.12	0.181	5	67	0.03	0.4	0.00	0.33
(8 fl oz)	248	0.0	<0.1	<0.1	0.1	0	278	25	2.78	0.079	0.1	104		0.03	0.06	5.0	14263
clam & tomato jce, cnd	80	145.1	1.0	18.2		0.3	601	20	37	1.79	0.125	18	7	0.07	0.3	50.80	0.42
5.5 fl oz	166	0.3	0.1	<0.1	<0.1	0	149	129	1.00	0.578	0.3	357		0.05	0.14	26.6	14187
Clearfruit Drinks, avg for 4 flvrs, Shasta[1] - 8 fl oz	90		0.0	22.6	22.6	0.0	0	<1					<1				
(8 fl oz)	250	0.0				0		<0.01				<1					SHST1
cranberry apple jce drink, bottled	164	202.9	0.2	41.9		0.2	5	17	5	0.10	0.441	0	78	0.01	0.1	0.00	0.14
8 fl oz	245	0.0	0.0	0.0	0.0	0	66	7	0.15	0.017	0.0	7	0.0	0.05	0.05	0.0	14238
cranberry apple raspberry jce, Min Maid Jce To Go - 8 fl oz	120			32.0	31.0		25	0					0	0.00			
(8 fl oz)	250						0										COLA52
cranberry apricot jce drink, bottled	157	204.6	0.5	39.7		0.2	5	22	7	0.10	0.306	56	0	0.01	0.3	0.00	0.09
8 fl oz	245	0.0	0.0	0.0	0.0	0	149	12	0.37	0.037	0.0	1134		0.02	0.05	2.5	14240
cranberry grape jce drink, bottled	137	209.7	0.5	34.3		0.2	7	20	7	0.10	0.387	0	78	0.02	0.3	0.00	0.13
8 fl oz	245	0.2	0.1	<0.1	0.1	0	59	10	0.02	0.017	0.0	12		0.04	0.07	2.5	14241
cranberry grape jce, Tropicana	170		0.0	41.0	41.0		10						60				
8 fl oz	245	0.0					10										TROP4
cranberry jce cocktail, bottled	144	216.3	0.0	36.4		0.3	5	8	5	0.18	0.488	0	90	0.02	0.1	0.00	0.14
8 fl oz	253	0.3	<0.1	<0.1	0.1	0	46	5	0.38	0.046	0.0	10	0.0	0.02	0.05	0.0	14242
from frzn conc	138	214.8	0.0	35.0		0.3	8	13	5	0.10	0.103	3	25	0.02	<0.1	0.00	0.35
8 fl oz	250	0.0	0.0	0.0	0.0	0	35	3	0.23	0.025	0.0	25		0.02	0.04	0.0	14431

	KCAL	H₂O (g)	PRO (g)	CHO (g)	SUGR (g)	DFIB (g)	Na (mg)	Ca (mg)	Mg (mg)	Zn (mg)	Mn (mg)	A (mcg RAE)	C (mg)	B-1 (mg)	NIA (mg)	B-12 (mcg)	PANT (mg)
	WT (g)	FAT (g)	SFA (g)	MUFA (g)	PUFA (g)	CHOL (mg)	K (mg)	P (mg)	Fe (mg)	Cu (mg)	Se (mcg)	A (IU)	E (mg ATE)	B-2 (mg)	B-6 (mg)	FOL (mcg DFE)	REF
low cal, bottled[2]	45	225.6	0.0	11.1		0.0	7	21	5	0.05	0.405	0	76	0.02	0.1	0.00	0.13
8 fl oz	237	0.0	0.0	0.0	0.0	0	52	2	0.09	0.033	0.0	9	0.0	0.02	0.05	0.0	14243
Tropicana	140		0.0	34.0	34.0		35						60				
8 fl oz	253	0.0															TROP5
cranberry medley, Tropicana	120		<1.0	29.0	26.0		20						60				
8 fl oz	253	0.0					200		2.00								TROP6
cranberry orange lemon jce, Mad River - *8 fl oz (240 ml)*	98			25.0	24.0		22						9				
	250						28					0					COLA54
Everfresh, avg for 13 flvrs, Shasta - *8 fl oz*	125		0.0	31.4	31.4	0.0	2	<1					<1				
	250	0.0				0			<0.01			<1					SHST2
avg for 8 flvrs, Shasta[3]	178		0.0	44.6	44.6	0.0	20	<1					<1				
11.5 fl oz	360	0.0				0			<0.01			<1					SHST3
fruit punch jce (100% fruit jce), jce box, Minute Maid - *6.8 fl oz*	110		2.0	27.0	24.0		25	20					72	0.15	0.4		
	211	0.0					480							0.08	60.0		MNTM4
fruit punch jce drink, from frzn conc - *8 fl oz*	124	216.5	0.2	30.3		0.2	12	17	10	0.55	0.149	0	14	<0.01	0.1	0.00	0.07
	248	0.5	0.1	0.1	0.1	0	191	0	0.57	0.060	0.0	15		0.16	0.03	0.0	14406
rtd, Capri Sun All Natural	99	182.9	0.0	26.3	25.2	0.0	21	2					3				
6.8 fl oz	210	0.0	0.0			0	25	2	0.06			8					14272
fruit punch, Min Maid Juice To Go	100			28.0	27.0		80	0					60	0.00			
8 fl oz (240 ml)	250						0										COLA55
grape jce, cnd/bottled	154	212.8	1.4	37.8		0.3	8	23	25	0.13	0.911	0	<1	0.07	0.7	0.00	0.10
8 fl oz	253	0.2	0.1	<0.1	0.1	0	334	28	0.61	0.071	0.3	20	0.0	0.09	0.16	7.6	09135
from frzn conc, sweetened	128	217.3	0.5	31.9		0.3	5	10	10	0.10	0.443	0	60	0.04	0.3	0.00	0.06
8 fl oz	250	0.2	0.1	<0.1	0.1	0	53	10	0.25	0.033	0.3	20	0.1	0.07	0.11	2.5	09137
jce box, Minute Maid	110		2.0	27.0	24.0		20	350					72	0.15	0.4		
6.8 fl oz	215	0.0					480							0.08	60.0		MNTM5
grape jce drink, cnd	125	217.5	0.3	32.3		0.3	3	8	10	0.08	0.270	0	40	0.03	0.3	0.00	0.03
8 fl oz	250	0.0	0.0	0.0	0.0	0	88	10	0.25	0.035	0.3	5	0.0	0.03	0.05	2.5	14282
grapefruit blend, ruby red w/Ca, refrig, Minute Maid - *8 fl oz*	110		2.0	27.0	24.0		25	350					72	0.15	0.4		
	247	0.0					480							0.08	60.0		MNTM6
grapefruit jce, cnd	94	222.5	1.3	22.1		0.2	2	17	25	0.22	0.049	0	72	0.10	0.6	0.00	0.32
8 fl oz	247	0.2	<0.1	<0.1	0.1	0	378	27	0.49	0.094	0.2	17	0.1	0.05	0.05	24.7	09123
cnd, sweetened	115	218.5	1.5	27.8		0.3	5	20	25	0.15	0.050	0	67	0.10	0.8	0.00	0.33
8 fl oz	250	0.2	<0.1	<0.1	0.1	0	405	28	0.90	0.120	0.3	0	0.1	0.06	0.05	25.0	09124
from frzn conc	101	220.6	1.4	24.0		0.2	2	20	27	0.12	0.049	0	83	0.10	0.5	0.00	0.47
8 fl oz	247	0.3	<0.1	<0.1	0.1	0	336	35	0.35	0.082	0.2	22	0.1	0.05	0.11	9.9	09126
from frzn conc, Min Maid	100		1.0	25.0	20.0		0	100					84				
8 fl oz	247	0.0					370										MNTM7
raw pink	96	222.3	1.2	22.7			2	22	30	0.12	0.049	54	94	0.10	0.5	0.00	0.47
8 fl oz	247	0.2	<0.1	<0.1	0.1	0	400	37	0.49	0.082		1087		0.05	0.11	24.7	09404
raw white	96	222.3	1.2	22.7		0.2	2	22	30	0.12	0.049	2	94	0.10	0.5	0.00	0.47
8 fl oz	247	0.2	<0.1	<0.1	0.1	0	400	37	0.49	0.082	0.2	25	0.1	0.05	0.11	24.7	09128
ruby red w/Ca, Tropicana	90		1.0	22.0	17.0		0	400	24				72	0.09	0.4		
8 fl oz	247	0.0					300							0.03	0.08	24.0	TROP8
kiwi strawberry jce, Snapple	119	218.2	0.2	29.3	23.1		7										
8 fl oz	248	0.0															14123
lemon jce, cnd/bottled	3	13.9	0.1	1.0		0.1	3	2	1	0.01	0.003	<1	4	0.01	<0.1	0.00	0.01
1 T	15	<0.1	<0.1	<0.1	<0.1	0	15	1	0.02	0.006	<0.1	2	<0.1	<0.01	0.01	1.5	09153
frzn, single-strength	54	225.4	1.1	15.9		1.0	2	20	20	0.12	0.073	2	77	0.14	0.3	0.00	0.30
1 cup	244	0.8	0.1	<0.1	0.2	0	217	20	0.29	0.073	0.2	32	0.2	0.03	0.15	24.4	09154
raw	12	42.6	0.2	4.1		0.2	0	3	3	0.02	0.004	<1	22	0.01	<0.1	0.00	0.05
yield from 1 lemon (1.5 fl oz)	47	0.0	0.0	0.0	0.0	0	58	3	0.01	0.014	<0.1	9	<0.1	<0.01	0.02	6.1	09152b
raw	61	221.4	0.9	21.1		1.0	2	17	15	0.12	0.020	2	112	0.07	0.2	0.00	0.25
8 fl oz	244	0.0	0.0	0.0	0.0	0	303	15	0.07	0.071	0.2	49	0.2	0.02	0.12	31.7	09152a
lime jce, cnd/bottled	6	28.5	0.1	2.1		0.1	5	4	2	0.02	0.002	<1	2	0.01	<0.1	0.00	0.02
1 fl oz	31	0.1	<0.1	<0.1	<0.1	0	23	3	0.07	0.009	<0.1	5	<0.1	<0.01	0.01	2.5	09161
raw	10	34.3	0.2	3.4		0.2	0	3	2	0.02	0.003	<1	11	0.01	<0.1	0.00	0.05
yield from 1 lime (1.2 fl oz)	38	<0.1	<0.1	<0.1	<0.1	0	41	3	0.01	0.011	<0.1	4	<0.1	<0.01	0.02	3.0	09160b
raw	66	221.9	1.1	22.2		1.0	2	22	15	0.15	0.020	2	72	0.05	0.2	0.00	0.34
8 fl oz	246	0.2	<0.1	<0.1	0.1	0	268	17	0.07	0.074	0.2	25	0.2	0.02	0.11	19.7	09160a

	KCAL	H₂0 (g)	PRO (g)	CHO (g)	SUGR (g)	DFIB (g)	Na (mg)	Ca (mg)	Mg (mg)	Zn (mg)	Mn (mg)	A (mcg RAE)	C (mg)	B-1 (mg)	NIA (mg)	B-12 (mcg)	PANT (mg)
	WT (g)	FAT (g)	SFA (g)	MUFA (g)	PUFA (g)	CHOL (mg)	K (mg)	P (mg)	Fe (mg)	Cu (mg)	Se (mcg)	A (IU)	E (mg ATE)	B-2 (mg)	B-6 (mg)	FOL (mcg DFE)	REF
mixed berry jce, jce box, Min Maid - *6.8 fl oz*	100		0.0	25.0	23.0		25	100					60				
	215	0.0															MNTM8
mixed veg & fruit jce drink *8 fl oz*	273	177.3	0.5	69.4		0.7	50	17	10	0.15		258	62	0.05	0.2	0.00	
	248	0.1	<0.1	<0.1	<0.1	0	446	25	0.32	0.047	0.7	5166	<0.1	0.04	0.11	2.5	14119
orange apricot jce drink, cnd *8 fl oz*	128	216.8	0.8	31.8		0.3	5	13	10	0.13	0.010	73	50	0.05	0.5	0.00	0.19
	250	0.3	<0.1	0.1	0.1	0	200	20	0.25	0.088	0.0	1450	0.0	0.03	0.07	15.0	14327
orange banana jce w/Ca, Tropicana - *8 fl oz*	140		2.0	32.0	26.0		0	350	24				72	0.06	0.4		
	247	0.0					490							0.07	0.20	60.0	TROP10
orange cranberry jce w/Ca, refrig, Min Maid - *8 fl oz*	130		1.0	31.0	29.0		25	350	24				72	0.12	0.4		
	248	0.0					320							0.08	40		MNTM9
orange grapefruit jce, cnd *8 fl oz*	106	218.9	1.5	25.4		0.2	7	20	25	0.17	0.042	15	72	0.14	0.8	0.00	0.35
	247	0.2	<0.1	<0.1	<0.1	0	390	35	1.14	0.188	0.2	294	0.2	0.07	0.06	34.6	09217
orange jce, cnd *8 fl oz*	105	221.6	1.5	24.5		0.5	5	20	27	0.17	0.035	22	86	0.15	0.8	0.00	0.37
	249	0.3	<0.1	0.1	0.1	0	436	35	1.10	0.142	0.2	436	0.2	0.07	0.22	44.8	09207
orange jce, from frzn conc *8 fl oz*	112	219.4	1.7	26.8		0.5	2	22	25	0.12	0.035	10	97	0.20	0.5	0.00	0.39
	249	0.1	<0.1	<0.1	<0.1	0	473	40	0.25	0.110	0.2	194	0.5	0.04	0.11	109.6	09215
country style, Min Maid *8 fl oz*	110		0.0	27.0	24.0		0	20					96	0.15			
	249	0.0					480								60		MNTM15
low acid, Min Maid *8 fl oz*	110		0.0	27.0	24.0		0	20					96	0.15			
	249	0.0					480								60		MNTM22
pulp free, Min Maid *8 fl oz*	110		0.0	27.0	24.0		5	20					96	0.15			
	249	0.0					480								60		MNTM25
w/Ca, Min Maid *8 fl oz*	120		0.0	27.0	24.0		0	350					96	0.15			
	249	0.0					480								60		MNTM10
w/vit C, E, & Zn, Min Maid *8 fl oz*	120		0.0	27.0	24.0		0	20	24		1.5		144	0.15	0.4		
	249	0.0					480						20		0.08	60	MNTM13
orange jce, jce box, Min Maid *6.8 fl oz*	100		0.0	23.0	20.0		25	100					60	0.12			
	212	0.0					400								40		MNTM21
orange jce, refrig, country style, Min Maid - *8 fl oz*	110		2.0	27.0	24.0		25	20	24				72	0.15	0.4		
	248	0.0					480							0.08	60		MNTM16
grove made, Simply Orange *8 fl oz*	110		2.0	26.0	22.0		0	20	24				72	0.15	0.4		
	248	0.0					450							0.08	60		MNTM18
home squeezed style, Min Maid *8 fl oz*	110		2.0	27.0	24.0		25	20	24				72	0.15	0.4		
	248	0.0					480							0.08	60		MNTM20
home squeezed style w/Ca, Min Maid - *8 fl oz*	110		2.0	27.0	24.0		20	350					72	0.15	0.4		
	248	0.0					480							0.08	60		MNTM19
low acid, Min Maid *8 fl oz*	110		2.0	27.0	24.0		25	20	24				72	0.15	0.4		
	248	0.0					480							0.08	60		MNTM23
original, Simply Orange *8 fl oz*	110		2.0	26.0	22.0		0	20	24				72	0.15	0.4		
	248	0.0					450							0.08	60		MNTM24
pulp free, Min Maid *8 fl oz*	110		2.0	27.0	24.0		25	20					72	0.15	0.4		
	248	0.0					480							0.08			MNTM26
w/Ca, Minute Maid *8 fl oz*	110		2.0	27.0	24.0		25	350	24				72	0.15	0.4		
	248	0.0					480							0.08	60		MNTM11
w/Ca, Simply Orange *8 fl oz*	110		2.0	26.0	22.0		0	350	24				72	0.15	0.4		
	248	0.0					450							0.08	60		MNTM12
w/Ca, Tropicana *8 fl oz*	110		3.0	26.0	39.0		0	600	40				102	0.15	0.8		
	248	0.0					450							0.07	0.12	60.0	TROP18
w/vit A, C, E, Tropicana - *8 fl oz*	110		1.0	27.0	23.0		15	100					90				
	248	0.0					430					500	6.0			60.0	TROP17
w/vit C, E, & Zn, Min Maid *8 fl oz*	110		2.0	27.0	24.0		20	20	24		1.5		144	0.15	0.4		
	248	0.0					480						20		0.08	60	MNTM14
orange jce, raw *8 fl oz*	112	219.0	1.7	25.8		0.5	2	27	27	0.12	0.035	25	124	0.22	1.0	0.00	0.47
	248	0.5	0.1	0.1	0.1	0	496	42	0.50	0.109	0.2	496	0.2	0.07	0.10	74.4	09206
orange kiwi passion jce, Tropicana - *8 fl oz*	100		<1.0	26.0	23.0		15	20					6				
	247	0.0					300										TROP11
orange passion jce w/Ca, from frzn conc, Min Maid - *8 fl oz*	130		0.0	31.0	29.0		5	350	24				72	0.15	0.4		
	249	0.0					300							0.08	40		MNTM28
w/Ca, refrig, Min Maid *8 fl oz*	130		1.0	31.0	29.0		25	350	24				72	0.15	0.4		
	248	0.0					300							0.08	40		MNTM29

	KCAL	H₂0 (g)	PRO (g)	CHO (g)	SUGR (g)	DFIB (g)	Na (mg)	Ca (mg)	Mg (mg)	Zn (mg)	Mn (mg)	A (mcg RAE)	C (mg)	B-1 (mg)	NIA (mg)	B-12 (mcg)	PANT (mg)
	WT (g)	FAT (g)	SFA (g)	MUFA (g)	PUFA (g)	CHOL (mg)	K (mg)	P (mg)	Fe (mg)	Cu (mg)	Se (mcg)	A (IU)	E (mg ATE)	B-2 (mg)	B-6 (mg)	FOL (mcg DFE)	REF
orange peach mango jce, Tropicana - 8 fl oz	110		<1.0	27.0	26.0		20	20				6					
	247	0.0					300										TROP12
orange pineapple jce w/Ca, Tropicana - 8 fl oz	130		2.0	31.0	25.0		0	350	24				72	0.09	0.4		
	247	0.0					480							0.07	0.12	60.0	TROP13
orange ruby red jce w/Ca, Tropicana - 8 fl oz	110		2.0	26.0	22.0		0	350	24				72	0.15	0.8		
	247	0.0					450							0.07	0.12	60.0	TROP14
orange, strawbry, ban jce, from frzn conc, Trop Twister - 8 fl oz	474	129.7	1.0	115.3	90.8		64					26					
	248	1.0															14139
w/Ca, refrig, Min Maid 8 fl oz	130		1.0	31.0	28.0		25	350	24				72	0.12	0.4		
	247	0.0					340							0.08		40	MNTM30
orange strawberry jce w/Ca, Tropicana - 8 fl oz	130		2.0	30.0	24.0		0	350	24				72	0.09	0.4		
	247	0.0					450							0.07	0.12	60.0	TROP15
orange tangerine jce w/Ca, from frzn conc, Minute Maid - 8 fl oz	110		0.0	27.0	24.0		0	350	24				96	0.15	0.4		
	247	0.0					450							0.08			MNTM31
w/Ca, refrig, Min Maid 8 fl oz	100		2.0	27.0	24.0		20	350	24				72	0.15	0.4		
	247	0.0					450							0.08		60	MNTM32
w/Ca, Tropicana 8 fl oz	110		2.0	25.0	22.0		0	350	24				30	0.15	0.8		
	247	0.0					450							0.07	0.12	60.0	TROP16
orange tropical jce, jce box, Minute Maid - 6.8 fl oz	110		0.0	27.0	25.0		20	100	16				60				
	212	0.0					190									16	MNTM33
papaya nectar, cnd 8 fl oz	143	212.6	0.4	36.3		1.5	13	25	8	0.38	0.033	15	8	0.02	0.4	0.00	0.14
	250	0.4	0.1	0.1	0.1	0	78	0	0.85	0.033	0.8	278	<0.1	0.01	0.02	5.0	09229
passion fruit jce, purple, raw 8 fl oz	126	211.5	1.0	33.6		0.5	15	10	42	0.12		89	74	0.00	3.6	0.00	
	247	0.1	<0.1	<0.1	0.1	0	687	32	0.59	0.131	0.2	1771	0.1	0.32	0.12	17.3	09232
yellow, raw 8 fl oz	148	208.0	1.7	35.7		0.5	15	10	42	0.15		299	45	0.00	5.5	0.00	
	247	0.4	<0.1	0.1	0.3	0	687	62	0.89	0.124	0.2	5953	0.1	0.25	0.15	19.8	09233
peach nectar, cnd 8 fl oz	134	213.2	0.7	34.7		1.5	17	12	10	0.20	0.047	32	13	0.01	0.7	0.00	0.17
	249	<0.1	<0.1	<0.1	<0.1	0	100	15	0.47	0.172	0.5	642	<0.1	0.03	0.02	2.5	09251
pear nectar, cnd 8 fl oz	150	210.0	0.3	39.4		1.5	10	13	8	0.18	0.075	0	3	<0.01	0.3	0.00	0.06
	250	<0.1	<0.1	<0.1	<0.1	0	33	8	0.65	0.168	1.3	3	0.3	0.03	0.04	2.5	09262
pineapple grapefruit jce, cnd, Dole 6 fl oz can	100		1.0	24.0	19.0	0.0	15	20					60				
	188	0.0	0.0			0	260		0.36			0					DOLE17
pineapple grapefruit jce drink, cnd 8 fl oz	118	219.8	0.5	29.0		0.3	35	18	15	0.15	1.033	5	115	0.08	0.7	0.00	0.13
	250	0.3	<0.1	<0.1	0.1	0	153	15	0.78	0.113	0.0	88	0.0	0.04	0.11	27.5	14334
pink, cnd, Dole 6 fl oz	100		0.0	25.0	24.0		15	0					60				
	188	0.0	0.0			0	95		0.00			0					DOLE16
pineapple jce, cnd 8 fl oz	140	213.8	0.8	34.5		0.5	3	43	33	0.28	2.475	0	27	0.14	0.6	0.00	0.25
	250	0.2	<0.1	<0.1	0.1	0	335	20	0.65	0.225	0.3	13	<0.1	0.06	0.24	57.5	09273
from frzn conc 8 fl oz	130	216.3	1.0	31.9		0.5	3	28	23	0.28	2.475	3	30	0.18	0.5	0.00	0.31
	250	0.1	<0.1	<0.1	<0.1	0	340	20	0.75	0.225	0.3	25	<0.1	0.05	0.19	27.5	09275
pineapple orange banana jce, cnd, Dole - 6 fl oz can	100		1.0	25.0	18.0	0.0	15	20					60				
	188	0.0	0.0			0	290		0.36			0					DOLE20
pineapple orange jce, Dole 6 fl oz can	100		1.0	24.0	18.0	0.0	15	20					60				
	188	0.0	0.0			0	270		0.36			0					DOLE21
pineapple orange jce drink, cnd 8 fl oz	125	217.3	3.3	29.5		0.3	8	13	15	0.15	0.903	68	56	0.08	0.5	0.00	0.14
	250	0.0	0.0	0.0	0.0	0	115	10	0.68	0.103	0.0	1328	0.0	0.05	0.12	27.5	14341
prune jce, cnd 8 fl oz	182	208.0	1.6	44.7		2.6	10	31	36	0.54	0.387	0	10	0.04	2.0	0.00	0.27
	256	0.1	<0.1	0.1	<0.1	0	707	64	3.02	0.174	1.5	8	<0.1	0.18	0.56	0.0	09294
tangerine jce, cnd, sweetened 8 fl oz	125	216.6	1.2	29.9		0.5	2	45	20	0.07	0.092	52	55	0.15	0.2	0.00	0.31
	249	0.5	<0.1	<0.1	0.1	0	443	35	0.50	0.062	0.2	1046	0.2	0.05	0.08	12.5	09223
from frzn conc, sweetened 8 fl oz	111	212.3	1.0	26.7			2	19	19	0.07	0.089	70	58	0.13	0.2	0.00	0.30
	241	0.3	<0.1	<0.1	<0.1	0	272	19	0.24	0.060		1381		0.05	0.10	12.1	09225
raw 8 fl oz	106	219.6	1.2	24.9		0.5	2	44	20	0.07	0.091	52	77	0.15	0.2	0.00	0.31
	247	0.5	0.1	0.1	0.1	0	440	35	0.49	0.062	0.2	1037	0.2	0.05	0.10	12.4	09221
tomato jce 8 fl oz	41	228.2	1.8	10.3		1.0	877	22	27	0.34	0.187	68	44	0.11	1.6	0.00	0.61
	243	0.1	<0.1	<0.1	0.1	0	535	46	1.41	0.245	1.2	1351	2.2	0.08	0.27	48.6	11540
veg jce cocktail, cnd 8 fl oz	46	226.3	1.5	11.0		1.9	653	27	27	0.48	0.242	143	67	0.10	1.8	0.00	0.64
	242	0.2	<0.1	<0.1	0.1	0	467	41	1.02	0.484	1.2	2831	0.8	0.07	0.34	50.8	11578

[1] Values are averages for blackberry rush, cherry blast, peach fling, and strawberry watermelon.

[2] Sweetened with calcium saccharin and corn sweeteners.

[3] Values are averages for apple-strawberry, cranberry, grape drink, grape-strawberry, kiwi-strawberry, lemonade, orange drink, and tropical fruit punch.

	KCAL / WT (g)	H₂0 (g) / FAT (g)	PRO (g) / SFA (g)	CHO (g) / MUFA (g)	SUGR (g) / PUFA (g)	DFIB (g) / CHOL (mg)	Na (mg) / K (mg)	Ca (mg) / P (mg)	Mg (mg) / Fe (mg)	Zn (mg) / Cu (mg)	Mn (mg) / Se (mcg)	A (mcg RAE) / A (IU)	C (mg) / E (mg ATE)	B-1 (mg) / B-2 (mg)	NIA (mg) / B-6 (mg)	B-12 (mcg) / FOL (mcg DFE)	PANT (mg) / REF

15. FRUITS

Food	KCAL/WT	H₂0/FAT	PRO/SFA	CHO/MUFA	SUGR/PUFA	DFIB/CHOL	Na/K	Ca/P	Mg/Fe	Zn/Cu	Mn/Se	A-RAE/A-IU	C/E	B-1/B-2	NIA/B-6	B-12/FOL	PANT/REF
abiyuch, raw	79	91.1	1.7	20.1	9.7	6.0	23	9	27	0.35	0.207	6	62				
1/2 cup	114	0.1	<0.1				347	54	1.84	0.065		114					09427
acerola, raw	31	89.6	0.4	7.5		1.1	7	12	18	0.10		37	1644	0.02	0.4	0.00	0.30
1 cup	98	0.3	0.1	0.1	0.1	0	143	11	0.20	0.084	0.6	752	0.1	0.06	0.01	13.7	09001
apple, boiled w/o skin, cnd	91	146.2	0.4	23.3		4.1	2	9	5	0.07	0.202	3	<1	0.03	0.2	0.00	0.08
1 cup slices	171	0.6	0.1	<0.1	0.2	0	150	14	0.32	0.060	0.5	75	<0.1	0.02	0.08	1.7	09005
dried, sulfured	16	2.0	0.1	4.2		0.6	6	1	1	0.01	0.006	0	<1	0.00	0.1	0.00	0.02
1 ring	6	<0.1	<0.1	<0.1	<0.1	0	29	2	0.09	0.012	0.1	0	<0.1	0.01	0.01	0.0	09011
micro ckd w/o skin	95	143.9	0.5	24.5		4.8	2	9	5	0.07	0.241	3	1	0.03	0.1	0.00	0.08
1 cup slices	170	0.7	0.1	<0.1	0.2	0	158	14	0.29	0.078	0.5	68	<0.1	0.02	0.08	1.7	09006
raw w/skin	81	115.8	0.3	21.0		3.7	0	10	7	0.06	0.062	4	8	0.02	0.1	0.00	0.08
1 med (2 3/4″ dia)	138	0.5	0.1	<0.1	0.1	0	159	10	0.25	0.057	0.4	73	0.4	0.02	0.07	4.1	09003
raw w/o skin	73	108.1	0.2	19.0		2.4	0	5	4	0.05	0.029	3	5	0.02	0.1	0.00	0.07
1 med (2 3/4″ dia)	128	0.4	0.1	<0.1	0.1	0	145	9	0.09	0.040	0.4	56	0.1	0.01	0.06	0.0	09004
sliced, sweetened	137	168.0	0.4	34.1		3.5	6	8	4	0.06	0.312	6	1	0.02	0.1	0.00	0.06
1 cup slices	204	1.0	0.2	<0.1	0.3	0	139	10	0.47	0.108	0.6	104	<0.1	0.02	0.09	0.0	09007
applesauce, sweetened, cnd	194	202.9	0.5	50.8		3.1	8	10	8	0.10	0.191	3	4	0.03	0.5	0.00	0.13
1 cup	255	0.5	0.1	<0.1	0.1	0	156	18	0.89	0.110	0.8	28	<0.1	0.07	0.07	2.6	09020
unsweetened, cnd	105	215.6	0.4	27.5		2.9	5	7	7	0.07	0.183	2	3	0.03	0.5	0.00	0.23
1 cup	244	0.1	<0.1	<0.1	<0.1	0	183	17	0.29	0.063	0.7	71	<0.1	0.06	0.06	2.4	09019
applesauce, raspberry, w/Splenda,	54		0.2	14.0	9.0	1.5	10	60					5				
Musselman's - 4 oz	113	0.0	0.0			0			0.18			60					KNSE1
apricots, cnd, heavy syrup	214	200.4	1.3	55.3		4.1	28	23	21	0.26	0.132	160	7	0.05	1.1	0.00	0.24
1 cup whole	258	0.2	<0.1	0.1	<0.1	0	346	34	1.11	0.168		3199		0.06	0.14	5.2	09028
cnd, jce pack	117	211.4	1.5	30.1		3.9	10	29	24	0.27	0.127	207	12	0.04	0.8	0.00	0.22
1 cup halves	244	0.1	<0.1	<0.1	<0.1	0	403	49	0.73	0.132	0.7	4126	2.2	0.05	0.13	4.9	09024
cnd, light syrup	159	208.9	1.3	41.7		4.0	10	28	20	0.28	0.132	167	7	0.04	0.8	0.00	0.23
1 cup halves	253	0.1	<0.1	0.1	<0.1	0	349	33	0.99	0.200	0.8	3345	2.3	0.05	0.14	5.1	09026
cnd, water pack	50	212.1	1.6	12.4		2.5	25	18	20	0.25	0.120	207	4	0.05	1.0	0.00	0.21
1 cup whole	227	0.1	<0.1	<0.1	<0.1	0	350	36	1.23	0.154		4109		0.05	0.12	4.5	09023
dried, sulfured	313	40.2	4.4	81.4	69.5	9.5	13	72	42	0.51	0.306	234	1	0.02	3.4	0.00	0.67
1 cup halves	130	0.7	<0.1	0.1	0.1	0	1511	92	3.46	0.446	2.9	4685	5.7	0.10	0.19	13.0	09032
raw	74	133.8	2.2	17.2		3.7	2	22	12	0.40	0.122	203	16	0.05	0.9	0.00	0.37
1 cup halves (4.4 apricots)	155	0.6	<0.1	0.3	0.1	0	459	29	0.84	0.138	0.6	4049	1.4	0.06	0.08	14.0	09021
sweetened, frzn	237	177.4	1.7	60.7		5.3	10	24	22	0.24	0.121	203	22	0.05	1.9	0.00	0.48
1 cup	242	0.2	<0.1	0.1	<0.1	0	554	46	2.18	0.155	1.0	4066	2.2	0.10	0.15	4.8	09035
avocado, calif, raw	306	125.5	3.7	12.0		8.5	21	19	71	0.73	0.422	54	14	0.19	3.3	0.00	1.68
1 med	173	30.0	4.5	19.4	3.5	0	1097	73	2.04	0.460		1059	2.3	0.21	0.48	114.2	09038
avocado, florida, raw	340	242.4	4.8	27.1		16.1	15	33	103	1.28	0.517	94	24	0.33	5.8	0.00	2.95
1 med	304	27.0	5.3	14.8	4.5	0	1484	119	1.61	0.763		1860		0.37	0.85	161.1	09039
banana chips	147	1.2	0.7	16.6		2.2	2	5	22	0.21	0.442	1	2	0.02	0.2	0.00	0.18
1 oz	28	9.5	8.2	0.6	0.2	0	152	16	0.35	0.058	0.4	24	1.5	<0.01	0.07	4.0	19400
raw	109	87.6	1.2	27.6		2.8	1	7	34	0.19	0.179	5	11	0.05	0.6	0.00	0.31
1 med (7–7 7/8″ long)	118	0.6	0.2	<0.1	0.1	0	467	24	0.37	0.123	1.3	96	0.3	0.12	0.68	22.4	09040
blackberries, cnd, heavy syrup	236	192.2	3.4	59.1		8.7	8	54	44	0.46	1.784	28	7	0.07	0.7	0.00	0.39
1 cup	256	0.4	<0.1	<0.1	0.2	0	253	36	1.66	0.340	1.0	561	1.8	0.10	0.09	69.1	09046
raw	75	123.3	1.0	18.4		7.6	0	46	29	0.39	1.859	12	30	0.04	0.6	0.00	0.35
1 cup	144	0.6	<0.1	0.1	0.3	0	282	30	0.82	0.202	0.9	238	1.0	0.06	0.08	49.0	09042
unsweetened, frzn	97	124.1	1.8	23.7		7.6	2	44	33	0.38	1.847	9	5	0.04	1.8	0.00	0.23
1 cup	151	0.6	<0.1	0.1	0.4	0	211	45	1.21	0.181	0.9	172	1.1	0.07	0.09	51.3	09048
blueberries, cnd, heavy syrup	225	196.6	1.7	56.5		3.8	8	13	10	0.18	0.520	8	3	0.09	0.3	0.00	0.23
1 cup	256	0.8	0.1	0.1	0.4	0	102	26	0.84	0.136	1.0	164	2.6	0.14	0.09	5.1	09052
raw	81	122.7	1.0	20.5		3.9	9	9	7	0.16	0.409	7	19	0.07	0.5	0.00	0.13
1 cup	145	0.6	<0.1	0.1	0.2	0	129	15	0.25	0.088	0.9	145	1.5	0.07	0.05	8.7	09050
sweetened, frzn	186	178.0	0.9	50.5		4.8	2	14	5	0.14	0.603	5	2	0.05	0.6	0.00	0.29
1 cup	230	0.3	<0.1	<0.1	0.1	0	138	16	0.90	0.090	1.4	101	1.6	0.12	0.14	16.1	09055
boysenberries, cnd, heavy syrup	225	195.2	2.5	57.1		6.7	8	46	28	0.49	0.640	5	16	0.07	0.6	0.00	0.34
1 cup	256	0.3	<0.1	<0.1	0.2	0	230	26	1.10	0.179	1.0	102	1.8	0.07	0.10	87.0	09056

	KCAL	H₂O (g)	PRO (g)	CHO (g)	SUGR (g)	DFIB (g)	Na (mg)	Ca (mg)	Mg (mg)	Zn (mg)	Mn (mg)	A (mcg RAE)	C (mg)	B-1 (mg)	NIA (mg)	B-12 (mcg)	PANT (mg)
	WT (g)	FAT (g)	SFA (g)	MUFA (g)	PUFA (g)	CHOL (mg)	K (mg)	P (mg)	Fe (mg)	Cu (mg)	Se (mcg)	A (IU)	E (mg ATE)	B-2 (mg)	B-6 (mg)	FOL (mcg DFE)	REF
unsweetened, frzn	66	113.4	1.5	16.1		5.1	1	36	21	0.29	0.722	4	4	0.07	1.0	0.00	0.33
1 cup	132	0.3	<0.1	<0.1	0.2	0	183	36	1.12	0.106	0.8	88	0.6	0.05	0.07	83.2	09057
cantaloupe, raw	62	158.9	1.6	14.8		1.4	16	19	19	0.28	0.083	285	75	0.06	1.0	0.00	0.23
1 cup pieces	177	0.5	0.1	<0.1	0.2	0	547	30	0.37	0.074	0.7	5706	0.3	0.04	0.20	30.1	09181
carambola (star fruit), raw	30	82.7	0.5	7.1		2.5	2	4	8	0.10	0.075	23	19	0.03	0.4	0.00	
1 med (3 5/8" dia)	91	0.3	<0.1	<0.1	0.2	0	148	15	0.24	0.109	0.5	449	0.3	0.02	0.09	12.7	09060
carissa (natal plum), raw	12	16.8	0.1	2.7			1	2	3			<1	8	0.01	<0.1	0.00	
1 med	20	0.3				0	52	1	0.26	0.042		8		0.01			09061
casaba melon, raw	44	156.4	1.5	10.5		1.4	20	9	14	0.27		3	27	0.10	0.7	0.00	
1 cup pieces	170	0.2	<0.1	<0.1	0.1	0	357	12	0.68	0.068	0.5	51	0.3	0.03	0.20	28.9	09183
cherimoya, raw	115	123.8	2.6	27.6		3.6	6	12	25	0.28	0.129	0	18	0.14	0.9	0.00	0.37
1 cup diced	156	1.0				0	420	41	0.47	0.114		0		0.19	0.33	28.1	09062
cherries, sour, cnd, heavy syrup	233	193.7	1.9	59.6		2.8	18	26	15	0.15	0.184	92	5	0.04	0.4		0.27
1 cup	256	0.3	0.1	0.1	0.1	0	238	26	3.33	0.169	0.8	1828	0.3	0.10	0.11	20.5	09066
cnd, light syrup	189	200.6	1.9	48.6		2.0	18	25	15	0.18	0.184	91	5	0.04	0.4		0.26
1 cup	252	0.3	0.1	0.1	0.1	0	239	25	3.33	0.171		1830		0.10	0.11	20.2	09065
cnd, water pack	88	219.4	1.9	21.8	18.5	2.7	17	27	15	0.17	0.185	93	5	0.04	0.4		0.26
1 cup	244	0.2	0.1	0.1	0.1	0	239	24	3.34	0.171	0.7	1840	0.3	0.10	0.11	19.5	09064
raw	52	88.7	1.0	12.5		1.6	3	16	9	0.10	0.115	66	10	0.03	0.4	0.00	0.15
1cup	103	0.3	0.1	0.1	0.1	0	178	15	0.33	0.107	0.4	1321	0.1	0.04	0.05	8.2	09063
unsweetened, frzn	71	135.2	1.4	17.1		2.5	2	20	14	0.16	0.088	68	3	0.07	0.2	0.00	0.28
1 cup	155	0.7	0.2	0.2	0.2	0	192	25	0.82	0.140	0.6	1349	0.2	0.05	0.10	7.8	09068
cherries, sweet, cnd, heavy syrup	210	196.4	1.5	53.8		3.8	8	23	23	0.25	0.149	20	9	0.05	1.0	0.00	0.32
1 cup	253	0.4	0.1	0.1	0.1	0	367	46	0.89	0.359	0.8	390	0.2	0.10	0.08	10.1	09074
cnd, jce pack	135	212.4	2.3	34.5		3.8	8	35	30	0.25	0.153	15	6	0.05	1.0	0.00	0.32
1 cup	250	<0.1	<0.1	<0.1	<0.1	0	328	55	1.45	0.183	0.8	313	0.3	0.06	0.08	10.0	09072
cnd, light syrup	169	205.5	1.5	43.6		3.8	8	23	23	0.25	0.151	20	9	0.05	1.0	0.00	0.32
1 cup	252	0.4	0.1	0.1	0.1	0	373	45	0.91	0.365	0.8	396	0.3	0.10	0.08	10.1	09073
cnd, water pack	114	215.9	1.9	29.2		3.7	2	27	22	0.20	0.154	20	5	0.05	1.0	0.00	0.31
1 cup	248	0.3	0.1	0.1	0.1	0	325	37	0.89	0.186	0.7	397	0.3	0.10	0.07	9.9	09071
raw	84	94.5	1.4	19.4		2.7	0	18	13	0.07	0.108	13	8	0.06	0.5	0.00	0.15
1cup	117	1.1	0.3	0.3	0.3	0	262	22	0.46	0.111	0.7	250	0.2	0.07	0.04	4.7	09070
sweetened, frzn	231	195.6	3.0	57.9		5.4	3	31	26	0.10	0.282	23	3	0.07	0.5	0.00	0.33
1 cup	259	0.3	0.1	0.1	0.1	0	515	41	0.91	0.062	1.0	490	0.3	0.12	0.09	10.4	09076
crabapples, raw	84	86.8	0.4	21.9			1	20	8		0.127	2	9	0.03	0.1	0.00	
1 cup slices	110	0.3	0.1	<0.1	0.1	0	213	17	0.40	0.074		44		0.02			09077
cranberries, raw	47	82.2	0.4	12.0		4.0	1	7	5	0.12	0.149	2	13	0.03	0.1	0.00	0.21
1 cup whole	95	0.2	<0.1	<0.1	0.1	0	67	9	0.19	0.055	0.6	44	0.1	0.02	0.06	1.9	09078
cranberry orange relish, cnd	490	146.3	0.8	127.1		0.0	88	30	11			11	50	0.03	0.0	0.00	
1 cup	275	0.3	<0.1			0	105	22	0.55	0.110		193		0.06			09082
cranberry sce, jelled, cnd	86	34.6	0.1	22.2		0.6	17	2	2	0.03	0.034	1	1	0.01	0.1	0.00	
1/2" thick slice	57	0.1	<0.1	<0.1	<0.1	0	15	3	0.13	0.011	0.3	11	0.1	0.01	0.01	0.6	09081
currants, european black, raw	71	91.8	1.6	17.2			2	62	27	0.30	0.287	13	203	0.06	0.3	0.00	0.45
1 cup	112	0.5	<0.1	0.1	0.2	0	361	66	1.72	0.096		258	1.1	0.06	0.07		09083
currants, red & white, raw	63	94.0	1.6	15.5		4.8	1	37	15	0.26	0.208	7	46	0.04	0.1	0.00	0.07
1 cup	112	0.2	<0.1	<0.1	0.1	0	308	49	1.12	0.120	0.7	134	0.1	0.06	0.08	9.0	09084
currants, zante, dried[1]	408	27.7	5.9	106.7		9.8	12	124	59	0.95	0.675	6	7	0.23	2.3	0.00	0.06
1 cup	144	0.4	<0.1	0.1	0.3	0	1284	180	4.69	0.674	1.0	105	0.1	0.20	0.43	14.4	09085
custard apple (bullock's heart), raw	101	71.5	1.7	25.2		2.4	4	30	18			2	19	0.08	0.5	0.00	0.14
3.5 oz	100	0.6	0.2			0	382	21	0.71			33		0.10	0.22		09086
dates, dried	23	1.9	0.2	6.1		0.6	0	3	3	0.02	0.025	<1	0	0.01	0.2	0.00	0.06
1 date	8	<0.1	<0.1	<0.1	<0.1	0	54	3	0.10	0.024	0.2	4	<0.1	0.01	0.02	1.1	09087
dried fruit bar	81	3.2	0.4	18.1		0.8	18	7	5	0.04	0.042	1	16	0.01	<0.1	0.00	0.02
.81 oz bar	23	1.2	0.9	0.1	<0.1	0	32	13	0.18	0.039	0.6	27		0.01	0.07	0.9	19011
durian, raw/frzn	357	157.9	3.6	65.8		9.2	2	15	73	0.68	0.787	5	48	0.91	2.6	0.00	0.56
1 cup chopped	243	13.0				0	1059	92	1.04	0.503		109		0.49	0.77		09422
elderberries, raw	106	115.7	1.0	26.7		10.2	9	55	7	0.16		44	52	0.10	0.7	0.00	0.20
1 cup	145	0.7	<0.1	0.1	0.4	0	406	57	2.32	0.088	0.9	870	1.5	0.09	0.33	8.7	09088
feijoa, raw	25	43.3	0.6	5.3			2	9	5	0.02	0.043	0	10	<0.01	0.1	0.00	0.11
1 med	50	0.4				0	78	10	0.04	0.028		0		0.02	0.03	19.0	09334
figs, cnd, heavy syrup	25	21.4	0.1	6.4		0.6	0	8	3	0.03	0.024	1	<1	0.01	0.1	0.00	0.02
1 fig w/liquid	28	<0.1	<0.1	<0.1	<0.1	0	28	3	0.08	0.030	0.1	10	0.2	0.01	0.02	0.6	09092

	KCAL / WT (g)	H₂0 (g) / FAT (g)	PRO (g) / SFA (g)	CHO (g) / MUFA (g)	SUGR (g) / PUFA (g)	DFIB (g) / CHOL (mg)	Na (mg) / K (mg)	Ca (mg) / P (mg)	Mg (mg) / Fe (mg)	Zn (mg) / Cu (mg)	Mn (mg) / Se (mcg)	A (mcg RAE) / A (IU)	C (mg) / E (mg ATE)	B-1 (mg) / B-2 (mg)	NIA (mg) / B-6 (mg)	B-12 (mcg) / FOL (mcg DFE)	PANT (mg) / REF
dried	48	5.4	0.6	12.4		2.3	2	27	11	0.10	0.074	1	<1	0.01	0.1		0.08
1 fig	19	0.2	<0.1	<0.1	0.1	0	135	13	0.42	0.059	0.2	25	0.0	0.02	0.04	1.5	09094
raw	37	39.6	0.4	9.6		1.7	1	18	9	0.08	0.064	4	1	0.03	0.2		0.15
1 med (2 1/4" dia)	50	0.2	<0.1	<0.1	0.1	0	116	7	0.19	0.035	0.3	71	0.4	0.03	0.06	3.0	09089
Fruit by the Foot, Betty Crocker[2]	80		0.0	17.0	10.0	0.0	50	0					15				
.7 oz roll	21	1.5	0.0			0			0.00			0					GENM206
fruit cocktail, cnd, heavy syrup[3]	181	199.4	1.0	46.9		2.5	15	15	12	0.20	0.357	25	5	0.04	0.9	0.00	0.15
1 cup	248	0.2	<0.1	<0.1	0.1	0	218	27	0.72	0.171	1.2	508	0.7	0.05	0.12	7.4	09100
cnd, jce pack	109	207.2	1.1	28.1		2.4	9	19	17	0.21	0.346	36	6	0.03	1.0	0.00	0.15
1 cup	237	<0.1	<0.1	<0.1	<0.1	0	225	33	0.50	0.147	1.2	723	0.5	0.04	0.12	7.1	09097
cnd, water pack	76	215.1	1.0	20.2		2.4	9	12	17	0.21	0.356	31	5	0.04	0.9	0.00	0.15
1 cup	237	0.1	<0.1	<0.1	<0.1	0	223	26	0.59	0.168	1.2	593	0.7	0.03	0.12	7.1	09096
Fruit Gushers, all flvrs, Bty	90		0.0	20.0	13.0	0.0	55	0					15				
Crocker - .9 oz pouch	25	1.0	0.0			0			0.00			0					GENM207
fruit roll	74	2.3	0.2	17.7		0.8	13	7	4	0.04	0.039	1	1	0.01	<0.1	0.00	0.07
1 large roll (.74 oz)	21	0.6	0.1	0.3	0.1	0	62	7	0.21	0.036	0.6	24	0.1	<0.01	0.06	1.7	19014
berry, Fruit Roll-Ups	104	2.9	0.0	23.9	10.8		89						34				
2 rolls	28	1.0	0.3	0.5	<0.1						0.9						19269
Fruit Roll-Ups, Bty Crckr[4]	50		0.0	12.0	7.0	0.0	55	0					15				
.5 oz roll	14	1.0	0.0			0			0.00			0					GENM208
fruit salad, cnd, heavy syrup[5]	186	204.7	0.9	48.7		2.6	15	15	13	0.18	0.370	64	6	0.04	0.9	0.00	0.14
1 cup	255	0.2	<0.1	<0.1	0.1	0	204	23	0.71	0.163	1.3	1285	1.2	0.05	0.08	7.7	09105
cnd, jce pack	125	214.5	1.3	32.5		2.5	12	27	20	0.35	0.376	75	8	0.03	0.9	0.00	0.13
1 cup	249	0.1	<0.1	<0.1	<0.1	0	289	35	0.62	0.125		1494		0.03	0.07	7.5	09103
tropical, cnd, heavy syrup[6]	221	197.3	1.1	57.5		3.3	5	33	33	0.28		15	45	0.14	1.4	0.00	
1 cup	257	0.3	<0.1	<0.1	0.1	0	337	18	1.34	0.206	1.3	326	1.3	0.12	0.31	23.1	09325
Fruit Shapes, Betty Crocker[7]	80		0.0	21.0	14.0	0.0	50	0					60				
.9 oz pouch	25	0.0	0.0			0			0.00			0					GENM210
Bugs Bunny, ScoobyDoo!, Bty	100		0.0	24.0	16.0	0.0	60	0					60				
Crckr[7] - 10 pcs (large pouch)	30	0.0	0.0			0			0.00			0					GENM209
Fruitfield's Adult	100		0.0	23.0	15.0	0.0	80	100					18				
10 pieces	30	0.5	0.0			0			0.00			0					GENM211
Fruit Snacks, strawberry, Nabisco	90		1.0	21.0	16.0	0.0	15	0					0	15			
12 pieces	30	0.0	0.0	0.0	0.0	0			0.00				5.0				NBSC2
w/vit A,C,E, Farley	89	3.8	1.1	21.0			9						23				
1 pouch	26	0.0										1413	10.4				19272
gooseberries, cnd, light syrup	184	201.9	1.6	47.3		6.0	5	40	15	0.28	0.446	18	25	0.05	0.4	0.00	0.35
1 cup	252	0.5	<0.1	<0.1	0.3	0	194	18	0.83	0.547	1.0	348	0.9	0.13	0.03	7.6	09109
raw	66	131.8	1.3	15.3		6.5	2	38	15	0.18	0.216	23	42	0.06	0.5	0.00	0.43
1 cup	150	0.9	0.1	0.1	0.5	0	297	41	0.47	0.105	0.9	435	0.6	0.05	0.12	9.0	09107
grapefruit, cnd, jce pack	92	223.3	1.7	22.9		1.0	17	37	27	0.20	0.017	0	84	0.07	0.6	0.00	0.30
1 cup	249	0.2	<0.1	<0.1	0.1	0	421	30	0.52	0.092	2.2	0	0.6	0.04	0.05	22.4	09120
cnd, light syrup	152	212.3	1.4	39.2		1.0	5	36	25	0.20	0.018	0	54	0.10	0.6	0.00	
1 cup	254	0.3	<0.1	<0.1	0.1	0	328	25	1.02	0.168	2.3	0	0.6	0.05	0.05	22.9	09121
pink & red, raw	37	112.4	0.7	9.4		1.0	0	14	10	0.09	0.012	16	47	0.04	0.2	0.00	0.35
1/2 med (3 3/4" dia)	123	0.1	<0.1	<0.1	<0.1	0	159	11	0.15	0.054		319		0.02	0.05	14.8	09112
white, raw	39	106.8	0.8	9.9		1.3	0	14	11	0.08	0.015	1	39	0.04	0.3	0.00	0.33
1/2 med (3 3/4" dia)	118	0.1	<0.1	<0.1	<0.1	0	175	9	0.07	0.059	1.7	12	0.3	0.02	0.05	11.8	09116
grapes, american (slip skin), raw	62	74.8	0.6	15.8		0.9	2	13	5	0.04	0.661	5	4	0.08	0.3	0.00	0.02
1 cup	92	0.3	0.1	<0.1	0.1	0	176	9	0.27	0.037	0.2	92	0.3	0.05	0.10	3.7	09131
grapes, european, red/green, seedless, raw - 1 cup	114	128.9	1.1	28.4		1.6	3	18	10	0.08	0.093	6	17	0.15	0.5	0.00	0.04
	160	0.9	0.3	<0.1	0.3	0	296	21	0.42	0.144	0.3	117	1.1	0.09	0.18	6.4	09132
grapes, thompson seedless, cnd, heavy syrup - 1 cup	187	203.6	1.2	50.3		1.0	13	26	15	0.13	0.097	8	3	0.08	0.3	0.00	0.10
	256	0.3	0.1	<0.1	0.1	0	264	44	2.41	0.138	0.3	164	1.8	0.06	0.17	7.7	09134
groundcherries, raw[8]	74	119.6	2.7	15.7				13				50	15	0.15	3.9	0.00	
1 cup	140	1.0				0		56	1.40			1008		0.06			09138
guava, raw	46	77.5	0.7	10.7		4.9	3	18	9	0.21	0.130	36	165	0.05	1.1	0.00	0.14
1 med	90	0.5	0.2	<0.1	0.2	0	256	23	0.28	0.093	0.5	713	1.0	0.05	0.13	12.6	09139
guava, strawberry, raw	168	196.8	1.4	42.4		13.2	90	51	41			12	90	0.07	1.5	0.00	
1 cup	244	1.5	0.4	0.1	0.6	0	712	66	0.54			220		0.07			09140
honeydew melon, raw	62	158.7	0.8	16.2		1.1	18	11	12	0.12	0.032	4	44	0.14	1.1	0.00	0.37
1 cup pieces	177	0.2	<0.1	<0.1	0.1	0	480	18	0.12	0.073	0.7	71	0.3	0.03	0.10	10.6	09184

	KCAL / WT (g)	H₂O (g) / FAT (g)	PRO (g) / SFA (g)	CHO (g) / MUFA (g)	SUGR (g) / PUFA (g)	DFIB (g) / CHOL (mg)	Na (mg) / K (mg)	Ca (mg) / P (mg)	Mg (mg) / Fe (mg)	Zn (mg) / Cu (mg)	Mn (mg) / Se (mcg)	A (mcg RAE) / A (IU)	C (mg) / E (mg ATE)	B-1 (mg) / B-2 (mg)	NIA (mg) / B-6 (mg)	B-12 (mcg) / FOL (mcg DFE)	PANT (mg) / REF
jackfruit, raw	155	120.8	2.4	39.6		2.6	5	56	61	0.69	0.325	25	11	0.05	0.7	0.00	
1 cup slices	165	0.5	0.1	0.1	0.1	0	500	59	0.99	0.309	1.0	490	0.2	0.18	0.18	23.1	09144
java plum, raw	81	112.2	1.0	21.0			19	26	20			0	19	0.01	0.4	0.00	
1 cup	135	0.3				0	107	23	0.26			4		0.02	0.05		09145
jujube, dried	80	5.5	1.0	20.6			3	22	10	0.05	0.085		4			0.00	
1 oz	28	0.3				0	149	28	0.50	0.074				0.10			09147
raw	79	77.9	1.2	20.2			3	21	10	0.05	0.084	2	69	0.02	0.9	0.00	
3.5 oz	100	0.2				0	250	23	0.48	0.073		40		0.04	0.08		09146
kiwifruit (chinese gooseberry), raw	46	63.1	0.8	11.3		2.6	4	20	23	0.13		7	74	0.02	0.4	0.00	
1 med	76	0.3	<0.1	<0.1	0.2	0	252	30	0.31	0.119	0.5	133	0.9	0.04	0.07	28.9	09148
kumquats, raw	12	15.5	0.2	3.1		1.3	1	8	2	0.02	0.016	3	7	0.02	0.1	0.00	
1 med	19	<0.1	<0.1	<0.1	<0.1	0	37	4	0.07	0.020	0.1	57	<0.1	0.02	0.01	3.0	09149
lemon peel	3	4.9	0.1	1.0		0.6	0	8	1	0.02		<1	8	<0.01	<0.1	0.00	0.02
1 T	6	<0.1	<0.1	<0.1	<0.1	0	10	1	0.05	0.006	<0.1	3	<0.1	<0.01	0.01	0.8	09156
lemon, raw	17	51.6	0.6	5.4		1.6	1	15	5	0.03	0.017	1	31	0.02	0.1	0.00	0.11
1 med (2 1/8″ dia)	58	0.2	<0.1	<0.1	0.1	0	80	9	0.35	0.021	0.2	17	0.1	0.01	0.05	6.4	09150
lichis/litchees, dried	7	0.6	0.1	1.8		0.1	0	1	1	0.01	0.006	0	5	<0.01	0.1	0.00	
1 fruit	2	<0.1	<0.1	<0.1	<0.1	0	28	5	0.04	0.016	<0.1	0	<0.1	0.01	<0.01	0.3	09165
raw	6	7.8	0.1	1.6		0.1	0	0	1	0.01	0.005	0	7	<0.01	0.1	0.00	
1 med	10	<0.1	<0.1	<0.1	<0.1	0	16	3	0.03	0.014	0.1	0	0.1	0.01	0.01	1.3	09164
lime, raw	20	59.1	0.5	7.1		1.9	1	22	4	0.07	0.005	1	19	0.02	0.1	0.00	0.15
1 med (2″ dia)	67	0.1	<0.1	<0.1	<0.1	0	68	12	0.40	0.044	0.3	7	0.2	0.01	0.03	5.4	09159
loganberries, frzn	81	124.4	2.2	19.1		7.2	1	38	31	0.50	1.833	3	22	0.07	1.2	0.00	0.36
1 cup	147	0.5	<0.1	<0.1	0.3	0	213	38	0.94	0.172	0.9	51	3.2	0.05	0.10	38.2	09167
longans, dried	80	4.9	1.4	20.7			13	13	13	0.06	0.069	0	8	0.01	0.3	0.00	
1 oz	28	0.1				0	184	55	1.51	0.226		0		0.14			09173
raw	2	2.6	0.0	0.5		0.0	0	0	<1	<0.01	0.002		3	<0.01	<0.1		
1 med	3	<0.1				0	9	1	<0.01	0.005				<0.01			09172
loquats, raw	8	13.9	0.1	1.9		0.3	0	3	2	0.01	0.024	12	<1	<0.01	<0.1	0.00	
1 med	16	<0.1	<0.1	<0.1	<0.1	0	43	4	0.04	0.006	0.1	244	0.1	<0.01	0.02	2.2	09174
mammy apple (mamey), raw	431	729.3	4.2	105.8		25.4	127	93	135	0.85		102	118	0.17	3.4	0.00	0.87
1 med	846	4.2	1.2	1.7	0.7	0	398	93	5.92	0.728	5.1	1946	5.0	0.34	0.85	118.4	09175
mandarin oranges, cnd, jce pack	92	222.9	1.5	23.8		1.7	12	27	27	1.27	0.080	107	85	0.20	1.1	0.00	0.31
1 cup	249	0.1	<0.1	<0.1	<0.1	0	331	25	0.67	0.082	1.0	2121	1.2	0.07	0.10	12.5	09219
cnd, jce pack, Dole	52		0.6	12.4	9.8	0.7	6	7					9				
1/2 cup	122	0.0	0.0			0	104		0.61			1025					DOLE12
cnd, light syrup	154	209.3	1.1	40.8		1.8	15	18	20	0.60	0.081	106	50	0.13	1.1	0.00	0.32
1 cup	252	0.3	<0.1	<0.1	<0.1	0	197	25	0.93	0.111	1.0	2117	0.9	0.11	0.11	12.6	09220
cnd, light syrup, Dole	85		1.0	20.2	15.8	1.1	10	12					14				
7 oz can	198	0.0	0.0			0	168		0.99			1663					DOLE9
light syrup, Dole Fruit Bowl	70		0.0	18.0	17.0	0.0							18				
4 oz bowl	113	0.0	0.0			0	75										DOLE10
light syrup, Dole Fruit Bowl	120		<1.0	29.0	28.0	1.0	15	0					48				
1 cup	198	0.0	0.0			0	130		0.00			0					DOLE11
mango, raw	135	169.1	1.1	35.2		3.7	4	21	19	0.08	0.056	404	57	0.12	1.2	0.00	0.33
1 med	207	0.6	0.1	0.2	0.1	0	323	23	0.27	0.228	1.2	8061	2.3	0.12	0.28	29.0	09176
mangosteen, cnd, syrup	143	158.6	0.8	35.1		3.5	14	24	25	0.41	0.200		6	0.11	0.6	0.00	0.06
1 cup	196	1.1				0	94	16	0.59	0.135				0.11	0.04	60.8	09177
melon balls (cantaloupe & honeydew), frzn - *1 cup*	57	156.1	1.5	13.7		1.2	54	17	24	0.29	0.069	154	11	0.29	1.1	0.00	0.28
	173	0.4	0.1	<0.1	0.2	0	484	21	0.50	0.104		3069	0.3	0.04	0.18	45.0	09185
mixed fruit, cnd, heavy syrup[9]	184	205.4	0.9	47.8		2.6	10	3	13	0.18	0.984	26	176	0.04	1.5	0.00	0.15
1 cup	255	0.3	<0.1	<0.1	0.1	0	214	26	0.92	0.148		495		0.10	0.09	7.7	09187
dried (prunes, apricots, pears)	712	91.4	7.2	187.7		22.9	53	111	114	1.47	0.665	357	11	0.13	5.6	0.00	1.29
11 oz pkg	293	1.4	0.1	0.7	0.3	0	2332	226	7.94	1.128		7155		0.46	0.47	11.7	09188
light syrup, Dole Fruit Bowl	80		<1.0	19.0	17.0	1.0	10						24				
4 oz bowl	113	0.0	0.0			0	90										DOLE13
sweetened, frzn[10]	245	184.3	3.6	60.6		4.8	8	18	15	0.13	0.160	40	188	0.04	1.0	0.00	0.23
1 cup	250	0.5	0.1	0.1	0.2	0	328	30	0.70	0.085		805		0.09	0.06	20.0	09189
mulberries, raw	60	122.8	2.0	13.7		2.4	14	55	25	0.17		1	51	0.04	0.9	0.00	
1 cup	140	0.5	<0.1	0.1	0.3	0	272	53	2.59	0.084	0.8	35	0.6	0.14	0.07	8.4	09190
nectarine, raw	67	117.3	1.3	16.0		2.2	0	7	11	0.12	0.060	50	7	0.02	1.3	0.00	0.21
1 med (2 1/2″ dia)	136	0.6	0.1	0.2	0.3	0	288	22	0.20	0.099	0.5	1001	1.2	0.06	0.03	5.4	09191

	KCAL / WT (g)	H₂0 (g) / FAT (g)	PRO (g) / SFA (g)	CHO (g) / MUFA (g)	SUGR (g) / PUFA (g)	DFIB (g) / CHOL (mg)	Na (mg) / K (mg)	Ca (mg) / P (mg)	Mg (mg) / Fe (mg)	Zn (mg) / Cu (mg)	Mn (mg) / Se (mcg)	A (mcg RAE) / A (IU)	C (mg) / E (mg ATE)	B-1 (mg) / B-2 (mg)	NIA (mg) / B-6 (mg)	B-12 (mcg) / FOL (mcg DFE)	PANT (mg) / REF
oheloberries, raw	39	129.2	0.5	9.6			1	10	8			59	8	0.02	0.4	0.00	
1 cup	140	0.3				0	53	14	0.13			1162		0.05			09192
orange, all varieties, raw	62	113.6	1.2	15.4		3.1	0	52	13	0.09	0.033	13	70	0.11	0.4	0.00	0.33
1 med (2 5/8" dia)	131	0.2	<0.1	<0.1	<0.1	0	237	18	0.13	0.059	0.7	269	0.3	0.05	0.08	39.3	09200
CA navel, raw	64	121.5	1.4	16.3		3.4	1	56	14	0.08	0.038	13	80	0.12	0.4	0.00	0.35
1 med (2 7/8" dia)	140	0.2	<0.1	<0.1	<0.1	0	249	27	0.17	0.078		256		0.06	0.10	47.6	09202
CA valencia, raw	59	104.5	1.3	14.4		3.0	0	48	12	0.07	0.028	15	59	0.11	0.3	0.00	0.30
1 med (2 5/8" dia)	121	0.4	<0.1	0.1	0.1	0	217	21	0.11	0.045		278		0.05	0.08	47.2	09201
FL, raw	65	122.9	1.0	16.3		3.4	0	61	14	0.11	0.034	14	63	0.14	0.6	0.00	0.35
1 med (2 5/8" dia)	141	0.3	<0.1	0.1	0.1	0	238	17	0.13	0.055	0.7	282	0.3	0.06	0.07	24.0	09203
orange peel	6	4.4	0.1	1.5		0.6	0	10	1	0.02		1	8	0.01	0.1	0.00	0.03
1 T	6	<0.1	<0.1	<0.1	<0.1	0	13	1	0.05	0.006	0.1	25	<0.1	0.01	0.01	1.8	09216
papaya, raw	119	270.0	1.9	29.8		5.5	9	73	30	0.21	0.033	43	188	0.08	1.0	0.00	0.66
1 med (5 1/8" long × 3" dia)	304	0.4	0.1	0.1	0.1	0	781	15	0.30	0.049	1.8	863	3.4	0.10	0.06	115.5	09226
passion fruit (grandilla), purple, raw - *1 med*	17	13.1	0.4	4.2		1.9	5	2	5	0.02		6	5	0.00	0.3	0.00	
	18	0.1	<0.1	<0.1	0.1	0	63	12	0.29	0.015	0.1	126	0.2	0.02	0.02	2.5	09231
peach, cnd, heavy syrup	194	207.7	1.2	52.2		3.4	16	8	13	0.24	0.118	45	7	0.03	1.6	0.00	0.13
1 cup	262	0.3	<0.1	0.1	0.1	0	241	29	0.71	0.134	0.8	870	2.3	0.06	0.05	7.9	09241
cnd, jce pack	110	218.7	1.6	28.9		3.3	10	15	18	0.28	0.120	48	9	0.02	1.5	0.00	0.13
1 cup	250	0.1	<0.1	<0.1	<0.1	0	320	43	0.68	0.125	0.8	953	3.8	0.04	0.05	7.5	09238
cnd, light syrup	136	212.0	1.1	36.5		3.3	13	8	13	0.23	0.115	45	6	0.02	1.5	0.00	0.13
1 cup	251	0.1	<0.1	<0.1	<0.1	0	243	28	0.90	0.131	0.8	889	2.2	0.06	0.05	7.5	09240
cnd, water pack	59	227.2	1.1	14.9		3.2	7	5	12	0.22	0.117	66	7	0.02	1.3	0.00	0.12
1 cup	244	0.1	<0.1	0.1	0.1	0	242	24	0.78	0.132	0.7	1298	2.2	0.05	0.05	7.3	09237
dried, sulfured	382	50.9	5.8	98.1		13.1	11	45	67	0.91	0.488	173	8	<0.01	7.0	0.00	0.90
1 cup halves	160	1.2	0.1	0.4	0.6	0	1594	190	6.50	0.582	3.5	3461	0.0	0.34	0.11	0.0	09246
light syrup, Dole Fruit Bowl	70		<1.0	14.0	14.0	1.0	15						24				
4 oz bowl	113	0.0	0.0			0	90										DOLE14
raw	42	85.9	0.7	10.9		2.0	0	5	7	0.14	0.046	26	6	0.02	1.0	0.00	0.17
1 med (2 1/2" dia)	98	0.1	<0.1	<0.1	<0.1	0	193	12	0.11	0.067	0.4	524	0.7	0.04	0.02	2.9	09236
sliced, light syrup, Dole Fruit Bowl - *1 cup*	120		<1.0	29.0	27.0	2.0	15	0					48				
Bowl - 1 cup	198	0.0	0.0			0	150		0.00			200					DOLE15
spiced, cnd, heavy syrup	182	191.7	1.0	48.6		3.1	10	15	17	0.19		39	13	0.03	1.3	0.00	0.12
1 cup	242	0.2	<0.1	0.1	0.1	0	206	22	0.68	0.237	0.7	767	2.2	0.08	0.05	7.3	09243
sweetened, frzn	235	186.8	1.6	60.0		4.5	15	8	13	0.13	0.073	35	236	0.03	1.6	0.00	0.33
1 cup	250	0.3	<0.1	0.1	0.2	0	325	28	0.93	0.060	1.0	710	2.2	0.09	0.05	7.5	09250
pear, asian, raw	51	107.7	0.6	13.0		4.4	0	5	10	0.02	0.073	0	5	0.01	0.3	0.00	0.09
1 pear (2 1/2" long, 2 1/2" dia)	122	0.3	<0.1	0.1	0.1	0	148	13	0.00	0.061	0.7	0	0.6	0.01	0.03	9.8	09340
pear, cnd, heavy syrup	197	213.7	0.5	51.0		4.3	13	13	11	0.21	0.085	0	3	0.03	0.6	0.00	0.06
1 cup	266	0.3	<0.1	0.1	0.1	0	173	19	0.59	0.130	1.1	0	1.3	0.06	0.04	2.7	09257
cnd, jce pack	124	214.4	0.8	32.1		4.0	10	22	17	0.22	0.084	0	4	0.03	0.5	0.00	0.05
1 cup	248	0.2	<0.1	<0.1	<0.1	0	238	30	0.72	0.131	1.0	15	1.2	0.03	0.03	2.5	09254
cnd, light syrup	143	212.0	0.5	38.1		4.0	13	13	10	0.20	0.083	0	2	0.03	0.4	0.00	0.06
1 cup	251	0.1	<0.1	<0.1	<0.1	0	166	18	0.70	0.123	1.0	0	1.3	0.04	0.04	2.5	09256
cnd, water pack	71	224.0	0.5	19.1		3.9	5	10	10	0.22	0.083	0	2	0.02	0.1	0.00	0.05
1 cup	244	0.1	<0.1	<0.1	<0.1	0	129	17	0.51	0.124	1.0	0	1.2	0.02	0.03	2.4	09253
dried, sulfured	459	46.7	3.3	122.0		13.1	11	60	58	0.68	0.572	5	12	0.01	2.4	0.00	0.27
10 halves	175	1.1	0.1	0.2	0.3	0	933	103	3.68	0.649	7.9	5	0.0	0.25	0.13	0.0	09259
raw	98	139.1	0.6	25.1		4.0	0	18	10	0.20	0.126	2	7	0.03	0.2	0.00	0.12
1 med	166	0.7	<0.1	0.1	0.2	0	208	18	0.42	0.188	1.7	33	0.8	0.07	0.03	11.6	09252
persimmon, japanese, dried	93	7.8	0.5	25.0		4.9	1	9	11	0.14	0.473	10	0		0.1	0.00	
1 med	34	0.2				0	273	28	0.25	0.150		190		0.01			09264
raw	118	134.9	1.0	31.2		6.0	2	13	15	0.18	0.596	181	13	0.05	0.2	0.00	
1 med (2 1/2" dia)	168	0.3	<0.1	0.1	0.1	0	270	29	0.25	0.190	1.0	3641	1.0	0.03	0.17	13.4	09263
persimmon, raw	32	16.1	0.2	8.4			0	7					17			0.00	
1 med	25	0.1				0	78	7	0.63								09265
pineapple, cnd, heavy syrup	198	200.6	0.9	51.3		2.0	3	36	41	0.30	2.743	3	19	0.23	0.7	0.00	0.25
1 cup pieces	254	0.3	<0.1	<0.1	0.1	0	264	18	0.97	0.257	1.0	36	0.3	0.06	0.19	12.7	09270
cnd, jce pack	149	207.9	1.0	39.1		2.0	2	35	35	0.25	2.791	5	24	0.24	0.7	0.00	0.25
1 cup pieces	249	0.2	<0.1	<0.1	0.1	0	304	15	0.70	0.214	1.0	95	0.2	0.05	0.18	12.5	09268
jce pack, Dole Fruit Bowl	90		<1.0	24.0	21.0	2.0	15	0					30				
1 cup	198	0.0	0.0			0	150		0.00			0					DOLE19

	KCAL / WT (g)	H₂0 (g) / FAT (g)	PRO (g) / SFA (g)	CHO (g) / MUFA (g)	SUGR (g) / PUFA (g)	DFIB (g) / CHOL (mg)	Na (mg) / K (mg)	Ca (mg) / P (mg)	Mg (mg) / Fe (mg)	Zn (mg) / Cu (mg)	Mn (mg) / Se (mcg)	A (mcg RAE) / A (IU)	C (mg) / E (mg ATE)	B-1 (mg) / B-2 (mg)	NIA (mg) / B-6 (mg)	B-12 (mcg) / FOL (mcg DFE)	PANT (mg) / REF
jce pack, Dole Fruit Bowl	60		<1.0	16.0	14.0	1.0	10						24				
4 oz bowl	113	0.0	0.0			0	90										DOLE18
raw	76	134.1	0.6	19.2		1.9	2	11	22	0.12	2.556	2	24	0.14	0.7	0.00	0.25
1 cup pieces	155	0.7	<0.1	0.1	0.2	0	175	11	0.57	0.171	0.9	36	0.2	0.06	0.13	17.1	09266
pitanga (surinam cherry), raw	57	157.1	1.4	13.0			5	16	21			130	45	0.05	0.5		
1 cup	173	0.7				0	178	19	0.35			2595		0.07			09276
plum, cnd, heavy syrup	41	35.0	0.2	10.7		0.5	9	4	2	0.03	0.014	6	<1	0.01	0.1	0.00	0.03
1 plum w/liquid	46	<0.1	<0.1	<0.1	<0.1	0	42	6	0.39	0.017	0.1	119	0.3	0.02	0.01	1.4	09284
cnd, jce pack	27	38.6	0.2	7.0		0.5	0	5	4	0.05	0.015	23	1	0.01	0.2	0.00	0.03
1 plum w/liquid	46	<0.1	<0.1	<0.1	<0.1	0	71	7	0.16	0.025	0.1	464	0.3	0.03	0.01	1.4	09282
raw	36	56.2	0.5	8.6		1.0	0	3	5	0.07	0.032	11	6	0.03	0.3	0.00	0.12
1 med (2 1/8" dia)	66	0.4	<0.1	0.3	0.1	0	114	7	0.07	0.028	0.3	213	0.4	0.06	0.05	1.3	09279
pomegranate, raw	105	124.7	1.5	26.4		0.9	5	5	5	0.18		0	9	0.05	0.5	0.00	0.92
1 med (3 3/8" dia)	154	0.5	0.1	0.1	0.1	0	399	12	0.46	0.108	0.9	0	0.8	0.05	0.16	9.2	09286
prickly pear, raw	42	90.2	0.8	9.9		3.7	5	58	88	0.12		3	14	0.01	0.5	0.00	
1 med	103	0.5	0.1	0.1	0.2	0	227	25	0.31	0.082	0.6	53	<0.1	0.06	0.06	6.2	09287
prune, cnd, heavy syrup	90	60.8	0.7	23.9		3.3	3	15	13	0.16	0.084	34	2	0.03	0.7	0.00	0.09
5 prunes w/liquid	86	0.2	<0.1	0.1	<0.1	0	194	22	0.35	0.101		685		0.10	0.17	0.0	09288
dried	20	2.7	0.2	5.3		0.6	0	4	4	0.04	0.018	8	<1	0.01	0.2	0.00	0.04
1 prune	8	<0.1	<0.1	<0.1	<0.1	0	63	7	0.21	0.036	0.2	167	0.1	0.01	0.02	0.3	09291
dried, stewed	265	172.9	2.9	69.6		16.4	5	57	50	0.60	0.243	37	7	0.06	1.8	0.00	0.27
1 cup pitted	248	0.6	<0.1	0.4	0.1	0	828	87	2.75	0.479	2.5	759	<0.1	0.25	0.54	0.0	09292
puree	72	8.4	0.6	18.2	10.9	0.9	6	9				28	1	0.01	0.7		0.12
1 oz	28	0.1	<0.1			0	239	20	0.78			560					09423
pummelo, raw	72	169.3	1.4	18.3		1.9	2	8	11	0.15	0.032	0	116	0.06	0.4	0.00	
1 cup pieces	190	0.1				0	410	32	0.21	0.091		0		0.05	0.07		09295
quince, raw	52	77.1	0.4	14.1		1.7	4	10	7	0.04		2	14	0.02	0.2	0.00	0.07
1 med	92	0.1	<0.1	<0.1	<0.1	0	181	16	0.64	0.120	0.6	37	0.5	0.03	0.04	2.8	09296
raisins, CA seedless, Dole	130		1.0	31.0	29.0	2.0	10	20					<1				
1/4 cup	36	0.0	0.0			0	310		1.08			<1					DOLE22
Cinnaraisins, Dole	130		1.0	32.0	30.0	2.0	5	20									
1/4 cup	36	0.5	0.0			0	270		1.08			0					DOLE23
golden seedless	438	21.7	4.9	115.3		5.8	17	77	51	0.46	0.447	3	5	0.01	1.7	0.00	0.20
1 cup	145	0.7	0.2	<0.1	0.2	0	1082	167	2.60	0.526	1.0	64	1.0	0.28	0.47	4.4	09297
seeded	429	24.0	3.7	113.8		9.9	41	41	44	0.26	0.387	0	8	0.16	1.6	0.00	0.07
1 cup	145	0.8	0.3	<0.1	0.2	0	1196	109	3.76	0.438	0.9	0	1.0	0.26	0.27	4.4	09299
seedless	129	6.6	1.4	34.0		1.7	5	21	14	0.12	0.132	0	1	0.07	0.4	0.00	0.02
1.5 oz box (snack size)	43	0.2	0.1	<0.1	0.1	0	323	42	0.89	0.133	0.3	3	0.3	0.04	0.11	1.3	09298
rambutan, cnd, syrup pack	175	167.0	1.4	44.7		1.9	24	47	15	0.17	0.734	0	10	0.03	2.9	0.00	0.04
1 cup	214	0.4				0	90	19	0.75	0.141		6		0.05	0.04	17.1	09301
raspberries, cnd, heavy syrup	233	192.8	2.1	59.8		8.4	8	28	31	0.41	0.596	5	22	0.05	1.1	0.00	0.63
1 cup	256	0.3	<0.1	<0.1	0.2	0	241	23	1.08	0.146	1.0	84	1.2	0.08	0.11	28.2	09304
raw	60	106.5	1.1	14.2		8.4	0	27	22	0.57	1.246	9	31	0.04	1.1	0.00	0.30
1 cup	123	0.7	<0.1	0.1	0.4	0	187	15	0.70	0.091	0.7	160	0.6	0.11	0.07	32.0	09302
sweetened, frzn	258	181.9	1.8	65.4		11.0	3	38	33	0.45	1.625	8	41	0.05	0.6	0.00	0.38
1 cup	250	0.4	<0.1	<0.1	0.2	0	285	43	1.63	0.263	1.5	150	1.1	0.11	0.09	65.0	09306
rose apple, raw	25	93.0	0.6	5.7			0	29	5	0.06	0.029	17	22	0.02	0.8	0.00	
3.5 oz	100	0.3				0	123	8	0.07	0.016		339		0.03			09312
roselle, raw	28	49.4	0.5	6.4			3	123	29			8	7	0.01	0.2	0.00	
1 cup	57	0.4				0	119	21	0.84			164		0.02			09311
rowal, raw	127	81.4	2.6	27.2	16.1	7.1	5	17	36	0.49	0.177	22	29				
1/2 cup	114	2.3	0.3				149	59	2.51	1.208		437					09428
sapodilla, raw	141	132.6	0.7	33.9		9.0	20	36	20	0.17		5	25	0.00	0.3	0.00	0.43
1 med	170	1.9	0.3	0.9	<0.1	0	328	20	1.36	0.146	1.0	102	0.4	0.03	0.06	23.8	09313
sapote, raw	302	140.5	4.8	76.0		5.9	23	88	68			47	45	0.02	4.1	0.00	
1 med	225	1.4				0	774	63	2.25			923		0.05			09314
soursop, raw	149	182.6	2.3	37.9		7.4	32	32	47	0.23		0	46	0.16	2.0	0.00	0.57
1 cup	225	0.7	0.1	0.2	0.2	0	626	61	1.35	0.194	1.4	5	0.9	0.11	0.13	31.5	09315
strawberries, raw	43	131.9	0.9	10.1		3.3	1	20	14	0.19	0.418	1	82	0.03	0.3	0.00	0.49
1 cup whole	144	0.5	<0.1	0.1	0.3	0	239	27	0.55	0.071	1.0	39	0.2	0.10	0.08	25.9	09316
sweetened, frzn	199	199.0	1.3	53.6		4.8	3	28	15	0.13	0.635	3	101	0.04	0.7	0.00	0.28
1 cup	255	0.4	<0.1	<0.1	0.2	0	250	31	1.20	0.048	1.8	69	0.7	0.20	0.07	10.2	09319

	KCAL	H₂0 (g)	PRO (g)	CHO (g)	SUGR (g)	DFIB (g)	Na (mg)	Ca (mg)	Mg (mg)	Zn (mg)	Mn (mg)	A (mcg RAE)	C (mg)	B-1 (mg)	NIA (mg)	B-12 (mcg)	PANT (mg)
	WT (g)	FAT (g)	SFA (g)	MUFA (g)	PUFA (g)	CHOL (mg)	K (mg)	P (mg)	Fe (mg)	Cu (mg)	Se (mcg)	A (IU)	E (mg ATE)	B-2 (mg)	B-6 (mg)	FOL (mcg DFE)	REF
unsweetened, frzn	77	198.8	1.0	20.2		4.6	4	35	24	0.29	0.641	4	91	0.05	1.0	0.00	0.24
1 cup	221	0.2	<0.1	<0.1	0.1	0	327	29	1.66	0.108	1.5	99	0.6	0.08	0.06	37.6	09318
sugar apple, raw	146	113.5	3.2	36.6		6.8	14	37	33	0.16		0	56	0.17	1.4	0.00	0.35
1 med (2 7/8 dia)	155	0.4	0.1	0.2	0.1	0	383	50	0.93	0.133	0.9	9	0.9	0.18	0.31	21.7	09321
tamarind, raw	287	37.7	3.4	75.0		6.1	34	89	110	0.12		2	4	0.51	2.3	0.00	0.17
1 cup	120	0.7	0.3	0.2	0.1	0	754	136	3.36	0.103	1.6	36	0.8	0.18	0.08	16.8	09322
tangerine, raw	37	73.6	0.5	9.4		1.9	1	12	10	0.20	0.027	39	26	0.09	0.1	0.00	0.17
1 med (2 3/8" dia)	84	0.2	<0.1	<0.1	<0.1	0	132	8	0.08	0.024	0.4	773	0.2	0.02	0.06	16.8	09218
tropical fruit, jce pack, Dole	60		<1.0	16.0	14.0	2.0	10						24				
Fruit Bowl - *4 oz bowl*	113	0.0	0.0			0	160										DOLE33
	100		1.0	25.0	23.0	1.0	20	0					36				
1 cup	198	0.0	0.0			0	280		0.00			0					DOLE34
watermelon, raw	49	139.1	0.9	10.9		0.8	3	12	17	0.11	0.056	27	15	0.12	0.3	0.00	0.32
1 cup pieces	152	0.7	0.1	0.2	0.2	0	176	14	0.26	0.049	0.2	556	0.2	0.03	0.22	3.0	09326

[1] Dried black Corinth grapes; not related to European black, red, or white currants.
[2] Values apply to Berry Berry Twist, Berry Tie-Dye, Color by the Foot, Disney Dinosaurs, Disney Princess, Endless Party, Pokemon, Strawberry, and Watermelon.
[3] Peaches, pineapples, pears, grapes, and cherries.
[4] Values apply to Atlantis, Blastin Berry Hot Colors, California Punch, Cartoon Network, Disney Mickey, Monsters, 102 Dalmations, Rockin' Fruity Rainbow, Strawberry Sensation, Tropical Tie Dye, Watermelon Punch, and Wild Berry.
[5] Peaches, pears, apricots, pineapples, and cherries.
[6] Pineapples, papayas, bananas, guava puree, cherries, and passion fruit juice.
[7] Values apply to Bugs Bunny, Winnie the Pooh, Hawaiian Punch, Lucky Charms, Nintendo All Stars, Pokemon, Scooby Doo!, Shark Bites, and Trix.
[8] Roundish yellow berries 3/4 inches across, sweet and slightly acid; native to eastern and central North America.
[9] Peaches, pears, and pineapple.
[10] Peaches, sweet cherries, red sour cherries, red raspberries, boysenberries, and grapes.

16. GRAIN-BASED SNACK FOODS

	KCAL	H₂0 (g)	PRO (g)	CHO (g)	SUGR (g)	DFIB (g)	Na (mg)	Ca (mg)	Mg (mg)	Zn (mg)	Mn (mg)	A (mcg RAE)	C (mg)	B-1 (mg)	NIA (mg)	B-12 (mcg)	PANT (mg)
	WT (g)	FAT (g)	SFA (g)	MUFA (g)	PUFA (g)	CHOL (mg)	K (mg)	P (mg)	Fe (mg)	Cu (mg)	Se (mcg)	A (IU)	E (mg ATE)	B-2 (mg)	B-6 (mg)	FOL (mcg DFE)	REF
Bugels, baked, Betty Crocker	150		2.0	26.5	2.5	<0.5	440	0					0				
1 1/2 cups (1.06 oz)	35	4.0	0.8			0	25		0.54			0					GENM212
Bugles, Betty Crocker[1]	156		1.3	18.4	1.3	<0.2	315	48					2				
1 1/3 cups (1.06 oz)	30	8.5	7.0			0	31		1.05			120					GENM213
	220		2.0	25.4	2.3	<0.4	438	72					2				
1.5 oz pouch	42	12.2	9.9			0	38		1.58			144					GENM214
cereal bar, all flvrs, Nature's	120		1.0	25.0	13.0	2.0	65	0					0				
Choice - *1.3 oz bar*	37	1.5	0.0			0			0.36			0					BARB3
mixed berry, Kellogg's	137	5.4	1.6	26.9	12.4	0.7	110	14	10	1.52			0	0.37	5.0	0.00	0.00
Nutri-Grain - *1.3 oz bar*	37	2.8	0.6	1.9	0.4	0	70	36	1.81	0.037		750	0.0	0.41	0.52		18501
multigrain cherry, Nature's	120		1.0	25.0	13.0	2.0	65	0					0				
Choice - *1.3 oz bar*	37	1.5	0.0			0			0.36			0					NRCH1
oatmeal raisin, frosted, Elfin	140		2.0	23.0	9.0	<1.0	135	20		0.60			0	0.30	9.0	0.60	
Magic Bar - *1.2 oz bar*	34	5.0	1.0			0			1.80			50		0.26	0.20	0.0	KBLR1
cheese puffs/twists	157	0.4	2.2	15.3		0.3	298	16	5	0.11	0.020	7	<1	0.07	0.9	0.04	0.11
1 oz	28	9.8	1.9	5.7	1.3	1	47	31	0.67	0.018	0.9	75	1.5	0.10	0.04	51.0	19008
Cheetos cheese snacks	159		1.7	15.0	0.8	0.4	266	17					<1				
1 oz	28	10.2	2.4			2	266		0.46			27					FRTO1
Chex Mix	120	1.0	3.1	18.5		1.6	288	10	18	0.59	0.440	2	13	0.44	4.8	3.52	0.13
2/3 cup (1 oz)	28	4.9	1.6			0	76	53	7.00	0.127		41		0.14	0.44	24.1	19033
Chex Snack Mixes, Betty Crocker[2]	211		4.1	34.4	4.1	2.6	579	0					0				
1.7 oz pouch	49	7.6	1.3			0	100		0.26			0					GENM215
Combos (cheddar cheese pretzels),	139	0.5	3.0	20.0			335	59	7	0.22	0.134	1	0	0.09	1.0	0.04	0.14
M&M/Mars - *10 pieces (1.1 oz)*	30	5.1				2	39	43	0.28	0.036		20		0.17	0.01	2.4	19049
corn cake	35	0.4	0.7	7.5		0.2	44	2	10	0.18	0.163	1	0	0.01	0.3	0.00	0.07
.32 oz cake	9	0.2	<0.1	0.1	0.1	0	14	14	0.13	0.038	0.9	22	<0.1	<0.01	0.01	1.7	19419
corn chips	153	0.3	1.9	16.1		1.4	179	36	22	0.36	0.108	1	0	0.01	0.3	0.00	0.11
1 oz	28	9.5	1.3	2.7	4.7	0	40	52	0.37	0.046	1.9	27	0.4	0.04	0.07	5.7	19003
barbecue	148	0.3	2.0	15.9		1.5	216	37	22	0.30	0.219	9	<1	0.02	0.5	0.00	0.04
1 oz	28	9.3	1.3	2.7	4.6	0	67	59	0.44	0.047	1.2	173		0.06	0.07	11.1	19004
corn-based cones	145	0.6	1.6	17.8		0.3	290	1	3	0.06	0.025	5	0	0.09	0.4	0.00	0.06
1 oz	28	7.6	6.4	0.5	0.2	0	23	12	0.72	0.011	1.1	90		0.07	0.01	0.9	19005
nacho	152	0.5	1.8	16.2		0.3	270	10	7	0.14	0.022	7	<1	0.06	0.4	0.00	0.11
1 oz	28	9.0	7.6	0.6	0.2	1	35	22	0.36	0.017	1.1	89		0.03	0.03	1.4	19006
corn-based snack, onion flavor	142	0.6	2.2	18.5		1.1	278	8	8	0.09	0.057	2	1	0.06	0.9	0.00	0.07
1 oz	28	6.4	1.2	3.8	0.9	0	41	20	1.05	0.033	3.0	34	0.5	0.09	0.04	49.9	19007

	KCAL	H₂O (g)	PRO (g)	CHO (g)	SUGR (g)	DFIB (g)	Na (mg)	Ca (mg)	Mg (mg)	Zn (mg)	Mn (mg)	A (mcg RAE)	C (mg)	B-1 (mg)	NIA (mg)	B-12 (mcg)	PANT (mg)
	WT (g)	FAT (g)	SFA (g)	MUFA (g)	PUFA (g)	CHOL (mg)	K (mg)	P (mg)	Fe (mg)	Cu (mg)	Se (mcg)	A (IU)	E (mg ATE)	B-2 (mg)	B-6 (mg)	FOL (mcg DFE)	REF
crisped rice bar w/choc chips	113	2.0	1.4	20.4		0.6	78	6	13	0.24	0.280		0	0.15	2.0	0.00	0.00
1 oz bar	28	3.8	1.5	1.1	1.0	0	47	38	1.76	0.087	2.7	494		0.17	0.20	39.2	19010
Doo Dads, Nabisco	128	0.8	2.9	18.0		1.9	356	21	17	0.63	0.494		<1	0.10	1.5	<0.01	0.16
1/2 cup (1 oz)	28	5.2	1.0			<1	78	83	0.70	0.090		42		0.07	0.06	40.3	19032
Fritos corn chips	158		1.7	15.3	0.2	1.0	161	45					<1				
1 oz	28	10.2	1.4			<1	161		0.37			29					FRTO2
Funyuns onion flavored rings	140		1.8	18.3	0.5	0.6	271	8					<1				
1 oz	28	6.6	1.1			<1	271		0.80			44					FRTO3
Gardetto's Snackens³	214		4.6	31.0	1.8	1.4	466	0					0				
1.7 oz pouch	47	8.0	1.4			0	89		0.90			0					GENM216
granola bar, almond, hard	119	0.7	1.8	14.9		1.2	61	8	19	0.38	0.328	<1	0	0.07	0.1	0.00	0.11
.85 oz bar	24	6.1	3.0	1.9	0.9	0	66	55	0.60	0.030	3.6	9		0.02	0.01	2.9	19016
granola bar, choc chip, hard	105	0.6	1.8	17.3		1.1	83	18	17	0.46	0.362	<1	<1	0.04	0.1	<0.01	0.12
.85 oz bar	24	3.9	2.7	0.6	0.3	0	60	49	0.73	0.063	3.0	10		0.02	0.01	3.1	19017
soft	118	1.5	2.0	19.3		1.3	76	26	22	0.42	0.364	1	0	0.06	0.3	0.05	0.15
1 oz bar	28	4.6	2.9	1.0	0.6	<1	95	64	0.71	0.112	3.5	12		0.04	0.03	6.2	19404
soft w/choc coating	130	1.0	1.6	17.9		1.0	56	29	18	0.36	0.260	2	0	0.03	0.2	0.16	0.14
1 oz bar	28	7.0	4.0	2.2	0.5	1	88	56	0.65	0.098		11		0.07	0.03	7.3	19024
granola bar, choc, graham, & marshmallow, soft - *1 oz bar*	120	1.7	1.7	19.8		1.1	88	25	20	0.36	0.358	1	0	0.04	0.3	0.00	0.11
	28	4.3	2.6	0.8	0.7	<1	77	57	0.72	0.078	4.3	13		0.04	0.01	5.9	19405
granola bar, cinn & raisin, Nature's Choice - *.74 oz bar*	80		2.0	14.0	7.0	<1.0	0	20					0				
	21	2.0	0.0			0			0.36			0					BARB4
granola bar, crunchy, all flvrs, Nature Valley - *2 bars (1.5 oz)*	180		4.3	29.0	11.0	2.0	163	0					0				
	42	6.0	0.7			0	100		1.13			0					GENM217
granola bar, nut & raisin, soft - *1 oz bar*	127	1.7	2.2	17.8		1.6	71	24	25	0.45	0.336	1	0	0.05	0.7	0.07	0.12
	28	5.7	2.7	1.2	1.5	<1	110	67	0.61	0.106	4.3	11		0.05	0.03	8.4	19406
granola bar, peanut butter & choc chip, soft - *1 oz bar*	121	1.7	2.7	17.4		1.2	92	22	25	0.48	0.378	1	0	0.03	0.9	0.13	0.15
	28	5.6	1.6	2.3	1.3	<1	106	73	0.54	0.112		3		0.03	0.03	9.2	19027
granola bar, peanut butter, hard	116	0.6	2.4	15.0		0.7	68	10	13	0.30	0.221	<1	<1	0.05	0.5	0.00	0.09
.85 oz bar	24	5.7	0.8	1.7	2.9	0	70	33	0.58	0.052	3.6	4		0.02	0.02	4.3	19420
soft	119	2.0	2.9	18.0		1.2	115	25	24	0.52	0.392	1	0	0.06	0.9	0.06	0.15
1 oz bar	28	4.4	1.0	1.8	1.2	<1	81	70	0.60	0.185	5.3	4		0.04	0.03	9.0	19021
soft w/choc coating	188	1.2	3.8	19.8		1.0	71	40	25	0.54	0.500	2	<1	0.04	1.2	0.00	0.20
1.3 oz bar	37	11.5	6.3	2.4	0.7	4	125	84	0.54	0.120		9		0.08	0.04	9.3	19026
granola bar, peanut, hard	136	0.7	3.1	18.1		1.2	79	11	31	0.59	0.399	1	0	0.05	0.4	0.00	0.17
1 oz bar	28	6.1	0.7	1.6	3.4	0	86	85	0.71	0.079	4.3	9	0.3	0.02	0.02	6.5	19019
granola bar, plain, hard	132	1.1	2.8	18.0		1.5	82	17	27	0.57	0.498	2	<1	0.07	0.4	0.00	0.23
1 oz bar	28	5.5	0.7	1.2	3.4	0	94	78	0.83	0.110	4.5	42		0.03	0.02	6.4	19015
soft	124	1.8	2.1	18.8		1.3	78	29	21	0.42	0.428	0	0	0.08	0.1	0.11	0.15
1 oz bar	28	4.8	2.0	1.1	1.5	<1	91	64	0.72	0.076	4.5	0		0.05	0.03	6.7	19020
granola bar, raisin, soft	125	1.8	2.1	18.6		1.2	79	28	20	0.36	0.353	0	0	0.06	0.3	0.05	0.13
1 oz bar	28	5.0	2.7	0.8	0.9	<1	101	62	0.68	0.078	4.4	0		0.05	0.03	5.9	19022
Krispy Crunchy Puffs, corn, Tumaro's - *1 oz (22 chips)*	110		2.0	21.0	1.0	1.0	240	20					0				
	28	2.0	0.0			0			0.36			0					TUMO1
Milk 'n Cereal Bar, Chex - *1.4 oz bar*	160		6.0	26.0	13.0	0.0	150	250					9				
	40	4.0	1.5			0	105		5.40			750					GENM218
Cinn Toast Crunch	180		6.0	31.0	18.0	1.0	180	250					9				
1.6 oz bar	45	4.0	1.5			0	130		5.40			750					GENM219
Cocoa Puffs	160		6.0	26.0	16.0	1.0	130	250					9				
1.4 oz bar	40	4.0	1.5			0	135		5.40			750					GENM220
Honey Nut Cheerios	160		6.0	26.0	16.0	1.0	150	250					9				
1.4 oz bar	40	4.0	1.5			0	120		5.40			750					GENM221
oriental mix, rice-based	156	0.7	4.9	14.6		3.7	117	15	33	0.75	0.361	0	<1	0.09	0.9	0.00	0.13
1 oz	28	7.3	1.1	2.8	3.0	0	93	74	0.69	0.038	2.3	1	2.4	0.04	0.02	10.8	19031
popcorn, butter, popped, PopSecret	35		<1.0	4.0	0.0	<1.0	60	0					0				
1 cup	7	2.5	0.5			0	10		0.00			0					GENM222
popcorn cake	38	0.5	1.0	8.0		0.3	29	1	16	0.40	0.099	<1	0	0.01	0.6	0.00	0.04
.35 oz cake	10	0.3	<0.1	0.1	0.1	0	33	28	0.19	0.057	1.0	7	<0.1	0.02	0.02	1.8	19036
popcorn, caramel	122	0.8	1.1	22.4		1.5	58	12	10	0.16	0.062	2	0	0.02	0.6	<0.01	0.02
1 oz	28	3.6	1.0	0.8	1.3	1	31	24	0.49	0.034	1.0	14	0.3	0.02	0.01	0.6	19039
w/peanuts	113	0.9	1.8	22.9		1.1	84	19	23	0.35	0.217	1	0	0.01	0.6	0.00	0.07
1 oz (~2/3 cup)	28	2.2	0.3	0.8	0.9	0	101	36	1.11	0.084	1.1	18	0.4	0.04	0.05	4.5	19038

	KCAL	H₂0 (g)	PRO (g)	CHO (g)	SUGR (g)	DFIB (g)	Na (mg)	Ca (mg)	Mg (mg)	Zn (mg)	Mn (mg)	A (mcg RAE)	C (mg)	B-1 (mg)	NIA (mg)	B-12 (mcg)	PANT (mg)
	WT (g)	FAT (g)	SFA (g)	MUFA (g)	PUFA (g)	CHOL (mg)	K (mg)	P (mg)	Fe (mg)	Cu (mg)	Se (mcg)	A (IU)	E (mg ATE)	B-2 (mg)	B-6 (mg)	FOL (mcg DFE)	REF
popcorn, cheese	149	0.7	2.6	14.6		2.8	252	32	26	0.57	0.202	11	<1	0.04	0.4	0.15	0.13
1 oz (~2.6 cups)	28	9.4	1.8	2.7	4.4	3	74	102	0.64	0.040	3.4	69	<0.1	0.07	0.07	3.1	19040
popcorn, extra butter, popped,	40		<1.0	3.0	0.0	<1.0	70	0					0				
PopSecret - *1 cup*	7	3.0	0.5			0	10		0.00			0					GENM223
popcorn, light butter, popped,	20		<1.0	4.0	0.0	<1.0	50	0					0				
PopSecret - *1 cup*	5	1.0	0.0			0	15		0.00			0					GENM224
popcorn, plain, air-popped	108	1.2	3.4	22.1		4.3	1	3	37	0.98	0.267	3	0	0.06	0.6	0.00	0.12
1 oz (~3.5 cups)	28	1.2	0.2	0.3	0.5	0	85	85	0.75	0.119	2.8	56	<0.1	0.08	0.07	6.5	19034
oil-popped	142	0.8	2.6	16.2		2.8	251	3	31	0.75	0.249	2	<1	0.04	0.4	0.00	0.09
1 oz (~2.6 cups)	28	8.0	1.4	2.3	3.8	0	64	71	0.79	0.063	2.1	44	<0.1	0.04	0.06	4.8	19035
potato chips[4]	152	0.5	2.0	15.0		1.3	168	7	19	0.31	0.125	0	9	0.05	1.1	0.00	0.11
1 oz	28	9.8	3.1	2.8	3.5	0	361	47	0.46	0.087	2.3	0	1.4	0.06	0.19	12.8	19411
from dried potatoes	158	0.4	1.7	14.5		1.0	186	7	16	0.17	0.098	0	2	0.06	0.9	0.00	0.06
1 oz	28	10.9	2.7	2.1	5.7	0	286	45	0.43	0.045	2.3	0	1.4	0.03	0.04	2.0	19410
Lay's Classic	153		1.7	15.0	0.1	0.7	144	6					9				
1 oz	28	9.8	2.5			0	144		0.29			27					FRTO5
Ruffles	157		1.9	14.4	0.2	1.1	163	9					6				
1 oz	28	10.3	2.9						0.38								FRTO7
potato chips, barbeque	139	0.5	2.2	15.0		1.2	213	14	21	0.27	0.142	3	10	0.06	1.3	0.00	0.17
1 oz	28	9.2	2.3	1.9	4.6	0	357	53	0.55	0.102	2.3	62	1.4	0.06	0.18	23.5	19042
Lay's	151		1.8	15.3	2.2	1.2	180	8					8				
1 oz	28	9.2	2.3			<1	180		0.27			105					FRTO4
potato chips, cheese	141	0.5	2.4	16.4		1.5	225	20	21	0.26	0.126	3	15	0.04	1.4	0.00	0.22
1 oz	28	7.7	2.4	2.2	2.7	1	433	85	0.52	0.071		9		0.04	0.10	0.0	19421
from dried potatoes	156	0.5	2.0	14.3		1.0	214	31	15	0.18	0.016	<1	2	0.05	0.7	0.00	0.10
1 oz	28	10.5	2.7	2.1	5.3	1	108	46	0.45	0.016	2.3	<1		0.03	0.15	5.1	19412
potato chips, light	134	0.3	2.0	19.0		1.7	139	6	25	0.02	0.125	0	7	0.06	2.0	0.00	0.08
1 oz	28	5.9	1.2	1.4	3.1	0	494	55	0.38	0.170	2.3	0	0.8	0.08	0.19	7.7	19422
potato chips, reduced fat,	142	0.4	1.6	18.4		1.0	121	10	18	0.17	0.099	0	3	0.05	1.2	0.00	0.07
from dried potatoes - *1 oz*	28	7.3	1.5	1.7	3.8	0	285	44	0.43	0.040	2.3	0	1.4	0.02	0.22	6.5	19045
Ruffles	136		2.1	17.9	0.2	1.2	119	5					10				
1 oz	28	6.6	1.4			<1	119		0.41			<1					FRTO6
potato chips, sour cream & onion	151	0.5	2.3	14.6		1.5	177	20	21	0.28	0.115	4	11	0.05	1.1	0.28	0.23
1 oz	28	9.6	2.5	1.7	4.9	2	377	50	0.45	0.085	2.3	48		0.06	0.19	17.6	19043
from dried potatoes	155	0.6	1.9	14.5		0.3	204	18	16	0.20	0.115	3		0.05	0.7	0.00	0.23
1 oz	28	10.5	2.7	2.0	5.3	1	141	48	0.40	0.018		214		0.03	0.13	6.5	19046
Lay's	160		2.2	12.8	0.7	1.0	185	16					13				
1 oz	28	11.1	3.1			2			0.32			48					FRTO8
potato chips, Wow! Lay's	74		1.9	17.5	0.1	1.1	193	14					8				
1 oz	28	0.2	0.1			<1			0.45			1630					FRTO9
Ruffles	71		1.7	16.6	0.1	0.9	175	7					11				
1 oz	28	0.2	0.1			<1			0.26			2037					FRTO10
potato crisps, baked, cheddar &	119		1.7	22.0	2.3	1.6	217	41					3				
sour cream, Ruffles - *1 oz*	28	2.7	0.5			<1			0.57			0					FRTO14
Lay's	120		1.6	21.9	2.8	1.6	214	37					3				
1 oz	28	2.9	0.4			0			0.46			78					FRTO11
Lay's Original	113		2.0	23.0	1.8	1.6	149	39					2				
1 oz	28	1.5	0.3			<1			0.44			0					FRTO12
Ruffles	120		1.9	21.3		1.7	186	33									
1 oz	28	3.1	0.5						0.38								FRTO13
Potato Poppers, white cheddar,	110		2.0	20.0	1.0	0.0	360	20					0				
Simple Snacks - *1 oz (44 pieces)*	28	1.5	0.0			0			1.44			0					SMPL2
potato sticks	94	0.4	1.2	9.6		0.6	45	3	12	0.18	0.076	0	9	0.02	0.9	0.00	0.07
1/2 cup	18	6.2	1.6	1.1	3.2	0	223	31	0.41	0.057	1.5	0	0.9	0.02	0.06	7.2	19415
pretzel nuggets, honey mustard,	132		1.9	19.8	1.5	0.9	195	9									
Rold Gold - *1 oz*	28	5.0	0.9			<1			1.05								FRTO15
parmesan garlic, Rold Gold	131		1.9	19.2	1.1	0.9	353	17									
1 oz	28	5.2	0.9			1			1.16								FRTO16
pretzels	229	2.0	5.5	47.5		1.9	1029	22	21	0.51	1.073	0	0	0.28	3.2	0.00	0.17
10 twists (2.1 oz)	60	2.1	0.5	0.8	0.7	0	88	68	2.59	0.158	3.5	0	0.1	0.37	0.07	139.8	19047
butter flavored, Rold Gold	113		2.5	22.3	0.7	0.8	200	6									
1 oz	28	1.5	0.5			2			1.00								FRTO20

	KCAL	H2O (g)	PRO (g)	CHO (g)	SUGR (g)	DFIB (g)	Na (mg)	Ca (mg)	Mg (mg)	Zn (mg)	Mn (mg)	A (mcg RAE)	C (mg)	B-1 (mg)	NIA (mg)	B-12 (mcg)	PANT (mg)
	WT (g)	FAT (g)	SFA (g)	MUFA (g)	PUFA (g)	CHOL (mg)	K (mg)	P (mg)	Fe (mg)	Cu (mg)	Se (mcg)	A (IU)	E (mg ATE)	B-2 (mg)	B-6 (mg)	FOL (mcg DFE)	REF
choc coated	50	0.3	0.8	7.8			63	8	5	0.10	0.062	<1	<1		0.01	0.1		0.08
.39 oz pretzel	11	1.8	0.8	0.6	0.2	0	25	16	0.22	0.033		1		0.02	0.02	1.0	19048
whole wheat	206	2.2	6.3	46.3		4.4	116	16	17	0.35	1.517	0	1		0.25	3.7	0.00	0.46
2 oz	57	1.5	0.3	0.6	0.5	0	245	71	1.53	0.160		0		0.17	0.16	30.8	19050
pretzel snack mix, Rold Gold	144		2.4	16.4	1.2	1.2	322	13					<1					
1 oz	28	7.7	1.3			<1			0.88			0					FRTO17
pretzel tiny twists, Rold Gold	109		2.5	22.5	0.6	0.9	560	8										
Classic - 1 oz	28	1.0	0.2						1.91								FRTO19
honey mustard, Rold Gold	111		2.7	22.4	1.3	1.1	366	8										
Classic - 1 oz	28	1.2	0.2						1.04								FRTO18
rice cakes (brown rice)	35	0.5	0.7	7.3		0.4	29	1	12	0.27	0.336	<1	0	0.01	0.7	0.00	0.09
.32 oz cake	9	0.3	0.1	0.1	0.1	0	26	32	0.13	0.040	2.2	4	0.1	0.01	0.01	1.9	19051
buckwheat	34	0.5	0.8	7.2		0.3	10	1	14	0.23	0.556	0	0	<0.01	0.7	0.00	0.10
.32 oz cake	9	0.3	0.1	0.1	0.1	0	27	34	0.10	0.034	1.5	0		0.01	0.01	1.9	19052
corn	35	0.5	0.8	7.3		0.3	26	1	10	0.20	0.457	0	0	0.01	0.6	0.00	0.08
.32 oz cake	9	0.3	0.1	0.1	0.1	0	25	29	0.11	0.038		0		0.01	0.01	1.7	19413
multigrain	35	0.6	0.8	7.2		0.3	23	2	12	0.23	0.470	0	0	0.01	0.6	0.00	0.09
.32 oz cake	9	0.3	<0.1	0.1	0.1	0	26	33	0.18	0.038		0		0.02	0.01	1.8	19414
rye	35	0.6	0.7	7.2		0.4	10	2	13	0.27	0.268	0	0	0.01	0.6	0.00	0.10
.32 oz cake	9	0.3	0.1	0.1	0.1	0	28	34	0.16	0.035		<1		0.01	0.01	0.5	19416
sesame seed	35	0.5	0.7	7.3		0.5	20	1	12	0.27	0.387	0	<1	<0.01	0.6	0.00	0.13
.32 oz cake	9	0.3	<0.1	0.1	0.1	0	26	34	0.14	0.035	2.2	0		0.01	0.01	1.6	19053
Rice Krispies Treats, original,	90		1.0	18.0	8.0	0.0	100	0			1.50		0	0.15	2.0		
Kellogg's - 1.13 oz bar	32	2.0	0.5			0			0.36			200		0.17	0.20	24.0	KELL1
sesame sticks, wheat-based	153	0.6	3.1	13.2		0.8	422	48	13	0.33	0.256	1	0	0.03	0.4	0.00	0.07
1 oz	28	10.4	1.8	3.1	4.9	0	50	39	0.21	0.115	4.8	25	1.1	0.02	0.02	6.2	19418
Soy Crisps, GeniSoy[5]	120		6.0	18.0	16.0	2.0	110	30					0				
1 oz	28	2.5	0.0			0	220		0.54			0					GENI1
Soy Snappers, white cheddar, Simple	110		7.0	14.0	1.0	2.0	320	80					0				
Snacks - 1 oz (68 pieces)	28	2.0	0.0			0			1.80			100					SMPL1
Sunchips, multigrain	137		2.3	19.2	2.2	1.9	107	6					0				
1 oz	28	5.6	0.6			0			0.45			0					FRTO21
french onion	139		2.3	18.3	3.0	1.7	160	15					0				
1 oz	28	6.2	0.7			1			0.39								FRTO22
harvest cheddar	136		2.4	18.8	1.9	1.8	170	15					0				
1 oz	28	5.7	1.1			<1			0.34								FRTO23
taro chips	115	0.5	0.5	15.7		1.7	79	14	19	0.09	<0.001	0	1	0.04	0.1	0.00	0.15
10 chips (.8 oz)	23	5.7	1.5	1.0	3.0	0	174	30	0.28	0.064	0.4	0	1.1	0.01	0.10	4.6	19524
tortilla chips	142	0.5	2.0	17.8		1.8	150	44	25	0.43	0.108	3	0	0.02	0.4	0.00	0.22
1 oz	28	7.4	1.4	4.4	1.0	0	56	58	0.43	0.034	1.9	56	0.4	0.05	0.08	2.8	19056
nacho	141	0.5	2.2	17.7		1.5	201	42	23	0.34	0.116	7	1	0.04	0.4	0.01	0.08
1 oz	28	7.3	1.4	4.3	1.0	1	61	69	0.41	0.050	1.9	105		0.05	0.08	4.0	19057
nacho cheesier, Doritos Wow	85		2.4	17.9			222	41									
1.38 oz pkg	39	1.0	0.3				222		0.25								FRTO24
nacho, red fat	126	0.4	2.5	20.3		1.4	284	45	27		0.124	7	<1	0.06	0.1	0.00	
1 oz	28	4.3	0.8	2.5	0.6	1	77	90	0.46	0.041		108		0.08	0.07	7.4	19424
ranch	139	0.5	2.2	18.3		1.1	174	40	25	0.35	0.111	4	<1	0.03	0.4	0.00	0.17
1 oz	28	6.7	1.3	4.0	0.9	<1	69	68	0.41	0.033	1.9	73		0.07	0.06	4.8	19058
taco flavor	136	0.5	2.2	17.9		1.5	223	44	25	0.36	0.125	13	<1	0.07	0.6	0.00	0.08
1 oz	28	6.9	1.3	4.1	1.0	1	62	68	0.57	0.053	1.9	257		0.06	0.08	6.0	19063
Trail Mix bar, fruit 'n nut, Nature	140		3.0	24.0	12.0	2.0	95	0					0				
Valley - 1.2 oz bar	35	4.0	0.5			0			0.00			0					GENM225
Wahoos, original	140		1.0	18.3	2.3	0.0	343	0					0				
1 oz	28	7.7	0.8			0	32		0.09			0					GENM226

[1] Values are averages for chili con queso, nacho cheese, original, and smoking BBQ.

[2] Values are averages for Bold Party Blend, Cheddar Cheese, Honey Nut, Hot'n Spicy, Nacho Fiesta, Peanut Lovers, and Traditional.

[3] Values are averages for Deli-Style Mustard Pretzel Mix, Italian Cheese Blend, Original Recipe Snackens, reduced fat Original Recipe Snackens, and Special Italian Recipe.

[4] Values are for potato chips made with cottonseed oil. If partially hydrogenated soybean oil is used, saturated fat is 1.5 g, monounsaturated fat is 5.0 g, and polyunsaturated fat is 2.6 g.

[5] Values are averages for 7 flavors, apple cinnamon crunch, creamy ranch, deep sea salt, rich cheddar cheese, roasted garlic & onion, tangy salt 'n vinegar, and zesty barbeque.

						Minerals					Vitamins					
KCAL	H₂0 (g)	PRO (g)	CHO (g)	SUGR (g)	DFIB (g)	Na (mg)	Ca (mg)	Mg (mg)	Zn (mg)	Mn (mg)	A (mcg RAE)	C (mg)	B-1 (mg)	NIA (mg)	B-12 (mcg)	PANT (mg)
WT (g)	FAT (g)	SFA (g)	MUFA (g)	PUFA (g)	CHOL (mg)	K (mg)	P (mg)	Fe (mg)	Cu (mg)	Se (mcg)	A (IU ATE)	E (mg ATE)	B-2 (mg)	B-6 (mg)	FOL (mcg DFE)	REF

17. GRAIN PRODUCTS
17.1 BAGELS

blueberry, Lender's — *3.6 oz bagel (4" dia)*

KCAL/WT	H₂0/FAT	PRO/SFA	CHO/MUFA	SUGR/PUFA	DFIB/CHOL	Na/K	Ca/P	Mg/Fe	Zn/Cu	Mn/Se	A	C/E	B-1/B-2	NIA/B-6	B-12/FOL	PANT/REF
264	34.6	10.7	53.4	9.6	1.7	427	57					0	0.27	4.1	0.00	
102	1.5	0.3	0.4	0.5	0	158		1.84			0		0.20	0.06		18504

Lender's Big 'n Crusty — *3 oz bagel (3 " dia)*

214	29.2	7.9	45.9	9.5	1.7	409	11					0	0.46	3.4	0.00	
85	0.8	0.2	0.1	0.4	0	73		3.15			0		0.26	0.05		18502

refrig, Lender's Premium — *2.9 oz bagel (3 " dia)*

209	27.3	8.4	42.5	8.0	2.0	409	12					0	0.21	1.6	0.00	
81	1.3	0.3	0.3	0.4	0	131		1.64			0		0.14	0.05		18503

cinn raisin — *3.7 oz bagel (3 1/2" dia)*

288	33.6	10.3	58.0		2.4	338	20	29	1.19	0.920	4	1	0.40	3.2	0.00	0.53
105	1.8	0.3	0.2	0.7	0	155	105	3.99	0.171	32.6	77	0.2	0.29	0.07	144.9	18005a

4.6 oz bagel (4 1/2" dia)

359	41.9	12.8	72.3		3.0	422	25	37	1.48	1.148	5	1	0.50	4.0	0.00	0.67
131	2.2	0.4	0.2	0.9	0	194	131	4.98	0.214	40.6	96	0.2	0.36	0.08	180.8	18005b

egg — *3.7 oz bagel (4" dia)*

292	34.3	11.1	55.7		2.4	530	14	26	0.81	0.431	35	1	0.56	3.6	0.17	0.70
105	2.2	0.4	0.4	0.7	25	71	88	4.18	0.095	32.1	114		0.25	0.09	140.7	18003

oat bran — *3.7 oz bagel (4" dia)*

268	34.5	11.2	56.0		3.8	532	13	33	0.95	0.906	0	<1	0.35	3.1	0.00	0.47
105	1.3	0.2	0.3	0.5	0	121	116	3.23	0.159	35.9	4	0.1	0.35	0.05	111.3	18007

plain/onion/poppy seed/sesame seed — *3.7 oz bagel (4" dia)*

289	34.2	11.0	56.1		2.4	561	78	30	0.92	0.567	0	0	0.56	4.8	0.00	0.38
105	1.7	0.2	0.1	0.7	0	106	101	3.74	0.171	33.6	0	<0.1	0.33	0.05	140.7	18001

Toaster Bagel Shoppe, frzn[1] — *1.66 oz bagel*

130		3.7	24.3	7.7	<1.0	199	0					0				
47	2.0	0.8			<2		1.08				0					GENM227

[1] Values are averages for blueberry & cream cheese, cinnamon raisin, cream cheese, and strawberry & cream cheese.

17.2 BISCUITS

blueberry, from refrig dough, *Grands! - 2.15 oz biscuit*

KCAL/WT	H₂0/FAT	PRO/SFA	CHO/MUFA	SUGR/PUFA	DFIB/CHOL	Na/K	Ca/P	Mg/Fe	Zn/Cu	Mn/Se	A	C/E	B-1/B-2	NIA/B-6	B-12/FOL	PANT/REF
210		4.0	29.0	10.0	<1.0	510	40					0				
61	9.0	3.0			0		1.08				0					GENM228

buttermilk, from refrig dough, *1869 Brand - 1.1 oz biscuit*

100		2.0	12.0	1.0	0.0	320	0					0				
31	5.0	1.5			0		0.72				0					GENM229

Big Country — 1.2 oz biscuit

100		2.0	14.0	2.0	0.0	360	0					0				
34	4.0	1.0			0		0.72				0					GENM230

Grands! — 2 oz biscuit

190		4.0	24.0	4.0	<1.0	600	20					0				
58	9.0	2.5			0		1.44				0					GENM231

Hungry Jack — 1.2 oz biscuit

100		2.0	14.0	2.0	0.0	360	0					0				
34	4.5	1.0			0		0.72				0					GENM232

Pillsbury — 2.3 oz biscuit

150		4.0	29.0	3.0	<1.0	540	0					0				
64	2.0	0.0			0		1.80				0					GENM233

red fat, Grands! — 2 oz biscuit

170		4.0	26.0	4.0	<1.0	590	20					0				
58	6.0	1.5			0		1.44				0					GENM234

tender layer, Pillsbury — 2.3 oz biscuit

160		4.0	27.0	3.0	<1.0	520	0					0				
64	4.5	1.0			0		1.44				0					GENM249

buttermilk, refrig dough, Pillsbury *2.3 oz biscuit*

154	25.1	5.0	30.4			547										
64	1.4	0.3	0.6	0.3			1.55									18629

Pillsbury Grands — 2.2 oz biscuit

195	21.2	4.1	25.1			605										
61	8.7	2.4					1.55									18633

Pillsbury Hungry Jack — 1.2 oz biscuit

108	11.6	2.4	14.5			343										
34	4.6	0.9	2.8	0.2			0.85									18634

Butter Tastin Flaky, from refrig dough, Hungry Jack *- 1.2 oz bsct*

100		2.0	14.0	2.0	0.0	360	0					0				
34	4.5	1.0			0		0.72				0					GENM235

Butter Tastin, from refrig dough, Big Country *- 1.2 oz biscuit*

100		2.0	13.0	2.0	0.0	360	0					0				
34	4.0	1.0			0		0.72				0					GENM236

Grands! — 2 oz biscuit

190		4.0	23.0	5.0	<1.0	600	40					0				
58	9.0	2.5			0		1.44				0					GENM237

cinn & sugar, from refrig dough, Hungry Jack *- 1.2 oz biscuit*

110		2.0	17.0	5.0	<1.0	280	0					0				
35	4.0	1.0			0		0.72				0					GENM238

country, from refrig dough, Pillsbury *- 2.3 oz biscuit*

150		4.0	29.0	3.0	<1.0	540	0					0				
64	2.0	0.0			0		1.80				0					GENM239

extra rich, from refrig dough, Grands! *- 2.15 oz biscuit*

220		4.0	25.0	6.0	<1.0	570	40					0				
61	11.0	3.0			0		1.44				0					GENM240

	KCAL	H₂0 (g)	PRO (g)	CHO (g)	SUGR (g)	DFIB (g)	Na (mg)	Ca (mg)	Mg (mg)	Zn (mg)	Mn (mg)	A (mcg RAE)	C (mg)	B-1 (mg)	NIA (mg)	B-12 (mcg)	PANT (mg)
	WT (g)	FAT (g)	SFA (g)	MUFA (g)	PUFA (g)	CHOL (mg)	K (mg)	P (mg)	Fe (mg)	Cu (mg)	Se (mcg)	A (IU)	E (mg ATE)	B-2 (mg)	B-6 (mg)	FOL (mcg DFE)	REF
flaky, from refrig dough, Grands!	200		4.0	25.0	3.0	<1.0	580	0					0				
2.15 oz biscuit	61	9.0	2.0			0			1.44			0					GENM241
Hungry Jack	100		2.0	14.0	2.0	0.0	360	0					0				
1.2 oz biscuit	34	4.5	1.0			0			0.72			0					GENM242
golden corn, from refrig dough,	190		4.0	28.0	8.0	<1.0	610	40					0				
Grands! - *2.15 oz biscuit*	61	7.0	2.0			0			1.44			0					GENM243
homestyle, from refrig dough,	180		4.0	24.0	5.0	<1.0	600	40					0				
Grands! - *2 oz biscuit*	58	8.0	2.0			0			1.44			0					GENM244
honey butter, from refrig dough,	110		2.0	17.0	5.0	0.0	280	0					0				
Hungry Jack - *1.2 oz biscuit*	35	4.0	1.0			0			0.72			0					GENM245
mixed grain, refrig dough	116	16.6	2.7	20.9			295	7	13	0.26	0.290	0	0	0.17	1.5	0.00	0.14
1.6 oz biscuit (2 1/2″ dia)	44	2.5	0.6	1.3	0.4	0	201	104	1.21	0.051		0		0.09	0.03	58.5	18017
plain/buttermilk	186	13.6	3.2	24.7		0.7	537	25	9	0.24	0.200	1	0	0.22	1.7	0.07	0.15
1.8 oz med biscuit	51	8.4	1.3	3.5	3.2	1	114	219	1.68	0.042	9.6	1	1.5	0.15	0.02	48.5	18009
from mix	95	8.2	2.1	13.7		0.5	271	52	7	0.17	0.071	7	<1	0.10	0.9	0.06	0.16
1 oz biscuit	28	3.4	0.8	1.2	1.2	1	53	133	0.58	0.033	1.8	27		0.10	0.02	23.8	18011
from refrig dough, 12–28% fat	93	7.5	1.8	12.8		0.4	325	5	4	0.10	0.068	0	0	0.09	0.8	0.00	0.10
1 oz biscuit (2 1/2″ dia)	27	4.0	1.0	2.2	0.5	0	42	104	0.70	0.020	4.8	0	0.5	0.06	0.01	18.9	18015
from refrig dough, 2–12% fat	63	5.8	1.6	11.6		0.4	305	4	4	0.10	0.074	0	0	0.09	0.7	0.00	0.06
.7 oz biscuit (2 1/4″ dia)	21	1.1	0.3	0.6	0.2	0	39	98	0.65	0.019	3.7	0	0.1	0.05	0.01	23.9	18013
homemade	212	17.3	4.2	26.8		0.9	348	141	11	0.32	0.227	14	<1	0.21	1.8	0.05	0.17
2.1 oz biscuit (2 1/2″ dia)	60	9.8	2.6	4.2	2.5	2	73	98	1.74	0.049	11.7	49	0.8	0.19	0.02	57.0	18016
southern style flaky, from refrig	100		2.0	14.0	2.0	0.0	360	0					0				
dough, Hungry Jack - *1.2 oz bsct*	34	4.5	1.0			0			0.72			0					GENM246
southern style, from refrig dough,	100		2.0	14.0	2.0	0.0	360	0					0				
Big Country - *1.2 oz biscuit*	34	4.0	1.0			0			0.72			0					GENM247
Grands!	190		4.0	23.0	5.0	<1.0	600	40					0				
2 oz biscuit	58	9.0	2.5			0			1.44			0					GENM248
wheat, red fat, from refrig dough,	190		4.0	27.0	6.0	2.0	600	40					0				
Grands! - *2.15 oz biscuit*	61	7.0	2.0			0			1.44			0					GENM250

17.3 BREADS, QUICK

	KCAL	H₂0 (g)	PRO (g)	CHO (g)	SUGR (g)	DFIB (g)	Na (mg)	Ca (mg)	Mg (mg)	Zn (mg)	Mn (mg)	A (mcg RAE)	C (mg)	B-1 (mg)	NIA (mg)	B-12 (mcg)	PANT (mg)
banana, homemade w/marg	196	17.5	2.6	32.8		0.7	181	13	8	0.21	0.125	64	1	0.10	0.9	0.06	0.16
2.1 oz slice	60	6.3	1.3	2.7	1.9	26	80	35	0.84	0.043	7.3	296	1.1	0.12	0.09	28.8	18019
boston brown, cnd	88	21.2	2.3	19.5		2.1	284	32	28	0.23	0.459	12	0	0.01	0.5	<0.01	0.25
1.6 oz slice	45	0.7	0.1	0.1	0.3	<1	143	50	0.95	0.036	9.9	39	0.3	0.05	0.04	6.3	18021
brown bread w/raisins, cnd, B&M	130		3.0	29.0	16.0	2.0	360	40					0				
1/2″ slice (2 oz)	56	0.5	0.0			0			1.44			0					BUMO1
cornbread, from mix	188	19.1	4.3	28.9		1.4	467	44	12	0.38	0.130	26	<1	0.15	1.2	0.10	0.26
2.1 oz piece	60	6.0	1.6	3.1	0.7	37	77	226	1.14	0.037	5.9	123		0.16	0.06	51.6	18023
frzn, Marie Callender's	140		2.0	26.0	9.0	1.0	320	20					0				
2.3 oz piece	65	3.5	1.0			5			0.36			0					CNAG1
homemade w/2% milk	173	25.4	4.4	28.3			428	162	16	0.39	0.077	31	<1	0.19	1.5	0.10	0.22
2.3 oz piece	65	4.6	1.0	1.2	2.1	26	96	110	1.63	0.033	6.6	180		0.19	0.07	62.4	18024
hush puppy, homemade[1]	74	6.4	1.7	10.1		0.6	147	61	5	0.15	0.048	11	<1	0.08	0.6	0.04	0.08
.8 oz hush puppy	22	3.0	0.5	0.7	1.6	10	32	42	0.67	0.015	3.5	56	0.5	0.07	0.02	24.6	18270

[1] Small, fried ball of cornmeal dough (originally used to hush the hunger cries of hunting dogs in the southern US).

17.4 BREADS, YEAST

	KCAL	H₂0 (g)	PRO (g)	CHO (g)	SUGR (g)	DFIB (g)	Na (mg)	Ca (mg)	Mg (mg)	Zn (mg)	Mn (mg)	A (mcg RAE)	C (mg)	B-1 (mg)	NIA (mg)	B-12 (mcg)	PANT (mg)
bread crumbs, dry, grated	427	6.7	13.5	78.3		2.6	931	245	50	1.32	0.883	0	0	0.83	7.4	0.02	0.33
1 cup	108	5.8	1.3	2.6	1.2	0	239	159	6.61	0.179	40.7	1	0.6	0.47	0.11	181.4	18079
seasoned	440	6.7	17.0	84.5		5.0	3180	119	46	1.09	0.918	5	<1	0.19	3.3	0.05	0.35
1 cup	120	3.1	0.9	1.2	0.8	1	324	160	3.82	0.190	42.4	16		0.20	0.18	205.2	18376
breadcrumbs, garlic & herb,	100		4.0	18.0	1.0	1.0	530	40					0				
Progresso - *1/4 cup (1 oz)*	28	1.5	0.0			0			1.44			0					GENM391
italian style, Progresso	110		4.0	20.0	1.0	1.0	430	40					0				
1/4 cup (1 oz)	28	1.5	0.0			0			1.44			0					GENM392
parmesan, Progresso	110		4.0	19.0	2.0	1.0	870	40					0				
1/4 cup (1 oz)	28	1.5	0.0			0			1.08			0					GENM251

	KCAL / WT (g)	H₂0 (g) / FAT (g)	PRO (g) / SFA (g)	CHO (g) / MUFA (g)	SUGR (g) / PUFA (g)	DFIB (g) / CHOL (mg)	Na (mg) / K (mg)	Ca (mg) / P (mg)	Mg (mg) / Fe (mg)	Zn (mg) / Cu (mg)	Mn (mg) / Se (mcg)	A (mcg RAE) / A (IU)	C (mg) / E (mg ATE)	B-1 (mg) / B-2 (mg)	NIA (mg) / B-6 (mg)	B-12 (mcg) / FOL (mcg DFE)	PANT (mg) / REF
Progresso	110		4.0	19.0	1.0	1.0	210	40					0				
1/4 cup (1 oz)	28	1.5	0.0			0			1.44			0					GENM393
cracked wheat	65	9.0	2.2	12.4		1.4	135	11	13	0.31	0.343	0	0	0.09	0.9	<0.01	0.13
.9 oz slice	25	1.0	0.2	0.5	0.2	0	44	38	0.70	0.056	6.3	0	0.1	0.06	0.08	19.0	18025
croutons	122	1.7	3.6	22.1		1.5	209	23	9	0.27	0.150	0	0	0.19	1.6	0.00	0.13
1 cup	30	2.0	0.5	0.9	0.4	0	37	35	1.22	0.049	11.3	0		0.08	0.01	62.7	18242
parmesan italian style, Salad	30	0.3	0.8	4.7			80										
Crispins - 1 cup	7	0.9	0.1	0.4	0.2												18636
seasoned	186	1.4	4.3	25.4		2.0	495	38	17	0.38	0.206	4	0	0.20	1.9	0.06	0.33
1 cup	40	7.3	2.1	3.8	0.9	3	72	56	1.13	0.067	11.5	16	0.9	0.17	0.03	48.8	18243
seasoned, classic style, Pepperidge	33	0.2	1.0	4.3			97										
Farm - 1 cup	7	1.3	0.3														18626
egg	115	13.9	3.8	19.1		0.9	197	37	8	0.32	0.200	9	0	0.18	1.9	0.04	0.11
1.4 oz slice (5″ × 3″ × 1/2″)	40	2.4	0.6	0.9	0.4	20	46	42	1.22	0.065	12.0	30	0.2	0.17	0.03	52.0	18027
french, crusty, from refrig dough,	150		5.0	27.0	3.0	<1.0	370	0					0				
Pillsbury - 1/5 loaf (2.2 oz)	62	2.0	0.5			0			1.44			0					GENM252
french, refrig dough, Pillsbury	154	24.5	5.8	28.9			389										
2.2 oz slice	62	1.7	0.5	0.6	0.3				1.48								18631
french toast[1], frzn	126	31.0	4.4	18.9		0.6	292	63	10	0.45	0.145	32	<1	0.16	1.6	0.99	0.55
2.1 oz piece	59	3.6	0.9	1.2	0.7	48	79	82	1.30	0.050	9.9	110	0.4	0.22	0.29	42.5	18268
homemade w/2% milk	149	35.6	5.0	16.3			311	65	11	0.44	0.122	81	<1	0.13	1.1	0.20	0.36
2.3 oz piece	65	7.0	1.8	2.9	1.7	75	87	76	1.09	0.038	13.1	327		0.21	0.05	37.1	18269
french/vienna/sourdough	175	22.0	5.6	33.2		1.9	390	48	17	0.56	0.325	0	0	0.33	3.0	0.00	0.25
2.3 oz med slice (4″ × 2 1/2″ × 1 3/4″)	64	1.9	0.4	0.8	0.4	0	72	67	1.62	0.122	20.2	0	0.2	0.21	0.03	89.6	18029
garlic, frzn, Marie Callender's	190		4.0	23.0	5.0	2.0	330	20					0				
2 oz piece	57	8.0	6.0			<5			1.44			200					CNAG2
italian, frzn, Campione D'Italia	101	8.0	2.4	12.4		1.3	154										
Foods - 1 oz slice	28	4.7	0.8						0.30								18604
italian, frzn, Pepperidge Farm	186	14.6	4.2	20.8			200										
1.8 oz slice	50	9.6	2.4	3.9	1.8	6			1.19								18627
parmesan & romano, frzn, Marie	200		5.0	23.0	2.0	2.0	430	200					0				
Callender's - 2 oz piece	57	10.0	3.0			5			1.44			300					CNAG3
Health Nut, Arnold	120		5.0	21.0	3.0	2.0	230	40					0				
1.3 oz slice	38	2.0	0.0			0			1.44			0					ARNO1
honey wheat/multigrain, Healthy	60		3.0	12.0	2.0	2.0	120	100	16	0.30			0	0.15	2.0		
Choice - 1 oz slice	28	0.5	0.0	0.0	0.0	0		40	1.80	0.040		0		0.17		40.0	HLCH9
irish soda, homemade	82	8.5	1.9	15.9		0.7	113	23	7	0.16	0.101	14	<1	0.08	0.7	0.01	0.07
1 oz slice	28	1.4	0.3	0.6	0.4	5	75	32	0.76	0.037	4.5	55	0.3	0.08	0.02	20.7	18032
italian	81	10.7	2.6	15.0		0.8	175	23	8	0.26	0.139	0	0	0.14	1.3	0.00	0.11
1.1 oz slice (4 1/2″ × 3 1/4″ × 3/4″)	30	1.1	0.3	0.2	0.4	0	33	31	0.88	0.057	8.2	0	0.1	0.09	0.01	42.3	18033
mixed grain/whole grain/7-grain	65	9.8	2.6	12.1		1.7	127	24	14	0.33	0.386	0	<1	0.11	1.1	0.02	0.13
.92 oz slice	26	1.0	0.2	0.4	0.2	0	53	46	0.90	0.066	7.7	0	0.2	0.09	0.09	26.5	18035
oat bran	71	13.2	3.1	11.9		1.4	122	20	11	0.27	0.234	0	0	0.15	1.4	0.00	0.17
1.1 oz slice	30	1.3	0.2	0.5	0.5	0	44	42	0.94	0.041	9.0	2	0.2	0.10	0.02	36.0	18037
red cal	46	10.6	1.8	9.5		2.8	81	13	13	0.24	0.253	0	0	0.08	0.9	0.00	0.11
.81 oz slice	23	0.7	0.1	0.2	0.4	0	23	32	0.72	0.067	4.7	<1	0.1	0.05	0.02	20.2	18049
oatmeal	73	9.9	2.3	13.1		1.1	162	18	10	0.28	0.254	<1	0	0.11	0.8	0.01	0.09
.95 oz slice	27	1.2	0.2	0.4	0.5	0	38	34	0.73	0.056	6.6	4	0.2	0.06	0.02	23.5	18039
red cal	48	10.1	1.7	10.0			89	26	6	0.19	0.124	0	<1	0.08	0.7	0.02	0.10
.81 oz slice	23	0.8	0.1	0.2	0.3	0	29	23	0.53	0.023	5.3	1		0.06	0.01	16.1	18051
protein/gluten	47	7.6	2.3	8.3		0.6	104	24	12	0.35	0.280	0	0	0.07	0.8	0.00	0.08
.67 oz slice	19	0.4	0.1	<0.1	0.2	0	61	35	0.79	0.079	6.3	<1	0.1	0.07	0.01	28.7	18043
pumpernickel	65	9.9	2.3	12.4		1.7	174	18	14	0.38	0.339	0	0	0.09	0.8	0.00	0.11
.92 oz slice	26	0.8	0.1	0.2	0.3	0	54	46	0.75	0.075	6.4	0	0.1	0.08	0.03	29.1	18044
raisin	71	8.7	2.1	13.6		1.1	101	17	7	0.19	0.130	0	<1	0.09	0.9	0.00	0.10
.92 oz slice	26	1.1	0.3	0.6	0.2	0	59	28	0.75	0.051	5.2	0	0.1	0.10	0.02	32.2	18047
rice bran	66	11.1	2.4	11.7		1.3	119	19	22	0.35	0.428	0	0	0.18	1.8	0.00	0.21
.95 oz slice	27	1.2	0.2	0.4	0.5	0	58	48	0.97	0.050	7.7	1	0.2	0.08	0.07	24.3	18059
rye	83	11.9	2.7	15.5		1.9	211	23	13	0.36	0.264	0	<1	0.14	1.2	0.00	0.14
1.1 oz slice	32	1.1	0.2	0.4	0.3	0	53	40	0.91	0.060	9.9	2	0.1	0.11	0.02	35.5	18060
red cal	47	10.6	2.1	9.3		2.8	93	17	5	0.15	0.104	0	<1	0.08	0.6	0.01	0.07
.81 oz slice	23	0.7	0.1	0.2	0.2	0	23	18	0.71	0.031	6.4	1	0.1	0.06	0.02	15.2	18053

							Minerals					Vitamins					
	KCAL	H₂O (g)	PRO (g)	CHO (g)	SUGR (g)	DFIB (g)	Na (mg)	Ca (mg)	Mg (mg)	Zn (mg)	Mn (mg)	A (mcg RAE)	C (mg)	B-1 (mg)	NIA (mg)	B-12 (mcg)	PANT (mg)
	WT (g)	FAT (g)	SFA (g)	MUFA (g)	PUFA (g)	CHOL (mg)	K (mg)	P (mg)	Fe (mg)	Cu (mg)	Se (mcg)	A (IU)	E (mg ATE)	B-2 (mg)	B-6 (mg)	FOL (mcg DFE)	REF
Texas Toast, garlic, frzn,	160		3.0	15.0	2.0	0	240	20					0				
Pepperidge Farm - *1.4 oz slice*	40	10.0	1.5			0			0.90			200					PEPP1
wheat bran	89	13.6	3.2	17.2		1.4	175	27	29	0.49	0.600	0		0.14	1.6	0.00	0.19
1.3 oz slice	36	1.2	0.3	0.6	0.2	0	82	67	1.11	0.080	11.2	0	0.2	0.10	0.06	36.0	18066
wheat germ	73	10.4	2.7	13.5		0.6	155	25	8	0.27	0.237	0	<1	0.10	1.3	0.02	0.15
1 oz slice	28	0.8	0.2	0.4	0.2	0	71	34	0.97	0.057	7.6	<1	<0.1	0.11	0.02	33.9	18068
wheat/wheat berry	65	9.3	2.3	11.8		1.1	133	26	12	0.26	0.256	0		0.10	1.0	0.00	0.11
.88 oz slice	25	1.0	0.2	0.4	0.2	0	50	38	0.83	0.053	7.7	0	0.1	0.07	0.02	25.5	18064
red cal	46	9.9	2.1	10.0		2.8	118	18	9	0.26	0.196	0	<1	0.10	0.9	0.00	0.14
.81 oz slice	23	0.5	0.1	0.1	0.2	0	28	23	0.68	0.032	7.0	0	<0.1	0.07	0.03	23.2	18055
white	67	9.2	2.1	12.4		0.6	135	27	6	0.16	0.096	0	0	0.12	1.0	0.01	0.10
.88 oz slice	25	0.9	0.1	0.2	0.5	<1	30	24	0.76	0.032	7.1	0	0.1	0.09	0.02	34.5	18069
homemade w/2% milk	120	14.8	3.3	20.8		0.8	151	24	8	0.27	0.175	9	<1	0.17	1.5	0.03	0.16
1.5 oz thick slice	42	2.4	0.5	0.5	1.2	1	61	48	1.25	0.048	8.9	33	0.4	0.16	0.02	52.5	18073
homemade w/nonfat milk	121	15.3	3.4	23.6		0.9	148	14	7	0.26	0.202	5	0	0.19	1.6	0.01	0.12
1.6 oz thick slice	44	1.1	0.2	0.2	0.6	0	49	42	1.40	0.049	10.2	18	0.2	0.15	0.02	55.4	18071
red cal	48	9.9	2.0	10.2		2.2	104	22	5	0.31	0.090	<1	<1	0.09	0.8	0.06	0.11
.81 oz slice	23	0.6	0.1	0.2	0.1	0	17	28	0.73	0.076	5.0	1	<0.1	0.07	0.01	31.7	18057
whole grain/7-grain, Healthy Choice	80		4.0	18.0	3.0	3.0	170	150	24	0.60			0	0.23	3.0		
1.3 oz slice	38	1.0	0.0			0		60	2.70	0.080		0		0.26		60.0	HLCH8
whole wheat	69	10.6	2.7	12.9		1.9	148	20	24	0.54	0.651	0	0	0.10	1.1	<0.01	0.15
1 oz slice	28	1.2	0.3	0.5	0.3	0	71	64	0.92	0.080	10.2	0	0.2	0.06	0.05	14.0	18075
homemade	128	15.0	3.9	23.6		2.8	159	15	37	0.69	0.865	0	0	0.14	1.8	0.00	0.22
1.6 oz thick slice	46	2.5	0.4	0.5	1.4	0	144	86	1.43	0.116	17.8	0	0.6	0.10	0.09	32.7	18077

¹ White bread dipped in an egg and milk mixture and lightly fried in vegetable oil.

17.5 BREADSTICKS

breadsticks, from refrig dough,	140		4.0	25.0	3.0	<1.0	370	0					0				
Pillsbury - *2 pieces (1.8 oz)*	52	2.5	0.5			0			1.44			0					GENM253
garlic & herb, from refrig dough,	180		4.0	25.0	3.0	<1.0	580	0					0				
Pillsbury - *2 pieces (2.1 oz)*	60	7.0	1.5			0			1.44			100					GENM254
parmesan, garlic, & herb, from refrig	180		5.0	24.0	3.0	<1.0	570	40					0				
dough, Pillsbury - *2 pcs (2.1 oz)*	60	7.0	1.5			0			1.44			100					GENM255
plain	41	0.6	1.2	6.8		0.3	66	2	3	0.09	0.056	0	0	0.06	0.5	0.00	0.05
.35 oz breadstick (7 5/8″ × 5/8″)	10	1.0	0.1	0.4	0.4	0	12	12	0.43	0.019	3.8	0	0.1	0.06	0.01	18.6	18080
cornbread twists, from refrig	130		3.0	17.0	4.0	0.0	340	0					0				
dough, Pillsbury - *1.45 oz piece*	41	6.0	1.5			0			1.08			0					GENM256

17.6 CRACKERS

cheese crackers	71	0.4	1.4	8.3		0.3	141	21	5	0.16	0.089	4	0	0.08	0.7	0.07	0.07
.5 oz	14	3.6	1.3	1.7	0.4	2	21	31	0.68	0.030	1.2	23	0.4	0.06	0.08	16.9	18214
w/peanut butter filling	34	0.3	0.9	4.0		0.2	69	6	4	0.08	0.053	1	<1	0.03	0.5	<0.01	0.04
2 crackers w/filling	7	1.6	0.4	0.8	0.3	<1	17	23	0.20	0.016	1.3	22	0.3	0.02	0.10	9.2	18215
zesty, Snackwell's	129	0.6	2.2	23.1	2.1	0.6	315	13	10	0.45	0.000		<1	0.07	1.1	0.02	0.04
1.1 oz	30	3.0	0.7	0.8	0.4	1	47	60	0.95	0.010		48		0.10	0.03		18622
cracker pepper, Snackwell's	61	0.2	1.3	10.5	0.9	0.4	117	24	4	0.11			<1	0.04	0.8	0.00	
5 crackers (.49 oz)	14	1.5	0.3	0.6	0.2	0	16	45	0.51	0.024		<1	0.0	0.05	0.01		18645
crispbread, multigrain, whole	44	1.0	1.6	8.3	0.2	2.0	<1	6		0.40				0.18	0.2		
grain, Wasa - *.5 oz crispbread*	14	0.4	0.1	<0.1	0.1		67	49	0.30				<0.1	<0.01			WASA1
crispbread, oats, whole grain, Wasa	48	1.0	1.9	8.2	0.4	1.4	<1	14		0.30				<0.01	0.3		
.5 oz crispbread	14	0.7	0.2	0.2	0.2		61	48	0.30				0.1	<0.01			WASA2
crispbread, rye	37	0.6	0.8	8.2		1.7	26	3	8	0.24	0.248	0	0	0.02	0.1	0.00	0.07
1 crispbread	10	0.1	<0.1	<0.1	0.1	0	32	27	0.24	0.026	3.7	0	0.1	0.02	0.02	6.5	18216
fiber, whole grain, Wasa	31	0.6	1.4	4.7	0.3	2.5	<1	15		0.40				<0.01	0.5		
.35 oz crispbread	10	0.8	0.1	0.2	0.3		68	55	0.60				0.2	<0.01			WASA3
hearty, whole grain, Wasa	43	1.0	1.3	9.2	0.2	2.3	<1	7		0.40				<0.01	0.2		
.5 oz crispbread	14	0.2	0.1	<0.1	<0.1		65	47	0.40				<0.1	<0.01			WASA4

	KCAL	H₂0 (g)	PRO (g)	CHO (g)	SUGR (g)	DFIB (g)	Na (mg)	Ca (mg)	Mg (mg)	Zn (mg)	Mn (mg)	A (mcg RAE)	C (mg)	B-1 (mg)	NIA (mg)	B-12 (mcg)	PANT (mg)
	WT (g)	FAT (g)	SFA (g)	MUFA (g)	PUFA (g)	CHOL (mg)	K (mg)	P (mg)	Fe (mg)	Cu (mg)	Se (mcg)	A (IU)	E (mg ATE)	B-2 (mg)	B-6 (mg)	FOL (mcg DFE)	REF
sourdough, whole grain, Wasa	35	0.7	1.0	7.4	0.1	1.5	<1	4		0.20				<0.01	0.1		
.39 oz crispbread	11	0.2	0.2	<0.1	<0.1		43	30	0.20				<0.1	<0.01			WASA6
whole grain, Wasa	39	0.8	1.1	8.3	0.2	1.9	<1	5		0.30				<0.01	0.1		
.46 oz crispbread	13	0.2	0.1	<0.1	<0.1		57	44	0.30				<0.1	<0.01			WASA7
crispbread, sesame, whole grain, Wasa - .5 oz crispbread	56	0.8	1.8	8.5	0.3	0.8	<1	14		0.30				<0.01	0.4		
	14	1.6	0.4	0.5	0.5		35	32	0.30				<0.1	<0.01			WASA8
crispbread, soya & rye, whole grain, Wasa - .32 oz crispbread	27	0.4	1.0	5.4	0.2	1.4	<1	5									
	9	0.1	<0.1	<0.1	<0.1				0.30								WASA9
french onion crackers, Snackwell's	128	0.6	2.1	23.1	2.3	0.6	275	12	10	0.48			<1	0.07	1.1	0.02	
1.1 oz	30	3.0	0.5	0.7	0.4	1	44	68	0.94	0.011		7	0.0	0.09	0.03		18648
italian ranch crackers, Snackwell's	128	0.5	2.1	23.3	2.2	0.6	311	12	7	0.29			<1	0.07	1.1	0.02	
1.1 oz	30	3.0	0.6	0.8	0.4	1	42	68	0.95	0.000		11	0.0	0.09	0.02		18647
melba toast	20	0.3	0.6	3.8		0.3	41	5	3	0.10	0.057	0	0	0.02	0.2	0.00	0.03
1 toast (3 3/4″ × 1 3/4″ × 1/8″)	5	0.2	<0.1	<0.1	0.1	0	10	10	0.19	0.014	1.7	0	<0.1	0.01	<0.01	9.7	18220
rye/pumpernickel	19	0.2	0.6	3.9		0.4	45	4	2	0.07	0.037	0	0	0.02	0.2	0.00	0.02
1 toast	5	0.2	<0.1	<0.1	0.1	0	10	9	0.18	0.020	1.9	0	<0.1	0.01	<0.01	6.5	18221
wheat	19	0.3	0.6	3.8		0.4	42	2	3	0.08	0.053	0	0	0.02	0.3	0.00	0.02
1 toast	5	0.1	<0.1	<0.1	<0.1	0	7	8	0.23	0.013	2.8	0		0.01	0.01	10.4	18222
milk crackers	50	0.5	0.8	7.7		0.2	65	19	2	0.07	0.061	1	<1	0.06	0.5	0.01	0.04
1 cracker	11	1.7	0.3	0.7	0.6	1	13	33	0.39	0.025	1.7	3	0.3	0.05	<0.01	14.1	18223
Ritz Crackers, Nabisco	79	0.5	1.2	10.3	1.3	0.3	124	24	3	0.23			0	0.04	0.6	0.00	
1 cracker	16	3.7	0.6	2.9	0.3	0	15	48	0.65			0		0.05	0.01		18621
round crackers	71	0.5	1.1	8.7		0.2	120	17	4	0.10	0.079	0	0	0.06	0.6	0.00	0.04
.5 oz (~5 crackers)	14	3.6	0.5	1.5	1.4	0	19	32	0.51	0.030	0.9	0	0.6	0.05	0.01	17.2	18229
w/cheese filling	33	0.3	0.7	4.3		0.1	98	18	3	0.04	0.020	1	<1	0.03	0.3	0.01	0.04
2 crackers w/filling	7	1.5	0.4	0.8	0.2	<1	30	28	0.17	0.006	1.5	5	0.2	0.05	<0.01	9.3	18230
w/peanut butter filling - 2 crackers w/filling	34	0.2	0.8	4.1		0.2	66	7	4	0.07	0.054	0	0	0.03	0.4	<0.01	0.03
	7	1.7	0.4	0.9	0.3	0	16	17	0.21	0.018	0.3	0	0.3	0.02	0.01	8.3	18231
rusk	41	0.6	1.4	7.2			25	3	4	0.11	0.044	1	0	0.04	0.5	0.02	0.06
1 rusk	10	0.7	0.1	0.3	0.2	8	25	15	0.27	0.025	2.0	4		0.04	<0.01	10.3	18224
rye crackers w/cheese filling	34	0.3	0.6	4.3		0.3	73	16	3	0.05	0.044	2	<1	0.04	0.2	0.01	0.04
2 crackers w/filling	7	1.6	0.4	0.9	0.2	1	24	24	0.17	0.007	1.5	23		0.03	0.01	8.9	18225
rye wafers	84	1.3	2.4	20.1		5.7	199	10	30	0.70	1.342	0	<1	0.11	0.4	0.00	0.14
1 triple cracker	25	0.2	<0.1	<0.1	0.1	0	124	84	1.49	0.115	6.0	1	0.4	0.07	0.07	11.3	18226
seasoned	84	0.9	2.0	16.2		4.6	195	10	23	0.56	0.522	0	<1	0.07	0.5	0.00	0.12
1 triple cracker	22	2.0	0.3	0.7	0.8	0	100	68	0.67	0.109	7.2	2		0.05	0.04	11.4	18227
salsa crackers, Snackwell's	128	0.6	2.1	23.4	2.2	0.6	321	13	10	0.47			<1	0.07	1.1	0.01	
1.1 oz	30	3.0	0.5	0.7	0.4	1	41	66	0.94	0.011		14	0.0	0.09	0.02		18646
saltines	62	0.6	1.3	10.2		0.4	185	17	4	0.11	0.099	0	0	0.07	0.7	0.00	0.06
5 crackers (.49 oz)	14	1.7	0.4	0.9	0.2	0	18	15	0.77	0.028	1.7	0	0.2	0.07	0.01	26.8	18228
fat-free, low-Na	118	1.0	3.2	24.7		0.8	191	7	8	0.28	0.191	0	0	0.16	1.7	0.00	0.12
6 saltines (1.1 oz)	30	0.5	0.1	<0.1	0.2	0	35	34	2.32	0.044	6.4	0	<0.1	0.18	0.03	60.6	18457
Nabisco Original Premium	59	0.5	1.5	10.0		0.4	178	27	3				0	0.05	0.6		
5 crackers	14	1.4	0.3	0.8	0.2	0	14	14	0.73			0		0.06	0.01		18620
soda crackers	62	0.6	1.3	10.2		0.4	90	17	4	0.11	0.099	0	0	0.08	0.7	0.00	0.06
5 crackers (.5 oz)	14	1.7	0.4	0.9	0.2	0	103	15	0.77	0.028	2.8	0	0.2	0.07	0.01	26.8	18425
wheat crackers	67	0.4	1.2	9.2		0.6	113	7	9	0.23	0.253	0	0	0.07	0.7	0.00	0.07
.5 oz (~7 thin squares)	14	2.9	0.7	1.6	0.4	0	26	31	0.62	0.045	0.9	0	0.5	0.05	0.02	8.8	18232
Snackwell's	62	0.3	1.2	11.6	1.8	0.6	150	22	7	0.32			0	0.04			
5 crackers (.5 oz)	15	1.5					29	50	0.59	0.001		0	0.0	0.06			18652
w/cheese filling	35	0.2	0.7	4.1		0.2	64	14	4	0.06	0.076	1	<1	0.03	0.2	0.01	0.04
2 crackers w/filling	7	1.8	0.3	0.7	0.6	<1	21	27	0.18	0.011	1.7	5		0.03	0.02	6.7	18233
w/peanut butter filling	35	0.2	0.9	3.8		0.3	56	12	3	0.06	0.049	0	0	0.03	0.4	0.00	0.04
2 crackers w/filling	7	1.9	0.3	0.8	0.6	0	21	24	0.19	0.004	1.5	0		0.02	0.01	6.5	18234
Wheat Thins, Nabisco	136	0.7	2.4	20.0	2.6	0.9	168	23	15				0	0.09	1.2		
16 crackers (1 oz)	29	5.8	0.9	2.0	0.4	0	56	60	1.07			0		0.09	0.03		18624
whole wheat crackers	63	0.4	1.2	9.7		1.5	94	7	14	0.31	0.319	0	0	0.03	0.6	0.00	0.12
.5 oz (~3.5 crackers)	14	2.4	0.5	0.8	0.9	0	42	42	0.44	0.063	2.1	0	0.2	0.01	0.03	4.0	18235

	KCAL / WT (g)	H₂0 (g) / FAT (g)	PRO (g) / SFA (g)	CHO (g) / MUFA (g)	SUGR (g) / PUFA (g)	DFIB (g) / CHOL (mg)	Na (mg) / K (mg)	Ca (mg) / P (mg)	Mg (mg) / Fe (mg)	Zn (mg) / Cu (mg)	Mn (mg) / Se (mcg)	A (mcg RAE) / A (IU)	C (mg) / E (mg ATE)	B-1 (mg) / B-2 (mg)	NIA (mg) / B-6 (mg)	B-12 (mcg) / FOL (mcg DFE)	PANT (mg) / REF

17.7 ENGLISH MUFFINS

	KCAL/WT	H₂O/FAT	PRO/SFA	CHO/MUFA	SUGR/PUFA	DFIB/CHOL	Na/K	Ca/P	Mg/Fe	Zn/Cu	Mn/Se	A-RAE/A-IU	C/E	B-1/B-2	NIA/B-6	B-12/FOL	PANT/REF
mixed grain/granola	155	26.5	6.0	30.6		1.8	275	129	27	0.92	0.399	0	0	0.28	2.4	0.00	0.27
2.3 oz muffin	66	1.2	0.2	0.5	0.4	0	103	53	1.99	0.160	16.8	0	0.2	0.21	0.03	73.9	18260
plain	134	24.0	4.4	26.2		1.5	264	99	12	0.40	0.203	0	0	0.25	2.2	0.02	0.25
2 oz muffin	57	1.0	0.1	0.2	0.5	0	75	76	1.43	0.074	11.5	0	0.1	0.16	0.02	63.8	18258
Thomas'	132	24.3	5.0	26.0			210	76				0	<1				0.21
2 oz muffin	57	0.9	0.7	1.1	1.9				1.70			0	1.0				18639
raisin cinn/apple cinn	139	22.0	4.3	27.8		1.7	255	84	9	0.57	0.195	0	<1	0.22	2.0	0.00	0.30
2 oz muffin	57	1.5	0.2	0.3	0.8	0	119	39	1.38	0.062	9.1	1	0.2	0.17	0.04	65.6	18262
wheat	127	24.1	5.0	25.5		2.6	218	101	21	0.61	0.571	0	0	0.25	1.9	0.00	0.25
2 oz muffin	57	1.1	0.2	0.2	0.5	0	106	61	1.64	0.084	16.6	1	0.3	0.17	0.05	37.6	18264
whole wheat	134	30.2	5.8	26.7		4.4	420	175	47	1.06	1.181	0	0	0.20	2.3	0.00	0.46
2.3 oz muffin	66	1.4	0.2	0.3	0.6	0	139	186	1.62	0.140	26.6	0	0.5	0.09	0.11	32.3	18266

17.8 ETHNIC GRAIN PRODUCTS

	KCAL/WT	H₂O/FAT	PRO/SFA	CHO/MUFA	SUGR/PUFA	DFIB/CHOL	Na/K	Ca/P	Mg/Fe	Zn/Cu	Mn/Se	A-RAE/A-IU	C/E	B-1/B-2	NIA/B-6	B-12/FOL	PANT/REF
cellophane/long rice noodles,	491	18.8	0.2	120.5		0.7	14	35	4	0.57	0.140	0	0	0.21	0.3	0.00	0.14
chinese, dehydrated - 1 cup	140	0.1	<0.1	<0.1	<0.1	0	14	45	3.04	0.113	11.1	0	0.2	0.00	0.07	2.8	16082
chow mein noodles	237	0.3	3.8	25.9		1.8	198	9	23	0.63	0.611	2	0	0.26	2.7	0.00	0.24
1 cup	45	13.8	2.0	3.5	7.8	0	54	72	2.13	0.075	19.4	38	0.1	0.19	0.05	62.1	20113
eggroll wrapper	93	9.2	3.1	18.5		0.6	183	15	6	0.23	0.204	1	0	0.17	1.7	0.01	0.01
7" sq wrapper	32	0.5	0.1	0.1	0.2	3	26	26	1.08	0.047	9.0	4	<0.1	0.12	0.01	42.9	18368a
indian (navajo) fry bread	296	23.9	6.4	48.0		1.6	626	210	14	0.45	0.423	0	0	0.39	3.3	0.00	0.18
5" dia	90	8.6	2.1	3.6	2.3	0	67	141	3.24	0.092	21.0	0	0.7	0.27	0.02	105.3	18031
matzo	111	1.2	2.8	23.4		0.8	1	4	7	0.19	0.182	0	0	0.11	1.1	0.00	0.12
1 matzo (1 oz)	28	0.4	0.1	<0.1	0.2	0	31	25	0.88	0.017	10.3	0	<0.1	0.08	0.03	4.8	18217
egg	109	1.8	3.4	22.0		0.8	6	11	7	0.20	0.168	4	<1	0.22	1.4	0.05	0.12
1 matzo (1 oz)	28	0.6	0.2	0.2	0.1	23	42	41	0.76	0.043	7.8	12		0.17	0.02	6.7	18218
egg & onion	109	2.0	2.8	21.6		1.4	80	10	8	0.20	0.230	2	<1	0.16	1.4	0.06	0.16
1 matzo (1 oz)	28	1.1	0.3	0.3	0.3	13	23	25	1.22	0.022	10.2	7		0.12	0.03	73.4	18400
whole wheat	98	1.3	3.7	22.1		3.3	1	6	38	0.73	0.980	0	0	0.10	1.5	0.00	0.35
1 matzo (1 oz)	28	0.4	0.1	0.1	0.2	0	88	85	1.30	0.098	21.0	0	0.4	0.04	0.04	9.8	18219
phyllo dough	57	6.2	1.3	10.0		0.4	92	2	3	0.09	0.090	0	0	0.10	0.8	0.00	0.06
1 sheet	19	1.1	0.3	0.6	0.2	0	14	14	0.61	0.019	4.4	0	0.2	0.06	0.01	21.5	18338
pita bread, white	165	19.3	5.5	33.4		1.3	322	52	16	0.50	0.289	0	0	0.36	2.8	0.00	0.24
1 large pita (6 1/2" dia)	60	0.7	0.1	0.1	0.3	0	72	58	1.57	0.101	16.3	0	<0.1	0.20	0.02	87.0	18041
whole wheat	170	19.6	6.3	35.2		4.7	340	10	44	0.97	1.114	0	0	0.22	1.8	0.00	0.53
1 large pita (6 1/2" dia)	64	1.7	0.3	0.2	0.7	0	109	115	1.96	0.186	28.2	0	0.6	0.05	0.17	22.4	18042
pizza crust, from refrig dough,	150		5.0	27.0	4.0	<1.0	410	0				0					
Pillsbury - 1/5 crust (2 oz)	57	2.0	0.0			0			1.44			0					GENM257
rice noodles, ckd	192	129.9	1.6	43.8		1.8	33	7	5	0.44	0.201	0	0	0.03	0.1	0.00	0.02
1 cup	176	0.4	<0.1	<0.1	<0.1	0	7	35	0.25	0.067	7.9	0		0.01	0.01	5.3	20134
soba (japanese noodles), ckd	113	83.2	5.8	24.4			68	5	10	0.14	0.426	0	0	0.11	0.6	0.00	0.27
1 cup	114	0.1	<0.1	<0.1	<0.1	0	40	29	0.55	0.009		0		0.03	0.05	8.0	20115
somen (japanese noodles), ckd	231	119.5	7.0	48.5			283	14	4	0.39	0.442	0	0	0.04	0.2	0.00	0.30
1 cup	176	0.3	<0.1	<0.1	0.1	0	51	48	0.92	0.044		0		0.06	0.02	3.5	20117
taco shells, mini, Old El Paso	150		2.0	19.0	0.0	1.0	130	20				0					
7 shells (1.1 oz)	31	7.0	1.5			0			0.00			0					GENM258
regular, Old El Paso	150		2.0	20.0	0.0	1.0	135	20				0					
3 shells (1.1 oz)	32	7.0	2.0			0			0.00			0					GENM259
super size, Old El Paso	170		2.0	23.0	0.0	2.0	160	40				0					
2 shells (1.3 oz)	37	8.0	1.5			0			0.00			0					GENM260
white corn, regular, Old El Paso	150		2.0	20.0	0.0	1.0	140	20				0					
3 shells (1.1 oz)	32	7.0	2.0			0			0.00			0					GENM261
tortilla, corn	53	10.6	1.4	11.2		1.2	39	42	16	0.23	0.096	0	0	0.03	0.4	0.00	0.05
1 med (6" dia)	24	0.6	0.1	0.2	0.3	0	37	75	0.34	0.037	1.3	0	<0.1	0.02	0.05	43.9	18363
shelf-stable, Old El Paso	160		3.0	26.0	<1.0	0.0	370	80				0					
2 tortillas (1.8 oz)	50	4.5	1.0			0			1.44			0					GENM262

	KCAL / WT (g)	H₂O (g) / FAT (g)	PRO (g) / SFA (g)	CHO (g) / MUFA (g)	SUGR (g) / PUFA (g)	DFIB (g) / CHOL (mg)	Na (mg) / K (mg)	Ca (mg) / P (mg)	Mg (mg) / Fe (mg)	Zn (mg) / Cu (mg)	Mn (mg) / Se (mcg)	A (mcg RAE) / A (IU)	C (mg) / E (mg ATE)	B-1 (mg) / B-2 (mg)	NIA (mg) / B-6 (mg)	B-12 (mcg) / FOL (mcg DFE)	PANT (mg) / REF
taco shell	62	0.8	1.0	8.3		1.0	49	21	14	0.19	0.058	0	0	0.03	0.2	0.00	0.06
1 med (5″ dia)	13	3.0	0.4	1.2	1.1	0	24	33	0.33	0.016	1.6	0	0.5	0.01	0.04	23.1	18360
tortilla, flour	150	12.3	4.0	25.6		1.5	220	58	12	0.33	0.213	0	0	0.24	1.6	0.00	0.27
1 med (7–8″ dia)	46	3.3	0.8	1.7	0.5	0	60	57	1.52	0.123	10.8	0	0.4	0.13	0.02	92.5	18364
Mission Foods	146	17.1	4.4	25.3			249	97									
1 med (8″ dia)	51	3.1	0.4	1.4	0.5				1.01								18616
no lard, Pinata	100		3.0	20.0	0.0	1.0	120	0					0				
1.2 oz tortilla	35	1.5	0.0			0			1.08			0					PNTA1
refrig, Old El Paso	130		3.0	21.0	<1.0	0.0	310	60						0			
1.45 oz tortilla	41	4.0	1.0			0			1.08			0					GENM263
shelf-stable, Old El Paso	130		3.0	21.0	0.0	0.0	290	60						0			
1.45 oz tortilla	41	3.5	1.0			0			1.44			0					GENM264
tostada shells, Old El Paso	150		2.0	20.0	0.0	1.0	135	20						0			
3 shells (1.1 oz)	32	7.0	1.5			0			0.00			0					GENM265
wonton wrapper	23	2.3	0.8	4.6		0.1	46	4	2	0.06	0.051	<1	0	0.04	0.4	<0.01	<0.01
3 1/2″ sq wrapper	8	0.1	<0.1	<0.1	<0.1	1	7	6	0.27	0.012	2.3	1	<0.1	0.03	<0.01	10.7	18368b

17.9 MUFFINS

	KCAL / WT (g)	H₂O (g) / FAT (g)	PRO (g) / SFA (g)	CHO (g) / MUFA (g)	SUGR (g) / PUFA (g)	DFIB (g) / CHOL (mg)	Na (mg) / K (mg)	Ca (mg) / P (mg)	Mg (mg) / Fe (mg)	Zn (mg) / Cu (mg)	Mn (mg) / Se (mcg)	A (mcg RAE) / A (IU)	C (mg) / E (mg ATE)	B-1 (mg) / B-2 (mg)	NIA (mg) / B-6 (mg)	B-12 (mcg) / FOL (mcg DFE)	PANT (mg) / REF
blueberry, homemade w/2% milk	162	22.5	3.7	23.2			251	108	9	0.31	0.178	22	1	0.16	1.3	0.08	0.19
2 oz muffin	57	6.2	1.2	1.5	3.1	21	70	83	1.29	0.040	9.7	80		0.16	0.02	41.6	18278
corn	424	45.3	8.2	70.8		4.7	724	103	44	0.75	0.493	42	0	0.38	2.8	0.13	0.62
4.9 oz muffin	139	11.7	1.9	2.9	4.5	36	96	395	3.91	0.416	21.1	289	2.6	0.45	0.12	114.0	18279
from mix	91	8.6	2.1	13.9		0.7	225	21	6	0.18	0.063	12	<1	0.07	0.6	0.05	0.13
1 oz muffin	28	2.9	0.8	1.5	0.4	18	37	109	0.55	0.018	4.3	60		0.08	0.03	25.2	18280
homemade w/2% milk	180	18.8	4.0	25.2			333	148	13	0.35	0.106	26	<1	0.17	1.4	0.09	0.20
2 oz muffin (2 3/4″ × 2″)	57	7.0	1.3	1.7	3.5	24	83	101	1.49	0.034	7.6	137		0.18	0.05	53.0	18282
oat bran	375	48.7	9.7	67.1		6.4	546	88	218	2.56	3.656	0	0	0.36	0.6	0.01	1.40
4.9 oz muffin	139	10.3	1.5	2.4	5.7	0	705	523	5.84	0.459	15.3	0	1.8	0.13	0.22	105.6	18283
plain, homemade w/2% milk	169	21.5	3.9	23.6		1.5	266	114	10	0.32	0.169	23	<1	0.16	1.3	0.09	0.20
2 oz muffin	57	6.5	1.2	1.6	3.3	22	69	87	1.36	0.039	10.3	80		0.17	0.02	44.5	18273
toaster muffin, blueberry, toasted	103	8.2	1.5	17.6		0.6	158	4	5	0.15	0.146	28	0	0.06	0.6	<0.01	0.06
1 muffin	31	3.1	0.5	0.7	1.7	2	27	60	0.17	0.031	5.8	94	0.2	0.09	0.01	22.9	18386
frzn, Howard Johnson's Toastees	235	23.0	5.0	32.0			408	46									
1 muffin	71	9.7	1.5			21			1.69								18607
wheat bran raisin, toasted	106	9.2	1.9	18.9		2.8	179	13	7	0.15	0.147	17	0	0.07	0.8	0.01	0.06
1 muffin	34	3.2	0.5	0.8	1.7	3	60	97	0.96	0.041	6.9	58	0.4	0.10	0.02	11.2	18388

17.10 PANCAKES

	KCAL / WT (g)	H₂O (g) / FAT (g)	PRO (g) / SFA (g)	CHO (g) / MUFA (g)	SUGR (g) / PUFA (g)	DFIB (g) / CHOL (mg)	Na (mg) / K (mg)	Ca (mg) / P (mg)	Mg (mg) / Fe (mg)	Zn (mg) / Cu (mg)	Mn (mg) / Se (mcg)	A (mcg RAE) / A (IU)	C (mg) / E (mg ATE)	B-1 (mg) / B-2 (mg)	NIA (mg) / B-6 (mg)	B-12 (mcg) / FOL (mcg DFE)	PANT (mg) / REF
buttermilk, homemade	86	20.0	2.6	10.9			198	60	6	0.24	0.077	11	<1	0.08	0.6	0.07	0.16
4″ dia pancake	38	3.5	0.7	0.9	1.7	22	55	53	0.65	0.020	5.7	40		0.11	0.02	21.3	18390
Kellogg's Eggo	270	54.8	7.0	44.2	9.5	1.3	615	41	21	0.70			2	0.30	4.0	1.19	0.00
3 pancakes	116	7.8	1.7	3.4	2.5	13	119	396	3.60	0.000		1000	0.0	0.34	0.41		18499
mini, microwave, frzn, Hungry	270		5.0	45.0	12.0	<1.0	570	80					0				
Jack - 11 pancakes	112	8.0	1.5			10			1.80			0					GENM266
plain, from complete mix	74	20.1	2.0	13.9		0.5	239	48	8	0.15	0.103	4	<1	0.08	0.7	0.08	0.09
4″ pancake	38	1.0	0.2	0.3	0.3	5	67	127	0.59	0.036	5.1	12		0.08	0.03	21.7	18290
from incomplete mix	83	20.1	3.0	11.0		0.7	192	82	8	0.29	0.053	27	<1	0.08	0.5	0.13	0.19
4″ pancake	38	2.9	0.8	0.8	1.1	27	76	119	0.49	0.018	3.7	95		0.12	0.04	20.5	18292
frzn	94	18.5	2.1	17.9		0.7	209	25	6	0.27	0.105	12	<1	0.16	1.6	0.07	0.18
4″ pancake	41	1.4	0.3	0.5	0.4	4	30	153	1.43	0.016	6.4	41	0.2	0.19	0.03	30.8	18288
homemade	86	20.1	2.4	10.8			167	83	6	0.21	0.076	21	<1	0.08	0.6	0.08	0.15
4″ pancake	38	3.7	0.8	0.9	1.7	22	50	60	0.68	0.019	5.7	74		0.11	0.02	21.3	18293
microwave, frzn, Hungry Jack[1]	260		5.0	51.0	13.0	1.0	600	80					0				
3 pancakes	116	4.0	1.0			10			1.80			0					GENM267
mini, frzn, Krusteaz	116	26.1	3.6	21.7			290					3002					
1.9 oz	54	1.6	0.2	0.7	0.3				1.46								18611
whole wheat, from incomplete mix	92	23.2	3.7	12.9		1.2	252	110	20	0.46	0.680	28	<1	0.09	1.0	0.13	0.23
4″ pancake	44	2.9	0.8	0.8	1.1	27	123	164	1.37	0.035	8.5	99		0.23	0.05	15.4	18300

[1] Values are averages for blueberry, buttermilk, and original.

17.11 PASTA

Food	KCAL / WT (g)	H₂O (g) / FAT (g)	PRO (g) / SFA (g)	CHO (g) / MUFA (g)	SUGR (g) / PUFA (g)	DFIB (g) / CHOL (mg)	Na (mg) / K (mg)	Ca (mg) / P (mg)	Mg (mg) / Fe (mg)	Zn (mg) / Cu (mg)	Mn (mg) / Se (mcg)	A (mcg RAE) / A (IU)	C (mg) / E (mg ATE)	B-1 (mg) / B-2 (mg)	NIA (mg) / B-6 (mg)	B-12 (mcg) / FOL (mcg DFE)	PANT (mg) / REF
corn pasta, ckd	176	95.6	3.7	39.1		6.7	0	1	50	0.88	0.214	4	0	0.07	0.8	0.00	0.18
1 cup	140	1.0	0.1	0.3	0.5	0	43	106	0.35	0.090	3.9	80	0.5	0.03	0.08	8.4	20092
creste de gallo, parsley garlic,	210		8.0	41.0	2.0	4.0	0	20	60	1.20		0	0	0.23	3.0		
unckd, Eden Foods - 1/2 cup (1.9 oz)	55	1.0	0.0			0	150	100	1.80			0		0.07		18.0	EDEN5
egg pasta, homemade, ckd	74	39.2	3.0	13.4			47	6	8	0.25	0.104	10	0	0.10	0.7	0.06	0.13
2 oz	57	1.0	0.2	0.3	0.3	23	12	30	0.66	0.032		33		0.10	0.02	34.2	20097
refrig, ckd	75	39.1	2.9	14.2			3	3	10	0.32	0.128	3	0	0.12	0.6	0.08	0.10
2 oz	57	0.6	0.1	0.1	0.2	19	14	36	0.65	0.053		11		0.09	0.02	59.3	20094
gemelli, pesto, 50% whole wheat,	210		8.0	41.0	2.0	4.0	0	20	40	0.90			0	0.12	1.6		
unckd, Eden Foods - 1/2 cup (1.9 oz)	55	1.0	0.0			0	220	100	1.08			100		0.03		18.0	EDEN14
twisted pair (wheat & quinoa), unckd,	210		8.0	40.0	2.0	5.0	0	20	80	1.50			0	0.23	3.0		
Eden Foods - 1/2 cup (1.9 oz)	55	2.0	0.0			0	280	200	2.70			0		0.14		21.0	EDEN15
homemade pasta w/o egg, ckd	71	39.3	2.5	14.3			42	3	8	0.21	0.110	0	0	0.10	0.8	0.00	0.09
2 oz	57	0.6	0.1	0.1	0.3	0	11	23	0.64	0.034		0		0.08	0.02	34.8	20098
macaroni, enr, ckd	197	92.4	6.7	39.7		1.8	1	10	25	0.74	0.399	0	0	0.29	2.3	0.00	0.16
1 cup	140	0.9	0.1	0.1	0.4	0	43	76	1.96	0.137	29.8	0	0.2	0.14	0.05	172.2	20100
macaroni, protein-fortified, ckd	189	68.7	9.3	36.4			6	12	35	0.58	0.480	0	0	0.34	2.1	0.00	0.33
1 cup	115	0.2	<0.1	<0.1	0.1	0	48	58	0.83	0.097		0		0.19	0.07	151.8	20102
macaroni, veg, ckd	172	91.6	6.1	35.7		5.8	8	15	25	0.59	1.321	4	0	0.15	1.4	0.00	0.47
1 cup	134	0.1	<0.1	<0.1	0.1	0	42	67	0.66	0.123	26.5	71	0.1	0.08	0.03	142.0	20106
macaroni, whole wheat, ckd	174	94.0	7.5	37.2		3.9	4	21	42	1.13	1.931	0	0	0.15	1.0	0.00	0.59
1 cup	140	0.8	0.1	0.1	0.3	0	62	125	1.48	0.234	36.3	0	0.1	0.06	0.11	7.0	20108
noodles, egg, & spinach, ckd	211	109.6	8.1	38.8		3.7	19	30	38	1.01	0.507	16	0	0.39	2.4	0.22	0.37
1 cup	160	2.5	0.6	0.8	0.6	53	59	91	1.74	0.128	34.9	165	0.1	0.20	0.18	150.4	20112
noodles, egg, enr, ckd	213	109.9	7.6	39.7		1.8	11	19	30	0.99	0.419	10	0	0.30	2.4	0.14	0.23
1 cup	160	2.4	0.5	0.7	0.7	53	45	110	2.54	0.138	34.7	32	0.1	0.13	0.06	166.4	20110
ribbons, spinach, unckd, Eden Foods	210		8.0	41.0	2.0	4.0	30	20	60	1.20			0	0.23	3.0		
1/2 cup (1.9 oz)	55	1.0	0.0			0	390	100	1.80			0		0.07		18.0	EDEN20
ribbons, thick kluski, unckd, Eden	210		8.0	41.0	2.0	4.0	0	20	60	1.20			0	0.23	3.0		
Foods - 1/2 cup (1.9 oz)	55	1.0	0.0			0	150	100	1.80			0		0.07		18.0	EDEN21
rigatoni, endless tubes, unckd,	210		8.0	41.0	2.0	4.0	0	20	60	1.20			0	0.23	3.0		
Eden Foods - 1/2 cup (1.9 oz)	55	1.0	0.0			0	220	100	1.80			0		0.07		18.0	EDEN22
spaghetti, enr, ckd	197	92.4	6.7	39.7		2.4	1	10	25	0.74	0.399	0	0	0.29	2.3	0.00	0.16
1 cup	140	0.9	0.1	0.1	0.4	0	43	76	1.96	0.137	29.8	0	0.2	0.14	0.05	172.2	20121
kamut wheat, unckd, Eden Foods	190		10.0	38.0	2.0	6.0	0	0	60	2.25			0	0.23	3.0		
1.9 oz	55	1.5	0.0			0	240	250	2.70			0		0.10		13.0	EDEN27
parsley garlic, unckd, Eden Foods	210		8.0	41.0	2.0	4.0	0	20	60	1.20			0	0.23	3.0		
1.9 oz	55	1.0	0.0			0	150	100	1.80			0		0.07		18.0	EDEN28
spaghetti, protein-fortified, ckd	230	83.6	11.3	44.3		2.4	7	14	42	0.70	0.584	0	0	0.42	2.6	0.00	0.40
1 cup	140	0.3	<0.1	<0.1	0.1	0	59	70	1.01	0.118	35.3	0	0.1	0.23	0.09	184.8	20123
spaghetti, spinach, ckd	182	95.4	6.4	36.6			20	42	87	1.51	2.106	11	0	0.14	2.1	0.00	0.26
1 cup	140	0.9	0.1	0.1	0.4	0	81	151	1.46	0.287	30.9	213		0.14	0.13	16.8	20127
spaghetti, whole wheat, ckd	174	94.0	7.5	37.2		6.3	4	21	42	1.13	1.931	0	0	0.15	1.0	0.00	0.59
1 cup	140	0.8	0.1	0.1	0.3	0	62	125	1.48	0.234	36.3	0	0.1	0.06	0.11	7.0	20125
100%, unckd, Eden Foods	210		10.0	40.0	2.0	6.0	0	20	80	2.25			0	0.30	3.0		
1/2 cup (1.9 oz)	55	1.5	0.0			0	260	200	2.70			100		0.07		13.0	EDEN25
50%, unckd, Eden Foods	210		8.0	41.0	2.0	4.0	0	20	60	1.20			0	0.23	3.0		
1.9 oz	55	1.0	0.0			0	220	100	1.80			0		0.07		18.0	EDEN26
spinach pasta, refrig, ckd	74	39.1	2.9	14.3			3	10	14	0.36	0.180	6	0	0.10	0.6	0.08	0.13
2 oz	57	0.5	0.1	0.2	0.1	19	21	32	0.63	0.046		59		0.08	0.06	54.7	20096
spirals, kamut wheat & veg, unckd,	210		8.0	40.0	3.0	6.0	45	20	80	2.25			0	0.15	0.0		
Eden Foods - 1/2 cup (1.9 oz)	55	2.0	0.0			0	210	200	3.60			200		0.07		24.0	EDEN29
kamut wheat, unckd, Eden	190		10.0	33.0	2.0	6.0	0	0	60	2.25			0	0.23	3.0		
Foods - 1/2 cup 1.9 oz	55	1.5	0.0			0	240	250	2.70					0.10		13.0	EDEN30
mixed grain, unckd, Eden Foods	210		8.0	41.0	3.0	7.0	15	20	60	2.25			0	0.09	2.0		
1/2 cup (1.9 oz)	55	2.0	0.0			0	210	150	2.70			0		0.10		32.0	EDEN31
rye, unckd, Eden Foods	200		6.0	44.0	1.0	8.0	10	26	110	2.20			12	0.38	4.0		
1/2 cup (1.9 oz)	55	0.0	0.0			0	300	270	4.00			0		0.16		130.0	EDEN32

	KCAL / WT (g)	H₂O (g) / FAT (g)	PRO (g) / SFA (g)	CHO (g) / MUFA (g)	SUGR (g) / PUFA (g)	DFIB (g) / CHOL (mg)	Na (mg) / K (mg)	Ca (mg) / P (mg)	Mg (mg) / Fe (mg)	Zn (mg) / Cu (mg)	Mn (mg) / Se (mcg)	A (mcg RAE) / A (IU)	C (mg) / E (mg ATE)	B-1 (mg) / B-2 (mg)	NIA (mg) / B-6 (mg)	B-12 (mcg) / FOL (mcg DFE)	PANT (mg) / REF
sesame rice, unckd, Eden Foods	200		8.0	37.0	1.0	4.0	0	80	100	2.25			0	0.30	8.0		
1/2 cup (1.9 oz)	55	2.0	0.0			0	280	300	1.80			0		0.10		16.0	EDEN33
spinach, unckd, Eden Foods	210		8.0	41.0	2.0	4.0	30	20	60	1.20			0	0.23	3.0		
1/2 cup (1.9 oz)	55	1.0	0.0			0	320	100	1.80			0		0.07		18.0	EDEN34

17.12 ROLLS

	KCAL / WT (g)	H₂O / FAT	PRO / SFA	CHO / MUFA	SUGR / PUFA	DFIB / CHOL	Na / K	Ca / P	Mg / Fe	Zn / Cu	Mn / Se	A RAE / A IU	C / E	B-1 / B-2	NIA / B-6	B-12 / FOL	PANT / REF
crescent, from refrig dough, Grands!	270		5.0	29.0	5.0	<1.0	510	0					0				
2.6 oz roll	73	15.0	3.5			0			1.44			0					GENM268
from refrig dough, Pillsbury	110		2.0	11.0	2.0	0.0	220						0				
1 oz roll	28	6.0	1.5			0			0.72			0					GENM269
red fat, from refrig dough, Pillsbury	100		2.0	12.0	2.0	0.0	230	0					0				
1 oz roll	28	4.5	1.0			0			0.72			0					GENM270
dinner	84	8.9	2.4	14.1		0.8	146	33	6	0.22	0.130	0	<1	0.14	1.1	0.02	0.14
1 oz roll (2" sq, 2" high)	28	2.0	0.5	1.0	0.3	<1	37	32	0.88	0.043	7.6	0	0.2	0.09	0.02	39.5	18342a
egg	107	10.6	3.3	18.2		1.3	191	21	9	0.39	0.184	3	0	0.18	1.2	0.08	0.23
1.2 oz roll (2 1/2" dia)	35	2.2	0.6	1.0	0.4	18	36	35	1.23	0.047	10.4	9	0.3	0.18	0.02	49.4	18344
homemade w/2% milk	111	10.2	3.0	18.7		0.7	145	21	7	0.25	0.140	30	<1	0.14	1.2	0.05	0.16
1.2 oz roll (2 1/2")	35	2.6	0.6	1.0	0.7	12	53	44	1.04	0.040	8.0	118	0.3	0.14	0.02	43.1	18396
wheat, from refrig dough, Pillsbury - 1.4 oz roll	110		4.0	18.0	3.0	1.0	270	0					0				
	40	2.0	0.0			0			1.08			0					GENM271
white, from refrig dough, Pillsbury - 1.4 oz roll	110		4.0	18.0	3.0	<1.0	270	0					0				
	40	2.0	0.0			0			1.08			0					GENM272
frankfurter/hot dog regular size (1.5 oz)	123	14.6	3.7	21.6		1.2	241	60	9	0.27	0.141	0	<1	0.21	1.7	0.03	0.23
	43	2.2	0.5	0.4	1.1	0	61	38	1.36	0.049	11.4	0	0.7	0.13	0.02	61.5	18350b
foot long roll (3 oz)	258	27.4	7.2	43.3		2.6	448	102	20	0.66	0.401	0	<1	0.42	3.5	0.05	0.43
	86	6.3	1.5	3.2	1.0	1	114	100	2.69	0.131	23.4	0	0.8	0.27	0.05	121.3	18342b
french	105	13.2	3.3	19.1		1.2	231	35	8	0.34	0.212	0	0	0.20	1.7	0.00	0.17
1.3 oz roll	38	1.6	0.4	0.7	0.3	0	43	32	1.03	0.051	10.6	0	0.2	0.11	0.01	52.4	18349
hamburger	123	14.6	3.7	21.6		1.2	241	60	9	0.27	0.141	0	<1	0.21	1.7	0.03	0.23
1.5 oz roll	43	2.2	0.5	0.4	1.1	0	61	38	1.36	0.049	11.4	0	0.7	0.13	0.02	61.5	18350c
mixed grain	113	16.3	4.1	19.2		1.6	197	41	19	0.45	0.436	0	0	0.20	1.9	<0.01	0.21
1.5 oz roll	43	2.6	0.6	1.2	0.5	0	69	52	1.70	0.093	13.7	<1	0.2	0.13	0.04	61.1	18351
Wonder	117	14.7	3.5	21.9	4.8	1.1	256	37									
1.5 oz roll	43	1.8	0.4	0.4	0.9				0.95								18641
hard/kaiser	167	17.7	5.6	30.0		1.3	310	54	15	0.54	0.262	0	0	0.27	2.4	0.00	0.23
2 oz roll (3 1/2" dia)	57	2.5	0.3	0.6	1.0	0	62	57	1.87	0.093	22.3	0	0.2	0.19	0.02	86.1	18353
oat bran	78	14.5	3.1	13.3		1.4	136	28	11	0.34	0.249	0	0	0.15	1.6	0.00	0.14
1.2 oz roll	33	1.5	0.2	0.5	0.5	0	40	38	1.37	0.045	9.7	2	0.2	0.10	0.01	46.2	18345
rye	103	10.8	3.7	19.1		1.8	321	11	19	0.35	0.253	0	0	0.14	1.4	0.00	0.14
1.3 oz roll	36	1.2	0.2	0.4	0.3	0	65	57	0.97	0.072	10.0	3	0.1	0.10	0.02	47.2	18346
wheat	76	10.4	2.4	12.9		1.1	95	49	10	0.25	0.286	0	0	0.12	1.1	0.00	0.10
1 oz roll	28	1.8	0.4	0.9	0.3	0	32	29	0.99	0.042	9.2	0	0.3	0.08	0.02	21.3	18347
whole wheat	96	11.9	3.1	18.4		2.7	172	38	31	0.72	0.827	0	0	0.09	1.3	0.00	0.18
1.3 oz roll (2 1/2" dia)	36	1.7	0.3	0.4	0.8	0	98	81	0.87	0.086	17.8	0	0.5	0.05	0.07	10.8	18348

17.13 STUFFINGS & COATINGS

	KCAL / WT (g)	H₂O / FAT	PRO / SFA	CHO / MUFA	SUGR / PUFA	DFIB / CHOL	Na / K	Ca / P	Mg / Fe	Zn / Cu	Mn / Se	A RAE / A IU	C / E	B-1 / B-2	NIA / B-6	B-12 / FOL	PANT / REF
bread stuffing, from mix	178	64.8	3.2	21.7		2.9	543	32	12	0.28	0.169	78	0	0.14	1.5	0.01	0.08
1/2 cup	100	8.6	1.7	3.8	2.6	0	74	42	1.09	0.072	49.8	313	1.4	0.11	0.04	160.0	18082
chicken flvr stuffing mix, Stove Top - amt to make 1/2 cup	107	1.5	3.5	20.5	2.8	0.7	429	18					1	0.11	1.1		
	28	1.1	0.2			1	75	36	1.21			30		0.08			18567
cornbread stuffing from mix	179	64.9	2.9	21.9		2.9	455	26	13	0.23	0.114	80	1	0.12	1.2	0.01	0.06
1/2 cup	100	8.8	1.8	3.9	2.7	0	62	34	0.94	0.069	30.7	353	1.4	0.09	0.04	159.0	18085
pork coating, dry, original recipe, Shake 'n Bake - 1 oz	106	0.9	1.7	22.3			795										
	28	1.0															18637
sage & onion stuffing mix, Brownberry - 2.4 oz	255	4.2	8.9	47.2		3.6	1126										
	67	3.4	0.6	1.4	0.5				2.55								18603
seasoned stuffing mix, Orowheat	107	2.9	4.0	21.6		1.4	284	42									
1.1 oz	30	0.5	0.1	0.1	0.2				1.57								18625

	KCAL	H₂0 (g)	PRO (g)	CHO (g)	SUGR (g)	DFIB (g)	Na (mg)	Ca (mg)	Mg (mg)	Zn (mg)	Mn (mg)	A (mcg RAE)	C (mg)	B-1 (mg)	NIA (mg)	B-12 (mcg)	PANT (mg)
	WT (g)	FAT (g)	SFA (g)	MUFA (g)	PUFA (g)	CHOL (mg)	K (mg)	P (mg)	Fe (mg)	Cu (mg)	Se (mcg)	A (IU)	E (mg ATE)	B-2 (mg)	B-6 (mg)	FOL (mcg DFE)	REF
diced, Gerber Graduates	82	149.4	0.9	19.1	15.0	1.4	13	14	14	0.12	<0.001	103	53	0.02	0.8		
6 oz jar	170	<0.1	<0.1			<1	133	29	0.31	0.041		342		0.05	0.04		GERB313
Gerber 1st Foods	31	63.0	0.5	7.0	5.3	1.0	1	<1	5	0.07	0.036	50	16	0.01	0.5		
2.5 oz jar	71	<0.1					114	11	0.14	0.036		166		0.03	0.02		GERB315
Gerber 1st Foods, Tender	31	63.1	0.5	7.0	5.3	1.0	1	<1	5	0.06	0.038	50	16	0.01	0.5		
Harvest - 2.5 oz jar	71	<0.1					113	12	0.11	0.036		166		0.03	0.02		GERB316
plastic container, Gerber 2nd	62	83.3	0.7	14.6	11.4	1.3	5	7	10	0.10	0.059	94	16	0.01	0.6		
Foods - 3.5 oz pkg	99	<0.1					164	23	0.10	0.069		315		0.04	0.05		GERB317
toddler	87	148.6	0.9	20.1		1.4	9	10	14	0.20	0.085	12	53	0.02	0.8	0.00	0.29
6 oz jar	170	0.3	<0.1	0.1	0.1	0	141	29	0.34	0.051	0.7	235	2.2	0.03	0.07	8.5	03161
peach strawbry w/mxd grains,	83	92.3	1.6	19.0	9.8	1.5	7	12	18	0.33	0.294	27	16	0.04	0.6		
Grbr 2nd Fds, Tndr Hrvst - 4 oz jar	113	0.4					116	48	0.43	0.045		89		0.02	0.06		GERB314
pear, diced, Gerber Graduates	93	146.5	0.5	23.4	18.0	2.5	9	16	12	0.10	<0.001	<1	53	0.02	0.2		
6 oz jar	170	<0.1	<0.1			<1	90	23	0.27	0.062		<1		0.03	0.06		GERB319
Beech-Nut Baby's 1st/Gerber 1st	29	62.8	0.2	7.7		2.6	1	6	6	0.06		1	17	0.01	0.1	0.00	0.06
Fds/Heinz Beg-1 - 2.5 oz jar	71	0.1	<0.1	<0.1	<0.1	0	92	9	0.17	0.046	0.3	23	0.4	0.02	0.01	2.8	03132a
Beech-Nut Stage 1/Gerber 2nd	46	99.9	0.3	12.2		4.1	2	9	9	0.09		2	28	0.01	0.2	0.00	0.10
Fds/Heinz Str-2 - 4 oz jar	113	0.2	<0.1	<0.1	0.1	0	147	14	0.27	0.073	0.5	37	0.7	0.03	0.01	4.5	03132b
Beech-Nut Stage 3/Gerber 3rd	73	149.3	0.5	19.7		6.1	3	14	15	0.14		3	37	0.02	0.3	0.00	0.16
Fds/Heinz Jr-3 - 6 oz jar	170	0.2	<0.1	<0.1	<0.1	0	196	20	0.43	0.136	0.7	58	1.0	0.05	0.02	6.8	03133
Earth's Best	52	113.2	0.4	13.8		4.6	3	10	10	0.10		3	31	0.02	0.2	0.00	0.12
4.5 oz jar	128	0.3	<0.1	0.1	0.1	0	166	15	0.31	0.083	0.5	42	0.8	0.04	0.01	5.1	03132c
Gerber 1st Foods	40	60.7	0.3	9.7	6.0	2.1	<1	7	5	0.07	0.036	2	16	0.01	0.1		
2.5 oz jar	71	<0.1					83	9	0.07	0.057		8		0.02	0.01		GERB323
plastic container, Gerber 2nd	71	81.4	0.4	17.0	11.0	2.7	3	11	10	0.10	0.069	<1	16	0.01	0.3		
Foods - 3.5 oz pkg	99	<0.1					144	15	0.20	0.069		<1		0.03	0.03		GERB324
toddler	97	145.5	0.5	23.1		2.0	10	17	12	0.15	0.051	0	53	0.02	0.2	0.00	
6 oz jar	170	0.2	<0.1	0.1	0.1	0	87	22	0.34	0.068	0.7	0	0.9	0.03	0.07	1.7	03141
pear & pinaple, Bch-Nut Stg 2/	46	100.0	0.3	12.3		2.9	5	11	8	0.08		1	31	0.02	0.2	0.00	0.10
Grbr 2nd Fds/Heinz Str-2 - 4 oz jar	113	0.1	<0.1	<0.1	<0.1	0	131	10	0.28	0.158	0.5	33	0.7	0.03	0.02	3.4	03158
Gerber 3rd Fds	75	149.3	0.5	19.4		4.4	2	17	12	0.22		3	29	0.04	0.3	0.00	0.16
6 oz jar	170	0.3	<0.1	0.1	0.1	0	201	17	0.36	0.179	0.7	54	1.0	0.04	0.02	5.1	03159
pear & wild blueberry, Gerber 2nd	73	94.7	0.4	17.4	11.9	2.3	2	13	9	0.11	0.398	<1	16	0.02	0.2		
Foods, Tender Harvest - 4 oz jar	113	<0.1					163	18	0.19	0.097		<1		0.06	0.02		GERB318
pear & winter squash, Gerber 2nd	53	99.5	1.1	11.6	7.5	1.8	3	24	18	0.19	0.077	363	1	0.03	0.6		
Foods, Tender Harvest - 4 oz jar	113	<0.1					268	30	0.30	0.090		1211		0.05	0.12		GERB322
plums w/apples, Gerber 2nd Foods	60	97.8	0.4	14.3	11.2	0.5	3	7	6	0.08	0.068	91	<1	0.02	0.4		
4 oz jar	113	<0.1					127	10	0.14	0.034		302		0.03	0.06		GERB327
Gerber 3rd Foods	64	97.0	0.5	14.6	11.3	1.6	2	8	6	0.11	0.057	95	<1	0.02	0.3		
4 oz jar	113	<0.1					122	10	0.11	0.034		315		0.06	0.07		GERB328
plums w/tapioca, Gerber 2nd Fds/	80	90.4	0.1	22.3		1.4	7	7	5	0.09		6	1	0.01	0.2	0.00	0.12
Heinz Str-2 - 4 oz jar	113	0.0	0.0	0.0	0.0	0	96	7	0.23	0.042	0.5	107	0.7	0.03	0.03	1.1	03134
Gerber 3rd Foods	126	134.6	0.2	34.7		2.0	14	10	7	0.14		9	1	0.01	0.4	0.00	0.19
6 oz jar	170	0.0	0.0	0.0	0.0	0	141	10	0.37	0.065	0.7	160	1.0	0.05	0.05	1.7	03135
prunes, Gerber 1st Foods	72	52.7	0.7	17.1	9.2	1.8	4	15	12	0.14	0.085	106	<1	0.01	0.6		
2.5 oz jar	71	<0.1					210	21	0.21	0.071		353		0.11	0.09		GERB332
prunes w/apples, Gerber 2nd Fds	86	91.2	0.7	20.2	11.8	2.4	3	13	12	0.13	0.089	74	<1	0.02	0.6		
4 oz jar	113	<0.1					198	20	0.30	0.071		245		0.08	0.12		GERB331
prunes w/tapioca, Gerber 2nd Fds	79	90.7	0.7	20.9		3.1	6	17	11	0.10		26	1	0.02	0.6	0.00	0.16
4 oz jar	113	0.1	<0.1	0.1	<0.1	0	200	17	0.40	0.069	0.6	512	0.7	0.08	0.09	0.0	03136a
Heinz Str-2	84	96.4	0.7	22.2		3.2	6	18	12	0.11		28	1	0.03	0.6	0.0	0.17
4.5 oz jar	120	0.1	<0.1	0.1	<0.1	0	212	18	0.42	0.073	0.6	544	0.7	0.09	0.10	0.0	03136b
junior	119	136.2	1.0	31.8		4.6	3	26	17	0.17		34	1	0.04	0.9	0.0	0.24
6 oz jar	170	0.2	<0.1	0.1	<0.1	0	275	26	0.56	0.105	0.9	692	1.0	0.14	0.15	0.0	03137
tropical fruit blend, Gerber 2nd	84	91.6	0.7	19.9	15.4	1.6	4	8	25	0.15	0.198	378	16	0.02	0.8		
Foods, Tender Harvest - 4 oz jar	113	<0.1					264	20	0.30	0.095		1261		0.07	0.30		GERB353

18.7 MEATS

	KCAL	H₂0 (g)	PRO (g)	CHO (g)	SUGR (g)	DFIB (g)	Na (mg)	Ca (mg)	Mg (mg)	Zn (mg)	Mn (mg)	A (mcg RAE)	C (mg)	B-1 (mg)	NIA (mg)	B-12 (mcg)	PANT (mg)
beef, Bch-Nut Stg 1/Gerber 2	76	57.2	9.7	0.0		0.0	58	5	12	1.75		14	1	0.01	2.0	1.01	0.24
Fds/Heinz Str-2 - 2.5 oz jar	71	3.8	1.8	1.6	0.2	21	156	60	1.04	0.031	6.7	48	0.3	0.10	0.10	4.3	03002
Gerber 3rd Fds/Heinz Jr-3	75	56.7	10.3	0.0		0.0	47	6	6	1.42		13	1	0.01	2.3	1.04	0.25
2.5 oz jar	71	3.5	1.8	1.3	0.1	20	135	51	1.17	0.065	5.1	42	0.3	0.11	0.09	4.3	03003

	KCAL / WT (g)	H₂0 (g) / FAT (g)	PRO (g) / SFA (g)	CHO (g) / MUFA (g)	SUGR (g) / PUFA (g)	DFIB (g) / CHOL (mg)	Na (mg) / K (mg)	Ca (mg) / P (mg)	Mg (mg) / Fe (mg)	Zn (mg) / Cu (mg)	Mn (mg) / Se (mcg)	A (mcg RAE) / A (IU)	C (mcg) / E (mg ATE)	B-1 (mg) / B-2 (mg)	NIA (mg) / B-6 (mg)	B-12 (mcg) / FOL (mcg DFE)	PANT (mg) / REF
beef & beef gravy, Gerber 2nd Foods	121	88.9	13.3	4.7	0.2	1.2	48	10	15	3.37	<0.001	<1	1	0.02	2.7		
4 oz jar	113	5.5					211	120	1.47	0.064		<1		0.12	0.18		GERB249
chicken, Beech-Nut Stage 1/Gerber	92	55.0	9.7	0.1		0.0	33	45	9	0.86		11	1	0.01	2.3	0.28	0.48
2nd Fds/Heinz Str-2 - *2.5 oz jar*	71	5.6	1.4	2.5	1.4	43	100	69	0.99	0.032	7.8	38	0.3	0.11	0.14	7.1	03012
Gerber 3rd Fds/Heinz Jr-3	106	54.0	10.4	0.0		0.0	36	39	8	0.72		9	1	0.01	2.4	0.28	0.52
2.5 oz jar	71	6.8	1.8	3.1	1.7	42	87	64	0.70	0.032	7.3	28	0.3	0.12	0.13	7.8	03013
chicken & chicken gravy, Gerber 2nd	127	89.3	12.4	3.4	0.2	0.7	50	118	16	1.30	<0.001	<1	1	0.02	4.1		
Foods - *4 oz jar*	113	7.1					172	153	1.16	0.067		<1		0.14	0.16		GERB264
chicken sticks, Gerber Graduates	133	48.5	10.4	1.0		0.1	340	52	10	0.72		2	1	0.01	1.4	0.28	0.52
2.5 oz jar	71	10.2	2.9	4.4	2.1	55	75	86	1.11	0.032	7.3	8	0.3	0.14	0.07	7.8	03014
ham, Gerber 2nd Foods	79	56.4	9.9	0.0		0.0	29	4	9	1.60		8	1	0.10	1.9	0.07	0.36
2.5 oz jar	71	4.1	1.4	2.0	0.6	17	145	58	0.73	0.046	10.1	27	0.3	0.11	0.18	1.4	03008
junior	89	55.7	10.7	0.0		0.0	48	4	8	1.21		7	1	0.10	2.0	0.07	0.38
2.5 oz jar	71	4.8	1.6	2.3	0.6	21	149	63	0.72	0.048	10.7	23	0.3	0.14	0.14	1.4	03009
ham & ham gravy, Gerber 2nd Foods	107	91.0	12.8	4.2	0.3	0.8	41	7	16	2.15	<0.001	<1	<1	0.18	3.6		
4 oz jar	113	4.3					223	128	0.76	0.068		<1		0.16	0.25		GERB286
lamb, Bch-Nut Ste 1/Gerber 2nd	73	57.0	10.0	0.1		0.0	44	5	9	1.96		7	1	0.01	2.1	1.55	0.29
Fds/Heinz Str-2 - *2.5 oz jar*	71	3.3	1.6	1.3	0.1	27	146	69	1.06	0.039	6.0	23	0.3	0.14	0.11	1.4	03010
junior	80	56.5	10.8	0.0		0.0	52	5	7	1.85		6	1	0.01	2.3	1.61	0.30
2.5 oz jar	71	3.7	1.8	1.5	0.2	27	150	65	1.18	0.040	5.0	19	0.3	0.14	0.13	1.4	03011
lamb & lamb gravy, Gerber 2nd Foods	103	90.8	13.6	4.5	0.2	0.6	47	9	15	2.84	<0.001	<1	<1	0.02	2.8		
4 oz jar	113	3.4					188	115	1.12	0.071		<1		0.15	0.14		GERB289
meat sticks, Gerber Graduates	131	49.3	9.5	0.8		0.1	388	24	8	1.35		15	2	0.04	1.1	0.21	0.34
2.5 oz jar	71	10.4	4.1	4.6	1.1	50	81	73	0.98	0.048	9.4	49	0.3	0.12	0.06	6.4	03021
pork, strained	88	55.7	9.9	0.0		0.0	30	4	7	1.61		8	1	0.10	1.6	0.70	0.19
2.5 oz jar	71	5.0	1.7	2.5	0.6	34	158	67	0.71	0.051	9.2	27	0.3	0.14	0.15	1.4	03007
turkey, Bch-Nut Ste 1/Gerber 2nd	81	56.0	10.2	0.1		0.0	39	16	10	1.30		10	2	0.01	2.6	0.71	0.40
Fds/Heinz Str-2 - *2.5 oz jar*	71	4.1	1.4	1.5	1.0	42	164	89	0.85	0.028	11.7	33	0.3	0.15	0.13	7.8	03015
Gerber 3rd Foods	92	55.0	10.9	0.0		0.0	51	20	9	1.28		7	2	0.01	2.5	0.76	0.43
2.5 oz jar	71	5.0	1.6	1.9	1.2	38	128	67	0.96	0.031	12.1	23	0.3	0.18	0.12	8.5	03016
turkey & turkey gravy, Gerber 2nd	119	90.3	11.6	3.9	0.3	0.3	58	86	15	2.53	<0.001	<1	1	0.02	3.0		
Foods - *4 oz jar*	113	6.3					174	152	1.09	0.079		<1		0.18	0.17		GERB355
turkey sticks, Gerber Graduates	129	49.6	9.7	1.0		0.4	343	51	11	1.30		4	1	0.01	1.2	0.71	0.40
2.5 oz jar	71	10.1	2.9	3.3	2.6	46	65	73	0.88	0.028	7.2	13	0.3	0.11	0.05	7.8	03017
veal, Bch-Nut Stg 1/Gerber 2nd Fds/	72	57.4	9.6	0.0		0.0	45	5	9	1.42		10	2	0.01	2.5	0.92	0.31
Heinz Str-2 - *2.5 oz jar*	71	3.4	1.6	1.5	0.1	18	153	70	0.90	0.028	4.3	33	0.3	0.11	0.11	4.3	03005
junior	78	56.7	10.9	0.0		0.0	49	4	8	1.79		11	1	0.01	2.7	0.92	0.32
2.5 oz jar	71	3.6	1.7	1.5	0.1	19	168	70	0.89	0.053	3.7	36	0.3	0.13	0.08	5.0	03006
veal & veal gravy, Gerber 2nd Foods	109	91.0	11.9	4.7	0.2	0.7	52	8	14	2.35	<0.001	671	1	0.02	3.6		
4 oz jar	113	4.7					200	118	0.80	0.062		2235		0.15	0.20		GERB358

18.8 VEGETABLES

	KCAL / WT (g)	H₂0 (g) / FAT (g)	PRO (g) / SFA (g)	CHO (g) / MUFA (g)	SUGR (g) / PUFA (g)	DFIB (g) / CHOL (mg)	Na (mg) / K (mg)	Ca (mg) / P (mg)	Mg (mg) / Fe (mg)	Zn (mg) / Cu (mg)	Mn (mg) / Se (mcg)	A (mcg RAE) / A (IU)	C (mcg) / E (mg ATE)	B-1 (mg) / B-2 (mg)	NIA (mg) / B-6 (mg)	B-12 (mcg) / FOL (mcg DFE)	PANT (mg) / REF
beets, Gerber 2nd Fds/Heinz Str-2	38	101.8	1.5	8.7		2.1	94	16	16	0.14		2	3	0.01	0.1	0.00	0.11
4 oz jar	113	0.1	<0.1	<0.1	<0.1	0	206	16	0.36	0.079	0.1	37	0.6	0.05	0.03	35.0	03098
broccoli & carrots w/cheese,	51	101.4	1.8	8.4	1.4	1.1	51	33	10	0.23	0.170	755	5	0.02	0.3		
Gerber 3rd Foods - *4 oz jar*	113	1.1					114	47	0.23	0.023		2515		0.03	0.06		GERB253
broccoli cauliflower, Gerber 2nd	58	101.6	1.2	7.1	1.6	1.4	15	21	15	0.23	0.237	36	14	0.03	0.5		
Foods, Tender Harvest - *4 oz jar*	113	2.7					162	37	0.34	0.023		119		0.05	0.09		GERB254
butternut squash & corn, Gerber	57	98.6	2.3	10.5	3.3	2.3	6	36	29	0.34	0.136	158	6	0.07	0.6	0.00	0.35
2nd Foods - *4 oz jar*	113	0.7	0.1	0.2	0.3	0	398	40	0.45	0.113	0.7	3156	0.1	0.07	0.12	26.0	03114
Gerber 2nd Foods, Tender	55	97.7	1.4	13.0	4.1	1.7	2	16	22	0.23	0.113	344	1	0.03	0.7		
Harvest - *4 oz jar*	113	0.3					245	46	0.34	0.079		1146		0.08	0.08		GERB255
carrots, Beech-Nut Baby's	28	62.1	2.5	5.8		1.5	3	14	11	0.25		20	5	0.06	0.7	0.00	0.20
First/Gerber 1st Fds - *2.5 oz jar*	71	0.2	<0.1	<0.1	0.1	0	80	31	0.68	0.045	0.1	401	0.4	0.04	0.05	18.5	03121a
Beech-Nut Baby's First/Gerber	19	65.5	0.6	4.3		1.2	26	16	6	0.11		407	4	0.02	0.3	0.00	0.17
1st Fds/Heinz Beg-1 - *2.5 oz jar*	71	0.1	<0.1	<0.1	<0.1	0	139	14	0.26	0.029	0.1	8137	0.4	0.03	0.05	10.7	03099a
Beech-Nut Stage 1/Gerber 2nd Fds/	31	104.3	0.9	6.8		1.9	42	25	10	0.17		647	6	0.03	0.5	0.00	0.27
Heinz Str-2 - *4 oz jar*	113	<0.1	<0.1	<0.1	<0.1	0	221	23	0.42	0.046	0.2	12951	0.6	0.04	0.08	17.0	03099b
Beech-Nut Stage 3/Gerber 3rd Fds/	54	154.7	1.4	12.2		2.9	83	39	19	0.31		1005	9	0.04	0.8	0.00	0.47
Heinz Jr-3 - *6 oz jar*	170	0.3	0.1	<0.1	0.2	0	343	34	0.66	0.080	0.3	20077	0.9	0.07	0.14	28.9	03100
diced, Gerber Graduates	46	158.9	0.9	9.1	4.2	4.0	82	43	18	0.32	0.117	7741	<1	0.03	0.4		
6 oz jar	170	0.4	<0.1			<1	194	34	0.36	0.121		25803		0.03	0.09		GERB256

	KCAL	H₂O (g)	PRO (g)	CHO (g)	SUGR (g)	DFIB (g)	Minerals Na (mg)	Ca (mg)	Mg (mg)	Zn (mg)	Mn (mg)	Vitamins A (mcg RAE)	C (mg)	B-1 (mg)	NIA (mg)	B-12 (mcg)	PANT (mg)
	WT (g)	FAT (g)	SFA (g)	MUFA (g)	PUFA (g)	CHOL (mg)	K (mg)	P (mg)	Fe (mg)	Cu (mg)	Se (mcg)	A (IU)	E (mg ATE)	B-2 (mg)	B-6 (mg)	FOL (mcg DFE)	REF
Earth's Best	35	118.1	1.0	7.7		2.2	47	28	12	0.19		733	7	0.03	0.6	0.00	0.31
4.5 oz jar	128	0.1	<0.1	<0.1	0.1	0	251	26	0.47	0.052	0.3	14670	0.7	0.05	0.09	19.2	03099c
Gerber 1st Foods, Tender Harvest	24	64.7	0.6	5.0	2.9	1.6	31	18	8	0.14	0.064	2205	<1	0.02	0.3		
2.5 oz jar	71	0.2					162	22	0.14	0.028		7351		0.03	0.07		GERB260
carrots & brown rice, Gerber 2nd	49	101.6	0.9	9.6	3.5	1.8	35	20	13	0.23	0.249	2002	<1	0.02	0.4		
Foods, Tender Harvest - *4 oz jar*	113	1.1					156	32	0.23	0.045		6674		0.02	0.11		GERB257
corn, crmd, Bch-Nut Stg 2/Grbr	64	94.5	1.6	15.9		2.4	49	23	9	0.21		5	2	0.01	0.6	0.02	0.33
2nd Fds/Heinz Str-2 - *4 oz jar*	113	0.5	0.1	0.1	0.2	1	102	37	0.32	0.038	1.5	85	0.6	0.05	0.05	12.4	03119
Heinz Jr-3	111	138.4	2.4	27.7		3.6	88	31	14	0.39		7	4	0.02	0.9	0.03	0.56
6 oz jar	170	0.7	0.1	0.2	0.3	2	138	56	0.46	0.065	2.2	131	0.9	0.08	0.07	22.1	03120
garden veg, strained	42	101.7	2.6	7.7		1.7	40	32	24	0.29		342	6	0.07	0.9	0.00	0.29
4 oz jar	113	0.2	<0.1	<0.1	0.1	0	190	32	0.94	0.079	0.8	6856	0.6	0.08	0.11	45.2	03283
green beans, Bch-Nut Stg 1/Grbr	28	104.0	1.5	6.7		2.1	2	44	27	0.24		25	6	0.03	0.4	0.00	0.18
2nd Fds/Heinz Str-2 - *4 oz jar*	113	0.1	<0.1	<0.1	0.1	0	179	23	0.85	0.058	0.3	506	0.6	0.10	0.04	39.6	03091b
Beech-Nut Stage 3	43	157.3	2.0	9.7		3.2	3	111	37	0.32		37	14	0.04	0.5	0.00	0.26
6 oz jar	170	0.2	<0.1	<0.1	0.1	0	218	32	1.84	0.083	0.5	736	0.9	0.17	0.06	56.1	03092
diced, Gerber Graduates	43	158.3	2.0	8.9	2.0	3.6	75	61	23	0.29	0.299	148	4	0.04	0.4		
6 oz jar	170	<0.1	<0.1			<1	147	35	0.67	0.085		495		0.07	0.05		GERB282
Gerber 1st Fds/Heinz Beg-1	18	65.3	0.9	4.2		1.3	1	28	17	0.15		16	4	0.02	0.2	0.00	0.11
2.5 oz jar	71	0.1	<0.1	<0.1	<0.1	0	112	14	0.53	0.036	0.2	318	0.4	0.06	0.03	24.9	03091a
toddler	49	157.4	2.0	9.7		2.2	63	46	32	0.17	0.136	31	3	0.03	0.4	0.00	0.09
6 oz jar	170	0.3	0.1	<0.1	0.2	0	197	37	0.68	0.051	0.7	595	0.2	0.07	0.05	54.4	03093
green beans & potatoes, Gerber	71	97.4	2.5	10.5	2.7	1.6	20	68	23	0.34	0.316	5	1	0.05	0.5	0.17	0.32
2nd Fds - *4 oz jar*	113	2.1	1.3	0.6	0.1	6	167	69	0.57	0.045	0.8	96	0.1	0.12	0.09	11.3	03096
Gerber 2nd Foods, Tender	71	97.2	2.5	10.6	2.6	1.5	18	64	22	0.34	0.294	44	1	0.05	0.6		
Harvest - *4 oz jar*	113	2.1					148	69	0.45	0.045		146		0.10	0.09		GERB283
green beans, crmd, Gerber 3rd	54	154.5	1.7	12.2		2.7	20	54	12	0.27		14	5	0.04	0.4	0.09	0.31
Fds/Heinz Jr-3 - *6 oz jar*	170	0.7	0.1	0.1	0.4	2	111	32	0.44	0.100	0.7	255	0.9	0.09	0.02	68.0	03097
green beans w/rice, Gerber 3rd	47	100.7	1.4	10.2	1.7	1.6	5	27	19	0.23	0.305	62	<1	0.02	0.4		
Foods - *4 oz jar*	113	<0.1					125	28	0.57	0.057		208		0.07	0.05		GERB284
mixed veg, junior	70	152.0	2.4	13.9		2.6	61	19	19	0.46		357	4	0.05	1.1	0.00	0.44
6 oz jar	170	0.7	0.1	<0.1	0.3	0	289	43	0.70	0.070	1.2	7132	0.9	0.05	0.14	6.8	03282
diced, Gerber Graduates	77	149.5	3.1	15.9	3.8	4.6	92	41	24	0.76	0.220	4922	3	0.08	0.7		
6 oz jar	170	0.7	<0.1			<1	182	61	0.77	0.298		16407		0.06	0.10		GERB299
strained	46	101.5	1.4	9.0		1.7	15	15	11	0.17		226	2	0.02	0.4	0.00	0.28
4 oz jar	113	0.6	0.1	0.1	0.2	0	144	25	0.36	0.045	0.8	4510	0.6	0.03	0.06	4.5	03286
peas, Beech-Nut Stage 1/	45	98.9	4.0	9.2		2.4	5	23	17	0.40		32	8	0.09	1.2	0.00	0.32
Gerber 2nd Fds - *4 oz jar*	113	0.3	0.1	<0.1	0.2	0	127	49	1.08	0.072	0.1	638	0.6	0.07	0.08	29.4	03121b
toddler	109	143.8	6.6	17.5		6.6	82	36	32	0.85	0.255	26	10	0.17	1.4	0.00	0.59
6 oz jar	170	1.4	0.2	0.1	0.6	0	138	114	1.70	0.136	0.2	517	0.8	0.10	0.10	59.5	03122
peas, creamed, Heinz Str-2	60	97.7	2.5	10.1		2.1	16	15	18	0.44		5	2	0.10	0.9	0.09	0.34
4 oz jar	113	2.1	0.5	0.5	1.1	5	99	35	0.63	0.058	0.5	97	0.6	0.06	0.05	26.0	03125
peas w/rice, Gerber 3rd Foods	59	98.4	2.7	11.1	1.7	2.5	7	15	18	0.57	0.237	65	<1	0.08	0.9		
4 oz jar	113	0.5					88	54	0.90	0.113		218		0.06	0.08		GERB326
potatoes, Gerber 1st Foods	35	62.1	0.7	7.9	<0.1	0.7	4	5	7	0.07	0.036	<1	<1	0.02	0.4		
2.5 oz jar	71	<0.1					94	18	0.14	0.021		<1		0.01	0.04		GERB330
Gerber Graduate	65	111.1	1.3	15.1		1.2	73	5	19	0.22	0.090	0	13	0.03	0.4	0.00	0.39
4.5 oz jar	128	0.1	<0.1	<0.1	<0.1	0	141	29	0.26	0.090	1.0	0	<0.1	0.01	0.09	7.7	03112
spinach, creamed, Gerber 2nd	42	101.2	2.8	6.4		2.0	55	101	62	0.35		236	10	0.02	0.2	0.07	
Foods - *4 oz jar*	113	1.5	0.8	0.4	0.2	6	216	61	0.70	0.068	2.7	4712	0.6	0.12	0.08	68.9	03127
spring garden veg, Gerber 2nd	37	103.5	1.6	7.1	3.7	2.1	25	21	12	0.23	0.102	1778	<1	0.06	0.6		
Foods, Tender Harvest - *4 oz jar*	113	0.3					163	35	0.45	0.057		5926		0.06	0.14		GERB345
squash, Bch-Nut Baby's 1st /Grbr	17	65.8	0.6	4.0		1.5	1	17	9	0.10		72	5	0.01	0.3	0.00	0.16
1st Fds/Heinz Beg-1 - *2.5 oz jar*	71	0.1	<0.1	<0.1	0.1	0	127	11	0.21	0.038	0.1	1436	0.4	0.04	0.04	10.7	03104c
Beech-Nut Stage 1/Gerber 2nd	27	104.8	0.9	6.3		2.4	2	27	14	0.16		114	9	0.01	0.4	0.00	0.25
Fds/Heinz Str-2 - *4 oz jar*	113	0.2	<0.1	<0.1	0.1	0	202	17	0.34	0.061	0.2	2286	0.6	0.06	0.07	17.0	03104b
Earth's Best	31	118.7	1.0	7.2		2.7	3	31	15	0.18		129	10	0.01	0.5	0.00	0.28
4.5 oz jar	128	0.3	0.1	<0.1	0.1	0	229	19	0.38	0.069	0.3	2589	0.7	0.07	0.08	19.2	03104a
Gerber 3rd Foods	41	157.8	1.4	9.5		3.6	2	41	20	0.14		172	13	0.02	0.6	0.00	0.37
6 oz jar	170	0.3	0.1	<0.1	0.1	0	315	27	0.60	0.092	0.3	3424	0.9	0.11	0.12	25.5	03105
sweet peas, Gerber 1st Foods,	34	62.7	2.1	5.7	1.8	2.0	4	14	14	0.38	0.164	<1	1	0.05	0.6		
Tender Harvest - *2.5 oz jar*	71	0.3					72	42	0.72	0.061		<1		0.04	0.04		GERB347

	KCAL	H₂O (g)	PRO (g)	CHO (g)	SUGR (g)	DFIB (g)	Na (mg)	Ca (mg)	Mg (mg)	Zn (mg)	Mn (mg)	A (mcg RAE)	C (mg)	B-1 (mg)	NIA (mg)	B-12 (mcg)	PANT (mg)
	WT (g)	FAT (g)	SFA (g)	MUFA (g)	PUFA (g)	CHOL (mg)	K (mg)	P (mg)	Fe (mg)	Cu (mg)	Se (mcg)	A (IU)	E (mg ATE)	B-2 (mg)	B-6 (mg)	FOL (mcg DFE)	REF
sweet pot, Bch-Nut Baby's 1st/Grbr	40	60.2	0.8	9.4		1.1	14	11	9	0.15		229	7	0.02	0.3	0.00	0.28
1st Fds/Heinz Beg-1 - *2.5 oz jar*	71	0.1	<0.1	<0.1	<0.1	0	187	17	0.26	0.058	0.5	4571	0.4	0.02	0.07	7.1	03108c
Beech-Nut Stage 1/Gerber 2nd	64	95.8	1.2	14.9		1.7	23	18	15	0.24		364	11	0.03	0.4	0.00	0.44
Fds/Heinz Str-2 - *4 oz jar*	113	0.1	<0.1	<0.1	<0.1	0	297	27	0.42	0.092	0.8	7275	0.6	0.04	0.11	11.3	03108b
Beech-Nut Stage 3/Gerber 3rd	102	143.0	1.9	23.6		2.6	37	27	20	0.19		564	16	0.04	0.7	0.00	0.69
Fds/Heinz Jr-3 - *6 oz jar*	170	0.2	<0.1	<0.1	0.1	0	413	41	0.66	0.170	1.2	11281	0.9	0.06	0.19	17.0	03109
Earth's Best	73	108.5	1.4	16.9		1.9	26	20	17	0.27		412	13	0.04	0.5	0.00	0.50
4.5 oz jar	128	0.1	<0.1	<0.1	0.1	0	337	31	0.47	0.104	0.9	8241	0.7	0.04	0.12	12.8	03108a
Gerber 1st Foods, Tender	47	59.1	0.8	10.6	5.5	1.1	9	11	11	0.14	0.178	1916	<1	0.02	0.3		
Harvest - *2.5 oz jar*	71	<0.1					178	20	0.21	0.071		6388		0.03	0.07		GERB350

19. MEATS
19.1 BEEF

	KCAL	H₂O / WT	PRO / FAT	CHO / SFA	SUGR / MUFA	DFIB / PUFA	Na / CHOL	Ca / K	Mg / P	Zn / Fe	Mn / Cu	A / Se	C / A(IU)	B-1 / E	NIA / B-2	B-12 / B-6	PANT / FOL / REF
bottom sirloin tri-tip roast, 0″	184	51.8	23.7	0.0	0.0	0.0	50	7	22	4.14	0.000	0	0	0.08	3.0	2.48	<0.01
trim, lean & fat, roasted - *3 oz*	85	9.2	3.4	4.6	0.3	71	289	177	3.18	0.096	20.0	0	0.1	0.24	0.25	8.5	23544
lean, roasted	177	52.5	24.0	0.0	0.0	0.0	50	7	22	4.20		0	0	0.08	3.0	2.51	
3 oz	85	8.2	3.0	4.2	0.3	70	293	179	3.22	0.098	20.1	0	0.1	0.25	0.25	8.5	13985
bottom sirloin tri-tip steak, 0″	225	42.9	25.5	0.0	0.0	0.0	61	10	22	5.99	0.000	0	0	0.11	3.6	2.41	<0.01
trim, lean & fat, broiled - *3 oz*	85	12.9	4.9	6.6	0.5	58	371	225	3.09	0.134	8.8	0	0.1	0.24	0.38	8.5	23545
lean, broiled	213	43.9	26.1	0.0	0.0	0.0	62	10	22	6.17		0	0	0.11	3.7	2.45	
3 oz	85	11.2	4.1	5.9	0.4	57	382	231	3.18	0.138	8.5	0	0.1	0.25	0.39	8.5	13987
breakfast strips, ckd	153	8.9	10.6	0.5		0.0	766	3	9	2.17	0.006	0	0	0.03	2.2	1.17	0.12
3 slices (1.2 oz)	34	11.7	4.9	5.7	0.5	40	140	80	1.07	0.039	9.1	0	0.1	0.09	0.11	2.7	13345
brisket, cured, corned beef, ckd	213	50.8	15.4	0.4		0.0	964	7	10	3.89	0.019	0	0	0.02	2.6	1.39	0.36
3 oz	85	16.1	5.4	7.8	0.6	83	123	106	1.58	0.131	27.9	0	0.1	0.14	0.20	5.1	13347
brisket, flat half, 0″ trim,	183	49.1	25.9	0.0		0.0	53	4	20	5.19	0.014	0	0	0.06	3.2	2.19	0.31
lean & fat, braised - *3 oz*	85	8.0	2.8	3.5	0.3	81	246	211	2.34	0.102	21.1	0		0.18	0.26	6.8	13369
lean, braised	162	50.8	26.8	0.0		0.0	54	4	21	5.41	0.014	0	0	0.06	3.3	2.24	0.31
3 oz	85	5.3	1.7	2.4	0.2	81	253	218	2.41	0.105	21.4	0		0.19	0.26	6.8	13370
brisket, flat half, 1/4″ trim,	309	39.4	21.3	0.0		0.0	48	7	16	4.10	0.012	0	0	0.05	2.7	1.97	0.26
lean & fat, braised - *3 oz*	85	24.2	9.4	10.6	0.9	81	207	171	1.95	0.085	19.6	0		0.15	0.22	5.1	13026
lean, braised	189	50.1	26.8	0.0		0.0	54	4	21	5.41	0.014	0	0	0.06	3.3	2.24	0.31
3 oz	85	8.2	2.7	3.7	0.3	81	253	218	2.41	0.105	21.4	0		0.19	0.26	6.8	13028
brisket, point half, 0″ trim,	304	39.1	20.0	0.0		0.0	58	7	15	4.96	0.012	0	0	0.05	2.6	1.98	0.25
lean & fat, braised - *3 oz*	85	24.2	9.6	10.8	0.8	78	198	159	1.99	0.082	18.6	0		0.16	0.20	6.0	13371
lean, braised	207	47.3	23.8	0.0		0.0	65	5	19	6.28	0.014	0	0	0.06	3.0	2.19	0.29
3 oz	85	11.7	4.4	5.5	0.3	77	232	192	2.37	0.098	20.0	0		0.20	0.24	6.8	13372
brisket, point half, 1/4″ trim,	343	36.9	18.8	0.0		0.0	55	8	14	4.55	0.012	0	0	0.05	2.4	1.91	0.24
lean & fat, braised - *3 oz*	85	29.1	11.5	12.9	1.0	78	188	149	1.87	0.077	18.3	0		0.15	0.20	5.1	13030
lean, braised	222	47.8	23.8	0.0		0.0	65	5	19	6.28	0.014	0	0	0.06	3.0	2.19	0.29
3 oz	85	13.3	5.0	6.2	0.3	77	232	192	2.37	0.098	20.0	0		0.20	0.24	6.8	13032
brisket, whole (flat & pt hlvs), 0″	247	43.8	22.8	0.0		0.0	55	6	18	5.07	0.013	0	0	0.06	2.9	2.08	0.27
trim, lean & fat, braised - *3 oz*	85	16.6	6.4	7.4	0.6	79	220	184	2.15	0.092	19.8	0	0.2	0.17	0.23	6.0	13367
lean, braised	185	49.1	25.3	0.0		0.0	60	5	20	5.86	0.014	0	0	0.06	3.2	2.21	0.31
3 oz	85	8.6	3.1	4.0	0.3	79	242	205	2.39	0.101	20.8	0	0.1	0.19	0.25	6.8	13368
brisket, whole (flat & pt hlvs), 1/4″	327	38.1	20.0	0.0		0.0	52	7	15	4.34	0.012	0	0	0.05	2.6	1.94	0.25
trim, lean & fat, braised - *3 oz*	85	26.8	10.5	11.8	1.0	80	196	159	1.90	0.081	19.0	0	0.2	0.15	0.20	5.1	13022
lean, braised	206	48.9	25.3	0.0		0.0	60	5	20	5.86	0.014	0	0	0.06	3.2	2.21	0.31
3 oz	85	10.8	3.9	5.0	0.3	79	242	205	2.39	0.101	20.8	0	0.1	0.19	0.25	6.8	13024
chuck arm pot roast, choice, 0″	249	43.7	25.0	0.0		0.0	53	9	18	6.38	0.014	0	0	0.06	2.9	2.65	0.30
trim, lean & fat, braised - *3 oz*	85	15.8	6.1	6.7	0.6	85	223	201	2.85	0.123	21.4	0		0.20	0.26	8.5	13374
lean, braised	186	49.0	28.1	0.0		0.0	56	8	20	7.36	0.016	0	0	0.07	3.2	2.92	0.32
3 oz	85	7.4	2.7	3.1	0.3	86	246	228	3.22	0.139	22.7	0		0.25	0.28	9.4	13377
chuck arm pot roast, choice, 1/4″	296	39.8	22.9	0.0		0.0	50	9	16	5.70	0.014	0	0	0.06	2.7	2.48	0.27
trim, lean & fat, braised - *3 oz*	85	21.9	8.6	9.4	0.8	84	207	184	2.59	0.112	20.6	0	0.2	0.20	0.24	7.7	13036
lean, braised	191	48.7	28.1	0.0	0.0	0.0	56	8	20	7.36	0.016	0	0	0.07	3.2	2.89	0.32
3 oz	85	7.9	2.9	3.3	0.3	86	246	228	3.22	0.139	22.7	0	0.1	0.25	0.28	9.4	13044
chuck arm pot roast, select, 0″	221	46.1	25.6	0.0		0.0	54	9	19	6.56	0.014	0	0	0.06	2.9	2.69	0.30
trim, lean & fat, braised - *3 oz*	85	12.4	4.8	5.3	0.5	85	227	207	2.92	0.127	21.6	0		0.22	0.26	8.5	13375
lean, braised	168	50.6	28.1	0.0		0.0	56	8	20	7.36	0.016	0	0	0.07	3.2	2.89	0.32
3 oz	85	5.4	1.9	2.2	0.2	86	246	228	3.22	0.139	22.7	0		0.25	0.28	9.4	13378

| | KCAL | H₂0 (g) | PRO (g) | CHO (g) | SUGR (g) | DFIB (g) | Na (mg) | Ca (mg) | Mg (mg) | Zn (mg) | Mn (mg) | A (mcg RAE) | C (mg) | B-1 (mg) | NIA (mg) | B-12 (mcg) | PANT (mg) |
	WT (g)	FAT (g)	SFA (g)	MUFA (g)	PUFA (g)	CHOL (mg)	K (mg)	P (mg)	Fe (mg)	Cu (mg)	Se (mcg)	A (IU)	E (mg ATE)	B-2 (mg)	B-6 (mg)	FOL (mcg DFE)	REF
chuck arm pot roast, select, 1/4"	268	41.9	23.7	0.0		0.0	51	9	17	5.94	0.014	0	0	0.06	2.7	2.54	0.28
trim, lean & fat, braised - 3 oz	85	18.5	7.3	7.9	0.7	85	213	190	2.69	0.116	20.7	0	0.2	0.20	0.25	7.7	13038
lean, braised	175	49.6	28.1	0.0	0.0	0.0	56	8	20	7.36	0.016	0	0	0.07	3.2	2.89	0.32
3 oz	85	6.1	2.2	2.6	0.2	86	246	228	3.22	0.139	22.7	0	0.1	0.25	0.28	9.4	13046
chuck blade roast, choice, 0" trim,	296	39.9	22.9	0.0		0.0	55	11	17	7.23	0.014	0	0	0.06	2.1	1.96	0.26
lean & fat, braised - 3 oz	85	22.0	8.7	9.5	0.8	88	199	173	2.69	0.108	21.2	0		0.21	0.22	4.3	13380
lean, braised	225	45.9	26.4	0.0		0.0	60	11	20	8.73	0.015	0	0	0.07	2.3	2.10	0.30
3 oz	85	12.5	4.8	5.4	0.4	90	224	200	3.13	0.126	22.7	0		0.24	0.25	5.1	13383
chuck blade roast, choice, 1/4" trim,	309	39.1	22.2	0.0		0.0	54	11	16	6.92	0.013	0	0	0.06	2.0	1.93	0.26
lean & fat, braised - 3 oz	85	23.6	9.4	10.2	0.9	88	194	167	2.59	0.105	20.6	0	0.2	0.20	0.21	4.3	13052
lean, braised	224	46.4	26.4	0.0	0.0	0.0	60	11	20	8.73	0.015	0	0	0.07	2.3	2.10	0.30
3 oz	85	12.2	4.7	5.3	0.4	90	224	200	3.13	0.126	22.7	0	0.1	0.24	0.25	5.1	13060
chuck blade roast, select, 0" trim,	266	42.0	23.5	0.0		0.0	56	11	17	7.45	0.014	0	0	0.06	2.1	1.98	0.27
lean & fat, braised - 3 oz	85	18.4	7.3	8.0	0.7	88	203	177	2.75	0.111	21.3	0		0.21	0.22	4.3	13381
lean, braised	202	47.3	26.4	0.0		0.0	60	11	20	8.73	0.015	0	0	0.07	2.3	2.10	0.30
3 oz	85	9.9	3.9	4.3	0.3	90	224	200	3.13	0.126	22.7	0		0.24	0.25	5.1	13384
chuck blade roast, select, 1/4" trim,	277	41.4	22.9	0.0		0.0	55	11	17	7.23	0.014	0	0	0.06	2.1	1.96	0.26
lean & fat, braised - 3 oz	85	19.8	7.9	8.6	0.7	88	199	173	2.69	0.108	20.7	0	0.2	0.21	0.22	4.3	13054
lean, braised	201	47.9	26.4	0.0	0.0	0.0	60	11	20	8.73	0.015	0	0	0.07	2.3	2.10	0.30
3 oz	85	9.9	3.8	4.3	0.3	90	224	200	3.13	0.126	22.7	0	0.1	0.24	0.25	5.1	13062
chuck clod roast, choice, 0" trim,	184	51.3	20.9	0.0	0.0	0.0	60	7	17	5.06	0.001	0	0	0.07	2.8	2.42	0.01
lean & fat, roasted - 3 oz	85	10.4	3.6	5.0	0.4	57	309	179	2.57	0.081	24.6	0	0.1	0.20	0.22	7.7	23528
lean, roasted	145	54.7	22.1	0.0	0.0	0.0	63	6	19	5.43		0	0	0.07	2.9	2.52	
3 oz	85	5.7	1.7	3.0	0.2	54	328	190	2.72	0.085	25.5	0	0.1	0.21	0.23	7.7	13937
chuck clod roast, choice, 1/4" trim,	206	50.2	20.5	0.0	0.0	0.0	57	7	17	4.89	0.001	0	0	0.07	2.7	2.40	0.02
lean & fat, roasted - 3 oz	85	13.1	4.8	6.2	0.5	67	286	166	2.39	0.079	24.1	0	0.1	0.19	0.22	7.7	23529
lean, roasted	151	55.2	22.2	0.0	0.0	0.0	60	6	19	5.43		0	0	0.07	2.9	2.54	
3 oz	85	6.3	2.0	3.3	0.2	65	314	181	2.60	0.085	25.5	0	0.1	0.21	0.23	7.7	13938
chuck clod roast, select, 0" trim,	167	52.8	23.2	0.0	0.0	0.0	61	6	18	5.24	0.000	0	0	0.08	3.1	2.68	0.01
lean & fat, roasted - 3 oz	85	7.4	2.8	3.5	0.4	62	316	183	2.63	0.082	25.0	0	0.1	0.22	0.24	8.5	23531
lean, roasted	146	54.6	23.9	0.0	0.0	0.0	63	6	19	5.43		0	0	0.08	3.1	2.74	
3 oz	85	4.9	1.8	2.5	0.3	61	326	189	2.71	0.085	25.5	0	0.1	0.22	0.25	8.5	13940
chuck clod roast, select, 1/4" trim,	207	49.3	20.7	0.0	0.0	0.0	57	7	17	4.79	0.001	0	0	0.07	2.7	2.42	0.02
lean & fat, roasted - 3 oz	85	13.1	4.9	5.6	0.5	58	287	167	2.40	0.078	23.9	0	0.1	0.19	0.22	7.7	23532
lean, roasted	141	55.1	22.7	0.0	0.0	0.0	61	6	19	5.43		0	0	0.08	3.0	2.61	
3 oz	85	4.9	1.5	2.0	0.2	54	320	184	2.65	0.085	25.5	0	0.1	0.21	0.24	8.5	13941
chuck clod steak, choice, 0" trim,	196	47.8	23.9	0.0	0.0	0.0	46	7	18	5.75	0.001	0	0	0.07	2.3	2.38	0.01
lean & fat, braised - 3 oz	85	10.4	3.5	4.8	0.4	76	247	158	3.09	0.107	24.7	0	0.2	0.20	0.18	6.0	23533
lean, braised	164	50.5	25.1	0.0	0.0	0.0	47	6	19	6.13		0	0	0.07	2.4	2.47	
3 oz	85	6.3	1.8	3.0	0.2	76	258	166	3.26	0.113	25.5	0	0.2	0.21	0.18	6.0	13943
chuck clod steak, choice, 1/4" trim,	231	44.8	22.5	0.0	0.0	0.0	53	9	16	6.31	0.001	0	0	0.06	2.6	2.40	0.02
lean & fat, braised - 3 oz	85	15.0	5.5	6.8	0.6	83	221	200	2.82	0.122	23.7	0	0.1	0.20	0.23	7.7	23534
lean, braised	164	50.5	25.1	0.0	0.0	0.0	56	8	19	7.31		0	0	0.06	2.8	2.59	
3 oz	85	6.3	1.8	3.0	0.2	83	244	226	3.20	0.139	25.5	0	0.1	0.22	0.25	8.5	13944
chuck clod steak, select, 0" trim,	174	50.3	25.4	0.0	0.0	0.0	54	8	18	6.92	0.000	0	0	0.06	2.9	2.63	<0.01
lean & fat, braised - 3 oz	85	7.3	2.7	3.3	0.3	84	232	215	3.20	0.132	25.2	0	0.2	0.22	0.25	8.5	23536
lean, braised	162	51.2	25.8	0.0	0.0	0.0	54	8	19	7.07		0	0	0.06	2.9	2.66	
3 oz	85	5.8	2.1	2.7	0.3	84	236	219	3.26	0.134	25.5	0	0.2	0.23	0.26	8.5	13946
chuck clod steak, select, 1/4" trim,	230	45.4	21.9	0.0	0.0	0.0	43	7	16	4.98	0.001	0	0	0.06	2.2	2.24	0.02
lean & fat, braised - 3 oz	85	15.1	6.0	6.9	0.6	76	219	140	2.85	0.094	23.5	0	0.1	0.18	0.17	5.1	23537
lean, braised	156	51.8	24.7	0.0	0.0	0.0	44	6	19	5.80		0	0	0.07	2.4	2.43	
3 oz	85	5.5	2.1	2.8	0.3	75	245	157	3.26	0.107	25.5	0	0.1	0.21	0.18	6.0	13947
chuck, tender steak, choice, 0"	137	55.7	21.9	0.0	0.0	0.0	62	7	20	6.66	0.000	0	0	0.09	3.1	2.86	0.00
trim, lean & fat, broiled - 3 oz	85	4.9	1.5	2.3	0.3	55	249	199	2.57	0.103	21.4	0	0.1	0.19	0.27	6.8	23519
lean, broiled	137	55.8	21.9	0.0	0.0	0.0	62	7	20	6.66		0	0	0.09	3.1	2.86	
3 oz	85	4.8	1.5	2.3	0.3	55	249	199	2.57	0.103	21.4	0	0.1	0.19	0.27	6.8	13961
chuck, tender steak, select, 0"	135	57.0	22.2	0.0	0.0	0.0	58	6	20	6.64	0.000	0	0	0.10	3.1	2.91	<0.01
trim, lean & fat, broiled - 3 oz	85	4.5	1.8	2.2	0.3	51	249	184	2.38	0.095	21.5	0	0.1	0.20	0.28	6.8	23521
lean, broiled	133	57.2	22.2	0.0	0.0	0.0	58	6	20	6.66		0	0	0.10	3.1	2.91	
3 oz	85	4.3	1.7	2.1	0.3	50	249	184	2.38	0.095	21.5	0	0.1	0.20	0.28	6.8	13963
chuck, top blade, choice, 0" trim,	193	51.6	21.9	0.0	0.0	0.0	58	6	20	7.45	0.000	0	0	0.09	3.1	2.87	<0.01
lean & fat, broiled - 3 oz	85	11.0	3.5	5.3	0.4	49	255	183	2.35	0.094	16.9	0	0.2	0.19	0.27	6.8	23523

	KCAL / WT (g)	H₂O (g) / FAT (g)	PRO (g) / SFA (g)	CHO (g) / MUFA (g)	SUGR (g) / PUFA (g)	DFIB (g) / CHOL (mg)	Na (mg) / K (mg)	Ca (mg) / P (mg)	Mg (mg) / Fe (mg)	Zn (mg) / Cu (mg)	Mn (mg) / Se (mcg)	A (mcg RAE) / A (IU)	C (mg) / E (mg ATE)	B-1 (mg) / B-2 (mg)	NIA (mg) / B-6 (mg)	B-12 (mcg) / FOL (mcg DFE)	PANT (mg) / REF
lean, broiled	184	52.4	22.2	0.0	0.0	0.0	58	6	20	7.58		0	0	0.10	3.1	2.91	
3 oz	85	9.9	3.1	4.9	0.3	48	258	185	2.39	0.096	17.0	0	0.2	0.20	0.28	6.8	13965
chuck, top blade, select, 0″ trim,	170	53.4	21.8	0.0	0.0	0.0	57	6	20	7.38	0.000	0	0	0.12	3.4	3.15	<0.01
lean & fat, broiled - *3 oz*	85	8.5	3.0	3.6	0.3	57	253	180	2.33	0.094	16.9	0	0.1	0.19	0.40	7.7	23525
lean, broiled	156	54.7	22.2	0.0	0.0	0.0	58	6	20	7.58		0	0	0.12	3.4	3.21	
3 oz	85	6.8	2.3	2.8	0.3	56	258	184	2.38	0.095	17.0	0	0.1	0.19	0.41	7.7	13967
flank, choice, 0″ trim,	224	46.7	22.9	0.0	0.0	0.0	60	5	20	4.90	0.015	0	0	0.12	3.8	2.81	0.31
lean & fat, braised - *3 oz*	85	14.0	5.9	5.9	0.5	61	286	218	2.83	0.101	25.8	0		0.15	0.30	7.7	13066
lean & fat, broiled	192	50.7	22.5	0.0		0.0	69	6	20	3.96	0.014	0	0	0.09	4.2	2.71	0.30
3 oz	85	10.7	4.5	4.4	0.4	58	342	196	2.13	0.082	20.3	0		0.15	0.29	6.8	13067
lean, braised	201	48.7	23.8	0.0	0.0	0.0	61	5	20	5.14	0.016	0	0	0.12	3.9	2.90	0.32
3 oz	85	11.1	4.7	4.6	0.3	60	298	227	2.95	0.105	26.2	0	0.1	0.16	0.31	7.7	13069
lean, broiled	176	52.1	23.0	0.0		0.0	71	6	20	4.08	0.014	0	0	0.09	4.3	2.76	0.31
3 oz	85	8.6	3.7	3.5	0.3	57	352	201	2.18	0.084	20.6	0		0.16	0.29	6.8	13070
ground, 5% fat,	164	53.2	24.8	0.0	0.0	0.0	72	8	24	6.00	0.011	0	0	0.04	6.2	2.24	0.69
crumbles, pan-browned - *3 oz*	85	6.4	2.8	2.7	0.3	76	390	224	2.75	0.090	17.9	0	0.3	0.17	0.36	6.0	23560
loaf, baked	148	55.0	23.2	0.0	0.0	0.0	49	7	19	5.83	0.009	0	0	0.03	4.7	2.13	0.56
3 oz piece	85	5.4	2.4	2.3	0.3	62	268	169	2.59	0.066	19.0	0	0.3	0.15	0.30	5.1	23561
patty, broiled	145	56.1	22.3	0.0	0.0	0.0	55	6	19	5.47	0.012	0	0	0.04	5.0	2.10	0.54
3 oz patty	85	5.6	2.4	2.3	0.3	65	296	175	2.41	0.082	18.4	0	0.3	0.15	0.35	6.0	23558
patty, pan-broiled	139	56.9	21.9	0.0	0.0	0.0	60	8	20	5.48	0.010	0	0	0.04	5.3	2.64	0.53
3 oz patty	85	5.0	2.2	2.1	0.3	65	320	189	2.42	0.077	17.9	0	0.3	0.15	0.33	6.0	23559
ground, 10% fat,	196	49.8	24.2	0.0	0.0	0.0	74	14	23	5.81	0.011	0	0	0.04	5.8	2.30	0.69
crumbles, pan-browned - *3 oz*	85	10.2	4.1	4.4	0.4	76	368	213	2.62	0.084	18.1	0	0.4	0.16	0.36	6.8	23565
loaf, baked	182	52.1	22.6	0.0	0.0	0.0	52	11	18	5.65	0.009	0	0	0.03	4.4	2.13	0.53
3 oz piece	85	9.4	3.8	4.1	0.3	73	255	164	2.46	0.066	18.4	0	0.4	0.15	0.30	5.1	23566
patty, broiled	184	52.1	22.2	0.0	0.0	0.0	58	11	19	5.41	0.011	0	0	0.04	4.8	2.18	0.55
3 oz patty	85	10.0	4.0	4.3	0.3	72	283	172	2.30	0.077	18.4	0	0.4	0.15	0.34	6.8	23563
patty, pan-broiled	173	53.7	21.4	0.0	0.0	0.0	64	13	20	5.38	0.010	0	0	0.04	5.1	2.51	0.53
3 oz patty	85	9.1	3.7	3.9	0.3	70	309	184	2.35	0.073	17.6	0	0.3	0.15	0.32	6.8	23564
ground, 15% fat,	218	47.5	23.6	0.0	0.0	0.0	76	19	21	5.63	0.010	0	0	0.04	5.4	2.37	0.69
crumbles, pan-browned - *3 oz*	85	13.0	5.1	5.7	0.4	77	346	202	2.49	0.079	18.4	0	0.4	0.16	0.36	8.5	23570
loaf, baked	204	50.1	22.0	0.0	0.0	0.0	54	15	17	5.48	0.009	0	0	0.03	4.2	2.12	0.51
3 oz piece	85	12.2	4.8	5.3	0.3	77	243	158	2.33	0.067	17.9	0	0.4	0.15	0.29	5.1	23571
patty, broiled	213	49.3	22.0	0.0	0.0	0.0	61	15	18	5.36	0.010	0	0	0.04	4.6	2.24	0.56
3 oz patty	85	13.2	5.2	5.8	0.4	77	270	168	2.21	0.072	18.4	0	0.4	0.15	0.32	7.7	23568
patty, pan-broiled	197	51.5	20.9	0.0	0.0	0.0	67	17	19	5.27	0.010	0	0	0.04	4.9	2.39	0.53
3 oz patty	85	11.9	4.7	5.2	0.3	73	297	179	2.28	0.069	17.3	0	0.4	0.15	0.31	6.8	23569
ground, 20% fat,	231	46.4	23.0	0.0	0.0	0.0	77	24	20	5.44	0.010	0	0	0.04	5.0	2.43	0.69
crumbles, pan-browned - *3 oz*	85	14.8	5.7	6.5	0.4	76	323	192	2.36	0.074	18.5	0	0.4	0.16	0.36	9.4	23575
loaf, baked	216	49.0	21.5	0.0	0.0	0.0	57	20	16	5.30	0.008	0	0	0.04	3.9	2.11	0.48
3 oz piece	85	13.7	5.3	6.0	0.3	77	230	152	2.19	0.068	17.3	0	0.4	0.14	0.28	6.0	23576
patty, broiled	230	47.7	21.9	0.0	0.0	0.0	64	20	17	5.31	0.009	0	0	0.04	4.3	2.32	0.57
3 oz patty	85	15.1	5.9	6.7	0.4	77	258	165	2.11	0.068	18.3	0	0.4	0.15	0.31	8.5	23573
patty, pan-broiled	209	50.2	20.4	0.0	0.0	0.0	71	22	18	5.16	0.010	0	0	0.04	4.7	2.26	0.53
3 oz patty	85	13.5	5.3	6.0	0.3	73	285	174	2.20	0.065	16.9	0	0.4	0.15	0.30	7.7	23574
ground, 25% fat,	235	46.3	22.3	0.0	0.0	0.0	79	29	19	5.24	0.010	0	0	0.04	4.5	2.50	0.68
crumbles, pan-browned - *3 oz*	85	15.5	6.0	6.8	0.4	76	301	182	2.24	0.068	18.7	0	0.4	0.16	0.36	10.2	23580
loaf, baked	216	48.9	20.9	0.0	0.0	0.0	60	24	15	5.13	0.008	0	0	0.04	3.7	2.10	0.46
3 oz piece	85	14.0	5.4	6.2	0.3	70	218	146	2.07	0.068	16.7	0	0.4	0.14	0.27	6.0	23581
patty, broiled	236	47.2	21.7	0.0	0.0	0.0	66	26	17	5.26	0.009	0	0	0.04	4.1	2.39	0.57
3 oz patty	85	15.9	6.1	7.0	0.4	76	246	161	2.01	0.064	18.2	0	0.4	0.15	0.30	9.4	23578
patty, pan-broiled	211	49.9	19.9	0.0	0.0	0.0	74	27	18	5.06	0.010	0	0	0.04	4.5	2.14	0.53
3 oz patty	85	14.0	5.4	6.2	0.3	71	274	169	2.13	0.060	16.7	0	0.4	0.15	0.29	8.5	23579
ribs 6–9 (large end), choice,	316	39.2	19.4	0.0		0.0	54	9	17	4.90	0.011	0	0	0.06	3.1	1.98	0.31
0″ trim, lean & fat, rstd - *3 oz*	85	25.9	10.4	11.1	0.9	72	247	146	1.98	0.075	18.0	0		0.16	0.20	6.0	13386
lean, roasted	215	48.3	23.4	0.0		0.0	62	7	21	6.34	0.014	0	0	0.08	3.8	2.22	0.38
3 oz	85	12.8	5.1	5.3	0.4	69	303	178	2.40	0.089	19.4	0		0.19	0.22	7.7	13389
ribs 6–9 (large end), choice,	312	39.3	17.8	0.0		0.0	54	9	15	4.14	0.011	0	0	0.06	2.3	2.40	0.29
1/4″ trim, lean & fat, brld - *3 oz*	85	26.2	10.6	11.1	1.0	69	253	150	1.81	0.065	18.1	0		0.14	0.20	5.1	13103
lean & fat, roasted	326	38.6	19.0	0.0		0.0	54	9	16	4.74	0.011	0	0	0.06	3.0	1.96	0.31
3 oz	85	27.2	11.0	11.6	1.0	72	241	143	1.93	0.073	18.6	0		0.15	0.19	6.0	13104c

	KCAL / WT (g)	H₂O (g) / FAT (g)	PRO (g) / SFA (g)	CHO (g) / MUFA (g)	SUGR (g) / PUFA (g)	DFIB (g) / CHOL (mg)	Na (mg) / K (mg)	Ca (mg) / P (mg)	Mg (mg) / Fe (mg)	Zn (mg) / Cu (mg)	Mn (mg) / Se (mcg)	A (mcg RAE) / A (IU)	C (mg) / E (mg ATE)	B-1 (mg) / B-2 (mg)	NIA (mg) / B-6 (mg)	B-12 (mcg) / FOL (mcg DFE)	PANT (mg) / REF
lean, broiled	204	48.9	21.4	0.0		0.0	61	8	20	5.34	0.013	0	0	0.07	2.7	2.81	0.35
3 oz	85	12.5	5.1	5.0	0.5	65	316	184	2.18	0.077	18.6	0		0.16	0.22	6.0	13115
lean, roasted	213	48.9	23.4	0.0		0.0	62	7	21	6.34	0.014	0	0	0.08	3.8	2.22	0.38
3 oz	85	12.5	5.0	5.2	0.4	69	303	178	2.46	0.089	19.4	0		0.19	0.22	7.7	13116
ribs 6–9 (large end), prime,	351	36.2	17.3	0.0		0.0	52	9	15	4.04	0.011	0	0	0.06	2.2	2.34	0.28
1/4 trim, lean & fat, brld - *3 oz*	85	30.8	12.8	13.4	1.1	73	247	137	1.73	0.064	18.0	0		0.14	0.22	5.1	13109b
lean & fat, roasted	342	37.1	19.1	0.0		0.0	54	9	16	4.79	0.011	0	0	0.06	3.0	1.96	0.34
3 oz	85	28.8	12.0	12.6	1.0	72	243	144	1.95	0.074	18.5	0		0.15	0.19	6.0	13110
lean, broiled	250	45.4	20.9	0.0		0.0	60	7	20	5.31	0.014	0	0	0.08	2.6	2.77	0.35
3 oz	85	17.7	7.6	7.9	0.5	70	314	169	2.11	0.076	18.6	0		0.17	0.27	6.0	13121
lean, roasted	241	46.2	23.4	0.0		0.0	62	7	21	6.34	0.014	0	0	0.08	3.8	2.22	0.38
3 oz	85	15.6	6.7	6.9	0.5	69	303	178	2.40	0.089	19.4	0		0.19	0.22	7.7	13122
ribs 6–9 (large end), select,	326	38.6	19.0	0.0		0.0	54	9	16	4.74	0.011	0	0	0.06	3.0	1.96	0.31
1/4" trim, lean & fat, brld - *3 oz*	85	27.2	11.0	11.6	1.0	72	241	143	1.93	0.073	18.6	0		0.15	0.19	6.0	13104b
lean & fat, roasted	351	36.2	17.3	0.0		0.0	52	9	15	4.04	0.011	0	0	0.06	2.2	2.34	0.28
3 oz	85	30.8	12.8	13.4	1.1	73	247	137	1.73	0.064	18.0	0		0.14	0.22	5.1	13109c
lean, broiled	175	51.6	21.4	0.0		0.0	61	8	20	5.34	0.013	0	0	0.07	2.7	2.81	0.35
3 oz	85	9.3	3.8	3.7	0.3	65	316	184	2.18	0.077	18.6	0		0.16	0.22	6.0	13118
lean, roasted	187	50.5	23.4	0.0		0.0	62	7	21	6.34	0.014	0	0	0.08	3.8	2.22	0.38
3 oz	85	9.7	3.9	4.1	0.3	69	303	178	2.40	0.089	19.4	0		0.19	0.22	7.7	13119
ribs 10–12 (small end), choice,	265	43.4	21.0	0.0		0.0	54	11	20	5.04	0.012	0	0	0.08	3.6	2.55	0.26
0" trim, lean & fat, brld - *3 oz*	85	19.4	7.9	8.3	0.7	71	291	156	1.94	0.077	17.9	0		0.16	0.30	6.0	13392
lean, broiled	191	49.9	23.8	0.0		0.0	59	11	23	5.94	0.014	0	0	0.09	4.1	2.82	0.29
3 oz	85	9.9	4.0	4.2	0.3	68	335	177	2.18	0.085	18.6	0		0.19	0.34	6.8	13395
ribs 10–12 (small end), choice,	297	40.1	20.0	0.0		0.0	53	11	19	4.71	0.012	0	0	0.08	3.4	2.45	0.25
1/4" trim, lean & fat, brld - *3 oz*	85	23.5	9.5	10.1	0.8	71	274	148	1.85	0.073	18.4	0		0.15	0.28	6.0	13127
lean & fat, roasted	312	39.5	18.7	0.0		0.0	53	11	16	4.05	0.011	0	0	0.05	2.6	2.40	0.20
3 oz	85	25.7	10.4	11.1	0.9	71	267	151	2.00	0.065	18.9	0		0.14	0.20	5.1	13128
lean, broiled	198	48.7	23.8	0.0		0.0	59	11	23	5.94	0.014	0	0	0.09	4.1	2.82	0.29
3 oz	85	10.7	4.3	4.5	0.3	68	335	177	2.18	0.085	18.6	0		0.19	0.34	6.8	13139
lean, roasted	197	49.6	22.8	0.0		0.0	60	10	21	5.28	0.014	0	0	0.06	3.2	2.83	0.23
3 oz	85	11.1	4.4	4.8	0.4	67	338	189	2.47	0.076	19.4	0		0.16	0.24	6.8	13140
ribs 10–12 (small end), prime,	307	39.8	20.3	0.0		0.0	53	11	19	4.80	0.012	0	0	0.08	3.4	2.47	0.25
1/4" trim, lean & fat, brld - *3 oz*	85	24.4	10.1	10.6	0.9	71	279	150	1.88	0.074	18.3	0		0.16	0.29	6.0	13133
lean & fat, roasted	354	35.1	18.6	0.0		0.0	55	11	16	4.04	0.011	0	0	0.05	2.6	2.41	0.30
3 oz	85	30.5	12.6	13.3	1.1	71	270	150	1.64	0.065	18.8	0		0.14	0.26	5.1	13134
lean, broiled	221	47.4	23.8	0.0		0.0	59	11	23	5.94	0.014	0	0	0.09	4.1	2.82	0.29
3 oz	85	13.2	5.6	5.8	0.4	68	335	177	2.18	0.085	18.6	0		0.19	0.34	6.8	13145
lean, roasted	258	43.4	22.7	0.0		0.0	64	11	21	5.26	0.014	0	0	0.07	3.1	2.86	0.37
3 oz	85	17.9	7.6	7.8	0.5	68	343	186	1.96	0.076	19.4	0		0.16	0.31	6.8	13146
ribs 10–12 (small end), select,	242	44.9	21.2	0.0		0.0	54	11	20	5.08	0.012	0	0	0.08	3.6	2.56	0.26
0" trim, lean & fat, brld - *3 oz*	85	16.8	6.8	7.2	0.6	71	292	156	1.96	0.077	17.9	0		0.16	0.30	6.0	13393
lean, broiled	168	51.3	23.8	0.0		0.0	59	11	23	5.94	0.014	0	0	0.09	4.1	2.82	0.29
3 oz	85	7.4	3.0	3.1	0.2	68	335	177	2.18	0.085	18.6	0		0.19	0.34	6.8	13396
ribs 10–12 (small end), select,	273	41.7	20.3	0.0		0.0	53	11	19	4.80	0.012	0	0	0.08	3.4	2.47	0.25
1/4" trim, lean & fat, brld - *3 oz*	85	20.6	8.3	8.9	0.7	71	279	150	1.88	0.074	18.4	0		0.16	0.29	6.0	13130
lean & fat, roasted	281	42.6	19.1	0.0		0.0	54	11	17	4.17	0.011	0	0	0.05	2.7	2.44	0.20
3 oz	85	22.2	8.9	9.6	0.8	71	275	156	2.05	0.065	19.0	0		0.14	0.20	5.1	13131
lean, broiled	176	49.9	23.8	0.0		0.0	59	11	23	5.94	0.014	0	0	0.09	4.1	2.82	0.29
3 oz	85	8.2	3.3	3.5	0.2	68	335	177	2.18	0.085	18.6	0		0.19	0.34	6.8	13142
lean, roasted	173	52.5	22.8	0.0	0.0	0.0	60	10	21	5.28	0.014	0	0	0.06	3.2	2.83	0.23
3 oz	85	8.3	3.3	3.6	0.3	67	338	189	2.47	0.076	19.4	0	0.1	0.16	0.24	6.8	13143
ribs 6–12 (whole), choice, 1/4"	306	39.6	18.7	0.0		0.0	53	10	16	4.36	0.011	0	0	0.07	2.7	2.41	0.27
trim, lean & fat, broiled - *3 oz*	85	25.1	10.2	10.7	0.9	70	262	149	1.83	0.068	18.2	0		0.14	0.23	5.1	13075
lean, broiled	201	48.8	22.4	0.0		0.0	60	9	21	5.58	0.014	0	0	0.08	3.3	2.82	0.32
3 oz	85	11.7	4.8	4.8	0.4	65	324	181	2.18	0.080	18.6	0		0.17	0.27	6.0	13087
lean, roasted	207	49.2	23.2	0.0	0.0	0.0	61	9	21	5.91	0.014	0	0	0.07	3.5	2.47	0.32
3 oz	85	11.9	4.8	5.0	0.4	68	318	182	2.43	0.084	19.4	0	0.1	0.18	0.23	6.8	13088
ribs 6–12 (whole), prime, 1/4"	333	37.7	18.5	0.0		0.0	53	9	17	4.34	0.011	0	0	0.07	2.7	2.40	0.27
trim, lean & fat, broiled - *3 oz*	85	28.2	11.7	12.3	1.0	72	260	142	1.79	0.068	18.1	0		0.14	0.25	5.1	13081
lean & fat, roasted	348	36.2	18.9	0.0		0.0	54	9	16	4.48	0.011	0	0	0.06	2.8	2.15	0.31
3 oz	85	29.6	12.2	12.9	1.0	72	254	146	1.82	0.070	18.6	0		0.14	0.22	6.0	13082

	KCAL	H₂0 (g)	PRO (g)	CHO (g)	SUGR (g)	DFIB (g)	Na (mg)	Ca (mg)	Mg (mg)	Zn (mg)	Mn (mg)	A (mcg RAE)	C (mg)	B-1 (mg)	NIA (mg)	B-12 (mcg)	PANT (mg)
	WT (g)	FAT (g)	SFA (g)	MUFA (g)	PUFA (g)	CHOL (mg)	K (mg)	P (mg)	Fe (mg)	Cu (mg)	Se (mcg)	A (IU)	E (mg ATE)	B-2 (mg)	B-6 (mg)	FOL (mcg DFE)	REF
lean, broiled	238	46.2	22.1	0.0		0.0	60	9	21	5.57	0.014	0	0	0.08	3.2	2.79	0.32
3 oz	85	15.9	6.8	7.0	0.5	69	322	173	2.14	0.079	18.6	0		0.18	0.30	6.0	13093
lean, roasted	248	45.1	23.1	0.0		0.0	63	9	21	5.90	0.014	0	0	0.07	3.5	2.48	0.37
3 oz	85	16.5	7.1	7.3	0.5	69	320	181	2.22	0.083	19.4	0		0.18	0.26	7.7	13094
ribs 6–12 (whole), select, 1/4″	275	42.3	19.1	0.0		0.0	54	9	17	4.51	0.011	0	0	0.07	2.8	2.47	0.28
trim, lean & fat, broiled - 3 oz	85	21.4	8.7	9.1	0.8	70	269	152	1.87	0.070	18.3	0		0.14	0.23	5.1	13078
lean & fat, roasted	286	41.9	19.4	0.0		0.0	54	9	17	4.66	0.012	0	0	0.06	2.9	2.18	0.27
3 oz	85	22.5	9.1	9.7	0.8	71	260	151	2.02	0.071	18.8	0		0.15	0.20	6.0	13079
lean, broiled	175	50.9	22.4	0.0		0.0	60	9	21	5.58	0.014	0	0	0.08	3.3	2.82	0.32
3 oz	85	8.9	3.6	3.6	0.3	65	324	181	2.18	0.080	18.6	0		0.17	0.27	6.0	13090
lean, roasted	181	51.3	23.2	0.0		0.0	61	9	21	5.91	0.014	0	0	0.07	3.5	2.47	0.32
3 oz	85	9.1	3.6	3.9	0.3	68	318	182	2.43	0.084	19.4	0		0.18	0.23	6.8	13091
ribs, shortribs,	400	30.4	18.3	0.0		0.0	43	10	13	4.15	0.011	0	0	0.04	2.1	2.23	0.21
lean & fat, braised - 3 oz	85	35.7	15.1	16.0	1.3	80	190	138	1.96	0.084	17.7	0	0.2	0.13	0.19	4.3	13148
lean, braised	251	42.6	26.1	0.0		0.0	49	9	19	6.63	0.015	0	0	0.06	2.7	2.94	0.29
3 oz	85	15.4	6.6	6.8	0.5	79	266	200	2.86	0.091	18.8	0	0.1	0.17	0.24	6.0	13150
round, bottom, choice, 0″ trim,	193	47.6	26.3	0.0		0.0	43	4	20	4.56	0.015	0	0	0.06	3.4	2.07	0.35
lean & fat, braised - 3 oz	85	9.0	3.1	3.9	0.3	82	257	226	2.88	0.111	23.6	0		0.21	0.30	9.4	13401
lean & fat, roasted	173	50.8	24.1	0.0		0.0	55	4	24	3.87	0.013	0	0	0.07	3.4	2.28	0.30
3 oz	85	7.7	2.7	3.5	0.3	66	327	201	2.63	0.092	23.1	0		0.20	0.31	10.2	13402
lean, braised	181	48.6	26.9	0.0		0.0	43	4	21	4.66	0.015	0	0	0.06	3.5	2.10	0.36
3 oz	85	7.4	2.5	3.2	0.3	82	262	231	2.94	0.114	23.9	0		0.22	0.31	9.4	13410
lean, roasted	164	51.6	24.5	0.0		0.0	56	4	24	3.93	0.014	0	0	0.07	3.5	2.30	0.30
3 oz	85	6.6	2.2	3.0	0.3	66	332	203	2.66	0.093	23.3	0		0.20	0.31	10.2	13411
round, bottom, choice, 1/4″ trim,	241	43.7	24.4	0.0		0.0	43	5	19	4.17	0.014	0	0	0.06	3.2	2.00	0.32
lean & fat, braised - 3 oz	85	15.2	5.7	6.6	0.6	82	240	208	2.65	0.104	26.7	0	0.2	0.20	0.28	8.5	13162
lean & fat, roasted	221	46.5	22.5	0.0		0.0	54	5	21	3.57	0.013	0	0	0.07	3.2	2.18	0.27
3 oz	85	13.9	5.2	6.1	0.5	68	302	185	2.43	0.086	22.1	0		0.19	0.29	9.4	13400
lean, braised	187	48.3	26.9	0.0		0.0	43	4	21	4.66	0.015	0	0	0.06	3.5	2.10	0.36
3 oz	85	8.0	2.7	3.5	0.3	82	262	231	2.94	0.114	23.9	0		0.22	0.31	9.4	13170
lean, roasted	168	51.1	24.5	0.0		0.0	56	4	24	3.93	0.014	0	0	0.07	3.5	2.30	0.30
3 oz	85	7.0	2.4	3.2	0.3	66	332	203	2.66	0.093	23.3	0		0.20	0.31	10.2	13409
round, bottom, select, 0″ trim,	171	49.4	26.5	0.0		0.0	43	4	21	4.59	0.015	0	0	0.06	3.4	2.08	0.36
lean & fat, braised - 3 oz	85	6.4	2.3	2.8	0.2	82	258	228	2.90	0.112	23.7	0		0.22	0.31	9.4	13404
lean & fat, roasted	150	53.2	24.3	0.0		0.0	56	4	24	3.90	0.014	0	0	0.07	3.4	2.29	0.30
3 oz	85	5.1	1.7	2.3	0.2	66	330	202	2.64	0.093	23.2	0		0.20	0.31	10.2	13405
lean, braised	163	50.1	26.9	0.0		0.0	43	4	21	4.66	0.015	0	0	0.06	3.5	2.10	0.36
3 oz	85	5.4	1.8	2.3	0.2	82	262	231	2.94	0.114	23.9	0		0.22	0.31	9.4	13413
lean, roasted	145	53.6	24.5	0.0		0.0	56	4	24	3.93	0.014	0	0	0.07	3.5	2.30	0.30
3 oz	85	4.6	1.5	2.1	0.2	66	332	203	2.66	0.093	23.3	0		0.20	0.31	10.2	13414
round, bottom, select, 1/4″ trim,	220	45.4	24.5	0.0		0.0	43	5	20	4.21	0.014	0	0	0.06	3.2	2.01	0.33
lean & fat, braised - 3 oz	85	12.8	4.8	5.6	0.5	82	241	210	2.68	0.104	26.9	0		0.20	0.28	8.5	13164
lean & fat, roasted	199	48.8	22.8	0.0		0.0	54	5	22	3.62	0.013	0	0	0.07	3.2	2.19	0.28
3 oz	85	11.3	4.3	5.0	0.4	68	307	188	2.47	0.087	22.3	0		0.20	0.30	9.4	13403
lean, braised	167	49.8	26.9	0.0		0.0	43	4	21	4.66	0.015	0	0	0.06	3.5	2.10	0.36
3 oz	85	5.8	2.0	2.5	0.2	82	262	231	2.94	0.114	23.9	0		0.22	0.31	9.4	13172
lean, roasted	152	52.9	24.5	0.0		0.0	56	4	24	3.93	0.014	0	0	0.07	3.5	2.30	0.30
3 oz	85	5.3	1.8	2.4	0.2	66	332	203	2.66	0.093	23.3	0		0.20	0.31	10.2	13412
round, eye of, choice, 0″ trim,	153	54.2	24.5	0.0		0.0	53	4	23	4.00	0.014	0	0	0.08	3.2	1.84	0.38
lean & fat, roasted - 3 oz	85	5.4	2.0	2.3	0.2	59	333	190	1.65	0.084	22.6	0		0.14	0.32	6.0	13416
lean, roasted	149	54.6	24.6	0.0		0.0	53	4	23	4.03	0.014	0	0	0.08	3.2	1.84	0.39
3 oz	85	4.8	1.8	2.1	0.2	59	336	192	1.66	0.085	22.7	0		0.14	0.32	6.0	13419
round, eye of, choice, 1/4″ trim,	205	50.0	22.6	0.0		0.0	50	5	20	3.66	0.013	0	0	0.07	2.9	1.79	0.36
lean & fat, roasted - 3 oz	85	12.0	4.7	5.2	0.4	61	305	175	1.56	0.079	21.8	0		0.14	0.30	5.1	13178
lean, roasted	149	55.2	24.6	0.0		0.0	53	4	23	4.03	0.014	0	0	0.08	3.2	1.84	0.39
3 oz	85	4.8	1.8	2.1	0.2	59	336	192	1.66	0.085	22.7	0		0.14	0.32	6.0	13186
round, eye of, select, 0″ trim,	137	54.9	24.5	0.0		0.0	53	4	23	4.00	0.014	0	0	0.08	3.2	1.84	0.38
lean & fat, roasted - 3 oz	85	3.5	1.3	1.5	0.1	59	333	190	1.65	0.084	22.6	0		0.14	0.32	6.0	13417
lean, roasted	132	55.3	24.6	0.0		0.0	53	4	23	4.03	0.014	0	0	0.08	3.2	1.84	0.39
3 oz	85	3.0	1.1	1.3	0.1	59	336	192	1.66	0.085	22.7	0		0.14	0.32	6.0	13420
round, eye of, select, 1/4″ trim,	184	51.0	22.9	0.0		0.0	51	5	21	3.71	0.013	0	0	0.07	3.0	1.79	0.36
lean & fat, roasted - 3 oz	85	9.6	3.8	4.1	0.3	61	310	178	1.57	0.080	21.8	0		0.14	0.30	6.0	13180

	KCAL	H₂0 (g)	PRO (g)	CHO (g)	SUGR (g)	DFIB (g)	Na (mg)	Ca (mg)	Mg (mg)	Zn (mg)	Mn (mg)	A (mcg RAE)	C (mg)	B-1 (mg)	NIA (mg)	B-12 (mcg)	PANT (mg)
	WT (g)	FAT (g)	SFA (g)	MUFA (g)	PUFA (g)	CHOL (mg)	K (mg)	P (mg)	Fe (mg)	Cu (mg)	Se (mcg)	A (IU)	E (mg ATE)	B-2 (mg)	B-6 (mg)	FOL (mcg DFE)	REF
lean, roasted	136	55.3	24.6	0.0		0.0	53	4	23	4.03	0.014	0	0	0.08	3.2	1.84	0.39
3 oz	85	3.4	1.2	1.4	0.1	59	336	192	1.66	0.085	22.7	0		0.14	0.32	6.0	13188
round, full cut, choice, 1/4″ trim,	204	47.9	23.2	0.0		0.0	52	5	21	3.67	0.013	0	0	0.08	3.4	2.56	0.32
lean & fat, broiled - *3 oz*	85	11.6	4.4	5.0	0.5	68	333	202	2.15	0.085	23.0	0	0.2	0.18	0.32	7.7	13152
lean, broiled	162	51.4	24.8	0.0		0.0	54	4	24	3.94	0.014	0	0	0.09	3.6	2.69	0.35
3 oz	85	6.2	2.2	2.6	0.3	66	359	218	2.30	0.090	23.5	0	0.1	0.19	0.34	8.5	13156
round, full cut, select, 1/4″ trim,	190	49.4	23.3	0.0		0.0	53	5	22	3.68	0.013	0	0	0.08	3.4	2.57	0.33
lean & fat, broiled - *3 oz*	85	10.0	3.5	3.9	0.3	47	333	202	2.16	0.086	23.0	0		0.18	0.32	7.7	13154
lean, broiled	146	53.1	24.9	0.0		0.0	54	4	24	3.96	0.014	0	0	0.09	3.6	2.69	0.35
3 oz	85	4.4	1.6	1.9	0.2	66	360	218	2.30	0.091	23.5	0		0.19	0.35	8.5	13158
round, tip, choice, 0″ trim,	170	53.8	23.8	0.0		0.0	54	4	22	5.81	0.014	0	0	0.09	3.1	2.41	0.39
lean & fat, roasted - *3 oz*	85	7.6	2.8	3.1	0.3	70	319	200	2.43	0.104	23.2	0		0.22	0.33	6.8	13422
lean, roasted	153	55.3	24.4	0.0		0.0	55	4	23	6.01	0.014	0	0	0.09	3.2	2.46	0.40
3 oz	85	5.4	1.9	2.2	0.2	69	328	206	2.50	0.106	23.5	0		0.23	0.34	6.8	13425
round, tip, choice, 1/4″ trim,	210	50.2	22.6	0.0		0.0	53	5	20	5.43	0.014	0	0	0.08	3.0	2.33	0.37
lean & fat, roasted - *3 oz*	85	12.6	4.8	5.3	0.5	71	301	189	2.30	0.098	22.4	0	0.2	0.21	0.31	6.0	13194
lean, roasted	160	54.9	24.4	0.0	0.0	0.0	55	4	23	6.01	0.014	0	0	0.09	3.2	2.46	0.40
3 oz	85	6.2	2.2	2.5	0.2	69	328	206	2.50	0.106	23.5	0	0.1	0.23	0.34	6.8	13202
round, tip, prime, 1/4″ trim,	233	47.2	22.4	0.0		0.0	53	5	20	5.38	0.014	0	0	0.08	2.9	2.31	0.37
lean & fat, roasted - *3 oz*	85	15.2	5.9	6.4	0.6	71	298	187	2.30	0.098	22.3	0		0.20	0.31	6.0	13198
lean, roasted	181	51.9	24.4	0.0		0.0	55	4	23	6.01	0.014	0	0	0.09	3.2	2.46	0.40
3 oz	85	8.6	3.1	3.5	0.3	69	328	206	2.50	0.106	23.5	0		0.23	0.34	6.8	13206
round, tip, select, 0″ trim,	158	54.5	23.9	0.0		0.0	54	4	22	5.87	0.014	0	0	0.09	3.1	2.42	0.39
lean & fat, roasted - *3 oz*	85	6.2	2.3	2.5	0.2	69	321	201	2.45	0.105	23.2	0		0.22	0.33	6.8	13423
lean, roasted	145	55.7	24.4	0.0		0.0	55	4	23	6.01	0.014	0	0	0.09	3.2	2.46	0.40
3 oz	85	4.5	1.6	1.8	0.2	69	328	206	2.50	0.106	23.5	0		0.23	0.34	6.8	13426
round, tip, select, 1/4″ trim,	191	51.8	23.0	0.0	0.0	0.0	54	5	21	5.58	0.014	0	0	0.08	3.0	2.36	0.37
lean & fat, roasted - *3 oz*	85	10.3	3.9	4.3	0.4	70	308	193	2.35	0.100	22.5	0	0.1	0.21	0.32	6.8	13196
lean, roasted	153	55.3	24.4	0.0		0.0	55	4	23	6.01	0.014	0	0	0.09	3.2	2.46	0.40
3 oz	85	5.4	1.9	2.2	0.2	69	328	206	2.50	0.106	23.5	0	0.1	0.23	0.34	6.8	13204
round, top, choice, 0″ trim,	184	48.7	30.3	0.0		0.0	38	3	21	3.83	0.015	0	0	0.06	3.2	2.28	0.31
lean & fat, braised - *3 oz*	85	6.0	2.1	2.4	0.3	77	281	190	2.78	0.104	27.8	0		0.21	0.24	7.7	13430
lean, braised	176	49.4	30.7	0.0		0.0	38	3	22	3.88	0.015	0	0	0.06	3.2	2.30	0.31
3 oz	85	4.9	1.7	1.9	0.2	77	284	192	2.82	0.105	28.1	0		0.21	0.24	7.7	13436
round, top, choice, 1/4″ trim,	221	45.1	28.5	0.0		0.0	38	4	20	3.60	0.014	0	0	0.06	3.0	2.20	0.30
lean & fat, braised - *3 oz*	85	10.9	4.1	4.5	0.5	77	265	179	2.63	0.099	27.4	0		0.20	0.23	7.7	13429
lean & fat, broiled	190	49.4	25.6	0.0		0.0	51	6	25	4.48	0.014	0	0	0.09	4.9	2.06	0.39
3 oz	85	9.0	3.3	3.7	0.4	72	356	199	2.34	0.099	23.6	0		0.22	0.45	9.4	13210
lean & fat, panfried	235	43.7	27.5	0.0		0.0	58	5	27	3.63	0.016	0	0	0.09	4.3	2.75	0.36
3 oz	85	13.1	4.5	5.0	1.5	82	400	228	2.48	0.104	26.9	0	0.2	0.22	0.48	10.2	13211
lean, braised	181	48.4	30.7	0.0		0.0	38	3	22	3.88	0.015	0	0	0.06	3.2	2.30	0.31
3 oz	85	5.5	1.9	2.1	0.2	77	284	192	2.82	0.105	28.1	0		0.21	0.24	7.7	13435
lean, broiled	161	52.0	26.9	0.0		0.0	52	5	26	4.73	0.014	0	0	0.10	5.1	2.11	0.42
3 oz	85	5.0	1.7	1.9	0.2	71	376	209	2.45	0.105	23.9	0		0.23	0.48	10.2	13219
lean, panfried	193	47.2	29.8	0.0	0.0	0.0	60	4	30	3.93	0.017	0	0	0.09	4.7	2.92	0.39
3 oz	85	7.3	2.1	2.4	1.4	82	436	248	2.68	0.111	28.6	0	0.1	0.24	0.52	11.1	13220
round, top, prime, 1/4″ trim,	195	50.2	26.4	0.0		0.0	51	5	26	4.62	0.014	0	0	0.10	5.0	2.08	0.41
lean & fat, broiled - *3 oz*	85	9.1	3.3	3.6	0.4	71	367	205	2.41	0.103	23.6	0		0.22	0.47	10.2	13215
lean, broiled	183	51.3	26.9	0.0		0.0	52	5	26	4.73	0.014	0	0	0.10	5.1	2.11	0.42
3 oz	85	7.5	2.6	2.9	0.4	71	376	209	2.45	0.105	23.9	0		0.23	0.48	10.2	13224
round, top, select, 0″ trim,	170	49.7	30.3	0.0		0.0	38	3	21	3.83	0.015	0	0	0.06	3.2	2.28	0.31
lean & fat, braised - *3 oz*	85	4.5	1.6	1.8	0.2	77	281	190	2.78	0.104	27.8	0		0.21	0.24	7.7	13432
lean, braised	162	50.4	30.7	0.0		0.0	38	3	22	3.88	0.015	0	0	0.06	3.2	2.30	0.31
3 oz	85	3.4	1.2	1.3	0.2	77	284	192	2.82	0.105	28.1	0		0.21	0.24	7.7	13438
round, top, select, 1/4″ trim,	199	46.6	29.0	0.0		0.0	38	4	20	3.66	0.014	0	0	0.06	3.1	2.22	0.30
lean & fat, braised - *3 oz*	85	8.4	3.2	3.5	0.3	77	269	182	2.67	0.100	27.4	0		0.20	0.23	7.7	13431
lean & fat, broiled	175	51.0	25.6	0.0		0.0	51	6	25	4.48	0.014	0	0	0.09	4.9	2.06	0.39
3 oz	85	7.2	2.8	3.0	0.3	72	356	199	2.34	0.099	23.6	0		0.22	0.45	9.4	13213
lean, braised	167	49.3	30.7	0.0		0.0	38	3	22	3.88	0.015	0	0	0.06	3.2	2.30	0.31
3 oz	85	3.9	1.3	1.5	0.2	77	284	192	2.82	0.105	28.1	0		0.21	0.24	7.7	13437
lean, broiled	144	53.7	26.9	0.0		0.0	52	5	26	4.73	0.014	0	0	0.10	5.1	2.11	0.42
3 oz	85	3.1	1.1	1.2	0.1	71	376	209	2.45	0.105	23.9	0		0.23	0.48	10.2	13222

	KCAL / WT (g)	H₂0 (g) / FAT (g)	PRO (g) / SFA (g)	CHO (g) / MUFA (g)	SUGR (g) / PUFA (g)	DFIB (g) / CHOL (mg)	Na (mg) / K (mg)	Ca (mg) / P (mg)	Mg (mg) / Fe (mg)	Zn (mg) / Cu (mg)	Mn (mg) / Se (mcg)	A (mcg RAE) / A (IU)	C (mg) / E (mg ATE)	B-1 (mg) / B-2 (mg)	NIA (mg) / B-6 (mg)	B-12 (mcg) / FOL (mcg DFE)	PANT (mg) / REF
shank, crosscuts, choice, 1/4″ trim,	224	45.1	26.1	0.0		0.0	52	26	23	7.91	0.015	0	0	0.10	4.5	2.98	0.31
lean & fat, simmered - 3 *oz*	85	12.5	4.8	5.5	0.5	68	343	203	2.98	0.132	24.4	0		0.17	0.29	7.7	13226
lean, simmered	171	49.5	28.6	0.0		0.0	54	27	26	8.92	0.017	0	0	0.12	5.0	3.22	0.35
3 *oz*	85	5.4	1.9	2.4	0.2	66	380	224	3.28	0.146	25.5	0		0.18	0.31	8.5	13228
short loin porterhse stk, choice,	291	41.5	18.6	0.0	0.0	0.0	52	7	17	3.45	0.012	0	0	0.07	3.2	1.78	0.24
1/4″ trim, lean & fat, brld - 3 *oz*	85	23.4	9.1	10.5	0.9	65	214	148	2.24	0.099	16.4	0	0.2	0.18	0.28	6.0	13230
lean, broiled	183	51.1	22.1	0.0		0.0	59	5	21	4.30	0.014	0	0	0.09	3.9	1.93	0.29
3 *oz*	85	9.8	3.4	4.8	0.3	59	256	179	2.75	0.122	17.0	0	0.1	0.21	0.34	6.8	13232
short loin porterhse stk, select,	264	43.5	19.9	0.0	0.0	0.0	54	7	17	3.60	0.012	0	0	0.08	3.3	1.80	0.25
1/4″ trim, lean & fat, brld - 3 *oz*	85	19.8	8.0	8.8	0.8	56	221	154	2.33	0.103	16.5	0	0.2	0.18	0.29	6.0	13462
lean, broiled	173	51.6	23.1	0.0	0.0	0.0	59	5	21	4.30	0.014	0	0	0.09	3.9	1.93	0.29
3 *oz*	85	8.2	3.3	3.8	0.4	49	256	179	2.75	0.122	17.0	0	0.1	0.21	0.34	6.8	13469
short loin T-bone steak, choice, 1/4″	274	43.2	19.4	0.0	0.0	0.0	58	7	18	3.56	0.012	0	0	0.08	3.3	1.79	0.24
trim, lean & fat, broiled - 3 *oz*	85	21.2	8.3	9.6	0.8	58	234	154	2.56	0.101	10.0	0	0.2	0.18	0.28	6.0	13234
lean, broiled	174	52.2	22.8	0.0	0.0	0.0	65	5	22	4.34	0.014	0	0	0.09	3.9	1.93	0.28
3 *oz*	85	8.5	3.1	4.2	0.3	50	278	183	3.11	0.122	8.5	0	0.1	0.21	0.33	6.8	13236
short loin T-bone steak, select, 1/4″	239	46.0	20.8	0.0	0.0	0.0	56	5	20	3.80	0.012	0	0	0.08	3.5	1.84	0.25
trim, lean & fat, broiled - 3 *oz*	85	16.7	6.6	7.2	0.6	51	247	162	2.72	0.107	9.6	0	0.2	0.19	0.29	6.0	13476
lean, broiled	168	52.3	23.2	0.0	0.0	0.0	60	3	22	4.34	0.014	0	0	0.09	3.9	1.93	0.28
3 *oz*	85	7.6	2.8	3.3	0.3	45	278	183	3.11	0.122	8.5	0	0.1	0.21	0.33	6.8	13483
short loin, top, choice, 0″ trim,	194	49.2	23.7	0.0		0.0	57	7	22	4.31	0.014	0	0	0.08	4.4	1.68	0.31
lean & fat, broiled - 3 *oz*	85	10.2	4.0	4.2	0.3	65	327	180	2.05	0.089	19.2	0		0.16	0.35	6.8	13446
lean, broiled	178	50.6	24.3	0.0		0.0	58	7	23	4.44	0.014	0	0	0.08	4.5	1.70	0.31
3 *oz*	85	8.2	3.1	3.3	0.3	65	337	185	2.10	0.091	19.4	0		0.17	0.36	6.8	13449
short loin, top, choice, 1/4″ trim,	253	44.1	21.6	0.0		0.0	54	8	20	3.85	0.012	0	0	0.07	4.0	1.64	0.28
lean & fat, broiled - 3 *oz*	85	17.8	7.1	7.5	0.6	67	294	163	1.89	0.082	19.6	0		0.15	0.31	6.0	13264
lean, broiled	182	50.4	24.3	0.0		0.0	58	7	23	4.44	0.014	0	0	0.08	4.5	1.70	0.31
3 *oz*	85	8.6	3.3	3.5	0.3	65	337	185	2.10	0.091	19.4	0		0.17	0.36	6.8	13272
short loin, top, prime, 1/4″ trim,	275	42.7	21.6	0.0		0.0	54	8	20	3.85	0.012	0	0	0.07	4.0	1.64	0.28
lean & fat, broiled - 3 *oz*	85	20.2	8.2	8.6	0.7	67	294	163	1.89	0.082	19.5	0		0.15	0.31	6.0	13268
lean, broiled	208	48.6	24.3	0.0		0.0	58	7	23	4.44	0.014	0	0	0.08	4.5	1.70	0.31
3 *oz*	85	11.6	4.6	4.8	0.4	65	337	185	2.10	0.091	19.4	0		0.17	0.36	6.8	13276
short loin, top, select, 0″ trim,	169	50.8	23.9	0.0		0.0	57	7	22	4.34	0.014	0	0	0.08	4.4	1.69	0.31
lean & fat, broiled - 3 *oz*	85	7.5	2.9	3.1	0.3	65	330	182	2.07	0.089	19.3	0		0.16	0.35	6.8	13447
lean, broiled	156	51.9	24.3	0.0		0.0	58	7	23	4.44	0.014	0	0	0.08	4.5	1.70	0.31
3 *oz*	85	5.9	2.2	2.4	0.2	65	337	185	2.10	0.091	19.4	0		0.17	0.36	6.8	13450
short loin, top, select, 1/4″ trim,	226	46.2	22.0	0.0		0.0	54	8	20	3.95	0.013	0	0	0.07	4.1	1.65	0.28
lean & fat, broiled - 3 *oz*	85	14.6	5.8	6.1	0.5	67	301	167	1.92	0.083	19.7	0		0.15	0.32	6.0	13266
lean, broiled	164	51.6	24.3	0.0		0.0	58	7	23	4.44	0.014	0	0	0.08	4.5	1.70	0.31
3 *oz*	85	6.6	2.5	2.7	0.2	65	337	185	2.10	0.091	19.4	0		0.17	0.36	6.8	13274
skirt steak, inside, 0″ trim,	187	51.3	22.2	0.0	0.0	0.0	64	9	20	6.15	0.000	0	0	0.08	3.2	3.16	<0.01
lean & fat, broiled - 3 *oz*	85	10.2	4.0	5.1	0.4	51	246	196	2.35	0.079	16.8	0	0.1	0.16	0.27	6.0	23540
lean, broiled	174	52.5	22.7	0.0	0.0	0.0	65	9	20	6.32		0	0	0.08	3.2	3.23	
3 *oz*	85	8.6	3.3	4.4	0.3	50	251	201	2.41	0.081	16.9	0	0.1	0.16	0.28	6.0	13977
skirt steak, outside, 0″ trim,	217	48.6	20.0	0.0	0.0	0.0	78	9	20	4.68	0.000	0	0	0.10	3.6	3.54	0.01
lean & fat, broiled - 3 *oz*	85	14.6	6.0	7.2	0.6	50	322	182	2.19	0.074	15.8	0	0.1	0.16	0.41	6.0	23541
lean, broiled	198	50.3	20.6	0.0	0.0	0.0	80	9	21	4.86		0	0	0.10	3.7	3.66	
3 *oz*	85	12.2	5.1	6.3	0.5	49	334	188	2.26	0.076	15.9	0	0.1	0.17	0.42	6.8	13979
tenderloin, choice, 0″ trim,	207	48.4	23.0	0.0		0.0	52	6	24	4.51	0.014	0	0	0.10	3.2	2.13	0.31
lean & fat, broiled - 3 *oz*	85	12.2	4.7	4.8	0.5	72	338	193	2.89	0.145	20.3	0		0.24	0.36	6.0	13440
lean, broiled	180	50.8	24.0	0.0		0.0	54	6	26	4.75	0.014	0	0	0.11	3.3	2.18	0.32
3 *oz*	85	8.6	3.2	3.2	0.3	71	356	202	3.04	0.152	20.7	0		0.26	0.37	6.0	13443
tenderloin, choice, 1/4″ trim,	258	44.1	21.3	0.0		0.0	50	7	22	4.11	0.013	0	0	0.09	3.0	2.04	0.29
lean & fat, broiled - 3 *oz*	85	18.6	7.3	7.6	0.7	73	310	178	2.66	0.132	20.7	0		0.22	0.33	5.1	13241
lean & fat, roasted	288	40.2	20.1	0.0		0.0	55	8	22	3.37	0.014	0	0	0.13	3.3	2.83	0.33
3 *oz*	85	22.4	8.9	9.3	0.9	73	340	197	2.60	0.103	19.6	0		0.23	0.40	6.8	13242
lean, broiled	189	50.3	24.0	0.0		0.0	54	6	26	4.75	0.014	0	0	0.11	3.3	2.18	0.32
3 *oz*	85	9.5	3.6	3.6	0.4	71	356	202	3.04	0.152	20.7	0		0.26	0.37	6.0	13253
lean, roasted	196	48.0	23.6	0.0		0.0	61	7	27	4.07	0.016	0	0	0.15	3.9	3.29	0.40
3 *oz*	85	10.6	4.0	4.1	0.4	71	416	239	3.14	0.123	20.1	0		0.28	0.48	7.7	13254
tenderloin, prime, 1/4″ trim,	269	43.4	21.2	0.0		0.0	50	7	21	4.07	0.013	0	0	0.09	2.9	2.03	0.29
lean & fat, broiled - 3 *oz*	85	19.9	7.9	8.2	0.8	73	308	176	2.64	0.131	20.5	0		0.22	0.32	5.1	13247

	KCAL	H₂0 (g)	PRO (g)	CHO (g)	SUGR (g)	DFIB (g)	Na (mg)	Ca (mg)	Mg (mg)	Zn (mg)	Mn (mg)	A (mcg RAE)	C (mg)	B-1 (mg)	NIA (mg)	B-12 (mcg)	PANT (mg)
	WT (g)	FAT (g)	SFA (g)	MUFA (g)	PUFA (g)	CHOL (mg)	K (mg)	P (mg)	Fe (mg)	Cu (mg)	Se (mcg)	A (IU)	E (mg ATE)	B-2 (mg)	B-6 (mg)	FOL (mcg DFE)	REF
lean & fat, roasted	300	40.3	20.1	0.0		0.0	47	8	19	3.66	0.012	0	0	0.08	2.5	2.13	0.32
3 oz	85	23.7	9.5	9.8	0.9	75	281	169	2.60	0.118	19.4	0		0.23	0.28	6.0	13248
lean, broiled	197	49.9	24.0	0.0		0.0	54	6	26	4.75	0.014	0	0	0.11	3.3	2.18	0.32
3 oz	85	10.5	4.1	4.1	0.4	71	356	202	3.04	0.152	20.7	0		0.26	0.37	6.0	13259
lean, roasted	217	47.6	23.4	0.0		0.0	50	6	23	4.39	0.014	0	0	0.09	2.9	2.35	0.38
3 oz	85	13.0	5.1	5.0	0.5	73	334	201	.3.11	0.142	20.1	0	0.1	0.27	0.32	6.8	13260
tenderloin, select, 0″ trim,	195	49.2	23.1	0.0		0.0	53	6	25	4.54	0.014	0	0	0.10	3.2	2.13	0.31
lean & fat, broiled - 3 oz	85	10.6	4.1	4.2	0.4	72	341	194	2.92	0.145	20.4	0		0.25	0.36	6.0	13441
lean, broiled	170	51.3	24.0	0.0		0.0	54	6	26	4.75	0.014	0	0	0.11	3.3	2.18	0.32
3 oz	85	7.5	2.8	2.8	0.3	71	356	202	3.04	0.152	20.7	0		0.26	0.37	6.0	13444
tenderloin, select, 1/4″ trim,	230	46.4	21.8	0.0		0.0	51	7	22	4.22	0.013	0	0	0.10	3.0	2.07	0.29
lean & fat, broiled - 3 oz	85	15.2	6.0	6.3	0.6	73	318	182	2.72	0.135	20.8	0		0.23	0.33	5.1	13244
lean & fat, roasted	275	41.0	20.1	0.0		0.0	48	8	19	3.37	0.012	0	0	0.07	2.5	2.08	0.21
3 oz	85	21.0	8.3	8.8	0.8	73	277	170	2.60	0.103	19.7	0		0.22	0.21	6.0	13245
lean, broiled	169	51.9	24.0	0.0		0.0	54	6	26	4.75	0.014	0	0	0.11	3.3	2.18	0.32
3 oz	85	7.4	2.8	2.8	0.3	71	356	202	3.04	0.152	20.7	0		0.26	0.37	6.0	13256
lean, roasted	179	48.9	23.6	0.0		0.0	52	6	23	4.07	0.014	0	0	0.09	2.9	2.30	0.24
3 oz	85	8.8	3.3	3.4	0.4	71	332	203	3.14	0.123	20.1	0		0.26	0.25	7.7	13257
top sirloin, choice, 0″ trim,	195	49.7	24.8	0.0		0.0	54	9	26	5.28	0.014	0	0	0.10	3.5	2.36	0.31
lean & fat, broiled - 3 oz	85	9.8	3.9	4.2	0.4	76	328	199	2.74	0.119	27.1	0		0.24	0.37	8.5	13452
lean, broiled	170	51.9	25.8	0.0		0.0	56	9	27	5.54	0.014	0	0	0.11	3.6	2.42	0.33
3 oz	85	6.6	2.6	2.8	0.3	76	343	207	2.86	0.124	28.0	0		0.25	0.38	8.5	13455
top sirloin, choice, 1/4″ trim,	229	47.2	23.5	0.0		0.0	53	9	24	4.93	0.014	0	0	0.09	3.3	2.28	0.30
lean & fat, broiled - 3 oz	85	14.2	5.7	6.1	0.5	77	309	187	2.58	0.112	22.7	0	0.2	0.23	0.35	7.7	13280
lean & fat, panfried	277	41.2	23.9	0.0		0.0	60	10	24	4.59	0.014	0	0	0.10	3.2	2.79	0.32
3 oz	85	19.4	7.6	8.2	1.5	83	337	195	2.83	0.109	23.0	0	0.2	0.24	0.37	7.7	13281
lean, broiled	172	52.4	25.8	0.0		0.0	56	9	27	5.54	0.014	0	0	0.11	3.6	2.42	0.33
3 oz	85	6.8	2.6	2.9	0.3	76	343	207	2.86	0.124	28.0	0	0.1	0.25	0.38	8.5	13289
lean, panfried	202	47.5	27.6	0.0		0.0	65	9	28	5.44	0.016	0	0	0.12	3.7	3.14	0.37
3 oz	85	9.3	3.4	3.8	1.3	84	395	227	3.32	0.127	20.1	0	0.1	0.28	0.43	8.5	13290
top sirloin, select, 0″ trim,	166	52.0	25.2	0.0		0.0	55	9	26	5.40	0.014	0	0	0.10	3.6	2.39	0.32
lean & fat, broiled - 3 oz	85	6.4	2.6	2.8	0.2	76	334	203	2.79	0.122	27.5	0		0.25	0.37	8.5	13453
lean, broiled	153	53.0	25.8	0.0		0.0	56	9	27	5.54	0.014	0	0	0.11	3.6	2.42	0.33
3 oz	85	4.8	1.9	2.0	0.2	76	343	207	2.86	0.124	28.0	0		0.25	0.38	8.5	13456
top sirloin, select, 1/4″ trim,	208	48.9	23.8	0.0		0.0	54	9	25	5.02	0.014	0	0	0.09	3.4	2.30	0.31
lean & fat, broiled - 3 oz	85	11.8	4.7	5.1	0.5	77	314	190	2.62	0.114	22.9	0	0.2	0.23	0.35	7.7	13283
lean, broiled	158	53.5	25.8	0.0		0.0	56	9	27	5.54	0.014	0	0	0.11	3.6	2.42	0.33
3 oz	85	5.3	2.0	2.2	0.2	76	343	207	2.86	0.124	28.0	0	0.1	0.25	0.38	8.5	13292

19.2 GAME

	KCAL	H₂0 (g)	PRO (g)	CHO (g)	SUGR (g)	DFIB (g)	Na (mg)	Ca (mg)	Mg (mg)	Zn (mg)	Mn (mg)	A (mcg RAE)	C (mg)	B-1 (mg)	NIA (mg)	B-12 (mcg)	PANT (mg)
antelope, roasted	128	56.0	25.0	0.0		0.0	46	3	24	1.43	0.019	0	0	0.22			
3 oz	85	2.3	0.8	0.5	0.5	107	316	179	3.57	0.181	11.0	0		0.62			17145
bear, simmered	220	45.5	27.6	0.0		0.0	60	4	20	8.73		0	0	0.09	2.8	2.10	
3 oz	85	11.4	3.0	4.8	2.0	83	224	145	9.12	0.126	9.5	0	0.2	0.70	0.25	5.1	17147
beaver, roasted	180	49.2	29.6	0.0		0.0	50	19	25	1.93		0	3	0.04	1.9	7.06	0.79
3 oz	85	5.9	1.8	1.6	1.1	99	343	248	8.50	0.161	36.6	0	0.7	0.26	0.40	9.4	17151
beefalo, roasted	160	52.4	26.1	0.0		0.0	70	20		5.44		0	8	0.03	4.2	2.17	0.49
3 oz	85	5.4	2.3	2.3	0.2	49	390	213	2.59		11.1	0		0.09		15.3	17153
bison, chuck, shoulder clod, lean,	164	51.4	28.7	0.0	0.0	0.0	48	6	22	7.34	0.014	0	0	0.10	4.1	2.02	1.38
braised - 3 oz	85	4.6	2.0	1.8	0.2	94	269	203	4.13	0.177	35.4	0	0.2	0.40	0.39	17.9	17333
bison, ground, pan-broiled	202	50.6	20.2	0.0	0.0	0.0	62	11	19	4.37	0.009	0	0	0.11	4.7	1.94	0.97
3 oz	85	12.9	5.5	5.0	0.6	71	290	174	2.62	0.124	25.5	0	0.2	0.21	0.32	12.8	17331
bison, ribeye steak, lean, broiled	150	54.8	25.0	0.0	0.0	0.0	44	6	22	4.26	0.010	0	0	0.12	5.7	1.10	0.86
3 oz	85	4.8	2.1	1.9	0.2	67	315	202	2.45	0.171	35.8	0	0.2	0.26	0.40	15.3	17335b
	317	115.4	52.7	0.0	0.0	0.0	93	13	47	8.97	0.021	0	0	0.25	12.0	2.31	1.81
6.3 oz	179	10.1	4.3	4.0	0.5	141	664	426	5.16	0.360	75.4	0	0.4	0.55	0.85	32.2	17335a
bison, top round steak, lean,	148	55.3	25.7	0.0	0.0	0.0	35	4	24	3.22	0.009	0	0	0.14	5.5	1.54	1.23
broiled - 3 oz	85	4.2	1.7	1.5	0.2	72	325	218	2.99	0.179	34.9	0	0.2	0.31	0.56	16.2	17336b
	313	117.1	54.3	0.0	0.0	0.0	74	9	50	6.82	0.020	0	0	0.30	11.7	3.26	2.61
broiled - 6.3 oz	180	8.9	3.5	3.2	0.4	153	688	463	6.34	0.378	73.8	0	0.4	0.66	1.18	34.2	17336a
bison, top round, lean, raw	94	63.4	19.0	0.0			43	4	21	2.98	0.011	1	0	0.04	1.6	1.62	
3 oz	85	1.4	0.5	0.5	0.1	56	293	173	2.47	0.115	23.1	3	0.4	0.08	0.24		17266

Food	KCAL / WT (g)	H₂0 (g) / FAT (g)	PRO (g) / SFA (g)	CHO (g) / MUFA (g)	SUGR (g) / PUFA (g)	DFIB (g) / CHOL (mg)	Na (mg) / K (mg)	Ca (mg) / P (mg)	Mg (mg) / Fe (mg)	Zn (mg) / Cu (mg)	Mn (mg) / Se (mcg)	A (mcg RAE) / A (IU)	C (mg) / E (mg ATE)	B-1 (mg) / B-2 (mg)	NIA (mg) / B-6 (mg)	B-12 (mcg) / FOL (mcg DFE)	PANT (mg) / REF
bison, top sirloin steak, lean,	145	55.3	23.8	0.0	0.0	0.0	45	4	23	4.34	0.011	0	0	0.19	4.7	2.41	1.14
broiled - *3 oz*	85	4.8	2.1	1.9	0.2	73	329	215	2.95	0.179	35.0	0	0.2	0.38	0.47	15.3	17332a
	332	126.3	54.4	0.0	0.0	0.0	103	10	52	9.91	0.025	0	0	0.44	10.8	5.49	2.61
broiled - *6.8 oz*	194	11.0	4.7	4.3	0.5	167	751	491	6.73	0.409	79.9	0	0.4	0.87	1.08	34.9	17332b
boar, wild, roasted	136	54.3	24.1	0.0		0.0	51	14	23	2.56		0	0	0.26	3.6	0.60	
3 oz	85	3.7	1.1	1.5	0.5	65	337	114	0.95	0.048	11.1	0	0.2	0.12	0.36	5.1	17159
buffalo, water, roasted	111	58.5	22.8	0.0		0.0	48	13	28	2.16		0		0.03	5.3	1.49	0.14
3 oz	85	1.5	0.5	0.5	0.3	52	266	187	1.80	0.151	10.2	0		0.21	0.39	7.7	17161
caribou, roasted	142	53.1	25.3	0.0		0.0	51	19	23	4.47	0.074	0	3	0.21	4.9	5.64	2.28
3 oz	85	3.8	1.4	1.1	0.5	93	264	198	5.24	0.224	11.6	0	<0.1	0.77	0.27	4.3	17163
deer, all cuts, roasted	134	55.4	25.7	0.0		0.0	46	6	20	2.34	0.039	0	0	0.15	5.7		
3 oz	85	2.7	1.1	0.7	0.5	95	285	192	3.80	0.255	11.0	0		0.51			17165
deer, ground, pan-broiled	159	54.6	22.5	0.0	0.0	0.0	66	12	20	4.42	0.011	0	0	0.43	7.9	1.97	0.65
3 oz	85	7.0	3.4	1.6	0.4	83	309	194	2.85	0.085	8.8	0	0.6	0.28	0.40	6.8	17344
deer, loin steak, lean, broiled	128	57.0	25.7	0.0	0.0	0.0	48	5	26	3.09	0.025	0	0	0.24	9.1	1.56	0.74
3 oz	85	2.0	0.7	0.3	0.1	67	338	235	3.48	0.193	11.3	0	0.5	0.44	0.64	7.7	17345
deer, shoulder clod, lean, braised	162	50.8	30.8	0.0	0.0	0.0	44	5	24	7.34	0.022	0	0	0.13	6.3	2.60	0.87
3 oz	85	3.4	1.7	0.7	0.2	96	266	222	4.26	0.242	15.0	0	0.6	0.56	0.41	9.4	17346
deer, tenderloin, lean, broiled	127	57.1	25.4	0.0	0.0	0.0	48	4	28	3.39	0.019	0	0	0.22	7.5	3.08	0.73
3 oz	85	2.0	1.0	0.5	0.1	75	369	254	3.61	0.216	9.4	0	0.5	0.48	0.52	7.7	17347
deer, top round steak, lean, broiled - *3 oz*	129	56.2	26.7	0.0	0.0	0.0	38	3	26	3.12	0.015	0	0	0.21	7.1	1.93	0.77
	85	1.6	0.9	0.4	0.1	72	320	231	3.60	0.231	9.6	0	0.5	0.43	0.60	8.5	17348b
sep lean, broiled	155	67.4	32.1	0.0	0.0	0.0	46	4	31	3.74	0.018	0	0	0.26	8.6	2.32	0.92
3.6 oz	102	2.0	1.1	0.4	0.1	87	385	277	4.31	0.277	11.5	0	0.7	0.51	0.72	10.2	17348a
elk, ground, pan-broiled	164	54.5	22.6	0.0	0.0	0.0	72	9	20	5.58	0.009	0	0	0.11	4.5	2.18	0.89
3 oz	85	7.4	3.4	2.3	0.4	66	301	188	2.84	0.121	7.7	0	0.5	0.27	0.36	6.8	17339
elk, loin, lean, broiled	142	54.8	26.4	0.0	0.0	0.0	46	4	24	4.34	0.010	0	0	0.14	7.6	0.71	1.04
3 oz	85	3.3	1.3	0.9	0.2	64	343	218	3.37	0.147	8.9	0	0.5	0.28	0.40	7.7	17340a
	190	73.5	35.3	0.0	0.0	0.0	62	6	32	5.81	0.014	0	0	0.18	10.2	0.95	1.39
4 oz steak	114	4.4	1.7	1.2	0.2	86	461	292	4.51	0.197	12.0	0	0.6	0.38	0.54	10.3	17340b
elk, roasted	124	56.3	25.7	0.0		0.0	52	4	20	2.69	0.011	0	0				
3 oz	85	1.6	0.6	0.4	0.3	62	279	153	3.09	0.121	11.1	0					17167
elk, round, lean, broiled	133	55.6	26.3	0.0	0.0	0.0	43	4	24	4.79	0.013	0	0	0.15	6.1	1.28	1.04
3 oz	85	2.2	0.9	0.6	0.1	66	333	226	3.47	0.188	9.0	0	0.5	0.39	0.40	7.7	17341b
	275	115.2	54.5	0.0	0.0	0.0	90	9	49	9.93	0.026	0	0	0.32	12.6	2.64	2.15
6.2 oz steak	176	4.6	1.8	1.3	0.2	137	690	468	7.18	0.389	18.7	0	1.0	0.81	0.82	15.8	17341a
elk, tenderloin, lean, broiled	138	55.2	26.1	0.0	0.0	0.0	43	4	25	3.50	0.016	0	0	0.12	5.2	2.52	1.03
3 oz	85	2.9	1.1	0.8	0.1	61	333	242	3.46	0.297	8.9	0	0.5	0.31	0.41	7.7	17342b
	149	59.7	28.3	0.0	0.0	0.0	46	5	27	3.79	0.017	0	0	0.13	5.7	2.72	1.12
3.2 oz steak	92	3.1	1.2	0.9	0.1	66	361	262	3.74	0.321	9.7	0	0.5	0.34	0.45	8.3	17342a
emu, fan fillet, broiled	131	56.5	26.6	0.0	0.0	0.0	45	5	26	2.71	0.022	0	0	0.30	8.3	7.96	2.88
3 oz	85	2.0	0.5	0.8	0.3	70	337	231	3.88	0.197	39.2	0	0.2	0.51	0.78	7.7	05624
emu, flat fillet, raw	87	64.1	18.9	0.0	0.0	0.0	128	3	26	2.55	0.024	0	0	0.21	5.8	5.20	2.11
3 oz	85	0.6	0.2	0.3	0.1	60	204	195	4.25	0.174	26.8	0	0.2	0.35	0.49	10.2	05625
emu, full rump, broiled	143	52.7	28.6	0.0	0.0	0.0	94	6	29	3.67	0.031	3	0	0.37	9.0	1.87	3.10
3 oz	85	2.3	0.7	0.9	0.5	110	275	275	5.86	0.242	44.3	9	0.2	0.55	0.84	8.5	05627
emu, ground, pan-broiled	139	56.0	24.2	0.0	0.0	0.0	55	7	25	3.88	0.026	0	0	0.27	7.6	7.24	2.62
3 oz patty	85	4.0	1.1	1.7	0.6	74	319	229	4.26	0.202	37.0	0	0.2	0.46	0.71	7.7	05622
emu, inside drum, broiled	133	54.7	27.5	0.0	0.0	0.0	100	5	28	4.33	0.029	3	0	0.35	8.6	2.04	2.98
3 oz	85	1.7	0.6	0.7	0.3	77	265	261	6.18	0.231	42.2	9	0.2	0.53	0.81	8.5	05629
emu, outside drum, raw	88	63.6	19.6	0.0	0.0	0.0	85	3	25	3.83	0.021	0	0	0.22	6.2	5.88	2.13
3 oz	85	0.4	0.1	0.2	0.1	66	272	191	3.83	0.169	30.9	0	0.1	0.38	0.57	6.0	05630
emu, oyster, raw	120	61.7	19.4	0.0	0.0	0.0	128	3	26	5.10	0.023	0	0	0.23	6.4	5.75	2.33
3 oz	85	4.1	1.0	1.6	0.6	69	213	184	4.68	0.165	25.3	0	0.2	0.39	0.55	11.1	05631
emu, top loin, broiled	129	57.3	24.7	0.0	0.0	0.0	49	8	26	2.91	0.026	0	0	0.28	7.8	7.40	2.68
3 oz	85	2.7	0.7	1.1	0.4	75	318	233	4.31	0.238	37.0	0	0.2	0.47	0.72	7.7	05632
goat, roasted	122	58.0	23.0	0.0		0.0	73	14	0	4.48	0.036	0	0	0.08	3.4	1.01	
3 oz	85	2.6	0.8	1.2	0.2	64	344	171	3.17	0.258	10.0	0	<0.1	0.52	0.00	4.3	17169
horse, roasted	149	54.4	23.9	0.0		0.0	47	7	21	3.25	0.019	0	2	0.09	4.1	2.69	
3 oz	85	5.1	1.6	1.8	0.7	58	322	210	4.28	0.145	11.5	0		0.10	0.28		17171
moose, roasted	114	57.7	24.9	0.0		0.0	59	5	20	3.13	0.008	0	4	0.04	4.5	5.36	
3 oz	85	0.8	0.2	0.2	0.3	66	284	150	3.59	0.067	10.9	0	0.2	0.29	0.31	3.4	17173

	KCAL / WT (g)	H₂0 (g) / FAT (g)	PRO (g) / SFA (g)	CHO (g) / MUFA (g)	SUGR (g) / PUFA (g)	DFIB (g) / CHOL (mg)	Na (mg) / K (mg)	Ca (mg) / P (mg)	Mg (mg) / Fe (mg)	Zn (mg) / Cu (mg)	Mn (mg) / Se (mcg)	A (mcg RAE) / A (IU)	C (mg) / E (mg ATE)	B-1 (mg) / B-2 (mg)	NIA (mg) / B-6 (mg)	B-12 (mcg) / FOL (mcg DFE)	PANT (mg) / REF
muskrat, roasted	199	47.2	25.6	0.0		0.0	81	31	22	1.93	0.027	0	6	0.07	6.1	7.06	0.79
3 oz	85	10.0				103	272	230	6.04	0.161	12.6	0		0.60	0.40	9.4	17175
opossum, roasted	188	49.6	25.7	0.0		0.0	49	14	29	1.94		0	0	0.09	7.2	7.06	
3 oz	85	8.7	1.0	3.2	2.5	110	372	236	3.94	0.161	15.5	0	0.7	0.31	0.40	8.5	17176
ostrich, ground, pan-broiled	149	57.1	22.2	0.0	0.0	0.0	68	7	20	3.68	0.014	0	0	0.18	5.6	4.88	1.03
3 oz	85	6.0	1.5	1.8	0.6	71	275	190	2.92	0.116	28.5	0	0.2	0.23	0.43	11.9	05642
ostrich, inside leg, ckd	120	59.5	24.7	0.0	0.0	0.0	71	5	21	4.00	0.015	0	0	0.20	6.2	5.41	1.14
3 oz	85	1.6	0.6	0.6	0.3	62	299	207	2.65	0.126	31.0	0	0.2	0.25	0.47	13.6	05645
ostrich, inside strip, ckd	139	56.6	25.0	0.0	0.0	0.0	62	4	22	4.17	0.016	0	0	0.20	6.3	5.47	1.16
3 oz	85	3.6	1.5	1.5	0.6	82	311	215	4.08	0.130	32.2	0	0.2	0.26	0.48	13.6	05647
ostrich, outside strip, ckd	133	56.8	24.3	0.0	0.0	0.0	61	4	22	4.17	0.016	0	0	0.20	6.1	5.32	1.12
3 oz	85	3.3	1.2	1.4	0.4	79	312	216	3.66	0.131	32.3	0	0.2	0.25	0.46	13.6	05650
ostrich, oyster, ckd	135	57.4	24.5	0.0	0.0	0.0	69	5	25	4.20	0.020	0	0	0.20	6.1	5.37	1.13
3 oz	85	3.4	1.4	1.2	0.4	77	348	239	4.17	0.153	39.5	0	0.2	0.25	0.47	13.6	05652
ostrich, tip trimmed, ckd	123	58.2	24.2	0.0	0.0	0.0	68	5	21	4.12	0.016	0	0	0.20	6.1	5.31	1.12
3 oz	85	2.2	0.9	0.8	0.4	72	308	213	2.37	0.129	31.9	0	0.2	0.25	0.46	12.8	05656
ostrich, top loin, ckd	132	57.8	23.9	0.0	0.0	0.0	65	5	21	4.01	0.015	0	0	0.19	6.0	5.24	1.11
3 oz	85	3.3	1.1	1.1	0.3	79	300	208	2.81	0.126	31.1	0	0.2	0.25	0.46	12.8	05658
rabbit, domesticated,	167	51.5	24.7	0.0		0.0	40	16	18	1.93	0.027	0	0	0.08	7.2	7.06	0.79
roasted - *3 oz*	85	6.8	2.0	1.8	1.3	70	326	224	1.93	0.161	32.7	0		0.18	0.40	9.4	17178
stewed	175	50.0	25.8	0.0		0.0	31	17	17	2.01	0.027	0	0	0.05	6.1	5.53	0.57
3 oz	85	7.1	2.1	1.9	1.4	73	255	192	2.01	0.150	32.7	0	0.7	0.14	0.29	7.7	17179
rabbit, wild, stewed	147	52.2	28.1	0.0		0.0	38	15	26	2.02		0	0	0.02	5.4	5.53	
3 oz	85	3.0	0.9	0.8	0.6	105	292	204	4.12	0.150	12.9	0	0.7	0.06	0.29	6.8	17181
raccoon, roasted	217	46.2	24.8	0.0		0.0	67	12	26	1.93		0	0	0.50	4.0	7.06	
3 oz	85	12.3	3.5	4.4	1.8	82	338	222	6.04	0.161	15.3	0	0.7	0.44	0.40	9.4	17182
squirrel, roasted	147	52.8	26.2	0.0		0.0	101	3	24	1.51	0.027	0	0	0.05	3.9	5.53	0.79
3 oz	85	4.0	0.7	1.1	1.2	103	299	179	5.79	0.126	12.8	0	0.6	0.25	0.31	7.7	17184

19.3 LAMB, DOMESTIC US

	KCAL / WT (g)	H₂0 (g) / FAT (g)	PRO (g) / SFA (g)	CHO (g) / MUFA (g)	SUGR (g) / PUFA (g)	DFIB (g) / CHOL (mg)	Na (mg) / K (mg)	Ca (mg) / P (mg)	Mg (mg) / Fe (mg)	Zn (mg) / Cu (mg)	Mn (mg) / Se (mcg)	A (mcg RAE) / A (IU)	C (mg) / E (mg ATE)	B-1 (mg) / B-2 (mg)	NIA (mg) / B-6 (mg)	B-12 (mcg) / FOL (mcg DFE)	PANT (mg) / REF
foreshank, choice, 1/4" trim,	207	48.3	24.1	0.0		0.0	61	17	19	6.54	0.021	0	0	0.04	4.6	1.94	0.54
lean & fat, braised - *3 oz*	85	11.4	4.8	4.8	0.8	90	218	141	1.82	0.105	26.0	0	0.2	0.16	0.09	14.5	17008
lean, braised	159	52.5	26.4	0.0		0.0	63	17	20	7.36	0.024	0	0	0.03	4.3	1.92	0.54
3 oz	85	5.1	1.8	2.2	0.3	88	227	149	1.93	0.110	30.0	0	0.2	0.16	0.09	16.2	17010
ground, broiled	241	46.8	21.0	0.0		0.0	69	19	20	3.97	0.020	0	0	0.09	5.7	2.22	0.56
3 oz	85	16.7	6.9	7.1	1.2	82	288	171	1.52	0.109	23.5	0	0.2	0.21	0.12	16.2	17225
leg & shoulder, cubed,	190	47.8	28.6	0.0		0.0	60	13	24	5.59	0.027	0	0	0.06	5.1	2.32	0.50
lean, braised[1] - *3 oz*	85	7.5	2.7	3.0	0.7	92	221	174	2.38	0.120	32.4	0	0.2	0.20	0.10	17.9	17060
lean, broiled[2]	158	54.0	23.9	0.0		0.0	65	11	26	4.90	0.025	0	0	0.09	5.6	2.58	0.59
3 oz	85	6.2	2.2	2.5	0.6	77	285	190	1.99	0.128	26.9	0	0.2	0.26	0.12	19.6	17061
leg, shank half, choice, 1/4" trim,	191	51.6	22.4	0.0		0.0	55	9	21	3.96	0.021	0	0	0.09	5.6	2.27	0.60
lean & fat, roasted - *3 oz*	85	10.6	4.3	4.5	0.7	77	277	168	1.68	0.099	25.0	0	0.1	0.23	0.14	18.7	17016
lean, roasted	153	55.2	23.9	0.0		0.0	56	7	22	4.27	0.024	0	0	0.09	5.4	2.30	0.60
3 oz	85	5.7	2.0	2.5	0.4	74	291	177	1.75	0.103	26.9	0	0.2	0.24	0.14	20.4	17018
leg, sirloin half, choice, 1/4" trim,	248	46.0	20.9	0.0		0.0	58	9	19	3.51	0.019	0	0	0.09	5.6	2.15	0.57
lean & fat, roasted - *3 oz*	85	17.6	7.4	7.4	1.3	82	256	156	1.70	0.095	21.7	0	0.1	0.24	0.12	14.5	17020
lean, roasted	173	53.1	24.1	0.0		0.0	60	7	21	4.12	0.024	0	0	0.10	5.3	2.19	0.60
3 oz	85	7.8	2.8	3.4	0.5	78	283	173	1.87	0.101	26.2	0	0.1	0.26	0.14	17.9	17022
leg, whole (shank & sirloin), choice,	219	48.9	21.7	0.0		0.0	56	9	20	3.74	0.020	0	0	0.09	5.6	2.20	0.58
1/4" trim, lean & fat, rstd - *3 oz*	85	14.0	5.9	5.9	1.0	79	266	162	1.68	0.098	23.1	0	0.1	0.23	0.13	17.0	17012
lean, roasted	162	54.3	24.1	0.0		0.0	58	7	22	4.20	0.024	0	0	0.09	5.4	2.24	0.60
3 oz	85	6.6	2.3	2.9	0.4	76	287	175	1.80	0.102	25.6	0	0.2	0.25	0.14	19.6	17014
loin, choice, 1/4" trim,	269	43.8	21.4	0.0		0.0	65	17	20	2.96	0.019	0	0	0.09	6.0	2.10	0.54
lean & fat, broiled - *3 oz*	85	19.6	8.4	8.2	1.4	85	278	167	1.54	0.111	23.3	0	0.1	0.21	0.11	15.3	17024
lean & fat, roasted	263	44.6	19.2	0.0		0.0	54	15	20	2.90	0.017	0	0	0.09	6.0	1.88	0.55
3 oz	85	20.1	8.7	8.2	1.6	81	209	153	1.80	0.101	20.9	0	0.1	0.20	0.09	16.2	17025
lean, broiled	184	51.8	25.5	0.0		0.0	71	16	24	3.51	0.024	0	0	0.09	5.8	2.14	0.56
3 oz	85	8.3	3.0	3.6	0.5	81	320	192	1.70	0.123	27.9	0	0.1	0.24	0.14	20.4	17027
lean, roasted	172	53.3	22.6	0.0		0.0	56	14	23	3.45	0.022	0	0	0.09	5.8	1.84	0.58
3 oz	85	8.3	3.2	3.4	0.7	74	227	175	2.07	0.112	25.8	0	0.1	0.23	0.14	21.3	17028

		Minerals					Vitamins				
	KCAL	H₂O (g)	PRO (g)	CHO (g)	SUGR (g)	DFIB (g)	Na (mg)	Ca (mg)	Mg (mg)	Zn (mg)	Mn (mg)	A (mcg RAE)	C (mg)	B-1 (mg)	NIA (mg)	B-12 (mcg)	PANT (mg)
	WT (g)	FAT (g)	SFA (g)	MUFA (g)	PUFA (g)	CHOL (mg)	K (mg)	P (mg)	Fe (mg)	Cu (mg)	Se (mcg)	A (IU)	E (mg ATE)	B-2 (mg)	B-6 (mg)	FOL (mcg DFE)	REF

	KCAL / WT	H₂O / FAT	PRO / SFA	CHO / MUFA	SUGR / PUFA	DFIB / CHOL	Na / K	Ca / P	Mg / Fe	Zn / Cu	Mn / Se	A RAE / A IU	C / E	B-1 / B-2	NIA / B-6	B-12 / FOL	PANT / REF
rib, choice, 1/4" trim,	305	40.7	18.0	0.0		0.0	62	19	17	2.97	0.016	0	0	0.08	5.7	1.90	0.54
lean & fat, broiled - 3 oz	85	25.3	10.9	10.6	1.8	82	230	141	1.36	0.098	18.5	0	0.1	0.18	0.09	12.8	17031
lean & fat, roasted	316	43.2	12.3	0.0		0.0	48	13	15	2.30	0.014	0	0	0.09	5.2	1.78	0.53
3 oz	85	29.2	12.9	12.0	2.3	65	162	116	1.18	0.076	14.3	0	0.2	0.16	0.09	11.9	17029
lean, broiled	289	41.7	19.6	0.0		0.0	65	15	20	3.58	0.018	0	0	0.08	5.9	2.18	0.52
3 oz	85	22.8	9.7	9.3	1.8	83	235	156	1.64	0.105	21.0	0	0.1	0.20	0.09	12.8	17240
lean, roasted	290	42.2	18.5	0.0		0.0	63	19	17	3.08	0.018	0	0	0.08	5.7	1.89	0.54
3 oz	85	23.4	9.9	9.9	1.7	82	235	145	1.38	0.099	19.0	0	0.1	0.18	0.10	13.6	17241
shoulder, arm, choice 1/4" trim,	294	37.6	25.8	0.0		0.0	61	21	22	5.17	0.020	0	0	0.06	5.7	2.19	0.52
lean & fat, braised - 3 oz	85	20.4	8.4	8.7	1.5	102	260	175	2.03	0.118	31.6	0	0.1	0.21	0.09	15.3	17044
lean & fat, broiled	239	46.5	20.8	0.0		0.0	65	15	22	4.16	0.020	0	0	0.09	6.0	2.43	0.58
3 oz	85	16.6	7.1	6.8	1.3	82	263	167	1.78	0.113	23.5	0	0.1	0.23	0.10	15.3	17045
lean & fat, roasted	237	47.5	19.2	0.0		0.0	55	15	20	3.81	0.018	0	0	0.08	5.7	2.17	0.60
3 oz	85	17.2	7.4	7.1	1.4	78	220	156	1.73	0.096	21.6	0	0.1	0.21	0.10	17.0	17046
lean, braised	237	41.9	30.2	0.0		0.0	65	22	25	6.21	0.024	0	0	0.06	5.4	2.25	0.53
3 oz	85	12.0	4.3	5.2	0.8	103	287	197	2.30	0.131	32.1	0	0.2	0.23	0.11	18.7	17048
lean, broiled	170	52.9	23.6	0.0		0.0	70	14	26	4.87	0.024	0	0	0.09	5.8	2.55	0.60
3 oz	85	7.7	2.9	3.1	0.7	78	289	186	1.96	0.123	26.8	0	0.2	0.25	0.12	19.6	17049
lean, roasted	163	54.7	21.6	0.0		0.0	57	14	22	4.46	0.022	0	0	0.09	5.4	2.22	0.63
3 oz	85	7.9	3.1	3.2	0.7	73	235	172	1.90	0.102	24.7	0	0.1	0.23	0.12	21.3	17050
shoulder, blade, choice 1/4" trim,	293	38.4	24.2	0.0		0.0	64	23	20	5.83	0.023	0	0	0.05	5.1	2.41	0.52
lean & fat, braised - 3 oz	85	21.0	8.7	8.6	1.7	99	207	157	2.00	0.103	28.1	0	0.1	0.18	0.09	15.3	17052
lean & fat, broiled	236	47.5	19.6	0.0		0.0	70	20	20	4.78	0.020	0	0	0.08	5.4	2.32	0.57
3 oz	85	16.9	7.0	7.2	1.2	81	286	168	1.46	0.104	23.3	0	0.1	0.21	0.13	15.3	17053
lean & fat, roasted	239	47.5	18.9	0.0		0.0	56	18	19	4.74	0.019	0	0	0.08	5.0	2.27	0.59
3 oz	85	17.5	7.3	7.2	1.4	78	209	156	1.63	0.090	21.4	0	0.1	0.20	0.09	17.9	17054
lean, braised	245	42.2	27.5	0.0		0.0	67	24	22	6.85	0.027	0	0	0.05	4.8	2.50	0.52
3 oz	85	14.1	5.4	5.7	1.2	99	216	172	2.21	0.109	31.1	0	0.2	0.19	0.10	17.9	17056
lean, broiled	179	53.1	21.7	0.0		0.0	75	20	22	5.51	0.024	0	0	0.09	5.2	2.39	0.59
3 oz	85	9.6	3.4	4.2	0.6	77	313	184	1.54	0.110	26.3	0	0.1	0.22	0.14	17.9	17057
lean, roasted	178	53.4	20.9	0.0		0.0	58	18	21	5.51	0.022	0	0	0.08	4.6	2.33	0.61
3 oz	85	9.8	3.7	4.0	0.9	74	219	169	1.76	0.094	23.9	0	0.1	0.21	0.13	21.3	17058
shldr, whole (arm & blade), choice,	292	38.4	24.4	0.0		0.0	64	21	20	5.41	0.022	0	0	0.06	5.4	2.38	0.52
1/4" trim, lean & fat, braised - 3 oz	85	20.9	8.8	8.5	1.7	99	211	158	2.04	0.105	28.1	0	0.1	0.19	0.09	14.5	17036
lean & fat, broiled	236	46.8	20.8	0.0		0.0	66	18	22	4.86	0.020	0	0	0.08	5.5	2.52	0.57
3 oz	85	16.4	6.8	6.7	1.3	82	256	168	1.73	0.109	23.3	0	0.1	0.22	0.10	16.2	17037
lean & fat, roasted	235	47.8	19.1	0.0		0.0	56	17	20	4.45	0.019	0	0	0.08	5.2	2.24	0.60
3 oz	85	17.0	7.2	6.9	1.4	78	213	156	1.67	0.092	22.3	0	0.1	0.20	0.11	17.9	17038
lean, braised	241	42.5	27.9	0.0		0.0	67	22	23	6.39	0.027	0	0	0.05	5.1	2.47	0.53
3 oz	85	13.5	5.2	5.5	1.2	99	222	173	2.27	0.112	31.5	0	0.2	0.20	0.10	17.9	17040
lean, broiled	179	52.2	23.1	0.0		0.0	71	18	25	5.61	0.024	0	0	0.09	5.2	2.64	0.59
3 oz	85	8.9	3.3	3.6	0.8	79	275	184	1.86	0.116	26.6	0	0.2	0.24	0.12	19.6	17041
lean, roasted	173	53.8	21.2	0.0		0.0	58	16	21	5.13	0.022	0	0	0.08	4.9	2.30	0.62
3 oz	85	9.2	3.5	3.7	0.8	74	225	170	1.81	0.096	24.2	0	0.2	0.22	0.13	21.3	17042

[1] Domestic leg and shoulder, cubed.　　[2] Cubed for stew or kabobs.

19.4 LAMB, IMPORTED FROM AUSTRALIA

	KCAL / WT	H₂O / FAT	PRO / SFA	CHO / MUFA	SUGR / PUFA	DFIB / CHOL	Na / K	Ca / P	Mg / Fe	Zn / Cu	Mn / Se	A RAE / A IU	C / E	B-1 / B-2	NIA / B-6	B-12 / FOL	PANT / REF
foreshank, 1/8" trim,	201	51.4	21.1	0.0			79	14	18	5.92	0.009			0.07	4.3	2.55	0.53
lean & fat, braised - 3 oz	85	12.3	5.8	5.1	0.5	77	207	142	1.52	0.099	7.1			0.22	0.21		17287
lean, braised	140	56.9	23.4	0.0			85	12	19	6.74	0.009			0.08	4.6	2.72	0.56
3 oz	85	4.4	1.6	2.0	0.2	78	217	150	1.62	0.106	7.7			0.24	0.22		17289
leg, whole (shank & sirloin), 1/8"	207	50.7	21.4	0.0			60	9	20	3.77	0.012			0.11	4.6	2.58	0.78
trim, lean & fat, roasted - 3 oz	85	12.9	6.0	5.2	0.5	75	263	172	1.73	0.125	4.8			0.33	0.36		17291
lean, roasted	162	54.9	23.2	0.0			61	8	21	4.11	0.012			0.11	4.9	2.71	0.84
3 oz	85	6.9	2.8	2.8	0.3	76	277	182	1.83	0.134	5.0			0.36	0.39		17293
loin, 1/8" trim,	186	52.7	21.7	0.0			66	18	21	2.86	0.011			0.15	6.7	1.70	0.69
lean & fat, broiled - 3 oz	85	10.4	4.7	4.2	0.4	70	281	182	1.80	0.128	8.2			0.27	0.42		17311
lean, broiled	163	54.8	22.6	0.0			68	18	22	2.96	0.012			0.15	6.9	1.71	0.71
3 oz	85	7.4	3.1	3.0	0.3	69	289	187	1.85	0.133	8.8			0.28	0.44		17313

	KCAL / WT (g)	H₂0 / FAT (g)	PRO / SFA (g)	CHO / MUFA (g)	SUGR / PUFA (g)	DFIB / CHOL (g/mg)	Na / K (mg)	Ca / P (mg)	Mg / Fe (mg)	Zn / Cu (mg)	Mn / Se (mg/mcg)	A (mcg RAE) / A (IU)	C / E (mg / mg ATE)	B-1 / B-2 (mg)	NIA / B-6 (mg)	B-12 / FOL (mcg / mcg DFE)	PANT / REF (mg)
retail cuts, 1/8" trim,	218	49.9	20.8	0.0			65	14	19	3.98	0.011			0.10	4.6	2.44	0.69
lean & fat, ckd - *3 oz*	85	14.3	6.7	5.7	0.6	74	256	166	1.64	0.121	8.6			0.28	0.31		17281
lean, ckd	171	54.2	22.7	0.0			68	14	20	4.37	0.012			0.11	4.9	2.56	0.74
3 oz	85	8.2	3.4	3.3	0.4	74	270	176	1.74	0.130	9.4			0.31	0.33		17283
rib, 1/8" trim,	235	48.9	18.9	0.0			65	14	18	2.85	0.010			0.11	4.7	1.65	0.55
lean & fat, roasted - *3 oz*	85	17.2	8.3	6.7	0.6	68	240	155	1.42	0.111	7.7			0.23	0.32		17315
lean, roasted	179	54.2	20.9	0.0			70	13	20	3.15	0.011			0.12	5.1	1.67	0.59
3 oz	85	9.9	4.3	3.8	0.4	68	257	166	1.51	0.122	8.2			0.25	0.36		17317
shoulder, whole (arm & blade),	252	47.0	20.0	0.0			72	24	18	4.97	0.012			0.08	3.8	2.80	0.61
lean & fat, braised - *3 oz*	85	18.4	8.8	7.3	0.7	76	245	156	1.51	0.116	3.8			0.23	0.17		17319
lean, braised	132	61.5	16.5	0.0			75	15	18	4.14	0.011			0.10	3.9	2.56	0.67
3 oz	85	6.8	2.9	2.7	0.3	54	260	151	1.21	0.111	3.3			0.20	0.25		17320

19.5 LAMB, IMPORTED FROM NEW ZEALAND

	KCAL / WT (g)	H₂0 / FAT (g)	PRO / SFA (g)	CHO / MUFA (g)	SUGR / PUFA (g)	DFIB / CHOL (g/mg)	Na / K (mg)	Ca / P (mg)	Mg / Fe (mg)	Zn / Cu (mg)	Mn / Se (mg/mcg)	A (mcg RAE) / A (IU)	C / E (mg / mg ATE)	B-1 / B-2 (mg)	NIA / B-6 (mg)	B-12 / FOL (mcg / mcg DFE)	PANT / REF (mg)
foreshank,	219	48.2	22.9	0.0		0.0	40	12	13	4.08	0.020	0	0	0.06	5.2	2.07	0.35
lean & fat, braised - *3 oz*	85	13.5	6.6	5.2	0.6	87	100	149	1.76	0.087	4.5	0	0.2	0.28	0.07	0.9	17069
lean, braised	158	54.0	26.1	0.0		0.0	42	9	14	4.76	0.024	0	0	0.06	4.8	2.08	0.31
3 oz	85	5.1	2.2	2.0	0.3	86	106	156	1.89	0.095	5.2	0	0.2	0.31	0.08	0.9	17071
leg, whole (shank & sirloin),	209	49.2	21.1	0.0		0.0	37	9	17	3.04	0.020	0	0	0.10	6.5	2.21	0.47
lean & fat, roasted - *3 oz*	85	13.2	6.5	5.1	0.6	86	142	185	1.79	0.088	3.4	0	0.1	0.38	0.11	0.9	17073
lean, roasted	154	54.3	23.5	0.0		0.0	38	6	18	3.43	0.023	0	0	0.10	6.4	2.24	0.46
3 oz	85	6.0	2.6	2.3	0.3	85	156	199	1.90	0.094	3.6	0	0.2	0.43	0.12	0.0	17075
loin,	268	42.9	19.9	0.0		0.0	42	20	16	2.25	0.018	0	0	0.10	6.7	2.15	0.43
lean & fat, broiled - *3 oz*	85	20.3	10.2	7.8	0.9	95	135	177	1.74	0.093	1.7	0	0.1	0.31	0.09	0.9	17077
lean, broiled	169	51.7	24.9	0.0		0.0	47	18	19	2.80	0.024	0	0	0.11	6.7	2.19	0.39
3 oz	85	7.0	3.0	2.7	0.4	97	161	204	1.99	0.111	1.7	0	0.1	0.37	0.12	0.0	17079
retail cuts, trimmed,	259	43.5	20.8	0.0		0.0	39	14	16	2.97	0.020	0	0	0.10	6.6	2.39	0.49
lean & fat, ckd - *3 oz*	85	18.9	9.4	7.3	0.9	93	138	184	1.79	0.085	1.7	0	0.1	0.35	0.10	0.9	17063
lean, ckd	175	51.0	25.2	0.0		0.0	43	11	19	3.66	0.025	0	0	0.11	6.5	2.51	0.49
3 oz	85	7.5	3.3	3.0	0.4	93	160	209	2.00	0.097	1.7	0	0.2	0.43	0.12	0.0	17065
rib,	289	42.7	16.1	0.0		0.0	37	16	12	2.21	0.014	0	0	0.08	5.8	1.98	0.43
lean & fat, roasted - *3 oz*	85	24.4	12.3	9.4	1.1	85	105	145	1.45	0.060	1.5	0	0.1	0.23	0.07	0.9	17081
lean, roasted	167	54.7	20.8	0.0		0.0	41	12	14	2.92	0.020	0	0	0.09	5.2	1.94	0.38
3 oz	85	8.6	3.8	3.4	0.5	80	124	162	1.61	0.065	1.4	0	0.1	0.28	0.09	0.0	17083
shoulder, whole (arm & blade),	303	36.2	24.0	0.0		0.0	43	23	15	3.85	0.021	0	0	0.07	5.4	2.89	0.44
lean & fat, braised - *3 oz*	85	22.3	10.8	8.7	1.1	105	125	167	1.79	0.088	3.8	0		0.27	0.06	0.9	17085
lean, braised	242	40.7	29.0	0.0		0.0	48	23	17	4.76	0.027	0	0	0.07	5.0	3.15	0.43
3 oz	85	13.2	5.8	5.2	0.8	108	141	183	1.99	0.099	4.5	0		0.31	0.07	0.0	17087

19.6 PORK

	KCAL / WT (g)	H₂0 / FAT (g)	PRO / SFA (g)	CHO / MUFA (g)	SUGR / PUFA (g)	DFIB / CHOL (g/mg)	Na / K (mg)	Ca / P (mg)	Mg / Fe (mg)	Zn / Cu (mg)	Mn / Se (mg/mcg)	A (mcg RAE) / A (IU)	C / E (mg / mg ATE)	B-1 / B-2 (mg)	NIA / B-6 (mg)	B-12 / FOL (mcg / mcg DFE)	PANT / REF (mg)
arm, picnic,	280	40.5	23.8	0.0		0.0	75	15	16	3.55	0.012	3	<1	0.46	4.4	0.55	0.51
lean & fat, braised - *3 oz*	85	19.7	7.2	8.8	1.9	93	314	180	1.37	0.117	27.7	8	0.2	0.26	0.30	3.4	10075
lean & fat, roasted	269	44.2	19.9	0.0		0.0	60	16	14	2.93	0.028	2	<1	0.44	3.3	0.60	0.45
3 oz	85	20.4	7.5	9.1	2.0	80	276	194	1.00	0.094	28.6	7		0.26	0.30	3.4	10076
lean, braised	211	46.1	27.4	0.0		0.0	87	7	19	4.22	0.014	2	<1	0.51	5.0	0.60	0.57
3 oz	85	10.4	3.5	4.9	1.0	97	344	192	1.66	0.137	31.5	7	0.2	0.31	0.35	4.3	10078
lean, roasted	194	51.2	22.7	0.0		0.0	68	8	17	3.46	0.035	2	<1	0.49	3.7	0.66	0.50
3 oz	85	10.7	3.7	5.1	1.0	81	298	210	1.21	0.109	32.7	6		0.30	0.35	4.3	10079
arm, picnic, cured,	238	46.5	17.4	0.0		0.0	911	9	12	2.13	0.020	0	0	0.52	3.5	0.79	0.48
lean & fat, roasted - *3 oz*	85	18.1	6.5	8.6	2.0	49	219	188	0.81	0.096	28.6	0	0.2	0.16	0.24	2.6	10168
lean, roasted	145	54.3	21.2	0.0		0.0	1046	9	14	2.50	0.026	0	0	0.62	4.1	0.94	0.56
3 oz	85	6.0	2.0	2.7	0.7	41	248	207	0.92	0.109	35.1	0	0.2	0.19	0.31	3.4	10169
backribs, lean & fat, roasted	315	38.6	20.6	0.0		0.0	86	38	18	2.86	0.008	3	<1	0.36	3.0	0.54	0.49
3 oz	85	25.1	9.3	11.4	2.0	100	268	166	1.17	0.069	33.4	8		0.17	0.26	2.6	10193
bacon, canadian style, cured,	87	29.0	11.4	0.6		0.0	727	5	10	0.80	0.013	0	0	0.39	3.3	0.37	0.24
grilled - *2 slices*	47	4.0	1.3	1.9	0.4	27	183	139	0.39	0.025	11.6	0	0.1	0.09	0.21	1.9	10131
unheated	89	38.2	11.8	1.0		0.0	803	5	10	0.79	0.013	0	0	0.43	3.6	0.38	0.30
2 slices	57	4.0	1.3	1.8	0.4	29	196	139	0.39	0.026	14.3	0	0.1	0.10	0.22	2.3	10130
bacon, cured, broiled/pan fried	109	2.5	5.8	0.1		0.0	303	2	5	0.62	0.008	0	0	0.13	1.4	0.33	0.20
3 med slices	19	9.4	3.3	4.5	1.1	16	92	64	0.31	0.032	4.7	0	0.1	0.05	0.05	1.0	10124a

	KCAL / WT (g)	H₂O (g) / FAT (g)	PRO (g) / SFA (g)	CHO (g) / MUFA (g)	SUGR (g) / PUFA (g)	DFIB (g) / CHOL (mg)	Na (mg) / K (mg)	Ca (mg) / P (mg)	Mg (mg) / Fe (mg)	Zn (mg) / Cu (mg)	Mn (mg) / Se (mcg)	A (mcg RAE) / A (IU)	C (mg) / E (mg ATE)	B-1 (mg) / B-2 (mg)	NIA (mg) / B-6 (mg)	B-12 (mcg) / FOL (mcg DFE)	PANT (mg) / REF
	732	16.4	38.7	0.7		0.0	2027	15	30	4.14	0.052	0	0	0.88	9.3	2.22	1.34
4.48 oz (yield from 1 lb raw)	127	62.5	22.1	30.1	7.4	108	617	427	2.04	0.216	31.4	0	0.7	0.36	0.34	6.4	10124b
bacon, cured, raw	378	21.5	5.9	0.1		0.0	496	5	6	0.78	0.005	0	0	0.25	1.9	0.63	0.24
3 med slices	68	39.1	14.5	17.9	4.6	46	104	97	0.41	0.044	17.0	0	0.3	0.07	0.10	1.4	10123
blade roll, cured, sep lean & fat,	244	47.8	14.7	0.3		0.0	827	6	11	2.08	0.020	0	3	0.39	2.0	0.89	0.65
roasted - 3 oz	85	20.0	7.1	9.4	2.1	57	165	133	0.76	0.065	24.3	0	0.2	0.24	0.18	2.6	10171
boston blade (steaks & roasts),	271	41.1	24.4	0.0		0.0	60	27	15	4.27	0.012	3	<1	0.57	3.4	0.77	0.66
lean & fat, braised - 3 oz	85	18.5	6.7	8.2	1.7	96	331	152	1.56	0.128	36.3	9	0.2	0.31	0.23	1.7	10081
lean & fat, broiled	220	48.7	21.7	0.0		0.0	59	31	18	3.83	0.003	3	<1	0.59	3.5	0.90	0.62
3 oz	85	14.1	5.1	6.3	1.2	81	277	179	1.19	0.049	30.9	8	0.2	0.34	0.24	3.4	10082
lean & fat, roasted	229	48.8	19.6	0.0		0.0	57	24	15	3.37	0.010	2	1	0.54	3.5	0.75	0.57
3 oz	85	16.0	5.9	7.0	1.5	73	282	167	1.23	0.097	29.2	6	0.2	0.30	0.20	4.3	10083
lean, braised	232	44.2	26.4	0.0		0.0	64	25	17	4.73	0.014	3	<1	0.61	3.6	0.83	0.72
3 oz	85	13.2	4.7	5.9	1.1	99	350	155	1.74	0.140	39.6	8	0.2	0.34	0.25	1.7	10085
lean, broiled	193	51.1	22.7	0.0		0.0	63	28	20	4.27	0.008	2	<1	0.64	3.7	0.96	0.69
3 oz	85	10.7	3.8	4.8	0.9	80	292	187	1.33	0.050	33.4	7	0.2	0.37	0.26	4.3	10086
lean, roasted	197	51.8	20.6	0.0		0.0	75	23	22	3.60	0.013	3	1	0.95	4.2	0.99	0.92
3 oz	85	12.2	4.4	5.4	1.1	72	363	200	1.33	0.103	30.7	8	0.2	0.34	0.37	6.8	10087
breakfast strips, cured,	156	9.2	9.8	0.4		0.0	714	5	9	1.25	0.015	0	0	0.25	2.6	0.60	0.31
ckd - 3 slices (1.2 oz)	34	12.5	4.3	5.6	1.9	36	158	90	0.67	0.052	8.4	0	0.1	0.13	0.12	1.4	10129
raw	264	32.2	8.0	0.5		0.0	671	5	8	1.13	0.020	0	18	0.32	2.5	0.67	0.32
3 slices (2.4 oz)	68	25.3	8.8	11.4	3.8	47	139	93	0.64	0.043	17.0	0		0.12	0.14	2.0	10128
center loin (chops) w/bone,	210	48.8	23.7	0.0		0.0	50	22	16	1.84	0.013	2	1	0.65	3.9	0.43	0.60
lean & fat, braised - 3 oz	85	12.0	4.5	5.3	1.1	73	300	152	0.89	0.062	34.9	7		0.18	0.32	2.6	10037
lean & fat, broiled	204	49.0	24.4	0.0		0.0	49	28	21	1.92	0.003	3	<1	0.91	4.5	0.62	0.54
3 oz	85	11.1	4.1	5.0	0.8	70	304	197	0.68	0.039	37.7	8		0.24	0.36	5.1	10038
lean & fat, panfried	235	45.0	25.4	0.0		0.0	68	23	25	1.96	0.009	2	1	0.97	4.8	0.62	0.78
3 oz	85	14.1	5.1	6.0	1.6	78	361	220	0.77	0.064	33.2	7	0.2	0.26	0.40	5.1	10179
lean, braised	172	52.2	25.3	0.0		0.0	53	20	17	1.92	0.014	2	1	0.70	4.1	0.43	0.64
3 oz	85	7.1	2.6	3.2	0.5	72	312	154	0.96	0.065	37.3	6	0.2	0.19	0.34	2.6	10041
lean, broiled	172	52.0	25.7	0.0		0.0	51	26	23	2.02	0.009	2	<1	0.98	4.7	0.63	0.59
3 oz	85	6.9	2.5	3.1	0.5	70	319	205	0.72	0.038	40.2	7		0.26	0.40	5.1	10042
lean, panfried	197	48.3	27.4	0.0		0.0	73	20	27	2.07	0.010	2	1	1.06	5.1	0.65	0.85
3 oz	85	8.9	3.1	3.8	1.1	78	382	230	0.83	0.066	40.6	7	0.2	0.28	0.44	5.1	10176
center loin (roasts),	199	50.8	22.4	0.0		0.0	54	23	17	1.72	0.013	2	1	0.73	4.4	0.48	0.56
lean & fat, roasted - 3 oz	85	11.4	4.3	5.0	1.0	68	299	183	0.84	0.058	34.9	6		0.22	0.30	3.4	10039
lean, roasted	169	53.5	23.4	0.0		0.0	56	21	19	1.78	0.014	2	1	0.78	4.6	0.49	0.59
3 oz	85	7.7	2.8	3.4	0.6	67	308	186	0.88	0.060	36.7	6		0.23	0.32	3.4	10043
center rib (chops) w/bone,	213	48.4	22.7	0.0		0.0	34	21	15	1.71	0.009	2	<1	0.50	4.2	0.45	0.44
lean & fat, braised - 3 oz	85	12.8	5.0	5.8	1.1	62	329	150	0.77	0.061	34.9	6		0.20	0.27	1.7	10045
lean & fat, broiled	224	45.4	24.5	0.0		0.0	53	28	22	1.92	0.015	2	<1	0.88	4.9	0.62	0.56
3 oz	85	13.2	4.8	5.8	1.0	70	341	201	0.65	0.058	37.7	6		0.26	0.37	2.6	10046
lean, braised	175	51.8	24.1	0.0		0.0	35	19	16	1.79	0.009	2	<1	0.53	4.4	0.46	0.46
3 oz	85	8.0	3.1	3.8	0.6	60	344	152	0.82	0.064	37.3	5	0.2	0.21	0.29	1.7	10049
lean, broiled	186	48.4	26.1	0.0		0.0	55	26	24	2.02	0.017	2	<1	0.95	5.2	0.65	0.60
3 oz	85	8.3	2.9	3.8	0.5	69	357	208	0.70	0.060	40.2	5	0.2	0.28	0.40	2.6	10050
lean, panfried	190	51.7	23.5	0.0		0.0	44	4	23	1.82	0.006	2	<1	0.65	4.3	0.52	0.66
3 oz	85	10.0	3.7	4.5	1.3	60	386	201	0.66	0.059	35.6	5	0.2	0.29	0.33	6.8	10197
center rib (roasts),	217	47.6	23.3	0.0		0.0	39	24	18	1.75	0.009	2	<1	0.62	5.2	0.56	0.45
lean & fat, roasted - 3 oz	85	13.0	5.0	5.9	1.1	62	358	196	0.80	0.063	34.9	5		0.26	0.28	2.6	10047
lean, roasted	190		24.4	0.0		0.0	40	22	19	1.81	0.01	2	<1	0.64	5.5	0.58	0.46
3 oz	85	9.5	3.7	4.5	0.7	60	371	201	0.83	0.07	36.7	5		0.27	0.29	2.6	10051
ground, ckd	252	44.8	21.8	0.0		0.0	62	19	20	2.73	0.009	2	1	0.60	3.6	0.46	0.44
3 oz	85	17.7	6.6	7.9	1.6	80	308	192	1.10	0.037	30.1	7	0.2	0.19	0.33	5.1	10220
ham, cured (fully ckd ap),	102	62.5	15.7	0.0		0.0	1067	5	14	1.64	0.021	0	0	0.71	4.5	0.70	0.42
lean (4% fat), cnd - 3 oz	85	3.9	1.3	1.9	0.3	32	309	190	0.80	0.071	12.3	0	0.2	0.20	0.38	5.1	10137
lean (4% fat), cnd, roasted	116	59.0	18.0	0.4		0.0	965	5	18	1.90	0.020	0	0	0.88	4.2	0.60	0.48
3 oz	85	4.1	1.4	2.1	0.4	26	296	178	0.78	0.043	14.8	0	0.2	0.21	0.38	4.3	10138
lean (5% fat), roasted	123	57.5	17.8	1.3		0.0	1023	7	12	2.45	0.046	0	0	0.64	3.4	0.55	0.34
3 oz	85	4.7	1.5	2.2	0.5	45	244	167	1.26	0.067	16.6	0	0.2	0.17	0.34	2.6	10134
reg (11% fat), roasted	151	54.9	19.2	0.0		0.0	1275	7	19	2.10	0.035	0	0	0.62	5.2	0.60	0.61
3 oz	85	7.7	2.7	3.8	1.2	50	348	239	1.14	0.123	16.8	0	0.2	0.28	0.26	2.6	10136

	KCAL ⁄ WT (g)	H₂0 (g) ⁄ FAT (g)	PRO (g) ⁄ SFA (g)	CHO (g) ⁄ MUFA (g)	SUGR (g) ⁄ PUFA (g)	DFIB (g) ⁄ CHOL (mg)	Na (mg) ⁄ K (mg)	Ca (mg) ⁄ P (mg)	Mg (mg) ⁄ Fe (mg)	Zn (mg) ⁄ Cu (mg)	Mn (mg) ⁄ Se (mcg)	A (mcg RAE) ⁄ A (IU)	C (mg) ⁄ E (mg ATE)	B-1 (mg) ⁄ B-2 (mg)	NIA (mg) ⁄ B-6 (mg)	B-12 (mcg) ⁄ FOL (mcg DFE)	PANT (mg) ⁄ REF
reg (13% fat), cnd	162	56.6	14.4	0.0		0.0	1054	5	12	1.41	0.020	0	0	0.82	2.7	0.66	0.33
3 oz	85	11.0	3.6	5.3	1.2	33	269	149	0.71	0.057	25.3	0	0.2	0.20	0.41	4.3	10139
reg (13% fat), cnd, roasted	192	51.8	17.5	0.4		0.0	800	7	14	2.13	0.025	0	12	0.70	4.5	0.90	0.62
3 oz	85	12.9	4.3	6.0	1.5	53	303	207	1.16	0.111	30.5	0		0.22	0.26	4.3	10140
reg, center slice, lean & fat,	173	53.9	17.1	0.0		0.0	1178	6	14	1.60	0.026	0	0	0.72	4.1	0.68	0.42
unheated - *3 oz*	85	11.0	3.9	5.2	1.2	46	286	183	0.64	0.063	19.2	0		0.17	0.40	3.4	10142
whole, lean & fat, roasted	207	49.6	18.3	0.0		0.0	1009	6	16	1.97	0.012	0	0	0.51	3.8	0.54	0.39
3 oz	85	14.3	5.1	6.7	1.5	53	243	182	0.74	0.071	19.3	0	0.2	0.19	0.32	2.6	10151
whole, lean & fat, unheated	209	50.8	15.7	0.1		0.0	1091	6	13	1.50	0.024	0	30	0.66	3.8	0.63	0.40
3 oz	85	15.7	5.6	7.4	1.4	48	264	171	0.60	0.060	13.0	0		0.16	0.35	3.4	10150
whole, lean, roasted	133	55.9	21.3	0.0		0.0	1128	6	19	2.18	0.014	0	0	0.58	4.3	0.60	0.42
3 oz	85	4.7	1.6	2.2	0.5	47	269	193	0.80	0.074	21.6	0	0.2	0.22	0.40	3.4	10153
whole, lean, unheated	125	58.0	19.0	0.0		0.0	1289	6	15	1.73	0.030	0	0	0.79	4.5	0.74	0.46
3 oz	85	4.9	1.6	2.2	0.6	44	315	197	0.69	0.067	16.0	0	0.2	0.19	0.45	3.4	10152
ham patties, cured,	205	30.8	8.0	1.0		0.0	638	5	6	1.14	0.013	0	0	0.21	1.9	0.42	0.16
grilled - *2 oz patty*	60	18.5	6.7	8.8	2.0	43	146	61	0.97	0.060	12.7	0	0.2	0.11	0.10	1.8	10147
unheated	205	35.4	8.3	1.1		0.0	707	5	7	1.02	0.015	0	0	0.30	2.0	0.70	0.20
2.3 oz patty	65	18.3	6.6	8.6	2.0	46	155	97	0.68	0.046	10.3	0		0.10	0.10	2.0	10146
ham steak, extra lean, cured,	104	61.4	16.6	0.0		0.0	1079	3	16	1.72	0.031	0	27	0.68	4.3	0.67	0.53
unheated - *3 oz*	85	3.6	1.2	1.7	0.4	38	276	221	0.85	0.068	13.2	0		0.17	0.31	3.4	10149
leg (rump & shank half),	232	46.8	22.8	0.0		0.0	51	12	19	2.52	0.027	3	<1	0.54	3.9	0.58	0.52
lean & fat, roasted - *3 oz*	85	15.0	5.5	6.7	1.4	80	299	224	0.86	0.085	38.5	9	0.2	0.27	0.34	8.5	10009
lean, roasted	179	51.6	25.0	0.0		0.0	54	6	21	2.77	0.031	3	<1	0.59	4.2	0.61	0.57
3 oz	85	8.0	2.8	3.8	0.7	80	317	239	0.95	0.092	42.4	8	0.2	0.30	0.38	10.2	10011
loin blade (chops) w/bone,	275	44.1	18.6	0.0		0.0	47	26	13	2.78	0.009	2	1	0.40	3.1	0.55	0.48
lean & fat, braised - *3 oz*	85	21.6	8.1	9.3	2.0	72	258	138	0.94	0.072	30.6	7	0.2	0.20	0.25	1.7	10029
lean & fat, broiled	272	44.1	19.1	0.0		0.0	60	25	19	2.86	0.007	2	1	0.55	3.5	0.71	0.52
3 oz	85	21.1	7.9	9.1	1.9	73	292	180	0.79	0.071	31.5	7		0.25	0.32	3.4	10030
lean & fat, panfried	291	42.5	18.3	0.0		0.0	57	26	18	2.71	0.007	2	1	0.53	3.4	0.71	0.56
3 oz	85	23.6	8.6	10.0	2.6	72	282	175	0.75	0.068	29.7	7	0.2	0.25	0.29	3.4	10178
lean, braised	191	51.9	21.3	0.0		0.0	53	20	15	3.32	0.012	2	1	0.45	3.3	0.60	0.54
3 oz	85	11.1	4.0	4.8	0.9	71	277	137	1.15	0.082	36.0	6	0.2	0.23	0.30	2.6	10033
lean, broiled	199	50.9	21.6	0.0		0.0	68	20	22	3.37	0.008	2	1	0.63	3.9	0.80	0.59
3 oz	85	11.8	4.3	5.1	0.9	71	318	192	0.93	0.078	36.5	6		0.30	0.38	3.4	10034
lean, panfried	205	50.4	21.0	0.0		0.0	66	19	22	3.29	0.008	2	1	0.62	3.8	0.82	0.66
3 oz	85	12.8	4.4	5.3	1.7	70	310	188	0.91	0.077	36.0	6	0.2	0.30	0.35	3.4	10120
loin blade (roasts),	275	43.5	20.2	0.0		0.0	26	29	17	2.81	0.009	3	<1	0.45	3.6	0.62	0.41
lean & fat, roasted - *3 oz*	85	20.9	7.8	9.0	1.8	79	277	179	0.94	0.067	31.5	8		0.25	0.32	3.4	10031
lean, roasted	210	49.5	22.6	0.0		0.0	25	25	20	3.24	0.011	2	<1	0.49	4.0	0.68	0.45
3 oz	85	12.6	4.5	5.5	0.9	79	297	188	1.10	0.073	36.0	7		0.29	0.37	4.3	10035
loin, whole,	203	49.5	23.1	0.0		0.0	41	18	16	2.02	0.010	2	1	0.54	3.8	0.46	0.55
lean & fat, braised - *3 oz*	85	11.6	4.3	5.2	1.0	68	318	154	0.91	0.065	38.5	6	0.2	0.22	0.31	2.6	10021
lean & fat, broiled	206	49.2	23.2	0.0		0.0	53	16	24	2.03	0.008	2	1	0.75	4.3	0.60	0.59
3 oz	85	11.8	4.4	5.3	1.0	68	360	209	0.74	0.062	38.5	6	0.2	0.27	0.39	4.3	10022
lean & fat, roasted	211	48.9	23.0	0.0		0.0	50	16	22	1.97	0.009	3	1	0.84	4.7	0.60	0.65
3 oz	85	12.5	4.6	5.5	1.0	70	347	206	0.84	0.048	28.4	8	0.2	0.27	0.44	5.1	10023
lean, braised	173	52.2	24.3	0.0		0.0	43	15	17	2.11	0.011	2	1	0.56	3.9	0.47	0.58
3 oz	85	7.8	2.9	3.5	0.6	67	329	156	0.96	0.067	41.0	6	0.2	0.23	0.33	3.4	10025
lean, broiled	179	51.6	24.3	0.0		0.0	54	14	25	2.11	0.008	2	1	0.78	4.5	0.61	0.66
3 oz	85	8.3	3.1	3.8	0.7	67	372	215	0.77	0.064	41.0	6	0.2	0.29	0.42	5.1	10026
lean, roasted	178	51.9	24.3	0.0		0.0	49	15	24	2.15	0.014	2	1	0.86	5.0	0.62	0.66
3 oz	85	8.2	3.0	3.7	0.6	69	361	212	0.93	0.050	29.8	7	0.2	0.28	0.47	6.0	10027
rump,	214	48.3	24.5	0.0		0.0	53	10	23	2.40	0.020	3	<1	0.64	4.0	0.61	0.53
lean & fat, roasted - *3 oz*	85	12.1	4.5	5.4	1.2	82	318	231	0.89	0.088	39.8	8	0.2	0.28	0.27	2.6	10013
lean, roasted	175	51.8	26.3	0.0		0.0	55	6	25	2.56	0.022	3	<1	0.68	4.2	0.64	0.56
3 oz	85	6.9	2.4	3.2	0.6	82	332	242	0.97	0.093	41.8	8		0.30	0.29	2.6	10015
sausage, fresh, ckd	100	12.0	5.3	0.3		0.0	349	9	5	0.68	0.019	0	1	0.20	1.2	0.47	0.19
1.1 oz patty (3 7/8″ dia, 1/4″ thick)	27	8.4	2.9	3.8	1.0	22	97	50	0.34	0.038	4.9	0	<0.1	0.07	0.09	0.5	07064
Oscar Mayer, ckd	165	23.8	7.8	0.5	0.4	0.0	401	8	9	1.25		0					
2 links (1.7 oz)	48	14.6	5.1	7.1	1.8	37	114	76	0.83	0.154		0					07225
sausage w/beef, ckd	107	12.0	3.7	0.7		0.0	217	3	3	0.50	0.010	0	0	0.10	0.9	0.12	0.13
1.1 oz patty (3 7/8″ dia, 1/4″ thick)	27	9.8	3.5	4.6	1.1	19	51	29	0.31	0.011	3.9	0	0.1	0.04	0.01	0.5	07065

	KCAL / WT (g)	H_2O (g) / FAT (g)	PRO (g) / SFA (g)	CHO (g) / MUFA (g)	SUGR (g) / PUFA (g)	DFIB (g) / CHOL (mg)	Na (mg) / K (mg)	Ca (mg) / P (mg)	Mg (mg) / Fe (mg)	Zn (mg) / Cu (mg)	Mn (mg) / Se (mcg)	A (mcg RAE) / A (IU)	C (mg) / E (mg ATE)	B-1 (mg) / B-2 (mg)	NIA (mg) / B-6 (mg)	B-12 (mcg) / FOL (mcg DFE)	PANT (mg) / REF
shank,	246	45.7	21.5	0.0		0.0	50	13	19	2.60	0.024	3	<1	0.49	3.8	0.56	0.53
lean & fat, roasted - *3 oz*	85	17.1	6.3	7.7	1.6	78	287	218	0.83	0.083	36.8	8		0.26	0.34	4.3	10017
lean, roasted	183	51.4	24.0	0.0		0.0	54	6	21	2.93	0.029	2	<1	0.54	4.1	0.60	0.58
3 oz	85	8.9	3.1	4.3	0.8	78	306	236	0.94	0.092	42.3	7	0.2	0.29	0.39	5.1	10019
shoulder, whole,	248	46.6	19.8	0.0		0.0	58	20	15	3.15	0.019	2	<1	0.49	3.4	0.68	0.51
lean & fat, roasted - *3 oz*	85	18.2	6.7	8.0	1.7	77	280	180	1.12	0.096	28.4	7	0.2	0.28	0.24	4.3	10071
lean, roasted	196	51.5	21.5	0.0		0.0	64	15	17	3.54	0.022	2	1	0.53	3.6	0.73	0.55
3 oz	85	11.5	4.1	5.2	1.1	77	294	188	1.28	0.105	31.8	6	0.2	0.31	0.27	4.3	10073
sirloin (chops) w/bone,	208	49.9	21.6	0.0		0.0	43	15	16	2.08	0.011	2	1	0.56	3.2	0.48	0.55
lean & fat, braised - *3 oz*	85	12.8	4.7	5.6	1.2	70	276	148	0.99	0.049	34.4	6		0.22	0.35	2.6	10053
lean & fat, broiled	220	47.9	22.7	0.0		0.0	58	14	25	2.18	0.009	2	1	0.81	3.8	0.64	0.62
3 oz	85	13.7	5.0	5.9	1.3	73	326	209	0.84	0.049	40.5	7	0.2	0.29	0.46	4.3	10054
lean, braised	167	53.7	23.0	0.0		0.0	45	11	17	2.21	0.012	2	1	0.59	3.4	0.48	0.59
3 oz	85	7.7	2.7	3.4	0.7	69	286	150	1.08	0.050	36.2	6		0.24	0.38	2.6	10057
lean, broiled	181	51.5	24.2	0.0		0.0	61	11	26	2.33	0.009	2	1	0.87	4.0	0.67	0.67
3 oz	85	8.6	3.1	3.8	0.8	72	341	218	0.91	0.050	43.9	6	0.2	0.32	0.51	4.3	10058
sirloin (roasts),	222	47.9	23.2	0.0		0.0	51	20	20	2.07	0.003	2	<1	0.64	4.5	0.65	0.49
lean & fat, roasted - *3 oz*	85	13.6	4.8	6.0	1.2	74	298	187	0.88	0.071	34.3	7		0.27	0.33	5.1	10055
lean, roasted	184	51.5	24.5	0.0		0.0	54	17	21	2.18	0.024	2	<1	0.68	4.7	0.66	0.53
3 oz	85	8.7	3.1	3.8	0.7	73	311	194	0.95	0.073	36.6	6		0.28	0.36	5.1	10059
spareribs, sep lean & fat, braised	337	34.4	24.7	0.0		0.0	79	40	20	3.91	0.012	3	0	0.35	4.7	0.92	0.64
3 oz	85	25.8	9.5	11.5	2.3	103	272	222	1.57	0.121	31.8	9	0.2	0.32	0.30	3.4	10089
tenderloin,	171	51.9	25.4	0.0		0.0	54	4	30	2.46	0.010	2	1	0.82	4.3	0.83	0.76
lean & fat, broiled - *3 oz*	85	6.9	2.5	2.8	0.6	80	377	247	1.18	0.057	40.5	6		0.32	0.44	5.1	10221
lean & fat, roasted	147	55.6	23.6	0.0		0.0	47	5	23	2.21	0.032	2	<1	0.79	4.0	0.47	0.58
3 oz	85	5.1	1.8	2.1	0.5	67	368	218	1.23	0.041	40.3	6	0.2	0.33	0.35	5.1	10222
lean, broiled	159	53.0	25.9	0.0		0.0	55	4	31	2.51	0.010	2	1	0.84	4.4	0.85	0.78
3 oz	85	5.4	1.9	2.2	0.5	80	383	251	1.22	0.058	43.9	6		0.33	0.45	5.1	10223
lean, roasted	139	56.4	23.9	0.0		0.0	48	5	24	2.24	0.033	2	<1	0.80	4.0	0.47	0.58
3 oz	85	4.1	1.4	1.6	0.3	67	371	220	1.25	0.041	40.9	6	0.2	0.33	0.36	5.1	10061
top loin (chops),	198	49.5	23.6	0.0		0.0	36	18	16	1.79	0.009	2	<1	0.47	3.9	0.39	0.54
lean & fat, braised - *3 oz*	85	10.8	4.0	4.8	0.9	64	346	157	0.82	0.065	35.1	6		0.22	0.28	3.4	10063
lean & fat, broiled	195	49.6	25.5	0.0		0.0	54	25	23	1.95	0.003	2	<1	0.73	4.3	0.59	0.60
3 oz	85	9.5	3.4	4.4	0.6	69	344	202	0.67	0.059	38.4	5		0.26	0.32	6.8	10064
lean & fat, panfried	218	46.6	24.7	0.0		0.0	47	18	24	1.87	0.006	2	<1	0.68	4.6	0.55	0.69
3 oz	85	12.6	4.5	5.5	1.4	66	407	223	0.69	0.064	39.0	6	0.2	0.30	0.34	6.8	10186
lean, braised	172	51.9	24.7	0.0		0.0	36	20	17	1.85	0.009	2	<1	0.49	4.0	0.39	0.56
3 oz	85	7.3	2.7	3.4	0.5	62	358	158	0.86	0.066	36.8	5		0.23	0.29	4.3	10067
lean, broiled	173	51.6	26.5	0.0		0.0	55	26	24	2.02	0.017	2	<1	0.76	4.4	0.60	0.63
3 oz	85	6.6	2.3	3.1	0.4	68	357	208	0.70	0.060	40.2	5	0.2	0.27	0.34	7.7	10068
lean, panfried	191	49.0	25.9	0.0		0.0	48	19	26	1.95	0.007	2	<1	0.71	4.8	0.57	0.73
3 oz	85	8.9	3.1	3.9	1.1	65	425	230	0.72	0.065	38.9	5	0.2	0.32	0.36	6.8	10181
top loin (roasts),	192	50.3	24.5	0.0		0.0	37	4	20	1.88	0.003	2	<1	0.52	4.4	0.47	0.46
lean & fat, roasted - *3 oz*	85	9.7	3.5	4.5	0.7	66	291	183	0.68	0.016	38.9	7		0.25	0.32	6.8	10065
lean, roasted	165	52.9	25.7	0.0		0.0	38	4	21	1.96	0.009	2	<1	0.54	4.6	0.47	0.49
3 oz	85	6.1	2.2	2.9	0.4	66	301	188	0.90	0.014	41.0	7		0.27	0.34	7.7	10069

19.7 VEAL

	KCAL / WT (g)	H_2O (g) / FAT (g)	PRO (g) / SFA (g)	CHO (g) / MUFA (g)	SUGR (g) / PUFA (g)	DFIB (g) / CHOL (mg)	Na (mg) / K (mg)	Ca (mg) / P (mg)	Mg (mg) / Fe (mg)	Zn (mg) / Cu (mg)	Mn (mg) / Se (mcg)	A (mcg RAE) / A (IU)	C (mg) / E (mg ATE)	B-1 (mg) / B-2 (mg)	NIA (mg) / B-6 (mg)	B-12 (mcg) / FOL (mcg DFE)	PANT (mg) / REF
ground, broiled	146	56.7	20.7	0.0		0.0	71	14	20	3.29	0.030	0	0	0.06	6.8	1.08	0.99
3 oz	85	6.4	2.6	2.4	0.5	88	286	184	0.84	0.088	11.6	0	0.1	0.23	0.33	9.4	17143
leg (top round),	179	47.2	30.7	0.0		0.0	57	7	25	3.37	0.033	0	0	0.05	9.0	0.99	0.87
lean & fat, braised - *3 oz*	85	5.4	2.2	2.0	0.4	114	326	212	1.12	0.119	13.1	0	0.4	0.30	0.31	15.3	17095
lean & fat, breaded, panfried	194	43.6	23.2	8.4		0.3	386	33	26	2.34	0.115	9	0	0.14	8.8	1.05	0.91
3 oz	85	7.8	2.6	2.9	1.3	95	315	213	1.39	0.062	14.0	29	0.5	0.30	0.34	28.1	17096
lean & fat, panfried	179	49.6	27.0	0.0		0.0	65	5	26	2.75	0.026	0	0	0.06	10.2	1.23	0.99
3 oz	85	7.1	2.7	2.7	0.5	89	361	237	0.75	0.053	11.4	0	0.4	0.30	0.42	12.8	17097
lean & fat, roasted	136	56.2	23.5	0.0		0.0	58	5	24	2.58	0.026	0	0	0.05	8.4	0.99	0.84
3 oz	85	4.0	1.6	1.5	0.3	88	331	199	0.77	0.110	9.5	0	0.4	0.27	0.26	13.6	17098
lean, braised	173	47.8	31.2	0.0		0.0	57	8	26	3.43	0.034	0	0	0.05	9.1	1.01	0.88
3 oz	85	4.3	1.6	1.6	0.3	115	329	214	1.12	0.121	13.3	0	0.4	0.31	0.31	15.3	17100

	KCAL / WT (g)	H₂0 (g) / FAT (g)	PRO (g) / SFA (g)	CHO (g) / MUFA (g)	SUGR (g) / PUFA (g)	DFIB (g) / CHOL (mg)	Na (mg) / K (mg)	Ca (mg) / P (mg)	Mg (mg) / Fe (mg)	Zn (mg) / Cu (mg)	Mn (mg) / Se (mcg)	A (mcg RAE) / A (IU)	C (mg) / E (mg ATE)	B-1 (mg) / B-2 (mg)	NIA (mg) / B-6 (mg)	B-12 (mcg) / FOL (mcg DFE)	PANT (mg) / REF
lean, breaded, panfried	175	45.2	24.1	8.3		0.2	387	33	27	2.44	0.116	9	0	0.14	9.2	1.09	0.94
3 oz	85	5.3	1.4	1.8	1.1	96	326	219	1.39	0.063	11.5	29	0.5	0.31	0.36	28.9	17101
lean, pan fried	156	51.6	28.2	0.0		0.0	65	6	27	2.87	0.027	0	0	0.06	10.7	1.28	1.04
3 oz	85	3.9	1.1	1.4	0.3	91	376	247	0.74	0.054	8.8	0	0.4	0.31	0.43	13.6	17102
lean, roasted	128	57.0	23.9	0.0		0.0	58	5	24	2.62	0.026	0	0	0.05	8.6	1.00	0.85
3 oz	85	2.9	1.0	1.0	0.2	88	334	201	0.77	0.111	10.1	0	0.5	0.28	0.26	13.6	17103
leg & shoulder, cubed for stew,	160	50.4	29.7	0.0		0.0	79	25	24	5.11	0.034	0	0	0.06	7.1	1.42	1.01
lean, braised - 3 oz	85	3.7	1.1	1.2	0.4	123	291	203	1.22	0.130	12.9	0	0.4	0.34	0.32	13.6	17141
loin,	241	44.2	25.7	0.0		0.0	68	24	20	3.09	0.029	0	0	0.03	7.7	1.03	0.67
lean & fat, braised - 3 oz	85	14.6	5.7	5.7	1.0	100	238	187	0.93	0.077	11.2	0	0.3	0.26	0.22	11.9	17105
lean & fat, roasted	184	51.6	21.1	0.0		0.0	79	16	21	2.58	0.025	0	0	0.04	7.5	1.05	1.02
3 oz	85	10.5	4.5	4.1	0.7	88	276	180	0.74	0.094	9.4	0	0.4	0.24	0.29	12.8	17106
lean, braised	192	48.4	28.5	0.0		0.0	71	27	23	3.48	0.032	0	0	0.04	8.5	1.12	0.72
3 oz	85	7.8	2.2	2.8	0.7	106	252	201	0.94	0.084	12.2	0	0.4	0.29	0.24	12.8	17108
lean, roasted	149	54.9	22.4	0.0		0.0	82	18	22	2.75	0.026	0	0	0.05	8.0	1.11	1.08
3 oz	85	5.9	2.2	2.1	0.5	90	289	189	0.72	0.099	9.9	0	0.4	0.26	0.31	13.6	17109
rib,	213	45.3	27.6	0.0		0.0	81	19	21	4.73	0.032	0	0	0.04	6.4	1.23	0.91
lean & fat, braised - 3 oz	85	10.7	4.2	4.0	0.8	118	260	179	1.20	0.112	11.8	0	0.3	0.25	0.27	13.6	17111
lean & fat, roasted	194	50.9	20.4	0.0		0.0	78	9	19	3.48	0.026	0	0	0.04	5.9	1.24	1.09
3 oz	85	11.9	4.6	4.6	0.8	94	251	167	0.82	0.084	8.9	0	0.3	0.23	0.21	11.1	17112
lean, braised	185	47.7	29.3	0.0		0.0	84	20	22	5.08	0.034	0	0	0.05	6.7	1.30	0.96
3 oz	85	6.6	2.2	2.2	0.6	122	270	185	1.23	0.119	12.4	0	0.3	0.26	0.29	13.6	17114
lean, roasted	150	54.9	21.9	0.0		0.0	82	10	20	3.82	0.027	0	0	0.05	6.4	1.34	1.17
3 oz	85	6.3	1.8	2.3	0.6	98	264	176	0.82	0.090	9.4	0	0.3	0.25	0.23	11.9	17115
shoulder, arm,	201	47.0	28.6	0.0		0.0	74	24	25	4.94	0.031	0	0	0.05	8.6	1.46	1.11
lean & fat, braised - 3 oz	85	8.7	3.4	3.4	0.6	126	283	224	1.17	0.109	12.3	0	0.4	0.26	0.25	15.3	17123
lean & fat, roasted	156	55.0	21.6	0.0		0.0	77	22	22	3.55	0.026	0	0	0.05	6.8	1.30	0.99
3 oz	85	7.0	3.0	2.7	0.5	92	296	188	0.98	0.120	9.4	0	0.4	0.27	0.25	14.5	17124
lean, braised	171	49.5	30.4	0.0		0.0	77	26	26	5.30	0.032	0	0	0.05	9.1	1.55	1.18
3 oz	85	4.5	1.3	1.6	0.4	132	295	235	1.20	0.115	13.0	0	0.4	0.28	0.26	16.2	17126
lean, roasted	139	56.5	22.2	0.0		0.0	77	23	23	3.67	0.026	0	0	0.06	7.0	1.33	1.01
3 oz	85	4.9	2.0	1.8	0.4	93	303	192	0.99	0.124	9.6	0	0.4	0.28	0.26	14.5	17127
shoulder, blade,	191	48.4	26.6	0.0		0.0	83	32	22	5.95	0.031	0	0	0.05	4.7	1.64	1.29
lean & fat, braised - 3 oz	85	8.6	3.1	3.3	0.6	130	252	207	1.22	0.139	11.9	0	0.4	0.30	0.20	12.8	17129
lean & fat, roasted	158	55.7	21.4	0.0		0.0	85	24	20	4.74	0.026	0	0	0.06	4.9	1.71	1.17
3 oz	85	7.4	2.9	2.8	0.5	99	260	180	0.85	0.117	9.0	0	0.4	0.30	0.20	9.4	17130
lean, braised	168	50.4	27.8	0.0		0.0	86	34	24	6.28	0.032	0	0	0.05	4.8	1.71	1.35
3 oz	85	5.5	1.5	2.0	0.5	134	259	214	1.25	0.145	12.3	0	0.4	0.31	0.21	12.8	17132
lean, roasted	145	56.9	21.8	0.0		0.0	87	24	20	4.86	0.026	0	0	0.06	4.9	1.75	1.20
3 oz	85	5.8	2.2	2.1	0.5	101	264	183	0.85	0.120	9.1	0	0.4	0.31	0.20	9.4	17133
shoulder, whole (arm & blade),	194	47.9	27.3	0.0		0.0	81	30	23	5.60	0.031	0	0	0.05	5.5	1.56	1.30
lean & fat, braised - 3 oz	85	8.6	3.2	3.3	0.6	107	263	213	1.21	0.128	12.1	0	0.4	0.29	0.21	12.8	17117
lean & fat, roasted	156	55.5	21.5	0.0		0.0	82	23	21	4.35	0.026	0	0	0.06	5.4	1.55	1.11
3 oz	85	7.2	2.9	2.7	0.5	96	274	183	0.88	0.118	9.1	0	0.4	0.29	0.22	10.2	17118
lean, braised	169	50.0	28.6	0.0		0.0	82	31	24	5.95	0.032	0	0	0.05	5.7	1.65	1.37
3 oz	85	5.2	1.4	1.9	0.5	111	271	221	1.23	0.135	12.5	0	0.4	0.30	0.22	13.6	17120
lean, roasted	145	56.7	21.9	0.0		0.0	82	23	21	4.46	0.026	0	0	0.06	5.5	1.58	1.12
3 oz	85	5.6	2.1	2.0	0.5	97	278	185	0.88	0.121	9.3	0	0.4	0.29	0.22	11.1	17121
sirloin,	214	46.3	26.6	0.0		0.0	67	14	23	3.67	0.030	0	0	0.04	5.6	1.26	0.86
lean & fat, braised - 3 oz	85	11.2	4.4	4.4	0.7	92	273	207	1.02	0.109	11.9	0	0.3	0.30	0.30	12.8	17135
lean & fat, roasted	172	53.3	21.4	0.0		0.0	71	11	22	2.85	0.025	0	0	0.05	7.5	1.21	1.07
3 oz	85	8.9	3.8	3.5	0.6	87	298	190	0.78	0.110	9.4	0	0.4	0.30	0.27	12.8	17136
lean, braised	173	49.8	28.9	0.0		0.0	69	16	25	4.04	0.032	0	0	0.05	6.0	1.35	0.92
3 oz	85	5.5	1.5	2.0	0.5	96	288	220	1.05	0.117	12.8	0	0.4	0.32	0.32	13.6	17138
lean, roasted	143	55.9	22.4	0.0		0.0	72	12	23	3.01	0.026	0	0	0.05	7.9	1.27	1.12
3 oz	85	5.3	2.0	1.9	0.4	88	310	196	0.77	0.116	9.8	0	0.4	0.31	0.29	13.6	17139

19.8 INTERNAL ORGANS & OTHER CUTS

	KCAL / WT (g)	H₂0 / FAT	PRO / SFA	CHO / MUFA	SUGR / PUFA	DFIB / CHOL	Na / K	Ca / P	Mg / Fe	Zn / Cu	Mn / Se	A(RAE) / A(IU)	C / E	B-1 / B-2	NIA / B-6	B-12 / FOL	PANT / REF
belly, pork, raw	440	31.2	7.9	0.0		0.0	27	4	3	0.87	0.005	3	<1	0.34	3.9	0.71	0.22
3 oz	85	45.1	16.4	21.0	4.8	61	157	92	0.44	0.044	6.8	9	0.4	0.21	0.11	0.9	10005
brain, beef,	167	60.1	10.7	0.0		0.0	134	8	13	1.15	0.027	0	3	0.11	3.2	12.92	0.48
panfried - 3 oz	85	13.5	3.2	3.4	2.0	1696	301	328	1.89	0.187	22.1	0		0.22	0.33	5.1	13319

	KCAL	H_2O (g)	PRO (g)	CHO (g)	SUGR (g)	DFIB (g)	Minerals Na (mg)	Ca (mg)	Mg (mg)	Zn (mg)	Mn (mg)	Vitamins A (mcg RAE)	C (mg)	B-1 (mg)	NIA (mg)	B-12 (mcg)	PANT (mg)
	WT (g)	FAT (g)	SFA (g)	MUFA (g)	PUFA (g)	CHOL (mg)	K (mg)	P (mg)	Fe (mg)	Cu (mg)	Se (mcg)	A (IU)	E (mg ATE)	B-2 (mg)	B-6 (mg)	FOL (mcg DFE)	REF
simmered	136	62.3	9.4	0.0		0.0	102	8	12	1.06	0.030	0	1	0.07	1.9	7.31	0.48
3 oz	85	10.7	2.5	2.1	1.2	1746	204	299	1.88	0.204	18.7	0	2.0	0.14	0.20	6.0	13320
brain, lamb,	123	64.4	10.7	0.0		0.0	114	10	12	1.16	0.050	0	10	0.09	2.1	7.86	0.84
braised - *3 oz*	85	8.6	2.2	1.6	0.9	1737	174	286	1.43	0.179	10.2	0	1.3	0.20	0.09	4.3	17186
panfried	232	51.6	14.4	0.0		0.0	133	18	19	1.70	0.057	0	20	0.14	3.9	20.49	1.33
3 oz	85	18.9	4.8	3.4	1.9	2128	304	421	1.73	0.408	10.2	0		0.31	0.20	6.0	17187
brain, pork, braised	117	64.5	10.3	0.0		0.0	77	8	10	1.26	0.072	0	12	0.07	2.8	1.21	1.55
3 oz	85	8.1	1.8	1.5	1.2	2169	166	187	1.55	0.224	15.7	0		0.19	0.12	3.4	10097
brain, veal,	116	65.4	9.8	0.0		0.0	133	14	14	1.37	0.032	0	11	0.07	2.1	8.20	0.85
braised - *3 oz*	85	8.2	1.9	1.5	1.3	2635	182	327	1.42	0.221	9.4	0		0.17	0.14	2.6	17189
panfried	181	58.3	12.3	0.0		0.0	150	9	15	1.55	0.037	0	13	0.13	4.8	18.11	0.96
3 oz	85	14.2	3.4	3.6	2.1	1802	401	369	0.91	0.255	10.2	0		0.31	0.28	5.1	17190
chitterlings, pork, simmered	258	53.0	8.7	0.0		0.0	33	23	9	4.30	0.010	0	0	0.00	0.1	0.88	0.19
3 oz	85	24.4	8.6	8.2	6.1	122	7	40	3.15	0.198	33.1	0	0.2	0.07	0.01	2.6	10099
ears, pork, simmered	184	80.6	17.7	0.2		0.0	185	20	8	0.22	0.011	0	0	0.02	0.6	0.04	0.04
1 ear (3.9 oz)	111	12.0	4.3	5.5	1.3	100	44	27	1.67	0.007	4.9	0	0.3	0.08	0.01	0.0	10101
feet, pork,	173	58.3	11.5	0.0		0.0	785	27	3	1.05	0.014	0	0	0.01	0.3	0.53	0.27
cured, pickled - *3 oz*	85	13.7	4.7	6.4	1.5	78	200	29	0.53	0.043	6.5	0	0.2	0.04	0.32	3.4	10132
simmered	165	56.1	16.3	0.0		0.0	26	38	4	0.92	0.004	0	0	0.01	0.4	0.15	0.20
3 oz	85	10.5	3.6	4.9	1.1	85	124	41	0.40	0.037	4.0	0	0.2	0.05	0.08	0.9	10173
heart, beef, simmered	149	54.5	24.5	0.4		0.0	54	5	21	2.66	0.050	0	1	0.12	3.5	12.16	0.74
3 oz	85	4.8	1.4	1.1	1.2	164	198	213	6.38	0.629	33.2	0	0.6	1.31	0.18	1.7	13322
heart, lamb, braised	157	54.6	21.2	1.6		0.0	54	12	20	3.13	0.047	0	6	0.14	3.7	9.52	1.16
3 oz	85	6.7	2.7	1.9	0.7	212	160	216	4.69	0.519	40.0	0		1.01	0.26	1.7	17192
heart, pork, braised	191	87.8	30.4	0.5		0.0	45	9	31	3.99	0.094	9	3	0.72	7.8	4.89	3.19
1 heart (4.6 oz)	129	6.5	1.7	1.5	1.7	285	266	230	7.52	0.655	23.6	28		2.20	0.50	5.2	10104
heart, veal, braised	158	52.9	24.8	0.1		0.0	49	7	15	1.90	0.052	0	9	0.30	4.1	12.29	1.40
3 oz	85	5.7	1.5	1.2	1.5	150	169	213	3.67	0.367	44.5	0		0.79	0.18	1.7	17194
jowl, pork, raw	557	18.9	5.4	0.0		0.0	21	3	3	0.71	0.004	3	0	0.33	3.9	0.70	0.21
3 oz	85	59.2	21.5	28.0	6.9	77	126	73	0.36	0.034	1.3	8	0.2	0.20	0.08	0.9	10105
kidneys, beef, simmered	122	58.5	21.7	0.8		0.0	114	14	15	3.59	0.157	317	1	0.16	5.1	43.61	1.44
3 oz	85	2.9	0.9	0.6	0.6	329	152	260	6.21	0.578	238.7	1055	0.2	3.45	0.44	83.3	13324
kidneys, lamb, braised	116	59.9	20.1	0.8		0.0	128	15	17	3.23	0.122	116	10	0.30	5.1	67.07	1.73
3 oz	85	3.1	1.0	0.7	0.6	480	151	247	10.54	0.315	186.0	387		1.76	0.10	68.9	17196
kidneys, pork, braised	128	58.4	21.6	0.0		0.0	68	11	15	3.53	0.127	66	9	0.34	4.9	6.62	2.44
3 oz	85	4.0	1.3	1.3	0.3	408	122	204	4.50	0.581	264.8	221		1.35	0.39	34.9	10107
kidneys, veal, braised	139	57.5	22.4	0.0		0.0	94	25	20	3.61	0.108	171	7	0.16	3.9	31.37	0.73
3 oz	85	4.8	1.5	1.1	1.0	672	135	316	2.58	0.306	85.0	569		1.69	0.15	17.9	17198
liver, beef,	137	56.0	20.7	2.9		0.0	60	6	17	5.16	0.351	9072	20	0.17	9.1	60.35	3.88
braised - *3 oz*	85	4.2	1.6	0.6	0.9	331	200	343	5.75	3.835	47.4	30327		3.49	0.77	184.5	13326
panfried	184	47.3	22.7	6.7		0.0	90	9	20	4.63	0.360	9019	20	0.18	12.3	95.03	5.03
3 oz	85	6.8	2.3	1.4	1.5	410	309	392	5.34	3.796	48.5	30689	0.5	3.52	1.22	187.0	13327
liver, lamb,	187	48.2	26.0	2.2		0.0	48	7	19	6.71	0.442	6367	3	0.20	10.3	65.03	3.37
braised - *3 oz*	85	7.5	2.9	1.6	1.1	426	188	357	7.04	6.013	94.7	21203	0.6	3.43	0.42	62.1	17200
panfried	202	47.8	21.7	3.2		0.0	105	8	20	4.79	0.505	6615	11	0.30	14.2	72.85	5.38
3 oz	85	10.8	4.2	2.2	1.6	419	299	363	8.67	8.356	98.7	22098	0.6	3.90	0.81	340.0	17201
liver, pork, braised	140	54.7	22.1	3.2		0.0	42	9	12	5.71	0.255	4594	20	0.22	7.2	15.87	4.06
3 oz	85	3.7	1.2	0.5	0.9	302	128	205	15.23	0.539	57.4	15297	0.4	1.87	0.48	138.6	10111
liver, veal,	140	57.2	18.4	2.3		0.0	45	6	16	8.09	0.095	6856	26	0.11	7.2	31.03	1.94
braised - *3 oz*	85	5.9	2.2	1.3	0.9	477	174	271	2.23	6.758	43.4	22851	0.3	1.65	0.42	645.2	17203
panfried	208	45.1	25.3	3.3		0.0	112	10	22	6.69	0.175	4793	19	0.21	14.4	54.36	4.12
3 oz	85	9.7	3.6	2.1	1.5	281	372	373	4.45	8.400	45.1	15978	0.4	2.86	0.73	272.0	17204
lungs, beef, braised	102	64.9	17.3	0.0		0.0	86	9	9	1.39	0.013	10	28	0.03	2.1	2.20	0.53
3 oz	85	3.1	1.1	0.8	0.4	235	147	151	4.59	0.188	42.8	33		0.12	0.02	6.8	13329
lungs, lamb, braised	96	64.5	16.9	0.0		0.0	71	10	9	1.64	0.014	27	24	0.03	2.1	2.14	
3 oz	85	2.6	0.9	0.7	0.4	241	108	160	3.88	0.199	17.9	90		0.12	0.05	6.8	17206
lungs, pork, braised	84	68.0	14.1	0.0		0.0	69	7	10	2.08	0.013	0	7	0.07	1.2	1.73	0.56
3 oz	85	2.6	0.9	0.6	0.3	329	128	158	13.95	0.068	19.9	0	0.2	0.27	0.07	1.7	10113
lungs, veal, braised	88	66.0	15.9	0.0		0.0	48	6	7	1.02	0.013	0	29	0.03	1.9	2.02	
3 oz	85	2.2	0.8	0.6	0.3	224	121	197	3.07	0.188	16.8	0		0.11	0.05	6.8	17208
pancreas (sweetbread), beef,	230	47.3	23.0	0.0		0.0	51	14	18	3.91	0.177	0	17	0.15	3.4	14.11	3.61
braised[1] - *3 oz*	85	14.6	5.0	5.0	2.7	223	209	385	2.22	0.076	41.2	0		0.41	0.15	2.6	13332
pancreas (sweetbread), lamb,	199	50.7	19.4	0.0		0.0	44	10	16	2.28	0.037	0	17	0.02	2.2	4.71	0.72
braised[1] - *3 oz*	85	12.9	5.8	4.6	0.6	340	247	366	1.80	0.071	55.1	0		0.18	0.04	11.1	17211

	KCAL	H₂O (g)	PRO (g)	CHO (g)	SUGR (g)	DFIB (g)	Na (mg)	Ca (mg)	Mg (mg)	Zn (mg)	Mn (mg)	A (mcg RAE)	C (mg)	B-1 (mg)	NIA (mg)	B-12 (mcg)	PANT (mg)
	WT (g)	FAT (g)	SFA (g)	MUFA (g)	PUFA (g)	CHOL (mg)	K (mg)	P (mg)	Fe (mg)	Cu (mg)	Se (mcg)	A (IU)	E (mg ATE)	B-2 (mg)	B-6 (mg)	FOL (mcg DFE)	REF
pancreas (sweetbread), pork,	186	51.3	24.2	0.0		0.0	36	14	20	3.65	0.168	0	5	0.08	2.7	14.51	4.03
braised[1] - 3 oz	85	9.2	3.2	3.2	1.7	268	143	247	2.29	0.094	61.9	0		0.56	0.37	4.3	10116
pancreas (sweetbread), veal,	218	47.3	24.7	0.0		0.0	58	15	20	4.42	0.200	0		0.43	0.16	2.6	17213
braised[1] - 3 oz	85	12.4	4.3	4.3	2.3		236	435	2.02	0.086	33.2	0	5	0.16	3.5	14.73	
spleen, beef, braised	123	59.5	21.3	0.0		0.0	48	10	16	2.37	0.064	0	43	0.04	4.7	4.27	0.74
3 oz	85	3.6	1.2	1.0	0.3	295	241	259	33.46	0.785	77.7	0		0.26	0.03	3.4	13334
spleen, lamb, braised	133	56.4	22.5	0.0		0.0	49	11	18	3.35	0.053	0	22	0.04	5.0	4.50	
3 oz	85	4.1	1.3	1.1	0.3	327	211	290	32.87	0.118	42.3	0		0.27	0.07	3.4	17215
spleen, pork, braised	127	56.7	24.0	0.0		0.0	91	11	13	3.01	0.038	0	10	0.12	5.0	2.35	0.76
3 oz	85	2.7	0.9	0.7	0.2	428	193	241	18.90	0.113	42.2	0		0.22	0.05	3.4	10118
spleen, veal, braised	110	60.6	20.5	0.0		0.0	49	6	12	1.62	0.064	0	34	0.04	4.5	4.10	
3 oz	85	2.5	0.8	0.7	0.2	380	183	265	6.26	0.786	69.0	0		0.24	0.06	3.4	17217
stomach, pork, raw	133	62.6	14.0	0.0		0.0	44	9	8	1.71	0.009	0	0	0.07	3.8	0.84	0.54
3 oz	85	8.1	2.9	3.7	0.9	164	171	132	1.85	0.310	21.8	0	0.2	0.10	0.03	1.7	10119
tail, pork, simmered	337	39.7	14.5	0.0		0.0	21	12	6	1.39	0.005	0	0	0.06	1.0	0.47	0.36
3 oz	85	30.4	10.6	14.4	3.3	110	133	40	0.67	0.057	2.6	0	0.2	0.06	0.23	3.4	10175
thymus (sweetbread), beef,	271	44.9	18.6	0.0		0.0	99	9	9	1.87	0.084	0	26	0.07	1.6	1.28	1.68
braised[1] - 3 oz	85	21.2	7.3	7.3	4.0	250	368	309	1.27	0.037	18.4	0		0.19	0.07	0.9	13338
thymus (sweetbread), veal,	148	54.8	26.8	0.0		0.0	56	3	14	2.64	0.000	0	63	0.05	1.7	1.85	
braised[1] - 3 oz	85	3.6	1.3	1.3	0.7	399	291	582	1.71	0.000	83.4	0	0.7	0.14	0.08	0.9	17219
tongue, beef, simmered	241	47.6	18.8	0.3		0.0	51	6	14	4.08	0.022	0	<1	0.03	1.8	5.02	0.44
3 oz	85	17.6	7.6	8.0	0.7	91	153	121	2.88	0.187	14.5	0	0.3	0.30	0.14	4.3	13340
tongue, lamb, braised	234	49.2	18.3	0.0		0.0	57	9	14	2.54	0.028	0	6	0.07	3.1	5.36	0.29
3 oz	85	17.2	6.7	8.5	1.1	161	134	114	2.24	0.179	23.8	0		0.36	0.14	2.6	17221
tongue, pork, braised	230	48.4	20.5	0.0		0.0	93	16	17	3.85	0.009	0	1	0.27	4.5	2.03	0.43
3 oz	85	15.8	5.5	7.4	1.6	124	201	148	4.24	0.094	13.2	0		0.43	0.20	3.4	10122
tongue, veal, braised	172	54.5	22.0	0.0		0.0	54	8	15	3.83	0.040	0	5	0.06	1.2	4.51	0.63
3 oz	85	8.6	3.7	3.9	0.3	202	138	141	1.78	0.179	9.4	0		0.30	0.13	7.7	17223
tripe, beef, raw	83	69.2	12.4	0.0		0.0	39	8	7	2.10	0.009	0	3	0.01	0.1	1.31	0.48
3 oz	85	3.4	1.7	1.1	0.1	81	230	67	1.66	0.077	39.0	0	0.1	0.14	0.03	1.7	13341

[1] Organs sometimes referred to as "sweetbreads."

20. MEATS, LUNCHEON & SNACK
20.1 FRANKFURTERS & OTHER LUNCHEON-TYPE SAUSAGES

	KCAL	H₂O	PRO	CHO	SUGR	DFIB	Na	Ca	Mg	Zn	Mn	A	C	B-1	NIA	B-12	PANT
beef sausage, smoked, ckd	134	23.0	6.1	1.0		0.0	486	3	6	1.20	0.004	0	0	0.02	1.4	0.80	0.08
1.5 oz sausage	43	11.6	4.9	5.6	0.5	29	76	45	0.76	0.031	6.3	0		0.06	0.05	1.7	13357
beerwurst, pork & beef	155	31.8	7.8	2.1	0.0	0.5	410	15	11	1.24	0.087	2	<1	0.14	1.7	0.65	0.17
2 oz	56	12.6	4.7	5.7	1.2	35	137	76	0.97	0.058	9.7	6	0.1	0.10	0.13	2.8	07931
bockwurst (pork, veal, milk, eggs),	253	55.4	9.9	0.5	0.0	0.0	452	37	16	1.41	0.014	0	0	0.37	3.8	0.74	0.61
raw - 3.2 oz sausage	91	23.5	9.0	11.7	2.6	85	246	133	1.05	0.055	9.6	0	0.1	0.15	0.21	5.5	07006
bratwurst, beef & pork, smoked	195	37.4	8.1	1.7	0.0	0.0	560	5	10	1.63	0.027	0	0	0.25	2.1	1.76	0.46
2.3 oz	66	17.4	4.0	5.3	1.0	51	187	86	0.66	0.053	9.3	0	0.1	0.14	0.13	2.6	07922
chicken	148	59.0	16.3	0.0		0.0	60	9	19	1.20		25	2	0.06	6.3	0.29	0.81
3 oz	84	8.7	2.5	3.7	1.7	60	177	134	0.73	0.042		85	0.3	0.11	0.32	5.0	07923
pork, beef, turkey, lite, smoked	129	43.5	9.5	2.6	1.0	0.0	648	9	9	1.77	0.010	0	0	0.06	1.2	1.06	0.27
2.3 oz	66	8.9	3.2	4.7	0.6	37	162	87	0.62	0.042	13.3	1	<0.1	0.11	0.14	3.3	07924
pork, ckd	256	47.7	12.0	1.8		0.0	473	37	13	1.96	0.039	0	1	0.43	2.7	0.81	0.27
3 oz link (1/3 oz pkg)	85	22.0	7.9	10.4	2.3	51	180	127	1.10	0.077	18.0	0	0.2	0.16	0.18	1.7	07013
veal, ckd	288	44.9	11.8	0.0	0.0	0.0	50	9	13	1.72	0.041	0	0	0.05	4.6	0.82	0.80
3 oz	84	26.6	12.5	10.9	1.4	66	194	126	0.62	0.068	16.1	0	0.2	0.16	0.26	7.6	07910
brotwurst (pork & beef w/nfdm)	226	35.9	10.0	2.1	2.1	0.0	778	34	11	1.47	0.027	0	0	0.18	2.3	1.44	0.04
2.5 oz link (7/lb)	70	19.5	6.9	9.3	2.0	44	197	94	0.72	0.056	9.5	0	0.2	0.16	0.09	3.5	07015
chicken, beef & pork sausage,	181	50.8	11.4	6.9	1.6	0.0	869	84	12	2.25	0.013	0	0	0.08	1.6	1.34	0.35
skinless, smoked - 1 link	84	12.0	4.0	6.0	0.7	101	207	111	4.03	0.053	17.0	0	<0.1	0.14	0.18	5.0	07928
chorizo (pork & beef)	273	19.1	14.5	1.1		0.0	741	5	11	2.05	0.024	0	0	0.38	3.1	1.20	0.67
2.1 oz link (4" long)	60	23.0	8.6	11.0	2.1	53	239	90	0.95	0.048	12.7	0	0.1	0.18	0.32	1.2	07019
frankfurter, beef	141	22.4	4.8	1.7	1.5	0.0	490	6	6	1.06	0.035	0	0	0.02	1.0	0.74	0.10
1.5 oz frank	43	12.7	5.0	6.2	0.5	23	67	69	0.65	0.079	3.5	0	0.1	0.06	0.04	2.2	07022
bun length, Oscar Mayer	185	30.3	6.3	1.5	1.0	0.0	584	7	9	1.28		0	0				
2 oz frank	57	17.2	7.1	8.3	0.5	34	90	60	0.89	0.086		0				6.3	07242

	KCAL	H₂0 (g)	PRO (g)	CHO (g)	SUGR (g)	DFIB (g)	Na (mg)	Ca (mg)	Mg (mg)	Zn (mg)	Mn (mg)	A (mcg RAE)	C (mg)	B-1 (mg)	NIA (mg)	B-12 (mcg)	PANT (mg)
WT (g)	FAT (g)	SFA (g)	MUFA (g)	PUFA (g)	CHOL (mg)	K (mg)	P (mg)	Fe (mg)	Cu (mg)	Se (mcg)	A (IU)	E (mg ATE)	B-2 (mg)	B-6 (mg)	FOL (mcg DFE)	REF
fat free, Oscar Mayer	39	39.0	6.6	2.6	1.9	0.0	464	10	10	1.21			0				
1.8 oz frank	50	0.3	0.1	0.1	<0.1	15	234	65	0.98	0.080		0					07243
heated	170	27.1	6.0	2.0	1.8	0.0	600	6	7	1.22	0.040	0		0.02	1.2	0.86	0.13
1.8 oz frank	52	15.3	5.9	7.4	0.6	29	76	89	0.81	0.080	6.3	0	0.1	0.07	0.05	3.6	07945
Hormel Wrangler	162	31.7	7.0	1.2	0.9	0.0	557	8	8	1.29		2	11				
2 oz frank	56	14.4	5.9	7.3	0.5	38	96		1.01	0.056		7				6.2	07279
light, Oscar Mayer	110	38.1	6.1	2.3	1.2	0.0	615	12	10	1.20		0					
2 oz frank	57	8.5	3.6	4.3	0.6	28	229	93	0.89	0.120		0					07244
Oscar Mayer	147	23.9	5.1	1.1	0.7	0.0	461	5	6	0.99	0.009	0	0	0.02	1.0	0.73	0.10
1.6 oz frank	45	13.6	5.6	6.6	0.6	25	59	63	0.60	0.063	5.2	0	0.05	0.03	2.7		07241
frankfurter, beef & pork	135	25.2	5.2	0.7	0.0	0.0	504	10	5	0.83	0.014	8	1	0.09	1.2	0.59	0.16
1.6 oz frank	45	12.4	4.8	6.2	1.2	23	75	39	0.52	0.036	6.2	26	0.1	0.05	0.06	1.8	07023
frankfurter, cheese w/turkey, Oscar	143	23.8	5.4	1.3	0.8	0.0	514	74	11	0.83		0					
Mayer - *1.6 oz frank*	45	12.9	4.5	5.9	1.7	33	59	97	0.67	0.081		0					07245
frankfurter, chicken	116	25.9	5.8	3.1		0.0	617	43	5	0.47	0.007	18	0	0.03	1.4	0.11	0.37
1.6 oz frank	45	8.8	2.5	3.8	1.8	45	38	48	0.90	0.023	8.3	59	0.1	0.05	0.14	1.8	07024
frankfurter, meat, fat free, Oscar	37	39.4	6.3	2.2	1.1	0.0	487	8	11	0.60		0					
Mayer - *1.8 oz frank*	50	0.3	0.1	0.1	0.1	15	236	81	0.46	0.110		0		0.03	1.4	0.82	0.16
heated	145	30.1	5.1	2.5		0.0	527	51	8	0.56	0.027	0		0.03	1.4	0.82	0.16
1 frank	52	12.6	3.8	5.6	2.1	38	73	110	0.63	0.079	6.5	0	0.1	0.06	0.09	3.1	07949
unheated	151	29.3	5.3	2.2		0.0	567	51	8	0.62	0.023	0		0.03	1.4	0.82	0.16
1 frank	52	13.4	4.0	5.9	2.3	40	79	107	0.57	0.050	6.5	0	0.1	0.06	0.09	3.1	07950
frankfurter, pork	204	45.5	9.7	0.2	0.0	0.1	620	203	11	1.59	0.012	60	2	0.45	2.1	0.37	0.39
1 link	76	18.0	6.6	8.3	1.7	50	201	130	2.81	0.056	21.1	200	<0.1	0.14	0.24	2.3	07939
frankfurter, pork & beef w/am	141	22.6	6.0	0.6	0.6	0.0	465	25	6	0.97	0.014	16	0	0.11	1.2	0.74	0.33
chs (cheesefurter) - *1.5 oz frank*	43	12.4	4.5	5.9	1.3	29	89	77	0.46	0.030	4.9	68	0.1	0.07	0.06	1.3	07016
frankfurter, pork & turkey,	146	24.0	4.9	1.2	0.8	0.0	445	27	8	0.77	0.004	0	0	0.12	1.1	0.17	0.17
Oscar Mayer - *1.6 oz frank*	45	13.5	4.3	6.2	1.9	32	73	62	0.52	0.117	6.8	0		0.06	0.10	1.8	07240
small, Oscar Mayer	177	31.4	6.2	1.3	0.9	0.0	592	7	7	1.05		0					
6 small franks (2 oz)	57	16.4	6.4	8.2	1.5	31	91	55	0.58	0.063		0					07248
frankfurter, pork, turkey, & beef,	111	38.0	6.9	1.6	0.9	0.0	591	22	10	1.01		0					
light, Oscar Mayer - *2 oz frank*	57	8.5	3.0	3.9	1.2	35	226	96	0.73	0.114		0					07247
frankfurter, turkey	102	28.3	6.4	0.7		0.0	642	48	6	1.40	0.007	0	0	0.02	1.9	0.13	0.32
1.6 oz frank	45	8.0	2.7	2.5	2.3	48	81	60	0.83	0.045	6.9	0	0.3	0.08	0.10	3.6	07025
Butcher Boy Meats	134	33.1	7.5	2.6	1.4	0.1	651	83	8	1.61		8	<1	0.03	1.2	0.14	0.37
2 oz frank	56	10.2	3.3	3.1	2.8	58	106	138	1.02	0.055		166	0.0	0.08	0.12	3.9	07269
frankfurter, turkey & chicken,	85	30.1	5.0	2.4	0.7	0.0	511	59	10	0.84		0					
Louis Rich - *1.6 oz frank*	45	6.1	1.7	2.5	1.4	41	72	66	0.98	0.099		0					07253
frankfurter, turkey & chicken	90	28.8	5.7	2.3	0.8	0.0	482	109	10	0.81		0					
w/chs, Louis Rich - *1.6 oz frank*	45	6.5	2.3	2.8	1.3	42	71	92	0.95	0.090		0					07252
italian sausage, pork, ckd - *2.4 oz link*	216	33.5	13.4	1.0		0.0	618	16	12	1.60	0.055	0	1	0.42	2.8	0.87	0.30
	67	17.2	6.1	8.0	2.2	52	204	114	1.01	0.054	14.7	0	0.2	0.16	0.22	3.4	07089
sweet	125	60.1	13.5	1.8		0.0	479	21	10	1.28	0.006	1	<1	0.14	1.5	0.87	0.23
3 oz link	84	7.1	2.7	3.0	0.4	25	163	87	1.00	0.034	9.1	2	<0.1	0.11	0.16	3.4	07914
turkey, smoked	88	38.4	8.4	2.6	1.8	0.5	520	12	14	1.19	0.037	24	17	0.04	2.1	0.24	0.45
2 oz	56	4.9	1.9	1.3	0.9	30	110	104	5.38	0.062	12.4	81	0.2	0.10	0.21	4.5	07927
kielbasa, polish, turkey & beef, smoked - *2 oz*	127	34.7	7.3	2.2	0.0	0.0	672					0	8				
	56	9.9	3.5	4.6	1.3	39			0.69			0					07934
knockwurst/knackwurst (pork & beef) - *2.5 oz sausage*	221	39.8	8.0	2.3		0.0	670	8	8	1.20	0.015	0	0	0.25	2.0	0.85	0.23
	72	19.9	7.4	9.2	2.1	43	143	71	0.48	0.043	9.7	0	0.4	0.10	0.12	1.4	07038
polish sausage, beef w/chicken, hot - *5 pieces*	142	30.4	9.7	2.0	0.0	0.0	847	7	8	1.06	0.027	0	0	0.28	1.9	0.54	0.25
	55	10.7	4.4	5.3	0.4	36	130	75	0.48	0.050	9.7	0	<0.1	0.08	0.10	1.1	07915
pork	740	120.7	32.0	3.7		0.0	1989	27	32	4.38	0.111	0	2	1.14	7.8	2.22	1.02
8 oz sausage (10" long, 1 1/4" dia)	227	65.2	23.4	30.7	7.0	159	538	309	3.27	0.204	40.2	0		0.34	0.43	4.5	07059
pork & beef, smoked	238	43.0	9.2	1.9	0.0	0.0	644	5	9	1.60	0.028	0	0	0.20	2.5	1.15	0.33
2.7 oz	76	20.2	8.8	10.8	2.5	54	144	81	0.76	0.046	10.0	0	0.2	0.13	0.13	3.0	07916
pork & beef sausage w/cheddar cheese, smoked - *2.7 oz*	226	43.2	9.9	1.6	0.1	0.0	653	44	10	1.73	0.025	0	0	0.19	2.2	1.33	0.59
	77	19.9	8.1	10.5	2.3	49	159	137	0.56	0.054	5.8	0	0.1	0.12	0.10	2.3	07917
smoked sausage (smokie), beef, Oscar Mayer - *1.5 oz link*	127	24.2	5.3	0.8	0.6	0.0	416	5	6	1.27		0	0				
	43	11.5	4.8	5.5	0.4	27	74	99	0.75	0.086		0				4.7	07233
cheese, Oscar Mayer	130	23.6	5.5	0.8	0.6	0.0	450	19	7	0.84		69					
1.5 oz link	43	11.7	4.4	5.6	1.2	30	78	124	0.46	0.086		0					07234

	KCAL / WT (g)	H₂0 (g) / FAT (g)	PRO (g) / SFA (g)	CHO (g) / MUFA (g)	SUGR (g) / PUFA (g)	DFIB (g) / CHOL (mg)	Na (mg) / K (mg)	Ca (mg) / P (mg)	Mg (mg) / Fe (mg)	Zn (mg) / Cu (mg)	Mn (mg) / Se (mcg)	A (mcg RAE) / A (IU)	C (mg) / E (mg ATE)	B-1 (mg) / B-2 (mg)	NIA (mg) / B-6 (mg)	B-12 (mcg) / FOL (mcg DFE)	PANT (mg) / REF
pork	265	26.7	15.1	1.4		0.0	1020	20	13	1.92	0.011	0	1	0.48	3.1	1.11	0.53
2.4 oz link (4" long)	68	21.6	7.7	10.0	2.6	46	228	110	0.79	0.049	14.8	0	0.2	0.17	0.24	3.4	07074
pork & beef	228	35.5	9.1	1.0		0.0	643	7	8	1.43	0.025	0	0	0.18	2.2	1.03	0.30
2.4 oz link (4" long)	68	20.6	7.2	9.6	2.2	48	129	73	0.99	0.041	8.9	0	0.1	0.12	0.12	1.4	07075
pork & beef w/flour & nfdm	182	39.0	9.5	2.7		0.0	741	12	9	1.36	0.035	0	2	0.16	1.8	0.90	0.41
2.4 oz link (4" long)	68	14.6	5.3	6.8	1.5	59	105	75	1.05	0.061	10.8	0	0.1	0.12	0.09	1.4	07076
pork & beef w/nfdm	213	36.7	9.0	1.3		0.0	798	28	11	1.33	0.026	0	0	0.13	1.9	1.07	0.41
2.4 oz link (4" long)	68	18.8	6.6	8.6	2.1	44	194	93	1.00	0.061	9.5	0		0.15	0.12	1.4	07077
pork & turkey, Oscar Mayer	172	31.6	7.1	1.0	0.8	0.0	583	6	10	1.12		0		0			
Little Smokies - 6 links (2 oz)	57	15.4	5.4	7.3	1.6	36	99	121	0.67	0.114		0					07235
pork & turkey w/chs, Oscar Mayer	180	30.3	7.7	1.0	0.2	0.0	591	38	12	1.16		0		0			
Little Smokies - 6 links (2 oz)	57	16.1	6.4	7.5	1.6	38	87	141	0.71	0.171		0					07236
Smokie Links, Oscar Mayer	130	23.9	5.3	0.7	0.7	0.0	433	4	7	0.90		0		0			
1.5 oz link	43	11.7	4.0	5.7	1.2	27	77	103	0.50	0.108		0					07232
turkey, Louis Rich	90	38.7	8.3	1.8	1.6	0.0	530	15	12	1.20		0	0				
2 oz link	56	5.5	1.5	2.0	1.5	37	113	114	0.77	0.095		0				3.4	07268
turkey sausage,	129	35.3	8.6	0.9	0.0	0.0	328	18	14	1.19	0.037	0	17	0.04	2.1	0.24	0.45
breakfast, mild - 2 links (2 oz)	56	10.1	2.1	1.3	0.9	34	110	104	0.60	0.062	12.4	0	0.2	0.10	0.21	4.5	07919
hot, smoked	88	38.4	8.4	2.6	1.8	0.5	520	12	14	1.19	0.037	24	17	0.04	2.1	0.24	0.45
2 oz	56	4.9	1.9	1.3	0.9	30	110	104	5.38	0.062	12.4	81	0.2	0.10	0.21	4.5	07929
vienna sausage, beef & pork, cnd	45	9.6	1.6	0.3		0.0	152	2	1	0.26	0.005	0	0	0.01	0.3	0.16	0.06
.6 oz sausage (2" long, 7/8" dia)	16	4.0	1.5	2.0	0.3	8	16	8	0.14	0.005	2.7	0	<0.1	0.02	0.02	0.6	07083

20.2 LUNCH MEATS & SPREADS

	KCAL / WT (g)	H₂0 (g) / FAT (g)	PRO (g) / SFA (g)	CHO (g) / MUFA (g)	SUGR (g) / PUFA (g)	DFIB (g) / CHOL (mg)	Na (mg) / K (mg)	Ca (mg) / P (mg)	Mg (mg) / Fe (mg)	Zn (mg) / Cu (mg)	Mn (mg) / Se (mcg)	A (mcg RAE) / A (IU)	C (mg) / E (mg ATE)	B-1 (mg) / B-2 (mg)	NIA (mg) / B-6 (mg)	B-12 (mcg) / FOL (mcg DFE)	PANT (mg) / REF
barbeque loaf	40	14.9	3.6	1.5		0.0	307	13	4	0.57	0.009	1	0	0.08	0.5	0.39	0.36
.8 oz slice	23	2.0	0.7	1.0	0.2	9	76	30	0.27	0.016	4.9	16		0.06	0.06	2.1	07001
beef,	37	19.3	5.7	0.5		0.0	352	2	6	1.10	0.008	0	0	0.02	1.3	0.48	0.17
chopped, smoked - 1 oz slice	28	1.2	0.5	0.5	0.1	13	106	51	0.80	0.007	5.5	0		0.05	0.10	2.2	13358
jellied lunch meat	31	20.9	5.3	0.0		0.0	370	3	5	0.99	0.015	0	0	0.04	1.4	1.44	0.19
1 oz slice	28	0.9	0.4	0.4	<0.1	10	113	39	0.97	0.034	4.6	0		0.08	0.07	2.0	13353
loaf lunch meat	86	14.7	4.0	0.8		0.0	372	3	4	0.71	0.013	0	0	0.03	1.0	1.09	0.15
1 oz slice	28	7.3	3.1	3.4	0.2	18	58	33	0.65	0.034	6.2	0	0.1	0.06	0.05	1.4	07042
sandwich steaks, flaked, chpd	173	31.4	9.2	0.0	0.0	0.0	38	7	9	2.03	0.010	0	0	0.02	2.6	1.52	0.20
formed, thinly sliced - 2 oz steak	56	15.1	6.5	6.2	0.3	40	130	74	1.04	0.035	7.3	0	0.1	0.09	0.14	3.9	13342
smoked, sliced, Carl Buddig	79	39.6	11.0	0.3		0.0	816	8							0.05	2.2	
2 oz	57	3.7	1.5		0.2	38	192		1.29					0.14			07272
thin sliced lunch meat	37	12.2	5.9	1.2		0.0	302	2	4	0.84	0.008	0	0	0.02	1.1	0.54	0.12
5 slices (.7 oz)	21	0.8	0.3	0.4	<0.1	9	90	35	0.57	0.007	5.9	0	<0.1	0.04	0.07	2.3	07043
beef pastrami	98	13.1	4.8	0.9		0.0	344	3	5	1.19	0.004	0	0	0.03	1.4	0.49	0.08
1 oz slice	28	8.2	2.9	4.1	0.3	26	64	42	0.53	0.022	2.9	0	0.1	0.05	0.05	2.0	13355
smoked, Carl Buddig	80	39.8	11.2	0.6		0.0	602	10							0.05	2.3	
2 oz	57	3.7	1.7		0.2	37	208		1.40					0.13			07274
berliner, pork & beef	53	14.0	3.5	0.6	0.5	0.0	298	3	3	0.57	0.009	0	0	0.09	0.7	0.61	0.16
.8 oz slice	23	4.0	1.4	1.8	0.4	11	65	30	0.26	0.018	3.2	0	<0.1	0.05	0.05	1.2	07004
blood sausage (blood pudding)	95	11.8	3.7	0.3	0.3	0.0	170	2	2	0.33	0.003	0	0	0.02	0.3	0.25	0.15
.9 oz slice	25	8.6	3.3	4.0	0.9	30	10	6	1.60	0.010	3.0	0	0.1	0.03	0.01	1.3	07005
bologna,	22	21.8	3.5	1.7	0.6	0.0	274	4	6	0.32				0			
fat free, Oscar Mayer - 1 oz slice	28	0.2	0.1	0.1	<0.1	7	44	43	0.26	0.056		0					07203
wisconsin-made ring, Oscar Mayer	175	30.6	6.6	1.5	1.2	0.0	463	8	8	1.04	0.027	0	0	0.16	1.5	0.71	
2 oz	56	15.9	6.2	7.9	1.1	35	78	59	0.65	0.073		0		0.08	0.08		07206
bologna, beef	87	15.5	3.4	0.2		0.0	275	3	3	0.60	0.008	0	0	0.01	0.7	0.40	0.08
1 oz slice	28	8.0	3.4	3.9	0.3	16	44	25	0.46	0.008	3.2	0	0.1	0.03	0.04	1.4	07007
light, Oscar Mayer	56	18.2	3.3	1.6	0.6	0.0	322	4	4	0.53		0	0				
1 oz slice	28	4.1	1.6	2.0	0.1	12	44	50	0.34	0.059		0				3.6	07202
Oscar Mayer	88	15.2	3.1	0.7	0.4	0.0	330	3	4	0.57		0	0	0.01	0.7	0.40	0.08
1 oz slice	28	8.1	3.6	4.3	0.3	18	47	31	0.38	0.031		0		0.03	0.05	3.6	07201
bologna, beef & pork	87	15.2	3.3	0.8	1.2	0.0	285	3	3	0.54	0.011	0	0	0.05	0.7	0.37	0.08
1 oz slice	28	7.9	3.0	3.7	0.7	15	50	25	0.42	0.022	3.2	0	0.1	0.04	0.05	1.4	07008
bologna, chicken, pork, & beef,	89	15.0	3.1	0.7	0.4	0.0	289	19	6	0.40				0			
Oscar Mayer - 1 oz slice	28	8.2	2.9	4.1	1.1	29	43	56	0.50	0.056		0					07200

	KCAL / WT (g)	H_2O (g) / FAT (g)	PRO (g) / SFA (g)	CHO (g) / MUFA (g)	SUGR (g) / PUFA (g)	DFIB (g) / CHOL (mg)	Na (mg) / K (mg)	Ca (mg) / P (mg)	Mg (mg) / Fe (mg)	Zn (mg) / Cu (mg)	Mn (mg) / Se (mcg)	A (mcg RAE) / A (IU)	C (mg) / E (mg ATE)	B-1 (mg) / B-2 (mg)	NIA (mg) / B-6 (mg)	B-12 (mcg) / FOL (mcg DFE)	PANT (mg) / REF
bologna, pork	69	17.0	4.3	0.2		0.0	332	3	4	0.57	0.010	0	0	0.15	1.1	0.26	0.20
1 oz slice	28	5.6	1.9	2.7	0.6	17	79	39	0.22	0.022	3.6	0	0.1	0.04	0.08	1.4	07010
bologna, pork & turkey, lite	118	36.3	7.3	1.9	0.0	0.0	401	27	10	0.41	0.087	1	0	0.09	1.7	0.16	0.19
2 oz	56	9.0	3.1	4.2	1.7	44	77	53	0.64	0.046	3.1	1	0.1	0.05	0.09	10.1	07936
bologna, pork, chicken, & beef, light, Oscar Mayer - *1 oz slice*	57	18.1	3.2	1.6	0.7	0.0	313	14	6	0.45	0.043	0	0	0.04	0.9	0.08	0.10
	28	4.1	1.6	2.0	0.4	16	46	52	0.39	0.056	1.6	0		0.03	0.05	5.0	07205
bologna, pork, turkey, & beef	94	12.9	3.3	1.9	0.4	0.0	299	9	4	0.63	0.075	0	3	0.04	0.9	0.31	0.10
1 oz	28	8.3	3.3	3.6	0.7	21	63	36	0.34	0.026	3.5	0	0.0	0.04	0.11	1.1	07937
bologna, turkey	56	18.5	3.9	0.3		0.0	249	24	4	0.49	0.004	0	0	0.02	1.0	0.08	0.20
1 oz slice	28	4.3	1.4	1.4	1.2	28	56	37	0.43	0.009	3.6	0	0.2	0.05	0.06	2.0	07011
Louis Rich	52	18.9	3.2	1.4	0.3	0.0	302	35	6	0.52		0	0					
1 oz slice	28	3.7	1.1	1.5	1.0	19	43	55	0.46	0.050		0				1.7	07255
braunschweiger (pork liver sausage)	65	8.6	2.4	0.6		0.0	206	2	2	0.51	0.028	760	0	0.04	1.5	3.62	0.61
.6 oz slice (2 1/2" dia, 1/4" thick)	18	5.8	2.0	2.7	0.7	28	36	30	1.68	0.043	10.4	2529	0.1	0.27	0.06	7.9	07014
saren tube, Oscar Mayer	191	27.8	8.0	1.3	0.4	0.1	626	5	7	1.77	0.050		5	0.13	4.6	10.37	1.61
2 oz	56	17.1	6.1	8.7	2.1	90	103	109	5.45	0.224		9335		0.87	0.19	34.2	07208
sliced, Oscar Mayer	93	14.1	4.0	0.7	0.3	0.1	325	3	4	0.95	0.041	1322	3	0.06	2.6	5.26	0.97
1 oz	28	8.2	3.1	4.3	1.0	50	57	56	2.94	0.140		4404		0.45	0.09	13.2	07207
chicken breast, baked/grilled, Louis Rich - *2 slices (1.6 oz)*	44	32.8	8.9	1.7	0.3	0.0	514	4	14	0.40			0					
	45	0.2	0.1	0.1	<0.1	23	131	127	0.58	0.108		0					07249
fat-free, mesquite flavor, sliced *2 slices*	34	32.2	7.1	0.9	0.1	0.0	437	2	15	0.25	0.014	0	0	0.01	1.2	0.03	0.08
	42	0.2	0.1	0.1	<0.1	15	133	108	0.13	0.097	2.6	0	<0.1	0.01	0.05	0.4	07932
fat-free, oven-roasted, sliced *2 slices*	33	32.2	7.1	0.9	0.0	0.0	457	3	4	0.13	0.018	0	0	0.01	1.4	0.04	0.10
	42	0.2	0.1	<0.1	<0.1	15	28	25	0.13	0.014	3.2	0	<0.1	0.01	0.06	0.4	07933
fat free, roasted, Oscar Mayer *4 slices (1.8 oz)*	44	39.4	9.5	0.9	0.5	0.0	646	6	19	0.31			0					
	52	0.3	0.1	0.1	<0.1	23	164	133	0.69	0.120		0					07210
honey glazed, Oscar Mayer *4 slices (1.8 oz)*	57	36.6	10.3	2.0	2.2	0.0	748	5	19	0.36			0					
	52	0.8	0.2	0.3	0.1	28	171	150	0.59	0.088		0				2.1	07209
roasted, Louis Rich *1 oz*	28	20.6	5.1	0.7	0.4	0.0	333	2	7	0.20			0					
	28	0.6	0.2	0.2	0.1	14	74	74	0.32	0.064		0					07250
chicken roll, breast meat, oven-roasted - *2 oz*	75	40.9	8.2	1.0	0.2	0.0	494	3	10	0.36	0.010	0	0	0.02	3.7	0.13	0.32
	56	4.3	1.4	1.6	0.8	22	181	68	0.18	0.039	6.6	0	<0.1	0.03	0.17	1.7	07935
light meat *2 slices (2 oz)*	88	39.1	11.1	1.4		0.0	333	25	11	0.41	0.007	14	0	0.04	3.0	0.09	0.22
	57	4.2	1.1	1.7	0.9	29	130	89	0.55	0.023	7.1	47	0.2	0.07	0.12	1.1	07017
chicken spread, cnd - *1 oz*	45	16.3	5.1	1.1	0.1	0.1	205	5	3	0.33	0.003	9	0	<0.01	0.8	0.04	0.12
	28	5.0	0.9	1.4	0.7	16	30	25	0.25	0.011	3.1	28	0.1	0.03	0.04	0.9	07018
rts, Libby's Spreadables *4.2 oz*	171	87.0	5.8	11.9			552										
	118	11.1	2.3	3.5	4.2	31						0					22697
chicken, smoked, light & dark, Carl Buddig - *2 oz*	94	38.9	10.2	0.4		0.0	544	71						0.04	3.8		
	57	5.8	1.5		1.2	30	146		0.89					0.14			07271
chicken, white meat, roasted, Louis Rich - *1 oz*	36	20.0	4.8	0.6	0.3	0.0	335	5	7	0.32			0					
	28	1.6	0.4	0.7	0.3	17	85	69	0.44	0.064		0					07251
corned beef, cnd - *.7 oz slice*	53	12.1	5.7	0.0		0.0	211	3	3	0.75	0.003	0	0	<0.01	0.5	0.34	0.13
	21	3.1	1.3	1.3	0.1	18	29	23	0.44	0.013	9.0	0	<0.1	0.03	0.03	1.9	13348
chopped, pressed, Carl Buddig *2 oz*	81	39.4	11.0	0.6		0.0	765	10						0.05	2.4		
	57	3.9	1.6		0.2	37	201		1.37					0.14			07270
jellied loaf *1 oz slice*	43	19.3	6.4	0.0		0.0	267	3	3	1.15	0.009	0	0	0.00	0.5	0.36	0.05
	28	1.7	0.7	0.8	0.1	13	28	20	0.57	0.017	4.8	0	0.1	0.03	0.03	2.2	07020
ham & cheese loaf *1 oz slice*	73	16.2	4.7	0.4		0.0	376	16	4	0.56	0.008	6	0	0.17	1.0	0.23	0.15
	28	5.7	2.1	2.6	0.6	16	82	71	0.25	0.022	9.7	21	0.1	0.05	0.07	0.8	07032
Oscar Mayer *1 oz slice*	66	16.9	3.9	1.1	0.9	0.0	327	19	5	0.51	0.005	0	0	0.16	1.0	0.21	0.12
	28	5.1	1.8	2.3	0.5	17	74	76	0.24	0.034		0		0.05	0.07	0.8	07211
ham & cheese spread *1 oz (~2T)*	69	16.8	4.6	0.6		0.0	339	62	5	0.64	0.010	26	0	0.09	0.6	0.21	0.17
	28	5.3	2.4	2.0	0.4	17	46	140	0.22	0.026	9.5	86		0.06	0.04	0.9	07033
ham, baked, 96% fat free, water added, Oscar Mayer - *.7 oz slice*	22	15.6	3.4	0.4	0.2	0.0	261	2	7	0.38			0	0				
	21	0.7	0.2	0.2	0.3	10	56	49	0.27	0.050		0				0.8	07213
ham, boiled, water added, Oscar Mayer - *.7 oz slice*	22	15.7	3.5	0.3	0.1	0.0	283	2	7	0.39			0					
	21	0.8	0.3	0.4	0.1	10	59	50	0.31	0.050		0					07214
ham, chopped, cnd - *.7 oz slice*	50	12.8	3.4	0.1		0.0	287	1	3	0.38	0.005	0	<1	0.11	0.7	0.15	0.06
	21	4.0	1.3	1.9	0.4	10	60	29	0.20	0.011	3.9	0	0.1	0.03	0.07	0.2	07026
Oscar Mayer *1 oz*	50	18.3	4.6	1.0	0.6	0.0	350	3	6	0.63			0	0				
	28	3.1	1.1	1.6	0.4	17	73	61	0.36	0.067		0				0.8	07212

	KCAL	H₂O (g)	PRO (g)	CHO (g)	SUGR (g)	DFIB (g)	Minerals Na (mg)	Ca (mg)	Mg (mg)	Zn (mg)	Mn (mg)	Vitamins A (mcg RAE)	C (mg)	B-1 (mg)	NIA (mg)	B-12 (mcg)	PANT (mg)
	WT (g)	FAT (g)	SFA (g)	MUFA (g)	PUFA (g)	CHOL (mg)	K (mg)	P (mg)	Fe (mg)	Cu (mg)	Se (mcg)	A (IU)	E (mg ATE)	B-2 (mg)	B-6 (mg)	FOL (mcg DFE)	REF
packaged	64	17.8	4.8	0.0		0.0	384	2	4	0.54	0.011	0	0	0.18	1.1	0.26	0.08
1 oz slice	28	4.8	1.6	2.3	0.6	14	89	43	0.23	0.017	4.9	0		0.06	0.10	0.3	07027
ham, honey, water added, Oscar	23	15.3	3.5	0.7	0.7		262	2	7	0.44			0				
Mayer - .7 oz slice	21	0.7	0.2	0.4	0.1	9	59	54	0.28	0.048		0					07215
ham, minced	55	12.0	3.4	0.4		0.0	261	2	3	0.40	0.007	0		0.15	0.9	0.20	0.04
.7 oz slice	21	4.3	1.5	2.0	0.5	15	65	33	0.17	0.017	4.2	0		0.04	0.05	0.2	07030
ham salad spread	61	17.7	2.5	3.0		0.0	259	2	3	0.31	0.004	0		0.12	0.6	0.22	0.09
1 oz (~2T)	28	4.4	1.4	2.0	0.8	10	43	34	0.17	0.020	5.0	0	0.5	0.03	0.04	0.3	07031
ham, sliced,	37	19.7	5.4	0.3		0.0	400	2	5	0.54	0.009	0	0	0.26	1.4	0.21	0.13
lean (5% fat) - 1 oz slice	28	1.4	0.5	0.7	0.1	13	98	61	0.21	0.020	4.5	0	0.1	0.06	0.13	1.1	07028
reg (11% fat)	51	18.1	4.9	0.9		0.0	369	2	5	0.60	0.009	0	0	0.24	1.5	0.23	0.13
1 oz slice	28	3.0	0.9	1.4	0.3	16	93	69	0.28	0.028	4.6	0	0.1	0.07	0.10	0.8	07029
ham, smoked, fat free, 40% water,	34	37.2	6.9	0.9	0.5	0.0	509	5	13	0.74		0					
Oscar Mayer - 3 slices (1.7 oz)	47	0.3	0.1	0.1	0.1	18	110	93	0.43	0.094		0					07217
sliced, Carl Buddig	93	38.2	10.5	0.6		0.0	787	9						0.43	2.9		
2 oz	57	5.3	1.8		0.6	31	194		1.16					0.20			07275
water added, Oscar Mayer	21	15.9	3.5	0.0	0.0	0.0	255	2	7	0.38			0				
.7 oz slice	21	0.8	0.3	0.4	0.1	10	56	49	0.27	0.050		0					07216
headcheese (pork)	59	18.1	4.5	0.1		0.0	352	4	3	0.36	0.005	0	0	0.01	0.3	0.29	0.06
1 oz slice	28	4.4	1.4	2.3	0.5	23	9	17	0.33	0.034	<0.1	0	0.1	0.05	0.05	0.6	07034
Oscar Mayer	52	18.9	4.4	0.0		0.0	300	6	3	0.33			0	0.01	0.3	0.27	0.06
1 oz slice	28	3.8	1.2	1.9	0.4	25	8	18	0.46	0.056		28		0.05	0.04	0.3	07218
honey loaf (pork & beef)	35	19.7	4.4	1.5		0.0	370	5	5	0.68	0.008	0	0	0.13	0.9	0.30	0.18
1 oz slice	28	1.3	0.4	0.6	0.1	10	96	40	0.38	0.017	7.9	0	0.1	0.07	0.09	2.2	07035
honey roll sausage (beef)	42	14.9	4.3	0.5		0.0	304	2	4	0.75	0.009	0	0	0.02	1.0	0.54	0.11
.8 oz slice	23	2.4	0.9	1.1	0.1	12	67	32	0.51	0.023	3.6	0	<0.1	0.04	0.06	0.9	07088
kielbasa/kolbassy (pork & beef)	81	14.0	3.4	0.6		0.0	280	11	4	0.53	0.010	0	0	0.06	0.7	0.42	0.21
w/nfdm - .9 oz slice	26	7.1	2.6	3.4	0.8	17	70	38	0.38	0.026	4.6	0	0.1	0.06	0.05	1.3	07037
lebanon bologna (beef)	45	14.6	4.4	0.6	0.6	0.0	312	4	4	0.90	0.009	1	0	0.02	0.9	0.63	0.10
.8 oz slice	23	3.0	1.3	1.4	0.1	14	72	39	0.53	0.019	3.1	5	0.1	0.04	0.07	1.2	07039
liver cheese (pork liver)	116	20.4	5.8	0.8		0.0	466	3	5	1.41	0.076	1996	1	0.08	4.5	9.33	1.34
1.3 oz slice	38	9.7	3.4	4.7	1.3	66	86	79	4.12	0.146	13.9	6646		0.85	0.18	39.5	07040
pork fat wrapped, Oscar Mayer	114	20.4	5.9	0.8	0.5	0.0	430	3	5	1.50	0.074	1687	1	0.08	4.6	9.23	1.42
1.3 oz slice	38	9.7	3.5	4.9	1.3	79	82	89	4.79	0.198		8590		0.84	0.17	42.9	07220
liver pate,	57	18.6	3.8	1.9		0.0	109	3	4	0.61	0.046	62	3	0.01	2.1	2.29	0.74
chicken, cnd - 1 oz (2 T)	28	3.7	1.1	1.5	0.7	111	27	50	2.61	0.051	13.1	205	0.3	0.40	0.07	91.0	07053
goose, smoked, cnd	131	10.5	3.2	1.3		0.0	198	20	4	0.26	0.034	284	0	0.02	0.7	2.66	0.34
1 oz (~2T)	28	12.4	4.1	7.3	0.2	43	39	57	1.56	0.113	12.5	945		0.08	0.02	17.0	07054
truffle flavor	183	29.0	6.3	3.5			452	39	7	1.60	0.067	2523	1	0.02	1.8	1.79	0.67
2 oz	56	16.0	5.7	7.6	1.9	59	77	112	2.21	0.224	23.3	8400		0.34	0.03	33.6	07942
unspecified, cnd	90	15.3	4.0	0.4		0.0	198	20	4	0.81	0.034	281	1	0.01	0.9	0.91	0.34
1 oz (~2T)	28	7.9	2.7	3.5	0.9	72	39	57	1.56	0.113	11.8	936		0.17	0.02	17.0	07055
liverwurst/liver sausage (pork)	59	9.4	2.5	0.4		0.0	155	5	2	0.41	0.028	1495	0	0.05	0.8	2.42	0.53
.6 oz slice (2 1/2" dia, 1/4" thick)	18	5.1	1.9	2.4	0.5	28	31	44	1.15	0.043	10.4	4980		0.19	0.03	5.4	07041
liverwurst spread	166	29.4	6.8	3.2	0.9	1.4	385	12	7	1.27	0.085	2252	2	0.15	2.4	7.40	1.62
4 T	55	14.0	5.0	7.3	1.4	65	94	127	4.87	0.132	31.9	7500		0.57	0.10	16.5	07911
luncheon loaf, spiced, Oscar Mayer	66	16.4	3.8	2.0	1.3	0.0	343	31	7	0.55			0				
1 oz slice	28	4.7	1.5	2.1	0.8	19	76	55	0.38	0.647		0					07221
luxury loaf (pork)	39	19.1	5.2	1.4		0.0	343	10	6	0.85	0.011	0	0	0.20	1.0	0.38	0.14
1 oz slice	28	1.3	0.4	0.7	0.1	10	106	52	0.29	0.028	6.0	0		0.08	0.09	0.6	07060
macaroni & cheese loaf, chicken,	87	21.9	4.5	4.5	0.0	0.0	1	46	10	0.57	0.105	0	6	0.09	1.1	0.26	0.20
pork, & beef - 1 slice	38	5.7	2.1	2.9	0.6	17	119	66	0.46	0.042	8.7	0	<0.1	0.09	0.13	9.1	07940
mortadella (beef & pork)	47	7.8	2.5	0.5		0.0	187	3	2	0.32	0.005	0	0	0.02	0.4	0.22	0.07
.5 oz slice	15	3.8	1.4	1.7	0.5	8	24	15	0.21	0.009	3.4	0	<0.1	0.02	0.02	0.5	07050
mother's loaf (pork)	59	11.5	2.5	1.6		0.0	237	9	3	0.30	0.014	0	<1	0.12	0.7	0.22	0.10
.7 oz slice	21	4.7	1.7	2.2	0.5	9	47	27	0.28	0.019	7.4	0		0.04	0.04	1.7	07061
old fashioned loaf, Oscar Mayer	65	16.5	3.7	2.2	1.3	0.0	332	32	6	0.52			0				
1 oz slice	28	4.6	1.6	2.2	0.7	17	82	58	0.37	0.039		0					07222
olive loaf, chicken, pork, &	74	16.1	2.8	1.9	0.9	0.0	369	31	8	0.29			0				
turkey, Oscar Mayer - 1 oz slice	28	6.1	2.0	3.1	0.7	20	52	37	0.49	0.062		0					07223
pork	66	16.3	3.3	2.6		0.0	416	31	5	0.39	0.010	3	0	0.08	0.5	0.35	0.22
1 oz slice	28	4.6	1.6	2.2	0.5	11	83	36	0.15	0.014	4.6	56	0.1	0.07	0.06	0.6	07051

							Minerals					Vitamins					
	KCAL	H₂0 (g)	PRO (g)	CHO (g)	SUGR (g)	DFIB (g)	Na (mg)	Ca (mg)	Mg (mg)	Zn (mg)	Mn (mg)	A (mcg RAE)	C (mg)	B-1 (mg)	NIA (mg)	B-12 (mcg)	PANT (mg)
	WT (g)	FAT (g)	SFA (g)	MUFA (g)	PUFA (g)	CHOL (mg)	K (mg)	P (mg)	Fe (mg)	Cu (mg)	Se (mcg)	A (IU)	E (mg ATE)	B-2 (mg)	B-6 (mg)	FOL (mcg DFE)	REF
pastrami, beef, 98% fat-free	54	42.4	11.2	0.9	0.0	0.0	576	5	10	2.43	0.007	0	20	0.05	2.9	1.00	0.17
6 slices	57	0.7	0.0	0.3	<0.1	27	130	86	1.58	0.045	5.9	0	0.1	0.10	0.10	4.0	07925
peppered loaf (pork & beef)	41	18.9	4.8	1.3	1.3	0.0	426	15	6	0.90	0.034	0	0	0.11	0.9	0.6	0.15
1 oz slice	28	1.8	0.6	0.8	0.1	13	110	48	0.30	0.034	5.9	0	0.1	0.08	0.08	0.6	07056
pepperoni, pork & beef	27	1.5	1.2	0.2		0.0	112	1	1	0.14	0.002	0	0	0.02	0.3	0.14	0.10
.2 oz slice (1 3/8" dia, 1/8" thick)	6	2.4	0.9	1.2	0.2	4	19	7	0.08	0.004	1.3	0	<0.1	0.01	0.01	0.2	07057
turkey, Hormel Pillow Pak	73	14.4	9.3	1.1	0.0	0.0	557	8	12	1.29		5	0				
~1 oz	30	3.5	1.1	1.5	1.1	37	135		0.81	0.060		15				1.2	07278
pickle & pimento loaf, chicken, Oscar Mayer - 1 oz slice	75	15.6	2.7	2.5	1.9	0.0	357	31	8	0.33			0				
	28	6.0	2.0	2.9	0.8	22	49	42	0.61	0.078		0					07224
pork	73	16.0	3.2	1.7		0.0	389	27	5	0.39	0.008	1	0	0.08	0.6	0.33	0.22
1 oz slice	28	5.9	2.2	2.7	0.7	10	95	39	0.29	0.035	4.1	20	0.1	0.07	0.05	1.4	07058
picnic loaf (pork & beef)	65	16.9	4.2	1.3		0.0	326	13	4	0.61	0.008	0	0	0.10	0.6	0.42	0.19
1 oz slice	28	4.7	1.7	2.2	0.5	11	75	35	0.29	0.020	10.0	0		0.07	0.08	0.6	07062
pork & beef loaf, Dutch Brand	108	22.1	4.6	2.8		0.0	401	3	6	0.52	0.013	12	<1	0.16	1.6	0.28	0.26
1.3 oz slice	38	8.7	3.4	4.4	1.2	23	75	58	0.06	0.027	7.2	41	<0.1	0.07	0.10	1.9	07021
pork & beef lunch meat	201	28.1	7.2	1.3		0.0	737	5	8	0.95	0.017	0	0	0.18	1.6	0.73	0.36
2 oz slice	57	18.3	6.6	8.6	2.1	31	115	49	0.49	0.023	16.3	0	0.1	0.09	0.11	3.4	07047
pork & beef luncheon sausage	60	13.5	3.5	0.4		0.0	272	3	3	0.56	0.010	0	0	0.05	0.8	0.45	0.09
.8 oz slice (4" dia, 1/8" thick)	23	4.8	1.8	2.3	0.5	15	56	28	0.33	0.018	3.5	0		0.04	0.05	0.7	07090
New England Brand	37	15.4	4.0	1.1		0.0	281	2	4	0.62	0.008	0	0	0.15	0.8	0.31	0.16
.8 oz slice (4" dia, 1/8" thick)	23	1.7	0.6	0.8	0.2	11	74	31	0.22	0.023	4.4	0	<0.1	0.06	0.08	1.6	07091
pork lunch meat, cnd	70	10.8	2.6	0.4		0.0	271	1	2	0.31	0.005	0	<1	0.08	0.7	0.19	0.10
.7 oz slice	21	6.4	2.3	3.0	0.7	13	45	17	0.15	0.008	5.9	0	0.1	0.04	0.04	1.3	07045
poultry (chicken/turkey) salad spread - 1 oz (~2T)	57	18.8	3.3	2.1		0.0	107	3	3	0.29	0.003	12	<1	0.01	0.5	0.11	0.08
	28	3.8	1.0	0.9	1.8	9	52	9	0.17	0.009	3.1	39	0.6	0.02	0.03	1.4	07067
roast beef spread	127	35.2	8.7	2.1	0.4	0.1	413	13	14	3.47		0	<1	0.01	2.4	1.36	
4 T	57	9.3	3.6	3.2	0.2	40	148	66	1.17	0.058	12.9	1	0.1	0.13	0.09	4.6	07912
salami, beef	78	11.7	4.3	0.1	0.1	0.0	382	3	3	0.50	0.011	0	0	0.02	0.7	0.70	0.22
.8 oz slice (4" dia, 1/8" thick)	23	7.4	2.0	2.2	0.2	16	64	26	0.43	0.028	3.4	0	<0.1	0.04	0.04	0.5	07068
salami, beef & pork	58	13.9	3.2	0.5		0.0	245	3	3	0.49	0.013	0	0	0.05	0.8	0.84	0.20
.8 oz slice (4" dia, 1/8" thick)	23	4.6	1.9	2.1	0.5	15	46	26	0.61	0.053	3.4	0	<0.1	0.09	0.05	0.5	07069
salami, beef cotto, Oscar Mayer	95	29.7	6.5	0.9	0.5	0.0	602	3	8	0.96			0				
2 slices (1.6 oz)	46	7.2	3.1	3.2	0.4	38	95	103	1.25	0.106							07226
salami, beerwurst, beef	76	12.2	2.9	0.4		0.0	236	2	3	0.56	0.006	0	0	0.02	0.8	0.45	0.08
.8 oz slice (4" dia, 1/8" thick)	23	6.9	3.0	3.2	0.3	14	40	22	0.35	0.009	3.7	0	<0.1	0.03	0.04	0.7	07002
Oscar Mayer	104	28.9	6.2	0.9	0.5	0.0	566	4	8	0.94			0				
2 slices (1.6 oz)	46	8.4	2.9	4.1	0.9	32	98	106	0.54	0.110		0					07228
pork	55	14.1	3.3	0.5		0.0	285	2	3	0.40	0.007	0	0	0.13	0.7	0.20	0.11
.8 oz slice (4" dia, 1/8" thick)	23	4.3	1.4	2.1	0.5	14	58	24	0.17	0.012	4.8	0		0.04	0.08	0.7	07003
salami, cotto (beef, pork, chkn), Oscar Mayer - 2 slices (1.6 oz)	113	27.9	6.2	1.0	0.7	0.0	504	35	13	0.91			0				
	46	9.3	3.9	4.7	0.8	37	100	114	1.33	0.193		0					07227
salami, dry/hard, Oscar Mayer	99	10.3	7.0	0.4	0.1	0.0	534	3	6	0.85	0.011	1	0	0.15	1.4	0.51	0.29
3 slices (1 oz)	27	7.7	3.0	4.1	0.8	26	96	49	0.49	0.051		9		0.07	0.12	0.8	07230
pork	41	3.6	2.3	0.2		0.0	226	1	2	0.42	0.007	0	<0.1	0.03	0.06	0.2	0.11
.4 oz slice (3 1/8" dia, 1/16" thick)	10	3.4	1.2	1.6	0.4	8	38	23	0.13	0.016	2.5	0		0.03	0.06	0.2	07071
pork & beef	42	3.5	2.3	0.3		0.0	186	1	2	0.32	0.004	0	<0.1	0.06	0.5	0.19	0.11
.4 oz slice (3 1/8" dia, 1/16" thick)	10	3.4	1.2	1.7	0.3	8	38	14	0.15	0.008	2.6	0		0.03	0.05	0.2	07072
salami, genoa, Oscar Mayer	105	10.6	5.6	0.3	0.1	0.0	493	5	6	0.91	0.012		0	0.17	1.2	0.36	
3 slices (1 oz)	27	9.0	3.3	4.5	0.7	28	90	55	0.50	0.068		0		0.08	0.09		07229
salami, italian, pork - 1 oz	119	9.7	6.1	0.3	0.3	0.0	529	3	6	1.18	0.020	0	0	0.26	1.6	0.78	0.30
	28	10.4	3.7	5.1	1.0	22	95	64	0.43	0.045	7.1	0	0.1	0.09	0.15	0.6	07926
pork & beef, dry, sliced, 50% less Na - 5 slices	98	11.3	6.1	1.8	0.0	0.0	262	2	5	0.90	0.011	0	0	0.17	1.4	0.53	0.30
	28	7.4	2.7	3.7	0.6	25	106	40	0.42	0.022	7.3	0	0.1	0.08	0.14	0.6	07941
salami, pork & beef, less Na - 3.5 oz	399	33.7	15.0	6.6	6.2	0.2	623	94	31	3.08	0.057	4	1	0.74	4.8	1.76	0.86
	100	30.5	10.6	13.3	3.1	90	1372	272	1.55	0.088	14.6	12	0.2	0.34	0.49	8.0	07913
salami, turkey - 2 slices (2 oz)	112	37.5	9.3	0.3		0.0	572	11	9	1.03	0.007	0	0	0.04	2.0	0.12	0.29
	57	7.9	2.3	2.6	2.0	47	139	60	0.92	0.029	7.5	0	0.3	0.10	0.14	2.3	07070
cotto, Louis Rich	42	20.0	4.2	0.3	0.1	0.0	285	9	6	0.66			0				
1 oz	28	2.7	0.8	1.1	0.7	22	62	76	0.46	0.101							07267
Louis Rich	41	20.1	4.3	0.1	0.1	0.0	281	11	6	0.65			0				
1 oz	28	2.6	0.8	0.9	0.7	21	60	74	0.35	0.053		0					07266

	KCAL / WT (g)	H₂0 (g) / FAT (g)	PRO (g) / SFA (g)	CHO (g) / MUFA (g)	SUGR (g) / PUFA (g)	DFIB (g) / CHOL (mg)	Na (mg) / K (mg)	Ca (mg) / P (mg)	Mg (mg) / Fe (mg)	Zn (mg) / Cu (mg)	Mn (mg) / Se (mcg)	A (mcg RAE) / A (IU)	C (mg) / E (mg ATE)	B-1 (mg) / B-2 (mg)	NIA (mg) / B-6 (mg)	B-12 (mcg) / FOL (mcg DFE)	PANT (mg) / REF
sandwich spread,	67	17.1	2.2	3.4		0.1	287	3	2	0.29	0.007	1	0	0.05	0.5	0.32	0.12
pork & beef - 1 oz (~2T)	28	4.9	1.7	2.2	0.7	11	31	17	0.22	0.037	2.7	25	0.5	0.04	0.03	0.6	07073
pork, chicken, & beef, Oscar	71	17.8	2.0	4.6	2.4	0.1	246	8	4	0.26			0				
Mayer - 1 oz	30	5.0	1.7	2.2	0.7	14	35	21	0.24	0.054		30					07231
Spam, lite (pork & chicken), cnd,	107	36.8	8.5	0.8	0.7	0.0	578	22	10	1.23		0	22				
Hormel - 2 oz	56	7.8	2.5	3.9	0.8	42	258		0.78	0.056		0				1.7	07277
reg (pork & ham), cnd, Hormel	174	29.5	7.4	1.7		0.0	767	8	8	1.01		0	<1				
2 oz	56	15.3	5.5	7.7	1.7	39	128		0.50	0.056		0				1.7	07276
swisswurst, pork & beef w/swiss	236	42.6	9.8	1.8	0.0	0.0	637	57	10	1.73	0.025	77	0	0.19	2.2	1.33	0.59
cheese, smoked - 2.7 oz	77	21.1	8.1	10.5	2.3	47	159	137	0.55	0.054	5.8	257	0.1	0.12	0.10	2.3	07920
thuringer (cervelat),	77	11.7	3.6	0.1		0.0	286	3	3	0.59	0.011	0	0	0.03	1.0	1.27	0.23
beef & pork - .8 oz slice	23	6.8	2.8	3.0	0.3	17	62	26	0.58	0.035	4.7	0	<0.1	0.08	0.06	0.5	07078
beef, Oscar Mayer	142	24.2	6.7	0.9	0.5	0.0	655	4	7	1.08	0.015	0	0	0.07	2.0	2.53	
2 slices (1.6 oz)	46	12.4	5.4	5.9	0.5	37	107	56	1.15	0.087				0.15	0.12	2.3	07237
Oscar Mayer	140	24.5	6.9	0.4	0.2	0.0	658	4	7	0.98	0.014	0	0	0.11	2.0	1.73	0.25
2 slices (1.6 oz)	46	12.3	4.9	5.6	1.0	39	105	60	1.03	0.078				0.13	0.14	2.3	07238
turkey breast	23	15.1	4.7	0.0		0.0	301	1	4	0.24	0.003	0	0	0.01	1.7	0.42	0.12
.7 oz slice (3 1/2" sq)	21	0.3	0.1	0.1	0.1	9	58	48	0.08	0.011	6.5	0	<0.1	0.02	0.08	0.8	07079
roasted, fat free, Louis Rich	24	21.4	4.2	1.3	0.5	0.0	334	3	8	0.24			0				
1 oz	28	0.2	0.1	0.1	<0.1	9	57	65	0.31	0.070		0					07259
turkey breast, smoked,	52	41.4	10.8	1.2	0.3	0.0	721	9	15	0.49			0				
fat free, Louis Rich - 2 oz	56	0.4	0.1	0.1	0.1	23	161	169	0.63	0.112		0					07262
fat free, Oscar Mayer	42	40.3	7.7	1.9	0.6	0.0	569	5	16	0.44			0				
4 slices (1.8 oz)	52	0.3	0.1	0.1	0.1	16	113	126	0.40	0.135		0					07239
lemon pepper flvr, 97% fat free	27	20.6	5.9	0.4	0.0	0.0	325						0				
1 slice	28	0.2	0.1	0.1	0.1	13						0					07943
Louis Rich	42	33.4	8.9	0.7	0.1	0.0	540	7	14	0.43			0				
2 slices (1.6 oz)	45	0.5	0.1	0.1	0.1	19	140	143	0.66	0.077		0					07261
turkey, ham (cured thigh meat)	73	40.7	10.8	0.2		0.0	568	6	9	1.68	0.009	0	0	0.03	2.0	0.14	0.48
2 slices	57	2.9	1.0	0.7	0.9	32	185	109	1.57	0.063	20.5	0	0.4	0.14	0.14	3.4	07080
10% water added, Louis Rich	32	20.5	5.1	0.3	0.3	0.0	316	1	6	0.73			0				
1 oz	28	1.1	0.3	0.3	0.2	19	81	82	0.36	0.070		0					07264
turkey, honey roasted, fat free,	57	40.3	10.8	2.5	2.2	0.0	661	8	16	0.56			0				
Louis Rich - 2 oz	56	0.4	0.1	0.1	0.1	22	147	155	0.62	0.123		0					07258
turkey pastrami	80	40.3	10.5	0.9		0.0	596	5	8	1.23	0.007	0	0	0.03	2.0	0.14	0.33
2 slices	57	3.5	1.0	1.2	0.9	31	148	114	0.95	0.029	9.2	0	0.1	0.14	0.15	2.9	07052
turkey roll, light & dark meat	85	40.0	10.3	1.2		0.0	334	18	10	1.14	0.007	0	0	0.05	2.7	0.13	0.32
2 slices	57	4.0	1.2	1.3	1.0	31	154	96	0.77	0.040	16.6	0	0.2	0.16	0.15	2.9	07082
light meat	84	40.8	10.7	0.3		0.0	279	23	9	0.89	0.007	0	0	0.05	4.0	0.14	0.24
2 slices	57	4.1	1.2	1.4	1.0	25	143	104	0.73	0.023	12.7	0	0.1	0.13	0.18	2.3	07081
turkey, smoked, sliced, Carl Buddig	91	38.9	10.0	1.0		0.0	625	34						0.10	3.3		
2 oz	57	5.2	1.8		1.5	32	188		1.05					0.18			07273
yachtwurst w/pistachio nuts	150	32.6	8.3	0.8	0.0	0.0	524	11					0	0			
2 oz	56	12.7	4.4			36			0.56				0				07930

20.3 MEAT-BASED SNACKS

	KCAL / WT (g)	H₂0 (g) / FAT (g)	PRO (g) / SFA (g)	CHO (g) / MUFA (g)	SUGR (g) / PUFA (g)	DFIB (g) / CHOL (mg)	Na (mg) / K (mg)	Ca (mg) / P (mg)	Mg (mg) / Fe (mg)	Zn (mg) / Cu (mg)	Mn (mg) / Se (mcg)	A (mcg RAE) / A (IU)	C (mg) / E (mg ATE)	B-1 (mg) / B-2 (mg)	NIA (mg) / B-6 (mg)	B-12 (mcg) / FOL (mcg DFE)	PANT (mg) / REF
bacon & beef sticks	146	6.0	8.1	0.2	0.2	0.0	398	4	5	0.90	0.011	0	0	0.17	1.4	0.53	0.30
1 oz	28	12.4	4.5	6.1	1.2	29	108	40	0.52	0.022	7.3	0	0.1	0.08	0.14	0.6	07921
beef, dried	35	11.9	6.1	0.3		0.0	729	1	7	1.10	0.009	0	0	0.02	1.1	0.56	0.13
5 slices (.7 oz)	21	0.8	0.3	0.3	<0.1	9	93	37	0.95	0.034	13.0	0	<0.1	0.04	0.07	2.3	13350
beef jerky, chopped & formed	82	4.7	6.6	2.2		0.4	443	4	10	1.62	0.022	0	0	0.03	0.3	0.20	0.03
1 large piece (.7 oz)	20	5.1	2.2	2.3	0.2	10	119	81	1.08	0.045	2.1	0	0.1	0.03	0.04	26.8	19002
beef sticks, smoked	110	3.8	4.3	1.1			296	14	4	0.48	0.017	3	1	0.03	0.9	0.20	0.07
.7 oz stick	20	9.9	4.2	4.1	0.9	27	51	36	0.68	0.026		50		0.09	0.04	0.20	19407
pork skins	155	0.5	17.4	0.0		0.0	521	9	3	0.16	0.020	11	<1	0.03	0.4	0.18	0.12
1 oz	28	8.9	3.2	4.2	1.0	27	36	24	0.25	0.027	11.6	37	0.2	0.08	0.01	0.0	19041
barbecue	153	0.6	16.4	0.5			756	12	0	0.20	0.021	18	<1	0.02	1.0	0.04	0.12
1 oz	28	9.0	3.3	4.3	1.0	33	51	62	0.29	0.099		189		0.12	0.04	8.8	19408
summer sausage sticks, pork & beef	121	10.3	5.5	0.5	0.0	0.1	420	23	4	0.64	0.009	64	0	0.07	0.8	0.49	0.22
w/cheddar cheese - 1 oz	28	10.7	3.0	3.9	0.9	25	58	50	0.64	0.020	2.1	212	<0.1	0.05	0.04	2.0	07918

	KCAL	H₂0 (g)	PRO (g)	CHO (g)	SUGR (g)	DFIB (g)	Na (mg)	Ca (mg)	Mg (mg)	Zn (mg)	Mn (mg)	A (mcg RAE)	C (mg)	B-1 (mg)	NIA (mg)	B-12 (mcg)	PANT (mg)
	WT (g)	FAT (g)	SFA (g)	MUFA (g)	PUFA (g)	CHOL (mg)	K (mg)	P (mg)	Fe (mg)	Cu (mg)	Se (mcg)	A (IU)	E (mg ATE)	B-2 (mg)	B-6 (mg)	FOL (mcg DFE)	REF

21. MEAT SUBSTITUTES & SOY PRODUCTS
21.1 MEAT SUBSTITUTES

	KCAL/WT	H₂O/FAT	PRO/SFA	CHO/MUFA	SUGR/PUFA	DFIB/CHOL	Na/K	Ca/P	Mg/Fe	Zn/Cu	Mn/Se	A-RAE/A-IU	C/E	B-1/B-2	NIA/B-6	B-12/FOL	PANT/REF
bacon, simulated meat product	50	7.8	1.7	1.0		0.4	234	4	3	0.07	0.033	1	0	0.70	1.2	0.00	0.02
3 strips (.6 oz)	16	4.7	0.7	1.1	2.5	0	27	11	0.39	0.017	1.2	14	1.1	0.08	0.08	6.7	16104
Beef Style, smoked, Worthington	135	30.2	11.2	6.7	2.0	0.6	507	21		0.44			0	2.21	6.6	2.31	
2 oz	57	7.0	1.0	1.8	3.8	<1	186		2.60			0		0.25	0.45		WRTH1
Big Franks, cnd, Loma Linda/	118	29.4	12.1	1.5	0.2	1.5	224	10		1.20				0.28	5.8	2.94	1.61
Worthington - 1.8 oz frank	51	7.1	0.8	1.5	3.7	0	61	85	0.99					0.68	0.67		22126
Bolono, Worthington	83	38.1	11.0	2.8	0.7	2.0	656	38		0.51			0	0.32	3.3	0.86	
2 oz	57	3.1	0.8	1.0	1.6	1	104	95	1.80			0		0.09	0.36		WRTH5
bratwurst, frzn, Boca	130		11.0	3.0	1.0	2.0	870	20					0				
2.5 oz bratwurst	71	7.0	0.5			0			1.44			0					BOCA1
Breakfast Links,	90		10.0	5.0	3.0	2.0	380	80					0				
frzn, Boca - 2 links (1.6 oz)	45	3.0	0.0			0			1.44			0					BOCA2
frzn, Morningstar Farms	78	28.8	8.7	3.1	0.4	1.8	302	12		0.39			0	0.36	7.6	3.32	
1.6 oz link	45	3.4	0.3	0.8	1.5	1	49		1.74			0		0.15	0.50		WRTH6
Breakfast Patty,	80		8.0	5.0	1.0	3.0	260	60					0				
frzn, Boca - 1.3 oz patty	38	4.0	0.0			0			1.44			0					BOCA3
frzn, Morningstar Farms	79	20.4	9.9	3.7	0.6	2.0	259	18	1	0.37	0.010		0	5.38	1.8	1.50	0.07
1.3 oz patty	38	2.8	0.5	0.7	1.3	1	102	106	1.92	0.010		0	0.3	0.13	0.19		22122
Natural Touch	78	21.4	8.2	4.1	0.6	1.5	247	12		0.63			0				
1.3 oz patty	38	3.2	0.4	0.9	1.7	1	162		0.87			0					WRTH8
Breakfast Strips, frzn, Morningstar	56	6.7	2.0	2.3	0.1	0.9	234	7		0.09			0	0.67	0.8	0.54	
Farms - .6 oz strip	16	4.4	0.7	1.0	2.6	<1	16	46	0.17			0		0.05	0.09		WRTH11
buffalo wings, meatless, frzn,	208	42.2	12.2	18.3	1.8	2.6	634	33		0.66			0	0.33	2.8	3.07	
Morningstar Farms - 3 oz	85	9.5	1.3	2.3	5.0	2	297		2.91			22		0.21	0.37		WRTH12
burger, all am classic, frzn, Boca	110		14.0	6.0	0.0	4.0	370	150					0				
2.5 oz patty	71	4.0	1.0			<5			1.80			0					BOCA4
burger, Better 'n Burgers, frzn,	91	60.6	13.9	7.5	0.5	4.3	383	87	16	0.75	0.224		0	0.26	4.1	0.00	1.13
Morningstar Farms - 3 oz patty	85	0.5	0.1	0.3	0.2	0	434	181	2.90	0.239		0	<0.1	0.55	0.20	245.7	22121
Burger Crumbles, frzn, Morningstar	116	33.1	11.1	3.3	0.6	2.5	238	40	1	0.82	0.048		0	4.96	1.5	2.18	<0.01
Farms - 1/2 cup (~2 oz)	55	6.5	1.6	2.3	2.5	0	89	87	3.20	0.051		0	0.3	0.18	0.27		22120
burger, grilled vegetable, frzn,	80		13.0	6.0	<1.0	5.0	300	100					2				
Boca - 2.5 oz patty	71	1.0	0.0			0			1.80			0					BOCA5
burger, Grillers, frzn,	140	35.6	15.2	5.5	0.8	2.0	273	39		0.79			0	11.00	4.1	2.89	
Mrngstr Frms - 2.3 oz patty	64	6.3	1.1	1.6	3.2	2	116	119	2.66			0		0.25	0.52		WRTH64
burger, Grillers Prime, frzn,	160	39.7	16.9	4.2	0.1	2.0	365	25		0.87			0	0.23			
Mrngstr Frms - 2.5 oz patty	71	8.4	1.0	3.6	3.8	1	159		1.44			0		0.15			WRTH63
burger, ground, frzn, Boca	70		11.0	7.0	0.0	4.0	220	80					0				
1/2 cup (2 oz)	57	0.5	0.0			0			1.44			0					BOCA6
burger, Harvest Burger, frzn, Green	138	58.5	18.0	7.0		5.7	411	102	70	8.07			0	0.32	6.3	0.00	
Giant - 3.2 oz patty	90	4.1	1.0	2.1	0.3	0	432	225	3.85	0.441	9.0	0	1.6	0.20	0.39	21.6	22125
burger, Harvest Original,	139	57.6	17.3	8.6	0.4	4.4	345	68		7.91			4	0.18	7.7	1.39	0.72
Morningstar Farms - 3.2 oz patty	90	3.9	1.6	2.4	0.4	<1	454	214	3.68			130		0.19	0.39		WRTH13
burger, original vegan, frzn, Boca	90		13.0	6.0	0.0	4.0	350	80					0				
2.5 oz patty	71	1.0	0.0			0			1.80			0					BOCA7
burger, portabella & rstd peppers,	117	40.4	11.0	9.6	1.6	3.0	463	29		0.71			3	0.00			
frzn, Mrngstr Frms - 2.4 oz patty	67	3.9	0.5	1.0	2.1	2	253	135	1.21			0		0.09			WRTH14
burger, rstd garlic, frzn, Boca	100		14.0	7.0	<1.0	5.0	400	100					1				
2.5 oz patty	71	2.0	0.5			<5			1.80			0					BOCA8
burger, rstd onion, frzn, Boca	90		13.0	8.0	<1.0	5.0	460	80					1				
2.5 oz patty	71	1.0	0.0			0			1.80			0					BOCA9
burger, salsa, frzn, Boca	90																
2.5 oz patty	71	1.0	0.0			<5											BOCA10
burger, spicy black bean, frzn,	115	47.1	11.8	15.2	1.4	4.8	499	56	44	0.93	0.850		0	8.06	0.0	0.07	0.41
Morningstar Farms - 2.8 oz patty	78	0.8	0.2	0.2	0.4	1	269	150	1.84	0.172		139	0.4	0.14	0.21		22123
burger, tex mex, frzn, Natural Touch	118	41.4	9.1	17.3	4.1	1.8	323	28		0.91			1				
2.5 oz patty	71	1.4	0.2	0.4	0.7	1	296		1.85			0					WRTH16
burger, thai, frzn, Natural Touch	103	43.9	10.0	7.4	1.2	2.8	403	25		0.67				0.01			
2.4 oz patty	67	3.8	0.4	0.9	1.7	1	309		1.49			114		0.18			WRTH17

	KCAL	H₂0 (g)	PRO (g)	CHO (g)	SUGR (g)	DFIB (g)	Na (mg)	Ca (mg)	Mg (mg)	Zn (mg)	Mn (mg)	A (mcg RAE)	C (mg)	B-1 (mg)	NIA (mg)	B-12 (mcg)	PANT (mg)
	WT (g)	FAT (g)	SFA (g)	MUFA (g)	PUFA (g)	CHOL (mg)	K (mg)	P (mg)	Fe (mg)	Cu (mg)	Se (mcg)	A (IU)	E (mg ATE)	B-2 (mg)	B-6 (mg)	FOL (mcg DFE)	REF
burger, tom & basil pizza, frzn,	128	40.8	10.5	7.8	1.8	3.2	259	67		0.79			21	0.00			
Morningstar Farms - *2.4 oz patty*	67	6.1	1.6	1.4	2.1	7	229		1.41			268		0.21			WRTH18
burger, vegan, frzn, Natural Touch	91	60.6	13.9	7.5	0.5	4.3	383	87	16	0.75	0.224	0	0	0.26	4.1	0.00	1.13
3 oz patty	85	0.5	0.1	0.3	0.2	0	434	181	2.90	0.239		0	<0.1	0.55	0.20	245.7	22128
burger, Vege-Burger, Loma	63	39.7	12.2	2.1	0.5	1.5	132	9		0.72		0		0.12	0.7	3.60	0.32
Linda - *1.9 oz patty*	55	0.7	0.1	0.1	0.4	0	40	44	0.62			0		0.10	0.25		WRTH109
burger, Veggie Patty, garden,	108	41.5	11.9	9.2	1.2	2.2	426	15		0.70		0	7.50	0.0			
frzn, Mrngstr Frms - *2.4 oz patty*	67	2.6	0.5	0.6	1.4	2	142	110	1.19			182		0.08			WRTH114
burger, vegetarian, frzn,	61	39.0	10.1	3.5	0.3	1.5	263	5		0.66		0		0.13	1.0	3.05	
Worthington - *1.9 oz patty*	55	1.6	0.3	0.3	1.0	0	17	54	1.27			0		0.11	0.21		WRTH20
Chicken Style, Worthington	91	38.1	9.7	2.3	0.3	0.9	245	295		0.46				0.42	4.5	2.14	
2 oz	57	4.7	0.7	1.0	2.6	<1	260		2.68			0		0.15	0.31		WRTH21
Chicken Supreme, Loma Linda	89	1.4	15.2	6.2	0.6	3.5	671	41		0.58				0.53	4.1	1.75	1.57
.9 oz	26	0.3	0.1	0.1	0.1	<1	398	136	1.54			0		0.29	0.30		WRTH22
Chic-Ketts, Worthington	112	31.9	14.3	2.5	0.5	2.5	406	12		0.73				0.08	2.5	1.26	
1.9 oz	55	5.0	0.8	1.2	3.0	<1	42	71	1.71			0		0.13	0.11		WRTH23
Chick'n patty, spicy, frzn, Boca	150		13.0	12.0	1.0	2.0	470	60					0				
2.5 oz patty	71	6.0	0.5			<5			1.08			0					BOCA11
Chik, diced, Worthington	50	41.8	9.5	2.1	0.2	0.8	216	29		0.41				0.13	2.7	1.71	
1.9 oz piece	55	0.4	0.0	0.0	0.0	1	130		1.91			0		0.15	0.17		WRTH27
sliced, Worthington	82	68.4	15.5	3.5	0.3	1.3	353	47		0.67				0.21	4.4	2.80	
3.2 oz piece	90	0.7	0.0	0.0	0.0	1	212		3.13			0		0.25	0.27		WRTH28
Chik Nuggets, frzn, Morningstar	184	45.7	13.3	17.6	1.7	4.1	615	17		0.83				0.65	2.6	1.55	
Farms - *3 oz*	86	6.7	0.6	1.1	2.7	1	301		1.35			0		0.19	0.24		WRTH25
Loma Linda	255	39.9	13.6	12.8	0.9	11.1	402	39		0.59				0.83	7.0	4.96	2.22
3 oz	85	16.6	2.2	4.3	8.2	1	211		1.97			0		0.54	0.95		WRTH24
Chik Patty, frzn, Morningstar Farms	150	39.5	9.7	13.4	1.4	2.9	488	26		0.57				0.78	2.3	2.47	
2.5 oz patty	71	6.3	0.7	1.3	2.6	1	209		0.99			0		0.12	0.18		WRTH26
Chik'n, fried w/gravy, Loma Linda	153	52.1	12.0	4.9	0.5	2.0	425	32		0.46				0.63	5.3	3.23	0.39
2.8 oz	80	9.4	1.4	2.4	4.8	1	72		2.48			0		0.27	0.32		WRTH29
Chik'n Nuggets, frzn, Boca	190		16.0	16.0	2.0	2.0	570	80					0				
4 nuggets (3.1 oz)	87	7.0	2.0			0			1.80			0					BOCA12
Chik'n patty, original, frzn, Boca	150		13.0	12.0	1.0	2.0	470	60					0				
2.5 oz patty	71	6.0	0.5			<5			1.08			0					BOCA13
Chik'n, rstd herb, Natural Touch	110	39.8	12.8	8.9	1.0	2.2	355	27		0.85				0.49			
2.4 oz	67	2.5	0.3	0.9	0.8	<1	218		1.64			0		0.21			WRTH30
ChikStiks, Worthington	105	26.6	9.9	3.6	0.4	2.0	293	23		0.44				0.67	7.1	2.75	
1.7 oz	47	5.6	0.8	1.2	2.8	1	100		2.69			0		0.21	0.49		WRTH31
chili, low fat, Worthington	166	185.8	15.2	23.9	2.7	7.1	890	37		1.41				0.12	0.0	0.00	
8.1 oz	230	1.1	0.2	0.2	0.5	0	569	236	2.46			758		0.13	0.30		WRTH32
vegetarian, Natural Touch	176	182.1	16.4	25.6	3.9	12.6	1144	40		0.61				0.00	0.0	0.00	
8.1 oz	230	0.9	0.2	0.2	0.5	1	645	237	3.68			469		0.15			WRTH33
Worthington	287	166.9	23.9	25.1	3.0	7.9	1078	42		1.91				0.29	2.3	3.75	0.16
8.1 oz	230	10.1	1.6	2.0	6.6	0	306	177	0.76			193		0.19	0.85		WRTH34
Choplets, Worthington	95	68.2	17.8	3.7	0.4	2.6	509	8		0.96				0.02	0.0	0.00	
3.2 oz piece	92	0.9	0.1	0.1	0.5	0	23	70	0.30			0		0.05	0.06		WRTH35
corn dog, frzn, MeatFree,	162	34.6	8.1	22.5	5.8	1.4	486	9		0.32				0.11	0.0	0.00	
Mrngstr Frms - *2.5 oz corn dog*	71	4.4	0.8	1.4	2.5	0	63	111	0.67			0		0.23	0.04		WRTH36
Loma Linda	162	34.6	8.1	22.5	5.8	1.4	486	9		0.32				0.11	0.0	0.00	
2.5 oz dog	71	4.4	0.8	1.4	2.5	0	63	111	0.67			0		0.23	0.04		WRTH39
mini, frzn, MeatFree, Mrngstr	172	37.1	10.4	22.0	4.1	1.6	543	18		0.60				0.24			
Frms - *2.7 oz corn dog*	76	4.7	0.5	1.9	1.3	<1	86	134	0.48			0		0.15			WRTH37
veggie, Natural Touch	156	35.2	8.2	22.2	4.7	2.7	533	10		0.60				0.29			
2.5 oz corn dog	71	3.8	0.5	0.9	2.0	0	72	81	2.04			0		0.14			WRTH38
Corned Beef Style, Worthington	143	30.6	10.5	5.5	1.4	0	466	19		0.48				13.13	5.5	2.06	
2 oz	57	8.7	1.3	2.0	4.8	<1	133		2.59			0		0.23	0.38		WRTH40
Country Stew, Worthington	205	196.6	12.9	18.6	2.8	3.7	742	34		1.17				1.94	5.2	3.67	
8.5 oz	240	8.8	0.9	1.7	4.2	1	264	151	3.95			2158		0.19	0.89		WRTH41
Crispy Chik patty, Worthington	151	38.6	9.8	15.0	1.1	1.1	396	32		0.54				2.37	4.2	2.21	
2.5 oz patty	71	5.8	0.7	1.4	2.9	1	172		1.97			0		0.19	0.29		WRTH42
Cutlets, Worthington	68	44.0	12.6	2.8	0.3	2.1	279	4		0.69				0.01	0.0	0.00	
2.2 oz piece	61	0.7	0.1	0.1	0.5	0	23	39	0.27			0		0.01	0.04		WRTH43

	KCAL / WT (g)	H₂0 (g) / FAT (g)	PRO (g) / SFA (g)	CHO (g) / MUFA (g)	SUGR (g) / PUFA (g)	DFIB (g) / CHOL (mg)	Na (mg) / K (mg)	Ca (mg) / P (mg)	Mg (mg) / Fe (mg)	Zn (mg) / Cu (mg)	Mn (mg) / Se (mcg)	A (mcg RAE) / A (IU)	C (mg) / E (mg ATE)	B-1 (mg) / B-2 (mg)	NIA (mg) / B-6 (mg)	B-12 (mcg) / FOL (mcg DFE)	PANT (mg) / REF
Deli Franks, frzn, Morningstar Farms	112	23.2	10.4	3.7	0.9	2.7	431	17	4	0.38	0.008		0	0.14	0.0	0.01	0.02
1.6 oz frank	45	6.2	0.9	2.0	3.3	<1	50	42	0.61	0.012		0	1.3	0.02	0.01		22119
Dinner Cuts, cnd, Loma Linda	70	49.4	13.0	2.8	0.3	1.6	333	7		0.69			0	0.01	0.0	0.00	0.05
2.4 oz piece	67	0.8	0.4	0.2	0.2	0	26	49	0.94			0		0.05	0.03		WRTH44
Dinner Roast, Worthington	181	52.4	13.6	5.8	1.1	2.6	570	39		0.78			0	2.13	6.6	1.48	
3 oz	85	11.5	2.1	4.6	4.8	1	128	112	2.28			0		0.26	0.60		WRTH45
english muffin w/egg & patty, frzn, Mrngstar Farms	239	86.3	21.8	31.9	4.1	5.3	650	135		1.31			0	6.83	9.3	1.32	1.38
5.2 oz sandwich	146	2.7				3	282	324	4.07			227		0.76	0.10		WRTH9
english muffin w/egg, patty, & chs, frzn, Mrngstr Frms	273	101.5	28.4	33.4	5.0	6.8	998	147		2.45			0	4.33	7.5	1.32	1.38
6 oz sandwich	171	2.9				6	307	532	2.03			273		0.74	0.10		WRTH10
Fillets, Worthington	189	46.9	16.6	10.1	0.9	4.5	642	54		1.09			0	0.44	10.6	2.75	
3 oz	85	9.2	1.8	3.3	4.1	1	132	128	2.10			0		0.14	0.36		WRTH48
FriChik, low fat, Worthington	84	65.5	11.9	3.5	0.0	0.9	355	18		0.59			0	0.26	5.6	3.94	
3 oz	85	2.4	0.4	0.7	1.3	<1	177		3.82			0		0.18	0.29		WRTH49
Worthington	144	63.6	12.3	3.6	0.1	0.9	343	44		0.59			0	0.20	3.2	2.66	
3.2 oz piece	90	9.0	1.1	2.1	4.7	1	180		3.05			0		0.18	0.19		WRTH50
FriPats, Worthington	133	36.5	15.2	5.0	0.9	1.8	338	66		0.78			0	2.70	7.8	1.08	
2.3 oz	64	5.8	0.9	1.4	3.3	2	117	120	3.05			0		0.19	0.65		WRTH51
Garden Vege Patties, frzn, Morningstar Farms	119	40.1	11.2	10.2	0.8	4.0	382	48	29	0.58	0.336		0	6.47	0.0	0.00	1.20
2.4 oz patty	67	3.8	0.5	1.1	2.2	1	180	124	1.21	0.429	30.6	766	1.0	0.10	0.00	28.8	22118
frzn, Natural Touch	119	40.1	11.2	10.2	0.8	4.0	382	48	29	0.58	0.336		0	6.47	0.0	0.00	1.20
2.4 oz patty	67	3.8	0.5	1.1	2.2	1	180	124	1.21	0.429		766	1.0	0.10	0.00		22127
Golden Croquettes, Worthington	212	43.3	14.7	14.1	2.9	2.3	521	37		0.79			0	0.66	6.8	1.57	
3 oz	85	10.8	1.5	2.7	5.7	1	141		1.96			0		0.22	0.49		WRTH52
gravy mix, brown, Natural Touch	19	0.5	0.7	3.8			349	4		0.06			0	0.20			
.2 oz	6	0.1				0	13		0.24			0		0.02			WRTH53
chicken style, Natural Touch	18	0.5	1.1	3.2			430	2		0.11			0	0.04			
.2 oz	6	0.1				<1	33		0.32			0		0.02			WRTH54
country style, Natural Touch	21	0.5	0.6	3.6			347	1		0.05			0	0.05			
.2 oz	6	0.5				0	11		0.26			0		0.02			WRTH55
mushroom, Natural Touch	16	0.4	0.7	2.8			290	3		0.08			0	0.05			
.2 oz	5	0.2				<1	32		0.41			0		0.04			WRTH56
onion, Natural Touch	16	0.4	0.6	2.9			270	2		0.09			0	0.05			
.2 oz	5	0.2				<1	32		0.24			0		0.03			WRTH57
Gravy Quik, brown, Loma Linda	19	0.5	0.7	3.8			349	4		0.06			0	0.20			
.2 oz	6	0.1				0	13		0.24			0		0.02			WRTH58
chicken style, Loma Linda	18	0.5	1.1	3.2			430	2		0.11			0	0.04			
.2 oz	6	0.1				<1	33		0.32			0		0.02			WRTH59
country style, Loma Linda	21	0.5	0.6	3.6			347	1		0.05			0	0.05			
.2 oz	6	0.5				0	11		0.26			0		0.02			WRTH60
mushroom, Loma Linda	16	0.4	0.7	2.8			290	3		0.08			0	0.05			
.2 oz	5	0.2				<1	33		0.41			0		0.04			WRTH61
onion, Loma Linda	16	0.4	0.6	2.9			270	2		0.09			0	0.05			
.2 oz	5	0.2				<1	32		0.24			0		0.03			WRTH62
Ground Meatless, frzn, Morningstar Farms - *1.9 oz*	61	39.3	10.4	3.7	0.5	1.9	254	22		0.75			0	0.46	6.4	2.13	
	55	0.5	0.1	0.1	0.3	0	134	109	0.69			0		0.12	0.36		WRTH65
Leanies, Worthington	100	21.8	7.8	2.5	0.5	1.5	431	29		0.33			0	0.13	0.7	0.84	
1.4 oz	40	6.6	1.3	2.9	3.5	1	40	83	0.75			0		0.05	0.18		WRTH67
Lentil Rice Loaf, Natural Touch	162	57.3	7.9	15.8	1.3	2.8	323	17		1.24			0	0.05	0.0	0.07	
3.2 oz	90	7.4	1.1	1.3	4.7	2	130	207	1.30			0		0.20	0.03		WRTH68
Linketts, cnd, Loma Linda	73	21.4	7.5	1.6	0.1	1.0	143	4		0.53			0	0.11	1.2	1.83	0.71
1.2 oz link	35	4.1	0.6	1.0	2.5	<1	20	40	0.42			0		0.23	0.30		WRTH69
Little Links, cnd, Loma Linda	102	27.6	8.9	2.5	0.4	1.9	217	9		0.59			0	0.18	1.3	1.71	1.00
1.6 oz link	46	6.2	0.9	1.7	3.6	<1	26	47	0.46			0		0.51	0.46		WRTH70
meat extender, simulated meat product - *1 oz*	89	2.1	10.8	10.9		5.0	3	58	61	0.63	0.077	1	0	0.20	6.2	1.70	0.42
	28	0.8	0.1	0.2	0.5	0	539	181	3.40	0.086	2.1	9		0.25	0.38	56.1	16106
meatballs, veggie, frzn, Morningstar Farms - *3 oz*	233	40.0	23.1	8.7	1.8	2.4	616	42		1.19			0	0.87	4.0	3.29	1.24
	86	11.7	1.4	2.6	5.1	1	198		2.06			0		0.34	0.50		WRTH71
Multigrain Cutlets, Worthington	73	48.6	12.1	4.2	0.2	3.4	274	7		0.84			0	0.02	0.0	0.00	
2.5 oz	72	0.9	0.4	0.1	0.4	0	23	61	0.64			0		0.02	0.03		WRTH72
	99	67.5	16.7	5.6	0.3	2.9	350	9		1.07			0	0.03	0.0	0.00	
3.2 oz cutlet	92	1.2	0.4	0.2	0.5	0	29	79	0.82			0		0.03	0.04		WRTH73

	KCAL / WT (g)	H₂0 (g) / FAT (g)	PRO (g) / SFA (g)	CHO (g) / MUFA (g)	SUGR (g) / PUFA (g)	DFIB (g) / CHOL (mg)	Na (mg) / K (mg)	Ca (mg) / P (mg)	Mg (mg) / Fe (mg)	Zn (mg) / Cu (mg)	Mn (mg) / Se (mcg)	A (mcg RAE) / A (IU)	C (mg) / E (mg ATE)	B-1 (mg) / B-2 (mg)	NIA (mg) / B-6 (mg)	B-12 (mcg) / FOL (mcg DFE)	PANT (mg) / REF
Nine Bean Loaf, Natural Touch	154	59.3	8.2	15.0	1.6	4.3	319	34		1.01			1	0.04	0.0		
3.2 oz	91	6.8	1.2	2.3	3.3	2	208	184	0.84			476		0.15			WRTH74
Numete, Worthington	136	31.7	6.6	5.8	1.1	2.3	284	11		0.67			0	0.13	2.0	0.26	
1.9 oz	55	9.6	2.4	4.4	2.7	0	165	100	1.28			0		0.04	0.20		WRTH75
Nuteena, Loma Linda	79	33.5	11.8	2.5	0.2	0.8	245	9		1.28			0	0.19	7.7	1.14	1.36
1.9 oz	55	2.4	0.3	0.6	1.5	<1	51	70	0.74			0		0.41	0.14		WRTH76
Ocean Platter, Loma Linda	90	1.5	14.0	7.8	0.6	3.6	412	52		0.56			0	2.79	2.6	1.61	1.44
1.1 oz	31	0.3	0.1	0.1	0.2	1	414	157	1.40			0		0.18	0.40		WRTH77
Okara Patty, Natural Touch	118	39.3	11.9	6.1	0.8	2.8	300	19		0.85			0				
2.3 oz patty	64	5.1	0.5	2.9	1.4	1	243		1.22			0				WRTH78
Patty Mix, Loma Linda	92	1.2	14.2	7.5	0.4	4.3	559	50		0.52			0	0.53	1.7	5.51	1.65
.9 oz	26	0.5	0.1	0.2	0.2	1	419	155	1.67			0		0.22	0.49		WRTH79
pizza, veggie supreme, frzn, Morningstar Farms - 4.6 oz	283	67.3	13.0	38.9	3.9	3.9	523	65		1.28				0.73			
	130	8.4	4.4	1.5	1.4	14	190		3.95			299		0.40			WRTH80
Prime Stakes, Worthington	121	68.5	9.2	6.1	0.1	1.3	388	25		0.53			0	0.29	6.4	1.44	
3.2 oz piece	92	6.6	1.0	1.8	3.6	1	88		2.19			0		0.21	0.40		WRTH81
Prosage Links, Worthington	64	30.4	9.1	2.3	0.3	1.3	369	12		0.45			0	6.52	3.9	3.41	
1.6 oz link	45	2.1	0.4	0.6	1.1	1	48	62	2.74			0		0.14	0.33		WRTH82
Prosage Patty, Worthington	80	21.2	9.7	2.5	0.2	1.9	305	16		0.49			0	0.50	2.6	1.51	
1.3 oz patty	38	3.4	0.5	0.8	2.0	1	74	103	1.50			0		0.12	0.27		WRTH83
Prosage Roll, Worthington	143	29.9	10.8	3.3	0.1	1.9	367	15		0.42			0	0.68	1.6	0.75	
1.9 oz roll	55	9.7	1.9	3.2	4.6	1	77	51	2.00			0		0.20	0.24		WRTH84
Protose, Worthington	136	28.4	13.7	5.0	0.5	2.6	316	8		0.83			0	0.08	2.8	1.26	
1.9 oz	55	6.8	1.0	3.1	2.4	<1	73	80	2.10			0		0.04	0.24		WRTH85
Redi-Burger, cnd, Loma Linda	126	55.2	18.5	7.0	1.0	3.6	440			1.46			0	0.14	1.9	1.39	1.58
3 oz patty	85	2.7	0.4	0.5	1.5	<1	142	135	0.98			0		0.28	0.45		WRTH88
salami, meatless, Worthington	121	32.6	12.5	2.9	0.4	2.1	817	26		0.52			0	0.76	5.5	0.65	
2 oz	57	6.7	0.7	1.1	4.8	1	99	77	1.22			0		0.20	0.27		WRTH89
sandwich spread, cnd, Loma Linda	85	38.4	4.2	6.7	0.9	1.5	245	18		0.58			0	0.19	2.5	3.61	1.08
1.9 oz	55	4.6	0.9	2.1	1.4	<1	133	75	0.94			161		0.23	0.46		WRTH90
Saucettes, Worthington	86	23.4	5.6	2.2	0.1	1.1	196	16		0.34			0	0.44	1.2	0.35	
1.3 oz	38	6.1	1.0	1.5	3.6	1	26	59	0.89			0		0.09	0.13		WRTH91
Sausage Crumbles, frzn, Morningstar Farms - 1.9 oz	93	34.2	11.2	5.1	1.1	1.4	404	30		0.76			0	5.64	6.6	4.66	
	55	3.1	0.5	0.7	1.9	1	94	98	1.16			0		0.15	0.38		WRTH87
sausage, Italian, frzn, Boca	130		11.0	6.0	4.0	3.0	990	40						0			
2.5 oz sausage	71	6.0	0.0			0			1.44			200					BOCA14
simulated meat product	64	12.6	4.6	2.5		0.7	222	16	9	0.37	0.181	8	0	0.59	2.8	0.00	0.08
.9 oz link	25	4.5	0.7	1.1	2.3	0	58	56	0.93	0.063	1.9	160	0.5	0.10	0.21	6.5	16107b
simulated meat product	97	19.2	7.0	3.7		1.1	337	24	14	0.55	0.276	12	0	0.89	4.3	0.00	0.12
1.3 oz patty	38	6.9	1.1	1.7	3.5	0	88	86	1.41	0.095	2.8	243	0.8	0.15	0.31	9.9	16107a
smoked, frzn, Boca	130		12.0	7.0	2.0	2.0	890	20						1			
2.5 oz sausage	71	5.0	0.5			0			1.44			0					BOCA15
Savory Dinner Loaf, Loma Linda	91	1.5	13.8	7.4	0.5	4.6	602	48		0.43			0	0.23	2.1	4.94	1.87
.9 oz	26	0.6	0.2	0.1	0.4	1	412	157	1.47			0		0.40	0.64		WRTH92
Savory Slices, Worthington	152	54.7	12.6	6.7	0.8	0.0	461	64		0.50			0	0.00	4.3	1.59	
3 oz	84	8.3	1.2	2.2	4.6	1	76		2.48			0		0.16	0.25		WRTH93
Stakelets, Worthington	150	40.8	14.0	6.8	0.8	3.0	462	61		0.86			0	1.26	6.6	1.58	
2.5 oz piece	71	7.4	1.3	2.5	3.6	1	136	149	0.61			0		0.16	0.26		WRTH98
Stripples, Worthington	56	6.7	2.0	2.3	0.1	0.9	234	7		0.09			0	0.67	0.8	0.54	
.6 oz piece	16	4.4	0.7	1.0	2.6	<1	16	46	0.17			0		0.05	0.08		WRTH99
Super Links, Worthington	104	30.0	6.9	2.6	0.3	0.9	338	16		0.44			0	0.15	0.8	2.65	
1.7 oz link	48	7.3	1.0	1.5	4.0	1	36	45	1.56			0		0.12	0.24		WRTH100
Swiss Stake w/gravy, cnd, Loma Linda - 3.2 oz	129	65.2	9.3	9.7	0.8	3.2	438	19		0.62			0	1.17	14.1	5.26	4.66
	92	5.8	0.8	1.5	3.4	1	208	129	0.96			0		0.81	1.02		WRTH101
Tender Bits, cnd, Loma Linda	116	59.3	13.0	7.2	0.5	3.6	518	11		0.81			0	0.26	6.4	0.11	1.55
3 oz	85	3.9	0.6	1.0	2.3	0	55	75	0.97			0		0.45	0.12		WRTH102
Tender Rounds, cnd, Loma Linda	116	55.4	13.1	5.8	1.3	1.4	311	20		0.70			0	0.83	2.3	1.44	0.40
2.8 oz	80	4.5	0.5	1.1	2.3	<1	85		1.32			0		0.19	0.17		WRTH103
Tuno, cnd, Worthington	84	38.5	6.8	3.8	0.1	1.8	371	35		0.65			0	0.25	3.9	1.90	
1.9 oz	55	4.6	0.7	1.0	3.0	<1	63	86	2.26			0		0.09	0.22		WRTH104
frzn, Worthington	83	38.4	6.8	3.0	0.1	2.0	300	28		0.51			0	0.26	4.6	1.99	
1.9 oz	55	5.6	0.9	1.3	3.2	<1	46	86	1.81			0		0.06	0.32		WRTH105

	KCAL / WT (g)	H₂0 (g) / FAT (g)	PRO (g) / SFA (g)	CHO (g) / MUFA (g)	SUGR (g) / PUFA (g)	DFIB (g) / CHOL (mg)	Na (mg) / K (mg)	Ca (mg) / P (mg)	Mg (mg) / Fe (mg)	Zn (mg) / Cu (mg)	Mn (mg) / Se (mcg)	A (mcg RAE) / A (IU)	C (mg) / E (mg ATE)	B-1 (mg) / B-2 (mg)	NIA (mg) / B-6 (mg)	B-12 (mcg) / FOL (mcg DFE)	PANT (mg) / REF
Natural Touch	57	42.2	7.3	2.2	0.0	1.7	359	29		0.57			0				
1.9 oz	55	2.1	0.8	0.3	0.9	0	69		1.09			0					WRTH106
Turkee Slices, Worthington	193	59.8	12.7	5.3	1.2	0.0	531	142		0.60			0	3.22	5.6	4.55	
3.3 oz	94	13.6	2.0	3.9	7.8	1	55		3.87			0		0.24	0.29		WRTH107
Turkey Style, smoked, Worthington	141	31.1	9.9	4.6	1.5	0.0	489	116		0.41			0	12.36	6.6	3.76	
2 oz	57	9.2	1.2	2.4	4.9	<1	66		3.27			0		0.19	0.46		WRTH108
Vegetable Skallops, Worthington	86	62.1	16.8	4.0	0.3	2.4	390	6		0.89			0	0.01	0.0	0.00	
3 oz	85	1.0	0.1	0.1	0.4	0	13	44	0.07			0		0.03	0.01		WRTH110
Vegetable Steaks, Worthington	83	51.4	15.2	3.7	0.4	1.6	310	5		0.81			0	0.23	3.4	3.27	
2.5 oz piece	72	0.8	0.3	0.2	0.3	0	23	56	2.81			0		0.20	0.23		WRTH111
Veggie Dog, frzn, Morningstar Farms	77	36.9	11.2	6.3	2.3	1.1	606	9		0.57			0	0.19	0.0	0.00	
2 oz veggie dog	57	0.7	0.1	0.1	0.3	<1	69	73	0.83			0		0.11	0.04		WRTH112
Veggie Medley, Natural Touch	124	39.8	10.6	10.9	1.1	0.8	261	20		0.85		0					
2.4 oz	67	4.2	0.4	2.3	1.0	1	233		1.25			0					WRTH113
Veja-Links, low fat, Worthington	38	22.6	4.9	1.3	0.2	0.3	218	10		0.16			0	0.10	2.2	1.39	
1.1 oz link	31	1.5	0.2	0.4	0.9	1	24		1.23			0		0.12	0.12		WRTH115
Worthington	49	21.9	4.5	1.3	0.2	0.3	180	11		0.16			0	0.13	2.0	1.57	
1.1 oz link	31	2.7	0.4	0.6	1.5	1	21		1.29			0		0.11	0.12		WRTH116
Wham, Worthington	82	28.1	8.0	2.5	1.3	0.5	317	45		0.36			0	3.58	5.2	1.96	
1.6 oz	45	5.2	0.8	1.2	2.9	<1	92		1.85			0		0.32	0.44		WRTH117

21.2 SOY PRODUCTS

	KCAL / WT (g)	H₂0 (g) / FAT (g)	PRO (g) / SFA (g)	CHO (g) / MUFA (g)	SUGR (g) / PUFA (g)	DFIB (g) / CHOL (mg)	Na (mg) / K (mg)	Ca (mg) / P (mg)	Mg (mg) / Fe (mg)	Zn (mg) / Cu (mg)	Mn (mg) / Se (mcg)	A (mcg RAE) / A (IU)	C (mg) / E (mg ATE)	B-1 (mg) / B-2 (mg)	NIA (mg) / B-6 (mg)	B-12 (mcg) / FOL (mcg DFE)	PANT (mg) / REF
cultured soy[1], apricot mango, Silk	160		4.0	30.0	20.0	1.0	20	500				2					
6 oz container	170	2.0	0.0			0			0.00			400					WHWA37
banana strawberry, Silk	160		4.0	30.0	20.0	1.0	20	500					1				
6 oz container	170	2.0	0.0			0			0.00			0					WHWA38
black cherry, Silk	160		4.0	29.0	20.0	1.0	20	500					0				
6 oz container	170	2.0	0.0			0			0.00			50					WHWA39
blueberry, Silk	160		4.0	29.0	21.0	1.0	20	500					0				
6 oz container	170	2.0	0.0			0			0.00			0					WHWA4
key lime, Silk	170		4.0	30.0	21.0	1.0	20	500					0				
6 oz container	170	2.0	0.0			0			0.00			0					WHWA5
lemon kiwi, Silk	160		4.0	31.0	22.0	1.0	20	500					0				
6 oz container	170	2.0	0.0			0			0.00			0					WHWA6
lemon, Silk	160		4.0	31.0	22.0	1.0	20	500					0				
6 oz container	170	2.0	0.0			0			0.00			0					WHWA7
mixed berry, Silk	160		4.0	31.0	22.0	1.0	20	500					0				
6 oz container	170	2.0	0.0			0			0.00			0					WHWA8
peach, Silk	170		4.0	32.0	25.0	1.0	20	500					0				
6 oz container	170	2.0	0.0			0			0.00			100					WHWA9
plain, Silk	120		5.0	22.0	12.0	1.0	30	700					0				
8 oz	227	2.5	0.0			0			0.90			50					WHWA10
raspberry, Silk	160		4.0	30.0	22.0	1.0	20	500					0				
6 oz container	170	2.0	0.0			0			0.00			0					WHWA11
strawberry, Silk	160		4.0	31.0	22.0	1.0	20	500					3				
6 oz container	170	2.0	0.0			0			0.00			0					WHWA12
van, Silk	120		4.0	23.0	16.0	1.0	20	500					0				
6 oz container	170	2.0	0.0			0			0.72			50					WHWA13
fuyu (salted & fermented tofu)	13	7.7	0.9	0.6			316	5	6	0.17	0.129	1	<1	0.02	<0.1	0.00	0.01
.4 oz block	11	0.9	0.1	0.2	0.5	0	8	8	0.22	0.041	1.9	18		0.01	0.01	3.2	16132
prep w/Ca sulfate	13	7.7	0.9	0.6			316	135	6	0.17	0.129	1	<1	0.02	<0.1	0.00	0.01
.4 oz block	11	0.9	0.1	0.2	0.5	0	8	8	0.22	0.041	1.9	18		0.01	0.01	3.2	16432
koyadufu (dried tofu),	82	1.0	8.1	2.5		1.2	1	62	10	0.83	0.627	4	<1	0.08	0.2	0.00	0.07
frzn - .6 oz piece	17	5.2	0.7	1.1	2.9	0	3	82	1.65	0.200	9.2	88		0.05	0.05	15.6	16128
prep w/Ca sulfate, frzn	82	1.0	8.1	2.5		0.2	1	363	31	0.83	0.627	4	<1	0.08	0.2	0.00	0.07
.6 oz piece	17	5.2	0.7	1.1	2.9	0	3	82	1.65	0.200	9.2	88		0.05	0.05	15.6	16428
miso	567	114.0	32.5	76.9		14.9	10029	182	116	9.13	2.362	11	0	0.27	2.4	0.00	0.71
1 cup (9.7 oz)	275	16.7	2.4	3.7	9.4	0	451	421	7.54	1.202	4.4	239	<0.1	0.69	0.59	90.8	16112
natto	371	96.3	31.0	25.1		9.5	12	380	201	5.30	2.674	0	23	0.28	0.0	0.00	0.38
1 cup (6.2 oz)	175	19.3	2.8	4.3	10.9	0	1276	305	15.05	1.167	15.4	0	<0.1	0.33	0.23	14.0	16113

	KCAL / WT (g)	H₂O (g) / FAT (g)	PRO (g) / SFA (g)	CHO (g) / MUFA (g)	SUGR (g) / PUFA (g)	DFIB (g) / CHOL (mg)	Na (mg) / K (mg)	Ca (mg) / P (mg)	Mg (mg) / Fe (mg)	Zn (mg) / Cu (mg)	Mn (mg) / Se (mcg)	A (mcg RAE) / A (IU)	C (mg) / E (mg ATE)	B-1 (mg) / B-2 (mg)	NIA (mg) / B-6 (mg)	B-12 (mcg) / FOL (mcg DFE)	PANT (mg) / REF
tempeh	320	99.0	30.8	15.6			15	184	134	1.89	2.158	0	0	0.13	4.4	0.13	0.46
1 cup (5.9 oz)	166	17.9	3.7	5.0	6.4	0	684	442	4.48	0.930	0.0	0		0.59	0.36	39.8	16114
brown rice, organic, Silk	140		12.0	13.0	2.0	5.0	0	20					0				
1/3 block (2.7 oz)	76	5.0	0.5			0			1.44			0					WHWA22
ckd	197	59.6	18.2	9.4			14	96	77	1.57	1.285			0.05	2.1	0.14	0.45
3.5 oz	100	11.4	3.4	3.7	2.6		401	253	2.13	0.540	0.0			0.36	0.20	21.0	16174
five grain, organic, Silk	140		12.0	15.0	2.0	4.0	0	20					0				
1/3 block (2.7 oz)	76	4.0	0.5			0			1.80			0					WHWA23
organic, Silk	150		16.0	10.0	0.0	6.0	0	20					0				
1/3 block (2.7 oz)	76	6.0	1.0			0			1.80			0					WHWA24
sea veggie, organic, Silk	120		12.0	11.0	0.0	8.0	25	100					0				
1/3 block (2.7 oz)	76	3.0	0.0			0			2.70			0					WHWA25
tofu, baked, garlic herb italian,	120		13.0	3.0	0.0	1.0	240	40					1				
Silk - *1 piece (~1.7 oz)*	~49	6.0	1.0			0			1.44			1250					WHWA26
hickory smoke bbq, Silk	75		8.0	4.0	3.0	1.0	140	60					0				
1 piece (~1.7 oz)	~49	3.0	0.5			0			0.72			0					WHWA27
roma tomato basil, Silk	100		8.0	3.0	1.0	2.0	220	60					0				
1 piece (~1.7 oz)	~49	6.0	0.5			0			0.72			0					WHWA28
teriyaki oriental, Silk	120		13.0	3.0	0.0	1.0	240	40					1				
1 piece (~1.7 oz)	~49	6.0	1.0			0			1.44			1250					WHWA29
thai style, Silk	120		13.0	3.0	0.0	1.0	240	40					1				
1 piece (~1.7 oz)	~51	6.0	1.0			0			1.44			1250					WHWA30
zesty lemon pepper, Silk	120		8.0	3.0	0.5	1.0	100	60					0				
1 piece (~1.7 oz)	~49	8.0	1.0			0			0.72			0					WHWA31
tofu, extra firm,	90		10.0	1.0	0.0	1.0	10	100					0				
organic, Silk - *1/5 block (~1.7 oz)*	~49	6.0	1.0			0			1.80			0					WHWA32
prep w/nigari	87	73.3	9.5	1.8	0.5	0.4	9	94	65	1.02	0.862	1	<1	0.04	0.3	0.00	0.06
1/5 block (3.2 oz)	91	5.7	0.8	1.2	3.2		121	147	1.56	0.166	10.2	9		0.04	0.04	23.7	16159
silken, lite, Mori-Nu	32	76.4	5.9	0.8	0.4	0.0	82	36	8	0.22		0	0	0.03	0.1	0.00	
1 slice (3 oz)	84	0.6	0.1	0.1	0.3	0	48	70	0.66	0.108		0	<0.1	0.02	0.00		16165
silken, Mori-Nu	46	74.0	6.2	1.7	0.8	0.1	53	26	23	0.50		0	0	0.07	0.2	0.00	
1 slice (3 oz)	84	1.6	0.3	0.3	0.9	0	129	84	1.00	0.168		0	0.1	0.03	0.01		16163
tofu, firm,	90		10.0	1.0	0.0	1.0	10	100					0				
organic, Silk - *1/5 block (~1.7 oz)*	~49	6.0	1.0			0			1.80			0		*			WHWA33
prep w/Ca sulfate	97	105.4	10.1	3.7	0.8	0.5	10	204	58	1.27	0.912	0	<1	0.12	<0.1	0.00	0.08
1/2 cup (4.4 oz)	126	5.6	0.8	1.2	3.2	0	222	185	1.83	0.302	11.8	~10		0.13	0.08	41.6	16126
prep w/Ca sulfate, raw	183	88.0	19.9	5.4		2.9	18	861	73	1.98	1.488	10	<1	0.20	0.5	0.00	0.17
1/2 cup (4.4 oz)	126	11.0	1.6	2.4	6.2	0	299	239	3.35	0.476	21.9	209		0.13	0.12	36.5	16426
prep w/nigari	178	86.8	15.5	5.4		0.7	2	421	65	2.03	1.283		<1	0.05	0.8	0.00	0.05
1/4 block (4.3 oz)	122	12.2	1.8	2.7	6.9	0	178	282	3.36	0.400	20.5			0.09	0.05	26.8	16160
prep w/nigari, Wildwood	80		12.0	3.0			24	300		0.40			1				
3 oz	85	3.0				0	325	120	1.00			30		0.18			WLWD2
silken, lite, Mori-Nu	31	76.8	5.3	0.9	0.4	0.0	71	30	8	0.28		0	0	0.03	0.1	0.00	
1 slice (3 oz)	84	0.7	0.1	0.1	0.4	0	53	68	0.63	0.102		0	<0.1	0.02	0.00		16164
silken, Mori-Nu	52	73.4	5.8	2.0	1.1	0.1	30	27	23	0.51		0	0	0.08	0.2	0.00	
1 slice (3 oz)	84	2.3	0.3	0.5	1.2	0	163	76	0.87	0.171		0	0.2	0.03	0.01		16162
tofu, fried	35	6.6	2.2	1.4		0.5	2	48	8	0.26	0.194	0	0	0.02	<0.1	0.00	0.02
.5 oz piece	13	2.6	0.4	0.6	1.5	0	19	37	0.63	0.052	3.7	0	<0.1	0.01	0.01	3.5	16129
tofu, medium, prep w/Ca, Wildwood	100		14.0	5.0			45	60		0.60			4				
3 oz	85	4.0				0	450	160	2.00			50		0.27			WLWD1
tofu, okara	94	99.6	3.9	15.3			11	98	32	0.68	0.493	0	0		0.1	0.00	0.11
1 cup (4.3 oz)	122	2.1	0.2	0.4	0.9	0	260	73	1.59	0.244	12.9	0		0.02	0.14	31.7	16130
tofu prep w/Ca sulfate, fried	35	6.6	2.2	1.4		0.5	2	125	12	0.26	0.194	0	0	0.02	<0.1	0.00	0.02
.5 oz piece	13	2.6	0.4	0.6	1.5	0	19	37	0.63	0.052	3.7	0		0.01	0.01	3.5	16429
tofu, red fat, organic, Silk	90		10.0	4.0	0.0	2.0	5	40					0				
1/5 block (~1.8 oz)	~51	4.0	0.0			0			1.44			0					WHWA36
tofu, soft,	90		10.0	1.0	0.0	1.0	10	100					0				
organic, Silk - *1/5 block (~1.7 oz)*	~49	6.0	1.0			0			1.80			0					WHWA34
prep w/Ca sulfate & nigari	71	101.2	7.6	2.1	0.8	0.2	9	129	31	0.74	0.451	0	<1	0.05	0.6	0.00	0.06
1/4 block (4.1 oz)	116	4.3	0.6	0.9	2.4	0	139	107	1.29	0.182	10.3	8	<0.1	0.04	0.06	51.0	16127b
prep w/Ca sulfate, raw	151	216.4	16.2	4.5	1.7	0.5	20	275	67	1.59	0.965	0	<1	0.12	1.3	0.00	0.13
1 cup (8.7 oz)	248	9.2	1.3	2.0	5.2	0	298	228	2.75	0.389	22.1	17	<0.1	0.09	0.13	109.1	16127a

	KCAL / WT (g)	H₂0 (g) / FAT (g)	PRO (g) / SFA (g)	CHO (g) / MUFA (g)	SUGR (g) / PUFA (g)	DFIB (g) / CHOL (mg)	Na (mg) / K (mg)	Ca (mg) / P (mg)	Mg (mg) / Fe (mg)	Zn (mg) / Cu (mg)	Mn (mg) / Se (mcg)	A (mcg RAE) / A (IU)	C (mg) / E (mg ATE)	B-1 (mg) / B-2 (mg)	NIA (mg) / B-6 (mg)	B-12 (mcg) / FOL (mcg DFE)	PANT (mg) / REF
silken, Mori-Nu	46	74.8	4.0	2.4	1.1	0.1	4	26	24	0.44		0	0	0.08	0.3	0.00	
1 slice (3 oz)	84	2.3	0.3	0.4	1.3	0	151	52	0.69	0.174		0	0.2	0.03	0.01		16161
tofu, transitional firm, organic,	90		10.0	1.0	0.0	1.0	10	100				0					
Silk - 1/5 block (~1.7 oz)	~49	6.0	1.0			0			1.80			0					WHWA35

[1] Cultured soy is a yogurt-like product.

22. MILKS, MILK BEVERAGES, & YOGURT
22.1 COW MILK

	KCAL / WT	H₂0 / FAT	PRO / SFA	CHO / MUFA	SUGR / PUFA	DFIB / CHOL	Na / K	Ca / P	Mg / Fe	Zn / Cu	Mn / Se	A-RAE / A-IU	C / E	B-1 / B-2	NIA / B-6	B-12 / FOL	PANT / REF
buttermilk, cultured	98	220.8	8.1	11.7		0.0	257	284	27	1.03	0.005	20	2	0.08	0.1	0.54	0.67
8 fl oz	245	2.2	1.3	0.6	0.1	10	370	218	0.12	0.027	4.9	81	0.1	0.38	0.08	12.3	01088
buttermilk, dry	25	0.2	2.2	3.2		0.0	34	77	7	0.26	0.001	3	<1	0.03	0.1	0.25	0.21
1 T	7	0.4	0.2	0.1	<0.1	4	103	61	0.02	0.007	1.3	14	<0.1	0.10	0.02	3.1	01094
condensed, sweetened, cnd	123	10.4	3.0	20.8		0.0	49	108	10	0.36	0.002	29	1	0.03	0.1	0.17	0.23
1 fl oz	38	3.3	2.1	0.9	0.1	13	142	97	0.07	0.006	5.7	125	0.1	0.16	0.02	4.2	01095
evaporated, nonfat, cnd	25	25.3	2.4	3.6		0.0	37	93	9	0.29	0.002	38	<1	0.01	0.1	0.08	0.24
1 fl oz	32	0.1	<0.1	<0.1	<0.1	1	106	62	0.09	0.005	0.8	125	<0.1	0.10	0.02	2.9	01097
evaporated, whole, cnd	42	23.3	2.1	3.2		0.0	33	82	8	0.24	0.002	21	1	0.01	0.1	0.05	0.20
1 fl oz	32	2.4	1.4	0.7	0.1	9	95	64	0.06	0.005	0.7	77	0.1	0.10	0.02	2.5	01096b
	169	93.3	8.6	12.7		0.0	134	329	30	0.97	0.008	83	2	0.06	0.2	0.20	0.80
4 fl oz	126	9.5	5.8	2.9	0.3	37	382	256	0.24	0.020	2.9	306	0.2	0.40	0.06	10.1	01096a
lowfat, 1% fat	102	219.8	8.0	11.7		0.0	124	300	34	0.95	0.005	144	2	0.10	0.2	0.90	0.79
8 fl oz	244	2.6	1.6	0.7	0.1	10	381	234	0.12	0.024	5.4	500	0.1	0.41	0.10	12.2	01082
pro fortified	118	218.3	9.7	13.6		0.0	143	349	39	1.11	0.005	150	3	0.11	0.2	1.06	0.92
8 fl oz	246	2.9	1.8	0.8	0.1	10	443	273	0.15	0.025	6.2	499		0.47	0.12	14.8	01084
w/nfdm	105	220.0	8.5	12.2		0.0	127	314	34	0.98	0.005	145	2	0.10	0.2	0.93	0.82
8 fl oz	245	2.4	1.5	0.7	0.1	10	397	245	0.12	0.025	5.6	500	0.1	0.42	0.11	12.3	01083
nonfat	86	222.5	8.4	11.9		0.0	127	301	27	0.98	0.005	149	2	0.09	0.2	0.93	0.81
8 fl oz	245	0.4	0.3	0.1	<0.1	5	407	247	0.10	0.027	5.1	500	0.1	0.34	0.10	12.3	01085
pro fortified	101	219.8	9.7	13.7		0.0	145	352	39	1.11	0.005	150	3	0.11	0.2	1.06	0.92
8 fl oz	246	0.6	0.4	0.2	<0.1	5	448	276	0.15	0.027	5.9	499		0.48	0.12	14.8	01087
w/nfdm	91	221.4	8.7	12.3		0.0	130	316	37	1.00	0.005	149	2	0.10	0.2	0.96	0.83
8 fl oz	245	0.6	0.4	0.2	<0.1	5	419	255	0.12	0.027	5.4	500	0.1	0.43	0.11	12.3	01086
nonfat, dry	109	0.9	10.8	15.6		0.0	161	377	33	1.22	0.006	2	2	0.12	0.3	1.21	1.07
1/4 cup	30	0.2	0.1	0.1	<0.1	6	538	290	0.10	0.012	8.2	11	<0.1	0.47	0.11	15.0	01091
Ca reduced[1]	100	1.4	10.1	14.7		0.0	646	79	17	1.14	0.002	1	2	0.05	0.2	1.13	0.94
1 oz	28	0.1	<0.1	<0.1	<0.1	1	193	287	0.09	0.005	7.7	2	<0.1	0.47	0.08	14.2	01093
inst[2]	326	3.6	31.9	47.5		0.0	500	1120	106	4.01	0.018	646	5	0.38	0.8	3.63	2.94
1 1/3 cups (3.2 oz pkt)	91	0.7	0.4	0.2	<0.1	16	1552	896	0.28	0.037	24.8	2157	<0.1	1.59	0.31	45.5	01092
reduced fat, 2% fat	122	217.7	8.1	11.7		0.0	122	298	34	0.95	0.005	137	2	0.10	0.2	0.88	0.78
8 fl oz	244	4.7	2.9	1.4	0.2	20	376	232	0.12	0.020	5.4	500	0.2	0.40	0.10	12.2	01079
pro fortified	138	215.8	9.7	13.5		0.0	145	352	39	1.11	0.005	138	3	0.11	0.2	1.06	0.92
8 fl oz	246	4.9	3.0	1.4	0.2	20	448	276	0.15	0.020	6.4	499		0.48	0.13	14.8	01081
w/nfdm	125	217.7	8.5	12.2		0.0	127	314	34	0.98	0.005	137	2	0.10	0.2	0.93	0.82
8 fl oz	245	4.7	2.9	1.4	0.2	20	397	245	0.12	0.020	5.6	500	0.2	0.42	0.11	12.3	01080
whole,	149	214.7	8.0	11.4		0.0	120	290	32	0.93	0.010	73	2	0.09	0.2	0.88	0.77
3.3% fat - 8 fl oz	244	8.1	5.1	2.4	0.3	34	371	227	0.12	0.024	4.9	307	0.2	0.40	0.10	12.2	01077
3.7% fat	156	214.0	8.0	11.3		0.0	120	290	32	0.93	0.010	81	4	0.09	0.2	0.88	0.76
8 fl oz	244	8.9	5.6	2.6	0.3	34	368	227	0.12	0.024	4.9	337	0.2	0.39	0.10	12.2	01078
low sodium	149	215.2	7.6	10.9		0.0	7	246	12	0.93	0.010	73	2	0.05	0.1	0.88	0.74
8 fl oz	244	8.4	5.3	2.4	0.3	34	617	210	0.12	0.024	4.9	317	0.2	0.26	0.08	12.2	01089
whole, dry	159	0.8	8.4	12.3		0.0	119	292	27	1.07	0.013	82	3	0.09	0.2	1.04	0.73
1/4 cup	32	8.5	5.4	2.5	0.2	31	426	248	0.15	0.026	5.2	295	0.3	0.39	0.10	11.8	01090

[1] Not fortified with vitamin A. [2] Reconstitutes to 1 quart of fluid nonfat milk.

22.2 COW MILK BEVERAGES

	KCAL / WT	H₂0 / FAT	PRO / SFA	CHO / MUFA	SUGR / PUFA	DFIB / CHOL	Na / K	Ca / P	Mg / Fe	Zn / Cu	Mn / Se	A-RAE / A-IU	C / E	B-1 / B-2	NIA / B-6	B-12 / FOL	PANT / REF
carob flavored mix in whole milk	195	215.0	8.2	22.5		1.0	133	292	33	0.92	0.005	69	2	0.09	0.3	0.87	0.77
8 fl oz	256	8.2	5.1	2.4	0.3	33	369	228	0.67	0.023	5.1	307		0.39	0.12	12.8	14169
choc malted milk, whole milk	236	214.8	9.1	30.0		0.3	172	305	48	1.09	0.143	3	3	0.13	0.6	0.90	0.91
8 fl oz	265	9.0	5.3	2.4	0.4	34	501	265	0.61	0.066	6.4	326	0.3	0.44	0.14	15.9	14318

| | KCAL | H_2O (g) | PRO (g) | CHO (g) | SUGR (g) | DFIB (g) | Na (mg) | Ca (mg) | Mg (mg) | Zn (mg) | Mn (mg) | A (mcg RAE) | C (mg) | B-1 (mg) | NIA (mg) | B-12 (mcg) | PANT (mg) |
	WT (g)	FAT (g)	SFA (g)	MUFA (g)	PUFA (g)	CHOL (mg)	K (mg)	P (mg)	Fe (mg)	Cu (mg)	Se (mcg)	A (IU)	E (mg ATE)	B-2 (mg)	B-6 (mg)	FOL (mcg DFE)	REF
choc malted milk, whole milk	233	215.0	9.1	29.3		0.3	246	384	53	1.17	0.143	832	34	0.74	11.0	0.90	0.91
w/added nutrients - 8 fl oz	265	8.9	5.3	2.4	0.4	34	623	313	3.82	0.159	6.4	3090	0.3	1.27	1.03	31.8	14316
choc milk,	158	211.3	8.1	26.1		1.3	153	288	33	1.03	0.193	148	2	0.10	0.3	0.85	0.76
1% fat milk - 8 fl oz	250	2.5	1.5	0.8	0.1	8	425	258	0.60	0.163	4.8	500	0.1	0.42	0.10	12.5	01104
2% fat milk	180	209.0	8.0	26.0		1.3	150	285	33	1.03	0.188	140	2	0.09	0.3	0.85	0.75
8 fl oz	250	5.0	3.1	1.5	0.2	18	423	255	0.60	0.158	4.8	500	0.1	0.41	0.10	12.5	01103
prep from powdered mix	63	185.2	5.3	10.6		0.4	171	192	47	0.82	0.157	73	<1	0.02	0.3	0.51	0.46
w/aspartame - 6 fl oz	204	0.6	0.4	0.1	<0.1	2	479	182	1.65	0.182	3.3	245		0.41	0.02	8.2	14423
whole milk	208	205.8	7.9	25.9		2.0	150	280	33	1.03	0.193	70	2	0.09	0.3	0.83	0.74
8 fl oz	250	8.5	5.3	2.5	0.3	30	418	253	0.60	0.163	4.8	303	0.2	0.41	0.10	12.5	01102
whole milk w/choc powder	226	215.0	8.8	30.9		1.3	165	301	53	1.28	0.157	69	2	0.10	0.3	0.88	0.77
8 fl oz	266	8.8	5.5	2.6	0.3	32	497	255	0.80	0.176	5.3	311		0.43	0.10	13.3	14177
whole milk w/choc syrup	257	226.2	8.8	36.4		0.8	147	296	56	1.21	0.158	71	2	0.10	0.3	0.87	0.77
8 fl oz	282	8.6	5.1	2.3	0.3	34	454	276	0.93	0.220	5.4	319	0.3	0.41	0.10	14.1	14182
cocoa (hot choc), homemade	193	202.4	9.8	29.5		2.0	128	315	70	1.48	0.285	135	3	0.10	0.4	0.93	0.82
2% milk - 8 fl oz	250	5.8	3.6	1.7	0.2	20	500	293	1.15	0.303	6.8	515	0.3	0.44	0.12	15.0	01105
prep w/water from mix	103	178.0	3.1	22.5		2.5	148	97	25	0.45	0.078	0	<1	0.03	0.2	0.37	0.25
1 oz pkt in 6 fl oz water	206	1.2	0.7	0.4	<0.1	2	202	89	0.35	0.093	0.8	4		0.16	0.03	0.0	14194
prep w/wtr from mix w/	54	177.4	2.2	10.8		1.3	173	90	33	0.58	0.102	12	<1	0.04	0.2	0.36	0.57
aspartame - 1 pkt in 6 fl oz wtr	192	0.2	0.0	0.1	<0.1		405	134	0.77	0.119	4.0	42	0.1	0.21	0.05	1.9	14390
eggnog, nonalcoholic	343	188.9	9.7	34.4		0.0	137	330	48	1.17	0.013	226	4	0.09	0.3	1.14	1.06
8 fl oz	254	19.0	11.3	5.7	0.9	150	419	277	0.51	0.033	10.7	894	0.6	0.48	0.13	2.5	01057
mix in whole milk	261	214.6	8.2	38.9		0.8	163	291	33	0.92	0.005	68	2	0.09	0.2	0.87	0.76
8 fl oz	272	8.4	5.1	2.5	0.3	33	370	228	0.38	0.024	4.9	307		0.39	0.10	13.6	14245
Instant Breakfast, van, powder in	250		12.5	39.0		0.0	240	500	100	3.75	0.500		30	0.38	5.0	1.50	2.50
2% milk, Carnation - 9 fl oz	280	4.6	3.2			21	630	500	4.50	0.500		2250	5.0	0.51	0.50	100.0	NEST6
w/o sugar, van, powder in 2%	190		12.5	24.0		0.0	216	500	100	3.75	0.500		30	0.38	5.0	1.50	2.50
milk, Carnation - 9 fl oz	264	4.6	3.2			21	630	500	4.50	0.500		2250	5.0	0.51	0.50	100.0	NEST5
malted milk, whole milk	239	214.9	10.4	27.5		0.0	225	355	53	1.14	0.101	13	3	0.20	1.3	1.03	0.91
8 fl oz	265	9.8	5.7	2.6	0.6	37	530	305	0.27	0.066	7.2	368	0.3	0.59	0.19	21.2	14312
whole milk w/added nutrients	233	215.2	9.9	28.6		0.0	207	371	48	1.09	0.101	670	30	0.72	10.5	1.03	0.91
8 fl oz	265	8.7	5.2	2.4	0.4	37	575	307	3.66	0.085	7.2	2555	0.3	1.15	0.87	21.2	14310
strawberry flavored milk, mix in	234	215.2	8.0	32.7		0.0	128	293	32	0.93	0.005	69	2	0.09	0.2	0.88	0.77
whole milk - 8 fl oz	266	8.2	5.1	2.4	0.3	32	370	229	0.21	0.024	4.8	309		0.42	0.10	13.3	14351

22.3 COW MILK MIXES

| | KCAL | H_2O (g) | PRO (g) | CHO (g) | SUGR (g) | DFIB (g) | Na (mg) | Ca (mg) | Mg (mg) | Zn (mg) | Mn (mg) | A (mcg RAE) | C (mg) | B-1 (mg) | NIA (mg) | B-12 (mcg) | PANT (mg) |
	WT (g)	FAT (g)	SFA (g)	MUFA (g)	PUFA (g)	CHOL (mg)	K (mg)	P (mg)	Fe (mg)	Cu (mg)	Se (mcg)	A (IU)	E (mg ATE)	B-2 (mg)	B-6 (mg)	FOL (mcg DFE)	REF
carob mix	45	0.3	0.2	11.2		1.0	12	4	1	0.01	0.008	0	0	<0.01	0.1	0.00	<0.01
1 T	12	<0.1	<0.1	<0.1	<0.1	0	12	1	0.55	0.007	0.2	0		<0.01	0.01	0.0	14168
choc milk mix	77	0.2	0.7	19.9		1.3	46	8	22	0.34	0.156	<1	<1	0.01	0.1	0.00	0.01
2–3 hp t	22	0.7	0.4	0.2	<0.1	0	130	28	0.69	0.155	0.6	4	0.1	0.03	<0.01	1.3	14175
malted	79	0.3	1.1	18.4		0.2	53	13	15	0.17	0.132	3	<1	0.04	0.4	0.04	0.14
3 hp t (.7 oz)	21	0.8	0.5	0.2	0.1	1	130	37	0.48	0.042	1.6	19	0.1	0.04	0.03	4.2	14317
malted w/added nutrients	80	0.7	1.8	17.1		0.1	85	79	14	0.15	0.089	662	27	0.62	10.2	0.16	0.14
4–5 hp t (.7 oz)	21	0.6	0.3	0.2	0.1	4	203	79	3.49	0.059	2.2	2222	0.1	0.75	0.76	9.7	14309b
w/aspartame	63	2.7	5.3	10.5		0.3	164	185	44	0.76	0.153	72	<1	0.02	0.3	0.50	0.45
.75 oz pkt	21	0.5	0.4	0.1	<0.1	2	470	179	1.62	0.168	3.2	242	<0.1	0.41	0.02	8.8	14422
cocoa mix	101	0.4	3.0	22.1		0.3	141	91	23	0.41	0.075	<1	<1	0.03	0.2	0.37	0.25
1 oz pkt (3–4 hp t)	28	1.1	0.7	0.4	<0.1	1	199	88	0.33	0.080	0.8	4	<0.1	0.16	0.03	0.0	14192
no sugar added, Carnation	55	0.5	4.3	8.4	6.7	0.8	142	123	27	0.60	0.095	0	<1	0.06	0.2	0.45	0.50
.53 oz pkt	15	0.4	0.2	0.1		3	288	135	0.39	0.101		0	<0.1	0.22	0.05	5.9	14198
rich choc, Carnation	112	0.4	1.3	24.2	20.8	0.7	102	40		0.36	0.158	0	0	0.03	0.2	0.10	0.25
1 oz pkt	28	1.1	0.3	0.3	0.3	2	194	71	0.28	0.169		0	<0.1	0.12	0.03	2.0	14197
w/marshmallows, Carnation	112	0.5	1.3	24.3	20.9	0.5	96	41	16	0.20	0.060	0	0	0.03	0.1	0.12	0.28
1 oz pkt	28	1.0	0.4	0.3	0.4	2	142	58	0.24	0.080		0	<0.1	0.12	0.03	1.1	14195
eggnog mix, nonalcoholic	109	0.1	0.1	27.3		0.9	43	1	0	0.02	0.000	1	0	<0.01	<0.1	0.02	1.72
2 rd t	28	0.3	0.1	0.1	<0.1	7	1	3	0.25	0.006	0.1	10	<0.1	<0.01	<0.01	0.6	14244
malted milk	87	0.4	2.4	15.9		0.1	104	63	20	0.21	0.089	17	1	0.11	1.1	0.16	0.14
3 hp t (.7 oz)	21	1.7	0.9	0.4	0.3	4	159	75	0.15	0.042	2.2	61	0.1	0.19	0.09	9.7	14311
w/added nutrients	80	0.7	1.8	17.1		0.1	85	79	14	0.15	0.089	662	27	0.62	10.2	0.16	0.14
4–5 hp t (.7 oz)	21	0.6	0.3	0.2	0.1	4	203	79	3.49	0.059	2.2	2222	0.1	0.75	0.76	9.7	14309c
strawberry flavored mix	85	0.1	0.0	21.8		0.0	8	0	0	0.00	0.000	0	<1	<0.01	<0.1	0.00	0.00
2–3 hp t (.8 oz)	22	<0.1	<0.1	<0.1	<0.1	0	1	0	0.10	0.004	<0.1	0	0	0.02	<0.01	0.0	14350

	KCAL	H₂0 (g)	PRO (g)	CHO (g)	SUGR (g)	DFIB (g)	Na (mg)	Ca (mg)	Mg (mg)	Zn (mg)	Mn (mg)	A (mcg RAE)	C (mg)	B-1 (mg)	NIA (mg)	B-12 (mcg)	PANT (mg)
	WT (g)	FAT (g)	SFA (g)	MUFA (g)	PUFA (g)	CHOL (mg)	K (mg)	P (mg)	Fe (mg)	Cu (mg)	Se (mcg)	A (IU)	E (mg ATE)	B-2 (mg)	B-6 (mg)	FOL (mcg DFE)	REF

22.4 COW MILK YOGURT

Food																	
custard style, fruit flavors,	190		7.0	32.0	28.0	0.0	90	300	16				0				
Yoplait - *6 oz*	170	3.5	2.0			15	310	150	0.00			750		0.26			GENM275
fruit flavors w/Trix, Yoplait	120		4.0	23.0	19.0	0.0	55	100					0				
4 oz	113	1.5	1.0			5	170	100	0.00			500					GENM276
fruit flavors, Yoplait Expresse	70		2.0	11.0	10.0	0.0	40	100					0				
2.3 oz tube	64	1.5	1.0			5	120	60	0.00			0		0.07			GENM277
Yoplait Go-Gurt	70		3.0	11.0	10.0	0.0	40	100					0				
2.3 oz tube	64	2.0	1.0			5	125	60				0		0.07			GENM278
Yoplait Yumsters	120		5.0	21.0	18.0	0.0	60	200					0				
4 oz	113	2.0	1.5			10	210		0.00			500					GENM279
light, fruit flavors, Yoplait	100		5.0	19.0	14.0	0.0	85	200	16				0				
6 oz	170	0.0	0.0			<5	250	150	0.00			750		0.17			GENM280
low fat, banana/strawberry, Colombo	230		7.0	47.0	42.0	0.0	90	200	24				0				
Classic - *8 oz*	227	2.0	1.0			10	330	150	0.00			0		0.26			GENM283
lowfat (1%), strawberry, Breyers	218	173.7	8.6	41.3	39.5	0.5	118	284					0		1.20		
8 oz container	227	1.8	1.1			20	436	202	0.23			77		0.43			01195
Breyers Light N'Lively	135	91.6	4.0	27.4	24.5	0.3	56	114					0		0.58		
4.4 oz container	125	1.0	0.6			11	189	84	0.14			38		0.18			01196
Breyers Smooth & Creamy	232	169.8	8.6	45.2	39.0	0.7	125	245					0		1.18		
8 oz container	227	2.0	1.1			20	402	177	0.30			70		0.41			01197
lowfat, french van, Colombo	180		8.0	32.0	26.0	0.0	120	250	24				0				
8 oz	227	2.5	1.5			15	370	200	0.00			0		0.34			GENM281
lowfat, fruit flavor	238	168.2	11.0	42.2		0.0	148	384	36	1.86	0.148	36	2	0.09	0.2	1.18	1.23
8 oz container	227	3.2	2.1	0.9	0.1	14	490	302	0.16	0.182	7.0	136		0.45	0.10	22.7	01122
lowfat, fruit on the bottom,	210		9.0	40.0	38.0	0.0	140	300					1	0.12		1.20	
strawberry, Dannon - *8 oz*	227	2.0	1.0			10	460	250	0.00			0		0.54	0.08		DANN6
lowfat, lemon/van, Colombo Classic	180		8.0	32.0	26.0	0.0	120	250	24				0				
8 oz	227	2.0	1.5			15	370	200	0.00			0		0.34			GENM284
lowfat, plain	143	193.1	11.9	16.0		0.0	159	415	39	2.02	0.009	34	2	0.10	0.3	1.27	1.34
8 oz container	227	3.5	2.3	1.0	0.1	14	531	327	0.18	0.030	7.5	150	0.1	0.49	0.11	25.0	01117
Colombo	130		10.0	16.0	10.0	0.0	125	300	24				0				
8 oz	227	2.5	1.5			15	440	200	0.00			0		0.34			GENM285
Dannon	150		12.0	18.0	17.0	0.0	190	350					0	0.00			
8 oz	227	3.5	2.0			20	580		0.00			100		0.00			DANN7
lowfat, strawberry, Colombo	190		9.0	31.0	27.0	0.0	130	300					0				
8 oz	227	3.0	2.0			20	400		0.00			0		0.34			GENM282
w/vit D, Dannon Danimals	90		4.0	16.0	15.0	0.0	55	100					0				
Drinkable - *3.1 fl oz (372 ml)*	88	1.5	1.0			5	180		0.00			0					DANN4
lowfat, van	193	179.3	11.2	31.3		0.0	150	388	36	1.88	0.009	30	2	0.10	0.2	1.20	1.25
8 oz container	227	2.8	1.8	0.8	0.1	11	497	306	0.16	0.030	11.1	123	0.1	0.46	0.10	25.0	01119
Dannon	230		11.0	36.0	35.0	0.0	170	350					0	0.00		0.00	
8 oz	227	3.5	2.0			15	520		0.00			100		0.00	0.00		DANN8
w/vit D, Dannon Danimals	110		5.0	20.0	18.0	0.0	75	150					0				
4 oz	113	1.5	1.0			5	230		0.00			0					DANN5
lowfat, various flavors, Colombo	220		7.0	42.0	36.0	0.0	115	200	24				0				
Classic[1] - *8 oz*	227	2.0	1.5			15	340	150	0.00			0		0.26			GENM286
lowfat, whpd, orange cream, Dannon	120		4.0	20.0	18.0		65	100						0.06		0.48	0.40
4 oz	113	2.5	1.5			10	190	100				300		0.17			DANN9
nonfat, fr van w/aspartame & fruc,	100		8.0	16.0	10.0	0.0	125	200								0.90	
Dannon Light 'n Fit Creamy - *6 oz*	170	0.0	0.0			<5	330	200						0.34			DANN12
nonfat, plain	127	193.5	13.0	17.4		0.0	175	452	43	2.20	0.011	5	2	0.11	0.3	1.38	1.46
8 oz container	227	0.4	0.3	0.1	<0.1	5	579	356	0.20	0.034	8.2	16	<0.1	0.53	0.12	27.2	01118
Colombo	100		10.0	16.0	10.0	0.0	125	300	32				0				
8 oz	227	0.0	0.0			10	440	250	0.00			0		0.43			GENM287
nonfat, strawberry w/aspartame,	125	195.2	7.7	22.5	17.5	0.0	102	216					1		0.93		
Breyers Light - *8 oz container*	227	0.5	0.2			11	331	154	0.25			9		0.32			01198
w/vit A & D, aspartame, & fructose,	120		8.0	22.0	16.0	0.0	160	250					2	0.00		0.90	0.80
Dannon Light 'n Fit - *8 oz*	227	0.0	0.0			<5	390	200				500		0.43			DANN11
nonfat, van, Colombo	160		8.0	32.0	28.0	0.0	140	250	24				0				
8 oz	227	0.0	0.0			5	410	200	0.00			0		0.34			GENM288

	KCAL / WT (g)	H₂O (g) / FAT (g)	PRO (g) / SFA (g)	CHO (g) / MUFA (g)	SUGR (g) / PUFA (g)	DFIB (g) / CHOL (mg)	Na (mg) / K (mg)	Ca (mg) / P (mg)	Mg (mg) / Fe (mg)	Zn (mg) / Cu (mg)	Mn (mg) / Se (mcg)	A (mcg RAE) / A (IU)	C (mg) / E (mg ATE)	B-1 (mg) / B-2 (mg)	NIA (mg) / B-6 (mg)	B-12 (mcg) / FOL (mcg DFE)	PANT (mg) / REF
Dannon	110		5.0	22.0	19.0	0.0	75	150				0		0.06		0.48	0.00
4 oz	113	0.0	0.0			<5	190	0						0.17	0.04		DANN10
nonfat, various flavors, Colombo	120		7.0	21.0	15.0	0.0	110	350	16				0				
Light² - 8 oz	227	0.0	0.0			5	320	200	0.00			0		0.26			GENM289
raspberry, Dannon La Crème	140		5.0	20.0	18.0	0.0	85	150								0.60	
4 oz	113	5.0	3.0			20	240	150				200		0.26			DANN3
whole, plain	138	199.5	7.9	10.6		0.0	104	275	27	1.34	0.009	66	1	0.07	0.2	0.84	0.88
8 oz container	227	7.4	4.8	2.0	0.2	30	352	216	0.11	0.020	5.0	279	0.2	0.32	0.07	15.9	01116
wild berries, Dannon Frusion	270		8.0	53.0	50.0	0.0	170	250				0		0.09		0.90	0.80
Smoothie - 9.8 fl oz bottle	278	3.5	2.0			15	420	250	0.00			100		0.43	0.08		DANN2

¹ Values are averages for 14 flavors, apricot, banana/strawberry, blackberry, blueberry, black cherry parfait, cherry, fruit burst, lemon, peach, raspberry, strawberry, strawberry kiwi, vanilla, and white chocolate raspberry.

² Values are averages for 12 flavors, blueberry, cherry vanilla, key lime pie, lemon meringue, mixed berries, peach, raspberry, strawberry, strawberry/banana, strawberry colada, vanilla, and white chocolate raspberry.

22.5 OTHER MAMMAL MILKS

	KCAL / WT (g)	H₂O (g) / FAT (g)	PRO (g) / SFA (g)	CHO (g) / MUFA (g)	SUGR (g) / PUFA (g)	DFIB (g) / CHOL (mg)	Na (mg) / K (mg)	Ca (mg) / P (mg)	Mg (mg) / Fe (mg)	Zn (mg) / Cu (mg)	Mn (mg) / Se (mcg)	A (mcg RAE) / A (IU)	C (mg) / E (mg ATE)	B-1 (mg) / B-2 (mg)	NIA (mg) / B-6 (mg)	B-12 (mcg) / FOL (mcg DFE)	PANT (mg) / REF
goat milk	168	212.4	8.7	10.9		0.0	122	327	34	0.73	0.044	137	3	0.12	0.7	0.17	0.76
8 fl oz	244	10.1	6.5	2.7	0.4	27	498	271	0.12	0.112	3.4	451	0.2	0.34	0.11	2.4	01106
human milk	172	215.3	2.5	16.9		0.0	42	79	7	0.42	0.064	153	12	0.03	0.4	0.12	0.55
8 fl oz	246	10.8	4.9	4.1	1.2	34	125	34	0.07	0.128	4.4	593	2.2	0.09	0.03	12.3	01107
preterm	165	216.2	3.5	16.3		0.0	61	61	7.6	0.84	0.001		27	0.05	0.4	0.12	0.44
8 fl oz	246	9.6					140	31	0.30	0.16	3.6	959	1.8	0.12	0.04	8.1	RSSP4
term	167	222.4	2.6	17.7			44	69	8.6	0.30	0.001		10	0.05	0.4	0.12	0.44
8 fl oz	246	9.6					130	34	0.07	0.06	3.7	554	1.8	0.09	0.05	12.3	RSSP5
indian buffalo milk	237	203.5	9.2	12.6		0.0	127	412	76	0.54	0.044	129	6	0.13	0.2	0.88	0.47
8 fl oz	244	16.8	11.2	4.4	0.4	46	434	285	0.29	0.112		434		0.33	0.06	14.6	01108
sheep milk	265	197.7	14.7	13.1		0.0	108	473	44	1.32	0.044	108	10	0.16	1.0	1.74	1.00
8 fl oz	245	17.2	11.3	4.2	0.8	66	336	387	0.25	0.113	4.2	360		0.87	0.15	17.2	01109

22.6 OTHER (NON-DAIRY) MILKS

	KCAL / WT (g)	H₂O (g) / FAT (g)	PRO (g) / SFA (g)	CHO (g) / MUFA (g)	SUGR (g) / PUFA (g)	DFIB (g) / CHOL (mg)	Na (mg) / K (mg)	Ca (mg) / P (mg)	Mg (mg) / Fe (mg)	Zn (mg) / Cu (mg)	Mn (mg) / Se (mcg)	A (mcg RAE) / A (IU)	C (mg) / E (mg ATE)	B-1 (mg) / B-2 (mg)	NIA (mg) / B-6 (mg)	B-12 (mcg) / FOL (mcg DFE)	PANT (mg) / REF
almond milk, choc, Almond Breeze	110		1.0	22.0	20.0	1.0	150	200				0					
8 fl oz (240ml)	245	3.0	0.0			0	210		0.72			500	15.0				BLDM2
choc w/soy pro, Almond Breeze	140		4.0	22.0	20.0	2.0	150	200				0					
8 fl oz (240 ml)	245	4.5	0.0			0	220		1.44			500	15.0				BLDM1
van, Almond Breeze	90		1.0	16.0	15.0	<1.0	150	200				0					
8 fl oz (240 ml)	245	2.5	0.0			0	180		0.36			500	15.0				BLDM4
van, Naturally Almond	90		2.0	15.0	9.0	<1.0	100	20				0					
8 fl oz (240 ml)	245	2.5	0.0			0			1.08			0					BLDM5
van w/soy pro, Almond Breeze	120		4.0	16.0	15.0	1.0	150	200				0					
8 fl oz (240 ml)	245	4.5	0.0			0	190		1.08			500	15.0				BLDM3
Better Than Milk,	75		0.0	16.0	4.0	1.0	155	300					12			1.80	
rice original powder - 2 T	19	1.2	0.2	0.1	0.9	0	4		0.36			500	4.5		0.30	60.0	BTTR5
rice van powder	75		0.0	15.0	5.0	1.0	117	300					12			1.80	
2 T	19	1.9	0.3	1.4	0.2	0	6		0.36			500	4.5		0.30	60.0	BTTR6
soy carob powder	99		4.0	16.0	9.0	3.0	268	300					12			1.80	
2 1/2 T	25	3.5	0.6	0.7	2.2	0	188		0.90			500	4.5		0.30	60.0	BTTR3
soy chocolate powder	111		3.0	22.0	19.0	2.0	220	300					12			1.80	
3 T	30	1.7	0.3	0.4	0.8	0	143		1.44			500	4.5		0.30	60.0	BTTR4
soy original powder	100		2.0	16.0	5.0	0.0	100	80					0			0.60	
2 T	23	2.5	0.0	1.9	0.2	0	250		0.00			0					BTTR1
soy van powder	81		6.3	8.0	8.0	1.0	180	300					6			0.60	
2 3/4 T	20	2.2	0.2	0.4	1.6	0	148		1.26			500	3.0				BTTR2
Rice Dream (rice beverage),	120	217.5	0.4	24.8		0.0	86	20	10	0.25	0.123	0	1	0.08	1.9	0.00	0.14
cnd, Imagine Foods - 8 fl oz	~245	2.0	0.2	1.3	0.3	0	69	34	0.20	0.123		5	1.8	0.01	0.04	90.7	14342
enr, Imagine Foods	120		1.0	25.0	11.0		90	300	13	0.29				0.12	0.8	1.50	0.23
8 fl oz	~245	2.0	0.0			0	60	150				500	0.8		0.08		IMAG1
Soy Dream, enr, Imagine Foods	130		7.0	17.0	9.0		140	300	40	0.60				0.15	0.8	3.00	0.40
8 fl oz	~245	4.0	0.5			0	240	250	1.80	0.200		500	5.0	0.07	0.12	60.0	IMAG2
Imagine Foods	130		7.0	17.0	9.0		140	40	40	0.60				0.15	0.8		0.40
8 fl oz	~245	4.0	0.5			0	240	100	1.80	0.200				0.07	0.12	60.0	IMAG3
soy milk	81	228.5	6.7	4.4		3.2	29	10	47	0.56	0.417	5	0	0.39	0.4	0.00	0.12
8 fl oz	245	4.7	0.5	0.8	2.0	0	345	120	1.42	0.294	3.2	78	<0.1	0.17	0.10	4.9	16120

	KCAL / WT (g)	H₂0 (g) / FAT (g)	PRO (g) / SFA (g)	CHO (g) / MUFA (g)	SUGR (g) / PUFA (g)	DFIB (g) / CHOL (mg)	Na (mg) / K (mg)	Ca (mg) / P (mg)	Mg (mg) / Fe (mg)	Zn (mg) / Cu (mg)	Mn (mg) / Se (mcg)	A (mcg RAE) / A (IU)	C (mg) / E (mg ATE)	B-1 (mg) / B-2 (mg)	NIA (mg) / B-6 (mg)	B-12 (mcg) / FOL (mcg DFE)	PANT (mg) / REF
EdenBlend	120		7.0	18.0	8.0	0.0	85	32	40	0.90			0	0.09	0.4	0.00	0.20
8 fl oz (240 ml)	245	3.0	0.5	0.5	2.0	0	270	100	1.08	0.200		0	0.0	0.10	0.08	26.0	EDEN6
organic, Silk	100		7.0	8.0	4.0	0.0	75	300		0.60			0				3.00
8 fl oz (240 ml)	245	4.0	0.0			0	280		1.08			500		0.51		24.0	WHWA19
original, Edensoy	130		10.0	13.0	7.0	0.0	105	80		0.90			0		0.15	0.8		0.60
8 fl oz (240 ml)	245	5.0	0.5	1.0	3.0	0	440	150	1.44	0.300		0		0.07	0.16	40.0	EDEN12
original, Edensoy Extra	130		11.0	13.0	7.0	3.0	100	200	60	0.90			0		0.15	0.8	3.00	0.60
8 fl oz (240 ml)	245	4.0				0	440	150	1.80	0.339		1500		0.07	0.16	40.0	EDEN7
original, Edensoy Light	100		5.0	14.0	5.0	0.0	85	80	33	0.60					0.10	0.9	0.00	0.20
8 fl oz (240 ml)	245	2.0	0.0	0.5	1.0	0	210	70	1.00	0.100				0.05	0.10	48.0	EDEN9
soy milk, carob, Edensoy	170		7.0	27.0	13.0	0.0	95	75	58	0.80			0		0.26	2.0		0.58
8 fl oz (240 ml)	245	4.0	0.5	1.0	2.0	0	350	125	1.30	0.170				0.08	0.16	80.0	EDEN11
soy milk, chai, Silk	130		6.5	20.0	15.0	1.0	125	300		0.90			0				0.90
8 fl oz (240 ml)	245	3.0	0.0			0			1.08			300		0.34			WHWA14
soy milk, choc, Silk	140		5.0	23.0	19.0	0.0	100	300		0.60			0				3.00
8 fl oz (240 ml)	245	3.5	0.0			0	350		1.44			500		0.51		24.0	WHWA15
soy milk, coffee, Silk Soylatte	220		7.0	38.0	31.0	0.0	70	400		1.20							1.20
11 fl oz container (330 ml)	337	5.0	0.5			0	350		1.44			400		0.51		24.0	WHWA16
soy milk, mocha, Silk	170		5.0	29.0	23.0	0.0	50	300		0.90			0				0.90
8 fl oz (240 ml)	245	3.5	0.0			0	245		1.08			300		0.34		16.0	WHWA17
soy milk, nog, Silk	90		3.0	15.0	12.0	0.0	75	20					0				
4 fl oz (120 ml)	123	2.0	0.0			0			0.72			0					WHWA18
soy milk, spice, Silk Soylatte	200		8.0	27.0	25.0	0.0	200	300		0.90			0				3.00
11 fl oz container (330 ml)	337	6.0	0.5			0	490		1.80			500		0.51		32.0	WHWA20
soy milk, van, Edensoy	150		7.0	24.0	15.0	1.0	85	60	40	0.60			0		0.12	1.2		0.80
8 fl oz (240 ml)	245	3.0	0.0	0.5	2.0	0	320	100	0.72	0.070				0.07	0.12	40.0	EDEN13
Edensoy Extra	150		7.0	23.0	15.0	1.0	90	200	40	0.60			0		0.12	1.2	3.00	0.80
8 fl oz (240 ml)	245	3.0	0.0	0.5	2.0	0	310	100	1.11			1500		0.07	0.12	40.0	EDEN8
Edensoy Light	120		4.0	20.0	10.0	0.0	85	75	32	0.30			0		1.00	1.7	0.00	0.18
8 fl oz (240 ml)	245	2.0	0.0	0.3	1.0	0	200	64	0.50	0.050				0.05	0.10	69.0	EDEN10
Silk	100		6.0	10.0	6.0	0.0	95	300		0.60			0				3.00
8 fl oz (240 ml)	245	3.5	0.0			0	280		1.08			500		0.51		24.0	WHWA21
soy milk powder,	128	1.8	6.2	12.7	5.0	3.9	130	100		0.65			6	0.13	0.0	1.45	0.28
all purpose, Soyagen - *1 oz*	28	5.8	0.8	1.1	3.5	0	318	194	1.85			773		0.08	0.09		WRTH95
carob, Soyagen	132	1.2	5.7	13.9	8.2	2.5	159	54		0.51			3	0.06	0.0	0.50	0.11
1 oz	28	6.0	0.8	1.0	3.5	0	275	116	1.45			899		0.02	0.08		WRTH96
no sucrose, Soyagen	131	1.2	6.2	13.3	4.2	2.8	137	46		0.36			5	0.08	0.0	1.56	0.16
1 oz	28	5.9	0.8	1.0	3.3	0	296	167	1.90			908		0.09	0.08		WRTH97
soy protein shake mix, GeniSoy[1]	127		14.0	17.3	14.0	1.0	173	250	100	3.75				15	0.38	5.0	1.50	2.50
1 scoop	35	0.0					123	250	4.50	0.500	50.0	1250	20.0	0.43	0.50	100.0	GENI8
Vitamite 100	110		3.0	14.0	4.0	0.0	120	300					0		0.15		1.80	1.00
8 fl oz	~245	5.0	1.5	3.5		0	170	150	0.36			500		0.26	0.20		DIHL1

[1] Values are averages for 3 flavors, vanilla, chocolate, and strawberry.

23. NUTS & SEEDS
23.1 NUTS & NUT PRODUCTS

	KCAL / WT (g)	H₂0 (g) / FAT (g)	PRO (g) / SFA (g)	CHO (g) / MUFA (g)	SUGR (g) / PUFA (g)	DFIB (g) / CHOL (mg)	Na (mg) / K (mg)	Ca (mg) / P (mg)	Mg (mg) / Fe (mg)	Zn (mg) / Cu (mg)	Mn (mg) / Se (mcg)	A (mcg RAE) / A (IU)	C (mg) / E (mg ATE)	B-1 (mg) / B-2 (mg)	NIA (mg) / B-6 (mg)	B-12 (mcg) / FOL (mcg DFE)	PANT (mg) / REF
acorn flour, full-fat	142	1.7	2.1	15.5			0	12	31	0.18	0.494	1	0	0.04	0.7	0.00	0.26
1 oz	28	8.6	1.1	5.4	1.6	0	202	29	0.34	0.173		14		0.04	0.20	32.3	12060
acorns,	144	1.4	2.3	15.2			0	15	23	0.19	0.386	0	0	0.04	0.7	0.00	0.27
dried - *1 oz*	28	8.9	1.2	5.6	1.7	0	201	29	0.29	0.232		0		0.04	0.20	32.6	12059
raw	110	7.9	1.7	11.6			0	12	18	0.14	0.379	1	0	0.03	0.5	0.00	0.20
1 oz	28	6.8	0.9	4.3	1.3	0	153	22	0.22	0.176		11		0.03	0.15	24.7	12058
almond butter	101	0.2	2.4	3.4		0.6	2	43	48	0.49	0.377	0	<1	0.02	0.5	0.00	0.04
1 T	16	9.5	0.9	6.1	2.0	0	121	84	0.59	0.144		0	3.2	0.10	0.01	10.4	12195
almond paste	130	4.0	2.6	13.6		1.4	3	49	37	0.42	0.243	0	<1	0.02	0.4	0.00	0.03
1 oz	28	7.9	0.7	5.1	1.7	0	89	73	0.45	0.129	1.2	1	5.7	0.12	0.01	20.7	12071
almonds, barbeque, Blue Diamond	170		6.0	5.0	1.0	3.0	140	80					0				
28 pieces (1 oz)	28	16.0	1.0			0			1.08			0	10.5				BLDM6
dry roasted	169	0.7	6.3	5.5	1.4	3.3	0	75	81	1.00	0.743	0	0	0.02	1.1	0.00	0.06
1 oz (~22 nuts)	28	15.0	1.1	9.5	3.6	0	211	139	1.28	0.332	1.2	<1	7.5	0.24	0.04	9.4	12063
honey roasted	168	0.5	5.2	7.9		3.9	37	75	68	0.74	0.568	0	<1	0.03	0.8	0.00	0.07
1 oz	28	14.1	1.3	9.2	3.0	0	159	113	0.80	0.275		0		0.27	0.02	9.1	12206

	KCAL / WT (g)	H_2O (g) / FAT (g)	PRO (g) / SFA (g)	CHO (g) / MUFA (g)	SUGR (g) / PUFA (g)	DFIB (g) / CHOL (mg)	Na (mg) / K (mg)	Ca (mg) / P (mg)	Mg (mg) / Fe (mg)	Zn (mg) / Cu (mg)	Mn (mg) / Se (mcg)	A (mcg RAE) / A (IU)	C (mg) / E (mg ATE)	B-1 (mg) / B-2 (mg)	NIA (mg) / B-6 (mg)	B-12 (mcg) / FOL (mcg DFE)	PANT (mg) / REF
oil roasted	172	0.8	6.0	5.0	1.3	3.0	0	82	78	0.87	0.697	0	0	0.03	1.0		0.06
1 oz (22 nuts)	28	15.6	1.2	9.9	3.8	0	198	132	1.04	0.271	1.2	<1	7.4	0.22	0.03	7.7	12065
smokehouse, Blue Diamond	170		6.0	5.0	1.0	3.0	150	80					0				
28 pieces (1 oz)	28	16.0	1.0			0			1.08			0	10.5				BLDM7
sugar-coated	16	0.1	0.3	2.5		0.2	1	4	3	0.03		0	0	<0.01	<0.1	0.00	
1 piece	3.5	0.7	0.1	0.4	0.1	0	9	6	0.07	0.011	0.1	0	0.1	0.01	<0.01	0.7	19858
beechnuts, dried	163	1.9	1.8	9.5			11	0	0	0.10	0.380	0	4	0.09	0.2	0.00	0.26
1 oz	28	14.2	1.6	6.2	5.7	0	288	0	0.70	0.190		0		0.11	0.19	32.0	12077
brazilnuts, dried	186	0.9	4.1	3.6		1.5	1	50	64	1.30	0.219	0	<1	0.28	0.5	0.00	0.07
1 oz (6–8 nuts)	28	18.8	4.6	6.5	6.8	0	170	170	0.96	0.502	839.2	0	2.2	0.03	0.07	1.1	12078
butternuts, dried	174	0.9	7.1	3.4		1.3	0	15	67	0.89	1.860	2	1	0.11	0.3	0.00	0.18
1 oz (~9 nuts)	28	16.2	0.4	3.0	12.1	0	119	126	1.14	0.128	4.9	35	1.0	0.04	0.16	18.7	12084
cashew butter	94	0.5	2.8	4.4		0.3	2	7	41	0.83	0.130	0	0	0.05	0.3	0.00	0.19
1 T	16	7.9	1.6	4.7	1.3	0	87	73	0.80	0.350	1.8	0	0.2	0.03	0.04	10.9	12088
cashews, dry roasted	163	0.5	4.3	9.3		0.9	5	13	74	1.59	0.234	0	0	0.06	0.4	0.00	0.35
1 oz	28	13.1	2.6	7.7	2.2	0	160	139	1.70	0.629	3.3	0	0.2	0.06	0.07	19.6	12085
oil roasted	164	1.0	4.8	8.5	1.4	0.9	4	12	77	1.52	0.473	0	<1	0.10	0.5	0.00	0.25
1 oz (18 nuts)	28	13.5	2.4	7.3	2.4	0	179	151	1.72	0.579	5.8	0	0.4	0.06	0.09	7.1	12086
raw	160	1.5	5.2	7.7	1.7	0.9	3	10	83	1.64	0.469	0	<1	0.12	0.3	0.00	0.24
1 oz	28	13.3	2.4	7.2	2.4	0	187	168	1.89	0.622	5.6	0	0.4	0.02	0.12	7.1	12087
chestnuts, chinese,	43	17.5	0.8	9.5			1	3	16	0.17	0.311	2	7	0.03	0.2	0.00	0.11
boiled & steamed - 1 oz	28	0.2	<0.1	0.1	0.1	0	87	19	0.27	0.071		39		0.03	0.08	13.0	12095
dried	103	2.5	1.9	22.6			1	8	39	0.40	0.737	5	17	0.07	0.4	0.00	0.26
1 oz	28	0.5	0.1	0.3	0.1	0	206	44	0.65	0.167		93		0.08	0.19	31.2	12094
raw	64	12.5	1.2	13.9			1	5	24	0.25	0.454	3	10	0.05	0.2	0.00	0.16
1 oz	28	0.3	<0.1	0.2	0.1	0	127	27	0.40	0.103		57		0.05	0.12	19.3	12093
roasted	68	11.4	1.3	14.8			1	5	26	0.26	0.484	0	11	0.04	0.4	0.00	0.17
1 oz	28	0.3	<0.1	0.2	0.1	0	135	29	0.43	0.110		1		0.03	0.12	20.4	12096
chestnuts, european,	37	19.3	0.6	7.9			8	13	15	0.07	0.242	<1	8	0.04	0.2	0.00	0.09
boiled & steamed - 1 oz	28	0.4	0.1	0.1	0.2	0	203	28	0.49	0.134		5		0.03	0.07	10.8	12101
dried	106	2.7	1.8	21.9		3.3	10	19	21	0.10	0.369	0	4	0.08	0.2	0.00	0.25
1 oz	28	1.3	0.2	0.4	0.5	0	280	50	0.67	0.184	0.5	0	0.3	0.10	0.19	30.9	12099
raw	60	13.8	0.7	12.9		2.3	1	8	9	0.15	0.270	<1	12	0.07	0.3	0.00	0.14
1 oz	28	0.6	0.1	0.2	0.3	0	147	26	0.29	0.127		8		0.05	0.11	17.6	12097
roasted	69	11.5	0.9	15.0		1.4	1	8	9	0.16	0.335	<1	7	0.07	0.4	0.00	0.16
1 oz (3 nuts)	28	0.6	0.1	0.2	0.2	0	168	30	0.26	0.144	0.3	7	0.3	0.05	0.14	19.8	12167
chestnuts, japanese,	16	24.4	0.2	3.6			1	3	5	0.11	0.163	<1	3	0.04	0.2	0.00	0.02
boiled & steamed - 1 oz	28	0.1	<0.1	<0.1	<0.1	0	34	7	0.15	0.058		4		0.02	0.03	4.8	12203
dried	102	2.8	1.5	23.1			10	20	33	0.73	1.052	1	17	0.23	1.0	0.00	0.14
1 oz	28	0.4	0.1	0.2	0.1	0	218	48	0.96	0.372		24		0.11	0.19	30.9	12175
raw	44	17.4	0.6	9.9			4	9	14	0.31	0.451	1	7	0.10	0.4	0.00	0.06
1 oz	28	0.2	<0.1	0.1	<0.1	0	93	20	0.41	0.159		10		0.05	0.08	13.3	12202
roasted	57	14.1	0.8	12.8			5	10	18	0.41	0.585	1	8	0.13	0.2	0.00	0.13
1 oz	28	0.2	<0.1	0.1	0.1	0	121	26	0.60	0.207		21			0.12	16.7	12204
coconut cream,	792	129.4	8.7	16.0		5.3	10	26	67	2.30	3.130	0	7	0.07	2.1	0.00	0.63
raw[1] - 8 fl oz	240	83.2	73.8	3.5	0.9	0	780	293	5.47	0.907		0	1.8	0.00	0.11	55.2	12115
sweetened, cnd[1]	568	210.8	8.0	24.7		6.5	148	3	50	1.78	2.412	0	5	0.07	0.1	0.00	0.48
8 fl oz	296	52.5	46.5	2.2	0.6	0	299	65	1.51	0.699	16.3	0	2.2	0.12	0.09	41.4	12116
coconut, dried	187	0.9	2.0	6.9		4.6	10	7	26	0.57	0.778	0	<1	0.02	0.2	0.00	0.23
1 oz	28	18.3	16.2	0.8	0.2	0	154	58	0.94	0.226	5.2	0	0.4	0.03	0.09	2.6	12108
creamed	194	0.5	1.5	6.1			10	7	26	0.58	0.789	0	<1	0.02	0.2	0.00	0.23
1 oz	28	19.6	17.4	0.8	0.2	0	156	59	0.95	0.229		0		0.03	0.09	2.6	12177
sweetened, flaked, cnd	505	26.5	3.8	46.6		5.1	23	16	56	1.81	2.475	0	0	0.03	0.3	0.00	0.72
4 oz	114	36.1	32.0	1.5	0.4	0	369	117	2.10	0.351		0	0.8	0.02	0.27	8.0	12110
sweetened, flaked,	134	4.4	0.9	13.5		1.2	73	4	14	0.50	0.677	0	0	0.01	0.1	0.00	0.20
packaged - 1 oz	28	9.1	8.1	0.4	0.1	0	90	28	0.51	0.085	4.6	0	0.2	0.01	0.07	2.3	12109
sweetened, shredded	466	11.7	2.7	44.3		4.2	244	14	47	1.69	2.302	0	1	0.03	0.4	0.00	0.67
1 cup	93	33.0	29.3	1.4	0.4	0	313	100	1.79	0.291	15.5	0	1.3	0.02	0.25	7.4	12179
toasted	168	0.3	1.5	12.6			10	8	26	0.58	0.794	0	<1	0.02	0.2	0.00	0.23
1 oz	28	13.3	11.8	0.6		0	157	60	0.96	0.230		0		0.03	0.09	2.6	12114
coconut milk,	445	164.7	4.6	6.4			29	41	104	1.27	1.736	0	2	0.05	1.4	0.00	0.35
cnd[2] - 8 fl oz	226	48.2	42.7	2.0	0.5	0	497	217	7.46	0.504		0		0.00	0.06	31.6	12118

	KCAL	H_2O (g)	PRO (g)	CHO (g)	SUGR (g)	DFIB (g)	Na (mg)	Ca (mg)	Mg (mg)	Zn (mg)	Mn (mg)	A (mcg RAE)	C (mg)	B-1 (mg)	NIA (mg)	B-12 (mcg)	PANT (mg)
	WT (g)	FAT (g)	SFA (g)	MUFA (g)	PUFA (g)	CHOL (mg)	K (mg)	P (mg)	Fe (mg)	Cu (mg)	Se (mcg)	A (IU)	E (mg ATE)	B-2 (mg)	B-6 (mg)	FOL (mcg DFE)	REF
frzn[2]	485	171.4	3.9	13.4			29	10	77	1.42	1.942	0	3	0.06	1.6	0.00	0.39
8 fl oz	240	49.9	44.3	2.1	0.5	0	557	142	1.94	0.564		0		0.00	0.07	33.6	12176
raw[2]	552	162.3	5.5	13.3		5.3	36	38	89	1.61	2.198	0	7	0.06	1.8	0.00	0.44
8 fl oz	240	57.2	50.7	2.4	0.6	0	631	240	3.94	0.638	14.9	0	1.8	0.00	0.08	38.4	12117
coconut, raw	159	21.1	1.5	6.9		4.1	9	6	14	0.50	0.675	0	1	0.03	0.2	0.00	0.14
1.6 oz piece (2″× 2″× 1/2″)	45	15.1	13.4	0.6	0.2	0	160	51	1.09	0.196	4.5	0	0.3	0.01	0.02	11.7	12104
coconut water[3]	46	228.0	1.7	8.9		2.6	252	58	60	0.24	0.341	0	6	0.07	0.2	0.00	0.10
8 fl oz	240	0.5	0.4	<0.1	<0.1	0	600	48	0.70	0.096	2.4	0	0.0	0.14	0.08	7.2	12119
cornuts	124	0.4	2.4	20.8		2.0	156	3	32	0.50	0.129	0	0	0.01	0.5	0.00	0.10
1 oz	28	4.0	0.7	2.1	0.9	0	79	78	0.47	0.033	4.2	0	0.3	0.04	0.06	0.0	19009
barbeque	124	0.5	2.6	20.3		2.4	277	5	31	0.53	0.138	5	<1	0.10	0.4	0.00	0.11
1 oz	28	4.1	0.7	2.1	0.9	0	81	80	0.48	0.039		96		0.04	0.05	0.0	19401
nacho	124	0.6	2.7	20.3		2.3	180	10	31	0.51	0.116	1	4	0.10	0.3	0.00	0.15
1 oz	28	4.0	0.7	2.1	0.9	1	88	88	0.48	0.043		11		0.02	0.06	4.3	19402
filberts (hazelnuts),	178	1.5	4.2	4.7	1.2	2.7	0	32	46	0.69	1.751	1	2	0.18	0.5	0.00	0.26
dried - 1 oz (20 nuts)	28	17.2	1.3	12.9	2.2	0	193	82	1.33	0.489	1.1	11	4.3	0.03	0.16	32.0	12120
dry roasted	183	0.7	4.3	5.0	1.4	2.7	0	35	49	0.71	1.573	1	1	0.10	0.6	0.00	0.26
1 oz	28	17.7	1.3	13.2	2.4	0	214	88	1.24	0.496	1.2	17	4.4	0.03	0.18	24.9	12122
ginkgo nuts,	31	20.7	0.6	6.3		2.6	87	1	5	0.06	0.019	5	3	0.04	1.0	0.00	0.03
cnd - 1 oz (14 nuts)	28	0.5	0.1	0.2	0.2	0	51	15	0.08	0.047	0.1	96	1.0	0.02	0.06	9.4	12129
dried	99	3.5	2.9	20.5			4	6	15	0.19	0.062	16	8	0.12	3.3	0.00	0.38
1 oz	28	0.6	0.1	0.2	0.2	0	283	76	0.45	0.152		309			0.18	30.1	12128
raw	52	15.6	1.2	10.7			2	1	8	0.10	0.032	8	4	0.06	1.7	0.00	0.05
1 oz	28	0.5	0.1	0.2	0.2	0	145	35	0.28	0.078		158		0.03	0.09	15.3	12127
hickorynuts, dried	186	0.8	3.6	5.2		1.8	0	17	49	1.22	1.307	2	1	0.25	0.3	0.00	0.49
1 oz (~9-10 nuts)	28	18.2	2.0	9.2	6.2	0	124	95	0.60	0.209	2.3	37	1.5	0.04	0.05	11.3	12130
macadamia nuts,	204	0.5	2.2	3.8	1.2	2.3	1	20	33	0.37	0.861	0	<1	0.20	0.6	0.00	0.17
dry roasted - 1 oz (10-12 nuts)	28	21.6	3.4	16.8	0.4	0	103	56	0.75	0.162	1.0	0	0.2	0.02	0.10	2.8	12132
raw	204	0.4	2.2	3.9	1.3	2.4	1	24	37	0.37	1.171	0	<1	0.34	0.7	0.00	0.21
1 oz (10-12 nuts)	28	21.5	3.4	16.7	0.4	0	104	53	1.05	0.214	1.0	0	0.2	0.05	0.08	3.1	12131
mixed nuts,	168	0.5	4.9	7.2		2.6	3	20	64	1.08	0.549	<1	<1	0.06	1.3	0.00	0.34
dry roasted[4] - 1 oz	28	14.6	2.0	8.9	3.1	0	169	123	1.05	0.363		4	1.7	0.06	0.08	14.2	12135
oil roasted[5]	175	0.6	4.8	6.1		2.8	3	31	67	1.44	0.536	<1	<1	0.14	1.4	0.00	0.35
1 oz	28	16.0	2.5	9.0	3.8	0	165	132	0.91	0.471		5	1.7	0.06	0.07	23.5	12137
w/o peanuts, oil roasted	174	0.9	4.4	6.3		1.6	3	30	71	1.32	0.439	<1	<1	0.14	0.6	0.00	0.27
1 oz	28	15.9	2.6	9.4	3.2	0	154	127	0.73	0.509		6	1.7	0.14	0.05	15.9	12138
peanut butter,	100		4.0	13.0	5.0	0	220	40				0	5					
85% less fat, Wonder - 2 T	32	2.5	0.0			0				0.36		0					WNDR2
chunk style/crunchy	188	0.4	7.7	6.9		2.1	156	13	51	0.89	0.597	0	0	0.04	4.4	0.00	0.31
2 T	32	16.0	3.1	7.5	4.5	0	239	101	0.61	0.165	2.4	0		0.04	0.14	29.4	16097
creamy, Skippy	190		7.0	7.0	3.0	2.0	150	0				0			4.0		
2 T	32	17.0	3.5			0				0.36		0	3.0				UNLV76
creamy/smooth	190	0.4	8.1	6.2		1.9	149	12	51	0.93	0.143	0	0	0.03	4.3	0.00	0.26
2 T	32	16.3	3.3	7.8	4.4	0	214	118	0.59	0.044	2.4	0	3.2	0.03	0.15	23.7	16098
super chunk, Skippy	190		7.0	7.0	3.0	2.0	140	0				0			4.0		
2 T	32	17.0	3.5			0				0.36		0	3.0				UNLV77
peanut butter spread, red fat,	190		7.0	15.0	5.0	2.0	190	0	60	0.90		0			5.0		
creamy, Skippy - 2 T	36	12.0	2.5			0			0.72	0.200		0			0.12	24.0	UNLV74
reduced fat, super chunk,	190		7.0	14.0	4.0	2.0	170	0	60	0.90		0			5.0		
Skippy - 2 T	35	12.0	2.5			0			0.72	0.200		0			0.12	24.0	UNLV75
peanut flour,	93	2.2	14.8	9.8		4.5	51	40	105	1.45	1.389	0	0	0.20	7.7	0.00	0.78
defatted - 1 oz	28	0.2	<0.1	0.1	<0.1	0	366	215	0.60	0.510	2.0	0	<0.1	0.14	0.14	70.3	16099
lowfat	121	2.2	9.6	8.9		4.5	0	37	14	1.70	1.199	0	0	0.13	3.3	0.00	0.44
1 oz	28	6.2	0.9	3.1	2.0	0	385	144	1.34	0.578	2.0	0		0.05	0.09	37.7	16100
peanut spread, crunch, Doubly	210		7.0	12.0	8.0	2.0	135	20				0			3.0		
Delicious - 2 T	35	15.0	3.5			0				0.72		0					UNLV78
morsels, Double Delicious	210		7.0	12.0	8.0	2.0	130	0				0			3.0		
Delicious - 2 T	35	15.0	3.5			0				0.72		0					UNLV79
peanuts, all types,	89	11.7	3.8	6.0		2.5	210	15	29	0.51	0.286	0	0	0.07	1.5	0.00	0.23
boiled - 1/2 cup (33 nuts)	28	6.2	0.9	3.1	1.9	0	50	55	0.28	0.140	1.2	0	0.9	0.02	0.06	21.0	16088
dry roasted	166	0.4	6.7	6.1		2.3	230	15	50	0.94	0.591	0	0	0.12	3.8	0.00	0.40
1 oz (28 nuts)	28	14.1	2.0	7.0	4.4	0	187	101	0.64	0.190	2.1	0	2.1	0.03	0.07	41.1	16090

	KCAL	H_2O (g)	PRO (g)	CHO (g)	SUGR (g)	DFIB (g)	Na (mg)	Ca (mg)	Mg (mg)	Zn (mg)	Mn (mg)	A (mcg RAE)	C (mg)	B-1 (mg)	NIA (mg)	B-12 (mcg)	PANT (mg)
	WT (g)	FAT (g)	SFA (g)	MUFA (g)	PUFA (g)	CHOL (mg)	K (mg)	P (mg)	Fe (mg)	Cu (mg)	Se (mcg)	A (IU)	E (mg ATE)	B-2 (mg)	B-6 (mg)	FOL (mcg DFE)	REF
oil roasted	837	2.8	37.9	27.3		13.2	624	127	266	9.55	2.969	0	0	0.36	20.6	0.00	2.00
1 cup halves & whole	144	71.0	9.9	35.2	22.4	0	982	744	2.64	1.872	10.8	0	10.7	0.16	0.37	181.4	16089
unroasted/raw	161	1.8	7.3	4.6		2.4	5	26	48	0.93	0.548	0	0	0.18	3.4	0.00	0.50
1 oz	28	14.0	1.9	6.9	4.4	0	200	107	1.30	0.324	2.0	0	2.6	0.04	0.10	68.0	16087
peanuts, spanish,	164	0.5	7.9	4.9		2.5	123	28	48	0.57	0.668	0	0	0.09	4.2	0.00	0.39
oil roasted - *1 oz*	28	13.9	2.1	6.3	4.8	0	220	110	0.65	0.187	2.1	0		0.02	0.07	35.7	16092
unroasted/raw	162	1.8	7.4	4.5		2.7	6	30	53	0.60	0.748	0	0	0.19	4.5	0.00	0.50
1 oz	28	14.1	2.2	6.3	4.9	0	211	110	1.11	0.255	2.0	0		0.04	0.10	68.0	16091
peanuts, valencia,	167	0.6	7.7	4.6		2.5	219	15	45	0.87	0.488	0	0	0.03	4.1	0.00	0.39
oil roasted - *1 oz*	28	14.5	2.2	6.5	5.0	0	174	90	0.47	0.238	2.1	0		0.04	0.07	35.7	16094
unroasted/raw	162	1.2	7.1	5.9		2.5	0	18	52	0.95	0.561	0	0	0.18	3.7	0.00	0.51
1 oz	28	13.5	2.1	6.1	4.7	0	94	95	0.59	0.332	2.1	0		0.09	0.10	69.7	16093
peanuts, virginia,	164	0.6	7.3	5.6		2.5	123	24	53	1.88	0.569	0	0	0.08	4.2	0.00	0.39
oil roasted - *1 oz*	28	13.8	1.8	7.2	4.2	0	185	143	0.47	0.361	2.1	0		0.03	0.07	35.4	16096
unroasted/raw	160	2.0	7.1	4.7		2.4	3	25	48	1.26	0.481	0	0	0.19	3.5	0.00	0.50
1 oz	28	13.8	1.8	7.2	4.2	0	196	108	0.72	0.315	2.0	0		0.04	0.10	67.8	16095
pecans,	196	1.0	2.6	3.9	1.1	2.7	0	20	34	1.28	1.276	1	<1	0.19	0.3	0.00	0.24
dried - *1 oz (20 halves)*	28	20.4	1.8	11.6	6.1	0	116	79	0.72	0.340	1.7	22	1.1	0.04	0.06	6.2	12142
dry roasted	201	0.3	2.7	3.8	1.2	2.7	0	20	37	1.44	1.115	2	<1	0.13	0.3	0.00	0.20
1 oz	28	21.1	1.8	12.5	5.8	0	120	83	0.79	0.331	1.1	40	1.1	0.03	0.05	4.5	12143
oil roasted	203	0.3	2.6	3.7	1.1	2.7	0	19	34	1.27	1.049	1	<1	0.13	0.3	0.00	0.21
1 oz (15 halves)	28	21.3	2.1	11.6	6.7	0	111	75	0.70	0.340	1.7	29	1.5	0.13	0.05	4.3	12144
pilinuts, dried	204	0.8	3.1	1.1			1	41	86	0.84	0.656	1	<1	0.26	0.1	0.00	0.14
1 oz (15 nuts)	28	22.6	8.8	10.6	2.2	0	144	163	1.00	0.272		12		0.03	0.03	17.0	12145
pine nuts,	160	1.9	6.8	4.0		1.3	1	7	66	1.20	1.218	<1	1	0.23	1.0	0.00	0.06
pignolia, dried - *1 oz (15–16 nuts)*	28	14.4	2.2	5.4	6.1	0	170	144	2.61	0.291	4.7	8	1.0	0.05	0.03	16.2	12147
pinyon, dried	178	1.7	3.3	5.5		3.0	20	2	66	1.21	1.228	<1	1	0.35	1.2	0.00	0.06
1 oz	28	17.3	2.7	6.5	7.3	0	178	10	0.87	0.293		8		0.06	0.03	16.4	12149
pistachios,	158	1.1	5.8	7.9	2.2	2.9	0	30	34	0.62	0.340	8	1	0.25	0.4	0.00	0.15
dried - *1 oz (47 nuts)*	28	12.6	1.5	6.6	3.8	0	291	139	1.18	0.369	2.0	157	1.3	0.05	0.48	14.5	12151
dry roasted	162	0.6	6.1	7.8	2.2	2.9	3	31	34	0.65	0.361	8	1	0.24	0.4	0.00	0.15
1 oz (47 nuts)	28	13.0	1.6	6.9	3.9	0	295	137	1.19	0.376	2.3	151	1.2	0.04	0.48	14.2	12152
soy nut butter, creamy/chunky, no	160		8.0	5.0	1.0	5.0	160	60					0				
added sugar, IM Healthy - *2 T*	32	13.0	1.5			0			1.26			0					SYNT1
creamy/chunky, original, IM	170		8.0	10.0	3.0	1.0	170	50					1				
Healthy - *2 T*	32	11.0	1.5			0			0.36			0					SYNT4
creamy/chunky w/honey, IM	170		7.0	12.0	2.0	2.0	150	30					1				
Healthy - *2 T*	32	11.0	1.5			0			0.54			0					SYNT3
creamy/crunchy, Wonder	170		8.0	10.0	3.0	1.0	170	60					0				
2 T	32	11.0	1.5			0			0.36			0					WNDR1
creamy w/choc, IM Healthy	190		7.0	12.0	6.0	1.0	50	30					0				
2 T	32	14.0	2.0			0			0.54			0					SYNT2
roasted, Natural Touch	186	0.4	6.7	11.6	2.7	2.5	133	5		0.53			<1	0.00	0.0		
1.1 oz	32	12.5	1.9	2.8	6.6	1	118	81	0.79			0		0.01			WRTH94
soy nuts,	130		9.0	8.0	3.0	5.0	170	40					1				
bbq, Simple Snacks - *1 oz*	28	9.0	1.0			0			1.80			100					SMPL4
choc covered, GeniSoy	200		9.0	23.0	16.0	2.0	190	200	80	3.75			15	0.38	5.0	1.50	2.50
1 oz	28	8.0	3.0			0	190	200	4.50	0.500		1250	7.5	0.43	0.50	100.0	GENI3
dry roasted	774	1.4	68.1	56.3		13.9	3	241	392	8.20	3.756	2	8	0.73	1.8	0.00	0.81
1 cup	172	37.2	5.4	8.2	21.0	0	2346	1116	6.79	1.856	33.2	40		1.30	0.39	352.6	16111
flavored, GeniSoy[6]	190		9.0	24.0	18.0	2.0	90	100	40	3.75			15	0.38	5.0	1.50	2.50
1 oz	28	7.0	3.5			0	190	150	4.50	0.500		1250	7.5	0.43	0.50	100.0	GENI4
honey rstd, Simple Snacks	110		8.0	11.0	5.0	5.0	90	40					1				
1 oz	28	7.0	1.0			0			1.08			100					SMPL5
lightly salted, Simple Snacks	100		9.0	9.0	3.0	5.0	100	40					1				
1 oz	28	6.0	1.0			0			1.08			100					SMPL3
roasted	810	3.4	60.6	57.7		30.4	280	237	249	5.40	3.712	17	4	0.17	2.4	0.00	0.78
1 cup	172	43.7	6.3	9.6	24.7	0	2528	624	6.71	1.424	32.9	344	3.4	0.25	0.36	362.9	16110
unsalted, GeniSoy	190		9.0	23.0	16.0	2.0	130	150	60	3.75			15	0.38	5.0	1.50	2.50
1 oz	28	7.0	3.0			0	180	200	4.50	0.500		1250	7.5	0.43	0.50	100.0	GENI5
w/praline coating, GeniSoy	190		9.0	24.0	18.0	1.0	90	150	40	3.75			15	0.38	5.0	1.50	2.50
1 oz (55 nuts)	28	7.0	3.0			0	150	150	4.50	0.500		1250	7.5	0.43	0.50	100.0	GENI2

	KCAL / WT (g)	H₂0 (g) / FAT (g)	PRO (g) / SFA (g)	CHO (g) / MUFA (g)	SUGR (g) / PUFA (g)	DFIB (g) / CHOL (mg)	Na (mg) / K (mg)	Ca (mg) / P (mg)	Mg (mg) / Fe (mg)	Zn (mg) / Cu (mg)	Mn (mg) / Se (mcg)	A (mcg RAE) / A (IU)	C (mg) / E (mg ATE)	B-1 (mg) / B-2 (mg)	NIA (mg) / B-6 (mg)	B-12 (mcg) / FOL (mcg DFE)	PANT (mg) / REF
trail mix,	115	2.6	1.8	18.6			3	16	27	0.33	0.274	1	2	0.13	0.4		0.35
tropical - *1 oz*	28	4.8	2.4	0.7	1.5	0	201	53	0.75	0.150		14		0.03	0.09	11.9	19061
w/choc chips	137	1.9	4.0	12.7			34	31	46	0.89	0.301	1	<1	0.12	1.2	0.00	0.27
1 oz	28	9.0	1.7	3.8	3.2	1	184	110	0.96	0.239		12		0.06	0.07	18.4	19062
walnuts,	175	1.3	6.8	2.8	0.3	1.9	1	17	57	0.96	1.105	1	<1	0.02	0.1	0.00	0.47
black, dried - *1 oz*	28	16.7	1.0	4.3	9.9	0	148	145	0.88	0.386	4.8	11	1.3	0.04	0.17	8.8	12154
english/persian, dried	185	1.2	4.3	3.9	0.7	1.9	1	28	45	0.88	0.968	1	<1	0.10	0.6	0.00	0.16
1 oz (14 halves)	28	18.5	1.7	2.5	13.4	0	125	98	0.82	0.450	1.3	12	0.8	0.04	0.15	27.8	12155
wheat-base formulated nuts,	183	0.6	3.7	5.9		1.5	26	6	17	0.84	1.970	0	<1	0.11	0.4	0.00	0.09
flavored[7] - *1 oz*	28	17.7	2.7	7.3	6.9	0	91	104	0.74	0.051		<1		0.09	0.10	35.4	12200
macadamia flavored[8]	175	0.9	3.2	7.9		1.5	13	6	16	0.83	1.461	0	<1	0.06	0.3	0.00	0.09
1 oz	28	16.0	2.4	6.7	6.2	0	74	85	0.57	0.051		<1		0.06	0.07	26.6	12199
unflavored[9]	176	0.7	3.9	6.7		1.5	143	7	16	0.83	2.245	0	<1	0.09	0.4	0.00	0.09
1 oz	28	16.4	2.5	6.7	6.4	0	90	105	0.68	0.051		<1		0.09	0.11	40.3	12140

[1] Liquid expressed from grated coconut.
[2] Liquid expressed from grated coconut and coconut water.
[3] Liquid from the coconut center.
[4] Cashews, almonds, peanuts, filberts, and pecans.
[5] Cashews, peanuts, brazilnuts, filberts, almonds, and pecans.
[6] Values are averages for 3 flavors, deep sea salted, old hickory smoked, and zesty barbeque.

[7] Hydrogenated soybean oil, wheat germ, sugar, sodium caseinate, soy protein, natural and artificial flavors, and artificial color.
[8] Hydrogenated soybean oil, wheat germ, sugar, wheat starch, sodium caseinate, soy protein, natural and artificial flavor.
[9] Hydrogenated soybean oil, wheat germ, fructose, wheat starch, sodium caseinate, soy protein, and salt.

23.2 SEEDS & SEED PRODUCTS

	KCAL / WT (g)	H₂0 (g) / FAT (g)	PRO (g) / SFA (g)	CHO (g) / MUFA (g)	SUGR (g) / PUFA (g)	DFIB (g) / CHOL (mg)	Na (mg) / K (mg)	Ca (mg) / P (mg)	Mg (mg) / Fe (mg)	Zn (mg) / Cu (mg)	Mn (mg) / Se (mcg)	A (mcg RAE) / A (IU)	C (mg) / E (mg ATE)	B-1 (mg) / B-2 (mg)	NIA (mg) / B-6 (mg)	B-12 (mcg) / FOL (mcg DFE)	PANT (mg) / REF
breadfruit seeds,	48	16.8	1.5	9.1		1.4	7	17	14	0.24	0.037	3	2	0.08	1.5	0.00	0.23
boiled - *1 oz*	28	0.7	0.2	0.1	0.3	0	248	35	0.17	0.303		67		0.05	0.08	13.9	12003
raw	54	16.0	2.1	8.3		1.5	7	10	15	0.26	0.040	4	2	0.14	0.1	0.00	0.25
1 oz	28	1.6	0.4	0.2	0.8	0	267	50	1.04	0.325		73		0.09	0.09	15.0	12001
roasted	59	14.1	1.8	11.4		1.7	8	24	18	0.29	0.046	4	2	0.12	2.1	0.00	0.29
1 oz	28	0.8	0.2	0.1	0.4	0	307	50	0.26	0.375		83		0.07	0.12	16.7	12158
cottonseed flour,	94	2.0	14.1	10.2			10	134	203	3.29	0.604	6	1	0.59	1.1	0.00	0.13
lowfat - *1 oz*	28	0.4	0.1	0.1	0.2	0	499	450	3.57	0.332		122		0.11	0.22	64.6	12008
partially defatted	18	0.3	2.0	2.0		0.2	2	24	36	0.58	0.107	1	<1	0.11	0.2	0.00	0.02
1 T	5	0.3	0.1	0.1	0.1	0	89	80	0.63	0.059	0.3	22	<0.1	0.02	0.04	11.5	12007
cottonseed kernels, roasted	51	0.5	3.3	2.2		0.6	3	10	44	0.60	0.218	2	1	0.08	0.3	0.00	0.05
1 T	10	3.6	1.0	0.7	1.8	0	135	80	0.54	0.120		44	<0.1	0.03	0.08	23.3	12160
cottonseed meal, partially defatted	104	0.3	13.9	10.9			10	143	215	3.49	0.641	7	1	0.63	1.2	0.00	0.13
1 oz	28	1.4	0.3	0.2	0.6	0	530	477	3.78	<0.001		130		0.12	0.23	68.6	12011
flaxseeds	59	1.1	2.3	4.1		3.3	4	24	43	0.50	0.394	0	<1	0.02	0.2	0.00	0.18
1 T	12	4.1	0.4	0.8	2.7	0	82	60	0.75	0.125	0.7	0	0.6	0.02	0.11	33.4	12220
lotus seeds,	94	4.0	4.4	18.3			1	46	60	0.30	0.657	1	0	0.18	0.5	0.00	0.24
dried - *1 oz (42 seeds)*	28	0.6	0.1	0.1	0.3	0	388	177	1.00	0.099		14		0.04	0.18	29.5	12013
raw	25	21.8	1.2	4.9			0	12	16	0.08	0.176	<1	0	0.05	0.1	0.00	0.06
1 oz	28	0.2	<0.1	<0.1	0.1	0	104	48	0.27	0.027		4		0.01	0.05	7.9	12205
poppy seed filling, Solo	120	9.6	1.7	20.9			27	116									
2 T	36	3.2	0.4	0.5	2.0												19251
pumpkin & squash seed kernels,	153	2.0	7.0	5.0		1.1	5	12	152	2.11	0.856	5	1	0.06	0.5	0.00	0.10
dried - *1 oz (142 seeds)*	28	13.0	2.5	4.0	5.9	0	229	333	4.24	0.393	1.6	108	0.3	0.09	0.06	16.4	12014
roasted	148	2.0	9.3	3.8		1.1	5	12	151	2.11	0.855	5	1	0.06	0.5	0.00	0.10
1 oz	28	11.9	2.3	3.7	5.4	0	229	332	4.24	0.392	1.6	108	0.3	0.09	0.03	16.2	12016
safflower seed kernels, dried	147	1.6	4.6	9.7			1	22	100	1.43	0.571	1	0	0.33	0.6	0.00	1.14
1 oz	28	10.9	1.0	1.4	8.0	0	195	183	1.39	0.495		14		0.12	0.33	45.4	12021
safflower seed meal, partially	97	1.8	10.1	13.8			1	22	99	1.42	0.566	1	0	0.33	0.6	0.00	1.13
defatted - *1 oz*	28	0.7	0.1	0.1	0.4	0	19	181	1.38	0.491		14		0.12	0.33	45.1	12022
sesame butter (tahini), from	89	0.5	2.6	3.2		1.4	17	64	14	0.69	0.218	<1	0	0.18	0.8	0.00	0.10
roasted & toasted kernels - *1 T*	15	8.1	1.1	3.0	3.5	0	62	110	1.34	0.242	0.3	10	0.3	0.07	0.02	14.7	12166
from unroasted kernels	85	0.4	2.5	2.5		1.3	0	20	49	1.46	0.204	<1	0	0.22	0.8	0.00	0.10
1 T	14	7.9	1.1	3.0	3.5	0	64	111	0.89	0.208		9		0.02	0.02	13.7	12171
sesame butter paste	95	0.3	2.9	4.1		0.9	2	154	58	1.17	0.406	<1	0	0.04	1.1	0.00	0.01
1 T	16	8.1	1.1	3.1	3.6	0	93	105	3.07	0.674	0.9	8	0.4	0.03	0.13	16.0	12169
sesame flour,	149	0.3	8.7	7.5			12	45	102	3.02	0.422	1	0	0.76	3.8	0.00	0.83
high fat - *1 oz*	28	10.5	1.5	4.0	4.6	0	120	229	4.30	0.431		20		0.08	0.04	8.8	12170

	KCAL / WT (g)	H₂O (g) / FAT (g)	PRO (g) / SFA (g)	CHO (g) / MUFA (g)	SUGR (g) / PUFA (g)	DFIB (g) / CHOL (mg)	Na (mg) / K (mg)	Ca (mg) / P (mg)	Mg (mg) / Fe (mg)	Zn (mg) / Cu (mg)	Mn (mg) / Se (mcg)	A (mcg RAE) / A (IU)	C (mg) / E (mg ATE)	B-1 (mg) / B-2 (mg)	NIA (mg) / B-6 (mg)	B-12 (mcg) / FOL (mcg DFE)	PANT (mg) / REF
lowfat	94	2.0	14.2	10.1			11	42	96	2.84	0.396	1	0	0.71	3.6		0.78
1 oz	28	0.5	0.1	0.2	0.2	0	113	215	4.03	0.404		18		0.08	0.04	8.2	12033
partially defatted	108	1.9	11.4	10.0			12	43	103	3.03	0.398	1	0	0.72	3.6	0.00	0.78
1 oz	28	3.4	0.5	1.2	1.4	0	120	230	4.05	0.406		20		0.08	0.04	8.2	12032
sesame meal, partially defatted	161	1.4	4.8	7.4			11	43	98	2.90	0.405	1	0	0.73	3.6	0.00	0.80
1 oz	28	13.6	1.9	5.1	6.0	0	115	219	4.12	0.413		19		0.08	0.04	8.5	12034
sesame seeds, kernels,	47	0.4	2.1	0.8		0.9	3	10	28	0.82	0.114	<1	0	0.06	0.4	0.00	0.05
dried - 1 T	8	4.4	0.6	1.7	1.9	0	33	62	0.62	0.117	0.1	5	0.2	0.01	0.01	7.7	12201
toasted	161	1.4	4.8	7.4		4.8	11	37	98	2.90	0.405	1	0	0.34	1.5	0.00	0.19
1 oz	28	13.6	1.9	5.1	6.0	0	115	219	2.21	0.413	0.5	19	0.6	0.13	0.04	27.2	12029
sesame seeds, whole,	52	0.4	1.6	2.1		1.1	1	88	32	0.70	0.221	0	0	0.07	0.4	0.00	<0.01
dried - 1 T	9	4.5	0.6	1.7	2.0	0	42	57	1.31	0.367	0.5	1	0.2	0.02	0.07	8.7	12023
roasted & toasted	160	0.9	4.8	7.3		4.0	3	280	101	2.03	0.708	0	0	0.23	1.3	0.00	0.01
1 oz	28	13.6	1.9	5.1	6.0	0	135	181	4.18	0.700	1.6	3		0.07	0.23	27.8	12024
sunflower seed butter	93	0.2	3.1	4.4			0	20	59	0.85	0.338	<1	<1	0.05	0.9		1.13
1 T	16	7.6	0.8	1.5	5.0	0	12	118	0.76	0.293		8		0.05	0.13	37.9	12040
sunflower seed flour, partially	13	0.3	1.9	1.4		0.2	0	5	14	0.20	0.079	<1	<1	0.13	0.3	0.00	0.26
defatted - 1 T	4	0.1	<0.1	<0.1	<0.1	0	3	28	0.26	0.069	2.3	2	0.1	0.01	0.03	8.9	12041
sunflower seed kernels,	821	7.7	32.8	27.0		15.1	4	167	510	7.29	2.909	4	2	3.30	6.5	0.00	9.71
dried - 1 cup w/o hulls	144	71.4	7.5	13.6	47.1	0	992	1015	9.75	2.523	85.7	72	72.4	0.36	1.11	326.9	12036
dry roasted	165	0.3	5.5	6.8		3.1	1	20	37	1.50		0	<1	0.09	2.0	0.00	2.00
1 oz	28	14.1	1.5	2.7	9.3	0	241	327	1.08	0.519	22.5	0	14.3	0.07	0.23	67.2	12037
oil roasted	174	0.7	6.1	4.2		1.9	1	16	36	1.48	0.590	1	<1	0.09	1.2	0.00	1.97
1 oz	28	16.3	1.7	3.1	10.8	0	137	323	1.90	0.511	22.2	14	14.3	0.08	0.22	66.3	12038
toasted	175	0.3	4.9	5.8		3.3	1	16	37	1.50	0.599	0	<1	0.09	1.2	0.00	2.00
1 oz	28	16.1	1.7	3.1	10.6	0	139	328	1.93	0.520		0		0.08	0.23	67.5	12039
watermelon seeds, dried	158	1.4	8.0	4.3			28	15	146	2.90	0.458	0	0	0.05	1.0	0.00	0.10
1 oz (95 large seeds)	28	13.4	2.8	2.1	8.0	0	184	214	2.06	0.194		0		0.04	0.03	16.4	12174

24. POULTRY
24.1 CHICKEN, BROILER/FRYER PARTS

	KCAL / WT (g)	H₂O (g) / FAT (g)	PRO (g) / SFA (g)	CHO (g) / MUFA (g)	SUGR (g) / PUFA (g)	DFIB (g) / CHOL (mg)	Na (mg) / K (mg)	Ca (mg) / P (mg)	Mg (mg) / Fe (mg)	Zn (mg) / Cu (mg)	Mn (mg) / Se (mcg)	A (mcg RAE) / A (IU)	C (mg) / E (mg ATE)	B-1 (mg) / B-2 (mg)	NIA (mg) / B-6 (mg)	B-12 (mcg) / FOL (mcg DFE)	PANT (mg) / REF
back w/skin, flour coated & fried	238	31.7	20.0	4.7			65	17	17	1.78	0.036	27	0	0.08	5.3	0.20	0.79
1/2 back (2.5 oz)	72	14.9	4.0	5.9	3.5	64	163	120	1.17	0.066	17.1	89		0.17	0.22	14.4	05050
breast w/skin, flour coated & fried	218	55.5	31.2	1.6		0.1	74	16	29	1.08	0.025	15	0	0.08	13.5	0.33	0.98
1/2 breast (3.5 oz)	98	8.7	2.4	3.4	1.9	87	254	228	1.17	0.056	23.4	49		0.13	0.57	6.9	05059
roasted	193	61.2	29.2	0.0		0.0	70	14	26	1.00	0.018	27	0	0.06	12.5	0.31	0.92
1/2 breast (3.5 oz)	98	7.6	2.1	3.0	1.6	82	240	210	1.05	0.049	24.2	91	0.3	0.12	0.55	3.9	05060
stewed	202	72.8	30.1	0.0		0.0	68	14	24	1.07	0.020	28	0	0.05	8.6	0.23	0.60
1/2 breast (3.9 oz)	110	8.2	2.3	3.2	1.7	83	196	172	1.01	0.048	24.0	90	0.3	0.13	0.32	3.3	05061
breast w/o skin, flour coated &	161	51.8	28.8	0.4			68	14	27	0.93	0.018	6	0	0.07	12.7	0.32	0.89
fried - 1/2 breast (3 oz)	86	4.1	1.1	1.5	0.9	78	237	212	0.98	0.046	22.5	20	0.4	0.11	0.55	3.4	05063
roasted	142	56.1	26.7	0.0		0.0	64	13	25	0.86	0.015	5	0	0.06	11.8	0.29	0.83
1/2 breast (3 oz)	86	3.1	0.9	1.1	0.7	73	220	196	0.89	0.042	23.7	18	0.2	0.10	0.52	3.4	05064
stewed	143	64.9	27.5	0.0		0.0	60	12	23	0.92	0.017	6	0	0.04	8.0	0.22	0.54
1/2 breast (3.4 oz)	95	2.9	0.8	1.0	0.6	73	178	157	0.84	0.041	21.2	18	0.3	0.11	0.31	2.9	05065
drumstick w/skin, flour coated &	120	27.8	13.2	0.8		0.0	44	6	11	1.42	0.014	12	0	0.04	3.0	0.16	0.60
fried - 1.7 oz drumstick	49	6.7	1.8	2.7	1.6	44	112	86	0.66	0.039	9.0	41		0.11	0.17	5.4	05068
roasted	112	32.6	14.1	0.0		0.0	47	6	12	1.49	0.011	16	0	0.04	3.1	0.17	0.63
1.8 oz drumstick	52	5.8	1.6	2.2	1.3	47	119	91	0.69	0.040	9.7	52	0.1	0.11	0.18	4.2	05069
stewed	116	37.1	14.4	0.0		0.0	43	6	11	1.51	0.011	15	0	0.03	2.4	0.13	0.49
2 oz drumstick	57	6.1	1.7	2.3	1.4	47	105	80	0.76	0.040	9.7	52	0.2	0.11	0.11	4.0	05070
drumstick w/o skin, roasted	76	29.4	12.4	0.0		0.0	42	5	11	1.40	0.009	8	0	0.03	2.7	0.15	0.57
1.6 oz drumstick	44	2.5	0.7	0.8	0.6	41	108	81	0.57	0.035	8.4	26	0.1	0.10	0.17	4.0	05073
leg w/skin, flour coated & fried	284	61.9	30.1	2.8		0.1	99	15	27	3.00	0.036	31	0	0.10	7.3	0.35	1.34
4 oz leg	112	16.2	4.4	6.4	3.7	105	261	204	1.60	0.095	23.3	103		0.26	0.38	14.6	05077
roasted	264	69.4	29.6	0.0		0.0	99	14	26	2.96	0.024	47	0	0.08	7.1	0.34	1.32
4 oz leg	114	15.3	4.2	6.0	3.4	105	257	198	1.52	0.088	23.6	154	0.3	0.24	0.38	8.0	05078
stewed	275	80.0	30.2	0.0		0.0	91	14	25	3.04	0.024	46	0	0.07	5.7	0.25	1.02
4.4 oz leg	125	16.2	4.5	6.3	3.6	105	220	174	1.69	0.089	23.6	155	0.3	0.24	0.23	7.5	05079
leg w/o skin, stewed	187	67.1	26.5	0.0		0.0	79	11	21	2.81	0.019	18	0	0.06	4.8	0.23	0.92
3.6 oz leg	101	8.1	2.2	3.0	1.9	90	192	150	1.41	0.078	26.8	61	0.3	0.22	0.21	8.1	05083
neck w/skin, flour coated & fried	120	17.1	8.6	1.5			30	11	7	1.11	0.019	21	0	0.03	1.9	0.09	0.35
1.3 oz neck	36	8.5	2.3	3.5	2.0	34	65	48	0.87	0.047	6.7	68		0.09	0.09	5.4	05086

	KCAL	H₂O (g)	PRO (g)	CHO (g)	SUGR (g)	DFIB (g)	Na (mg)	Ca (mg)	Mg (mg)	Zn (mg)	Mn (mg)	A (mcg RAE)	C (mg)	B-1 (mg)	NIA (mg)	B-12 (mcg)	PANT (mg)
	WT (g)	FAT (g)	SFA (g)	MUFA (g)	PUFA (g)	CHOL (mg)	K (mg)	P (mg)	Fe (mg)	Cu (mg)	Se (mcg)	A (IU)	E (mg ATE)	B-2 (mg)	B-6 (mg)	FOL (mcg DFE)	REF
simmered	94	23.5	7.5	0.0		0.0	20	10	5	1.03	0.017	18	0	0.02	1.3	0.05	0.20
1.3 oz neck	38	6.9	1.9	2.7	1.5	27	41	46	0.87	0.037	6.6	61	0.1	0.09	0.04	1.1	05087
neck w/o skin, simmered	32	12.1	4.4	0.0		0.0	12	8	3	0.68	0.009	6	0	0.01	0.7	0.03	0.12
.63 neck	18	1.5	0.4	0.5	0.4	14	25	23	0.47	0.023	3.7	22	<0.1	0.05	0.03	1.1	05090
thigh w/skin, flour coated & fried	162	33.6	16.6	2.0		0.1	55	9	16	1.56	0.022	18	0	0.06	4.3	0.19	0.73
2.2 oz thigh	62	9.3	2.5	3.6	2.1	60	147	116	0.92	0.055	12.3	61		0.15	0.20	9.3	05093
roasted	153	36.8	15.5	0.0		0.0	52	7	14	1.46	0.013	31	0	0.04	3.9	0.18	0.69
2.2 oz thigh	62	9.6	2.7	3.8	2.1	58	138	108	0.83	0.048	12.1	102	0.2	0.13	0.19	4.3	05094
stewed	158	42.9	15.8	0.0		0.0	48	7	13	1.53	0.013	31	0	0.04	3.3	0.13	0.53
2.4 oz thigh	68	10.0	2.8	4.0	2.2	57	116	95	0.93	0.048	12.2	103	0.2	0.13	0.12	4.1	05095
thigh w/o skin, roasted	109	32.7	13.5	0.0		0.0	46	6	12	1.34	0.011	10	0	0.04	3.4	0.16	0.62
1.8 oz thigh	52	5.7	1.6	2.2	1.3	49	124	95	0.68	0.042	15.1	34	0.1	0.12	0.18	4.2	05098
wing w/skin, flour coated & fried	103	15.6	8.4	0.8		0.0	25	5	6	0.56	0.009	12	0	0.02	2.1	0.09	0.28
1.1 oz wing	32	7.1	1.9	2.8	1.6	26	57	48	0.40	0.020	6.8	40		0.04	0.13	2.6	05102
roasted	99	18.7	9.1	0.0		0.0	28	5	6	0.62	0.006	16	0	0.01	2.3	0.10	0.30
1.2 oz wing	34	6.6	1.9	2.6	1.4	29	63	51	0.43	0.019	7.5	54	0.1	0.04	0.14	1.0	05103
stewed	100	24.9	9.1	0.0		0.0	27	5	6	0.65	0.007	16	0	0.02	1.8	0.07	0.20
1.4 oz wing	40	6.7	1.9	2.6	1.4	28	56	48	0.45	0.018	7.4	53	0.1	0.04	0.09	1.2	05104

24.2 CHICKEN, BROILERS/FRYERS

	KCAL	H₂O (g)	PRO (g)	CHO (g)	SUGR (g)	DFIB (g)	Na (mg)	Ca (mg)	Mg (mg)	Zn (mg)	Mn (mg)	A (mcg RAE)	C (mg)	B-1 (mg)	NIA (mg)	B-12 (mcg)	PANT (mg)
dark meat w/skin,	215	49.8	22.1	0.0		0.0	74	13	19	2.12	0.018	51	0	0.06	5.4	0.25	0.94
roasted - *3 oz*	85	13.4	3.7	5.3	3.0	77	187	143	1.16	0.065	17.2	171		0.18	0.26	6.0	05037
stewed	198	53.5	20.0	0.0		0.0	60	12	15	1.92	0.016	48	0	0.04	3.8	0.17	0.66
3 oz	85	12.5	3.5	4.9	2.8	70	141	113	1.11	0.058	15.6	158		0.15	0.14	5.1	05038
dark meat w/o skin,	203	47.3	24.6	2.2		0.0	82	15	21	2.47	0.028	20	0	0.08	6.0	0.28	1.07
fried - *3 oz*	85	9.9	2.7	3.7	2.4	82	215	159	1.27	0.076	17.4	67		0.21	0.31	7.7	05044
roasted	174	53.6	23.3	0.0		0.0	79	13	20	2.38	0.018	19	0	0.06	5.6	0.27	1.03
3 oz	85	8.3	2.3	3.0	1.9	79	204	152	1.13	0.068	15.3	61	0.2	0.19	0.31	6.8	05045
stewed	163	56.0	22.1	0.0		0.0	63	12	17	2.26	0.017	18	0	0.05	4.0	0.19	0.76
3 oz	85	7.6	2.1	2.8	1.8	75	154	122	1.16	0.064	14.7	59	0.2	0.17	0.18	6.0	05046
light & dark meat w/skin,	246	42.0	19.2	8.0		0.3	248	18	18	1.42	0.048	24	0	0.10	6.0	0.24	0.76
batter dipped & fried - *3 oz*	85	14.7	3.9	6.0	3.5	74	157	132	1.16	0.061	21.7	79	1.1	0.16	0.26	21.3	05007
flour coated & fried	229	44.5	24.3	2.7		0.1	71	14	21	1.73	0.029	23	0	0.07	7.6	0.26	0.92
3 oz	85	12.7	3.5	5.0	2.9	77	199	162	1.17	0.064	18.4	76	0.5	0.16	0.35	9.4	05008
roasted	203	50.5	23.2	0.0		0.0	70	13	20	1.65	0.017	41	0	0.05	7.2	0.26	0.88
3 oz	85	11.6	3.2	4.5	2.5	75	190	155	1.07	0.056	20.3	137	0.2	0.14	0.34	4.3	05009
stewed	186	54.3	21.0	0.0		0.0	57	11	16	1.50	0.016	37	0	0.04	4.8	0.17	0.57
3 oz	85	10.7	3.0	4.2	2.3	66	141	118	0.99	0.048	15.3	124	0.2	0.13	0.19	4.3	05010
light & dark meat w/o skin,	186	48.9	26.0	1.4		0.1	77	14	23	1.90	0.024	15	0	0.07	8.2	0.29	0.99
flour coated & fried - *3 oz*	85	7.8	2.1	2.8	1.8	80	218	174	1.15	0.064	20.8	50	0.4	0.17	0.41	6.0	05012
roasted	162	54.2	24.6	0.0		0.0	73	13	21	1.79	0.016	14	0	0.06	7.8	0.28	0.94
3 oz	85	6.3	1.7	2.3	1.4	76	207	166	1.03	0.057	18.7	45	0.2	0.15	0.40	5.1	05013
stewed	150	56.8	23.2	0.0		0.0	60	12	18	1.69	0.016	13	0	0.04	5.2	0.19	0.63
3 oz	85	5.7	1.6	2.0	1.3	71	153	128	0.99	0.052	17.8	43	0.2	0.14	0.22	5.1	05014
light meat w/skin,	209	46.5	25.9	1.5		0.1	65	14	23	1.07	0.022	17	0	0.06	10.2	0.28	0.82
flour coated & fried - *3 oz*	85	10.3	2.8	4.1	2.3	74	203	181	1.03	0.049	24.7	58	0.5	0.11	0.46	7.7	05031
roasted	189	51.4	24.7	0.0		0.0	64	13	21	1.05	0.015	28	0	0.05	9.5	0.27	0.79
3 oz	85	9.2	2.6	3.6	2.0	71	193	170	0.97	0.045	20.5	94		0.10	0.44	2.6	05032
stewed	171	55.4	22.2	0.0		0.0	54	11	17	0.97	0.015	25	0	0.03	5.9	0.17	0.45
3 oz	85	8.5	2.4	3.3	1.8	63	142	124	0.83	0.037	18.0	82	0.2	0.10	0.23	2.6	05033
light meat w/o skin,	163	51.1	27.9	0.4		0.0	69	14	25	1.08	0.017	8	0	0.06	11.4	0.31	0.88
fried - *3 oz*	85	4.7	1.3	1.7	1.1	77	224	196	0.97	0.046	22.3	26		0.11	0.54	3.4	05040
roasted	147	55.0	26.3	0.0		0.0	65	13	23	1.05	0.014	8	0	0.06	10.6	0.29	0.83
3 oz	85	3.8	1.1	1.3	0.8	72	210	184	0.90	0.043	20.7	25	0.2	0.10	0.51	3.4	05041
stewed	135	57.8	24.5	0.0		0.0	55	11	19	1.01	0.015	7	0	0.04	6.6	0.20	0.49
3 oz	85	3.4	1.0	1.1	0.7	65	153	135	0.79	0.037	19.0	23	0.2	0.10	0.28	2.6	05042

24.3 CHICKEN, ROASTERS

	KCAL	H₂O (g)	PRO (g)	CHO (g)	SUGR (g)	DFIB (g)	Na (mg)	Ca (mg)	Mg (mg)	Zn (mg)	Mn (mg)	A (mcg RAE)	C (mg)	B-1 (mg)	NIA (mg)	B-12 (mcg)	PANT (mg)
dark meat w/o skin, roasted	151	57.0	19.8	0.0		0.0	81	9	17	1.81	0.016	14	0	0.05	4.9	0.23	0.87
3 oz	85	7.4	2.1	2.8	1.7	64	190	145	1.13	0.060	16.7	46		0.16	0.26	6.0	05120
light & dark meat w/skin, roasted	190	52.8	20.4	0.0		0.0	62	10	17	1.23	0.015	21	0	0.05	6.3	0.23	0.78
3 oz	85	11.4	3.2	4.6	2.5	65	179	152	1.07	0.049	20.1	71	0.2	0.12	0.30	4.3	05112

	KCAL	H₂0 (g)	PRO (g)	CHO (g)	SUGR (g)	DFIB (g)	Minerals Na (mg)	Ca (mg)	Mg (mg)	Zn (mg)	Mn (mg)	Vitamins A (mcg RAE)	C (mg)	B-1 (mg)	NIA (mg)	B-12 (mcg)	PANT (mg)
	WT (g)	FAT (g)	SFA (g)	MUFA (g)	PUFA (g)	CHOL (mg)	K (mg)	P (mg)	Fe (mg)	Cu (mg)	Se (mcg)	A (IU)	E (mg ATE)	B-2 (mg)	B-6 (mg)	FOL (mcg DFE)	REF
light & dark meat w/o skin, roasted	142	57.3	21.3	0.0		0.0	64	10	18	1.29	0.014	10	0	0.05	6.7	0.25	0.83
3 oz	85	5.6	1.5	2.1	1.3	64	195	163	1.03	0.048	20.9	35		0.12	0.35	4.3	05114
light meat w/o skin, roasted	130	57.7	23.1	0.0		0.0	43	11	20	0.66	0.013	7	0	0.05	8.9	0.26	0.77
3 oz	85	3.5	0.9	1.3	0.8	64	201	184	0.92	0.036	21.9	21	0.2	0.08	0.46	2.6	05118

24.4 CHICKEN, STEWERS

dark meat w/o skin, stewed	219	46.8	23.9	0.0		0.0	81	10	19	2.65	0.020	37	0	0.11	3.9	0.21	0.86
3 oz	85	13.0	3.5	4.5	3.1	81	173	159	1.39	0.122	18.5	123		0.29	0.20	6.8	05132
light & dark meat w/skin, stewed	242	45.1	22.8	0.0		0.0	62	11	17	1.50	0.018	33	0	0.08	4.9	0.20	0.64
3 oz	85	16.0	4.3	6.1	3.6	67	155	153	1.16	0.085	16.7	111	0.2	0.20	0.21	4.3	05124
light & dark meat w/o skin, stewed	201	47.9	25.9	0.0	0.0	0.0	66	11	19	1.75	0.019	29	0	0.10	5.4	0.22	0.73
3 oz	85	10.1	2.6	3.4	2.4	71	172	173	1.22	0.099	21.4	95	0.3	0.24	0.26	5.1	05126
light meat w/o skin, stewed	181	49.1	28.1	0.0		0.0	49	12	20	0.71	0.017	19	0	0.08	7.3	0.23	0.59
3 oz	85	6.8	1.7	2.3	1.6	60	169	191	1.01	0.072	24.4	62		0.17	0.33	3.4	05130

24.5 CHICKEN, UNSPECIFIED TYPES

bites, frzn, Country Skillet	270		12.0	18.0	2.0	1.0	720	20					0				
5 pieces (3.2 oz)	91	16.0	3.0			20			1.44			0					CNAG4
breast, crispy baked, frzn,	180		16.0	16.0	2.0	1.0	500	0					0				
Butterball - 3.5 oz	99	6.0	2.0			45			0.72			0					CNAG12
breast, italian style, frzn,	190		17.0	16.0	0.0	1.0	710	0					1				
Butterball - 3.5 oz	99	6.0	2.0			55			0.72			0					CNAG13
breast, lemon pepper, frzn,	200		16.0	16.0	2.0	<1.0	420	0					1				
Butterball - 3.5 oz	99	7.0	2.5			50			0.36			0					CNAG14
breast, parmesan, frzn, Butterball	200		17.0	16.0	5.0	<1.0	650	20					1				
3.5 oz	99	7.0	3.0			55			0.36			0					CNAG15
breast patty, fat-free, baked,	100		9.0	15.0	3.0	1.0	400	0					0				
frzn, Banquet - 2.6 oz patty	74	0.0	0.0			20			0.36			0					CNAG5
grilled honey bbq, frzn, Banquet	110		13.0	3.0	2.0	0.0	440	40					0				
2.6 oz patty	74	5.0	2.0			40			0.72			0					CNAG6
grilled honey mustard, frzn,	120		13.0	5.0	3.0	0.0	500	40					0				
Banquet - 2.6 oz patty	74	5.0	2.0			25			0.72			0					CNAG7
breast, southwestern, frzn,	170		17.0	13.0	0.0	2.0	590	0					1				
Butterball - 3.5 oz	99	6.0	2.0			35			0.72			100					CNAG16
breast tenders, fat-free, baked,	120		13.0	16.0	0.0	2.0	480	0					0				
frzn, Banquet - 3 pieces (3 oz)	99	0.0	0.0			30			0.72			0					CNAG8
frzn, Country Skillet	240		11.0	16.0	1.0	1.0	450	20					0				
3 pieces (3 oz)	85	14.0	4.0			25			0.72			0					CNAG9
original, frzn, Banquet	250		12.0	15.0	1.0	<1.0	480	0					1				
3 pieces (3.1 oz)	89	15.0	3.5			40			0.72			0					CNAG10
southern, frzn, Banquet	260		12.0	16.0	1.0	1.0	460	0					1				
3 pieces (3.1 oz)	89	16.0	4.0			40			0.72			0					CNAG11
chunks, frzn, Country Skillet	270		12.0	18.0	2.0	1.0	720	20					0				
5 chunks (3.4 oz)	95	16.0	3.0			20			1.44			0					CNAG17
southern fried, frzn, Country	270		11.0	17.0	4.0	1.0	550	20					0				
Skillet - 5 chunks (3.4 oz)	95	18.0	4.0			20			1.08			0					CNAG18
cnd w/broth	234	97.5	30.9	0.0		0.0	714	20	17	2.00	0.021	50	3	0.02	9.0	0.41	1.21
5 oz can	142	11.3	3.1	4.5	2.5	88	196	158	2.24	0.065	22.4	166	0.3	0.18	0.50	5.7	05277
fried, country, frzn, Banquet	270		14.0	13.0	1.0	1.0	620	80					4				
3 oz	85	18.0	5.0			65			0.72			0					CNAG34
frzn, Country Skillet	270		14.0	13.0	1.0	1.0	620	80					4				
3 oz	85	18.0	5.0			65			0.72			0					CNAG35
honey bbq, skinless, frzn,	230		18.0	9.0	1.0	1.0	480	20					2				
Banquet - 3 oz	85	13.0	3.0			55			0.36			0					CNAG36
hot 'n spicy, frzn, Banquet	260		14.0	13.0	1.0	1.0	730	20					4				
3 oz	85	18.0	5.0			65			0.72			0					CNAG37
original, frzn, Banquet	290		14.0	15.0	1.0	1.0	630	20					4				
3 oz	85	18.0	5.0			65			0.72			0					CNAG38
skinless, frzn, Banquet	220		18.0	7.0	1.0	2.0	480	20					2				
3 oz	85	13.0	3.0			65			0.36			0					CNAG39

	KCAL	H₂0 (g)	PRO (g)	CHO (g)	SUGR (g)	DFIB (g)	Na (mg)	Ca (mg)	Mg (mg)	Zn (mg)	Mn (mg)	A (mcg RAE)	C (mg)	B-1 (mg)	NIA (mg)	B-12 (mcg)	PANT (mg)
	WT (g)	FAT (g)	SFA (g)	MUFA (g)	PUFA (g)	CHOL (mg)	K (mg)	P (mg)	Fe (mg)	Cu (mg)	Se (mcg)	A (IU)	E (mg ATE)	B-2 (mg)	B-6 (mg)	FOL (mcg DFE)	REF
southern, frzn, Banquet	280		14.0	15.0	1.0	1.0	700	40					4				
3 oz	85	18.0	5.0			65			0.72			0					CNAG40
nuggets, breast, frzn, Banquet	280		11.0	13.0	2.0		500	0					0				
7 nuggets (3.1 oz)	89	20.0	5.0			40			0.72			0					CNAG19
frzn, Country Skillet	280		14.0	16.0	2.0	1.0	610	20					0				
10 nuggets (3.4 oz)	95	17.0	4.0			25			1.44			0					CNAG20
original, frzn, Banquet	270		14.0	12.0	2.0	1.0	540	0					0				
6 nuggets (3 oz)	85	19.0	4.0			35			1.08			0					CNAG21
southern, frzn, Banquet	270		12.0	16.0	4.0	2.0	570	20					1				
5 nuggets (3 oz)	85	18.0	4.0			35			1.08			0					CNAG22
patty, frzn, Country Skillet	190		9.0	12.0	3.0	1.0	490	0					0				
2.5 oz patty	71	11.0	2.5			20			1.08			0					CNAG23
original, frzn, Banquet	190		7.0	10.0	2.0	1.0	440	0					0				
2.3 oz patty	64	14.0	3.0			30			0.72			0					CNAG24
southern fried, frzn, Country Skillet - 2.5 oz patty	190		9.0	12.0	3.0	1.0	440	0					1				
	71	12.0	2.5			20			1.08			0					CNAG25
southern, frzn, Banquet	190		8.0	10.0	<1.0	<1.0	430	0					1				
2.3 oz patty	64	13.0	3.0			25			0.72			0					CNAG26
tenders breast, baked, frzn, Butterball - 3 pieces (3.1 oz)	170		14.0	15.0	2.0	1.0	410	0					0				
	88	6.0	2.0			35			0.36			0					CNAG27
tenders, hckry smkd grld, frzn, Butterball - 4 pcs w/sce (4.3 oz)	160		17.0	12.0	9.0	1.0	570	20					2				
	121	5.0	1.5			50			0.72			0					CNAG28
oriental grilled, frzn, Butterball	160		17.0	12.0	10.0	1.0	560	0					1				
4 pieces w/sce (4.3 oz)	121	5.0	2.0			45			0.72			0					CNAG29
wings, firehouse, frzn, Banquet	190		14.0	1.0	0.0	0.0	650	0					0				
2 big wings (4 oz)	113	14.0	4.0			70			0.36			0					CNAG30
honey bbq, frzn, Banquet	380		21.0	15.0	4.0	1.0	570	40					1				
4 wings (4 oz)	113	26.0	10.0			70			0.36			0					CNAG31
hot 'n spicy, frzn, Banquet	290		18.0	9.0	0.0	<1.0	450	20					1				
4 wings (4 oz)	113	20.0	5.0			90			0.72			0					CNAG32
smokehouse, frzn, Banquet	200		14.0	4.0	3.0	0.0	300	0					0				
2 big wings (4 oz)	113	14.0	4.0			70			0.36			0					CNAG33

24.6 TURKEY, ROASTERS

	KCAL	H₂0 (g)	PRO (g)	CHO (g)	SUGR (g)	DFIB (g)	Na (mg)	Ca (mg)	Mg (mg)	Zn (mg)	Mn (mg)	A (mcg RAE)	C (mg)	B-1 (mg)	NIA (mg)	B-12 (mcg)	PANT (mg)
	WT (g)	FAT (g)	SFA (g)	MUFA (g)	PUFA (g)	CHOL (mg)	K (mg)	P (mg)	Fe (mg)	Cu (mg)	Se (mcg)	A (IU)	E (mg ATE)	B-2 (mg)	B-6 (mg)	FOL (mcg DFE)	REF
breast w/skin, roasted	130	57.5	24.7	0.0		0.0	45	13	24	1.50	0.020	0	0	0.03	5.9	0.31	0.56
3 oz	85	2.7	0.7	1.0	0.6	77	237	184	1.33	0.065	25.9	0		0.11	0.43	5.1	05218
breast w/o skin, roasted	141	59.3	17.1	0.1		0.0	54	14	19	1.90	0.025	102	<1	0.05	3.4	1.45	0.81
3 oz	85	7.5	2.1	2.7	1.9	62	227	151	1.61	0.101	19.7	340		0.18	0.34	20.4	05229
dark meat w/skin, roasted	155	55.1	23.5	0.0		0.0	65	23	20	3.26	0.020	0	0	0.04	2.8	0.31	1.02
3 oz	85	6.0	1.8	1.9	1.6	99	201	162	1.98	0.178	33.2	0		0.20	0.28	7.7	05208
dark meat w/o skin, roasted	138	56.4	24.5	0.0		0.0	67	22	20	3.51	0.021	0	0	0.04	3.0	0.33	1.15
3 oz	85	3.7	1.2	0.8	1.1	95	209	167	2.05	0.190	34.8	0		0.21	0.32	8.5	05212
leg w/skin, roasted	417	160.8	69.8	0.0		0.0	196	56	59	10.02	0.061	0	0	0.13	8.0	0.91	3.03
8.6 oz leg w/o bone	245	13.3	4.1	3.9	3.6	172	617	490	6.35	0.571	97.3	0		0.63	0.83	22.1	05222
light meat w/skin, roasted	139	56.6	24.5	0.0		0.0	48	15	22	1.77	0.020	0	0	0.03	5.3	0.31	0.55
3 oz	85	3.9	1.1	1.4	0.9	81	223	174	1.37	0.078	25.4	0		0.12	0.42	5.1	05206
light meat w/o skin, roasted	119	58.3	25.7	0.0		0.0	48	13	24	1.77	0.021	0	0	0.03	5.9	0.33	0.61
3 oz	85	1.0	0.3	0.2	0.3	73	235	184	1.33	0.073	27.3	0		0.12	0.48	5.1	05210
skin, roasted	102	18.9	7.1	0.0		0.0	21	12	6	0.70	0.007	0	0	0.01	0.9	0.07	0.09
1.2 oz (yield from 1 lb of turkey)	34	7.9	2.1	3.4	1.8	49	62	51	0.63	0.044	52.1	0		0.05	0.02	1.4	05204
wing w/skin, roasted	186	56.1	24.9	0.0		0.0	66	26	18	2.93	0.022	0	0	0.03	3.3	0.32	0.54
3.2 oz wing w/o bone	90	8.9	2.4	3.3	2.1	104	176	149	1.63	0.139	25.3	0		0.14	0.38	5.4	05226

24.7 TURKEY, YOUNG HEN

	KCAL	H₂0 (g)	PRO (g)	CHO (g)	SUGR (g)	DFIB (g)	Na (mg)	Ca (mg)	Mg (mg)	Zn (mg)	Mn (mg)	A (mcg RAE)	C (mg)	B-1 (mg)	NIA (mg)	B-12 (mcg)	PANT (mg)
	WT (g)	FAT (g)	SFA (g)	MUFA (g)	PUFA (g)	CHOL (mg)	K (mg)	P (mg)	Fe (mg)	Cu (mg)	Se (mcg)	A (IU)	E (mg ATE)	B-2 (mg)	B-6 (mg)	FOL (mcg DFE)	REF
dark meat w/skin, roasted	197	50.7	23.3	0.0		0.0	61	26	20	3.49	0.020	0	0	0.05	3.1	0.29	0.95
3 oz	85	10.9	3.3	3.5	2.9	71	235	167	1.94	0.118	31.6	0		0.19	0.26	6.8	05240
dark meat w/o skin, roasted	163	53.3	24.2	0.0		0.0	64	26	21	3.73	0.020	0	0	0.05	3.2	0.31	1.05
3 oz	85	6.6	2.2	1.5	2.0	68	248	173	1.98	0.126	34.8	0		0.20	0.29	7.7	05244
light & dark meat w/skin, roasted - 3 oz	185	51.9	23.9	0.0		0.0	54	22	21	2.47	0.019	0	0	0.05	4.5	0.29	0.71
	85	9.2	2.7	3.0	2.4	66	240	173	1.51	0.073	26.7	0		0.14	0.34	6.0	05232

	KCAL / WT (g)	H₂0 (g) / FAT (g)	PRO (g) / SFA (g)	CHO (g) / MUFA (g)	SUGR (g) / PUFA (g)	DFIB (g) / CHOL (mg)	Na (mg) / K (mg)	Ca (mg) / P (mg)	Mg (mg) / Fe (mg)	Zn (mg) / Cu (mg)	Mn (mg) / Se (mcg)	A (mcg RAE) / A (IU)	C (mg) / E (mg ATE)	B-1 (mg) / B-2 (mg)	NIA (mg) / B-6 (mg)	B-12 (mcg) / FOL (mcg DFE)	PANT (mg) / REF
light & dark meat w/o skin, roasted - 3 oz	149	54.8	24.9	0.0		0.0	57	21	22	2.58	0.019	0	0	0.05	4.8	0.31	0.77
	85	4.7	1.5	1.0	1.3	62	254	180	1.50	0.074	29.2	0		0.15	0.37	6.0	05234
light meat w/skin, roasted 3 oz	176	52.8	24.3	0.0		0.0	49	20	22	1.68	0.018	0	0	0.04	5.6	0.29	0.52
	85	8.0	2.3	2.7	1.9	63	243	177	1.18	0.037	24.2	0		0.11	0.39	5.1	05238
light meat w/o skin, roasted 3 oz	137	55.9	25.4	0.0		0.0	51	18	24	1.67	0.017	0	0	0.05	6.0	0.31	0.56
	85	3.2	1.0	0.6	0.9	58	258	185	1.11	0.033	27.3	0		0.11	0.44	5.1	05242

24.8 TURKEY, YOUNG TOM

	KCAL / WT (g)	H₂0 (g) / FAT (g)	PRO (g) / SFA (g)	CHO (g) / MUFA (g)	SUGR (g) / PUFA (g)	DFIB (g) / CHOL (mg)	Na (mg) / K (mg)	Ca (mg) / P (mg)	Mg (mg) / Fe (mg)	Zn (mg) / Cu (mg)	Mn (mg) / Se (mcg)	A (mcg RAE) / A (IU)	C (mg) / E (mg ATE)	B-1 (mg) / B-2 (mg)	NIA (mg) / B-6 (mg)	B-12 (mcg) / FOL (mcg DFE)	PANT (mg) / REF
dark meat w/skin, roasted 3 oz	157	53.6	24.4	0.0		0.0	70	30	20	3.88	0.019	0	0	0.06	3.0	0.32	1.13
	85	5.9	2.0	1.3	1.8	75	249	174	1.98	0.139	34.8	0		0.22	0.31	8.5	05268
dark meat w/o skin, roasted 3 oz	184	51.3	23.4	0.0		0.0	68	30	20	3.61	0.019	0	0	0.05	2.9	0.31	1.02
	85	9.2	2.8	2.9	2.5	77	235	167	1.92	0.131	33.7	0		0.21	0.28	7.7	05264
young tom, light & dark meat w/skin, roasted - 3 oz	172	52.6	23.9	0.0		0.0	61	23	21	2.57	0.017	0	0	0.05	4.2	0.31	0.75
	85	7.7	2.2	2.5	2.0	70	240	173	1.51	0.080	29.3	0		0.16	0.36	6.0	05256
young tom, light & dark meat w/o skin, roasted - 3 oz	143	55.3	25.0	0.0		0.0	63	21	22	2.69	0.017	0	0	0.06	4.5	0.32	0.82
	85	4.0	1.3	0.8	1.1	65	256	182	1.51	0.081	31.3	0		0.16	0.40	6.8	05258
young tom, light meat w/skin, roasted - 3 oz	162	53.7	24.2	0.0		0.0	57	18	23	1.79	0.016	0	0	0.05	5.1	0.31	0.54
	85	6.5	1.8	2.3	1.6	64	244	178	1.20	0.041	26.1	0		0.11	0.41	5.1	05262
young tom, light meat w/o skin, roasted - 3 oz	131	56.6	25.4	0.0		0.0	58	15	24	1.79	0.016	0	0	0.06	5.6	0.32	0.59
	85	2.5	0.8	0.4	0.7	59	262	187	1.16	0.036	27.3	0		0.11	0.47	5.1	05266

24.9 TURKEY, UNSPECIFIED TYPES

	KCAL / WT (g)	H₂0 (g) / FAT (g)	PRO (g) / SFA (g)	CHO (g) / MUFA (g)	SUGR (g) / PUFA (g)	DFIB (g) / CHOL (mg)	Na (mg) / K (mg)	Ca (mg) / P (mg)	Mg (mg) / Fe (mg)	Zn (mg) / Cu (mg)	Mn (mg) / Se (mcg)	A (mcg RAE) / A (IU)	C (mg) / E (mg ATE)	B-1 (mg) / B-2 (mg)	NIA (mg) / B-6 (mg)	B-12 (mcg) / FOL (mcg DFE)	PANT (mg) / REF
bacon, Louis Rich .5 oz	35	8.3	2.1	0.3	0.3	0.0	170	6	3	0.35		0	0				
	14	2.8	0.7	1.1	0.7	13	29	28	0.20	0.035		0				1.1	07254
breast w/skin, prebasted, roasted 3 oz	107	60.3	18.8	0.0		0.0	337	8	18	1.30	0.013	0	0	0.05	7.7	0.27	0.42
	85	2.9	0.8	1.0	0.7	36	211	182	0.56	0.035	21.8	0		0.11	0.27	4.3	05293
cnd w/broth 5 oz can	231	93.8	33.6	0.0		0.0	663	17	28	3.37	0.024	0	3	0.02	9.4	0.40	0.97
	142	9.7	2.8	3.2	2.5	94	318	230	2.64	0.105	36.8	0	0.4	0.24	0.47	8.5	05284
diced, seasoned 1 oz	39	20.3	5.3	0.3		0.0	241	0	5	0.57	0.004	0	0	0.01	1.4	0.07	0.17
	28	1.7	0.5	0.6	0.4	16	88	68	0.51	0.018	7.4	0		0.03	0.08	1.4	05285
ground, ckd 2.9 oz patty	193	48.7	22.4	0.0		0.0	88	21	20	2.35	0.016	0	0	0.04	4.0	0.27	0.67
	82	10.8	2.8	4.0	2.6	84	221	161	1.58	0.074	30.5	0	0.3	0.14	0.32	5.7	05306
nuggets/sticks, breaded, Louis Rich 3 pieces (3 oz)	235	43.1	12.2	13.1	0.0	0.4	577	8	18	1.56		0	0				
	85	14.9	2.9	7.0	4.7	34	150	167	0.74	0.247		0					07265
patties, breaded/battered & fried 3.3 oz patty	266	46.7	13.2	14.8		0.5	752	13	14	1.35	0.072	10	0	0.09	2.2	0.21	0.49
	94	16.9	4.4	7.0	4.4	58	259	254	2.07	0.066	18.7	35	2.2	0.18	0.19	39.5	05292
roast, boneless, frzn, seasoned, roasted - 3 oz	132	57.7	18.1	2.6		0.0	578	4	19	2.16	0.013	0	0	0.04	5.3	1.29	0.69
	85	4.9	1.6	1.0	1.4	45	253	207	1.39	0.051	31.0	0	0.3	0.14	0.23	4.3	05296
sticks, breaded/battered & fried 2.25 oz stick	179	31.6	9.1	10.9			536	9	10	0.93	0.053	8	0	0.06	1.3	0.15	0.34
	64	10.8	2.8	4.4	2.8	41	166	150	1.41	0.047	13.2	26		0.12	0.13	27.5	05300
thigh w/skin, prebasted, roasted 11.1 oz thigh (w/o bone)	493	221.7	59.0	0.0		0.0	1372	25	53	12.94	0.047	0	0	0.26	7.6	0.75	2.55
	314	26.8	8.3	7.9	7.4	195	757	537	4.74	0.436	87.6	0		0.80	0.72	18.8	05294

24.10 OTHER POULTRY

	KCAL / WT (g)	H₂0 (g) / FAT (g)	PRO (g) / SFA (g)	CHO (g) / MUFA (g)	SUGR (g) / PUFA (g)	DFIB (g) / CHOL (mg)	Na (mg) / K (mg)	Ca (mg) / P (mg)	Mg (mg) / Fe (mg)	Zn (mg) / Cu (mg)	Mn (mg) / Se (mcg)	A (mcg RAE) / A (IU)	C (mg) / E (mg ATE)	B-1 (mg) / B-2 (mg)	NIA (mg) / B-6 (mg)	B-12 (mcg) / FOL (mcg DFE)	PANT (mg) / REF
cornish game hen, w/skin, roasted - 3 oz	221	49.9	18.9	0.0		0.0	54	11	15	1.27	0.013	27	<1	0.06	5.0	0.24	0.50
	85	15.5	4.3	6.8	3.1	111	208	124	0.77	0.052	13.2	90	0.2	0.17	0.26	1.7	05308
w/o skin, roasted 3 oz	114	61.1	19.8	0.0		0.0	54	11	16	1.30	0.013	17	1	0.06	5.3	0.26	0.47
	85	3.3	0.8	1.1	0.8	90	213	127	0.65	0.050	17.7	55	0.2	0.19	0.30	1.7	05310
duck, w/skin, roasted - 3 oz	286	44.1	16.1	0.0		0.0	50	9	14	1.58	0.016	54	0	0.15	4.1	0.26	0.93
	85	24.1	8.2	11.0	3.1	71	173	133	2.30	0.193	17.0	179	0.6	0.23	0.15	5.1	05140
w/o skin, roasted 3 oz	171	54.6	20.0	0.0		0.0	55	10	17	2.21	0.016	20	0	0.22	4.3	0.34	1.28
	85	9.5	3.5	3.1	1.2	76	214	173	2.30	0.196	19.0	65	0.6	0.40	0.21	8.5	05142
goose, w/skin, roasted - 3 oz	259	44.2	21.4	0.0		0.0	60	11	19	2.23	0.020	18	0	0.07	3.5	0.35	1.30
	85	18.6	5.8	8.7	2.1	77	280	230	2.41	0.224	18.5	60	1.5	0.27	0.31	1.7	05147
w/o skin, roasted 3 oz	202	48.6	24.6	0.0		0.0	65	12	21	2.69	0.020	10	0	0.08	3.5	0.42	1.56
	85	10.8	3.9	3.7	1.3	82	330	263	2.44	0.235	21.7	34		0.33	0.40	10.2	05149
guinea hen, w/o skin, raw 3 oz	94	63.3	17.5	0.0		0.0	59	9	20	1.02	0.015	10	1	0.06	7.5	0.31	0.80
	85	2.1	0.5	0.6	0.5	54	187	144	0.65	0.037	14.9	35		0.10	0.40	5.1	05152
pheasant, w/skin, raw - 3 oz	154	57.6	19.3	0.0		0.0	34	10	17	0.82	0.014	45	5	0.06	5.5	0.65	0.79
	85	7.9	2.3	3.7	1.0	60	207	182	0.98	0.055	13.3	150	0.3	0.12	0.56	5.1	05153

	KCAL	H₂0 (g)	PRO (g)	CHO (g)	SUGR (g)	DFIB (g)	Na (mg)	Ca (mg)	Mg (mg)	Zn (mg)	Mn (mg)	A (mcg RAE)	C (mg)	B-1 (mg)	NIA (mg)	B-12 (mcg)	PANT (mg)
	WT (g)	FAT (g)	SFA (g)	MUFA (g)	PUFA (g)	CHOL (mg)	K (mg)	P (mg)	Fe (mg)	Cu (mg)	Se (mcg)	A (IU)	E (mg ATE)	B-2 (mg)	B-6 (mg)	FOL (mcg DFE)	REF
w/o skin, raw	113	61.9	20.0	0.0		0.0	31	11	17	0.82	0.014	43	5	0.07	5.7	0.71	0.82
3 oz	85	3.1	1.1	1.0	0.5	56	223	196	0.98	0.059	13.8	140		0.13	0.63	5.1	05154
quail, w/o skin, raw	114	59.5	18.5	0.0		0.0	43	11	21	2.30	0.016	14	6	0.24	7.0	0.40	0.67
3 oz	85	3.9	1.1	1.1	1.0	60	201	261	3.83	0.505	14.8	48		0.24	0.45	6.0	05158
squab (pigeon), w/o skin, raw	121	61.9	14.9	0.0		0.0	43	11	21	2.30	0.016	24	6	0.24	5.8	0.40	0.67
3 oz	85	6.4	1.7	2.3	1.4	77	201	261	3.83	0.505	11.5	80		0.24	0.45	6.0	05161

24.11 INTERNAL ORGANS

	KCAL	H₂0	PRO	CHO	SUGR	DFIB	Na	Ca	Mg	Zn	Mn	A	C	B-1	NIA	B-12	PANT
	WT	FAT	SFA	MUFA	PUFA	CHOL	K	P	Fe	Cu	Se	A(IU)	E	B-2	B-6	FOL	REF
giblets, chicken,	235	40.7	27.7	3.7		0.0	96	15	21	5.33	0.189	3045	7	0.08	9.3	11.31	3.79
fried - *3 oz*	85	11.4	3.2	3.8	2.9	379	281	243	8.77	0.359	88.6	10140		1.30	0.52	322.2	05021
simmered	133	57.5	22.0	0.8		0.0	49	10	17	3.88	0.145	1897	7	0.07	3.5	8.62	2.52
3 oz	85	4.1	1.3	1.0	0.9	334	134	195	5.47	0.217	79.6	6316	1.1	0.81	0.29	319.6	05022
giblets, turkey, simmered	142	55.5	22.6	1.8		0.0	50	11	14	3.13	0.149	1541	1	0.04	3.8	20.43	2.94
3 oz	85	4.3	1.3	1.0	1.0	355	170	173	5.70	0.332	188.5	5131	1.2	0.77	0.28	293.3	05172
gizzard, chicken, simmered	130	57.2	23.1	1.0		0.0	57	9	17	3.72	0.053	48	1	0.02	3.4	1.65	0.61
3 oz	85	3.1	0.9	0.8	0.9	165	152	132	3.53	0.094	80.3	160	1.0	0.21	0.10	45.1	05024
gizzard, turkey, simmered	139	55.6	25.0	0.5		0.0	46	13	16	3.54	0.083	48	1	0.03	2.6	1.62	0.72
3 oz	85	3.3	0.9	0.6	1.0	197	179	109	4.62	0.147	79.5	157	0.1	0.28	0.10	44.2	05174
heart, chicken, simmered	157	55.1	22.4	0.1		0.0	41	16	17	6.21	0.091	7	2	0.06	2.4	6.20	2.26
3 oz	85	6.7	1.9	1.7	2.0	206	112	169	7.68	0.427	6.8	24		0.63	0.27	68.0	05026
heart, turkey, simmered	150	54.6	22.7	1.7		0.0	47	11	19	4.48	0.078	7	1	0.06	2.8	6.08	2.31
3 oz	85	5.2	1.5	1.0	1.5	192	156	174	5.86	0.533	7.3	24	0.1	0.75	0.27	67.2	05176
liver, chicken, simmered	133	58.1	20.7	0.7		0.0	43	12	18	3.69	0.252	4179	13	0.13	3.8	16.48	4.60
3 oz	85	4.6	1.6	1.1	0.8	536	119	265	7.20	0.315	85.2	13919	1.2	1.48	0.49	654.5	05028
liver, duck, raw	116	61.0	15.9	3.0		0.0	119	9	20	2.61	0.219	10186	4	0.48	5.5	45.90	5.26
3 oz	85	3.9	1.2	0.6	0.5	438	196	229	25.95	5.068	57.0	33921		0.76	0.65	627.3	05143
liver, goose, raw	113	61.0	13.9	5.4		0.0	119	37	20	2.61	0.000	7913	4	0.48	5.5	45.90	5.26
3 oz	85	3.6	1.4	0.7	0.2	438	196	222	25.95	6.394	57.9	26348		0.76	0.65	627.3	05150
liver, turkey, simmered	144	55.7	20.4	2.9		0.0	54	9	13	2.63	0.215	3211	2	0.04	5.0	40.38	5.07
3 oz	85	5.1	1.6	1.3	0.9	532	165	231	6.63	0.476	85.6	10694	2.5	1.21	0.44	566.1	05178

25. SALAD DRESSINGS
25.1 LOW & REDUCED CALORIE

	KCAL	H₂0	PRO	CHO	SUGR	DFIB	Na	Ca	Mg	Zn	Mn	A	C	B-1	NIA	B-12	PANT
	WT	FAT	SFA	MUFA	PUFA	CHOL	K	P	Fe	Cu	Se	A(IU)	E	B-2	B-6	FOL	REF
blue cheese, chunky, fat free,	35		0.0	7.0	1.0	1.0	290	20							0		
Wish-Bone - *2 T (30 ml)*	~32	0.0	0.0			0			0.00			0	1.8				UNLV113
Wish-Bone Just 2 Good!	45		1.0	6.0	2.0	0.0	320	0							0		
2 T	~32	2.0	0.0			0			0.00			0	1.8				UNLV1
caesar, classic, low fat, Wish-Bone	40		1.0	5.0	2.0	0.0	310	0							0		
Just 2 Good! - *2 T*	32	2.0	0.5			5			0.00			0	1.8				UNLV127
creamy, Wish-Bone Just 2 Good!	45		1.0	7.0	2.0	0.0	310	0							0		
2 T (30 ml)	~32	2.0	0.5			10			0.00			0	1.8				UNLV115
creamy rstd garlic, fat free,	40		0.0	9.0	4.0		280										
Wish-Bone - *2 T (30 ml)*	~32	0.0	0.0			0											UNLV104
french	21	11.1	0.0	3.5		0.0	126	2	0	0.03		10	0	0.00	0.0	0.00	0.00
1 T	16	0.9	0.1	0.2	0.5	0	13	2	0.06	0.002	0.3	208	0.2	0.00	0.00	0.0	04020
french style, deluxe, Wish-Bone	45		0.0	7.0	6.0	<1.0	230	0							0		
Just 2 Good! - *2 T*	33	2.0	0.0			0			0.00			400	1.8				UNLV117
french, sweet & spicy, Wish-Bone	50		0.0	9.0	5.0	0.0	240	0							0		
Just 2 Good! - *2 T (30 ml)*	~32	2.0	0.0			0			0.00			0	1.8				UNLV118
honey dijon, fat free, Wish-Bone	45		1.0	10.0	9.0	0.0	270	0							0		
2 T	~32	0.0	0.0			0			0.00			0	1.8				UNLV119
Wish-Bone Just 2 Good!	50		0.0	8.0	5.0	0.0	250								0		
2 T (30 ml)	~32	2.0	0.0			0			0.00			0	1.8				UNLV120
italian	16	12.3	0.0	0.7		0.0	118	0	0	0.02		0	0	0.00	0.0	0.00	0.00
1 T	15	1.5	0.2	0.3	0.9	1	2	1	0.03	0.001	0.2	0	0.2	0.00	0.00	0.0	04021
country w/herbs, Wish-Bone	30		0.0	3.0	2.0	0.0	290	0							0		
Just 2 Good! - *2 T (30 ml)*	~32	2.0	0.0			0			0.00			0	1.8				UNLV121
fat free, Kraft Free	20	26.9	0.5	3.6	2.2	0.2	430	14					<1				
2 T	33	0.3	0.2			1	38	68	0.08			52					04121
fat free, Wish-Bone	20		0.0	5.0	3.0	0.0	390	0							0		
2 T	~32	0.0	0.0			0			0.00			0	1.8				UNLV159

	KCAL / WT (g)	H₂O / FAT (g)	PRO / SFA (g)	CHO / MUFA (g)	SUGR / PUFA (g)	DFIB (g) / CHOL (mg)	Na / K (mg)	Ca / P (mg)	Mg / Fe (mg)	Zn / Cu (mg)	Mn / Se (mcg)	A (mcg RAE) / A (IU)	C / E (mg ATE)	B-1 / B-2 (mg)	NIA / B-6 (mg)	B-12 (mcg) / FOL (mcg DFE)	PANT (mg) / REF
Light Done Right, Kraft	53	22.6	0.3	2.5	1.5	0.4	228	9					1				
2 T	31	4.5	0.4			<1	28	8	0.10			55					04118
Wish-Bone Just 2 Good!	35			5.0	4.0	0.0	480	0					0				
2 T (30 ml)	~32	2.0	0.0			0			0.00			0	1.8				UNLV122
parmesan basil italian, Wish-Bone	40		1.0	6.0	2.0	0.0	320	0					0				
Just 2 Good! - 2 T (30 ml)	~32	2.0	0.5			5			0.00			0	1.8				UNLV140
ranch, fat free, Kraft Free	48	22.3	0.2	10.7	2.1	0.2	354	9					<1				
2 T	35	0.4	0.1			<1	31	28	0.02			3					04119
fat free, Wish-Bone	30			7.0	2.0	<1.0	280	20					0				
2 T	33	0.0	0.0			0			0.00			0	1.8				UNLV123
Light Done Right, Kraft	77	18.4	0.4	3.2	1.3	0.2	303	8					<1				
2 T	30	6.8	0.6			8	40	47	0.06			12					04117
Wish-Bone Just 2 Good!	40			5.0	3.0	0.0	270	0					0				
2 T (30 ml)	~32	2.0	0.0			0			0.00			0	1.8				UNLV124
russian	23	10.4	0.1	4.4		0.0	139	3	0	0.02		<1	1	<0.01	<0.1	0.02	0.02
1 T	16	0.6	0.1	0.1	0.4	1	25	6	0.10	0.002	0.3	9	0.1	<0.01	<0.01	0.5	04022
thousand island	24	10.4	0.1	2.4		0.2	150	2	<1	0.02		2	0	<0.01	<0.1	0.03	0.03
1 T	15	1.6	0.2	0.4	0.9	2	17	3	0.09	0.002	0.2	48	0.2	<0.01	<0.01	0.9	04023
fat free, Wish-Bone	35		0.0	9.0	6.0	<1.0	290	0					0				
2 T	~32	0.0	0.0			0			0.00			0	1.8				UNLV125
Wish-Bone Just 2 Good!	60		0.0	9.0	5.0	0.0	290	0					0				
2 T (30 ml)	~32	2.0	0.0			5			0.00			0	1.8				UNLV126
vinaigrette, red wine, fat free, Wish-Bone	35		0.0	7.0	6.0	0.0	230	0					0				
- 2 T (30 ml)	~32	0.0	0.0			0			0.00				0.0				UNLV105

25.2 REGULAR

	KCAL / WT (g)	H₂O / FAT (g)	PRO / SFA (g)	CHO / MUFA (g)	SUGR / PUFA (g)	DFIB (g) / CHOL (mg)	Na / K (mg)	Ca / P (mg)	Mg / Fe (mg)	Zn / Cu (mg)	Mn / Se (mcg)	A (mcg RAE) / A (IU)	C / E (mg ATE)	B-1 / B-2 (mg)	NIA / B-6 (mg)	B-12 (mcg) / FOL (mcg DFE)	PANT (mg) / REF
blue (bleu) cheese/roquefort	76	4.8	0.7	1.1		0.0	164	12	0	0.04		9	<1	<0.01	<0.1	0.04	0.06
1 T	15	7.8	1.5	1.8	4.2	3	6	11	0.03	0.002	0.2	32	1.4	0.02	0.01	1.2	04539
blue cheese, chunky, Wish-Bone	170		1.0	2.0	1.0	0.0	280	0					0				
2 T (30ml)	~30	17.0	2.5			10			0.00			0					UNLV156
caesar, classic, Wish-Bone	110		1.0	2.0	1.0	0.0	390	0					0				
2 T (30 ml)	~30	10.0	<0.1			0			0.00			0					UNLV177
creamy, Wish-Bone	180		1.0	1.0	1.0	0.0	290	0					0				
2 T (30 ml)	~30	18.0	2.5			10			0.00			0					UNLV176
Deli Blend, Hellmann's/Best Foods	0		0.0	2.0	1.0	0.0	100	0					0				
1 T	15	6.0	0.5			10			0.00								UNLV50
french	69	6.1	0.1	2.8		0.0	219	2	0	0.01		10	<0.01	<0.1	0.02	0.03	
1 T	16	6.6	1.5	1.3	3.5	0	13	2	0.06	0.002	0.3	208	1.3	<0.01	<0.01	0.6	04120
deluxe, Wish-Bone	120		0.0	5.0	4.0	0.0	170	0					0				
2 T (30 ml)	~32	11.0	1.5			0			0.00			0					UNLV175
homemade	88	3.4		0.5		0.0	92	1		0.00		4	<1	<0.01	<0.1	0.00	0.00
1 T	14	9.8	1.8	2.9	4.7	0	3	<1	0.03		0.2	72	1.1	<0.01	0.00	0.0	04133
sweet 'n spicy, Wish-Bone	140		0.0	6.0	5.0	0.0	330	0					0				
2 T (30 ml)	~32	12.0	1.5			0			0.00			0					UNLV174
homemade, ckd	25	11.1	0.7	2.4		0.0	117	13	1	0.06		8	<1	0.01	<0.1	0.06	0.00
1 T	16	1.5	0.5	0.6	0.3	9	19	14	0.08	0.002	0.3	28	0.2	0.02	<0.01	1.4	04134
italian	69	5.6	0.1	1.5		0.0	116	1	<1	0.02		1	0	<0.01	<0.1	0.02	0.03
1 T	15	7.1	1.0	1.6	4.1	0	2	1	0.03	0.001	0.2	11	1.5	<0.01	<0.01	0.7	04114
creamy, Wish-Bone	110		1.0	4.0	2.0		240	0					0				
2 T	~30	10.0	1.5			0			0.00			0					UNLV18
house, Wish-Bone	110		0.0	3.0	2.0	0.0	280	0					0				
2 T (30 ml)	~30	10.0	1.5			<5			0.00			100					UNLV173
Wish-Bone	80		0.0	3.0	2.0	0.0	490	0					0				
2 T (30 ml)	~30	8.0	1.0			0			0.00			0					UNLV172
Wish-Bone Robusto	90		0.0	4.0	3.0	0.0	550	0					0				
2 T (30 ml)	~30	8.0	1.0			0			0.00			0					UNLV171
zesty, Kraft	109	16.3	0.1	1.8	1.3	0.2	505	1					<1				
2 T	31	11.1	1.2			0	9	4	0.05			11					04116
mayonnaise type	57	5.9	0.1	3.5		0.0	105	2	<1	0.03		10	0	<0.01	<0.1	0.03	0.04
2 T	15	4.9	0.7	1.3	2.6	4	1	4	0.03	0.001	0.2	32	0.6	<0.01	<0.01	0.9	04018
oriental, Wish-Bone	60		0.0	5.0	3.0	0.0	440	0					0				
2 T (30 ml)	~30	4.0	0.5			0			0.00			100					UNLV170

	KCAL	H₂0 (g)	PRO (g)	CHO (g)	SUGR (g)	DFIB (g)	Na (mg)	Ca (mg)	Mg (mg)	Zn (mg)	Mn (mg)	A (mcg RAE)	C (mg)	B-1 (mg)	NIA (mg)	B-12 (mcg)	PANT (mg)
	WT (g)	FAT (g)	SFA (g)	MUFA (g)	PUFA (g)	CHOL (mg)	K (mg)	P (mg)	Fe (mg)	Cu (mg)	Se (mcg)	A (IU)	E (mg ATE)	B-2 (mg)	B-6 (mg)	FOL (mcg DFE)	REF
ranch,	148	10.7	0.4	1.3	1.2	0.1	287	8					<1				
Kraft - 2 T	29	15.6	2.4			8	14	26	0.05			11					04115
Wish-Bone	160		0.0	1.0	1.0		200	20					0				
2 T (30 ml)	~30	17.0	2.5			10			0.00			0					UNLV158
russian	74	5.2	0.2	1.6		0.0	130	3	<1	0.06		5	1	0.01	0.1	0.05	0.06
1 T	15	7.6	1.1	1.8	4.4	3	24	6	0.09	0.002	0.2	104	1.5	0.01	<0.01	1.5	04015
Wish-Bone	110		0.0	15.0	7.0	0.0	350	0					0				
2 T (30 ml)	~30	6.0	1.0			0			0.00			0					UNLV168
sesame seed	66	5.9	0.5	1.3		0.2	150	3	0	0.02		5	0	0.00	0.0	0.00	0.00
1 T	15	6.8	0.9	1.8	3.8	0	24	6	0.09		0.2	104	0.8	0.00	0.00	0.0	04016
sun-dried tomato, Wish-Bone	50		0.0	2.0	1.0	0.0	280	0					0				
2 T (30 ml)	~30	5.0	0.5			0			0.00			0					UNLV178
thousand island	60	7.4	0.1	2.4		0.0	112	2	<1	0.02		3	0	<0.01	<0.1	0.03	0.04
1 T	16	5.7	1.0	1.3	3.2	4	18	3	0.10	0.002	0.3	51	0.2	<0.01	<0.01	1.0	04017
Wish-Bone	140		0.0	18.0	6.0	0.0		0					0				
2 T (30 ml)	~30	12.0	1.5			10			0.00			0					UNLV166
vinaigrette, balsamic, Wish-Bone	60		0.0	3.0	2.0	0.0	280	0					0				
2 T (30 ml)	~32	5.0	0.5			0			0.00			0					UNLV165
vinaigrette, berry, Wish-Bone	50		0.0	2.0	2.0	0.0	130	0					0				
2 T (30 ml)	~32	4.5	0.5			0			0.00			0					UNLV164
vinaigrette, olive oil, Wish-Bone	60		0.0	4.0	3.0	0.0	250	0					0				
2 T (30 ml)	~32	5.0	0.5			0			0.00			0					UNLV163
vinaigrette, red wine, Wish-Bone	90		0.0	9.0	8.0	0.0	230	0					0				
2 T (30 ml)	~32	5.0	0.5			0			0.00			0					UNLV162
vinaigrette, rstd garlic, Wish-Bone	60		0.0	3.0	2.0	0.0	290	0					0				
2 T (30 ml)	~32	5.0	0.5			0			0.00			100					UNLV161
vinaigrette, white wine, Wish-Bone	60		0.0	4.0	2.0	0.0	250	0					0				
2 T (30 ml)	~32	4.5	0.5			0			0.00			0					UNLV160
vinegar & oil, homemade	72	7.6	0.0	0.4		0.0	0	0	0	0.00		0	0	0.00	0.0	0.00	0.00
1 T	16	8.0	1.5	2.4	3.9	0	1	0	0.00	0.000	0.3	0	1.4	0.00	0.00	0.0	04135

26. SAUCES, GRAVIES, & CONDIMENTS
26.1 CONDIMENT SAUCES

	KCAL	H₂0 (g)	PRO (g)	CHO (g)	SUGR (g)	DFIB (g)	Na (mg)	Ca (mg)	Mg (mg)	Zn (mg)	Mn (mg)	A (mcg RAE)	C (mg)	B-1 (mg)	NIA (mg)	B-12 (mcg)	PANT (mg)
	WT (g)	FAT (g)	SFA (g)	MUFA (g)	PUFA (g)	CHOL (mg)	K (mg)	P (mg)	Fe (mg)	Cu (mg)	Se (mcg)	A (IU)	E (mg ATE)	B-2 (mg)	B-6 (mg)	FOL (mcg DFE)	REF
barbeque sce	7	7.5	0.2	1.2		0.1	76	2	2	0.02	0.028	4	1	<0.01	0.1	0.00	0.03
1 pkt	9	0.2	<0.1	0.1	0.1	0	16	2	0.08	0.019	0.1	81	0.1	<0.01	0.01	0.4	06150
hickory smoke, Kraft	39	23.0	0.2	8.9	7.4	0.3	418	5					<1				
2 T	34	0.1	0.0			0	28	3	0.21			114					06308
original, Bulls-Eye	63	19.2	0.4	15.2	11.5		302										
2 T	36	0.1															06140
original, Kraft	39	23.0	0.2	8.9	7.4	0.3	424	5					<1				
2 T	34	0.1	0.0			0	28	3	0.21			114					06307
original recipe, Texas Best	42	23.0	0.6	4.0	2.8		315										
Kraft	32	2.7	0.6			0											06141
catsup (ketchup)	16	10.0	0.2	4.1		0.2	178	3	3	0.03	0.020	8	2	0.01	0.2	0.00	0.02
1 T	15	0.1	<0.1	<0.1	<0.1	0	72	6	0.11	0.031	0.1	152	0.2	0.01	0.03	2.3	11935
Dijonnaise, Hellmann's/Best Foods	5		0.0	1.0	0.0	0.0	70	0					0				
1 t	5	0.0	0.0			0			0.00			0					UNLV52
hoisin sce	35	7.1	0.5	7.1		0.4	258	5	4	0.05	0.041	<1	<1	<0.01	0.2	0.00	0.01
1 T	16	0.5	0.1	0.2	0.3	<1	19	6	0.16	0.020	0.3	2	0.0	0.03	0.01	3.7	06175
honey mustard dressing,	10		0.0	1.0	1.0		20										
Hellmann's/Best Foods - 1 t	5	0.0															UNLV56
horseradish (prepared sce)	7	12.8	0.2	1.7		0.5	47	8	4	0.12	0.019	0	4	<0.01	0.1	0.00	0.01
1 T	15	0.1	<0.1	<0.1	<0.1	0	37	5	0.06	0.009	0.4	<1	<0.1	<0.01	0.01	8.6	02055
jalapeno relish, Old El Paso	5		0.0	1.0	0.0	0.0	110	0					0				
1 T	15	0.0	0.0			0			0.00			0					GENM290
mustard (prepared sce)	3	4.1	0.2	0.4		0.2	56	4	2	0.03	0.015	<1	<1	<0.01	<0.1	0.00	0.02
1 t	5	0.2	<0.1	0.1	<0.1	0	8	4	0.09	0.007	1.8	7	0.1	<0.01	<0.01	0.4	02046
deli, Hellmann's/Best Foods	0		0.0	0.0	0.0	0.0	50	0					0				
1 t	5	0.0	0.0			0			0.00			0					UNLV51
pepper sce, Tabasco	1	4.5	0.1	0.0		0.0	30	1	1	0.01	0.005	4	<1	<0.01	<0.1	0.00	0.01
1 t	4.7	<0.1	<0.1	<0.1	<0.1	0	6	1	0.05	0.004		77		<0.01	0.01	0.0	06169

	KCAL / WT (g)	H₂0 (g) / FAT (g)	PRO (g) / SFA (g)	CHO (g) / MUFA (g)	SUGR (g) / PUFA (g)	DFIB (g) / CHOL (mg)	Na (mg) / K (mg)	Ca (mg) / P (mg)	Mg (mg) / Fe (mg)	Zn (mg) / Cu (mg)	Mn (mg) / Se (mcg)	A (mcg RAE) / A (IU)	C (mg) / E (mg ATE)	B-1 (mg) / B-2 (mg)	NIA (mg) / B-6 (mg)	B-12 (mcg) / FOL (mcg DFE)	PANT (mg) / REF
pepper/hot sce	1	4.2	0.0	0.1		0.1	124	0	<1	0.01	0.002	1	4	<0.01	<0.1	0.00	0.01
1 t	4.7	<0.1	<0.1	<0.1	<0.1	0	7	1	0.02	0.001	0.0	14		<0.01	0.01	0.3	06168
picante sce, mild/med/hot, Thick 'n Chunky, Old El Paso[1] - *2 T*	10		0.0	2.0	1.0	0.0	230	0					0				
	30	0.0	0.0			0					0.00	100					GENM291
Ortega	10	26.8	0.4	2.0	0.2	0.0	252	13	5	0.05	0.047		1	0.02	0.3	0.00	0.08
2 T	30	0.1	<0.1	<0.1	<0.1	0	80	8	0.15	0.031		83	0.4	0.01	0.04	3.0	06157
plum sce	35	10.2	0.2	8.1		0.1	102	2	2	0.04	0.022	<1	<1	<0.01	0.2	0.00	0.01
1 T	19	0.2	<0.1	<0.1	0.1	0	49	4	0.27	0.015	0.1	8	<0.1	0.02	0.01	1.1	06151
salsa	4	14.5	0.2	1.0		0.3	69	5	2	0.04	0.016	5	2	0.01	0.1	0.00	0.02
1 T	16	<0.1	<0.1	<0.1	<0.1	0	34	4	0.16	0.051	0.1	96	0.1	0.01	0.02	2.6	06164
Old El Paso[2]	10		0.0	2.0	<0.3	<0.3	147	6					2				
2 T	30	0.0	0.0			0					0.00	75					GENM292
salsa, brava, hot, La Victoria	2	4.4	0.1	0.3	0.2	0.0	32	1					<1				
1 T	5	0.1				0					0.03	103					06261
salsa, chunky chili dip, cnd, La Victoria - *2 T*	9	27.2	0.2	2.0		0.2	148	4					3				
	30	<0.1									0.01	63					06139
salsa, green chili, mild, La Victoria - *2 T*	8	27.6	0.4	1.3	0.5	0.1	172	5					4				
	30	0.1									0.27	137					06269
salsa, green jalapena, La Victoria	10	27.4	0.3	1.4	0.6	0.3	180	5					4				
2 T	30	0.3				0					0.12	85					06273
salsa, picante, med, La Victoria - *2 T*	8	27.5	0.4	1.5	0.9	0.2	150	4					2				
	30	0.1				0					0.02	140					06266
mild, La Victoria	8	27.5	0.4	1.4	0.9	0.1	179	5					2				
2 T	30	0.1				0					0.03	124					06265
salsa, ranchera, hot, La Victoria	9	27.3	0.4	1.6	0.8	0.1	169	5					1				
2 T	30	0.1				0					0.04	357					06263
salsa, red jalapena, La Victoria	12	26.6	0.4	2.2	1.2	0.4	146	6					10				
2 T	30	0.2				0					0.05	744					06274
salsa, suprema, med, La Victoria - *2 T*	8	27.6	0.3	1.4	1.0	0.2	165	3					2				
	30	0.1				0					0.02	97					06268
mild, La Victoria	8	27.4	0.2	1.6	0.9	0.2	176	5					4				
2 T	30	0.1				0					0.05	182					06267
salsa, thick 'n chunky, Old El Paso[3]	10		0.0	2.6	1.0	0.0	230	0					0				
2 T	30	0.0	0.0			0					0.00	100					GENM293
hot, La Victoria	8	27.5	0.5	1.4	1.0	0.2	131	3					2				
2 T	30	0.1				0					0.02	157					06272
medium, La Victoria	8	27.6	0.4	1.3	0.9	0.3	158	6					4				
2 T	30	0.1				0					0.05	173					06271
mild, La Victoria	8	27.6	0.3	1.5	1.1	0.2	156	5					4				
2 T	30	0.1				0					0.04	230					06270
salsa, victoria, hot, La Victoria	7	27.7	0.3	1.3	0.6	0.2	162	2					4				
2 T	30	0.1				0					0.01	52					06262
soy sauce, made w/hydrolyzed veg protein - *1 T*	7	13.6	0.4	1.4		0.1	1024	1	1	0.06	0.064	0	0	0.01	0.5	0.00	0.05
	18	<0.1	<0.1	<0.1	<0.1	0	27	17	0.27	0.017	0.1	0	0.0	0.02	0.03	2.3	16125
made w/soy (tamari) *1 T*	11	11.9	1.9	1.4		0.1	1005	4	7	0.08	0.090	0	0	0.01	0.7	0.00	0.07
	18	<0.1	<0.1	<0.1	<0.1	0	38	23	0.43	0.024	0.1	0	0.0	0.03	0.04	3.2	16124
made w/soy & wheat (shoyu) *1 T*	8	11.4	0.8	1.4		0.1	914	3	5	0.06	0.068	0	0	0.01	0.5	0.00	0.05
	16	<0.1	<0.1	<0.1	<0.1	0	29	18	0.32	0.018	0.1	0	0.0	0.02	0.03	2.6	16123
stir-fry sce, Chef-Mate *1 T*	16	11.1	0.2	2.3	0.9	0.0	233	2	2	0.02	0.020		1	<0.01	0.1	0.00	0.01
	15	0.6	0.1	0.2	0.3	0	8	5	0.11	0.006		4	<0.1	0.01	0.01	0.6	06130
taco sce, green, med, La Victoria *1 T*	5	13.6	0.1	0.9	0.4	0.1	95	1					1				
	15	0.1				0					0.01	12					06260
green, mild, La Victoria *1 T*	5	13.6	0.1	0.9	0.4	0.1	95	1					1				
	15	0.1				0					0.01	12					06259
Old El Paso[1] *1 T*	5		0.0	1.0	0.0	0.0	88	0					0				
	15	0.0	0.0			0					0.00	0					GENM294
red, med, La Victoria *1 T*	7	14.0	0.2	1.3	1.0	0.1	105	3					3				
	16	0.1				0					0.03	256					06258
red, mild, La Victoria *1 T*	7	14.0	0.2	1.3	1.0	0.1	105	3					3				
	16	0.1				0					0.03	256					06257
tartar sce, Hellmann's/Best Foods *2 T*	80		0.0	3.0	2.0	0.0	300	0					0				
	30	7.0	1.0			10					0.00	0					UNLV95

	KCAL / WT (g)	H₂O (g) / FAT (g)	PRO (g) / SFA (g)	CHO (g) / MUFA (g)	SUGR (g) / PUFA (g)	DFIB (g) / CHOL (mg)	Na (mg) / K (mg)	Ca (mg) / P (mg)	Mg (mg) / Fe (mg)	Zn (mg) / Cu (mg)	Mn (mg) / Se (mcg)	A (mcg RAE) / A (IU)	C (mg) / E (mg ATE)	B-1 (mg) / B-2 (mg)	NIA (mg) / B-6 (mg)	B-12 (mcg) / FOL (mcg DFE)	PANT (mg) / REF
low fat, Hellmann's/Best Foods	40		0.0	7.0	5.0		360										
2 T	32	1.5	0.0	0.5	1.0	0											UNLV96
teriyaki sce,	15	12.2	1.1	2.9		0.0	690	5	11	0.02	0.000	0	0	0.01	0.2	0.00	0.04
bottled - 1 T	18	0.0	0.0	0.0	0.0	0	41	28	0.31	0.018	0.2	0	0.0	0.01	0.02	3.6	06112
Chef-Mate	21	11.0	0.1	3.7	2.8	0.0	159	1	1	0.02	0.018	0		0.01	0.1	0.00	0.01
1 T	16	0.6	0.1	0.2	0.3	0	8	3	0.09	0.007		0	<0.1	<0.01	<0.01	0.5	06129
dry mix	130	0.5	4.1	27.6		0.9	4784	112	83	0.14	0.000	0	0	0.04	1.3	0.00	0.28
1 pkt	46	0.9	0.1	0.2	0.5	0	215	213	2.79	0.138		0		0.09	0.14	27.6	06111

[1] Values are averages for mild, medium, and hot.
[2] Values are averages for green chili salsa, mild homestyle salsa, medium homestyle salsa, and salsa verde.
[3] Values are averages for extra mild, mild, medium, and hot.

26.2 ENTRÉE SAUCES

	KCAL / WT (g)	H₂O (g) / FAT (g)	PRO (g) / SFA (g)	CHO (g) / MUFA (g)	SUGR (g) / PUFA (g)	DFIB (g) / CHOL (mg)	Na (mg) / K (mg)	Ca (mg) / P (mg)	Mg (mg) / Fe (mg)	Zn (mg) / Cu (mg)	Mn (mg) / Se (mcg)	A (mcg RAE) / A (IU)	C (mg) / E (mg ATE)	B-1 (mg) / B-2 (mg)	NIA (mg) / B-6 (mg)	B-12 (mcg) / FOL (mcg DFE)	PANT (mg) / REF
alfredo & mushroom sce, Five	80		2.0	3.0	1.0	0.0	380	60				0					
Brothers - 1/2 cup	~48	7.0	3.0			25				0.00		200					UNLV19
alfredo sce, creamy garlic, Bertolli	110		2.0	3.0	1.0	0.0	360	40				0					
1/2 cup	~60	10.0	4.0			30				0.00		200					UNLV21
alfredo sce mix, Knorr	60		2.0	7.0	3.0	0.0	680	20				0					
2 T (1/2 cup prep)	15	3.0	1.0			<5				0.00		0					UNLV66
béarnaise sce mix	91	1.4	3.5	14.9			848	41	7	0.18	0.025	<1	<1	0.03	0.2	0.10	0.10
1 pkt	25	2.3	0.3	1.0	0.8	<1	73	37	0.13	0.025		1		0.05	0.01	3.3	06102
carbonara sce mix, Knorr	70		3.0	7.0	3.0	0.0	650	40				0					
2 T (1/2 cup prep)	16	3.0	1.0			5				0.00		0					UNLV67
creamy cheddar sce mix, Knorr	50		2.0	6.0	2.0	0.0	600	40				0					
2 T (1/2 cup prep)	12	2.0	1.0			<5				0.00		0					UNLV68
creamy clam sce, Progresso	110		5.0	8.0	0.0	0.0	440	0				0					
1/2 cup	120	6.0	1.5			10				0.72		0					GENM297
creole sce, Chef-Mate	25	55.3	0.9	3.7	2.9	0.8	339	35	9	0.10	0.104	0		0.03	0.5	0.00	0.16
1/2 cup	62	0.7	0.1	0.2	0.3	0	187	17	0.31	0.059		234	0.6	0.02	0.07		06903
curry sce mix	149	1.5	3.3	17.7			1428	62	14	0.32	0.035	2	1	0.04	0.3	0.14	0.14
1 pkt	35	8.1	1.2	3.5	3.0	<1	123	52	1.09	0.035		36		0.07	0.02	3.2	06104
enchilada sce,	30		<1.0	3.0	<1.0	0.0	330	0				0					
green chili, Old El Paso - 1/4 cup	61	1.5	0.0			0				0.00		500					GENM295
La Victoria	20	55.1	0.2	2.8	0.6	0.4	395	7					3				
1/2 cup	60	0.9				0				0.07		1386					06275
mild/med/hot, Old El Paso	20		0.0	3.0	<1.0	0.0	220	0					1				
1/4 cup	60	1.0	0.0			0				0.00		200					GENM296
Ortega	15	26.6	0.4	2.0	0.2	0.3	77	7	5	0.06	0.050		2	0.02	0.3	0.00	0.08
2 T	30	0.6	0.1	0.2	0.3	0	83	11	0.31	0.031		123	0.0	0.01	0.04	2.4	06153
fish sce	10	20.2	1.4	1.0		0.0	2192	12	50	0.06	0.066	0	<1	<0.01	0.7	0.14	0.03
1 fl oz (1.5 T)	28	<0.1	<0.1	<0.1	<0.1	0	82	2	0.22	0.014	2.6	1	<0.1	0.02	0.11	14.5	06179
garlic herb sce mix, Knorr	60		1.0	8.0	2.0	0.0	900	0				0					
2 T (1/2 cup prep)	15	3.0	0.5			0				0.00		0					UNLV54
guava sce	86	213.2	0.8	22.6		8.6	10	17	17	0.40	0.257	33	348	0.06	1.0	0.00	
1 cup	238	0.3	0.1	<0.1	0.1	0	536	26	0.43	0.183	1.2	674	0.0	0.03	0.21	11.9	09143
hollandaise sce mix,	10		0.0	2.0	0.0	0.0	105	0				0					
Knorr - 1 t (2 T prep)	2.5	0.0	0.0			0				0.00		0					UNLV55
w/butter	188	0.7	3.7	10.9		0.4	1241	98	6	0.54	0.034	173	<1	0.03	<0.1	0.61	0.68
1 pkt	34	15.7	9.2	4.7	0.7	40	99	100	0.71	0.102		578	0.3	0.14	0.41	16.7	06155
w/veg oil	94	1.3	3.4	15.6		0.3	650	64	7	0.23	0.025	<1	<1	0.03	0.2	0.20	0.20
1 pkt	25	2.3	0.5	1.0	0.7	<1	94	53	0.08	0.025		2		0.10	0.03	3.5	06154
hot dog sce, chili, Chef-Mate	69	47.2	2.7	9.2	1.1	1.7	399	20	13	0.55	0.129		<1	0.05	0.7	0.13	0.14
1/4 cup	63	2.4	1.0	1.0	0.2	4	149	40	0.98	0.069		423	0.3	0.05	0.07	22.1	06156
italian sce, Chef-Mate	61	47.1	1.0	11.5	3.5	0.9	304	34	20	0.26	0.254		4	0.08	1.1	0.00	0.34
1/4 cup	62	1.2	0.2	0.7	0.2	0	377	43	0.38	0.150		244	1.2	0.05	0.17	16.1	06181
lemon sce, Chef-Mate	43	21.5	0.1	10.2	7.8	0.0	3	1	1	0.01	0.010		3	<0.01	<0.1	0.00	0.01
2 T	32	0.2	<0.1	0.1	0.1	0	6	1	0.12	0.008		0	<0.1	<0.01	<0.01		06905
lobster sce, Progresso	100		3.0	6.0	3.0	2.0	430	20				0					
1/2 cup	123	7.0	1.0			5				1.08		300					GENM298
mole poblano,	205	89.4	4.4	16.2		5.3	168	30	40	0.58	0.293	0		0.03	2.1		0.30
homemade - 1/2 cup	125	13.7					408	103	2.31	0.236				0.00	0.31	35.0	06136

Food	KCAL / WT (g)	H₂O / FAT (g)	PRO / SFA (g)	CHO / MUFA (g)	SUGR / PUFA (g)	DFIB (g) / CHOL (mg)	Na / K (mg)	Ca / P (mg)	Mg / Fe (mg)	Zn / Cu (mg)	Mn (mg) / Se (mcg)	A (mcg RAE) / A (IU)	C (mg) / E (mg ATE)	B-1 / B-2 (mg)	NIA (mg) / B-6 (mg)	B-12 (mcg) / FOL (mcg DFE)	PANT (mg) / REF
La Victoria	240	3.5	8.3	28.4	11.0	9.2	1847	58					0				
2 oz	57	10.3				0			1.59			11742					06276
mushroom sce mix	98	1.0	4.0	15.3			1744	3	5	0.25	0.028	0	0	0.03	1.3	0.00	0.64
1 pkt	28	2.7	0.4	1.1	1.0	0	121	37	0.28	0.168		0		0.14	0.03	7.6	06106
oyster sce	9	14.4	0.2	2.0		0.1	492	6	1	0.02	0.010	1	<1	<0.01	0.3	0.07	<0.01
1 T	18	<0.1	<0.1	<0.1	<0.1	0	10	4	0.03	0.03	0.8	4	<0.1	0.02	<0.01	2.7	06176
parma rosa sce mix, Knorr	60		2.0	8.0	2.0	0.0	640	40					2				
2 T (1/2 cup prep)	15	2.5	0.5			0			0.36			100					UNLV65
pasta sce w/cheese, avg for 5 flvrs,	92		2.6	3.0	1.0	0.0	412	60					0				
Ragu Cheese Creations[1] - (1/4 cup)	62	7.9	3.3			24			0.00			180					UNLV169
pesto sce mix	15		<1.0	3.0	2.0	0.0	490	0					0				
Knorr - 2 t (1/4 cup prep)	5	0.0	0.0			0			0.00			200					UNLV72
red bell pepper, Knorr	20		<1.0	4.0	1.0	<1.0	480	0					6				
2/3 T (1/4 cup prep)	7	0.0	0.0			0			0.00			200					UNLV70
sundried tomato, Knorr	35		1.0	7.0	3.0	<1.0	630	0					2				
1 T (1/4 cup prep)	11	0.0	0.0			0			0.36			100					UNLV71
red clam sce, Progresso	60		4.0	8.0	4.0	1.0	350	20					0				
1/2 cup	125	1.0	0.0			10			0.72			200					GENM300
sofrito, homemade	244	61.4	13.2	5.6		1.8	1179	21	26	1.45	0.197		21	0.29	3.0		0.61
1/2 cup	103	18.7					413	143	0.97	0.170			0.22	0.37	44.3	06142
stroganoff sce mix	161	2.1	5.6	26.5		0.5	1863	307	19	1.10	0.184	11	<1	0.84	0.6	0.28	0.60
1 pkt	46	4.4	2.8	1.2	0.1	12	398	126	1.33	0.070		222		0.48	0.05	3.7	06109
sweet & sour glaze, Chef-Mate	51	18.5	0.1	12.5	8.3		229	15	6	0.06	0.247		3	0.02	0.1	0.00	0.04
2 T	32	<0.1	<0.1	<0.1	<0.1	0	72	7	0.36	0.049		48	<0.1	0.01	0.03	2.6	06131
sweet & sour sce, Chef-Mate	40	23.5	0.2	8.2	6.9	0.3	116	6	2	0.03	0.096		0	<0.01	0.1	0.00	0.02
2 T	33	0.8	0.1	0.2	0.4	0	22	3	0.28	0.016		25	0.1	0.01	0.01	0.7	06132
sweet & sour sce mix	222	0.3	0.6	54.8		1.1	587	31	7	0.07	0.000	0	0	0.01	0.6	0.00	0.51
1 pkt	57	0.1	<0.1	<0.1	<0.1	0	50	34	1.22	0.021		0	0.0	0.07	0.29	1.7	06110
tomato basil sce mix, Knorr	70		2.0	14.0	7.0	1.0	630	20					6				
3 T (1/2 cup prep)	20	1.0	0.0			0			0.36			500					UNLV73
tomato sce, Bertolli (5 flvrs)[2] - 1/2 cup	82		3.2	10.8	9.0	3.0	530	88					11				
	126	2.9	0.2			1			1.08			750					UNLV167
Eden Foods	80		3.0	12.0	6.0	3.0	320	80	32	0.00			2	2.00			
1/2 cup	125	2.5	0.0			0	530	60	1.08	0.000		2000	8.00				EDEN23
Eden Foods, no salt added	80		3.0	12.0	6.0	3.0	10	40	32				12	0.09	1.6		
1/2 cup	125	2.5	0.0			0	530	60	1.44			2000	0.03				EDEN24
Prego Traditional 100% Natural	263	192.0	4.3	40.0	20.3	7.8	1075						26				
1 cup	250	9.8	2.2			0						1418					06932
Ragu Chicken Tonight Cacciatore	70		2.0	9.0	8.0	2.0	576						0				
1/2 cup	126	1.3	0.0			0						500					UNLV188
Ragu Chunky Gardenstyle (8 flvrs)[3]	108		2.4	17.4	12.1	2.1	546	48					6				
1/2 cup	128	3.1	0.3			0			1.08			594					UNLV198
Ragu Express (3 flvrs)[4]	200		7.0	36.0	6.0	2.0	580	20					0				
1 container	~105	3.0	0.5			0			1.80			300					UNLV197
Ragu Hearty Meat (2 flvrs)[5]	135		6.0	8.0	6.5	2.0	600	30					6				
1/2 cup	124	8.5	2.8			18			0.90			450					UNLV20
Ragu Light (2 flvrs)[6]	48		2.0	9.5	7.5	2.0	370	40					5				
1/2 cup	~105	0.0	0.0			0			0.90			400					UNLV153
Ragu Old World Style (5 flvrs)[7]	76		2.2	7.6	6.4	2.0	774	40					3				
1/2 cup	125	3.6	0.4			2			0.72			400					UNLV157
Ragu Old World Style, smooth	160	211.0	3.8	24.2	10.8	5.3	1513										
1 cup	250	5.3	0.7	1.1	2.6				2.05			1293					06933
Ragu Pizza Quick (3 flvrs)[8]	43		1.3	4.7	3.0	1.0	410	20					1				
1/4 cup	63	2.0	0.2			2			0.36			300					UNLV196
Ragu Robusto (10 flvrs)[9]	87		2.7	10.4	8.6	2.3	607	49					6				
1/2 cup	129	3.9	0.8			2			1.08			500					UNLV154
tomato sce, cnd	74	218.2	3.3	17.6		3.4	1482	34	47	0.61	0.537	120	32	0.16	2.8	0.00	0.76
1 cup	245	0.4	0.1	0.1	0.2	0	909	78	1.89	0.480	1.5	2399	3.4	0.14	0.38	22.1	11549
marinara	143	217.2	3.6	20.6		4.0	1030	55	43	0.43	0.550	48	20	0.14	2.7	0.00	0.75
1 cup	250	5.2	0.7	2.2	1.8	0	738	80	1.80	0.280	1.5	938	3.1	0.10	0.29	25.0	06931
marinara, Progresso	100		4.0	12.0	2.0	3.0	590	80					0				
1/2 cup	124	4.0	1.0			<5			1.08			750					GENM299

	KCAL / WT (g)	H₂0 (g) / FAT (g)	PRO (g) / SFA (g)	CHO (g) / MUFA (g)	SUGR (g) / PUFA (g)	DFIB (g) / CHOL (mg)	Na (mg) / K (mg)	Ca (mg) / P (mg)	Mg (mg) / Fe (mg)	Zn (mg) / Cu (mg)	Mn (mg) / Se (mcg)	A (mcg RAE) / A (IU)	C (mg) / E (mg ATE)	B-1 (mg) / B-2 (mg)	NIA (mg) / B-6 (mg)	B-12 (mcg) / FOL (mcg DFE)	PANT (mg) / REF
oven rstd garlic & vidalia onion, Five Brothers - 1/2 cup	80		3.0	12.0	10.0	3.0	480	80					18				
	127	1.5	0.0			0			1.08			750					UNLV155
spanish style 1 cup	81	217.4	3.5	17.7		3.4	1152	41	46	0.83	0.527	120	21	0.18	3.2	0.00	0.69
	244	0.7	0.1	0.1	0.3	0	900	117	8.49	0.390	1.5	2403		0.15	0.43	34.2	11649
w/herbs & cheese 1 cup	144	203.6	5.2	25.0		5.4	1325	90	46	0.88	0.459	120	24	0.19	2.9		0.67
	244	4.7	1.5	0.9	2.0	7	869	132	2.12	0.425	2.2	2408		0.30	0.05	19.5	11555
w/mushrooms 1 cup	86	215.5	3.6	20.7		3.7	1107	32	47	0.51	0.461	118	30	0.18	3.1	0.00	0.90
	245	0.3	<0.1	<0.1	0.1	0	931	78	2.18	0.488		2340		0.26	0.33	22.1	11551
w/tomato pieces 1 cup	78	217.4	3.2	17.3		3.4	37	24	49	0.46	0.537	98	52	0.18	2.9	0.00	0.53
	244	1.0	0.1	0.1	0.4	0	910	102	1.66	0.034	1.5	1954		0.24	0.38	22.0	11559
w/onions 1 cup	103	210.9	3.8	24.4		4.4	1350	42	47	0.56	0.737	105	31	0.18	3.0	0.00	0.90
	245	0.5	0.1	0.1	0.2	0	1012	96	2.28	0.443	2.0	2083		0.33	0.65	53.9	11553
w/onions, green peppers, & celery 1 cup	103	220.7	2.4	21.9		3.5	1365	33	53	0.70	0.610	103	33	0.17	2.7	0.00	0.55
	250	1.9	0.3	0.3	0.8	0	995	95	1.90	0.495	1.5	2025	3.7	0.30	0.49	35.0	11557
white clam sce, authentic, Progresso 1/2 cup	150		9.0	5.0	<1.0	0.0	710	40					1				
	124	10.0	1.5			20			1.80			200					GENM301
white sce,[10] med, homemade - 1/2 cup	184	93.6	4.8	11.5		0.3	443	148	18	0.51	0.054	35	1	0.09	0.5	0.35	0.41
	125	13.3	3.6	5.5	3.6	9	195	123	0.41	0.020	5.1	691	1.7	0.23	0.05	12.5	06166
thick, homemade 1/2 cup	233	86.4	5.0	14.5		0.4	466	139	18	0.50	0.084	43	1	0.11	0.7	0.33	0.39
	125	17.3	4.3	7.3	4.9	8	186	120	0.63	0.026	6.5	841	2.3	0.24	0.05	18.8	06167
thin, homemade 1/2 cup	131	100.8	4.7	9.3		0.1	410	158	19	0.53	0.030	25	1	0.07	0.3	0.38	0.42
	125	8.4	2.7	3.3	2.0	10	204	126	0.26	0.016	4.1	504	0.9	0.23	0.05	8.8	06165

[1] Values are averages for classic alfredo, double cheddar, lite parmesan alfredo, parmesan and mozzarella, and roasted garlic parmesan.
[2] Values are averages for five cheese, marinara with burgundy wine, mushroom and garlic, summer tomato and basil, and summer vegetables.
[3] Values are averages for mushrooms and green pepper; mama's special garden sauce; roasted red pepper and onion; sundried tomato and sweet basil; super chunky mushroom; super vegetable primavera; tomato, basil, and Italian cheese; and tomato, garlic, and onions.
[4] Values are averages for meat flavored tomato, sweet tomato & garlic, and traditional tomato.
[5] Values are averages for classic Italian meat and mama's meat sauce.
[6] Values are averages for roasted garlic primavera and tomato and basil.
[7] Values are averages for flavored with meat, marinara, traditional, with meat, and with mushrooms.
[8] Values are averages for garlic and basil, pepperoni, and traditional.
[9] Values are averages for beef with mushroom; chopped tomato, olive oil, and garlic; parmesan and romano cheese; roasted garlic; sautéed beef, onions, & garlic; sautéed onion and garlic; sautéed onion and mushroom; seven herb tomato; six cheese; and sweet Italian sausage and cheese.
[10] Ingredients are lowfat milk margarine, flour, and salt.

26.3 GRAVIES

	KCAL / WT (g)	H₂0 (g) / FAT (g)	PRO (g) / SFA (g)	CHO (g) / MUFA (g)	SUGR (g) / PUFA (g)	DFIB (g) / CHOL (mg)	Na (mg) / K (mg)	Ca (mg) / P (mg)	Mg (mg) / Fe (mg)	Zn (mg) / Cu (mg)	Mn (mg) / Se (mcg)	A (mcg RAE) / A (IU)	C (mg) / E (mg ATE)	B-1 (mg) / B-2 (mg)	NIA (mg) / B-6 (mg)	B-12 (mcg) / FOL (mcg DFE)	PANT (mg) / REF
au jus, cnd 10.5 oz can	48	281.6	3.6	7.5		0.0	149	12	6	2.98	0.596	0	3	0.06	2.7	0.30	0.06
	298	0.6	0.3	0.2	<0.1	0	241	89	1.79	0.298	1.2	0		0.18	0.03	6.0	06114
au jus gravy mix 1 t	9	0.1	0.3	1.4			348	4	2	0.02	0.008	<1	<1	0.01	0.1	0.01	<0.01
	3	0.3	0.1	0.1	<0.1	<1	8	5	0.28	0.004	0.2	<1		0.01	0.01	2.4	06115
Knorr 1 t (1/4 cup prep)	10		0.0	2.0	0.0	0.0	250	0					0				
	3.5	0.0	0.0			0			0.00			0					UNLV38
beef, cnd 10.3 oz can	154	254.6	10.9	14.0		1.2	1630	17	6	2.91	0.582	0	0	0.09	1.9	0.29	0.06
	291	6.9	3.4	2.8	0.2	9	236	87	2.04	0.291	2.9	0	0.2	0.10	0.03	5.8	06116
glass jar, Pepperidge Farm 1/6 jar	26	53.0	1.8	3.7			379										
	60	0.4	0.1	0.2	<0.1	3						0					06746
brown, cnd, Heinz Home Style Savory 1/4 cup	25	53.9	0.9	3.4			352										
	60	0.8	0.3	0.3	<0.1	2						0					06579
brown gravy mix 1 T	22	0.3	0.6	3.6		0.1	291	8	2	0.07	0.025	<1	<1	0.01	0.2	0.04	0.01
	6	0.6	0.2	0.3	<0.1	<1	16	12	0.10	0.011	0.4	2	<0.1	0.02	0.01	2.6	06118
classic, Knorr 2 t (1/2 cup prep)	20		<1.0	3.0	1.0	0.0	380	0					0				
	6	0.5	0.0			0			0.00			0					UNLV39
mushroom (hunter), Knorr 1 T (1/4 cup prep)	20		<1.0	3.0	<1.0	0.0	300	0					0				
	6	0.5	0.0			0			0.00			0					UNLV40
w/onion (lyonnaise), Knorr 2 T (1/4 cup prep)	20		<1.0	4.0	<1.0	0.0	300	0					0				
	6	0.5	0.5			0			0.00			0					UNLV41
chicken, cnd 10.5 oz can	235	254.3	5.8	16.2		1.2	1719	60	6	2.38	0.596	331	0	0.05	1.3	0.30	0.06
	298	17.0	4.2	7.6	4.5	6	325	86	1.40	0.298	2.4	1100	0.5	0.13	0.03	6.0	06119
chicken gravy mix 1 T (amt for 1 serving)	30	0.3	0.9	5.0			332	12	3	0.11	0.018	3	<1	0.02	0.3	0.04	0.10
	8	0.8	0.2	0.4	0.2	2	32	20	0.11	0.009	0.4	25		0.05	0.02	10.9	06120
roasted, Knorr 1 T (1/4 cup prep)	25		1.0	4.0	<1.0	0.0	340	0					0				
	7	0.5	0.0			0			0.00			0					UNLV47
country sausage, Chef-Mate 1/4 cup	96	46.7	2.9	3.9	0.5	0.4	236	4	3	0.34	0.020		<1	0.10	0.7	0.21	0.10
	62	7.7	2.0	2.9	2.2	13	48	25	0.34	0.024		0	0.2	0.04	0.04		06800

	KCAL / WT (g)	H₂0 (g) / FAT (g)	PRO (g) / SFA (g)	CHO (g) / MUFA (g)	SUGR (g) / PUFA (g)	DFIB (g) / CHOL (mg)	Na (mg) / K (mg)	Ca (mg) / P (mg)	Mg (mg) / Fe (mg)	Zn (mg) / Cu (mg)	Mn (mg) / Se (mcg)	A (mcg RAE) / A (IU)	C (mg) / E (mg ATE)	B-1 (mg) / B-2 (mg)	NIA (mg) / B-6 (mg)	B-12 (mcg) / FOL (mcg DFE)	PANT (mg) / REF
mushroom, cnd	149	265.2	3.8	16.3		1.2	1699	21	6	2.09	0.894	0	0	0.10	2.0	0.00	3.28
10.5 oz can	298	8.1	1.2	3.5	3.0	0	316	45	1.97	0.298	5.7	0		0.19	0.06	35.8	06121
peppercorn gravy mix, classic, Knorr	20		<1.0	4.0	<1.0	0.0	380	0					0				
2 t (1/4 cup prep)	6	0.5	0.0			0			0.00			0					UNLV80
pork gavy mix	25	0.3	0.6	4.3		0.2	359	9	2	0.07	0.021	2	<1	0.01	0.2	0.03	0.02
amt to make 1 serving	7	0.6	0.3	0.3	<0.1	1	16	13	0.26	0.010	0.4	8	<0.1	0.02	0.01	2.8	06124
roasted, Knorr	25		<1.0	4.0	<1.0	0.0	230	0					0				
1 T (1/4 cup prep)	7	0.0	0.0			0			0.00			0					UNLV81
turkey, cnd	8	13.2	0.4	0.8		0.1	86	1	<1	0.12	0.030	0	0	<0.01	0.2	0.01	<0.01
1 T	15	0.3	0.1	0.1	0.1	<1	16	4	0.10	0.015	0.1	0	<0.1	0.01	<0.01	0.3	06125
turkey gravy mix	26	0.3	0.7	4.6			307	10	3	0.09	0.015	1	<1	0.01	0.2	0.04	0.07
amt to make 1 serving	7	0.5	0.1	0.2	0.2	1	30	18	0.23	0.009	0.4	2		0.03	0.01	6.5	06126
roasted, Knorr	25		<1.0	4.0	<1.0	0.0	370	0					0				
1 T (1/4 cup prep)	7	0.5	0.0			0			0.00			0					UNLV99
roasted, Knorr	25		<1.0	4.0	<1.0	0.0	370	0					0				
1 T (1/4 cup prep)	7	0.5	0.0			0			0.00			0					UNLV99

26.4 OLIVES

black (manzanillo/mission), cnd	4	2.6	0.0	0.2		0.1	28	3	<1	0.01	0.001	1	<1	<0.01	<0.1	0.00	<0.01
1 small	3.2	0.3	<0.1	0.3	<0.1	0	<1	<1	0.11	0.008	<0.1	13	0.1	0.00	<0.01	0.0	09193a
1 large	445	3.5	0.0	0.3		0.1	38	4	<1	0.01	0.001	1	<1	<0.01	<0.1	0.00	<0.01
	4.4	0.3	<0.1	0.3	<0.1	0	<1	<1	0.15	0.011	<0.1	18	0.1	0.00	<0.01	0.0	09193b
green (sevailano/ascolano), cnd	7	7.0	0.1	0.5		0.2	75	8	<1	0.02	0.002	1	<1	<0.01	<0.1	0.00	<0.01
1 jumbo	8	0.6	0.1	0.4	<0.1	0	1	<1	0.28	0.019	0.1	29	0.2	0.00	<0.01	0.0	09194b
1 super colossal	12	12.7	0.1	0.8		0.4	135	14	1	0.03	0.003	3	<1	<0.01	<0.1	0.00	<0.01
	15	1.0	0.1	0.8	0.1	0	1	<1	0.50	0.034	0.1	52	0.5	0.00	<0.01	0.0	09194a

26.5 PICKLES

pickle, dill	5	27.5	0.2	1.2		0.4	385	3	3	0.04	0.005	5	1	<0.01	<0.1	0.00	0.02
1 spear	30	0.1	<0.1	<0.1	<0.1	0	35	6	0.16	0.024	0.0	99	<0.1	0.01	<0.01	0.3	11937a
1 large (4" long)	24	123.8	0.8	5.6		1.6	1731	12	15	0.19	0.020	22	3	0.02	0.1	0.00	0.07
	135	0.3	0.1	<0.1	0.1	0	157	28	0.72	0.107	0.0	444	0.2	0.04	0.02	1.4	11937b
pickle relish, hamburger	157	74.6	0.8	42.1		3.9	1337	5	9	0.13	0.018	16	3	0.02	0.8	0.00	0.01
1/2 cup	122	0.7	0.1	0.3	0.2	0	93	21	1.39	0.101	0.0	326		0.05	0.02	1.2	11958
pickle relish, hot dog	111	87.4	1.8	28.5		1.8	1331	6	23	0.26	0.018	10	1	0.05	0.6	0.00	0.01
1/2 cup	122	0.6	0.1	0.3	0.1	0	95	49	1.53	0.100	0.0	204		0.05	0.02	1.2	11944
pickle relish, sweet	20	9.3	0.1	5.3		0.2	122	0	1	0.02	0.002	1	<1	0.00	<0.1	0.00	<0.01
1 T	15	0.1	<0.1	<0.1	<0.1	0	4	2	0.13	0.013	0.0	23	<0.1	<0.01	<0.01	0.2	11945
pickle, sour	7	61.2	0.2	1.5		0.8	785	0	3	0.01	0.007	5	1	0.00	0.0	0.00	0.02
1 med (3 3/4" long)	65	0.1	<0.1	<0.1	0.1	0	15	9	0.26	0.055	0.0	94	0.1	0.01	0.01	0.7	11941
pickle, sweet (gherkin)	18	9.8	0.1	4.8		0.2	141	1	1	0.01	0.002	1	<1	<0.01	<0.1	0.00	0.02
1 small (2 1/2" long)	15	<0.1	<0.1	<0.1	<0.1	0	5	2	0.09	0.016	0.0	19	<0.1	<0.01	<0.01	0.2	11940a
1 large (3" long)	41	22.8	0.1	11.1		0.4	329	1	1	0.03	0.005	2	<1	<0.01	0.1	0.00	0.04
	35	0.1	<0.1	<0.1	<0.1	0	11	4	0.21	0.037	0.0	44	0.1	0.01	0.01	0.4	11940b

27. SOUPS
27.1 CONDENSED

beef broth/consommé	72	275.9	13.0	4.3		0.0	1550	21	0	0.89	0.894	0	2	0.05	1.7	0.00	0.12
10.5 oz can	298	0.0	0.0			0	373	77	1.28	0.596	6.3	0		0.07	0.06	6.0	06032
celery, crm of	220	259.1	4.0	21.4		1.8	2309	98	15	0.37	0.610	177	1	0.07	0.8	0.12	2.81
10.8 oz can	305	13.6	3.4	3.1	6.1	34	299	92	1.53	0.345	5.5	744	0.5	0.12	0.03	6.1	06010
cheese	378	240.7	13.2	25.6		2.5	2331	346	9	1.56	0.624	131	0	0.04	1.0	0.00	0.22
11 oz can	312	25.4	16.2	7.2	0.7	72	374	331	1.81	0.312	11.2	2643	0.5	0.33	0.06	9.4	06011
chicken, crm of	284	249.3	8.3	22.5		0.6	2397	82	6	1.53	0.915	393	<1	0.07	2.0	0.21	0.52
10.8 oz can	305	17.9	5.1	8.0	3.6	24	214	92	1.46	0.305	19.2	1360	0.4	0.15	0.04	3.1	06016
mushroom, crm of	314	247.7	4.9	22.6		0.9	2111	79	12	1.43	0.610	0	3	0.07	2.0	0.31	0.61
10.8 oz can	305	23.1	6.3	4.4	10.8	3	204	104	1.28	0.305	3.7	0	3.2	0.20	0.03	9.2	06043
tomato	207	247.8	5.0	40.3		1.2	1690	34	18	0.58	0.610	85	162	0.21	3.4	0.00	0.37
10.8 oz can	305	4.7	0.9	1.0	2.3	0	641	82	4.27	0.610	1.2	1693	6.2	0.12	0.27	36.6	06159

	KCAL / WT (g)	H₂0 (g) / FAT (g)	PRO (g) / SFA (g)	CHO (g) / MUFA (g)	SUGR (g) / PUFA (g)	DFIB (g) / CHOL (mg)	Na (mg) / K (mg)	Ca (mg) / P (mg)	Mg (mg) / Fe (mg)	Zn (mg) / Cu (mg)	Mn (mg) / Se (mcg)	A (mcg RAE) / A (IU)	C (mg) / E (mg ATE)	B-1 (mg) / B-2 (mg)	NIA (mg) / B-6 (mg)	B-12 (mcg) / FOL (mcg DFE)	PANT (mg) / REF

27.2 CONDENSED, PREPARED WITH MILK

	KCAL/WT	H₂0/FAT	PRO/SFA	CHO/MUFA	SUGR/PUFA	DFIB/CHOL	Na/K	Ca/P	Mg/Fe	Zn/Cu	Mn/Se	A RAE/A IU	C/E	B-1/B-2	NIA/B-6	B-12/FOL	PANT/REF
asparagus, crm of	161	213.3	6.3	16.4		0.7	1042	174	20	0.92	0.379	62	4	0.10	0.9	0.50	0.52
1 cup (8 fl oz)	248	8.2	3.3	2.1	2.2	22	360	154	0.87	0.139		600	0.8	0.28	0.06	29.8	06201
celery, crm of	164	214.4	5.7	14.5		0.7	1009	186	22	0.20	0.253	114	1	0.07	0.4	0.50	1.51
1 cup (8 fl oz)	248	9.7	3.9	2.5	2.7	32	310	151	0.69	0.154	4.7	461	1.0	0.25	0.06	7.4	06210
cheese	231	206.9	9.5	16.2		1.0	1019	289	20	0.68	0.259	359	1	0.06	0.5	0.43	0.48
1 cup (8 fl oz)	251	14.6	9.1	4.1	0.5	48	341	251	0.80	0.141	7.0	1242	0.3	0.33	0.08	10.0	06211
chicken, crm of	191	210.4	7.5	15.0		0.2	1047	181	17	0.67	0.379	179	1	0.07	0.9	0.55	0.57
1 cup (8 fl oz)	248	11.5	4.6	4.5	1.6	27	273	151	0.67	0.139		714	0.2	0.26	0.07	7.4	06216
clam chowder, new england	164	211.4	9.5	16.6		1.5	992	186	22	0.79	0.253	50	3	0.07	1.0	10.24	0.69
1 cup (8 fl oz)	248	6.6	3.0	2.3	1.1	22	300	156	1.49	0.139	12.9	164	0.1	0.24	0.13	9.9	06230
mushroom, crm of	203	209.7	6.1	15.0		0.5	918	179	20	0.64	0.253	45	2	0.08	0.9	0.50	0.62
1 cup (8 fl oz)	248	13.6	5.1	3.0	4.6	20	270	156	0.60	0.139	4.0	154	1.3	0.28	0.06	9.9	06243
onion, crm of	186	209.6	6.8	18.4		0.7	1004	179	22	0.62	0.248	52	2	0.10	0.6	0.50	0.69
1 cup (8 fl oz)	248	9.4	4.0	3.3	1.6	32	310	154	0.69	0.149		451	0.1	0.27	0.07	22.3	06246
oyster stew	135	217.9	6.1	9.8		0.0	1041	167	20	10.34	0.370	56	4	0.07	0.3	2.62	0.49
1 cup (8 fl oz)	245	7.9	5.0	2.1	0.3	32	235	162	1.05	1.605		225		0.23	0.06	9.8	06248
pea, green	239	197.9	12.6	32.2		2.8	970	173	56	1.75	0.660	66	3	0.15	1.3	0.43	0.56
1 cup (8 fl oz)	254	7.0	4.0	2.2	0.5	18	376	239	2.01	0.391		356	0.2	0.27	0.10	7.6	06249
potato, crm of	149	214.9	5.8	17.2		0.5	1061	166	17	0.67	0.379	52	1	0.08	0.6	1.04	1.69
1 cup (8 fl oz)	248	6.4	3.8	1.7	0.6	22	322	161	0.55	0.263		444	0.1	0.24	0.09	9.9	06253
shrimp, crm of	164	214.3	6.8	13.9		0.2	1037	164	22	0.79	0.397	79	1	0.06	0.5	1.04	0.55
1 cup (8 fl oz)	248	9.3	5.8	3.7	0.3	35	248	146	0.60	0.136	7.9	312	0.9	0.23	0.45	9.9	06256
tomato	161	209.8	6.1	22.3		2.7	744	159	22	0.30	0.253	74	68	0.13	1.5	0.45	0.55
1 cup (8 fl oz)	248	6.0	2.9	1.6	1.1	17	449	149	1.81	0.263	2.2	848	2.6	0.25	0.16	19.8	06359
tomato bisque	198	204.6	6.3	29.4		0.5	1109	186	25	0.63	0.259	63	7	0.11	1.3	0.43	0.50
1 cup (8 fl oz)	251	6.6	3.1	1.9	1.2	23	605	173	0.88	0.141		879		0.27	0.14	22.6	06358

27.3 CONDENSED, PREPARED WITH WATER

	KCAL/WT	H₂0/FAT	PRO/SFA	CHO/MUFA	SUGR/PUFA	DFIB/CHOL	Na/K	Ca/P	Mg/Fe	Zn/Cu	Mn/Se	A RAE/A IU	C/E	B-1/B-2	NIA/B-6	B-12/FOL	PANT/REF
asparagus, crm of	85	224.0	2.3	10.7		0.5	981	29	5	0.88	0.376	37	3	0.05	0.8	0.05	0.12
1 cup (8 fl oz)	244	4.1	1.0	1.0	1.9	5	173	39	0.81	0.124		444	0.7	0.08	0.01	22.0	06401
bean w/franks	188	207.6	10.0	22.0			1093	88	48	1.18	0.788	43	1	0.11	1.0	0.08	0.10
1 cup (8 fl oz)	250	7.0	2.1	2.7	1.7	13	478	165	2.35	0.395	8.5	870		0.07	0.13	30.0	06406
bean w/pork	172	212.9	7.9	22.8		8.6	951	81	46	1.04	0.670	46	2	0.09	0.6	0.05	0.10
1 cup (8 fl oz)	253	5.9	1.5	2.2	1.8	3	402	132	2.05	0.402	8.1	888	0.1	0.03	0.04	32.9	06404
beef broth/bouillon/consommé	29	231.9	5.4	1.8		0.0	636	10	0	0.36	0.366	0	1	0.02	0.7	0.00	0.05
1 cup (8 fl oz)	241	0.0	0.0	0.0	0.0	0	154	31	0.53	0.246		0		0.03	0.02	2.4	06432
beef mushroom	73	225.9	5.8	6.3		0.2	942	5	10	1.46	0.488	0	5	0.04	1.0	0.20	0.22
1 cup (8 fl oz)	244	3.0	1.5	1.2	0.1	7	154	34	0.88	0.244		0		0.06	0.05	9.8	06547
beef noodle	83	224.5	4.8	9.0		0.7	952	15	5	1.54	0.273	32	<1	0.07	1.1	0.20	0.20
1 cup (8 fl oz)	244	3.1	1.1	1.2	0.5	5	100	46	1.10	0.139	7.3	630	<0.1	0.06	0.04	29.3	06409
black bean	116	215.6	5.6	19.8		4.4	1198	44	42	1.41	0.642	25	1	0.08	0.5	0.02	0.20
1 cup (8 fl oz)	247	1.5	0.4	0.5	0.5	0	274	106	2.15	0.385	1.0	506	0.1	0.05	0.09	24.7	06402
cheese	156	217.7	5.4	10.5		1.0	958	141	5	0.64	0.257	296	0	0.02	0.4	0.00	0.10
1 cup (8 fl oz)	247	10.5	6.7	3.0	0.3	30	153	136	0.74	0.128	4.4	1087		0.14	0.02	4.9	06411
chicken & dumplings	96	221.2	5.6	6.0		0.5	860	14	5	0.36	0.489	27	0	0.02	1.8	0.17	0.14
1 cup (8 fl oz)	241	5.5	1.3	2.5	1.3	34	116	60	0.63	0.123	11.8	518	0.1	0.07	0.04	2.4	06412
chicken broth	38	230.3	4.8	0.9		0.0	763	10	2	0.24	0.245	0	0	0.01	3.3	0.24	0.05
1 cup (8 fl oz)	240	1.4	0.4	0.6	0.3	0	206	72	0.50	0.122	0.0	0	<0.1	0.07	0.02	4.8	06413
chicken, crm of	117	221.1	3.4	9.3		0.2	986	34	2	0.63	0.376	163	<1	0.03	0.8	0.10	0.20
1 cup (8 fl oz)	244	7.4	2.1	3.3	1.5	10	88	37	0.61	0.124		561	0.2	0.06	0.02	2.4	06416
chicken gumbo	56	229.0	2.6	8.4		2.0	954	24	5	0.37	0.251	7	5	0.02	0.7	0.02	0.20
1 cup (8 fl oz)	244	1.4	0.3	0.7	0.3	5	76	24	0.90	0.124	8.1	137	<0.1	0.05	0.06	4.9	06417
chicken mushroom	132	219.6	4.4	9.3		0.2	942	29	10	0.98	0.244	56	0	0.02	1.6	0.05	0.24
1 cup (8 fl oz)	244	9.2	2.4	4.0	2.3	10	154	27	0.88	0.244		1135		0.11	0.05	0.0	06549
chicken noodle[1]	75	221.7	4.0	9.4		0.7	1106	17	5	0.39	0.289	36	<1	0.05	1.4	0.14	0.17
1 cup (8 fl oz)	241	2.5	0.7	1.1	0.6	7	55	36	0.77	0.193	6.3	711	0.1	0.06	0.03	36.2	06419
chicken rice	60	226.1	3.5	7.2		0.7	815	17	0	0.27	0.366	34	<1	0.02	1.1	0.14	0.17
1 cup (8 fl oz)	241	1.9	0.5	0.9	0.4	7	101	22	0.75	0.118	4.8	660	0.1	0.02	0.02	0.0	06423

	KCAL / WT (g)	H₂0 (g) / FAT (g)	PRO (g) / SFA (g)	CHO (g) / MUFA (g)	SUGR (g) / PUFA (g)	DFIB (g) / CHOL (mg)	Na (mg) / K (mg)	Ca (mg) / P (mg)	Mg (mg) / Fe (mg)	Zn (mg) / Cu (mg)	Mn (mg) / Se (mcg)	A (mcg RAE) / A (IU)	C (mg) / E (mg ATE)	B-1 (mg) / B-2 (mg)	NIA (mg) / B-6 (mg)	B-12 (mcg) / FOL (mcg DFE)	PANT (mg) / REF
chicken veg	75	223.3	3.6	8.6		1.0	945	17	7	0.36	0.366	133	1	0.04	1.2	0.12	0.17
1 cup (8 fl oz)	241	2.8	0.8	1.3	0.6	10	154	41	0.87	0.123	5.3	2656	0.1	0.06	0.05	4.8	06425
chili beef	170	211.7	6.7	21.5		9.5	1035	43	30	1.40	1.050	75	4	0.06	1.1	0.33	0.50
1 cup (8 fl oz)	250	6.6	3.4	2.8	0.3	13	525	148	2.13	0.395	6.0	1510	0.2	0.08	0.16	17.5	06426
clam chowder, manhattan	78	224.2	2.2	12.2		1.5	578	27	12	0.98	0.378	51	4	0.03	0.8	4.05	0.00
1 cup (8 fl oz)	244	2.2	0.4	0.4	1.3	2	188	41	1.63	0.132	9.3	964	0.7	0.04	0.10	9.8	06428
clam chowder, new england	95	220.9	4.8	12.4		1.5	915	44	7	0.76	0.251	0	2	0.02	1.0	8.00	0.32
1 cup (8 fl oz)	244	2.9	0.4	1.2	1.1	5	146	54	1.49	0.124	10.2	7	0.1	0.04	0.08	4.9	06430
minestrone	82	220.1	4.3	11.2		1.0	911	34	7	0.75	0.366	118	1	0.05	0.9	0.00	0.34
1 cup (8 fl oz)	241	2.5	0.6	0.7	1.1	2	313	55	0.92	0.123		2338	0.1	0.04	0.10	50.6	06440
mushroom barley	73	225.5	1.9	11.7		0.7	891	12	10	0.49	0.122	10	0	0.02	0.9	0.00	0.12
1 cup (8 fl oz)	244	2.3	0.4	1.0	0.7	0	93	61	0.51	0.244		198		0.09	0.17	4.9	06442
mushroom, crm of	129	220.4	2.3	9.3		0.5	881	46	5	0.59	0.251	0	1	0.05	0.7	0.05	0.29
1 cup (8 fl oz)	244	9.0	2.4	1.7	4.2	2	100	49	0.51	0.124	1.5	0	1.2	0.09	0.01	4.9	06443
onion	58	224.3	3.8	8.2		1.0	1053	27	2	0.60	0.246	0	1	0.03	0.6	0.00	0.00
1 cup (8 fl oz)	241	1.7	0.3	0.7	0.7	0	67	12	0.67	0.123	4.3	0	0.3	0.02	0.05	14.5	06445
onion, crm of	107	220.8	2.8	12.7		1.0	927	34	5	0.15	0.244	15	1	0.05	0.5	0.05	0.29
1 cup (8 fl oz)	244	5.3	1.5	2.1	1.5	15	120	37	0.63	0.146		295		0.08	0.02	7.3	06446
oyster stew	58	228.6	2.1	4.1			981	22	5	10.29	0.366	19	3	0.02	0.2	2.19	0.12
1 cup (8 fl oz)	241	3.8	2.5	0.9	0.2	14	48	48	0.99	1.593		70		0.04	0.01	2.4	06448
pea, green	165	208.7	8.6	26.5		2.8	918	28	40	1.70	0.658	10	2	0.11	1.2	0.00	0.13
1 cup (8 fl oz)	250	2.9	1.4	1.0	0.4	0	190	125	1.95	0.378	9.3	203	0.1	0.07	0.05	2.5	06449
pea, split w/ham	190	206.9	10.3	28.0		2.3	1007	23	48	1.32	0.670	23	2	0.15	1.5	0.25	0.25
1 cup (8 fl oz)	253	4.4	1.8	1.8	0.6	8	400	213	2.28	0.369		445		0.08	0.07	2.5	06451
pepperpot	104	217.3	6.4	9.4		0.5	971	24	5	1.23	0.612	43	1	0.05	1.2	0.17	0.34
1 cup (8 fl oz)	241	4.6	2.0	2.0	0.4	10	152	41	0.89	0.123	4.3	865	0.1	0.05	0.06	9.6	06452
potato, crm of [2]	73	225.7	1.8	11.5		0.5	1000	20	2	0.63	0.376	71	0	0.03	0.5	0.05	0.83
1 cup (8 fl oz)	244	2.4	1.2	0.6	0.4	5	137	46	0.49	0.251		288	<0.1	0.04	0.04	2.4	06453
scotch broth	80	221.1	5.0	9.5		1.2	1012	14	5	1.59	0.366	108	1	0.02	1.2	0.27	0.24
1 cup (8 fl oz)	241	2.6	1.1	0.8	0.6	5	159	55	0.84	0.246	4.3	2179	0.1	0.05	0.07	9.6	06455
shrimp, crm of	90	225.0	2.8	8.2		0.2	976	17	10	0.76	0.366	37	0	0.02	0.4	0.59	0.15
1 cup (8 fl oz)	244	5.2	3.2	1.5	0.2	17	59	32	0.54	0.122	5.6	159	0.8	0.03	0.05	4.9	06456
stockpot	99	223.7	4.9	11.5			1047	22	5	1.16	0.257	200	2	0.04	1.2	0.00	0.35
1 cup (8 fl oz)	247	3.9	0.9	1.0	1.8	5	237	54	0.86	0.128		3979		0.05	0.09	9.9	06460
tomato	85	220.5	2.0	16.6		0.5	695	12	7	0.24	0.251	34	66	0.09	1.4	0.00	0.15
1 cup (8 fl oz)	244	1.9	0.4	0.4	1.0	0	264	34	1.76	0.251	0.5	688	2.5	0.05	0.11	14.6	06559
tomato beef w/noodles	139	211.5	4.5	21.2		1.5	917	17	7	0.76	0.251	27	0	0.08	1.9	0.20	0.20
1 cup (8 fl oz)	244	4.3	1.6	1.7	0.7	5	220	56	1.12	0.124	4.9	534	0.8	0.09	0.09	29.3	06461
tomato bisque	124	215.3	2.3	23.7		0.5	1047	40	10	0.59	0.257	44	6	0.07	1.1	0.00	0.12
1 cup (8 fl oz)	247	2.5	0.5	0.7	1.1	5	417	59	0.82	0.128		721		0.07	0.09	14.8	06558
tomato rice	119	217.6	2.1	21.9		1.5	815	22	5	0.52	0.385	37	15	0.06	1.1	0.00	0.12
1 cup (8 fl oz)	247	2.7	0.5	0.6	1.4	2	331	35	0.79	0.128	2.2	756	0.8	0.05	0.08	14.8	06463
turkey noodle	68	226.9	3.9	8.6		0.7	815	12	5	0.59	0.251	15	<1	0.07	1.4	0.15	0.17
1 cup (8 fl oz)	244	2.0	0.6	0.8	0.5	5	76	49	0.95	0.124	10.7	293	0.1	0.06	0.04	31.7	06465
turkey veg	72	223.9	3.1	8.6		0.5	906	17	5	0.60	0.246	123	0	0.03	1.0	0.17	0.48
1 cup (8 fl oz)	241	3.0	0.9	1.3	0.7	2	176	41	0.77	0.123		2444	0.1	0.04	0.05	4.8	06466
veg beef [3]	78	223.5	5.6	10.2		0.5	791	17	5	1.54	0.315	95	2	0.04	1.0	0.32	0.41
1 cup (8 fl oz)	244	1.9	0.9	0.8	0.1	5	173	41	1.12	0.183	4.4	1891	0.3	0.05	0.08	9.8	06471
veg vegetarian	72	222.5	2.1	12.0		0.5	822	22	7	0.46	0.460	149	1	0.05	0.9	0.00	0.34
1 cup (8 fl oz)	241	1.9	0.3	0.8	0.7	0	210	34	1.08	0.123	4.3	3005	0.8	0.05	0.06	9.6	06468
veg w/beef broth	82	220.5	3.0	13.1		0.5	810	17	7	0.80	0.337	104	2	0.05	1.0	0.00	0.34
1 cup (8 fl oz)	241	1.9	0.4	0.6	0.8	2	193	39	0.96	0.154	2.7	2089	0.3	0.05	0.06	9.6	06472

[1] Includes chicken alphabet, chicken noodle-o's, chicken with stars, and curly noodle with chicken.
[2] Includes vichyssoise.
[3] Includes beef, beef vegetables, and barley and vegetable beef.

27.4 DEHYDRATED

	KCAL / WT (g)	H₂0 (g) / FAT (g)	PRO (g) / SFA (g)	CHO (g) / MUFA (g)	SUGR (g) / PUFA (g)	DFIB (g) / CHOL (mg)	Na (mg) / K (mg)	Ca (mg) / P (mg)	Mg (mg) / Fe (mg)	Zn (mg) / Cu (mg)	Mn (mg) / Se (mcg)	A (mcg RAE) / A (IU)	C (mg) / E (mg ATE)	B-1 (mg) / B-2 (mg)	NIA (mg) / B-6 (mg)	B-12 (mcg) / FOL (mcg DFE)	PANT (mg) / REF
beef broth cube	6	0.1	0.6	0.6		0.0	864	2	2	0.01	0.014	1	0	0.01	0.1	0.04	0.01
1 cube (amt for 6 fl oz)	3.6	0.1	0.1	0.1	<0.1	<1	15	8	0.08	0.000	1.0	2	<0.1	0.01	0.01	1.2	06076
beef noodle	30	0.5	1.6	4.5		0.2	774	4	7	0.07	0.064	<1	<1	0.09	0.5	<0.01	<0.01
1 pkt	9	0.6	0.2	0.2	0.1	1	60	29	0.25	0.028	3.3	6	<0.1	0.05	0.03	18.3	06077

							Minerals					Vitamins					
	KCAL / WT (g)	H₂0 (g) / FAT (g)	PRO (g) / SFA (g)	CHO (g) / MUFA (g)	SUGR (g) / PUFA (g)	DFIB (g) / CHOL (mg)	Na (mg) / K (mg)	Ca (mg) / P (mg)	Mg (mg) / Fe (mg)	Zn (mg) / Cu (mg)	Mn (mg) / Se (mcg)	A (mcg RAE) / A (IU)	C (mg) / E (mg ATE)	B-1 (mg) / B-2 (mg)	NIA (mg) / B-6 (mg)	B-12 (mcg) / FOL (mcg DFE)	PANT (mg) / REF
beefy mushroom, Lipton Recipe Secrets - *amt for 1 serving*	33 / 11	0.4 / 0.4	0.9 / 0.1	6.6 /	1.6 /	0.1 / <1	645 /	11 /	/ 0.10	/	/	/ 1	<1 /	<0.01 / 0.01	0.1 /	/ 0.0	/ 06722
beefy onion, Lipton Recipe Secrets *amt for 1 serving*	25 / 8	0.3 / 0.6	0.5 / 0.1	4.7 /	0.5 /	0.4 / 0	607 /	11 /	/ 0.12	/	/	/ 0	1 /	0.01 / 0.02	0.1 /	/	/ 06724
broccoli & cheese, Lipton Cup-A-Soup *amt for 1 serving*	67 / 16	0.6 / 2.9	1.8 / 0.8	8.9 /	2.1 /	0.7 / 3	545 /	46 /	/ 0.16	/	/	/ 47	3 /	<0.01 / 0.01	0.1 /	/ 3.7	/ 06286
cheese broccoli, Knorr *1/4 cup (1 cup prep)*	100 / 27	/ 2.5	3.0 / 1.0	17.0 /	5.0 /	<1.0 / <5	900 /	20 /	/ 0.36	/	/	/ 100	1 /	/	/	/	/ UNLV42
chicken broth cube *1 cube (amt for 6 fl oz)*	10 / 4.8	0.1 / 0.2	0.7 / 0.1	1.1 / 0.1	/ 0.1	0.0 / 1	1152 / 18	9 / 9	3 / 0.09	0.01 / 0.000	0.018 / 1.3	3 / 12	<1 /	0.01 / 0.02	0.2 / <0.01	0.01 / 1.5	0.03 / 06081
chicken broth, fat free, Lipton Cup A Soup - *amt for one serving*	18 / 6	0.2 / 0.1	1.2 / <0.1	3.2 /	0.2 /	0.0 / <1	442 /	2 /	/ 0.09	/	/	/ 1	<1 /	<0.01 / <0.01	0.2 /	/ 0.0	/ 06297
w/pasta, Lipton Cup-A-Soup *amt for 1 serving*	45 / 13	/ 0.0	2.0 / 0.0	8.0 /	/	/ 0	440 /	/	/ 0.36	/	/	/	/	0.06 / 0.03	0.8 /	/ 16.0	/ UNLV194
chicken, crm of, Lipton Cup-A-Soup *amt for 1 serving*	68 / 17	0.7 / 2.2	0.8 / 0.3	11.7 /	2.0 /	0.5 / 1	636 /	19 /	/ 0.07	/	/	/ 25	<1 /	0.06 / 0.05	0.6 /	/ 0.0	/ 06290
chicken flavor mushroom, Knorr *1 T (1 cup prep)*	25 / 10	/ 0.5	1.0 / 0.0	4.0 /	0.0 /	0.0 / 0	1190 /	0 /	/ 0.00	/	/	/ 0	0 /	/	/	/	/ UNLV43
chicken flvr noodle hearty hmstyl, Knorr - *3 T (1 cup prep)*	80 / 21	/ 1.5	3.0 / 0.5	13.0 /	2.0 /	1.0 / 15	860 /	0 /	/ 0.36	/	/	/ 0	0 /	/	/	/	/ UNLV44
chicken flavor noodle, Knorr Soup Cup - *1.1 oz container*	130 / 30	/ 2.0	5.0 / 1.0	23.0 /	6.0 /	0.0 / 20	910 /	0 /	/ 0.00	/	/	/ 0	0 /	/	/	/	/ UNLV45
chicken flvr rice, Knorr Soup Cup *1.41 oz container*	180 / 40	/ 2.0	4.0 / 0.5	32.0 /	8.0 /	1.0 / 0	990 /	0 /	/ 0.72	/	/	/ 1000	4 /	/	/	/	/ UNLV46
chicken noodle *amt for 1 serving*	43 / 11	0.4 / 1.0	1.5 / 0.2	6.7 / 0.4	0.8 / 0.3	0.2 / 8	418 / 24	3 / 21	5 / 0.36	0.16 / 0.026	0.058 / 7.0	3 / 11	<1 / 0.1	0.15 / 0.06	0.8 / 0.02	0.04 / 22.3	0.08 / 06128
hearty, Lipton Cup-A-Soup *amt for 1 serving*	61 / 16	0.6 / 1.2	2.6 / 0.4	10.2 /	0.2 /	0.3 / 14	591 /	6 /	/ 0.49	/	/	/ 41	<1 /	0.12 / 0.06	1.3 /	/	/ 06288
Lipton Soup Secrets *amt for 1 serving*	77 / 20	0.8 / 2.0	3.5 / 0.6	11.3 /	1.6 /	0.4 / 15	690 /	10 /	/ 0.68	/	/	/ 23	<1 /	0.24 / 0.08	1.6 /	/ 0.0	/ 06281
w/meat, Lipton *3 T*	80 / 20	/ 2.0	3.0 / 0.5	11.0 /	<1.0 /	/ 20	690 /	/	/ 0.72	/	/	/	/	0.23 / 0.10	1.6 /	/	/ UNLV193
w/meat, Lipton Cup-A-Soup *amt for 1 serving*	50 / 13	/ 1.0	2.0 / 0.0	8.0 /	/	/ 10	560 /	/	/ 0.36	/	/	/ 100	/	0.06 / 0.03	0.8 /	/ 16.0	/ UNLV192
chicken pasta, fat free, Lipton Cup-A-Soup - *amt for 1 serving*	44 / 13	0.5 / 0.3	2.1 / <0.1	8.3 /	0.2 /	0.2 / 0	449 /	3 /	/ 0.38	/	/	/ 1081	<1 /	0.08 / 0.03	0.7 /	/	/ 06298
chicken rice *amt for 1 serving*	59 / 16	0.6 / 1.4	2.4 / 0.3	9.1 / 0.6	/ 0.4	0.3 / 3	968 / 11	7 / 11	0 / 0.10	0.13 / 0.064	0.192 /	19 / 64	<1 / <0.1	0.01 / <0.01	0.4 / 0.02	0.08 / 0.5	0.08 / 06085
chicken supreme, hearty, Lipton Cup-A-Soup - *amt for 1 serving*	90 / 21	0.8 / 3.8	1.1 / 1.4	13.6 /	2.0 /	0.7 / 1	635 /	23 /	/ 0.19	/	/	/ 25	<1 /	0.06 / 0.05	0.6 /	/ 0.0	/ 06287
chicken veg, Lipton Cup-A-Soup *amt for 1 serving*	52 / 14	0.6 / 1.0	1.4 / 0.4	9.6 /	0.4 /	0.3 / 10	518 /	6 /	/ 0.39	/	/	/ 2023	<1 /	0.08 / 0.03	0.5 /	/	/ 06291
chicken w/pasta & beans, Lipton Kettle Creations - *amt for 1 serving*	124 / 35	1.4 / 1.5	5.4 / 0.3	22.6 /	1.6 /	3.0 / 7	815 /	44 /	/ 1.28	/	/	/ 543	2 /	0.24 / 0.16	1.8 /	/	/ 06300
chili rosa, Knorr Recipes Classics *1.5 T (1 cup prep)*	70 / 19	/ 2.0	2.0 / 1.0	11.0 /	2.0 /	<1.0 / <5	800 /	40 /	/ 0.72	/	/	/ 0	6 /	/	/	/	/ UNLV48
clam chowder, manhattan *amt for 1 cup (8 fl oz)*	66 / 19	0.8 / 1.6	2.1 / 0.3	10.9 / 0.7	/ 0.5	/ 0	1343 / 200	25 / 44	11 / 1.73	0.99 / 0.133	0.399 /	51 / 1020	4 /	0.03 / 0.04	0.9 / 0.11	4.37 / 10.1	0.13 / 06087
clam chowder, new england *amt for 1 cup (8 fl oz)*	96 / 23	0.8 / 3.7	2.8 / 0.6	13.1 / 1.7	/ 1.2	1.2 / 1	755 / 207	78 / 101	7 / 1.29	0.69 / 0.115	0.230 /	<1 / 9	2 /	0.02 / 0.16	0.9 / 0.07	8.97 / 3.5	0.30 / 06088
corn chowder, Knorr Soup Cup *1.3 oz container*	140 / 34	/ 2.5	3.0 / 0.0	28.0 /	6.0 /	2.0 / 0	890 /	0 /	/ 0.72	/	/	/ 100	5 /	/	/	/	/ UNLV49
creamy chicken vegetable, Lipton Cup-A-Soup - *amt for 1 serving*	80 / 19	/ 4.0	2.0 / 1.5	10.0 /	3.0 /	<1.0 /	590 /	/	/	/	/	/	/	/	/	/	/ UNLV200
extra noodle w/chicken broth, Lipton Soup Secrets - *3 T (8 fl oz prep)*	90 / 23	/ 1.5	3.0 / 0.5	15.0 /	1.0 /	<1.0 / 25	680 /	/	/ 0.72	/	/	/	/	0.38 / 0.14	1.6 /	/ 32.0	/ UNLV152
giggle noodle, Lipton Soup Secrets *2 T (8 fl oz prep)*	70 / 19	/ 2.0	2.0 / 0.5	11.0 /	2.0 /	1.0 / 15	680 /	/	/ 0.36	/	/	/	/	0.12 / 0.07	0.8 /	/ 16.0	/ UNLV199
golden onion, Lipton Recipe Secrets *1.7 T (8 fl oz prep)*	50 / 15	/ 1.5	1.0 /	10.0 /	1.0 /	/	640 /	/	/	/	/	/	/	/	/	/	/ UNLV187
green pea, Lipton Cup A Soup *1 pkt (6 fl oz prep)*	80 / 21	/ 1.0	4.0 / 0.0	12.0 /	1.0 /	3.0 / 0	520 /	/	/ 0.72	/	/	/	/	/	/	/	/ UNLV186

							Minerals					Vitamins					
	KCAL	H₂0 (g)	PRO (g)	CHO (g)	SUGR (g)	DFIB (g)	Na (mg)	Ca (mg)	Mg (mg)	Zn (mg)	Mn (mg)	A (mcg RAE)	C (mg)	B-1 (mg)	NIA (mg)	B-12 (mcg)	PANT (mg)
	WT (g)	FAT (g)	SFA (g)	MUFA (g)	PUFA (g)	CHOL (mg)	K (mg)	P (mg)	Fe (mg)	Cu (mg)	Se (mcg)	A (IU)	E (mg ATE)	B-2 (mg)	B-6 (mg)	FOL (mcg DFE)	REF
onion	49	0.6	1.3	11.7		1.3	3	36	13	0.26	0.194	0	11	0.07	0.1		0.19
dehydrated flakes - 1/4 cup	14	0.1	<0.1	<0.1	<0.1	0	227	42	0.22	0.058	0.7	0		0.01	0.22	23.2	11284
powder	24	0.3	0.7	5.6		0.4	4	25	8	0.16	0.026	0	1	0.03	<0.1	0.00	
1 T	7	0.1	<0.1	<0.1	<0.1	0	65	23	0.18	0.012	0.1	0	<0.1	<0.01	0.08	11.5	02026
oregano, ground	14	0.3	0.5	2.9		1.9	1	71	12	0.20	0.210	16	2	0.02	0.3	0.00	
1 T	4.5	0.5	0.1	<0.1	0.2	0	75	9	1.98	0.042	0.3	311	0.1	0.01	0.05	12.3	02027
paprika	20	0.7	1.0	3.8		1.4	2	12	13	0.28	0.058	209	5	0.04	1.1	0.00	0.12
1 T	7	0.9	0.1	0.1	0.6	0	162	24	1.63	0.042	0.3	4182	<0.1	0.12	0.28	7.3	02028
parsley,	4	0.1	0.3	0.7		0.4	6	19	3	0.06	0.137	15	2	<0.01	0.1	0.00	
dried - 1 T	1.3	0.1	<0.1	<0.1	<0.1	0	49	5	1.27	0.008	0.4	303	<0.1	0.02	0.01	2.3	02029
freeze-dried	4	<0.1	0.4	0.6		0.5	5	2	5	0.09	0.019		2	0.01	0.1	0.00	0.04
1/4 cup	1.4	0.1				0	88	8	0.75	0.006	0.5	885		0.03	0.02	2.7	11625
sprigs, raw	4	8.8	0.3	0.6		0.3	6	14	5	0.11	0.016	26	13	0.01	0.1	0.00	0.04
10 sprigs	10	0.1	<0.1	<0.1	<0.1	0	55	6	0.62	0.015	<0.1	520	0.2	0.01	0.01	15.2	11297
pepper, black	16	0.7	0.7	4.1		1.7	3	28	12	0.09	0.360	1	1	0.01	0.1	0.00	
1 T	6	0.2	0.1	0.1	0.1	0	81	11	1.85	0.072	0.2	12	0.1	0.02	0.02	0.6	02030
pepper, red/cayenne	17	0.4	0.6	3.0		1.4	2	8	8	0.13	0.106	110	4	0.02	0.5	0.00	
1 T	5	0.9	0.2	0.1	0.4	0	107	16	0.41	0.020	0.5	2205	0.3	0.05	0.13	5.6	02031
pepper, white	21	0.8	0.7	4.9		1.9	0	19	6	0.08	0.305	0	1	<0.01	<0.1	0.00	
1 T	7	0.2	<0.1	0.1	<0.1	0	5	12	1.02	0.065	0.2	0	0.2	0.01	0.01	0.7	02032
peppermint, raw	2	2.5	0.1	0.5		0.3	1	8	3	0.04	0.038	7	1	<0.01	0.1	0.00	0.01
2 T	3.2	<0.1	<0.1	<0.1	<0.1	0	18	2	0.16	0.011		136	<0.1	0.01	<0.01	3.6	02064
poppy seeds	47	0.6	1.6	2.1		0.9	2	127	29	0.90	0.601	0	<1	0.07	0.1	0.00	
1 T	9	3.9	0.4	0.6	2.7	0	62	75	0.83	0.144	0.1	0	0.2	0.02	0.04	5.1	02033
poultry seasoning[3]	11	0.3	0.4	2.4		0.4	1	37	8	0.12	0.254	5	<1	0.01	0.1	0.00	
1 T	3.7	0.3	0.1	<0.1	0.1	0	25	6	1.31	0.031	0.3	97	<0.1	0.01	0.05	5.1	02034
pumpkin pie spice[4]	19	0.5	0.3	3.9		0.8	3	38	8	0.13	0.887	1	1	0.01	0.1	0.00	
1 T	6	0.7	0.4	0.1	<0.1	0	37	7	1.10	0.027	0.5	15	<0.1	0.01	0.02	2.9	02035
rosemary,	11	0.3	0.2	2.1		1.4	2	42	7	0.11	0.062	5	2	0.02	<0.1	0.00	
dried - 1 T	3.3	0.5	0.2	0.1	0.1	0	32	2	0.97	0.018	0.2	103	0.1	0.01	0.06	10.1	02036
raw	2	1.2	0.1	0.4		0.2	0	5	2	0.02	0.016	2	<1	<0.01	<0.1	0.00	0.01
1 T	1.7	0.1	<0.1	<0.1	<0.1	0	11	1	0.11	0.005		50	<0.1	<0.01	0.01	1.9	02063
saffron	7	0.2	0.2	1.4		0.1	3	2	6	0.02	0.597	1	2	<0.01	<0.1	0.00	
1 T	2.1	0.1	<0.1	<0.1	<0.1	0	36	5	0.23	0.007	0.1	11	<0.1	0.01	0.02	2.0	02037
sage, ground	6	0.2	0.2	1.2		0.8	0	33	9	0.09	0.063	6	1	0.02	0.1	0.00	
1 T	2	0.3	0.1	<0.1	<0.1	0	21	2	0.56	0.015	0.1	118	<0.1	0.01	0.05	5.5	02038
salt (sodium chloride)[5]	0	<0.1	0.0	0.0		0.0	6976	4	<1	0.02	0.018	0	0	0.00	0.0	0.00	
1 T	18	0.0	0.0	0.0	0.0	0	1	0	0.06	0.005	<0.1	0	0.0	0.00	0.00	0.0	02047
canning & pickling, Morton	0		0.0	0.0			2358										
1 t	6	0.0					<1										MORT1
garlic, Morton	4		0.2	0.8			1525	13									
1 t	5	<0.1					12										MORT2
kosher, Morton	0		0.0	0.0			1960	3									
1 t	5	0.0															MORT3
Lite, Morton	0		0.0	<0.1			1182	2	4								
1 t	6	0.0					1518										MORT4
Morton[5]	0		0.0	<0.1			2346	2									
1 t	6	0.0					<1										MORT9
popcorn, Morton	0		0.0	0.0			2334	30									
1 t	6	0.0					<1										MORT6
seasoned, Morton	4		0.2	0.8			1550	16									
1 t	5	<0.1					13										MORT10
salt substitute,	<1		0.0	0.1			<1	28									
Morton - 1 t	5	0.0					2515	23									MORT7
seasoned, Morton	2		0.0	0.4			<1										
1 t	4	<0.1					1732										MORT8
savory, ground	12	0.4	0.3	3.0		2.0	1	94	17	0.19	0.268	11	2	0.02	0.2	0.00	
1 T	4.4	0.3	0.1			0	46	6	1.67	0.037	0.2	226			0.08		02039
shallots,	13	0.1	0.4	2.9			2	7	4	0.07	0.051	101	1	0.01	<0.1	0.00	0.05
freeze-dried - 1/4 cup	3.6	<0.1	<0.1	<0.1	<0.1	0	59	11	0.22	0.015	0.2	2020		<0.01	0.06	4.2	11640
raw, chopped	7	8.0	0.3	1.7			1	4	2	0.04	0.029	6	1	0.01	<0.1	0.00	0.03
1 T	10	<0.1	<0.1	<0.1	<0.1	0	33	6	0.12	0.009	0.1	119		<0.01	0.03	3.4	11677

	KCAL	H₂0 (g)	PRO (g)	CHO (g)	SUGR (g)	DFIB (g)	Na (mg)	Ca (mg)	Mg (mg)	Zn (mg)	Mn (mg)	A (mcg RAE)	C (mg)	B-1 (mg)	NIA (mg)	B-12 (mcg)	PANT (mg)
	WT (g)	FAT (g)	SFA (g)	MUFA (g)	PUFA (g)	CHOL (mg)	K (mg)	P (mg)	Fe (mg)	Cu (mg)	Se (mcg)	A (IU)	E (mg ATE)	B-2 (mg)	B-6 (mg)	FOL (mcg DFE)	REF
spearmint,	5	0.2	0.3	0.8		0.5	6	24	10	0.04	0.184	8	0	<0.01	0.1	0.00	0.02
dried - *1 T*	1.6	0.1	<0.1	<0.1	0.1 -	0	31	4	1.40	0.025		169	<0.1	0.02	0.04	8.5	02066
raw	5	9.8	0.4	1.0		0.8	3	23	7	0.12	0.127	23	2	0.01	0.1	0.00	0.03
2 T	11	0.1	<0.1	<0.1	<0.1	0	52	7	1.35	0.027		462	<0.1	0.02	0.02	12.0	02065
tarragon, ground	14	0.4	1.1	2.4		0.4	3	55	17	0.19	0.382	10	2	0.01	0.4	0.00	
1 T	4.8	0.3	0.1	<0.1	0.2	0	145	15	1.55	0.032	0.2	202	0.1	0.06	0.12	13.2	02041
Tender Quick (meat cure),	<1		0.0	0.1	0.1		1920	0									
Morton - *1 t*	5	0.0															MORT11
thyme,	12	0.3	0.4	2.7		1.6	2	81	9	0.27	0.338	8	2	0.02	0.2	0.00	
ground - *1 T*	4.3	0.3	0.1	<0.1	0.1	0	35	9	5.31	0.037	0.2	163	0.1	0.02	0.02	11.8	02042
raw	1	0.5	0.0	0.2		0.1	0	3	1	0.01	0.014	2	1	<0.01	<0.1	0.00	<0.01
1 t	0.8	<0.1	<0.1	<0.1	<0.1	0	5	1	0.14	0.004		38		<0.01	<0.01	0.4	02049
turmeric, ground	24	0.8	0.5	4.4		1.4	3	12	13	0.30	0.533	0	2	0.01	0.3	0.00	
1 T	7	0.7	0.2	0.1	0.1	0	172	18	2.82	0.041	0.3	0	<0.1	0.02	0.12	2.7	02043
vanilla extract[6]	37	6.8	0.0	1.6		0.0	1	1	2	0.01	0.030	0	0	<0.01	0.1	0.00	<0.01
1 T	13	<0.1	<0.1	<0.1	<0.1	0	19	1	0.02	0.009	0.0	0	0	0.01	<0.01	0.0	02050
imitation w/alcohol[6]	31	8.4	0.0	0.3		0.0	1	0	1	0.01	0.063	0	0	<0.01	<0.1	0.00	<0.01
1 T	13	0.0				0	13	3	0.02	0.003		0			<0.01	0.0	02051
imitation w/o alcohol	7	11.1	0.0	1.9		0.0	0	0	<1	<0.01	<0.001	0	0	<0.01	<0.1	0.00	<0.01
1 T	13	0.0	0.0	0.0	0.0	0	0	0	0.01	<0.001	0.0	0	0.0	<0.01	<0.01	0.0	02052

[1] Contains red pepper, cumin, oregano, salt, and garlic powder.
[2] Values apply to classic italiano, extra spicy, garlic & herb, lemon pepper, minced onion medley, onion & herb, original blend, table blend, and tomato basil garlic.
[3] Contains white pepper, sage, thyme, marjoram, savory, ginger, allspice, and nutmeg.

[4] Contains cinnamon, ginger, nutmeg, allspice, and cloves.
[5] Iodized salt contains 400 mcg iodine per teaspoon; non-iodized salt contains less than 100 mcg iodine per teaspoon.
[6] Contains 4.2 g alcohol (ethanol) in 1 tablespoon.

29. SUGARS, SYRUPS, & OTHER SWEETENERS

	KCAL	H₂0 (g)	PRO (g)	CHO (g)	SUGR (g)	DFIB (g)	Na (mg)	Ca (mg)	Mg (mg)	Zn (mg)	Mn (mg)	A (mcg RAE)	C (mg)	B-1 (mg)	NIA (mg)	B-12 (mcg)	PANT (mg)
apple butter	29	9.6	0.1	7.3	6.0	0.3	1	2	1	0.01	0.057	1	<1	<0.01	<0.1	0.00	0.01
1 T	17	0.0	0.0	0.0	0.0	0	15	2	0.05	0.014	0.1	20	<0.1	<0.01	0.01	0.2	19294
honey, strained	64	3.6	0.1	17.3		0.0	1	1	<1	0.05	0.017	0	<1	0.00	<0.1	0.00	0.01
1 T	21	0.0	0.0	0.0	0.0	0	11	1	0.09	0.008	0.2	0	0.0	0.01	<0.01	0.4	19296
jam/preserves	56	6.1	0.1	13.8	9.7	0.2	6	4	1	0.01	0.008	<1	2	0.00	<0.1	0.00	<0.01
1 T	20	<0.1	<0.1	<0.1	0.0	0	15	2	0.10	0.020	0.4	2	0.0	<0.01	<0.01	6.6	19297
apricot	48	6.9	0.1	12.9		0.2	8	4	1	0.01	0.008	2	2	0.00	<0.1	0.00	<0.01
1 T	20	<0.1	<0.1	<0.1	0.0	0	15	2	0.020	0.020	0.4	41	0.0	<0.01	<0.01	6.6	19719
jelly	54	5.5	<0.1	13.4	7.9	0.2	5	2	1	0.01	0.026	<1	<1	<0.01	<0.1	0.00	0.04
1 T	19	<0.1	<0.1	<0.1	<0.1	0	12	2	0.04	0.003	0.4	3	0.0	<0.01	<0.01	0.2	19300
marmalade, orange	49	6.6	0.1	13.3		0.0	11	8	<1	0.01	0.004	<1	1	<0.01	<0.01	0.00	
1 T	20	0.0	0.0	0.0	0.0	0	7	1	0.03	0.018	<0.1	9	0.0	<0.01	<0.01	7.2	19303
molasses	53	5.2	0.0	13.8		0.0	7	41	48	0.06	0.306	0	0	0.01	0.2	0.00	0.16
1 T	20	<0.1	<0.1	<0.1	<0.1	0	293	6	0.94	0.097	3.6	0	0.0	<0.01	0.13	0.0	19304
molasses, blackstrap	47	5.7	0.0	12.2		0.0	11	172	43	0.20	0.522	0	0	0.01	0.2	0.00	0.18
1 T	20	0.0	0.0	0.0	0.0	0	498	8	3.50	0.408	3.6	0	0.0	0.01	0.14	0.2	19305
Chatfield's	45		0.0	11.0	8.0	0.0	15	150				0					
1 T (15 ml)	~20	0.0	0.0	0.0	0.0	0			3.60			0					CHAT2
strawberry spread, Polaner All	42	7.5	0.1	10.3	7.6		4										
Fruit - *1 T*	18	0.0							3.60								19257
sugar, brown	34	0.1	0.0	8.8		0.0	4	8	3	0.02	0.029	0	0	<0.01	<0.1	0.00	0.01
1T	9	0.0	0.0	0.0	0.0	0	31	2	0.17	0.027	0.1	0	0.0	<0.01	<0.01	0.1	19334b
	545	2.3	0.0	141.1		0.0	57	123	42	0.26	0.464	0	0	0.01	0.1	0.00	0.16
1 cup unpacked	145	0.0	0.0	0.0	0.0	0	502	32	2.77	0.432	1.7	0	0.0	0.01	0.04	1.5	19334a
sugar, maple	100	2.3	0.0	25.8		0.0	3	26	5	1.72	1.254	<1	0	<0.01	<0.1	0.00	0.01
1 oz (~3.2 t)	28	0.1	<0.1	<0.1	<0.1	0	78	1	0.46	0.028	0.2	7	0.0	<0.01	<0.01	0.0	19340
sugar substitute, Equal, Nutrasweet	4	0.1	0.0	0.9		0.0	0	0	<1	0.00	0.000	0	0	0.00	0.0	0.00	0.00
1 pkt	1	<0.1	<0.1	<0.1	<0.1	0	<1	<1	<0.01	0.000	<0.1	0	0.0	0.00	0.00	0.0	19337a
	12	0.4	0.1	3.0		0.0	0	0	<1	0.00	0.000	0	0	0.00	0.0	0.00	0.00
1 t	3.5	<0.1	<0.1	<0.1	<0.1	0	<1	<1	<0.01	0.000	0.1	0	0.0	0.00	0.00	0.0	19337b
sugar, white, granulated	16	0.0	0.0	4.2		0.0	0	0	0	<0.01	<0.001	0	0	0.00	0.00	0.00	0.00
1 t	4.2	0.0	0.0	0.0	0.0	0	<1	<1	<0.01	0.002	<0.1	0	0.0	0.00	0.00	0.0	19335b
	23	0.0	0.0	6.0		0.0	0	0	0	<0.01	<0.001	0	0	0.00	0.00	0.00	0.00
1 pkt	6	0.0	0.0	0.0	0.0	0	<1	<1	<0.01	0.003	<0.1	0	0.0	<0.01	0.00	0.0	19335c

	KCAL	H₂0 (g)	PRO (g)	CHO (g)	SUGR (g)	DFIB (g)	Minerals — Na (mg)	Ca (mg)	Mg (mg)	Zn (mg)	Mn (mg)	Vitamins — A (mcg RAE)	C (mg)	B-1 (mg)	NIA (mg)	B-12 (mcg)	PANT (mg)
	WT (g)	FAT (g)	SFA (g)	MUFA (g)	PUFA (g)	CHOL (mg)	K (mg)	P (mg)	Fe (mg)	Cu (mg)	Se (mcg)	A (IU)	E (mg ATE)	B-2 (mg)	B-6 (mg)	FOL (mcg DFE)	REF
	774	0.0	0.0	199.8		0.0	2	2	0	0.06	0.014	0	0	0.00	0.0		0.00
1 cup	200	0.0	0.0	0.0	0.0	0	4	4	0.12	0.086	1.2	0	0.0	0.04	0.00	0.0	19335a
sugar, white, powdered	31	<0.1	0.0	8.0		0.0	0	0	0	<0.01	0.001	0	0	0.00	0.0		0.00
1 T	8	<0.1	<0.1	<0.1	<0.1	0	<1	<1	<0.01	0.003	<0.1	0	0.0	0.00	0.00	0.0	19336a
	467	0.4	0.0	119.4		0.0	1	1	0	0.04	0.008	0	0	0.00	0.0		0.00
1 cup	120	0.1	<0.1	<0.1	0.1	0	2	2	0.07	0.052	0.7	0	0.0	0.00	0.00	0.0	19336b
syrup, cane & 15% maple	56	4.8	0.0	15.0		0.0	21	3	1	0.13	0.114	0	0	<0.01	<0.1		<0.01
1 T	20	<0.1	<0.1	<0.1	<0.1	0	7	<1	0.16	0.004	0.1	0	0.0	<0.01	<0.01	0.0	19361
syrup, corn & sugar	64	3.1	0.0	16.8		0.0	14	5	2	0.01	0.018	0	0	<0.01	<0.1		0.01
1 T	20	0.0	0.0			0	13	2	0.15	0.012	0.2	0	0.0	0.01	<0.01	0.6	19362
syrup, corn, dark	56	4.6	0.0	15.3		0.0	31	4	2	0.01	0.020	0	0	<0.01	<0.1		<0.01
1 T	20	0.0	0.0	0.0	0.0	0	9	2	0.07	0.011	0.2	0	0.0	<0.01	<0.01	0.0	19349
syrup, corn, high fructose	53	4.6	0.0	14.4		0.0	0	0	0	<0.01	0.018	0	0	0.00	0.0		<0.01
1 T	19	0.0	0.0			0	0	0	0.01	0.006	0.1	0	0.0	<0.01	0.00	0.0	19351
syrup, corn, light (in color)	56	4.6	0.0	15.3		0.0	24	1	<1	0.01	0.018	0	0	<0.01	<0.1		<0.01
1 T	20	0.0	0.0	0.0	0.0	0	1	<1	0.01	0.002	0.1	0	0.0	<0.01	<0.01	0.0	19350
syrup, malt	76	5.1	1.5	17.1		0.0	8	15	17	0.03	0.024	0	0	<0.01	1.9		0.04
1 T	24	0.0	0.0	0.0	0.0	0	77	57	0.23	0.048	3.0	0	0.0	0.09	0.12	0.0	19352
syrup, maple	52	6.4	0.0	13.4	12.7	0.0	2	13	3	0.83	0.660	0	0	<0.01	<0.1		0.01
1 T	20	<0.1	<0.1	<0.1	<0.1	0	41	<1	0.24	0.015	0.1	0	0.0	<0.01	<0.01	0.0	19353
syrup, pancake/waffle	57	4.8	0.0	15.1		0.0	17	0	<1	0.01	0.018	0	0	<0.01	<0.1		<0.01
1 T	20	0.0	0.0	0.0	0.0	0	<1	2	0.02	0.043	0.1	0	0.0	<0.01	0.00	0.0	19129
butter maple/reg, Hungry Jack	208		0.0	52.0	28.0		90	0					0				
Microwave - *1/4 cup*	~80	0.0	0.0			0				0.00			0				GENM350
lite, butter maple/reg, Hungry	96		0.0	24.0	23.0	0.0	180	0					0				
Jack Microwave - *1/4 cup*	~60	0.0	0.0			0				0.00			0				GENM351
red cal	25	8.2	0.0	6.6		0.0	30	0	0	<0.01	0.013	0	0	<0.01	<0.1		<0.01
1 T	15	0.0	0.0	0.0	0.0	0	<1	6	<0.01	<0.001	0.1	0	0.0	<0.01	0.00	0.0	19128
w/2% maple syrup	53	6.0	0.0	13.9		0.0	12	1	<1	0.05	0.037	0	0	<0.01	<0.1		<0.01
1 T	20	<0.1	<0.1	<0.1	<0.1	0	1	2	0.01	0.009	0.1	0	0.0	<0.01	0.00	0.0	19360
w/butter	59	4.8	0.0	14.8		0.0	20	0	<1	0.01	0.017	3	0	<0.01	<0.1		<0.01
1 T	20	0.3	0.2	0.1	<0.1	1	1	2	0.02	0.042	0.1	12	<0.1	<0.01	0.00	0.0	19113
syrup, sorghum	61	4.3	0.0	15.7		0.0	2	32	21	0.09	0.321	0	0	0.02	<0.1		0.17
1 T	21	0.0	0.0	0.0	0.0	0	210	12	0.80	0.027	0.1	0	0.0	0.03	0.14	0.0	19355

30. VEGETABLES & VEGETABLE DISHES
30.1 FLOWER, STEM, & STALK VEGETABLES

	KCAL	H₂0	PRO	CHO	SUGR	DFIB	Na	Ca	Mg	Zn	Mn	A (RAE)	C	B-1	NIA	B-12	PANT
	WT	FAT	SFA	MUFA	PUFA	CHOL	K	P	Fe	Cu	Se	A (IU)	E	B-2	B-6	FOL	REF
artichoke (globe/french),	60	100.8	4.2	13.4		6.5	114	54	72	0.59	0.311	11	12	0.08	1.2		0.41
boiled - *1 med*	120	0.2	<0.1	<0.1	0.1	0	425	103	1.55	0.280	0.2	212	0.2	0.08	0.13	61.2	11008
frzn, boiled	36	69.2	2.5	7.3		3.7	42	17	25	0.29	0.218	6	4	0.05	0.7		0.16
2.8 oz (1/3 of 9 oz pkg)	80	0.4	0.1	<0.1	0.2	0	211	49	0.45	0.049	0.2	131	0.2	0.13	0.07	95.2	11010
asparagus,	22	83.0	2.3	3.8		1.4	10	18	9	0.38	0.137	24	10	0.11	1.0		0.14
boiled - *1/2 cup (6 spears)*	90	0.3	0.1	<0.1	0.1	0	144	49	0.66	0.101	1.5	485	0.3	0.11	0.11	131.4	11012
cnd	46	227.4	5.2	6.0		3.9	695	39	24	0.97	0.411	65	45	0.15	2.3		0.34
1 cup	242	1.6	0.4	<0.1	0.7	0	416	104	4.43	0.232	4.1	1285	1.0	0.24	0.27	232.3	11015
frzn, boiled	50	164.1	5.3	8.8		2.9	7	41	23	1.01	0.333	74	44	0.12	1.9		0.28
1 cup	180	0.8	0.2	<0.1	0.3	0	392	99	1.15	0.308	3.1	1472	2.3	0.19	0.04	243.0	11019
broccoli,	50	163.2	5.4	9.1		5.2	47	83	43	0.68	0.392	124	134	0.10	1.0		0.91
boiled - *1 med stalk*	180	0.6	0.1	<0.1	0.3	0	526	106	1.51	0.077	3.4	2498	3.0	0.20	0.26	90.0	11091
chopped, frzn, boiled	52	166.9	5.7	9.8		5.5	44	94	37	0.55	0.598	175	74	0.10	0.8		0.50
1 cup	184	0.2	<0.1	<0.1	0.1	0	331	101	1.12	0.079	5.5	3481	3.0	0.15	0.24	103.0	11093
raw, chopped	25	79.8	2.6	4.6		2.6	24	42	22	0.35	0.202	68	82	0.06	0.6		0.47
1 cup	88	0.3	<0.1	<0.1	0.1	0	286	58	0.77	0.040	2.6	1357	1.5	0.10	0.14	62.5	11090
spears, frzn, boiled	26	83.5	2.9	4.9		2.8	22	47	18	0.28	0.299	87	37	0.05	0.4		0.25
1/2 cup	92	0.1	<0.1	<0.1	<0.1	0	166	51	0.56	0.040	1.7	1741	0.9	0.07	0.12	27.6	11095
w/cheese sce, frzn, Green Giant	113	142.0	3.9	15.0			806						59				
1 cup	168	4.2	0.8	1.7	0.4							2268					22600
broccoli, chinese, boiled	19	82.3	1.0	3.3		2.2	6	88	16	0.34	0.232	72	25	0.08	0.4		0.14
1 cup	88	0.6	0.1	<0.1	0.3	0	230	36	0.49	0.054	1.1	1441	0.4	0.13	0.06	87.1	11969
cardoon, boiled[1]	22	93.5	0.8	5.3		1.7	176	72	43	0.18	0.133	6	2	0.02	0.3		0.10
3.5 oz	100	0.1	<0.1	<0.1	<0.1	0	392	23	0.73		1.0	118		0.03	0.04	22.0	11123

	KCAL / WT (g)	H₂O (g) / FAT (g)	PRO (g) / SFA (g)	CHO (g) / MUFA (g)	SUGR (g) / PUFA (g)	DFIB (g) / CHOL (mg)	Na (mg) / K (mg)	Ca (mg) / P (mg)	Mg (mg) / Fe (mg)	Zn (mg) / Cu (mg)	Mn (mg) / Se (mcg)	A (mcg RAE) / A (IU ATE)	C (mg) / E (mg ATE)	B-1 (mg) / B-2 (mg)	NIA (mg) / B-6 (mg)	B-12 (mcg) / FOL (mcg DFE)	PANT (mg) / REF
cauliflower,	14	57.7	1.1	2.5		1.7	9	10	6	0.11	0.086	1	27	0.03	0.3		0.31
boiled - 1/2 cup pieces	62	0.3	<0.1	<0.1	0.1	0	88	20	0.20	0.017	0.3	11	<0.1	0.03	0.11	27.3	11136
frzn, boiled	34	169.2	2.9	6.8		4.9	32	31	16	0.23	0.270	2	56	0.07	0.6	0.00	0.18
1 cup pieces	180	0.4	0.1	<0.1	0.2	0	250	43	0.74	0.043	1.1	40	0.1	0.10	0.16	73.8	11138
raw	25	91.9	2.0	5.2		2.5	30	22	15	0.28	0.156	1	46	0.06	0.5	0.00	0.65
1 cup pieces	100	0.2	<0.1	<0.1	0.1	0	303	44	0.44	0.042	0.6	19	<0.1	0.06	0.22	57.0	11135
w/cheese sce, frzn, Green Giant	60		2.0	7.0	4.0	1.0	510	60					15				
1/2 cup	99	2.5	0.5			<5			0.00			500					GENM353
cauliflower, green,	29	80.5	2.7	5.7		3.0	21	29	17	0.57	0.218	6	65	0.06	0.6	0.00	0.61
ckd - 1/5 head	90	0.3	<0.1	<0.1	0.1	0	250	51	0.65	0.036	0.7	127		0.09	0.19	36.9	11967
raw	20	57.5	1.9	3.9		2.0	15	21	13	0.41	0.158	5	56	0.05	0.5	0.00	0.45
1 cup pieces	64	0.2	<0.1	<0.1	0.1	0	192	40	0.47	0.026	0.4	97	<0.1	0.07	0.14	36.5	11965
celery,	27	141.2	1.2	6.0		2.4	137	63	18	0.21	0.159	11	9	0.06	0.5	0.00	0.29
diced, boiled - 1 cup	150	0.2	0.1	<0.1	0.1	0	426	38	0.63	0.054	1.5	198	0.5	0.07	0.13	33.0	11144
raw	6	37.9	0.3	1.5		0.7	35	16	4	0.05	0.041	3	3	0.02	0.1	0.00	0.07
1 med stalk (7.5" long)	40	0.1	<0.1	<0.1	<0.1	0	115	10	0.16	0.014	0.4	54	0.1	0.02	0.03	11.2	11143
fennel bulb, raw, sliced	27	78.5	1.1	6.3		2.7	45	43	15	0.17	0.166	6	10	0.01	0.6	0.00	0.20
1 cup	87	0.2				0	360	44	0.64	0.057	0.6	117		0.03	0.04	23.5	11957
kohlrabi, sliced, boiled	48	149.0	3.0	11.0		1.8	35	41	31	0.51	0.234	3	89	0.07	0.6	0.00	0.26
1 cup	165	0.2	<0.1	<0.1	0.1	0	561	74	0.66	0.218	1.3	58	2.8	0.03	0.25	19.8	11242
leeks,	38	112.6	1.0	9.4		1.2	12	37	17	0.07	0.306	2	5	0.03	0.2	0.00	0.09
boiled - 1 leek	124	0.2	<0.1	<0.1	0.1	0	108	21	1.36	0.077	0.6	57		0.02	0.14	29.8	11247
raw	54	73.9	1.3	12.6		1.6	18	53	25	0.11	0.428	4	11	0.05	0.4	0.00	0.07
1 leek (~1 cup)	89	0.3	<0.1	<0.1	0.1	0	160	31	1.87	0.107	0.9	85	0.8	0.03	0.21	57.0	11246
onion, green/spring (scallion),	32	89.8	1.8	7.3		2.6	16	72	20	0.39	0.160	19	19	0.06	0.5	0.00	0.08
raw, chopped - 1 cup	100	0.2	<0.1	<0.1	0.1	0	276	37	1.48	0.083	0.6	385	0.1	0.08	0.06	64.0	11291
pumpkin flowers,	20	127.6	1.5	4.4		1.2	8	50	34	0.13		117	7	0.02	0.4	0.00	
boiled - 1 cup	134	0.1	0.1	<0.1	<0.1	0	142	46	1.18	0.134	0.9	2324	0.1	0.04	0.07	54.9	11417
raw	5	31.4	0.3	1.1			2	13	8			32	9	0.01	0.2	0.00	
1 cup	33	<0.1	<0.1	<0.1	<0.1	0	57	16	0.23		0.2	643		0.02		19.5	11416
rhubarb,	278	162.7	0.9	74.9		4.8	2	348	29	0.19	0.175	7	8	0.04	0.5	0.00	0.12
ckd, sweetened, frzn - 1 cup	240	0.1	<0.1	<0.1	0.1	0	230	19	0.50	0.065	2.2	166	0.5	0.06	0.05	12.0	09310
raw	26	114.2	1.1	5.5		2.2	5	105	15	0.12	0.239	6	10	0.02	0.4	0.00	0.10
1 cup	122	0.2	0.1	<0.1	0.1	0	351	17	0.27	0.026	1.3	122	0.2	0.04	0.03	8.5	09307
raw, frzn	29	128.1	0.8	7.0		2.5	3	266	25	0.14	0.133	7	7	0.04	0.3	0.00	0.09
1 cup	137	0.2	<0.1	<0.1	0.1	0	148	16	0.40	0.032	1.5	147	0.3	0.04	0.03	11.0	09309
sesbania flower, steamed	23	97.0	1.2	5.4			11	23	12			0	38	0.05	0.3	0.00	
1 cup	104	0.1				0	111	22	0.58		0.7	0		0.04		59.3	11448

[1] Plant with edible stalks; related to the artichoke.

30.2 FRUIT (SEED-CONTAINING) VEGETABLES

	KCAL / WT (g)	H₂O (g) / FAT (g)	PRO (g) / SFA (g)	CHO (g) / MUFA (g)	SUGR (g) / PUFA (g)	DFIB (g) / CHOL (mg)	Na (mg) / K (mg)	Ca (mg) / P (mg)	Mg (mg) / Fe (mg)	Zn (mg) / Cu (mg)	Mn (mg) / Se (mcg)	A (mcg RAE) / A (IU)	C (mg) / E (mg ATE)	B-1 (mg) / B-2 (mg)	NIA (mg) / B-6 (mg)	B-12 (mcg) / FOL (mcg DFE)	PANT (mg) / REF
acorn squash,	83	219.8	1.6	21.5		6.4	7	64	64	0.27	0.358	32	16	0.25	1.3	0.00	0.74
boiled, mshd - 1 cup	245	0.2	<0.1	<0.1	0.1	0	644	66	1.37	0.127	1.0	632		0.02	0.29	27.0	11484
cubed, baked	115	169.9	2.3	29.9		9.0	8	90	88	0.35	0.496	43	22	0.34	1.8	0.00	1.03
1 cup	205	0.3	0.1	<0.1	0.1	0	896	92	1.91	0.176	1.4	877		0.03	0.40	39.0	11483
balsam pear (bitter melon/bitter	24	116.5	1.0	5.4		2.5	7	11	20	0.95	0.107	7	41	0.06	0.3	0.00	0.24
gourd) pods, boiled - 1 cup pieces	124	0.2	<0.1	<0.1	0.1	0	396	45	0.47	0.041	0.2	140	0.9	0.07	0.05	63.2	11025
breadfruit, raw	99	67.8	1.0	26.0		4.7	2	16	24	0.12	0.058	2	28	0.11	0.9	0.00	0.44
1/4 small	96	0.2	<0.1	<0.1	0.1	0	470	29	0.52	0.081	0.6	38	1.1	0.03	0.10	13.4	09059
butternut squash,	82	180.0	1.8	21.5			8	84	59	0.27	0.353	718	31	0.15	2.0	0.00	0.74
cubed, baked - 1 cup	205	0.2	<0.1	<0.1	0.1	0	582	55	1.23	0.133	1.0	14352		0.03	0.25	39.0	11486
mshd, frzn, boiled	94	210.7	3.0	24.1			5	46	22	0.29	0.415	401	8	0.12	1.1	0.00	0.37
1 cup	240	0.2	<0.1	<0.1	0.1	0	319	34	1.39	0.086	1.2	8014		0.09	0.17	38.4	11488
calabash (white-flowered) gourd,	22	139.2	0.9	5.4			3	35	16	1.02	0.096	0	12	0.04	0.6	0.00	0.21
cubed, boiled - 1 cup	146	<0.1	<0.1	<0.1	<0.1	0	248	19	0.37	0.038	0.3	0		0.03	0.06	5.8	11219
chayote, boiled[1]	38	149.5	1.0	8.1		4.5	2	21	19	0.50	0.270	3	13	0.04	0.7	0.00	0.65
1 cup pieces	160	0.8	0.1			0	277	46	0.35	0.176	0.5	75		0.06	0.19	28.8	11150
crookneck/straightneck squash,	25	122.6	1.2	5.3		2.5	3	27	27	0.38	0.204	22	11	0.07	0.6	0.00	0.13
raw, sliced - 1 cup	130	0.3	0.1	<0.1	0.1	0	276	42	0.62	0.133	0.3	439		0.06	0.14	29.9	11467
sliced, boiled	36	168.7	1.6	7.8		2.5	2	49	43	0.70	0.383	25	10	0.09	0.9	0.00	0.25
1 cup	180	0.6	0.1	<0.1	0.2	0	346	70	0.65	0.185	0.4	517	0.2	0.09	0.17	36.0	11468

	KCAL / WT (g)	H₂0 (g) / FAT (g)	PRO (g) / SFA (g)	CHO (g) / MUFA (g)	SUGR (g) / PUFA (g)	DFIB (g) / CHOL (mg)	Na (mg) / K (mg)	Ca (mg) / P (mg)	Mg (mg) / Fe (mg)	Zn (mg) / Cu (mg)	Mn (mg) / Se (mcg)	A (mcg RAE) / A (IU)	C (mg) / E (mg ATE)	B-1 (mg) / B-2 (mg)	NIA (mg) / B-6 (mg)	B-12 (mcg) / FOL (mcg DFE)	PANT (mg) / REF
sliced, cnd	28	207.4	1.3	6.4		3.0	11	26	28	0.63	0.210	13	6	0.03	0.9	0.00	0.10
1 cup	216	0.2	<0.1	<0.1	0.1	0	207	45	1.53	0.173	0.4	261	0.3	0.06	0.09	21.6	11471
sliced, frzn, boiled	48	177.1	2.5	10.6		2.7	12	38	52	0.65	0.505	19	13	0.07	0.8	0.00	0.20
1 cup	192	0.4	0.1	<0.1	0.2	0	486	79	1.00	0.140	0.6	374	0.5	0.09	0.19	25.0	11474
cucumber,	39	289.0	2.1	8.3		2.4	6	42	33	0.60	0.229	33	16	0.07	0.7	0.00	0.54
raw w/peel - *1 med 8 1/4" long*	301	0.4	0.1	<0.1	0.2	0	433	60	0.78	0.099	0.0	647	0.2	0.07	0.13	39.1	11205
raw w/o peel	24	193.9	1.1	5.0		1.4	4	28	24	0.28	0.171	8	6	0.04	0.2	0.00	0.57
1 med	201	0.3	0.1	<0.1	0.1	0	297	42	0.32	0.064	0.0	149	0.2	0.02	0.14	28.1	11206
dishcloth (towel) gourd, sliced,	100	150.0	1.2	25.5			37	16	36	0.30	0.397	23	10	0.08	0.5	0.00	0.89
boiled - *1 cup*	178	0.6	<0.1	0.1	0.3	0	806	55	0.64	0.151	0.4	463		0.07	0.18	21.4	11221
eggplant (aubergine),	28	90.9	0.8	6.6		2.5	3	6	13	0.15	0.135	3	1	0.08	0.6	0.00	0.07
boiled - *1 cup*	99	0.2	<0.1	<0.1	0.1	0	246	22	0.35	0.107	0.4	63	<0.1	0.02	0.09	13.9	11210
raw	21	75.5	0.8	5.0		2.1	2	6	11	0.11	0.107	3	1	0.04	0.5	0.00	0.21
1 cup	82	0.1	<0.1	<0.1	0.1	0	178	18	0.22	0.045	0.2	69	<0.1	0.03	0.07	15.6	11209
green beans (snap beans)[2],	44	111.5	2.4	9.9		4.0	4	58	31	0.45	0.368	41	12	0.09	0.8	0.00	0.09
boiled - *1 cup*	125	0.4	0.1	<0.1	0.2	0	374	49	1.60	0.129	0.5	833	0.2	0.12	0.07	41.3	11053
cnd	27	126.0	1.6	6.1		2.6	354	35	18	0.39	0.270	23	6	0.02	0.3	0.00	0.17
1 cup	135	0.1	<0.1	<0.1	0.1	0	147	26	1.22	0.051	0.5	471	0.2	0.08	0.05	43.2	11056
frzn, boiled	38	123.4	2.0	8.7		4.1	12	66	32	0.65	0.436	27	6	0.05	0.8	0.00	0.07
1 cup	135	0.2	<0.1	<0.1	0.1	0	170	42	1.19	0.082	0.5	541	0.2	0.12	0.08	31.1	11061
horseradish tree pods, sliced,	42	104.3	2.5	9.7		5.0	51	24	50	0.50	0.284	5	114	0.05	0.7	0.00	0.83
boiled - *1 cup*	118	0.2	<0.1	0.1	<0.1	0	539	58	0.53	0.092	0.8	83	0.1	0.08	0.13	35.4	11621
hubbard squash,	71	215.0	3.5	15.2		6.8	12	24	31	0.24	0.297	472	15	0.10	0.8	0.00	0.70
boiled, mshd - *1 cup*	236	0.9	0.2	0.1	0.4	0	505	33	0.66	0.111	0.7	9452	0.3	0.07	0.24	23.6	11491
cubed, baked	103	174.5	5.1	22.2			16	35	45	0.31	0.349	619	19	0.15	1.1	0.00	0.92
1 cup	205	1.3	0.3	0.1	0.5	0	734	47	0.96	0.092	1.2	12372		0.10	0.35	32.8	11490
kanpyo (dried gourd strips)	70	5.4	2.3	17.6			4	76	34	1.58	0.307	0	<1	0.00	0.8	0.00	0.69
1/2 cup	27	0.2	<0.1	<0.1	0.1	0	427	51	1.38	0.117	0.7	0		0.01	0.14	16.5	11237
okra (lady's finger/gumbo),	27	76.4	1.6	6.1		2.1	4	54	48	0.47	0.774	25	14	0.11	0.7	0.00	0.18
boiled - *8 pods (3" long)*	85	0.1	<0.1	<0.1	<0.1	0	274	48	0.38	0.073	0.6	489	0.6	0.05	0.16	39.1	11279
sliced, frzn	26	83.8	1.9	5.3		2.6	3	88	47	0.57	0.939	24	11	0.09	0.7	0.00	0.22
1/2 cup	92	0.3	0.1	<0.1	0.1	0	215	42	0.62	0.089	0.6	473	0.6	0.11	0.04	134.3	11281
peppers, ancho, dried	48	3.8	2.0	8.7		3.7	7	10	19	0.24	0.217	174	<1	0.03	1.1	0.00	0.34
1 pepper	17	1.4	0.1	0.1	0.8	0	410	34	1.86	0.086	0.5	3474	0.7	0.38	0.60	11.7	11978
peppers, banana, raw	12	42.2	0.8	2.5		1.6	6	6	8	0.12	0.046	8	38	0.04	0.6	0.00	0.12
1 med (4 1/2" long)	46	0.2	<0.1	<0.1	0.1	0	118	15	0.21	0.043	0.1	156	0.3	0.02	0.16	13.3	11976
peppers, chili, green,	5		0.0	1.0	0.0	1.0	110	40					6				
chopped, cnd, Old El Paso - *2 T*	30	0.0	0.0			0			0.00			0					GENM354
cnd	29	129.6	1.0	6.4		2.4	552	50	6	0.13		8	48	0.01	0.9	0.00	0.12
1 cup	139	0.4	<0.1	<0.1	0.2	0	157	15	1.85		0.4	175		0.04	0.17	75.1	11980
whole, cnd, Old El Paso	10		0.0	2.0	0.0	1.0	230	0					9				
1.2 oz pepper	35	0.0	0.0			0			0.00			200					GENM355
peppers, chili, green, hot,	15	67.5	0.7	3.7		0.9	856	5	10	0.12	0.101	23	50	0.01	0.6	0.00	0.02
cnd - *1 pepper*	73	0.1	<0.1	<0.1	<0.1	0	137	12	0.37	0.074	0.2	445	0.5	0.04	0.11	7.3	11329
raw	18	39.5	0.9	4.3		0.7	3	8	11	0.14	0.107	18	109	0.04	0.4	0.00	0.03
1 pepper	45	0.1	<0.1	<0.1	<0.1	0	153	21	0.54	0.078	0.2	347	0.3	0.04	0.13	10.4	11670
peppers, chili, red, hot,	15	67.5	0.7	3.7		0.9	856	5	10	0.12	0.101	434	50	0.01	0.6	0.00	0.02
cnd - *1 pepper*	73	0.1	<0.1	<0.1	<0.1	0	137	12	0.37	0.074	0.2	8681	0.5	0.04	0.11	7.3	11820
raw	18	39.5	0.9	4.3		0.7	3	8	11	0.14	0.107	242	109	0.04	0.4	0.00	0.03
1 pepper	45	0.1	<0.1	<0.1	<0.1	0	153	21	0.54	0.078	0.2	4838	0.3	0.04	0.13	10.4	11819
sun-dried	2	<0.1	0.1	0.3		0.1	0	0	<1	0.01	0.004	7	<1	<0.01	<0.1	0.00	<0.01
1 pepper	0.5	<0.1	<0.1	<0.1	<0.1	0	9	1	0.03	0.001	<0.1	132	<0.1	0.01	<0.01	0.3	11962
peppers, hungarian, raw	8	24.7	0.2	1.8			0	3	4	0.08	0.055	2	25	0.02	0.3	0.00	0.06
1 pepper	27	0.1	<0.1	<0.1	0.1	0	55	8	0.12	0.031	0.1	38		0.01	0.14	14.3	11981
peppers, jalapeno,	6	19.6	0.2	1.0		0.6	368	5	3	0.07	0.025	19	2	0.01	0.1	0.00	0.09
cnd - *1 pepper*	22	0.2	<0.1	<0.1	0.1	0	42	4	0.41	0.032	0.1	374	0.2	0.01	0.04	3.1	11632
pickled, sliced, cnd, Old El Paso	10		0.0	3.0	0.0	1.0	400	60					2				
2 T	31	0.0	0.0			0			0.00			100					GENM356
pickled, whole, cnd, Old El Paso	5		0.0	1.0	0.0	0.0	380	0					0				
2 peppers (.9 oz)	26	0.0	0.0			0			0.00			0					GENM357
raw	4	12.8	0.2	0.8		0.4	0	1	3	0.03	0.035	2	6	0.02	0.2	0.00	0.03
1 pepper	14	0.1	<0.1	<0.1	<0.1	0	30	4	0.10	0.019	<0.1	30	0.1	0.01	0.07	6.6	11979

	KCAL	H_2O (g)	PRO (g)	CHO (g)	SUGR (g)	DFIB (g)	Minerals Na (mg)	Ca (mg)	Mg (mg)	Zn (mg)	Mn (mg)	Vitamins A (mcg RAE)	C (mg)	B-1 (mg)	NIA (mg)	B-12 (mcg)	PANT (mg)
	WT (g)	FAT (g)	SFA (g)	MUFA (g)	PUFA (g)	CHOL (mg)	K (mg)	P (mg)	Fe (mg)	Cu (mg)	Se (mcg)	A (IU)	E (mg ATE)	B-2 (mg)	B-6 (mg)	FOL (mcg DFE)	REF
peppers, pasilla, dried	24	1.0	0.9	3.6		1.9	6	7	9	0.10	0.111	125	<1	0.01	0.5	0.00	0.11
1 pepper	7	1.1				0	156	19	0.69	0.030	0.2	2503		0.22	0.30	11.9	11982
peppers, pimiento, cnd	3	11.2	0.1	0.6		0.2	2	1	1	0.02	0.011	16	10	<0.01	0.1	0.00	<0.01
1 T	12	<0.1	<0.1	<0.1	<0.1	0	19	2	0.20	0.006	<0.1	319	0.1	0.01	0.03	0.7	11943
peppers, serrano, raw	2	5.5	0.1	0.4		0.2	1	1	1	0.02	0.011	3	3	<0.01	0.1	0.00	0.01
1 pepper	6	<0.1	<0.1	<0.1	<0.1	0	19	2	0.05	0.008	<0.1	57	<0.1	<0.01	0.03	1.4	11977
peppers, sweet (bell), green,	24	127.8	1.3	5.3		1.2	5	11	9	0.07	0.131	20	56	0.07	1.5	0.00	0.03
chpd, frzn, boiled - *1 cup pcs*	135	0.2	<0.1	<0.1	0.1	0	97	18	0.70	0.059	0.3	392		0.04	0.15	13.5	11338
cnd	25	127.8	1.1	5.5		1.7	1917	57	15	0.25	0.224	11	65	0.04	0.8	0.00	0.05
1 cup halves	140	0.4	0.1	<0.1	0.2	0	204	28	1.12	0.182	0.4	217		0.04	0.25	22.4	11335
raw	32	109.7	1.1	7.7		2.1	2	11	12	0.14	0.138	38	106	0.08	0.6	0.00	0.10
1 med (2 3/4″ long)	119	0.2	<0.1	<0.1	0.1	0	211	23	0.55	0.077	0.4	752	0.8	0.04	0.30	26.2	11333
sliced, boiled	38	124.0	1.2	9.0		1.6	3	12	14	0.16	0.155	41	100	0.08	0.6	0.00	0.11
1 cup	135	0.3	<0.1	<0.1	0.1	0	224	24	0.62	0.088	0.4	799	0.9	0.04	0.31	21.6	11334
peppers, sweet (bell), red,	24	127.8	1.3	5.3			5	11	9	0.07	0.131	225	56	0.07	1.5	0.00	0.03
chpd, frzn, boiled - *1 cup pcs*	135	0.2	<0.1	<0.1	0.1	0	97	18	0.70	0.059	0.3	4513		0.04	0.15	13.5	11918
raw	32	109.7	1.1	7.7		2.4	2	11	12	0.14	0.138	339	226	0.08	0.6	0.00	0.10
1 med (2 3/4″ long)	119	0.2	<0.1	<0.1	0.1	0	211	23	0.55	0.077	0.4	6783	0.8	0.04	0.30	26.2	11821
sliced, boiled	38	124.0	1.2	9.0		1.6	3	12	14	0.16	0.155	254	231	0.08	0.6	0.00	0.11
1 cup	135	0.3	<0.1	<0.1	0.1	0	224	24	0.62	0.088	0.4	5076	0.9	0.04	0.31	21.6	11823
peppers, sweet (bell), yellow, raw	50	171.2	1.9	11.8		1.7	4	20	22	0.32	0.218	22	341	0.05	1.7	0.00	0.31
1 large (3 3/4″ long)	186	0.4	0.1			0	394	45	0.86	0.199	0.6	443		0.05	0.31	48.4	11951
plantain, sliced, ckd	179	103.6	1.2	48.0		3.5	8	3	49	0.20		69	17	0.07	1.2	0.00	0.36
1 cup	154	0.3	0.1	<0.1	<0.1	0	716	43	0.89	0.102	2.2	1400	0.2	0.08	0.37	40.0	09278
pumpkin,	49	229.5	1.8	12.0		2.7	2	37	22	0.56	0.218	132	12	0.08	1.0	0.00	0.49
boiled, mshd - *1 cup*	245	0.2	0.1	<0.1	<0.1	0	564	74	1.40	0.223	0.5	2651	2.6	0.19	0.11	22.1	11423
cnd	83	220.4	2.7	19.8		7.1	12	64	56	0.42	0.365	2702	10	0.06	0.9	0.00	0.98
1 cup	245	0.7	0.4	0.1	<0.1	0	505	86	3.41	0.262	1.0	54037	2.6	0.13	0.14	29.4	11424
scallop squash,	23	122.4	1.6	5.0			1	25	30	0.38	0.204	8	23	0.09	0.8	0.00	0.13
raw, sliced - *1 cup*	130	0.3	0.1	<0.1	0.1	0	237	47	0.52	0.133	0.3	143		0.04	0.14	39.0	11475
sliced, boiled	29	171.0	1.9	5.9		3.4	2	27	34	0.43	0.230	7	19	0.09	0.8	0.00	0.14
1 cup	180	0.3	0.1	<0.1	0.1	0	252	50	0.59	0.149	0.4	153	0.2	0.05	0.15	37.8	11476
snow peas (edible podded peas),	67	142.3	5.2	11.3		4.5	6	67	42	0.59	0.269	11	77	0.20	0.9	0.00	1.08
boiled - *1 cup*	160	0.4	0.1	<0.1	0.2	0	384	88	3.15	0.123	1.1	210	0.6	0.12	0.23	46.4	11301
frzn, boiled	83	138.6	5.6	14.4		5.0	8	94	45	0.78	0.448	13	35	0.10	0.9	0.00	1.37
1 cup	160	0.6	0.1	0.1	0.3	0	347	93	3.84	0.144	1.3	267	0.3	0.19	0.28	56.0	11303
frzn, LaChoy	35		2.0	4.0	2.0	2.0	0	20					15				
3 oz (~42 pods)	85	1.5	0.0			0			0.72			200					CNAG41
raw	26	56.0	1.8	4.8		1.6	3	27	15	0.17	0.154	4	38	0.09	0.4	0.00	0.47
1 cup whole	63	0.1	<0.1	<0.1	0.1	0	126	33	1.31	0.050	0.4	91	0.2	0.05	0.10	26.5	11300
spaghetti squash, boiled/baked	42	143.1	1.0	10.0		2.2	28	33	17	0.31	0.169	9	5	0.06	1.3	0.00	0.55
1 cup	155	0.4	0.1	<0.1	0.2	0	181	22	0.53	0.054	0.5	171	0.2	0.03	0.15	12.4	11493
squash, summer (marrow)[3],	23	105.9	1.3	4.9		2.1	2	23	26	0.29	0.177	11	17	0.07	0.6	0.00	0.12
all varieties, raw, sliced - *1 cup*	113	0.2	<0.1	<0.1	0.1	0	220	40	0.52	0.086	0.2	221	0.1	0.04	0.12	29.4	11641
all varieties, sliced, boiled	36	168.7	1.6	7.8		2.5	2	49	43	0.70	0.383	25	10	0.08	0.9	0.00	0.25
1 cup	180	0.6	0.1	<0.1	0.2	0	346	70	0.65	0.185	0.4	517	0.2	0.07	0.12	36.0	11642
squash, winter, all varieties[4],	80	182.5	1.8	17.9		5.7	2	29	16	0.53	0.433	365	20	0.17	1.4	0.00	0.72
cubed, baked - *1 cup*	205	1.3	0.3	0.1	0.5	0	896	41	0.68	0.195	0.8	7292	0.2	0.05	0.15	57.4	11644
tomatillo, raw	11	31.2	0.3	2.0		0.6	0	2	7	0.07	0.052	2	4	0.01	0.6	0.00	0.05
1 med	34	0.3	<0.1	0.1	0.1	0	91	13	0.21	0.027	0.2	39	0.1	0.01	0.02	2.4	11954
tomato paste, cnd	139	125.5	6.2	32.8		7.0	150	60	87	1.36	0.884	207	72	0.26	5.5	0.00	1.28
6 oz can	170	0.9	0.1	0.1	0.4	0	1593	134	3.30	1.006	2.4	4157	7.3	0.32	0.65	37.4	11546
tomato puree, cnd	100	218.7	4.2	23.9		5.0	85	43	60	0.55	0.640	160	26	0.18	4.3	0.00	1.10
1 cup	250	0.4	0.1	0.1	0.2	0	1065	100	3.10	0.408	1.8	3188	6.3	0.14	0.38	27.5	11547
tomato, green, raw	30	114.4	1.5	6.3		1.4	16	16	12	0.09	0.123	39	29	0.07	0.6	0.00	0.62
1 med	123	0.2	<0.1	<0.1	0.1	0	251	34	0.63	0.111	0.5	790	0.5	0.05	0.10	11.1	11527
tomato, orange, raw	18	105.2	1.3	3.5		1.0	47	6	9	0.16	0.098	83	18	0.05	0.7	0.00	0.21
1 tomato	111	0.2	<0.1	<0.1	0.1	0	235	32	0.52	0.069	0.4	1661		0.04	0.07	32.2	11695
tomato, red,	65	221.2	2.6	14.0		2.4	26	14	34	0.26	0.317	89	55	0.17	1.8	0.00	0.71
boiled - *1 cup*	240	1.0	0.1	0.2	0.4	0	670	74	1.34	0.223	1.2	1783	0.9	0.14	0.23	31.2	11530
crushed, cnd, Eden Foods	20		1.0	3.0	2.0	1.0	0	20	16				9	0.06	0.8		
1/4 cup	61	0.0	0.0			0	170	60	0.72			750		0.07			EDEN35

	KCAL	H₂0 (g)	PRO (g)	CHO (g)	SUGR (g)	DFIB (g)	Na (mg)	Ca (mg)	Mg (mg)	Zn (mg)	Mn (mg)	A (mcg RAE)	C (mg)	B-1 (mg)	NIA (mg)	B-12 (mcg)	PANT (mg)
	WT (g)	FAT (g)	SFA (g)	MUFA (g)	PUFA (g)	CHOL (mg)	K (mg)	P (mg)	Fe (mg)	Cu (mg)	Se (mcg)	A (IU)	E (mg ATE)	B-2 (mg)	B-6 (mg)	FOL (mcg DFE)	REF
diced, cnd, Eden Foods	30		1.0	6.0	4.0	2.0	5	20	16				18	0.09	1.2		
1/2 cup	130	0.0	0.0			0	330		0.36			1000		0.03			EDEN36
raw	26	115.3	1.0	5.7		1.4	11	6	14	0.11	0.129	38	23	0.07	0.8	0.00	0.30
1 med (2 3/5" dia)	123	0.4	0.1	0.1	0.2	0	273	30	0.55	0.091	0.5	766	0.5	0.06	0.10	18.5	11529e
raw, chopped, sliced	26	115.3	1.0	5.7		1.4	11	6	14	0.11	0.129	38	23	0.07	0.8	0.000	0.30
1 cup	123	0.4	0.1	0.1	0.2	0	273	30	0.55	0.091	0.5	766	0.5	0.06	0.10	18.5	11529e
stewed[5]	80	81.4	2.0	13.2		1.7	460	26	15	0.18	0.195	33	18	0.11	1.1	0.00	0.26
1 cup	101	2.7	0.5	1.1	0.9	0	249	38	1.07	0.096	1.2	673	1.3	0.08	0.09	11.1	11660
stewed, cnd	71	232.1	2.4	17.3		2.6	564	84	31	0.43	0.150	69	29	0.12	1.8	0.00	0.29
1 cup	255	0.3	<0.1	0.1	0.1	0	607	51	1.86	0.286	1.5	1380	1.0	0.09	0.04	12.8	11533
sun-dried	139	7.9	7.6	30.1		6.6	1131	59	105	1.07	0.997	24	21	0.29	4.9	0.00	1.13
1 cup	54	1.6	0.2	0.3	0.6	0	1851	192	4.91	0.768	3.0	472	<0.1	0.26	0.18	36.7	11955
sun-dried, cnd, packed in oil	234	59.2	5.6	25.7		6.4	293	52	89	0.86	0.513	70	112	0.21	4.0	0.00	0.53
1 cup	110	15.5	2.1	9.5	2.3	0	1722	153	2.95	0.520	3.3	1415		0.42	0.35	25.3	11956
wedges in tomato jce, cnd	68	239.5	2.1	16.5			566	68	29	0.42	0.431	76	39	0.15	1.8	0.00	0.57
1 cup	261	0.4	0.1	0.1	0.2	0	655	60	1.20	0.271	1.3	1509		0.07	0.31	26.1	11535
whole, peeled, cnd	46	224.8	2.2	10.5		2.4	355	72	29	0.38	0.305	72	34	0.11	1.8	0.00	0.40
1 cup	240	0.3	<0.1	<0.1	0.1	0	530	46	1.32	0.264	1.7	1428	0.8	0.07	0.22	19.2	11531
w/green chili, cnd	36	227.1	1.7	8.7			966	48	27	0.31	0.318	48	15	0.08	1.5	0.00	0.36
1 cup	241	0.2	<0.1	<0.1	0.1	0	258	34	0.63	0.217	1.0	940		0.05	0.25	21.7	11537
tomato, red, cherry, raw	31	139.7	1.3	6.9		1.6	13	7	16	0.13	0.156	46	28	0.09	0.9	0.00	0.37
1 cup	149	0.5	0.1	0.1	0.2	0	331	36	0.67	0.110	0.6	928	0.6	0.07	0.12	22.4	11529a
tomato, red, italian, raw	13	58.1	0.5	2.9		0.7	6	3	7	0.06	0.065	19	12	0.04	0.4	0.00	0.15
1 tomato	62	0.2	<0.1	<0.1	0.1	0	138	15	0.28	0.046	0.2	386	0.2	0.03	0.05	9.3	11529d
tomato, red, plum, raw	13	58.1	0.5	2.9		0.7	6	3	7	0.06	0.065	19	12	0.04	0.4	0.00	0.15
1 tomato	62	0.2	<0.1	<0.1	0.1	0	138	15	0.28	0.046	0.2	386	0.2	0.03	0.05	9.3	11529c
tomato, yellow, raw	32	202.0	2.1	6.3		1.5	49	23	25	0.59	0.254	0	19	0.09	2.5	0.00	0.23
1 tomato	212	0.6	0.1	0.1	0.2	0	547	76	1.04	0.214	0.8	0		0.10	0.12	63.6	11696
waxgourd (chinese preserving melon), cubed, boiled - *1 cup*	23	168.1	0.7	5.3		1.8	187	32	18	1.03	0.098	0	18	0.06	0.7	0.00	0.21
	175	0.4	<0.1	0.1	0.2	0	9	30	0.67	0.039	0.4	0	0.7	<0.01	0.06	7.0	11594
yellow snap beans,	44	111.5	2.4	9.9		4.1	4	58	31	0.45	0.368	5	12	0.09	0.8	0.00	0.09
boiled - *1 cup*	125	0.4	0.1	<0.1	0.2	0	374	49	1.60	0.129	0.5	101	0.4	0.12	0.07	41.3	11724
cnd	27	126.0	1.6	6.1		1.8	339	35	18	0.39	0.270	7	6	0.02	0.3	0.00	0.17
1 cup	135	0.1	<0.1	<0.1	0.1	0	147	26	1.22	0.051	0.5	142	0.4	0.08	0.05	43.2	11932
frzn	38	123.4	2.0	8.7		4.1	12	66	32	0.65	0.436	8	6	0.05	0.5	0.00	0.07
1 cup	135	0.2	0.1	<0.1	0.1	0	170	42	1.19	0.082	0.5	151	0.2	0.12	0.08	31.1	11732
zucchini,	2	10.2	0.3	0.3		0.1	0	2	4	0.09	0.022	3	4	<0.01	0.1	0.00	0.04
baby, raw - *1 med*	11	<0.1	<0.1	<0.1	<0.1	0	50	10	0.09	0.011	<0.1	54		<0.01	0.02	2.2	11953
cnd, italian style	66	205.7	2.3	15.5			849	39	32	0.59	0.545	61	5	0.10	1.2	0.00	0.62
1 cup	227	0.2	0.1	<0.1	0.1	0	622	66	1.54	0.222	0.9	1224		0.09	0.35	68.1	11481
raw, sliced	16	107.7	1.3	3.3		1.4	3	17	25	0.23	0.144	19	10	0.08	0.5	0.00	0.09
1 cup	113	0.2	<0.1	<0.1	0.1	0	280	36	0.47	0.064	0.2	384	0.1	0.03	0.10	24.9	11477
sliced, boiled	29	170.5	1.2	7.1		2.5	5	23	40	0.32	0.320	22	8	0.07	0.9	0.00	0.21
1 cup	180	0.1	<0.1	<0.1	<0.1	0	455	72	0.63	0.155	0.4	432	0.2	0.07	0.14	30.6	11478
sliced, frzn, boiled	38	211.3	2.6	7.9		2.9	4	38	29	0.45	0.513	49	8	0.09	0.9	0.00	0.59
1 cup	223	0.3	0.1	<0.1	0.1	0	433	56	1.07	0.105	0.4	963	0.7	0.09	0.10	17.8	11480

[1] Also known as mango squash, miriliton, and vegetable pear.
[2] Includes Italian, green, and yellow varieties of beans.
[3] See also crookneck squash, scallop squash, and zucchini.
[4] See also acorn squash, butternut squash, hubbard squash, pumpkin, and spaghetti squash.
[5] Made with tomatoes, bread crumbs, margarine, sugar, onions, salt, and pepper.

30.3 LEAFY VEGETABLES

	KCAL	H₂0 (g)	PRO (g)	CHO (g)	SUGR (g)	DFIB (g)	Na (mg)	Ca (mg)	Mg (mg)	Zn (mg)	Mn (mg)	A (mcg RAE)	C (mg)	B-1 (mg)	NIA (mg)	B-12 (mcg)	PANT (mg)
	WT (g)	FAT (g)	SFA (g)	MUFA (g)	PUFA (g)	CHOL (mg)	K (mg)	P (mg)	Fe (mg)	Cu (mg)	Se (mcg)	A (IU)	E (mg ATE)	B-2 (mg)	B-6 (mg)	FOL (mcg DFE)	REF
amaranth leaves,	28	120.8	2.8	5.4			28	276	73	1.16	1.137	183	54	0.03	0.7	0.00	0.08
boiled - *1 cup*	132	0.2	0.1	0.1	0.1	0	846	95	2.98	0.209	1.2	3656		0.18	0.23	75.2	11004
raw	6	25.7	0.7	1.1			6	60	15	0.25	0.248	41	12	0.01	0.2	0.00	0.02
1 cup	28	0.1	<0.1	<0.1	<0.1	0	171	14	0.65	0.045	0.3	817		0.04	0.05	23.8	11003
arugula, raw	3	9.2	0.3	0.4		0.2	3	16	5	0.05	0.032	12	2	<0.01	<0.1	0.00	0.04
1/2 cup	10	0.1	<0.1	<0.1	<0.1	0	37	5	0.15	0.008	<0.1	237	<0.1	0.01	0.01	9.7	11959
balsam pear (bitter melon/bitter gourd) leafy tips, boiled - *1 cup*	20	51.4	2.1	3.9		1.1	8	24	55	0.17	0.311	50	32	0.09	0.6	0.00	0.03
	58	0.1	<0.1	<0.1	<0.1	0	349	45	0.59	0.117	0.5	1005	0.3	0.16	0.44	51.0	11023
beet greens, boiled	39	128.3	3.7	7.9		4.2	347	164	98	0.72	0.740	367	36	0.17	0.7	0.00	0.47
1/2 cup	144	0.3	<0.1	0.1	0.1	0	1309	59	2.74	0.361	1.3	7344	0.4	0.42	0.19	20.2	11087

	KCAL / WT (g)	H₂O (g) / FAT (g)	PRO (g) / SFA (g)	CHO (g) / MUFA (g)	SUGR (g) / PUFA (g)	DFIB (g) / CHOL (mg)	Na (mg) / K (mg)	Ca (mg) / P (mg)	Mg (mg) / Fe (mg)	Zn (mg) / Cu (mg)	Mn (mg) / Se (mcg)	A (mcg RAE) / A (IU)	C (mg) / E (mg ATE)	B-1 (mg) / B-2 (mg)	NIA (mg) / B-6 (mg)	B-12 (mcg) / FOL (mcg DFE)	PANT (mg) / REF
borage, boiled	25	91.9	2.1	3.6			88	102	57	0.22	0.385	219	33	0.06	0.9	0.00	0.05
3.5 oz	100	0.8	0.2	0.2	0.1	0	491	55	3.64	0.143	0.9	4385		0.17	0.09	10.0	11614
brussels sprouts, boiled - *1/2 cup*	30	68.1	2.0	6.8		2.0	16	28	16	0.26	0.177	28	48	0.08	0.5	0.00	0.20
	78	0.4	0.1	<0.1	0.2	0	247	44	0.94	0.065	1.2	561	0.7	0.06	0.14	46.8	11099
frzn, boiled	65	134.4	5.6	12.9		6.4	36	37	37	0.56	0.496	45	71	0.16	0.8	0.00	0.53
1 cup	155	0.6	0.1	<0.1	0.3	0	504	84	1.15	0.109	2.3	913	0.9	0.18	0.45	156.6	11101
cabbage, chinese, pak-choi, raw, shredded - *1/2 cup*	9	66.7	1.1	1.5		0.7	46	74	13	0.13	0.111	105	32	0.03	0.4	0.00	0.06
	70	0.1	<0.1	<0.1	0.1	0	176	26	0.56	0.015	0.4	2100	0.1	0.05	0.14	46.2	11116
shredded, boiled	20	162.4	2.7	3.0		2.7	58	158	19	0.29	0.245	218	44	0.05	0.7	0.00	0.13
1 cup	170	0.3	<0.1	<0.1	0.1	0	631	49	1.77	0.032	0.7	4366	0.2	0.11	0.28	69.7	11117
cabbage, chinese, pe-tsai, raw, shredded - *1/2 cup*	12	71.7	0.9	2.5		2.4	7	59	10	0.17	0.144	46	21	0.04	0.3	0.00	0.08
	76	0.2	<0.1	<0.1	0.1	0	181	22	0.24	0.027	0.5	912	0.1	0.04	0.18	60.0	11119
cabbage, chinese, pe-tsai, sliced, boiled - *1 cup*	17	113.3	1.8	2.9		2.0	11	38	12	0.21	0.182	57	19	0.05	0.6	0.00	0.10
	119	0.2	<0.1	<0.1	0.1	0	268	46	0.36	0.035	0.5	1151		0.05	0.21	63.1	11120
cabbage, green, raw, shredded - *1 cup*	18	64.5	1.0	3.8		1.6	13	33	11	0.13	0.111	5	23	0.04	0.2	0.00	0.10
	70	0.2	<0.1	<0.1	0.1	0	172	16	0.41	0.016	0.6	93	0.1	0.03	0.07	30.1	11109
shredded, boiled	17	70.2	0.8	3.3		1.7	6	23	6	0.07	0.088	5	15	0.04	0.2	0.00	0.10
1/2 cup	75	0.3	<0.1	<0.1	0.1	0	73	11	0.13	0.009	0.5	99	0.1	0.04	0.08	15.0	11110
cabbage, red, raw, shredded - *1 cup*	19	64.1	1.0	4.3		1.4	8	36	11	0.15	0.126	1	40	0.04	0.2	0.00	0.23
	70	0.2	<0.1	<0.1	0.1	0	144	29	0.34	0.068	0.6	28	0.1	0.02	0.15	14.7	11112
shredded, boiled	16	70.2	0.8	3.5		1.5	6	28	8	0.11	0.097	1	26	0.03	0.2	0.00	0.17
1/2 cup	75	0.2	<0.1	<0.1	0.1	0	105	22	0.26	0.052	0.5	20	0.1	0.02	0.11	9.8	11113
cabbage, savoy[1], raw, shredded - *1 cup*	19	63.7	1.4	4.3		2.2	20	25	20	0.19	0.126	35	22	0.05	0.2	0.00	0.13
	70	0.1	<0.1	<0.1	<0.1	0	161	29	0.28	0.043	0.6	700	0.1	0.02	0.13	56.0	11114
shredded, boiled	35	133.4	2.6	7.8		4.1	35	44	35	0.33	0.220	64	25	0.07	<0.1	0.00	0.13
1 cup	145	0.1	<0.1	<0.1	0.1	0	267	48	0.55	0.075	1.0	1289		0.03	0.22	66.7	11115
cabbage, swamp (skunk cabbage), chopped, boiled - *1 cup*	20	91.1	2.0	3.6		1.9	120	53	29	0.16	0.140	255	16	0.08	0.5	0.00	0.12
	98	0.2	<0.1	<0.1	0.1	0	278	41	1.29	0.021	0.9	5096	<0.1	0.08	0.08	34.3	11504
raw, chopped	11	51.8	1.5	1.8		1.2	63	43	40	0.10	0.090	176	31	0.02	0.5	0.00	0.08
1 cup	56	0.1				0	175	22	0.94	0.013	0.5	3528		0.06	0.05	31.9	11503
celtuce, raw	18	94.5	0.9	3.7		1.7	11	39	28	0.27	0.688	175	20	0.06	0.6	0.00	0.18
12 leaves	100	0.3				0	330	39	0.55	0.040	0.9	3500		0.07	0.05	46.0	11145
chard, swiss, chopped, boiled	35	162.1	3.3	7.2		3.7	313	102	151	0.58	0.585	275	32	0.06	0.6	0.00	0.29
1 cup	175	0.1	<0.1	<0.1	<0.1	0	961	58	3.96	0.285	1.6	5493	3.3	0.15	0.15	15.8	11148
chicory greens, raw, chopped	41	165.6	3.1	8.5		7.2	81	180	54	0.76	0.772	360	43	0.11	0.9	0.00	2.09
1 cup	180	0.5	0.1	<0.1	0.2	0	756	85	1.62	0.531	0.5	7200	4.1	0.18	0.19	198.0	11152
chicory, witloof, raw	8	42.5	0.4	1.8		1.4	1	9	5	0.07	0.045	<1	1	0.03	0.1	0.00	0.07
1/2 cup	45	<0.1	<0.1	<0.1	<0.1	0	95	12	0.11	0.023	0.1	13		0.01	0.02	16.7	11151
chrysanthemum leaves, raw, chopped	12	46.6	1.7	1.5		1.5	60	60	16	0.36	0.481	48	1	0.07	0.3	0.00	0.11
1 cup	51	0.3				0	289	28	1.17	0.070	0.2	954		0.07	0.09	90.3	11698
coleslaw, homemade[2]	41	48.9	0.8	7.4		0.9	14	27	6	0.12	0.058	32	20	0.04	0.2	0.00	0.08
1/2 cup	60	1.6	0.2	0.4	0.8	5	109	19	0.35	0.014	0.4	220		0.04	0.08	16.2	11159
collards, chopped, boiled - *1 cup*	49	174.5	4.0	9.3		5.3	17	226	32	0.80	1.074	296	35	0.08	1.1	0.00	0.41
	190	0.7	0.1	<0.1	0.3	0	494	49	0.87	0.061	2.1	5945	1.7	0.20	0.24	176.7	11162
chopped, frzn, boiled	61	150.4	5.0	12.1		4.8	85	357	51	0.46	1.127	508	45	0.08	1.1	0.00	0.20
1 cup	170	0.7	0.1	<0.1	0.4	0	427	46	1.90	0.094	2.6	10168	0.9	0.20	0.19	129.2	11164
coriander (cilantro) leaves, raw	5	18.4	0.4	0.7		0.6	9	13	5	0.10	0.085	67	5	0.01	0.2	0.00	0.11
9 pieces	20	0.1	<0.1	0.1	<0.1	0	104	10	0.35	0.045	0.2	1350	0.5	0.03	0.03	12.4	11165
cornsalad, raw[3]	12	52.0	1.1	2.0			2	21	7	0.33	0.201	199	21	0.04	0.2	0.00	0.02
1 cup	56	0.2				0	257	30	1.22	0.075	0.5	3972		0.05	0.15	7.8	11190
cowpeas, leafy tips, chopped, boiled	12	48.4	2.5	1.5			3	37	33	0.13	0.218	15	10	0.14	0.5	0.00	0.02
1 cup	53	0.1	<0.1	<0.1	<0.1	0	186	22	0.58	0.082	0.5	305		0.08	0.07	31.8	11202
dandelion greens, chopped, boiled - *1 cup*	35	94.3	2.1	6.7		3.0	46	147	25	0.29	0.242	614	19	0.14	0.5	0.00	0.06
	105	0.6	0.2	<0.1	0.3	0	244	44	1.89	0.121	0.3	12285	2.6	0.18	0.17	13.7	11208
raw, chopped	25	47.1	1.5	5.1		1.9	42	103	20	0.23	0.188	385	19	0.10	0.4	0.00	0.05
1 cup	55	0.4	0.1	<0.1	0.2	0	218	36	1.71	0.094	0.3	7700	1.4	0.14	0.14	14.9	11207
dock (sorrel), boiled - *3.5 oz*	20	93.6	1.8	2.9		2.6	3	38	89	0.17	0.303	174	26	0.03	0.4	0.00	0.04
	100	0.6				0	321	52	2.08	0.114	0.9	3474		0.09	0.10	8.0	11617
raw, chopped	29	123.7	2.7	4.3		3.9	5	59	137	0.27	0.464	266	64	0.05	0.7	0.00	0.05
1 cup	133	0.9				0	519	84	3.19	0.174	1.2	5320		0.13	0.16	17.3	11616
endive, raw, chopped	4	23.4	0.3	0.8		0.8	6	13	4	0.20	0.105	26	2	0.02	0.1	0.00	0.23
1/2 cup	25	<0.1	<0.1	<0.1	<0.1	0	79	7	0.21	0.025	<0.1	513	0.1	0.02	<0.01	35.5	11213

	KCAL (g) / WT (g)	H₂0 (g) / FAT (g)	PRO (g) / SFA (g)	CHO (g) / MUFA (g)	SUGR (g) / PUFA (g)	DFIB (g) / CHOL (mg)	Na (mg) / K (mg)	Ca (mg) / P (mg)	Mg (mg) / Fe (mg)	Zn (mg) / Cu (mg)	Mn (mg) / Se (mcg)	A (mcg RAE) / A (IU)	C (mg) / E (mg ATE)	B-1 (mg) / B-2 (mg)	NIA (mg) / B-6 (mg)	B-12 (mcg) / FOL (mcg DFE)	PANT (mg) / REF
eppaw, raw	150	60.0	4.6	31.7			12	110	32	1.15	1.094	0	13	0.11	0.3	0.00	1.17
1 cup	100	1.8				0	340	165	1.15	0.234	0.9	0		0.12	0.18	24.0	11618
fiddlehead ferns,	34	88.9	4.3	5.7			0	24	19	0.71	0.940	51	18	0.01	3.3	0.00	
frzn - 3.5 oz	100	0.4				0	129	58	0.73	0.220		1028		0.13			11996
raw, chopped	24	16.3	1.1	4.4		2.4	8	99	36	0.61	1.542	41	<1	0.01	1.1	0.00	0.31
1 cup	23	0.6				0	114	25	0.55	0.074	0.2	828		0.03	0.15	25.8	11985
garden cress,	31	124.9	2.6	5.1		0.9	11	82	35	0.20	0.502	520	31	0.08	1.1	0.00	0.22
boiled - 1 cup	135	0.8	<0.1	0.3	0.3	0	477	65	1.08	0.154	1.2	10395	0.9	0.22	0.21	50.0	11204
raw	16	44.7	1.3	2.8		0.6	7	41	19	0.12	0.277	233	35	0.04	0.5	0.00	0.12
1 cup	50	0.4	<0.1	0.1	0.1	0	303	38	0.65	0.085	0.5	4650	0.4	0.13	0.12	40.0	11203
garland chrysanthemum[4],	20	92.5	1.6	4.3		2.3	53	69	18	0.20	0.355	253	24	0.02	0.7	0.00	0.04
boiled - 1 cup pieces	100	0.1	<0.1	<0.1	<0.1	0	569	43	3.74	0.133	0.3	5050	2.5	0.16	0.12	50.0	11158
raw	5	23.1	0.4	1.1		0.7	13	14	4	0.05	0.093	184	9	0.01	0.2	0.00	0.01
1 cup pieces	25	<0.1				0	143	8	0.78	0.035	<0.1	3669		0.06	0.03	19.3	11157
grape leaves,	3	3.0	0.2	0.5			114	12	1	0.02	0.012	11	<1	<0.01	0.2	0.00	0.17
cnd - 1 leaf	4	0.1	<0.1	<0.1	<0.1	0	1	1	0.12	0.074	<0.1	210		0.01	0.01	3.1	11975
raw	13	10.3	0.8	2.4		1.5	1	51	13	0.09	0.400	189	2	0.01	0.3	0.00	0.03
1 cup	14	0.3	<0.1	<0.1	0.1	0	38	13	0.37	0.058	0.1	3779	0.3	0.05	0.06	11.6	11974
horseradish tree, leafy tips[5],	25	34.3	2.2	4.7		0.8	4	63	63	0.21	0.365	147	13	0.09	0.8	0.00	0.04
chopped, boiled - 1 cup	42	0.4	0.1	0.2	<0.1	0	144	28	0.97	0.036	0.4	2945	<0.1	0.21	0.39	9.7	11223
jute, potherb,	32	75.8	3.2	6.4		1.7	10	184	54	0.69	0.107	225	29	0.08	0.8	0.00	0.06
boiled - 1 cup	87	0.2	<0.1	<0.1	0.1	0	479	63	2.73	0.222	0.8	4511	0.6	0.17	0.50	90.5	11232
raw	10	24.6	1.3	1.6			2	58	18	0.22	0.034	78	10	0.04	0.4	0.00	0.02
1 cup	28	0.1	<0.1	<0.1	<0.1	0	157	23	1.33	0.071	0.3	1557		0.15	0.17	34.4	11231
kale,	36	118.6	2.5	7.3		2.6	30	94	23	0.31	0.541	481	53	0.07	0.7	0.00	0.06
chopped, boiled - 1 cup	130	0.5	0.1	<0.1	0.3	0	296	36	1.17	0.203	1.2	9620	1.1	0.09	0.18	16.9	11234
chopped, frzn, boiled	39	117.7	3.7	6.8		2.6	20	179	23	0.23	0.585	413	33	0.06	0.9	0.00	0.07
1 cup	130	0.6	0.1	<0.1	0.3	0	417	36	1.22	0.061	1.2	8260	0.2	0.15	0.11	18.2	11236
kale, scotch, chopped, boiled	36	118.6	2.5	7.3		1.6	59	172	74	0.31	0.542	130	69	0.07	1.0	0.00	0.06
1 cup	130	0.5	0.1	<0.1	0.3	0	356	49	2.51	0.203	1.2	2592		0.05	0.18	16.9	11623
lambsquarters, chopped, boiled	58	160.0	5.8	9.0		3.8	52	464	41	0.54	0.945	873	67	0.18	1.6	0.00	0.11
1 cup	180	1.3	0.1	0.2	0.6	0	518	81	1.26	0.355	1.6	17460	2.4	0.47	0.31	25.2	11245
lettuce, butterhead, raw, chopped[6]	7	52.6	0.7	1.3		0.6	3	18	7	0.09	0.073	27	4	0.03	0.2	0.00	0.10
1 cup	55	0.1	<0.1	<0.1	0.1	0	141	13	0.17	0.013	0.1	534	0.2	0.03	0.03	40.2	11250
lettuce, iceberg, raw, chopped[7]	7	52.7	0.6	1.1		0.8	5	10	5	0.12	0.083	9	2	0.03	0.1	0.00	0.03
1 cup	55	0.1	<0.1	<0.1	0.1	0	87	11	0.28	0.015	0.1	182	0.2	0.02	0.02	30.8	11252
lettuce, looseleaf (leaf), raw,	5	26.3	0.4	1.0		0.5	3	19	3	0.08	0.210	27	5	0.01	0.1	0.00	0.06
shredded - 1/2 cup	28	0.1	<0.1	<0.1	<0.1	0	74	7	0.39	0.012	0.1	532	0.1	0.02	0.02	14.0	11253
lettuce, romaine/cos, raw, shredded	4	26.6	0.5	0.7		0.5	2	10	2	0.07	0.178	36	7	0.03	0.1	0.00	0.05
1/2 cup	28	0.1	<0.1	<0.1	<0.1	0	81	13	0.31	0.010	0.1	728	0.1	0.03	0.01	38.1	11251
malbar spinach, boiled	10	40.7	1.3	1.2		0.9	24	55	21	0.13	0.112	26	3	0.05	0.3	0.00	0.06
1 cup	44	0.3				0	113	16	0.65	0.049	0.4	510		0.06	0.04	50.2	11986
mixed greens, chopped, cnd, Bush's	25		2.0	3.0	1.0	2.0	300	100					9				
1/2 cup	130	0.0	0.0			0			1.08			3500					BUSH1
mustard greens,	21	132.2	3.2	2.9		2.8	22	104	21	0.15	0.384	213	35	0.06	0.6	0.00	0.17
chopped, boiled - 1 cup	140	0.3	<0.1	0.2	0.1	0	283	57	0.98	0.118	0.8	4243	2.8	0.09	0.14	102.2	11271
chopped, frzn, boiled	29	140.7	3.4	4.7		4.2	38	152	20	0.30	0.441	336	21	0.06	0.4	0.00	0.02
1 cup	150	0.4	<0.1	0.2	0.1	0	209	36	1.68	0.087	0.9	6705	2.6		0.16	105.0	11273
mustard spinach (tendergreen),	29	170.1	3.1	5.0		3.6	25	284	13	0.20	0.486	738	117	0.07	0.8	0.00	0.21
chopped, boiled - 1 cup	180	0.4				0	513	32	1.44	0.090	1.1	14760		0.11	0.17	131.4	11275
raw, chopped	33	138.3	3.3	5.9		4.2	32	315	17	0.26	0.611	743	195	0.10	1.0	0.00	0.27
1 cup	150	0.5	<0.1	0.2	0.1	0	674	42	2.25	0.113	1.2	14850	2.6	0.14	0.23	238.5	11274
new zealand spinach,	22	170.6	2.3	4.0			193	86	58	0.56	0.947	326	29	0.05	0.7	0.00	0.46
chopped, boiled - 1 cup	180	0.3	<0.1	<0.1	0.1	0	184	40	1.19	0.139	1.6	6520		0.19	0.43	14.4	11277
raw, chopped	8	52.6	0.8	1.4			73	32	22	0.21	0.358	123	17	0.02	0.3	0.00	0.17
1 cup	56	0.1	<0.1	<0.1	<0.1	0	73	16	0.45	0.052	0.4	2464		0.07	0.17	8.4	11276
pumpkin leaves, boiled	15	65.7	1.9	2.4		1.9	6	31	27	0.14	0.252	88	1	0.05	0.6	0.00	0.03
1 cup	71	0.2	0.1	<0.1	<0.1	0	311	56	2.27	0.094	0.6	1757	0.7	0.10	0.14	17.8	11419
purslane, boiled	21	107.5	1.7	4.1			51	90	77	0.20	0.353	107	12	0.04	0.5	0.00	0.04
1 cup	115	0.2				0	561	43	0.89	0.131	1.0	2130		0.10	0.08	10.4	11428
radicchio, raw, shredded	9	37.3	0.6	1.8		0.4	9	8	5	0.25	0.055	<1	3	0.01	0.1	0.00	0.11
1 cup	40	0.1	<0.1	<0.1	<0.1	0	121	16	0.23	0.136	0.4	11	0.9	0.01	0.02	24.0	11952

	KCAL	H₂0 (g)	PRO (g)	CHO (g)	SUGR (g)	DFIB (g)	Na (mg)	Ca (mg)	Mg (mg)	Zn (mg)	Mn (mg)	A (mcg RAE)	C (mg)	B-1 (mg)	NIA (mg)	B-12 (mcg)	PANT (mg)
	WT (g)	FAT (g)	SFA (g)	MUFA (g)	PUFA (g)	CHOL (mg)	K (mg)	P (mg)	Fe (mg)	Cu (mg)	Se (mcg)	A (IU)	E (mg ATE)	B-2 (mg)	B-6 (mg)	FOL (mcg DFE)	REF
salsify (oyster plant/vegetable	92	109.4	3.7	20.7		4.2	22	63	24	0.41	0.284	0	6	0.08	0.5	0.00	0.37
oyster), sliced, boiled - *1 cup*	135	0.2	0.1	<0.1	0.1	0	382	76	0.74	0.095	0.8	0	0.3	0.23	0.29	20.3	11438
sauerkraut,	15		0.0	3.0	2.0	1.0	105	0					2				
bavarian, cnd, Bush's - *1/2 cup*	130	0.0	0.0			0			0.00			0					BUSH2
cnd	27	131.4	1.3	6.1		3.6	939	43	18	0.27	0.214	1	21	0.03	0.2		0.13
1 cup	142	0.2	<0.1	<0.1	0.1	0	241	28	2.09	0.136	0.9	26	0.1	0.03	0.18	34.1	11439
shredded, cnd, Bush's	5		0.0	1.0	0.0	1.0	180	0					2				
1/2 cup	130	0.0	0.0			0			0.36			200					BUSH3
spinach, au gratin, frzn, Budget	222	116.4	6.7	11.5		2.3	654	243					27				
Gourmet - *5.5 oz pkg*	155	16.6	7.6			42			1.95			7079					22603
boiled	41	164.2	5.3	6.8		4.3	126	245	157	1.37	1.683	738	18	0.17	0.9	0.00	0.26
1 cup	180	0.5	0.1	<0.1	0.2	0	839	101	6.43	0.313	2.7	14742	1.7	0.42	0.44	262.8	11458
cnd	49	196.4	6.0	7.3		5.1	58	272	163	0.98	1.278	939	31	0.03	0.8	0.00	0.10
1 cup	214	1.1	0.2	<0.1	0.4	0	740	94	4.92	0.385	3.0	18781	2.8	0.30	0.21	209.7	11461
creamed, frzn, Green Giant	80		3.0	9.0	5.0	1.0	510	100					5				
1/2 cup	109	3.0	1.0			0			0.36			4500					GENM358
creamed, frzn, Stouffer's	169	97.3	3.5	9.0		2.3	335	141									
4.4 oz (1/2 pkg)	125	13.1	3.7	2.8	4.5	16						4564					22602
frzn, boiled	27	85.5	3.0	5.1		2.9	82	139	66	0.67	0.895	370	12	0.06	0.4	0.00	0.08
1/2 cup	95	0.2	<0.1	<0.1	0.1	0	283	46	1.44	0.134	1.6	7395	0.9	0.16	0.14	102.6	11464
raw, chopped	7	27.5	0.9	1.1		0.8	24	30	24	0.16	0.269	101	8	0.02	0.2	0.00	0.02
1 cup	30	0.1	<0.1	<0.1	<0.1	0	167	15	0.81	0.039	0.3	2015	0.6	0.06	0.06	58.2	11457
sweet potato leaves, steamed	22	56.8	1.5	4.7		1.2	8	15	39	0.17	0.147	29	1	0.07	0.6	0.00	0.13
1 cup	64	0.2	<0.1	<0.1	0.1	0	305	38	0.38	0.021	0.6	586	0.6	0.17	0.10	31.4	11506
taro leaves, steamed	35	133.6	3.9	5.8		2.9	3	125	29	0.30	0.538	307	51	0.20	1.8	0.00	0.06
1 cup	145	0.6	0.1	<0.1	0.2	0	667	39	1.71	0.203	1.3	6145		0.55	0.10	69.6	11521
turnip greens	28	153.5	3.4	4.7		2.9	24	148	20	0.21	0.289	421	15	0.05	0.5	0.00	0.16
& turnips, frzn, boiled - *1 cup*	163		0.1	<0.1	0.1	0	101	28	2.17	0.067	1.5	8412	0.4	0.11	0.09	35.9	11577
chopped, boiled	29	134.2	1.6	6.3		5.0	42	197	32	0.20	0.485	396	39	0.06	0.6	0.00	0.39
1 cup	144	0.3	0.1	<0.1	0.1	0	292	42	1.15	0.364	1.3	7917	2.5	0.10	0.26	169.9	11569
chopped, frzn, boiled	49	148.3	5.5	8.2		5.6	25	249	43	0.67	0.779	654	36	0.09	0.8	0.00	0.11
1 cup	164	0.7	0.2	<0.1	0.3	0	367	56	3.18	0.246	2.0	13079	4.8	0.12	0.11	64.0	11575
cnd	16	110.8	1.6	2.8		2.0	324	138	23	0.27	0.324	209	18	0.01	0.4	0.00	0.05
1/2 cup	117	0.4	0.1	<0.1	0.1	0	165	25	1.77	0.097	0.8	4196		0.07	0.04	48.0	11570
raw, chopped	15	50.1	0.8	3.2		1.8	22	105	17	0.10	0.256	209	33	0.04	0.3	0.00	0.21
1 cup	55	0.2	<0.1	<0.1	0.1	0	163	23	0.61	0.193	0.7	4180	1.6	0.06	0.14	106.7	11568
vinespinach, raw	19	93.1	1.8	3.4			24	109	65	0.43	0.735	400	102	0.05	0.5	0.00	0.05
3.5 oz	100	0.3				0	510	52	1.20	0.107	0.8	8000		0.16	0.24	140.0	11587
watercress, raw, chopped	4	32.3	0.8	0.4		0.2	14	41	7	0.04	0.083	80	15	0.03	0.1	0.00	0.11
1 cup	34	<0.1	<0.1	<0.1	<0.1	0	112	20	0.07	0.026	0.3	1598	0.3	0.04	0.04	3.1	11591
winged bean leaves, raw	74	76.9	5.9	14.1			9	224	8	1.28	1.367	405	45	0.83	3.5	0.00	0.14
3.5 oz	100	1.1	0.3	0.3	0.2	0	176	63	4.00	0.456	0.9	8090		0.60	0.23	16.0	11597

[1] Similar to green cabbage except that leaves are wrinkled.
[2] Made with cabbage, celery, table cream, sugar, green pepper, lemon juice, onion, pimento, vinegar, salt, dry mustard, and white pepper.
[3] European plant used as an herb and as salad greens.
[4] Used as a cooked leafy vegetable, primarily in China and Japan.
[5] Leaves from a tree native to Africa and the East Indies.
[6] Includes Boston and Bibb lettuce.
[7] Includes crisphead lettuce.

30.4 LEGUMES (BEANS & PEAS)

	KCAL	H₂0 (g)	PRO (g)	CHO (g)	SUGR (g)	DFIB (g)	Na (mg)	Ca (mg)	Mg (mg)	Zn (mg)	Mn (mg)	A (mcg RAE)	C (mg)	B-1 (mg)	NIA (mg)	B-12 (mcg)	PANT (mg)
	WT (g)	FAT (g)	SFA (g)	MUFA (g)	PUFA (g)	CHOL (mg)	K (mg)	P (mg)	Fe (mg)	Cu (mg)	Se (mcg)	A (IU)	E (mg ATE)	B-2 (mg)	B-6 (mg)	FOL (mcg DFE)	REF
adzuki beans, mature,	294	152.5	17.3	57.0		16.8	18	64	120	4.07	1.318	0	0	0.26	1.6	0.00	0.99
boiled - *1 cup*	230	0.2	0.1			0	1224	386	4.60	0.685	2.8	14		0.15	0.22	278.3	16002
cnd, sweetened	702	120.1	11.2	162.8			645	65	92	4.62	1.492	0	0	0.30	1.9	0.00	1.12
1 cup	296	0.1	<0.1			0	352	219	3.34	0.784	9.5	15		0.17	0.25	316.7	16003
w/sugar (yokan)	36	5.0	0.5	8.5			12	4	3	0.01	0.020	0	0	<0.01	<0.1	0.00	0.01
1 slice	14	<0.1	<0.1			0	6	6	0.16	0.004	0.3	<1		<0.01	<0.01	1.1	16004
baked beans, cnd,	160		6.0	32.0	13.0	6.0	510	60					0				
barbecue, Bush's - *1/2 cup*	130	1.0	0.0			0			1.80			1500					BUSH4
bold & spicy, Bush's	120		6.0	24.0	9.0	5.0	550	40					0				
1/2 cup	130	0.5	0.0			0			1.80			300					BUSH5
boston recipe, Bush's	170		6.0	32.0	6.0	6.0	440	80					0				
1/2 cup	130	1.5	0.0			0			4.50			0					BUSH6

Columns span two header rows. Group headers: **Minerals** (Na, Ca, Mg, Zn, Mn / K, P, Fe, Cu, Se) and **Vitamins** (A, C, B-1, NIA, B-12, PANT / A, E, B-2, B-6, FOL, REF).

	KCAL / WT (g)	H$_2$O (g) / FAT (g)	PRO (g) / SFA (g)	CHO (g) / MUFA (g)	SUGR (g) / PUFA (g)	DFIB (g) / CHOL (mg)	Na (mg) / K (mg)	Ca (mg) / P (mg)	Mg (mg) / Fe (mg)	Zn (mg) / Cu (mg)	Mn (mg) / Se (mcg)	A (mcg RAE) / A (IU)	C (mg) / E (mg ATE)	B-1 (mg) / B-2 (mg)	NIA (mg) / B-6 (mg)	B-12 (mcg) / FOL (mcg DFE)	PANT (mg) / REF
country style, Bush's	170		7.0	33.0	16.0	7.0	680	60					1				
1/2 cup	130	1.0	0.0			0				1.80		0					BUSH7
homestyle, Bush's	150		6.0	28.0	8.0	8.0	480	40					0				
1/2 cup	130	1.5				5				1.44		800					BUSH8
in sweet sce w/pork	281	178.9	13.4	53.1		13.2	850	154	86	3.80	0.939	15	8	0.12	0.9	0.00	0.26
1 cup	253	3.7	1.4	1.6	0.5	18	673	266	4.20	0.253	11.9	288	1.4	0.15	0.22	93.6	16010
in tomato sce w/pork	248	183.9	13.1	49.1		12.1	1113	142	89	14.83	1.240	15	8	0.13	1.3	0.00	1.34
1 cup	253	2.6	1.0	1.1	0.3	18	759	296	8.30	0.643	11.9	314	1.4	0.12	0.17	58.2	16011
maple cured bacon, Bush's	150		7.0	28.0	11.0	7.0	620	60					1				
1/2 cup	130	1.0	0.5			0				1.80		0					BUSH9
onion, Bush's	150		7.0	26.0	6.0	6.0	500	40					0				
1/2 cup	130	1.5	0.0			0				1.80		100					BUSH10
original, Bush's	150		7.0	29.0	5.0	7.0	550	60					0				
1/2 cup	130	1.0	0.0			0				1.80		0					BUSH11
baked beans, homemade	382	164.9	14.0	54.1		13.9	1068	154	109	1.85	0.645	0	3	0.34	1.0	0.00	0.39
1 cup	253	13.0	4.9	5.4	1.9	13	906	276	5.03	0.402	14.4	0		0.12	0.23	121.4	16005
baked beans, vegetarian, cnd	236	184.5	12.2	52.1		12.7	1008	127	81	3.56	0.879	23	8	0.39	1.1	0.00	0.24
1 cup	254	1.1	0.3	0.1	0.5	0	752	264	0.74	0.523	11.9	434	1.3	0.15	0.34	61.0	16006
Bush's	130		5.0	24.0	4.0	6.0	550	40					0				
1/2 cup	130	0.0	0.0			0				0.54		800					BUSH12
black bean dip, cnd, Old El Paso	25		1.0	5.0	0.0	1.0	280	0					0				
2 T	30	0.0	0.0			0				0.36		0					GENM359
black beans, mature, boiled	227	113.1	15.2	40.8		15.0	2	46	120	1.93	0.764	0	0	0.42	0.9	0.00	0.42
1 cup	172	0.9	0.2	0.1	0.4	0	611	241	3.61	0.359	2.1	10		0.10	0.12	256.3	16015
black turtle beans, mature,	241	121.6	15.1	45.0		9.8	6	102	91	1.41	0.605	0	0	0.42	1.0	0.00	0.48
boiled - 1 cup	185	0.6	0.2	0.1	0.3	0	801	281	5.27	0.498	2.2	11	0.6	0.10	0.14	159.1	16017
cnd	218	181.5	14.5	39.7		16.6	922	84	84	1.30	0.559	0	6	0.34	1.5	0.00	0.44
1 cup	240	0.7	0.2	0.1	0.3	0	739	259	4.56	0.461	3.1	10		0.29	0.13	146.4	16018
w/kombu seaweed, cnd, Eden Foods	100		7.0	18.0	0.0	6.0	15	60	60	1.20			0	0.09	0.4		
1/2 cup	130	0.0	0.0			0	280	100	1.80			0		0.07			EDEN2
broadbeans (fava beans), mature,	187	121.6	12.9	33.4		9.2	9	61	73	1.72	0.716	2	1	0.16	1.2	0.00	0.27
boiled - 1 cup	170	0.7	0.1	0.1	0.3	0	456	213	2.55	0.440	4.4	26	0.2	0.15	0.12	176.8	16053
cnd	182	205.6	14.0	31.8		9.5	1160	67	82	1.59	0.737	3	5	0.05	2.5	0.00	0.30
1 cup	256	0.6	0.1	0.1	0.2	0	620	202	2.56	0.279	4.6	26		0.13	0.12	84.5	16054
falafel, homemade[1]	57	5.9	2.3	5.4			50	9	14	0.26	0.117	<1	<1	0.02	0.2	0.00	0.05
.6 oz patty (2 1/4" dia)	17	3.0	0.4	1.7	0.7	0	99	33	0.58	0.044	0.2	2		0.03	0.02	17.7	16138
chickpeas (garbanzo beans),	269	98.7	14.5	45.0		12.5	11	80	79	2.51	1.689	2	2	0.19	0.9	0.00	0.47
boiled - 1 cup	164	4.2	0.4	1.0	1.9	0	477	276	4.74	0.577	6.1	44	0.6	0.10	0.23	282.1	16057
cnd	286	167.3	11.9	54.3		10.6	718	77	70	2.54	1.450	2	9	0.07	0.3	0.00	0.72
1 cup	240	2.7	0.3	0.6	1.2	0	413	216	3.24	0.418	6.7	58		0.08	1.14	160.8	16058
hummus, commercial[2]	23	9.3	1.1	2.0		0.8	53	5	10	0.26	0.108	<1		0.03	0.1	0.00	0.02
1 T	14	1.3	0.2	0.6	0.5	0	32	25	0.34	0.074	0.4	4		0.01	0.03	11.6	16158
hummus, homemade[2]	26	9.7	0.7	3.0		0.8	37	8	4	0.17	0.085	<1	1	0.01	0.1	0.00	0.04
1 T	15	1.3	0.2	0.5	0.5	0	26	17	0.24	0.034	0.4	4	0.2	0.01	0.06	8.9	16137
w/kombu seaweed, cnd, Eden Foods	120		7.0	19.0	0.0	5.0	10	60	60	1.50			0	0.09	0.4		
1/2 cup	130	1.5	0.0			0	250	100	1.40			0		0.07			EDEN4
chili beans, cnd, Bush's	120		6.0	20.0		6.0	480	20					1				
1/2 cup	130	1.0				0				1.44		500					BUSH13
cowpeas (blackeye peas), immature[3],	160	124.5	5.2	33.5		8.3	7	211	86	1.70	0.944	66	4	0.17	2.3	0.00	0.25
boiled - 1 cup	165	0.6	0.2	0.1	0.3	0	690	84	1.85	0.219	4.1	1305	0.4	0.24	0.11	209.6	11192
frzn, boiled	224	112.4	14.4	40.4		10.9	9	39	85	2.41	1.345	7	4	0.44	1.2	0.00	0.36
1 cup	170	1.1	0.3	0.1	0.5	0	638	207	3.60	0.313	5.8	128	0.7	0.11	0.16	239.7	11196
cowpeas (blackeye peas), mature[3],	200	120.5	13.3	35.7		11.2	7	41	91	2.22	0.817	2	1	0.35	0.9	0.00	0.71
boiled - 1 cup	172	0.9	0.2	0.1	0.4	0	478	268	4.32	0.461	4.3	26	0.5	0.09	0.17	357.8	16063
cnd	185	191.1	11.4	32.7		7.9	718	48	67	1.68	0.679	2	6	0.18	0.8	0.00	0.46
1 cup	240	1.3	0.3	0.1	0.6	0	413	168	2.33	0.281	5.5	31		0.18	0.11	122.4	16064
cowpeas (blackeye peas), young pods w/seeds, boiled[3] - 1 cup	32	85.0	2.5	6.7			3	52	39	0.23	0.208	67	16	0.09	0.8	0.00	0.61
	95	0.3	0.1	<0.1	0.1	0	186	47	0.67	0.067	0.7	1330		0.09	0.12	24.7	11198
cowpeas, catjang, mature, boiled	200	119.2	13.9	34.7		6.2	32	44	164	3.20	0.809	2	1	0.28	1.2	0.00	0.66
1 cup	171	1.2	0.3	0.1	0.5	0	641	243	5.22	0.463	4.3	17		0.08	0.16	242.8	16061
cranberry (roman) beans, mature,	241	114.4	16.5	43.3		17.7	2	89	89	2.02	0.655	0	0	0.37	0.9	0.00	0.42
boiled - 1 cup	177	0.8	0.2	0.1	0.4	0	685	239	3.70	0.409	2.3	0		0.12	0.14	366.4	16020

	KCAL / WT (g)	H₂O (g) / FAT (g)	PRO (g) / SFA (g)	CHO (g) / MUFA (g)	SUGR (g) / PUFA (g)	DFIB (g) / CHOL (mg)	Na (mg) / K (mg)	Ca (mg) / P (mg)	Mg (mg) / Fe (mg)	Zn (mg) / Cu (mg)	Mn (mg) / Se (mcg)	A (mcg RAE) / A (IU)	C (mg) / E (mg ATE)	B-1 (mg) / B-2 (mg)	NIA (mg) / B-6 (mg)	B-12 (mcg) / FOL (mcg DFE)	PANT (mg) / REF
cnd	216	201.7	14.4	39.3		16.4	863	88	83	2.18	0.520	0	2	0.10	1.3	0.00	0.37
1 cup	260	0.7	0.2	0.1	0.3	0	676	224	4.03	0.369	8.1	0		0.10	0.14	200.2	16021
french beans, mature, boiled	228	117.8	12.5	42.5		16.6	11	112	99	1.13	0.676	0	2	0.23	1.0	0.00	0.39
1 cup	177	1.3	0.1	0.1	0.8	0	655	181	1.91	0.204	2.1	5		0.11	0.19	132.8	16023
great northern beans, mature, boiled - *1 cup*	209	122.1	14.7	37.3		12.4	4	120	89	1.56	0.917	0	2	0.28	1.2	0.00	0.47
	177	0.8	0.2	<0.1	0.3	0	692	292	3.77	0.437	7.3	2		0.10	0.21	180.5	16025
cnd	299	183.1	19.3	55.1		12.8	10	139	134	1.70	1.069	0	3	0.37	1.2	0.00	0.73
1 cup	262	1.0	0.3	<0.1	0.4	0	920	356	4.11	0.419	10.7	3		0.16	0.28	212.2	16026
hyacinth beans, immature, boiled	44	75.6	2.6	8.0			2	36	37	0.33	0.183	6	4	0.05	0.4	0.00	0.05
1 cup	87	0.2	0.1	0.1	<0.1	0	228	43	0.66	0.042	1.4	124		0.08	0.02	40.9	11225
hyacinth beans, mature, boiled	227	134.1	15.8	40.2			14	78	159	5.53	0.935	0	0	0.52	0.8	0.00	0.61
1 cup	194	1.1	0.2			0	654	233	8.89	0.662	5.4	0		0.07	0.07	7.8	16068
kidney beans, mature, all types, boiled - *1 cup*	225	118.5	15.3	40.4		11.3	4	50	80	1.89	0.844	0	2	0.28	1.0	0.00	0.39
	177	0.9	0.1	0.1	0.5	0	713	251	5.20	0.428	2.1	0	0.4	0.10	0.21	230.1	16028
all types, cnd	207	199.6	13.3	38.1		9.0	888	69	79	1.41	0.556	0	3	0.28	1.3	0.00	0.37
1 cup	256	0.8	0.1	0.1	0.4	0	658	269	3.15	0.384	3.1	0		0.18	0.18	125.4	16029c
CA red, boiled	207	199.6	13.3	38.1		9.0	888	69	79	1.41	0.556	0	3	0.28	1.3	0.00	0.37
1 cup	256	0.8	0.1	0.1	0.4	0	658	269	3.15	0.384	3.1	0		0.18	0.18	125.4	16029b
dark w/kombu seaweed, cnd, Eden Foods - *1/2 cup*	100		8.0	18.0	0.0	10.0	15	60	40	1.20			0	0.15	0.4		
	130	0.0	0.0			0	440	150	1.44					0.03			EDEN16
red, boiled	225	118.5	15.3	40.4		13.1	4	50	80	1.89	0.844	0	2	0.28	1.0	0.00	0.39
1 cup	177	0.9	0.1	0.1	0.5	0	713	251	5.20	0.428	2.1	0	0.1	0.10	0.21	230.1	16033
red, cnd	218	198.0	13.4	39.9		16.4	873	61	72	1.41	0.620	0	3	0.27	1.2	0.00	0.38
1 cup	256	0.9	0.1	0.1	0.5	0	658	241	3.23	0.384	3.1	0	0.1	0.23	0.06	130.6	16034
royal red, boiled	218	118.6	16.8	38.7		16.5	9	78	74	4.90	0.464	5		0.17	1.0	0.00	0.39
1 cup	177	0.3	<0.1	<0.1	0.2	0	669	251	4.90	0.464	2.1	5		0.12	0.18	131.0	16036
lentils, mature, boiled	230	137.9	17.9	39.9		15.6	4	38	71	2.51	0.978	0	3	0.33	2.1	0.00	1.26
1 cup	198	0.8	0.1	0.1	0.3	0	731	356	6.59	0.497	5.5	16	0.2	0.14	0.35	358.4	16070
lima beans, fordhook, frzn, boiled - *1/2 cup*	85	62.5	5.2	16.0		4.9	45	19	29	0.37	0.264	9	11	0.06	0.9	0.00	0.14
	85	0.3	0.1	<0.1	0.1	0	347	54	1.16	0.047	1.4	162	0.2	0.05	0.10	17.9	11038
lima beans, immature, baby, frzn, boiled - *1/2 cup*	95	65.1	6.0	17.5		5.4	26	25	50	0.50	0.732	7	5	0.06	0.7	0.00	0.16
	90	0.3	0.1	<0.1	0.1	0	370	101	1.76	0.177	1.5	150	0.6	0.05	0.10	14.4	11040
boiled	209	114.2	11.6	40.2		9.0	29	54	126	1.34	2.128	32	17	0.24	1.8	0.00	0.44
1 cup	170	0.5	0.1	<0.1	0.3	0	969	221	4.17	0.519	3.4	629	0.2	0.16	0.33	44.2	11032
lima beans, mature, baby, boiled - *1 cup*	229	122.2	14.6	42.4		14.0	5	53	96	1.87	1.065	0	0	0.29	1.2	0.00	0.86
	182	0.7	0.2	0.1	0.3	0	730	231	4.37	0.391	8.9	0		0.10	0.14	273.0	16075
large, boiled	216	131.2	14.7	39.3		13.2	4	32	81	1.79	0.970	0	0	0.30	0.8	0.00	0.79
1 cup	188	0.7	0.2	0.1	0.3	0	955	209	4.49	0.442	8.5	0	0.3	0.10	0.30	156.0	16072
large, cnd	190	185.8	11.9	35.9		11.6	810	51	94	1.57	0.875	0	0	0.13	0.6	0.00	0.62
1 cup	241	0.4	0.1	<0.1	0.2	0	530	178	4.36	0.434	10.8	0		0.08	0.22	120.5	16073
lupins, mature, boiled	198	118.0	25.8	16.4		4.6	7	85	90	2.29	1.122	0	2	0.22	0.6	0.00	0.31
1 cup	166	4.8	0.6	2.0	1.2	0	407	212	1.99	0.383	4.3	12		0.09	0.01	97.9	16077
mothbeans, mature, boiled	207	122.5	13.8	37.1			18	5	184	1.04	0.933	2	2	0.22	1.2	0.00	0.69
1 cup	177	1.0	0.2	0.1	0.5	0	538	266	5.56	0.290	5.0	18		0.04	0.16	253.1	16079
mung beans, mature, boiled	212	146.8	14.2	38.7		15.4	4	55	97	1.70	0.602	2	2	0.33	1.2	0.00	0.83
1 cup	202	0.8	0.2	0.1	0.3	0	537	200	2.83	0.315	5.1	48	1.0	0.12	0.14	321.2	16081
mungo beans, mature, boiled	189	130.5	13.6	33.0		11.5	13	95	113	1.49	0.742	4	2	0.27	2.7	0.00	0.78
1 cup	180	1.0	0.1	0.1	0.6	0	416	281	3.15	0.250	4.5	56	0.3	0.14	0.10	169.2	16084
navy beans, mature, baked w/sorghum, cnd, Eden Foods - *1/2 cup*	150		8.0	27.0	6.0	7.0	130	100	80	1.50			0	0.06	0.8		
	130	0.0	0.0			0	460	150	3.60					0.14			EDEN1
boiled	258	115.0	15.8	47.9		11.6	2	127	107	1.93	1.012	0	2	0.37	1.0	0.00	0.46
1 cup	182	1.0	0.3	0.1	0.4	0	670	286	4.51	0.537	10.6	4		0.11	0.30	254.8	16038
cnd	296	184.6	19.7	53.6		13.4	1174	123	123	2.02	0.983	0	2	0.37	1.3	0.00	0.45
1 cup	262	1.1	0.3	0.1	0.5	0	755	351	4.85	0.545	15.2	3	1.0	0.14	0.27	162.4	16039
w/kombu seaweed, cnd, Eden Foods *1/2 cup*	110		7.0	20.0	0.0	7.0	15	80	60	0.90			0	0.12	0.4		
	130	0.5	0.0			0	300	150	2.70					0.03			EDEN17
peas, green, boiled - *1 cup*	134	124.6	8.6	25.0		8.8	5	43	62	1.90	0.840	48	23	0.41	3.2	0.00	0.24
	160	0.4	0.1	<0.1	0.2	0	434	187	2.46	0.277	3.0	955	0.6	0.24	0.35	100.8	11305
cnd	117	138.9	7.5	21.4		7.0	428	34	29	1.21	0.515	65	16	0.21	1.2	0.00	0.22
1 cup	170	0.6	0.1	0.1	0.3	0	294	114	1.62	0.139	2.9	1306	0.6	0.13	0.11	74.8	11308
frzn, boiled	62	63.6	4.1	11.4		4.4	70	19	23	0.75	0.331	26	8	0.23	1.2	0.00	0.11
1/2 cup	80	0.2	<0.1	<0.1	0.1	0	134	72	1.26	0.111	0.8	534	0.1	0.08	0.09	47.2	11313

	KCAL / WT (g)	H₂0 (g) / FAT (g)	PRO (g) / SFA (g)	CHO (g) / MUFA (g)	SUGR (g) / PUFA (g)	DFIB (g) / CHOL (mg)	Na (mg) / K (mg)	Ca (mg) / P (mg)	Mg (mg) / Fe (mg)	Zn (mg) / Cu (mg)	Mn (mg) / Se (mcg)	A (mcg RAE) / A (IU)	C (mg) / E (mg ATE)	B-1 (mg) / B-2 (mg)	NIA (mg) / B-6 (mg)	B-12 (mcg) / FOL (mcg DFE)	PANT (mg) / REF
raw	117	114.3	7.9	21.0		7.4	7	36	48	1.80	0.595	46	58	0.39	3.0	0.00	0.15
1 cup	145	0.6	0.1	<0.1	0.3	0	354	157	2.13	0.255	2.6	928	0.6	0.19	0.25	94.3	11304
w/onions, red peppers, & garlic, cnd	57	98.6	3.5	10.5		2.3	290	17	17	0.74	0.306	25	13	0.11	0.8	0.00	0.10
1/2 cup	114	0.3	0.1	<0.1	0.1	0	139	62	1.37	0.113	1.5	494		0.08	0.11	33.1	11310
peas, split, mature, boiled	231	136.2	16.3	41.4		16.3	4	27	71	1.96	0.776	0	1	0.37	1.7	0.00	1.17
1 cup	196	0.8	0.1	0.2	0.3	0	710	194	2.53	0.355	1.2	14	0.8	0.11	0.09	127.4	16086
pigeon peas (red gram), immature,	170	109.9	9.1	29.8		9.5	8	63	61	1.25	0.690	11	43	0.54	3.3	0.00	0.96
boiled - 1 cup	153	2.1	0.6	<0.1	1.4	0	698	181	2.40	0.161	1.8	199	0.3	0.25	0.08	153.0	11345
pigeon peas (red gram), mature,	203	115.2	11.4	39.1		11.3	8	72	77	1.51	0.842	0	0	0.25	1.3	0.00	0.54
boiled - 1 cup	168	0.6	0.1	<0.1	0.3	0	645	200	1.86	0.452	4.9	5		0.10	0.08	186.5	16102
pink beans, mature, boiled	252	103.4	15.3	47.2		9.0	3	88	110	1.62	0.926	0	0	0.43	1.0	0.00	0.51
1 cup	169	0.8	0.2	0.1	0.4	0	859	279	3.89	0.458	2.4	0	0.7	0.11	0.30	283.9	16041
pinto beans, mature,	234	109.9	14.0	43.9		14.7	3	82	94	1.85	0.951	0	4	0.32	0.7	0.00	0.49
boiled - 1 cup	171	0.9	0.2	0.2	0.3	0	800	274	4.46	0.439	12.1	3	1.6	0.16	0.27	294.1	16043
cnd	206	186.1	11.7	36.6		11.0	706	103	65	1.66	0.550	2	2	0.24	0.7	0.00	0.33
1 cup	240	1.9	0.4	0.4	0.7	0	583	221	3.50	0.336	17.0	58	2.3	0.15	0.18	144.0	16044
w/kombu seaweed, cnd, Eden Foods	100		6.0	18.0	0.0	6.0	15	60	40	0.90			0	0.15	0.4	0.00	0.00
1/2 cup	130	0.0	0.0	0.0		0	350	100	1.80	0.000		0		0.03	0.00	0.0	EDEN18
refried beans[4],	237	191.4	13.8	39.1		13.4	753	88	83	2.95	0.396	0	15	0.07	0.8	0.00	0.24
cnd - 1 cup	252	3.2	1.2	1.4	0.4	20	673	217	4.18	0.421	3.3	0	0.0	0.04	0.36	27.7	16103
cnd, Old El Paso	100		6.0	17.0	1.0	6.0	570	40				0					0.00	
1/2 cup	120	0.5	0.0			0			1.80			0					GENM360
fat free, cnd, Old El Paso	100		6.0	18.0	1.0	6.0	480	40				0						
1/2 cup	124	0.0	0.0			0			1.80			0					GENM361
vegetarian, cnd, Old El Paso	100		6.0	17.0	2.0	6.0	490	40				0						
1/2 cup	118	1.0	0.0			0			1.80			0					GENM362
w/cheese, cnd, Old El Paso	130		7.0	18.0	1.0	6.0	500	80				0						
1/2 cup	120	3.5	1.5			5			1.80			0					GENM363
w/green chilies, cnd, Old El Paso	100		6.0	19.0	1.0	6.0	550	40				0						
1/2 cup	122	0.5	0.0			<5			1.80			0					GENM364
w/sausage, cnd, Old El Paso	200		7.0	14.0	1.0	4.0	360	40				0						
1/2 cup	118	13.0	5.0			10			1.80			0					GENM365
shellie (shell) beans, cnd	74	222.2	4.3	15.2		8.3	818	71	37	0.66	0.936	27	8	0.08	0.5	0.00	0.33
1 cup	245	0.5	0.1	<0.1	0.3	0	267	74	2.43	0.196	2.0	559	0.1	0.13	0.12	44.1	11050
soybeans, green, boiled	254	123.5	22.2	19.9		7.6	25	261	108	1.64	0.904	14	31	0.47	2.3	0.00	0.23
1 cup	180	11.5	1.3	2.2	5.4	0	970	284	4.50	0.211	2.5	281	<0.1	0.28	0.11	199.8	11451
soybeans, mature,	298	107.6	28.6	17.1		10.3	2	175	148	1.98	1.417	0	3	0.27	0.7	0.00	0.31
boiled - 1 cup	172	15.4	2.2	3.4	8.7	0	886	421	8.84	0.700	12.6	15	3.4	0.49	0.40	92.9	16109
raw	774	15.9	67.9	56.1		17.3	4	515	521	9.10	4.682	2	11	1.63	3.0	0.00	1.47
1 cup	186	37.1	5.4	8.2	20.9	0	3342	1309	29.20	3.084	33.1	45	3.6	1.62	0.70	697.5	16108
white beans, mature,	249	112.9	17.4	44.9		11.3	11	161	113	2.47	1.138	0	0	0.21	0.3	0.00	0.41
boiled - 1 cup	179	0.6	0.2	0.1	0.3	0	1004	202	6.62	0.514	2.3	0	0.4	0.08	0.17	145.0	16050
cnd	307	183.7	19.0	57.5		12.6	13	191	134	2.93	1.349	0	0	0.25	0.3	0.00	0.48
1 cup	262	0.8	0.2	0.1	0.3	0	1189	238	7.83	0.608	4.2	0		0.10	0.20	170.3	16051
small, boiled	254	113.2	16.1	46.2		18.6	4	131	122	1.95	0.913	0	0	0.42	0.5	0.00	0.45
1 cup	179	1.1	0.3	0.1	0.5	0	829	303	5.08	0.267	2.3	0		0.11	0.23	245.2	16046
winged beans, immature, boiled	24	55.9	3.3	2.0			2	38	19	0.17	0.098	2	6	0.05	0.4	0.00	0.03
1 cup	62	0.4	0.1	0.1	0.1	0	170	16	0.68	0.023	0.7	55		0.04	0.05	21.7	11596
winged beans, mature, boiled	253	115.6	18.3	25.7			22	244	93	2.48	2.062	0	0	0.51	1.4	0.00	0.27
1 cup	172	10.0	1.4	3.7	2.7	0	482	263	7.45	1.330	5.0	0		0.22	0.08	17.2	16136
yardlong bean, immature, sliced,	49	91.0	2.6	9.5			4	46	44	0.37	0.209	24	17	0.09	0.7	0.00	0.05
boiled[5] - 1 cup	104	0.1	<0.1	<0.1	<0.1	0	302	59	1.02	0.049	1.6	468		0.10	0.02	46.8	11200
yardlong bean, mature, boiled[5]	202	117.6	14.2	36.1		6.5	9	72	168	1.85	0.833	2	1	0.36	0.9	0.00	0.68
1 cup	171	0.8	0.2	0.1	0.3	0	539	310	4.51	0.385	4.8	27		0.11	0.16	249.7	16134
yellow beans, mature, boiled	255	111.5	16.2	44.7		18.4	9	110	131	1.88	0.805	0	3	0.33	1.3	0.00	0.41
1 cup	177	1.9	0.5	0.2	0.8	0	575	324	4.39	0.329	2.3	4		0.18	0.23	143.4	16048

[1] Made with broadbeans, soy oil, onions, flour, salt, garlic, coriander, and cumin.
[2] Made with chickpeas, lemon juice, tahini, olive oil, and garlic.
[3] Also called crowder peas and southern peas.
[4] Usually made from mashed pinto beans with the addition of lard.
[5] A type of Asian cowpea that grows up to 3 feet in length.

	KCAL	H₂O (g)	PRO (g)	CHO (g)	SUGR (g)	DFIB (g)	Na (mg)	Ca (mg)	Mg (mg)	Zn (mg)	Mn (mg)	A (mcg RAE)	C (mg)	B-1 (mg)	NIA (mg)	B-12 (mcg)	PANT (mg)
	WT (g)	FAT (g)	SFA (g)	MUFA (g)	PUFA (g)	CHOL (mg)	K (mg)	P (mg)	Fe (mg)	Cu (mg)	Se (mcg)	A (IU)	E (mg ATE)	B-2 (mg)	B-6 (mg)	FOL (mcg DFE)	REF

30.5 SPROUT & SHOOT VEGETABLES

	KCAL/WT	H₂O/FAT	PRO/SFA	CHO/MUFA	SUGR/PUFA	DFIB/CHOL	Na/K	Ca/P	Mg/Fe	Zn/Cu	Mn/Se	A/A	C/E	B-1/B-2	NIA/B-6	B-12/FOL	PANT/REF
alfalfa sprouts, raw	10	30.1	1.3	1.2		0.8	2	11	9	0.30	0.062	3	3	0.03	0.2	0.00	0.19
1 cup	33	0.2	<0.1	<0.1	0.1	0	26	23	0.32	0.052	0.2	51	<0.1	0.04	0.01	11.9	11001
bamboo shoots,	14	115.1	1.8	2.3		1.2	5	14	4	0.56	0.136	0	0	0.02	0.4	0.00	0.08
boiled - *1 cup*	120	0.3	0.1	<0.1	0.1	0	640	24	0.29	0.098	0.5	0		0.06	0.12	2.4	11027
cnd	25	123.6	2.3	4.2		1.8	9	10	5	0.85	0.206	0	1	0.03	0.2	0.00	0.12
1 cup	131	0.5	0.1	<0.1	0.2	0	105	33	0.42	0.149	0.7	10	0.5	0.03	0.18	3.9	11028
raw	41	137.4	3.9	7.9		3.3	6	20	5	1.66	0.396	2	6	0.23	0.9	0.00	0.24
1 cup	151	0.5	0.1	<0.1	0.2	0	805	89	0.76	0.287	1.2	30	1.5	0.11	0.36	10.6	11026
kidney bean sprouts, boiled	41	111.6	6.0	5.9			9	24	29	0.55	0.249	0	45	0.45	3.8	0.00	0.48
1 cup	125	0.7	0.1	0.1	0.4	0	243	48	1.11	0.218	0.8	3		0.34	0.12	58.8	11030
lentil sprouts, stir-fried	126	85.9	11.0	26.6			13	18	44	2.00	0.628	3	16	0.28	1.5	0.00	0.71
1 cup	125	0.6	0.1	0.1	0.3	0	355	191	3.88	0.421	0.8	51		0.11	0.21	83.8	11249
mung bean sprouts,	26	115.8	2.5	5.2		1.0	12	15	17	0.58	0.174	1	14	0.06	1.0	0.00	0.30
boiled - *1 cup*	124	0.1	<0.1	<0.1	<0.1	0	125	35	0.81	0.151	0.7	17	<0.1	0.13	0.07	36.0	11044
cnd	15	120.1	1.8	2.7		1.0	175	18	11	0.35	0.091	1	<1	0.04	0.3	0.00	0.18
1 cup	125	0.1	<0.1	<0.1	<0.1	0	34	40	0.54	0.196	0.8	29	<0.1	0.09	0.04	12.5	11626
raw	31	94.0	3.2	6.2		1.9	6	14	22	0.43	0.196	1	14	0.09	0.8	0.00	0.40
1 cup	104	0.2	<0.1	<0.1	0.1	0	155	56	0.95	0.171	0.6	22	<0.1	0.13	0.09	63.4	11043
stir-fried	62	104.5	5.3	13.1		2.4	11	16	41	1.12	0.362	2	20	0.17	1.5	0.00	0.69
1 cup	124	0.3	<0.1	0.1	0.1	0	272	98	2.36	0.316	0.7	38		0.22	0.16	86.8	11045
navy bean sprouts, boiled	98	95.0	8.8	18.8			18	20	139	1.21	0.558	0	22	0.48	1.6	0.00	1.07
1 cup	125	1.0	0.1	0.1	0.6	0	396	129	2.64	0.486	0.8	5		0.29	0.25	132.5	11047
pea sprouts, boiled	148	93.0	8.8	27.3			4	33	51	0.98	0.406	6	8	0.27	1.3	0.00	0.85
1 cup	125	0.6	0.1	0.1	0.3	0	335	30	2.09	0.025	0.8	134		0.36	0.16	45.0	11317
pokeberry shoots (poke), boiled	33	153.3	3.8	5.1		2.5	30	87	23	0.31	0.554	718	135	0.12	1.8	0.00	0.06
1 cup	165	0.7	0.2	<0.1	0.3	0	304	54	1.98	0.208	1.5	14355	1.4	0.41	0.18	14.9	11351
radish seed sprouts, raw	16	34.2	1.4	1.4			2	19	17	0.21	0.099	8	11	0.04	1.1	0.00	0.28
1 cup	38	1.0	0.3	0.2	0.4	0	33	43	0.33	0.046	0.2	149		0.04	0.11	36.1	11676
soy sprouts,	43	24.2	4.6	3.3		0.4	5	23	25	0.41	0.246	<1	5	0.12	0.4	0.00	0.33
raw - *1/2 cup*	35	2.3	0.3	0.5	1.3	0	169	57	0.74	0.149	0.2	4		0.04	0.06	60.2	11452
steamed	76	74.7	8.0	6.1		0.8	9	55	56	0.98	0.667	1	8	0.19	1.0	0.00	0.70
1 cup	94	4.2	0.6	0.9	2.4	0	334	127	1.23	0.310	0.6	10	<0.1	0.05	0.10	75.2	11453
stir-fried	156	84.0	16.4	11.8		1.0	18	103	120	2.63	1.416	1	15	0.53	1.4	0.00	1.48
1 cup	125	8.9	1.2	2.0	5.0	0	709	270	0.50	0.659	0.8	21		0.24	0.21	158.8	11454
taro shoots, sliced, ckd	20	133.4	1.0	4.5			3	20	11	0.76	0.182	4	26	0.05	1.1	0.00	0.11
1 cup	140	0.1	<0.1	<0.1	<0.1	0	482	36	0.57	0.132	1.4	71		0.07	0.16	4.2	11523

30.6 TUBER & ROOT VEGETABLES

	KCAL/WT	H₂O/FAT	PRO/SFA	CHO/MUFA	SUGR/PUFA	DFIB/CHOL	Na/K	Ca/P	Mg/Fe	Zn/Cu	Mn/Se	A/A	C/E	B-1/B-2	NIA/B-6	B-12/FOL	PANT/REF
arrowhead, boiled	9	9.2	0.5	1.9			2	1	6	0.03	0.034	0	<1	0.02	0.1	0.00	0.05
1 med	12	<0.1				0	106	24	0.15	0.016	0.1	0		0.01	0.02	1.1	11006
arrowroot, raw, sliced	78	96.9	5.1	16.1		1.6	31	7	30	0.76	0.209	1	2	0.17	2.0	0.00	0.35
1 cup	120	0.2	<0.1	<0.1	0.1	0	545	118	2.66	0.145	0.8	23		0.07	0.32	405.6	11697
beet (beetroot),	37	74.0	1.4	8.5		1.7	65	14	20	0.30	0.277	2	3	0.02	0.3	0.00	0.12
sliced, boiled - *1/2 cup*	85	0.2	<0.1	<0.1	0.1	0	259	32	0.67	0.063	0.6	30	0.3	0.03	0.06	68.0	11081
sliced, cnd	53	154.6	1.5	12.2		2.9	330	26	29	0.36	0.488	2	7	0.02	0.3	0.00	0.27
1 cup	170	0.2	<0.1	<0.1	0.1	0	252	29	3.09	0.100	0.9	19	0.5	0.07	0.10	51.0	11084
sliced, harvard, cnd	180	197.2	2.1	44.7		6.2	399	27	47	0.57	0.593	2	6	0.02	0.2	0.00	0.37
1 cup	246	0.1	<0.1	<0.1	<0.1	0	403	42	0.89	0.239	2.7	27		0.12	0.14	71.3	11605
sliced, pickled, cnd	148	185.9	1.8	37.0		5.9	599	25	34	0.59	0.499	2	5	0.02	0.6	0.00	0.31
1 cup	227	0.2	<0.1	<0.1	0.1	0	336	39	0.93	0.263	2.3	25		0.11	0.11	61.3	11609
burdock root, boiled	110	94.6	2.6	26.4		2.3	5	61	49	0.48	0.338	0	3	0.05	0.4	0.00	0.44
1 cup pieces	125	0.2	<0.1	<0.1	0.1	0	450	116	0.96	0.111	1.1	0	0.2	0.07	0.35	25.0	11105
butterbur (fuki), boiled	8	96.7	0.2	2.2			4	59	8	0.09	0.156	1	19	0.01	0.1	0.00	0.02
3.5 oz	100	<0.1				0	354	7	0.10	0.059	0.9	27		0.01	0.05	4.0	11107

	KCAL / WT (g)	H₂0 (g) / FAT (g)	PRO (g) / SFA (g)	CHO (g) / MUFA (g)	SUGR (g) / PUFA (g)	DFIB (g) / CHOL (mg)	Na (mg) / K (mg)	Ca (mg) / P (mg)	Mg (mg) / Fe (mg)	Zn (mg) / Cu (mg)	Mn (mg) / Se (mcg)	A (mcg RAE) / A (IU)	C (mg) / E (mg ATE)	B-1 (mg) / B-2 (mg)	NIA (mg) / B-6 (mg)	B-12 (mcg) / FOL (mcg DFE)	PANT (mg) / REF
carrots,	4	9.0	0.1	0.8		0.2	4	2	1	0.02	0.008	75	1	<0.01	0.1	0.00	0.02
baby, raw - *1 med*	10	0.1	<0.1	<0.1	<0.1	0	28	4	0.08	0.005	0.1	1501		<0.01	0.01	3.3	11960
honey glazed, frzn, Green Giant	90		<1.0	13.0	10.0	2.0	180	20				6000	0				
1 cup	115	3.5	0.5						0.00			6000					GENM366
raw	31	63.2	0.7	7.3		2.2	25	19	11	0.14	0.102	1012	7	0.07	0.7	0.00	0.14
1 large (7 1/2" long)	72	0.1	<0.1	<0.1	0.1	0	233	32	0.36	0.034	0.8	20253	0.3	0.04	0.11	10.1	11124
sliced, boiled	35	68.2	0.9	8.2		2.6	51	24	10	0.23	0.587	958	2	0.03	0.4	0.00	0.24
1/2 cup	78	0.1	<0.1	<0.1	0.1	0	177	23	0.48	0.105	0.6	19152	0.3	0.04	0.19	10.9	11125
sliced, cnd	37	135.7	0.9	8.1		2.2	353	37	12	0.38	0.657	1006	4	0.03	0.8	0.00	0.20
1 cup	146	0.3	0.1	<0.1	0.1	0	261	35	0.93	0.152	0.6	20110	0.6	0.04	0.16	13.1	11128
sliced, frzn	53	131.2	1.7	12.0		5.1	86	41	15	0.35	0.591	1292	4	0.04	0.6	0.00	0.24
1 cup	146	0.2	<0.1	<0.1	0.1	0	231	38	0.69	0.107	0.9	25845	0.6	0.05	0.19	16.1	11131
cassava, raw[1]	330	122.9	2.8	78.4		3.7	29	33	43	0.70	0.791	2	42	0.18	1.8	0.00	0.22
1 cup	206	0.6	0.2	0.2	0.1	0	558	56	0.56	0.206	1.4	52	0.4	0.10	0.18	55.6	11134
celeriac (celery root), boiled	42	143.1	1.5	9.1		1.9	95	40	19	0.31	0.149	0	6	0.04	0.7	0.00	0.31
1 cup pieces	155	0.3				0	268	102	0.67	0.067	0.6	0		0.06	0.16	4.7	11142
chicory root, raw	44	48.0	0.8	10.5			30	25	13	0.20	0.140	0	3	0.02	0.2	0.00	0.19
1 root	60	0.1	<0.1	<0.1	0.1	0	174	37	0.48	0.046	0.4	4		0.02	0.14	13.8	11154
garlic, raw	13	5.3	0.6	3.0		0.2	2	16	2	0.10	0.150	0	3	0.02	0.1	0.00	0.05
3 cloves	9	<0.1	<0.1	<0.1	<0.1	0	36	14	0.15	0.027	1.3	0	<0.1	0.01	0.11	0.3	11215
jerusalem artichoke (sunchoke), raw, sliced - *1 cup*	114	117.0	3.0	26.2		2.4	6	21	26	0.18	0.090	2	6	0.30	2.0	0.00	0.60
	150	<0.1	0.0	<0.1	<0.1	0	644	117	5.10	0.210	1.1	30	0.3	0.09	0.12	19.5	11226
jicama (yambean), boiled - *3.5 oz*	38	90.1	0.7	8.8			4	11	11	0.15	0.057	1	14	0.02	0.2	0.00	0.12
	100	0.1				0	135	16	0.57	0.046	0.7	19		0.03	0.04	8.0	11604
raw, sliced	46	108.1	0.9	10.6		5.9	5	14	14	0.19	0.072	1	24	0.02	0.2	0.00	0.16
1 cup	120	0.1	<0.1	<0.1	0.1	0	180	22	0.72	0.058	0.8	25	0.5	0.03	0.05	14.4	11603
lotus root, raw, sliced - *10 slices (2 1/2" dia)*	60	64.1	2.1	14.0		4.0	32	36	19	0.32	0.211	0	36	0.13	0.3	0.00	0.31
	81	0.1	<0.1	<0.1	<0.1	0	450	81	0.94	0.208	0.6	0		0.18	0.21	10.5	11254
sliced, boiled	59	72.5	1.4	14.3		2.8	40	23	20	0.29	0.196	0	24	0.11	0.3	0.00	0.27
10 slices (2 1/2" dia)	89	0.1	<0.1	<0.1	<0.1	0	323	69	0.80	0.193	0.5	0	<0.1	0.01	0.19	7.1	11255
mountain yam, hawaiian, cubed, steamed - *1 cup*	119	111.9	2.5	29.0			17	12	15	0.46	0.410	0	0	0.12	0.2	0.00	0.70
	145	0.1	<0.1	<0.1	0.1	0	718	58	0.62	0.187	1.3	0		0.02	0.30	17.4	11259
onion, chopped, boiled - *1 cup*	92	184.5	2.9	21.3		2.9	6	46	23	0.44	0.321	0	11	0.09	0.3	0.00	0.24
	210	0.4	0.1	0.1	0.2	0	349	74	0.50	0.141	1.3	0	0.3	0.05	0.27	31.5	11283
chopped, cnd	21	105.4	1.0	4.5		1.3	416	50	7	0.32	0.114	0	5	0.04	0.1	0.00	0.11
1/2 cup	112	0.1	<0.1	<0.1	<0.1	0	124	31	0.15	0.062	0.3	0	0.1	0.01	0.15	11.2	11285
chopped, frzn, boiled	29	96.9	0.8	6.9		1.9	13	17	6	0.07	0.075	2	3	0.02	0.1	0.00	0.10
1/2 cup	105	0.1	<0.1	<0.1	<0.1	0	113	20	0.32	0.020	0.4	36	0.2	0.03	0.07	13.7	11288
raw, chopped	61	143.5	1.9	13.8		2.9	5	32	16	0.30	0.219	0	10	0.07	0.2	0.00	0.17
1 cup	160	0.3	<0.1	<0.1	0.1	0	251	53	0.35	0.096	1.0	0	0.5	0.03	0.19	30.4	11282
onion rings, breaded, parfried, frzn, heated[2] - *10 med rings (2–3" dia)*	244	17.1	3.2	22.9		0.8	225	19	11	0.25	0.252	7	1	0.17	2.2	0.00	0.14
	60	16.0	5.2	6.5	3.1	0	77	49	1.01	0.048	2.1	135		0.08	0.05	61.8	11296
onions, welsh, raw[3]	34	90.5	1.9	6.5			17	18	23	0.52	0.137	58	27	0.05	0.4	0.00	0.17
3.5 oz	100	0.4	0.1	0.1	0.2	0	212	49	1.22	0.070	0.6	1160		0.09	0.07	16.0	11293
parsnip, boiled	130	124.4	2.1	31.2		6.4	16	59	46	0.42	0.470	0	21	0.13	1.2	0.00	0.94
1 parsnip (9" long)	160	0.5	0.1	0.2	0.1	0	587	110	0.93	0.221	2.7	0	1.6	0.08	0.15	92.8	11299
poi[4]	269	171.9	0.9	65.4		1.0	29	38	58	0.53	0.888	2	10	0.31	2.6	0.00	0.70
1 cup	240	0.3	0.1	<0.1	0.1	0	439	94	2.11	0.398	1.7	48	0.4	0.10	0.66	50.4	11349
potato, baked w/skin - *1 med potato (2 1/4" dia)*	161	129.6	4.3	36.6	2.0	3.8	17	26	48	0.62	0.379	2	17	0.11	2.4	0.00	0.65
	173	0.2	0.1	<0.1	0.1	0	926	121	1.87	0.204	0.7	17	0.1	0.08	0.54	48.4	11674
w/skin, microwaved	212	145.5	4.9	48.7		4.6	16	22	55	0.73	0.590	0	31	0.24	3.5	0.00	0.92
1 potato (2 1/2" dia)	202	0.2	0.1	<0.1	0.1	0	903	212	2.50	0.675	0.8	0		0.06	0.69	24.2	11675
w/o skin	145	117.7	3.1	33.6		2.3	8	8	39	0.45	0.251	0	20	0.16	2.2	0.00	0.87
1 potato (2 1/3" × 4 3/4")	156	0.2	<0.1	<0.1	0.1	0	610	78	0.55	0.335	0.5	0	0.1	0.03	0.47	14.0	11363
w/o skin, microwaved	156	114.7	3.3	36.3		2.5	11	8	39	0.51	0.265	0	24	0.20	2.5	0.00	0.93
1 potato (2 1/3" × 4 3/4")	156	0.2	<0.1	<0.1	0.1	0	641	170	0.64	0.370	0.6	0		0.04	0.50	18.7	11368
potato, boiled w/o skin	144	129.4	2.9	33.4		3.0	8	13	33	0.45	0.234	0	12	0.16	2.2	0.00	0.85
1 med potato (2 1/4–3 1/4" dia)	167	0.2	<0.1	<0.1	0.1	0	548	67	0.52	0.279	0.5	0	0.1	0.03	0.45	15.0	11367
potato, cnd w/o skin	108	151.7	2.5	24.5		4.1	394	9	25	0.50	0.175	0	9	0.12	1.6	0.00	0.64
1 cup	180	0.4	0.1	<0.1	0.2	0	412	50	2.27	0.103	1.6	0	0.1	0.02	0.34	10.8	11376
potato, raw w/skin	164	169.0	4.3	37.2	1.7	4.7	13	26	49	0.62	0.326	0	42	0.17	2.2	0.00	0.63
1 potato (2 1/4–3 1/4" dia)	213	0.2	0.1	<0.1	0.1	0	897	121	1.66	0.230	0.6	4	<0.1	0.07	0.63	34.1	11352

Columns grouped as **Minerals** (Na, Ca, Mg, Zn, Mn, K, P, Fe, Cu, Se) and **Vitamins** (A, C, B-1, NIA, B-12, PANT, A, E, B-2, B-6, FOL).

	KCAL	H₂0 (g)	PRO (g)	CHO (g)	SUGR (g)	DFIB (g)	Na (mg)	Ca (mg)	Mg (mg)	Zn (mg)	Mn (mg)	A (mcg RAE)	C (mg)	B-1 (mg)	NIA (mg)	B-12 (mcg)	PANT (mg)
	WT (g)	FAT (g)	SFA (g)	MUFA (g)	PUFA (g)	CHOL (mg)	K (mg)	P (mg)	Fe (mg)	Cu (mg)	Se (mcg)	A (IU)	E (mg ATE)	B-2 (mg)	B-6 (mg)	FOL (mcg DFE)	REF
potato, red-skinned,	123	105.8	3.2	27.0	2.0	2.5	11	12	39	0.55	0.239	1	17	0.10	2.2	0.00	0.47
baked w/skin - *1 small (1 3/4–2 1/2" dia)*	138	0.2	<0.1	<0.1	0.1	0	752	99	0.97	0.240	0.7	14	0.1	0.07	0.29	37.3	11358c
baked w/skin	154	132.6	4.0	33.9	2.5	3.1	14	16	48	0.69	0.299	2	22	0.12	2.8		0.59
1 med (2 1/4–3 1/4" dia)	173	0.3	<0.1	<0.1	0.1	0	943	125	1.21	0.301	0.9	17	0.1	0.09	0.37	46.7	11358b
baked w/skin	266	229.2	6.9	58.6	4.3	5.4	24	27	84	1.20	0.517	3	38	0.22	4.8	0.00	1.02
1 large (3–4 1/4" dia)	299	0.4	0.1	<0.1	0.1	0	1630	215	2.09	0.520	1.5	30	0.1	0.15	0.63	80.7	11358a
raw w/skin	153	172.4	4.0	33.9	2.1	3.6	13	21	47	0.70	0.300	0	42	0.17	2.4	0.00	0.59
1 potato (2 1/4–3 1/4" dia)	213	0.3	0.1	<0.1	0.1	0	969	130	1.55	0.285	1.1	15	<0.1	0.07	0.36	38.3	11355
potato, russet,	134	102.7	3.6	29.6		3.2	11	25	41	0.48	0.315	1	18	0.09	1.9	0.00	0.52
baked w/skin - *1 small (1 3/4–2 1/2" dia)*	138	0.2		<0.1	0.1	0	759	98	1.48	0.148	0.7	14	0.1	0.07	0.49	15.2	11356b
baked w/skin	168	128.8	4.5	37.1		4.0	14	31	52	0.61	0.394	2	22	0.12	2.3	0.00	0.66
1 med (2 1/4–3 1/4" dia)	173	0.2		<0.1	0.1	0	952	123	1.85	0.185	0.9	17	0.1	0.08	0.61	19.0	11356c
baked w/skin	290	222.6	7.9	64.1		6.9	24	54	90	1.05	0.682	3	39	0.20	4.0	0.00	1.14
1 large (3–4 1/4" dia)	299	0.4		<0.1	0.1	0	1645	212	3.20	0.320	1.5	30	0.1	0.14	1.06	32.9	11356a
raw w/skin	168	167.4	4.6	38.5	1.3	2.8	11	28	49	0.62	0.334	0	42	0.17	2.2	0.00	0.64
1 potato (2 1/4–3 1/4" dia)	213	0.2	<0.1	<0.1	0.1	0	888	117	1.83	0.219	0.9	2	<0.1	0.07	0.73	29.8	11353
potato, white-skinned,	130	104.1	2.9	29.1	2.1	2.9	10	14	37	0.48	0.261	1	17	0.07	2.1	0.00	0.53
baked w/skin - *1 small (1 3/4–2 1/2" dia)*	138	0.2	<0.1	<0.1	0.1	0	751	104	0.88	0.175	0.7	14	0.1	0.06	0.29	52.4	11357c
baked w/skin	163	130.5	3.6	36.5	2.6	3.6	12	17	47	0.61	0.327	2	22	0.08	2.6	0.00	0.66
1 med (2 1/4–3 1/4" dia)	173	0.3	<0.1	<0.1	0.1	0	941	130	1.11	0.220	0.9	17	0.1	0.07	0.37	65.7	11357b
baked w/skin	281	225.5	6.3	63.0	4.6	6.3	21	30	81	1.05	0.565	3	38	0.14	4.6	0.00	1.15
1 large (3–4 1/4" dia)	299	0.4	0.1	<0.1	0.1	0	1627	224	1.91	0.380	1.5	30	0.1	0.13	0.63	113.6	11357a
raw w/skin	149	173.8	3.6	33.5	2.4	5.1	13	19	45	0.62	0.309	0	42	0.07	2.3	0.00	0.60
1 potato (2 1/4–3 1/4" dia)	213	0.2	<0.1	<0.1	0.1	0	867	132	1.11	0.247	0.6	17	<0.1	0.07	0.43	38.3	11354
potato pancake, homemade[5]	207	35.9	4.7	21.8		1.5	386	18	25	0.63	0.312	5	17	0.10	1.6	0.14	0.56
1 pancake	76	11.6	2.3	3.5	5.0	73	597	84	1.19	0.279	3.5	109		0.13	0.29	17.5	11672
potato puffs, frzn, prep	284	67.7	4.3	39.0		4.1	955	38	24	0.38	0.347	1	9	0.25	2.8	0.00	0.84
1 cup (18 puffs)	128	13.7	6.5	5.6	1.0	0	486	61	2.00	0.077	0.5	20	0.1	0.09	0.30	21.8	11399
potato salad, homemade	358	190.0	6.7	27.9		3.3	1323	48	38	0.78	0.253	80	25	0.19	2.2	0.00	1.34
1 cup	250	20.5	3.6	6.2	9.3	170	635	130	1.63	0.295	10.3	393		0.15	0.35	17.5	11414
potatoes & broc w/cheddar chs sce,	280		13.0	41.0	8.0	6.0	550	200				100	12				
frzn, Healthy Choice - *1 entrée*	298	7.0	3.0			25			1.08			100					CNAG42
potatoes au gratin,	127	108.2	3.2	17.6		1.2	601	114	21	0.33	0.178	71	4	0.03	1.3	0.00	0.33
from mix - *1/6 of 5.5 oz pkg*	137	5.6	3.5	1.6	0.2	21	300	130	0.44	0.063	3.7	292		0.11	0.05	9.6	11385
from mix, Betty Crocker Specialty	150		3.0	23.0	3.0	1.0	620	60				200	0				
Potatoes - *1/2 cup prep*	~141	6.0	1.5			<5	320		0.00			200					GENM367
homemade[6]	323	181.3	12.4	27.6		4.4	1061	292	49	1.69	0.394	157	24	0.16	2.4	0.00	0.95
1 cup	245	18.6	11.6	5.3	0.7	56	970	277	1.57	0.392	6.6	647		0.28	0.43	31.9	11373
potatoes, cheesy scalloped, from mix,	150		3.0	20.0	3.0	1.0	540	60					0				
Bty Crckr Specialty Pot - *1/2 cup prep*	~143	6.0	1.5			<5	310		0.36			200					GENM368
potatoes, cottage fries, frzn,	109	26.5	1.7	17.0		1.6	23	5	11	0.21	0.152	0	5	0.06	1.2	0.00	0.35
heated - *10 pieces*	50	4.1	1.9	1.7	0.3	0	240	33	0.75	0.100	0.2	0		0.02	0.12	8.5	11407
potatoes, fries,	167	17.7	1.8	19.8		1.6	307	6	12	0.21	0.143	0	3	0.04	1.3	0.00	0.30
extruded, frzn, heated - *10 pieces*	50	9.4	3.0	5.7	0.7	0	270	48	0.83	0.020	0.3	0		0.02	0.11	11.0	11409
frzn, heated	100	28.6	1.6	15.6		1.6	15	4	11	0.20	0.131	0	5	0.06	1.0	0.00	0.17
10 pieces	50	3.8	0.6	2.4	0.4	0	209	41	0.62	0.059	0.2	0	0.1	0.01	0.15	6.0	11403
potatoes, hash brown, from mix, Bty	120		3.0	30.0		3.0	35	0					0				
Crckr Specialty Pot - *1/2 cup prep*	~78	0.0	0.0			0	540		0.36			0					GENM369
frzn, prep[7]	170	43.8	2.5	21.9		1.6	27	12	13	0.25	0.174	0	5	0.09	1.9	0.00	0.35
1/2 cup	78	9.0	3.5	4.0	1.0	0	340	56	1.18	0.119	0.2	0	0.1	0.02	0.10	5.5	11391
homemade[7]	326	96.0	3.8	33.3		3.1	37	12	31	0.47	0.237	0	9	0.12	3.1	0.00	0.78
1 cup	156	21.7	8.5	9.7	2.5	0	501	66	1.26	0.282	0.5	0	0.3	0.03	0.43	12.5	11370
w/butter sce, frzn, prep	135	48.4	1.9	18.3		2.9	77	25	11	0.25	0.185	20	3	0.04	1.1	0.00	0.28
1/2 cup	76	6.7	2.6	2.4	1.4	17	249	29	0.75	0.078	0.2	84		0.02	0.20	9.9	11393
potatoes, mshd, from flakes w/o milk	237	160.2	4.0	31.5		4.8	697	103	38	0.38	0.239	95	20	0.23	1.4	0.17	0.25
1 cup	210	11.8	7.2	3.3	0.5	29	489	118	0.46	0.034	2.9	378	1.5	0.11	0.02	14.7	11379
potatoes, mshd, from granules w/milk[8]	166	170.9	4.2	27.5		3.8	491	65	34	0.53	0.214	74	6	0.06	1.7	0.00	0.86
1 cup	210	4.6	1.4	1.4	1.3	4	704	92	1.26	0.254	2.3	317		0.11	0.42	14.7	11383
potatoes, mshd, from mix, four,	150		3.0	20.0	2.0	1.0	540	60					0				
cheese, Betty Crocker - *1/2 cup prep*	~105	7.0	2.0			<5	360		0.36			300					GENM370
from mix, Potato Buds	160		3.0	19.0	2.0	1.0	460	20					0				
1/2 cup prep	~105	8.0	1.5			<5	370		0.36			300					GENM371

	KCAL	H₂0 (g)	PRO (g)	CHO (g)	SUGR (g)	DFIB (g)	Na (mg)	Ca (mg)	Mg (mg)	Zn (mg)	Mn (mg)	A (mcg RAE)	C (mg)	B-1 (mg)	NIA (mg)	B-12 (mcg)	PANT (mg)
	WT (g)	FAT (g)	SFA (g)	MUFA (g)	PUFA (g)	CHOL (mg)	K (mg)	P (mg)	Fe (mg)	Cu (mg)	Se (mcg)	A (IU)	E (mg ATE)	B-2 (mg)	B-6 (mg)	FOL (mcg DFE)	REF
roasted garlic, Betty Crocker	150		3.0	19.0	2.0	2.0	400	40									
1/2 cup prep	~105	8.0	2.0			<5	350		0.00			300					GENM372
sour cream & chives, Betty Crocker	90		2.0	19.0	2.0	1.0	380	20					0				
1/2 cup prep	~105	1.0	0.5			<5	340		0.00			0					GENM373
w/beef gravy, Betty Crocker	170		3.0	24.0	2.0	2.0	760	40					0				
3/4 cup prep	~209	7.0	1.5			0	370		0.36			300					GENM374
potatoes, mshd, homemade w/whole	223	160.1	3.9	35.1		4.2	620	55	38	0.57	0.239	80	13	0.18	2.3	0.00	1.20
milk & butter[9] - 1 cup	210	8.9	2.2	3.7	2.5	4	607	97	0.55	0.288	1.1	384	0.6	0.08	0.47	16.8	11371
potatoes o'brien,	173	52.7	1.9	18.6		1.4	37	17	29	0.47	0.192	8	9	0.04	1.2	0.00	0.62
frzn, prep - 2/3 cup	85	11.2	2.8	5.0	3.0	0	402	79	0.82	0.205	1.0	160		0.11	0.32	10.2	11397
homemade[10]	157	154.4	4.6	30.0			421	70	35	0.58	0.235		32	0.15	2.0	0.00	0.85
1 cup	194	2.5	1.5	0.7	0.1	8	516	97	0.91	0.250	2.3	933		0.11	0.41	15.5	11671
potatoes, rstd w/garlic & herbs,	270		3.0	33.0	0.0	4.0	610	20					4				
frzn, Green Giant - 1 1/4 cup	154	14.0	2.5			0			1.08			0					GENM375
potatoes, scalloped (escalloped)[11],	127	108.5	2.9	17.5		1.5	467	49	19	0.34	0.248	48	5	0.03	1.4	0.00	0.45
from mix - 1/6 of 5.5 oz pkg	137	5.9	3.6	1.7	0.3	15	278	77	0.52	0.067	2.2	203	0.2	0.08	0.06	13.7	11387
homemade	211	198.3	7.0	26.4		4.7	821	140	47	0.98	0.407	78	26	0.17	2.6	0.00	1.26
1 cup	245	9.0	5.5	2.5	0.4	29	926	154	1.40	0.399	3.9	331		0.23	0.44	31.9	11372
potatoes, sour crm 'n chive, from mix,	160		3.0	22.0	5.0	2.0	600	60					0				
Bty Crckr Specialty Pot - 1/2 cup prep	~139	7.0	2.0			5	310		0.36			200					GENM376
potatoes, twice bkd bcn & cheddar, from	210		6.0	22.0	4.0	1.0	580	80					0				
mix, Bty Crckr Specialty Pot - 1/2 cup prep	~143	11.0	2.5			85	410		0.72			400					GENM377
radish, oriental[12],	314	22.8	9.2	73.5			322	730	197	2.47	0.625	0	0	0.31	3.9	0.00	2.15
dried - 1 cup	116	0.8	0.3	0.1	0.4	0	4053	237	7.81	1.892	0.8	0		0.79	0.72	342.2	11432
raw	61	319.8	2.0	13.9		5.4	71	91	54	0.51	0.128	0	74	0.07	0.7	0.00	0.47
1 radish 7" long	338	0.3	0.1	0.1	0.2	0	767	78	1.35	0.389	2.4	0	<0.1	0.07	0.16	94.6	11430
sliced, boiled	25	139.7	1.0	5.0		2.4	19	25	13	0.19	0.049	0	22	0.00	0.2	0.00	0.17
1 cup	147	0.4	0.1	0.1	0.2	0	419	35	0.22	0.148	1.0	0	0.0	0.03	0.06	25.0	11431
radish, red, raw, sliced	12	55.0	0.3	2.1		0.9	14	12	5	0.17	0.041	0	13	<0.01	0.2	0.00	0.05
1/2 cup	58	0.3	<0.1	<0.1	<0.1	0	135	10	0.17	0.023	0.4	5	<0.1	0.03	0.04	15.7	11429
radish, white icicle, raw, sliced[13]	7	47.7	0.6	1.3		0.7	8	14	5	0.07	0.017	0	15	0.02	0.2	0.00	0.09
1/2 cup	50	<0.1	<0.1	<0.1	<0.1	0	140	14	0.40	0.050	0.4	0		0.01	0.04	7.0	11637
rutabaga (swede), cubed, boiled	66	151.1	2.2	14.9		3.1	34	82	39	0.60	0.296	48	32	0.14	1.2	0.00	0.26
1 cup	170	0.4	<0.1	<0.1	0.2	0	554	95	0.90	0.070	1.2	954	0.3	0.07	0.17	25.5	11436
sweet potato, baked w/skin	117	83.0	2.0	27.7		3.4	11	32	23	0.33	0.638	1244	28	0.08	0.7	0.00	0.74
1 med (2" dia, 5" long)	114	0.1	<0.1	<0.1	0.1	0	397	63	0.51	0.237	0.8	24877	0.3	0.14	0.27	26.2	11508
boiled w/o skin, mshd	344	238.9	5.4	79.6		5.9	43	69	33	0.89	1.105	2798	56	0.17	2.1	0.00	1.74
1 cup	328	1.0	0.2	<0.1	0.4	0	604	89	1.84	0.528	2.3	55937	0.9	0.46	0.80	36.1	11510
candied, frzn, Green Giant	240		2.0	41.0	20.0	3.0	430	20					12				
3/4 cup	137	7.0	1.0			0			0.72			16500					GENM378
candied, homemade[14]	144	70.3	0.9	29.3		2.5	74	27	12	0.16	0.448	219	7	0.02	0.4	0.00	0.28
1 piece (2 1/2" long & 2" dia)	105	3.4	1.4	0.7	0.2	8	198	27	1.19	0.107	0.8	4398		0.04	0.04	11.6	11659
cnd, mshd	258	188.4	5.0	59.2		4.3	191	77	61	0.54	2.519	1928	13	0.07	2.4	0.00	1.31
1 cup	255	0.5	0.1	<0.1	0.2	0	536	133	3.39	0.709	2.0	38571	0.7	0.23	0.60	28.1	11514
cnd, syrup pack	212	142.0	2.5	49.7		5.9	76	33	24	0.31	1.205	702	21	0.05	0.7	0.00	0.79
1 cup	196	0.6	0.1	<0.1	0.3	0	378	49	1.86	0.327	1.6	14028	0.5	0.07	0.12	15.7	11647
cnd, vacuum packed	182	152.1	3.3	42.3		3.6	106	44	44	0.36	0.910	798	53	0.07	1.5	0.00	1.05
1 cup pieces	200	0.4	0.1	<0.1	0.2	0	624	98	1.78	0.278	1.4	15966	0.5	0.11	0.38	34.0	11512
cubed, baked, frzn	176	129.7	3.0	41.2		3.2	14	62	37	0.53	1.170	1445	16	0.12	1.0	0.00	0.99
1 cup	176	0.2	<0.1	<0.1	0.1	0	664	77	0.95	0.322	1.1	28882	0.5	0.10	0.33	38.7	11517
taro, sliced, ckd	187	84.2	0.7	45.7		6.7	20	24	40	0.36	0.593	0	7	0.14	0.7	0.00	0.44
1 cup	132	0.1	<0.1	<0.1	0.1	0	639	100	0.95	0.265	1.2	0	0.6	0.04	0.44	25.1	11519
taro, tahitian, sliced, ckd	60	118.5	5.7	9.4			74	204	70	0.14	0.230	121	52	0.06	0.7	0.00	0.17
1 cup	137	0.9	0.2	0.1	0.4	0	854	92	2.14	0.104	1.1	2417		0.27	0.16	9.6	11526
turnip,	48	215.3	1.6	11.3		4.6	115	51	18	0.46	0.230	0	27	0.06	0.7	0.00	0.33
boiled, mshd - 1 cup	230	0.2	<0.1	<0.1	0.1	0	311	44	0.51	0.147	1.4	0	0.1	0.05	0.15	20.7	11565a
cubed, boiled	33	146.0	1.1	7.6		3.1	78	34	12	0.31	0.156	0	18	0.04	0.5	0.00	0.22
1 cup	156	0.1	<0.1	<0.1	0.1	0	211	30	0.34	0.100	0.9	0	<0.1	0.04	0.10	14.0	11565b
frzn, boiled	36	146.0	2.4	6.8		3.1	56	50	22	0.31	0.156	2	6	0.05	0.9	0.00	0.22
1 cup	156	0.4	<0.1	<0.1	0.2	0	284	41	1.53	0.098	0.9	39	<0.1	0.04	0.10	12.5	11567
wasabi root, raw, sliced	142	89.9	6.2	30.6		10.0	22	166	90	2.11	0.508	3	54	0.17	1.0	0.00	0.26
1 cup	130	0.8				0	738	104	1.34	0.200	0.9	60		0.15	0.36	23.4	11990

	KCAL	H₂O (g)	PRO (g)	CHO (g)	SUGR (g)	DFIB (g)	Na (mg)	Ca (mg)	Mg (mg)	Zn (mg)	Mn (mg)	A (mcg RAE)	C (mg)	B-1 (mg)	NIA (mg)	B-12 (mcg)	PANT (mg)
	WT (g)	FAT (g)	SFA (g)	MUFA (g)	PUFA (g)	CHOL (mg)	K (mg)	P (mg)	Fe (mg)	Cu (mg)	Se (mcg)	A (IU)	E (mg ATE)	B-2 (mg)	B-6 (mg)	FOL (mcg DFE)	REF
yam, cubed, boiled/baked	158	95.4	2.0	37.5		5.3	11	19	24	0.27	0.505	0	16	0.13	0.8	0.00	0.42
1 cup	136	0.2	<0.1	<0.1	0.1	0	911	67	0.71	0.207	1.0	0	0.2	0.04	0.31	21.8	11602
yautia (tannier), raw, sliced	132	98.6	2.0	32.0		2.0	28	12	32	0.68	0.251	1	7	0.13	0.9	0.00	0.28
1 cup	135	0.5	0.1			0	807	69	1.32	0.347	0.9	15		0.05	0.32	23.0	11991

[1] This tuber is the source for tapioca.
[2] Breaded, then parboiled in vegetable oil.
[3] A small onion or shallot used in cookery; also called a cibol.
[4] A paste by baking, grinding, and fermenting taro roots; used in Hawaiian and other Pacific Island cuisine.
[5] Made with potatoes, eggs, onion, margarine, flour, and salt.
[6] Made with potatoes, whole milk, cheddar cheese, butter, flour, and salt.
[7] Panfried in vegetable oil.
[8] Whole milk, water, and margarine added.
[9] Whole milk and margarine added.
[10] Made with potatoes, whole milk, onions, green pepper, bread crumbs, salt, butter, and black pepper.
[11] Sliced potatoes baked in a milk or cream sauce with crumbs and seasoning until brown.
[12] Includes daikon (Japanese) and Chinese radishes.
[13] Large, white-skinned mild radish native to China and South Asia; vegetable of the turnip family.
[14] Made with canned sweet potato and syrup, brown sugar, butter, and salt.

30.7 VEGETABLE COMBINATIONS

	KCAL	H₂O (g)	PRO (g)	CHO (g)	SUGR (g)	DFIB (g)	Na (mg)	Ca (mg)	Mg (mg)	Zn (mg)	Mn (mg)	A (mcg RAE)	C (mg)	B-1 (mg)	NIA (mg)	B-12 (mcg)	PANT (mg)
	WT (g)	FAT (g)	SFA (g)	MUFA (g)	PUFA (g)	CHOL (mg)	K (mg)	P (mg)	Fe (mg)	Cu (mg)	Se (mcg)	A (IU)	E (mg ATE)	B-2 (mg)	B-6 (mg)	FOL (mcg DFE)	REF
broc, carrots, cauliflower, frzn,	25		2.0	4.0	2.0	2.0	30	0					18				
Green Giant Am Mixtures - *2/3 cup*	82	0.0	0.0			0		0.00				2000					GENM379
broc, carrots, water chestnuts, frzn	25		1.0	5.0	2.0	2.0	30	0					15				
Green Giant Am Mixtures - *2/3 cup*	82	0.0	0.0			0		0.00				2000					GENM380
broc, cauliflower, & carrots in chs	80		3.0	9.0	5.0	2.0	560	60					18				
sce, frzn, Green Giant - *2/3 cup*	122	3.0	0.5			<5		0.00				2000					GENM381
corn, southwestern style & rstd	80		2.0	17.0	4.0	2.0	125	0					6				
peppers, frzn, Green Giant - *3/4 cup*	99	0.5	0.0			0		0.00				200					GENM382
green bean casserole w/sce, frzn,	90		2.0	9.0	3.0	2.0	460	40									
Green Giant - *2/3 cup*	109	5.0	1.0			0		0.36				200	1				GENM383
mixed veg,	77	141.8	4.2	15.1		4.9	243	44	26	0.67	0.926	949	8	0.07	0.9	0.00	0.23
cnd[1] - *1 cup*	163	0.4	0.1	<0.1	0.2	0	474	68	1.71	0.119	0.5	18985	1.0	0.08	0.13	39.1	11581
frzn[2]	54	75.7	2.6	11.9		4.0	32	23	20	0.45	0.345	195	3	0.06	0.8	0.00	0.14
1/2 cup	91	0.1	<0.1	<0.1	0.1	0	154	46	0.75	0.076	0.3	3892	0.3	0.11	0.07	17.3	11584
Pasta Accents Vegs, creamy cheddar,	250		9.0	36.0	5.0	3.0	640	150					24				
frzn, Green Giant - *2 1/3 cups*	190	8.0	3.0			15		1.44				3000					GENM384
primavera, frzn, Green Giant	280		12.0	37.0	6.0	4.0	460	150					24				
2 1/4 cups	200	9.0	2.5			10		1.80				1500					GENM385
three cheese, frzn, Green Giant	120		4.0	19.0	4.0	2.0	520	80					12				
3/4 cup	122	3.5	1.0			5		0.36				200					GENM386
peas & carrots,	97	224.8	5.5	21.6		5.1	663	59	36	1.48	0.910	737	17	0.19	1.5	0.00	0.31
cnd - *1 cup*	255	0.7	0.1	0.1	0.3	0	255	117	1.91	0.263	2.3	14714		0.14	0.22	45.9	11318
frzn	38	68.6	2.5	8.1		2.5	54	18	13	0.36	0.162	310	6	0.18	0.9	0.00	0.13
1/2 cup	80	0.3	0.1	<0.1	0.2	0	126	39	0.75	0.061	0.9	6209	0.3	0.05	0.07	20.8	11323
peas & onions,	61	103.7	3.9	10.3		2.8	530	20	19	0.70	0.306	10	4	0.12	1.5	0.00	0.19
cnd - *1 cup*	120	0.5	0.1	<0.1	0.2	0	115	61	1.04	0.120	0.5	193		0.08	0.23	32.4	11324
frzn, boiled	81	158.7	4.6	15.5		4.0	67	25	23	0.52	0.299	31	12	0.27	1.9	0.00	0.16
1 cup	180	0.4	0.1	<0.1	0.2	0	211	61	1.69	0.113	0.7	625	0.3	0.12	0.16	36.0	11327
potatoes & broc w/cheddar chs	328	221.0	13.0	53.0	7.5	6.0	551	241					29				
sce, Healthy Choice - *10.5 oz pkg*	298	7.0	3.0	2.2	1.8	27		1.07				331					22604
potatoes, rstd w/broc, frzn, Green	120		4.0	19.0	4.0	2.0	520	80					12				
Giant - *3/4 cup*	122	3.5	1.0			5		0.36				200					GENM387
salad, all am toss, Dole Salad Kit	50		4.0	7.0	4.0	2.0	160	40					12				
3.5 oz	100	1.0	0.0			<5		0.72				2000					DOLE24
salad, caesar, Dole Salad Kit	170		3.0	7.0	2.0	2.0	380	60					15				
3.5 oz	100	15.0	2.5			10		1.08				1750					DOLE26
w/light dressing, Dole Salad Kit	100		3.0	8.0	2.0	1.0	370	60					18				
3.5 oz	100	7.0	1.5			10		1.08				1750					DOLE25
salad, classic greek marinade, Dole	100		2.0	5.0	3.0	1.0	340	40					15				
Salad Kit - *3.5 oz*	100	8.0	1.5			<5		0.72				1750					DOLE27
salad, creamy garlic caesar, Dole	170		3.0	8.0	7.0	1.0	390	60					18				
Salad Kit - *3.5 oz*	100	15.0	2.5			5		1.08				1750					DOLE28
salad, family caesar, Dole Salad Kit	170		3.0	8.0	1.0	2.0	440	60					15				
3.5 oz	100	15.0	2.5			10		1.08				1750					DOLE29
salad, mediterranean marinade, Dole	90		1.0	5.0	3.0	1.0	180	40					18				
Salad Kit - *3.5 oz*	100	8.0	1.0			0		0.72				2250					DOLE30

	KCAL	H₂O (g)	PRO (g)	CHO (g)	SUGR (g)	DFIB (g)	Na (mg)	Ca (mg)	Mg (mg)	Zn (mg)	Mn (mg)	A (mcg RAE)	C (mg)	B-1 (mg)	NIA (mg)	B-12 (mcg)	PANT (mg)
	WT (g)	FAT (g)	SFA (g)	MUFA (g)	PUFA (g)	CHOL (mg)	K (mg)	P (mg)	Fe (mg)	Cu (mg)	Se (mcg)	A (IU)	E (mg ATE)	B-2 (mg)	B-6 (mg)	FOL (mcg DFE)	REF
salad, sunflower ranch, Dole Salad	170		2.0	5.0	3.0	2.0	220	40					6				
Kit - *3.5 oz*	100	16.0	2.0			5	200		0.36			2000					DOLE31
salad, triple cheese toss, Dole	80		5.0	4.0	2.0	1.0	120	150					12				
Salad Kit - *3.5 oz*	100	5.0	3.0			15	180		0.72			2000					DOLE32
succotash (corn & lima beans),	221	131.3	9.7	46.8		8.6	33	33	102	1.21	1.476	29	16	0.32	2.5	0.00	1.09
boiled - *1 cup*	192	1.5	0.3	0.3	0.7	0	787	225	2.92	0.344	1.2	564		0.18	0.22	63.4	11496
cnd	161	209.0	6.6	35.6		6.6	564	28	48	1.28	0.933	18	12	0.07	1.6	0.00	0.79
1 cup	255	1.2	0.2	0.2	0.6	0	416	140	1.35	0.278	1.5	372	2.4	0.15	0.12	81.6	11499
frzn, boiled	158	126.0	7.3	33.9		7.0	77	26	39	0.77	0.476	20	10	0.13	2.2	0.00	0.39
1 cup	170	1.5	0.3	0.3	0.7	0	451	119	1.51	0.102	1.0	393	0.6	0.12	0.16	56.1	11502
w/cream style corn, cnd	205	207.9	7.0	46.8		8.0	652	29	3	1.14	1.716	19	17	0.07	1.6	0.00	0.58
1 cup	266	1.4	0.3	0.3	0.7	0	487	157	1.46	0.473	1.6	375		0.17	0.34	117.0	11497
vegetables alfredo w/sce, frzn,	70		4.0	9.0	4.0	3.0	440	80					18				
Green Giant - *3/4 cup*	109	2.5	1.0			5			0.36			2000					GENM388
vegetables teriyaki, frzn, Green	100		5.0	18.0	10.0	4.0	850	40					42				
Giant - *1 1/4 cups*	110	0.5	0.0			0			1.08			750					GENM389

30.8 OTHER VEGETABLES

	KCAL	H₂O (g)	PRO (g)	CHO (g)	SUGR (g)	DFIB (g)	Na (mg)	Ca (mg)	Mg (mg)	Zn (mg)	Mn (mg)	A (mcg RAE)	C (mg)	B-1 (mg)	NIA (mg)	B-12 (mcg)	PANT (mg)
	WT (g)	FAT (g)	SFA (g)	MUFA (g)	PUFA (g)	CHOL (mg)	K (mg)	P (mg)	Fe (mg)	Cu (mg)	Se (mcg)	A (IU)	E (mg ATE)	B-2 (mg)	B-6 (mg)	FOL (mcg DFE)	REF
corn pudding, homemade[1]	273	190.8	11.0	31.9			138	100	38	1.25	1.340	135	7	1.03	2.5	0.23	0.62
1 cup	250	13.3	6.3	4.3	1.7	250	403	143	1.40	0.108	13.0	658		0.32	0.30	62.5	11656a
corn, yellow,	9	5.6	0.3	2.0		0.2	1	0	3	0.04	0.016	1	<1	0.02	0.1	0.00	0.07
boiled - *1 baby ear*	8	0.1	<0.1	<0.1	<0.1	0	20	8	0.05	0.004	0.1	17	<0.1	0.01	<0.01	3.7	11168c
boiled	83	53.6	2.6	19.3		2.2	13	2	25	0.37	0.149	8	5	0.17	1.2	0.00	0.68
1 ear	77	1.0	0.2	0.3	0.5	0	192	79	0.47	0.041	0.6	167	0.1	0.06	0.05	35.4	11168b
boiled	177	114.1	5.4	41.2		4.6	28	3	52	0.79	0.318	18	10	0.35	2.6	0.00	1.44
1 cup	164	2.1	0.3	0.6	1.0	0	408	169	1.00	0.087	1.3	356	0.1	0.12	0.10	75.4	11168a
cnd	133	126.1	4.3	30.5		3.3	351	8	33	0.64	0.284	13	14	0.05	2.0	0.00	1.09
1 cup	164	1.6	0.3	0.5	0.8	0	320	107	1.41	0.095	1.1	256	0.2	0.13	0.08	80.4	11172
cnd, vacuum pack	83	80.4	2.5	20.4		2.1	286	5	24	0.48	0.070	13	9	0.04	1.2	0.00	0.71
1 cup	105	0.5	0.1	0.2	0.2	0	195	67	0.44	0.050	0.7	253	0.1	0.08	0.06	51.5	11176
cream style, cnd	184	201.5	4.5	46.4		3.1	730	8	44	1.36	0.100	13	12	0.06	2.5	0.00	0.46
1 cup	256	1.1	0.2	0.3	0.5	0	343	131	0.97	0.133	1.5	248	0.2	0.14	0.16	115.2	11174
frzn, boiled	66	62.9	2.3	16.0		2.0	4	3	16	0.33	0.104	9	3	0.07	1.1	0.00	0.15
1/2 cup	82	0.4	0.1	0.1	0.2	0	121	47	0.29	0.030	0.6	180	0.1	0.06	0.11	25.4	11179
w/red & green peppers,	170	175.9	5.3	41.2			788	11	57	0.84	0.098	27	20	0.05	2.2	0.00	1.01
cnd - *1 cup*	227	1.2	0.2	0.4	0.6	0	347	141	1.79	0.136	1.4	527		0.18	0.22	77.2	11184
fungi, cloud ears, dried	80	4.1	2.6	20.4		19.6	10	45	23	0.37	0.546	0	0	<0.01	1.8	0.00	0.13
1 cup	28	0.2				0	211	52	1.65	0.051	35.8	0		0.24	0.03	10.6	11988
hearts of palm (heart palm), cnd	41	131.7	3.7	6.7		3.5	622	85	55	1.68	2.035	0	12	0.02	0.6	0.00	0.18
1 cup	146	0.9	0.2	0.2	0.3	0	258	95	4.57	0.194	1.0	0		0.08	0.03	56.9	11961
hominy,	119	136.2	2.4	23.5		4.1	347	17	26	1.73	0.116	0	0	<0.01	0.1	0.00	0.25
white, cnd - *1 cup*	165	1.5	0.2	0.4	0.7	0	15	58	1.02	0.050	5.0	0	0.1	0.01	0.01	1.7	20030
yellow, cnd	115	132.0	2.4	22.8		4.0	336	16	26	1.68	0.112	10	0	<0.01	0.1	0.00	0.25
1 cup	160	1.4	0.2	0.4	0.6	0	14	56	0.99	0.048	4.8	176		0.01	0.01	1.6	20330
mushrooms, common white,	42	142.1	3.4	8.0		3.4	3	9	19	1.36	0.179	0	6	0.11	7.0	0.00	3.37
boiled - *1 cup pieces*	156	0.7	0.1	<0.1	0.3	0	555	136	2.71	0.786	18.6	0	0.2	0.47	0.15	28.1	11261
cnd	37	142.1	2.9	7.7		3.7	663	17	23	1.12	0.134	0	0	0.13	2.5	0.00	1.27
1 cup pieces	156	0.5	0.1	<0.1	0.2	0	201	103	1.23	0.367	6.4	0	0.2	0.03	0.10	18.7	11264
raw	18	64.3	2.0	2.9		0.8	3	4	7	0.51	0.078	0	2	0.06	2.8	0.03	1.02
1/2 cup pieces	70	0.2	<0.1	<0.1	0.1	0	259	73	0.73	0.344	6.2	0	0.1	0.30	0.07	8.4	11260
mushrooms, crimini, italian,	3	12.9	0.4	0.6	0.2	0.1	1	3	1	0.15	0.020	0	0	0.01	0.5	0.01	0.21
brown, raw - *1 piece*	14	<0.1	<0.1	<0.1	<0.1	0	63	17	0.06	0.070	3.6	0	<0.1	0.07	0.02	2.0	11266
mushrooms, enoki, raw	2	4.5	0.3	0.4		0.1	0	0	1	0.03	0.004	0	1	<0.01	0.2	0.00	0.05
1 large	5	<0.1	<0.1	<0.1	<0.1	0	19	6	0.04	0.003	0.8	<1		0.01	<0.01	1.5	11950
mushrooms, oyster, raw	55	129.9	6.1	9.2		3.6	46	9	30	1.15	0.210	3	0	0.08	5.3	0.00	1.91
1 large	148	0.8				0	764	209	2.58	0.537	27.2	71		0.53	0.18	69.6	11987
mushrooms, portabella, raw	29	100.3	2.8	5.6	2.0	1.7	7	9	12	0.66	0.156	0	0	0.08	5.0	0.06	1.65
1 med (3.9 oz)	110	<0.1	<0.1	<0.1	0.1	0	532	143	0.66	0.440	12.1	0	0.1	0.53	0.11	24.2	11265
mushrooms, shiitake,	40	60.1	1.1	10.3		1.5	3	2	10	0.96	0.147	0	<1	0.03	1.1	0.00	2.59
ckd - *4 mushrooms*	72	0.2	<0.1	<0.1	<0.1	0	84	21	0.32	0.645	17.9	0	0.1	0.12	0.11	15.1	11269
dried	44	1.4	1.4	11.3		1.7	2	2	20	1.15	0.176	0	1	0.05	2.1	0.00	3.28
4 mushrooms	15	0.1	<0.1	<0.1	<0.1	0	230	44	0.26	0.775	20.4	0	<0.1	0.19	0.14	24.5	11268

Food	KCAL / WT (g)	H₂O (g) / FAT (g)	PRO (g) / SFA (g)	CHO (g) / MUFA (g)	SUGR (g) / PUFA (g)	DFIB (g) / CHOL (mg)	Na (mg) / K (mg)	Ca (mg) / P (mg)	Mg (mg) / Fe (mg)	Zn (mg) / Cu (mg)	Mn (mg) / Se (mcg)	A (mcg RAE) / A (IU)	C (mg) / E (mg ATE)	B-1 (mg) / B-2 (mg)	NIA (mg) / B-6 (mg)	B-12 (mcg) / FOL (mcg DFE)	PANT (mg) / REF
mushrooms, straw, cnd	58	163.6	7.0	8.5		4.6	699	18	13	1.22	0.178	0	0	0.02	0.4	0.00	0.75
1 cup	182	1.2	0.2	<0.1	0.5	0	142	111	2.60	0.242	27.7	0		0.13	0.03	69.2	11989
nopales (prickly pear)², ckd - *1 cup*	22	140.5	2.0	4.9		3.0	30	244	70	0.31	0.608	34	8	0.02	0.4	0.00	0.22
	149	0.1	<0.1	<0.1	<0.1	0	291	24	0.75	0.073	1.0	684	<0.1	0.06	0.10	4.5	11964
raw, sliced	14	80.8	1.1	2.9		2.0	19	140	50	0.25	0.434	18	12	0.01	0.5	0.00	0.16
1 cup	86	0.1	<0.1	<0.1	<0.1	0	274	15	0.58	0.048	0.6	357	<0.1	0.04	0.06	2.6	11963
pepeao (jew's ear), dried - *1 cup*	72	2.7	1.2	19.4			17	27	35	1.80	0.276	0	<1	0.20	0.7	0.00	5.15
	24					0	170	28	1.47	1.217	31.9	0		0.08	0.23	38.4	11230
raw, sliced	25	91.7	0.5	6.7			9	16	25	0.65	0.100	0	1	0.08	0.1	0.00	1.97
1 cup	99	<0.1				0	43	14	0.55	0.441	11.0	0		0.20	0.09	18.8	11228
seaweed, agar, dried - *1 oz*	86	2.4	1.7	22.6		2.2	29	175	216	1.62	1.204	0	0	<0.01	0.1	0.00	0.85
	28	0.1	<0.1	<0.1	<0.1	0	315	15	5.99	0.171	2.1	0	1.4	0.06	0.08	162.4	11663
raw	3	9.1	0.1	0.7		0.1	1	5	7	0.06	0.037	0	0	<0.01	<0.1	0.00	0.03
2 T	10	<0.1	<0.1	<0.1	<0.1	0	23	<1	0.19	0.006	0.1	0	0.1	<0.01	<0.01	8.5	11442
seaweed, irish moss, raw	5	8.1	0.2	1.2		0.1	7	7	14	0.20	0.037	1	<1	<0.01	0.1	0.00	0.02
2 T	10	<0.1	<0.1	<0.1	<0.1	0	6	16	0.89	0.015	0.1	12	0.1	0.05	0.01	18.2	11444
seaweed, kelp (kombu/tangle), raw	4	8.2	0.2	1.0		0.1	23	17	12	0.12	0.020	1	<1	<0.01	<0.1	0.00	0.06
2 T	10	0.1	<0.1	<0.1	<0.1	0	9	4	0.29	0.013	0.1	12	0.1	0.02	<0.01	18.0	11445
seaweed, laver (nori), raw	4	8.5	0.6	0.5		0.0	5	7	<1	0.11	0.099	26	4	0.01	0.1	0.00	0.05
2 T (~4 sheets)	10	<0.1	<0.1	<0.1	<0.1	0	36	6	0.18	0.026	0.1	520	0.1	0.04	0.02	14.6	11446
seaweed, spirulina, dried - *1 cup*	44	0.7	8.6	3.6		0.5	157	18	29	0.30	0.285	4	2	0.36	1.9	0.00	0.52
	15	1.2	0.4	0.1	0.3	0	204	18	4.28	0.915	1.1	86	0.8	0.55	0.05	14.1	11667
raw	7	25.4	1.7	0.7			27	3	5	0.06	0.052	1	<1	0.06	0.3	0.00	0.09
1 oz	28	0.1	<0.1	<0.1	<0.1	0	36	3	0.78	0.167	0.2	16		0.10	0.01	2.5	11666
seaweed, wakame, raw	5	8.0	0.3	0.9		0.1	87	15	11	0.04	0.140	2	<1	0.01	0.2	0.00	0.07
2 T	10	0.1	<0.1	<0.1	<0.1	0	5	8	0.22	0.028	0.1	36	0.1	0.02	<0.01	19.6	11669
tree fern, chopped, ckd³	28	62.9	0.2	7.8		2.6	4	6	4	0.22	0.383	7	21	0.00	2.5	0.00	0.04
1/2 cup	71	<0.1	<0.1	<0.1	<0.1	0	4	3	0.11	0.143	0.6	142	0.5	0.21	0.13	10.7	11563
water chestnuts, chinese (matai)⁴, raw, sliced - *1/2 cup*	60	45.5	0.9	14.8		1.9	9	7	14	0.31	0.205	0	2	0.09	0.6	0.00	0.30
	62	0.1	<0.1	<0.1	<0.1	0	362	39	0.04	0.202	0.4	0	0.7	0.12	0.20	9.9	11588
sliced, cnd	35	60.5	0.6	8.7		1.8	6	3	4	0.27	0.113	0	1	0.01	0.3	0.00	0.15
1/2 cup	70	<0.1	<0.1	<0.1	<0.1	0	83	13	0.61	0.070	0.5	3	0.4	0.02	0.11	4.2	11590

[1] Made with yellow corn, whole milk, egg, sugar, butter, salt, and pepper.
[2] The pods of the prickly pear cactus are used as a vegetable; the leaves are used as a fruit. (See prickly pear in Section 15.)
[3] Trunk of *Cyathea medullaris* has a mucilaginous pulp used for food in Polynesia and New Zealand. The pulp is similar to sago.
[4] Round corm of a tule/bulrush.

31. MISCELLANEOUS FOOD INGREDIENTS

Food	KCAL / WT (g)	H₂O (g) / FAT (g)	PRO (g) / SFA (g)	CHO (g) / MUFA (g)	SUGR (g) / PUFA (g)	DFIB (g) / CHOL (mg)	Na (mg) / K (mg)	Ca (mg) / P (mg)	Mg (mg) / Fe (mg)	Zn (mg) / Cu (mg)	Mn (mg) / Se (mcg)	A (mcg RAE) / A (IU)	C (mg) / E (mg ATE)	B-1 (mg) / B-2 (mg)	NIA (mg) / B-6 (mg)	B-12 (mcg) / FOL (mcg DFE)	PANT (mg) / REF
baking choc (unsweetened)	146	0.4	2.9	7.9		4.3	4	21	87	1.12	0.537	1	0	0.02	0.3	0.00	0.06
1 oz sq	28	15.5	9.1	5.2	0.5	0	233	117	1.77	0.607	2.1	27	0.3	0.05	0.03	2.0	19078
liquid	134	0.3	3.4	9.6	0.0	5.1	3	15	75	1.04	0.468	<1	0	0.01	0.6	0.00	0.04
1 oz pkt	28	13.5	7.2	2.6	3.0	0	331	96	1.18	0.541	2.2	3	1.7	0.08	0.02	5.4	19077
mexican	121	0.5	1.0	21.9		1.1	1	10	27	0.36	0.127	<1	<1	0.02	0.5	0.00	0.05
1 oz	28	4.4	2.4	1.4	0.3	0	113	40	0.62	0.190	0.5	5	0.1	0.03	0.01	0.6	19124
baking powder, double-acting, Na Al sulfate - *1 t*	2	0.2	0.0	1.3		0.0	488	270	1	<0.01	<0.001	0	0	0.00	0.0	0.00	0.00
	4.6	0.0	0.0	0.0	0.0	0	1	101	0.51	<0.001	<0.1	0	0.0	0.00	0.00	0.0	18369
double-acting, straight phosphate *1 t*	2	0.2	0.0	1.1		0.0	363	339	2	<0.01	0.001	0	0	0.00	0.0	0.00	0.00
	4.6	0.0	0.0	0.0	0.0	0	<1	456	0.52	0.001	<0.1	0	0.0	0.00	0.00	0.0	18370
low Na *1 t*	5	0.3	0.0	2.3		0.1	5	217	1	0.04	0.021	0	0	0.00	0.0	0.00	0.00
	4.6	<0.1	<0.1	<0.1	<0.1	0	505	343	0.41	0.001	<0.1	0	<0.1	0.00	0.00	0.0	18371
baking soda (sodium bicarbonate)	0	<0.1	0.0	0.0		0.0	1259	0	0	0.00	0.000	0	0	0.00	0.0	0.00	0.00
1 t	5	0.0	0.0	0.0	0.0	0	0	0	0.00	0.000	<0.1	0	0.0	0.00	0.00	0.0	18372
carob powder, Chatfield's	90		1.0	20.0	12.0	2.0	10	100					0				
1/4 cup	30	0.0	0.0	0.0	0.0	0			0.72			0					CHAT1
cocoa, unsweetened powder	12	0.2	1.1	2.9		1.8	1	7	27	0.37	0.207	<1	0	<0.01	0.1	0.00	0.01
1 T	5	0.7	0.4	0.2	<0.1	0	82	40	0.75	0.205	0.8	1	<0.1	0.01	0.01	1.7	19165
european style, Hershey	20		1.0	3.0		1.0	0	0					0				
1 T	5	0.5	0.0			0			1.80			0					19171
processed w/alkali	12	0.1	1.0	3.0		1.6	1	6	26	0.34	0.202	<1	0	0.01	0.1	0.00	0.01
1 T	5	0.7	0.4	0.2	<0.1	0	135	39	0.84	0.195	0.7	1	<0.1	0.02	0.01	1.7	19166
cornstarch	488	10.6	0.3	116.8		1.2	12	3	4	0.08	0.068	0	0	0.00	0.0	0.00	0.00
1 cup	128	0.1	<0.1	<0.1	<0.1	0	4	17	0.60	0.064	3.6	0	0.0	0.00	0.00	0.0	20027

	KCAL	H₂0 (g)	PRO (g)	CHO (g)	SUGR (g)	DFIB (g)	Na (mg)	Ca (mg)	Mg (mg)	Zn (mg)	Mn (mg)	A (mcg RAE)	C (mg)	B-1 (mg)	NIA (mg)	B-12 (mcg)	PANT (mg)
	WT (g)	FAT (g)	SFA (g)	MUFA (g)	PUFA (g)	CHOL (mg)	K (mg)	P (mg)	Fe (mg)	Cu (mg)	Se (mcg)	A (IU)	E (mg ATE)	B-2 (mg)	B-6 (mg)	FOL (mcg DFE)	REF
cream of tartar (potassium acid	8	0.1	0.0	1.8		0.0	2	0	<1	0.01	0.006	0	0	0.00	0.00	0.00	0.00
tartrate) - *1 t*	3	0.0	0.0	0.0	0.0	0	495	<1	0.11	0.006	<0.1	0	0.0	0.00	0.00	0.00	18373
gelatin, dry, unsweetened	94	3.6	24.0	0.0		0.0	55	15	6	0.04	0.029	0	0	0.01	<0.1	0.00	0.00
1 oz pkt (4 T)	28	<0.1	<0.1	<0.1	<0.1	0	4	11	0.31	0.605	11.1	0	0.0	0.06	<0.01	8.4	19177a
pectin, unsweetened, dry	163	4.4	0.2	45.2		4.3	100	4	<1	0.24	0.035	0	0	<0.01	<0.1	0.00	0.06
1.75 oz pkt	50	0.2	<0.1	<0.1	<0.1	0	4	1	1.36	0.210	0.0	2	0.0	0.03	<0.01	0.5	19310
rennin, unsweetened	8	0.6	0.1	2.0		0.0	2579	370	2	0.63	0.089	0	0	0.00	0.00	0.00	0.00
.35 oz pkt	10	<0.1	<0.1	<0.1	<0.1	0	29	34	0.70	0.020	0.0	0	0.0	0.00	0.00	0.0	19225
soy protein concentrate,	94	1.6	16.5	8.8		1.6	255	103	40	1.25	1.188	0	0	0.09	0.2	0.00	0.02
acid wash - *1 oz*	28	0.1	<0.1	<0.1	0.1	0	128	238	3.06	0.277	0.2	0	0.04	0.04	96.4	16420
alcohol extraction	94	1.6	16.5	8.8		1.6	1	103	89	1.25	1.188	0	0	0.09	0.2	0.00	0.02
1 oz	28	0.1	<0.1	<0.1	0.1	0	624	238	3.06	0.277	0.2	0	0.0	0.04	0.04	96.4	16121
soy protein isolate	96	1.4	22.9	2.1		1.6	285	50	11	1.14	0.423	0	0	0.05	0.4	0.00	0.02
1 oz	28	1.0	0.1	0.2	0.5	0	23	220	4.11	0.453	0.2	0	0.0	0.03	0.03	49.9	16122
potassium type	96	1.4	22.9	2.1		1.6	14	50	11	1.14	0.423	0	0	0.05	0.4	0.00	0.02
1 oz	28	1.0	0.1	0.2	0.5	0	451	220	4.11	0.453	0.2	0	0.0	0.03	0.03	49.9	16422
ProPlus, Protein Tech	108	1.4	24.4	0.0			11	57		17.01		158	0	0.74	10.2	2.84	2.55
International - *1 oz*	28	1.1	0.1	0.2	0.5	0	454	227	5.10	0.851		527		0.28	0.74	56.7	16176
Supro, Protein Tech	110	1.3	24.9	0.0			337	57	11	1.13		0	0	0.06	0.1	0.00	0.06
International - *1 oz*	28	1.1	0.2	0.2	0.5	0	28	244	4.54	0.397		0		0.03		56.7	16175
soy protein powder, GeniSoy	100		25.0	0.0	0.0	0.0	290	250	100	3.75			15	0.38	5.0	1.50	2.50
1.1 oz scoop	30	0.0					90	300	4.50	0.500	50.0	1250	20.0	0.43	0.50	100.0	GENI7
tapioca, pearl, dry	544	16.7	0.3	134.8		1.4	2	30	2	0.18	0.167	0	0	0.01	0.0	0.00	0.21
1 cup	152	<0.1	<0.1	<0.1	<0.1	0	17	11	2.40	0.030	1.2	0	0.0	0.00	0.01	6.1	20068
vinegar,	10		0.0	2.0	2.0	0.0	0	0					0				
balsamic, Progresso - *1 T*	15	0.0	0.0			0			0.00			0					GENM390
cider	2	14.1	0.0	0.9		0.0	0	1	3	0.00	0.036	0	0.0	0.00	0.0	0.0	0.04
1 T	15	0.0	0.0	0.0	0.0	0	15	1	0.09	0.006	<0.1	0	0.0	0.00	0.00	0.0	02048
whey, acid,	193	2.0	6.7	41.9		0.0	552	1171	113	3.60	0.009	10	1	0.35	0.7	1.43	3.21
dry - *1 cup*	57	0.3	0.2	0.1	<0.1	2	1305	769	0.71	0.029	15.6	33	<0.1	1.17	0.35	18.8	01113
fluid	59	229.8	1.9	12.6		0	118	253	25	1.06	0.005	5	<1	0.10	0.2	0.44	0.94
1 cup	246	0.2	0.1	0.1	<0.1	2	352	192	0.20	0.007	4.4	17	<0.1	0.34	0.10	4.9	01112
whey, sweet,	512	4.6	18.7	108.0		0.0	1565	1154	255	2.86	0.013	13	2	0.75	1.8	3.44	8.15
dry - *1 cup*	145	1.6	1.0	0.4	<0.1	9	3016	1351	1.28	0.102	39.4	64	<0.1	3.20	0.85	17.4	01115
fluid	66	229.1	2.1	12.6		0.0	133	116	20	0.32	0.002	10	<1	0.09	0.2	0.69	0.94
1 cup	246	0.9	0.6	0.2	<0.1	5	396	113	0.15	0.010	4.7	39	<0.1	0.39	0.08	2.5	01114
yeast, baker's,	21	0.5	2.7	2.7		1.5	4	4	7	0.45	0.039	0	<1	0.17	2.8	<0.01	0.79
active dry - *.25 oz pkg*	7	0.3	<0.1	0.2	<0.1	0	140	90	1.16	0.035	1.7	<1	<0.1	0.38	0.11	163.8	18375
compressed	18	11.7	1.4	3.1		1.4	5	3	7	1.69	0.034	0	<1	0.32	2.1	<0.01	0.83
.6 oz cake	17	0.3	<0.1	0.2	<0.1	0	102	57	0.55	0.025	1.4	0	<0.1	0.19	0.07	133.5	18374

Column key (four lines per item):

Line	Energy / Proximates	Minerals	Vitamins
1	KCAL, H₂0 (g), PRO (g), CHO (g), SUGR (g), DFIB (g)	Na (mg), Ca (mg), Mg (mg), Zn (mg), Mn (mg)	A (mcg RAE), C (mg), B-1 (mg), NIA (mg), B-12 (mcg)
2	WT (g), FAT (g), SFA (g), MUFA (g), PUFA (g), CHOL (mg)	K (mg), P (mg), Fe (mg), Cu (mg), Se (mcg)	A (IU), E (mg ATE), B-2 (mg), B-6 (mg), FOL (mcg DFE)
3	HIS, ISO, LEU, LYS, MET, CYS, TAU (mg)	Cl (mg), I (mcg), Mo (mcg), Cr (mcg)	PANT (mg), E (IU), D (IU), K (mcg)
4	PHE, TYR, THR, TRY, VAL, ARG, CAR (mg)		BIO (mcg), CHLN (mg), INOS (mg), REF

32. SPECIAL DIETARY FOODS
32.1 FORMULAS & MEDICAL FOODS FOR INFANTS & CHILDREN

Alimentum, Ross[1] — *1 fl oz*

KCAL/WT/HIS/PHE	H₂0/FAT/ISO/TYR	PRO/SFA/LEU/THR	CHO/MUFA/LYS/TRY	SUGR/PUFA/MET/VAL	DFIB/CHOL/CYS/ARG	CAR	Na/K/Cl/	Ca/P/I/	Mg/Fe/Mo/	Zn/Cu/Cr/	Mn/Se	A/A/PANT/BIO	C/E/E/CHLN	B-1/B-2/D/INOS	NIA/B-6/K	B-12/FOL/REF
20	26.6	0.5	2.0		0.0		9	21	2	0.15	0.006	18	2	0.01	0.3	0.09
31	1.1	0.6	0.1	0.3	<1		23	15	0.36	0.015	0.5	60		0.02	0.01	
												0.2				
																03846

Compleat Pediatric, Novartis — *8 fl oz (250 ml)*

250		9.4	31.5		1.1		170	250	47	3.00	0.560		24	0.64	4.0	1.40
~248	9.7						380	250	3.30	0.300	13.0	830	3.6	0.50	0.62	88.0
						21		34	14	22.0		2.4	5	120	9.50	
						4						76	71	19		NVAR1

EleCare, Ross[2] — *5 fl oz (150 ml)*

152	124.2	4.6	16.2				68	164	12	1.67	0.159		14	0.32	2.5	0.64
~153	7.2						227	123	2.73	0.191	3.5	414	2.1	0.16	0.15	45.5
							91	11				1.7	3	64	9.09	
												6	12	8		RSSP1

EnfaCare Lipil, Mead Johnson[3] — *4.5 fl oz (135 ml)*

100	120.0	2.8	10.4				35	120	8	1.25	0.015		16	0.20	2.0	0.30
~139	5.3						105	66	1.80	0.120	2.8	450	2.7	0.20	0.10	26.0
44	154	162	270	210	63	6	78	21				0.9	4	80	8.00	
30	107	126	170		55	2						6	24	30		MDJN19

Enfalyte, Mead Johnson[4] — *5 fl oz (150 ml)*

19							172									
~167							147									
							240					0.0				
																MDJN20

Enfamil AR, Mead Johnson[5] — *5 fl oz (150 ml)*

100	133.0	2.5	11.0				40	78	8	1.00	0.015		12	0.08	1.0	0.30
~152	5.1						108	53	1.80	0.075		300	1.3	0.14	0.06	16.0
34	108	123	250	200	64		75	10				0.5	2	60	8.00	
12	120	110	147		69							3	12	6		MDJN21

Enfamil Human Milk Fortifier, pwdr, Mead Johnson[6] — *4 pkts (.13 oz)*

14		1.1	<0.4				16	90	1	0.72	0.010		12	0.15	3.0	0.18
4	1.0						29	50	1.44	0.044		950	3.1	0.22	0.12	25.0
							13					0.7	5	150	4.40	
												3				MDJN22

Enfamil, low Fe, Mead Johnson — *1 fl oz*

20	26.8	0.4	2.2		0.0		5	16	2	0.20	0.002	18	2	0.02	0.2	0.06
31	1.1	0.5	0.4	0.2	<1		22	11	0.14	0.015	0.5	60		0.03	0.01	
												0.1				
																03806

liquid conc, Mead Johnson — *1 fl oz*

41	23.7	0.9	4.5		0.0		11	32	3	0.41		37	5	0.03	0.4	0.12
31	2.2	0.9	0.8	0.4	<1		45	22	0.29	0.031	1.1	124		0.06	0.02	
																03807

powder, Mead Johnson — *1 scoop*

44	0.2	0.9	4.6		0.0		12	33	3	0.43		39	5	0.03	0.4	0.13
8	2.3	1.0	0.9	0.4	<1		46	22	0.30	0.032	1.2	129		0.06	0.03	
																03809

Enfamil Premature, 20 cal/fl oz, Mead Johnson[7] — *5 fl oz (150 ml)*

100	133.0	3.0	11.1				58	165	9	1.50	0.006		20	0.20	4.0	0.25
~153	5.1						98	83	0.50	0.120		1250	4.2	0.30	0.15	40.0
47	165	174	290	230	68		90	25				1.2	6	240	8.00	
32	115	135	182		59							4	20	44		MDJN23

24 cal/fl oz, Mead Johnson[7] — *4.2 fl oz (126 ml)*

100	108.0	3.0	11.1				58	165	9	1.50	0.006		20	0.20	4.0	0.25
~128	5.1						98	83	0.50	0.120		1250	4.2	0.30	0.15	40.0
47	165	174	290	230	68		90	25				1.2	6	240	8.00	
32	115	135	182		59							4	20	44		MDJN24

Enfamil w/Fe, Mead Johnson[8] — *1 fl oz*

20	26.8	0.4	2.2		0.0		5	16	2	0.20		18	2	0.02	0.2	0.06
31	1.1	0.5	0.4	0.2	<1		22	11	0.36	0.015	0.5	60		0.03	0.01	
																03803

liquid conc, Mead Johnson[8] — *1 fl oz*

41	23.7	0.9	4.5		0.0		11	32	3	0.41		37	5	0.03	0.4	0.12
31	2.2	0.9	0.8	0.4	<1		45	22	0.74	0.031	1.1	124		0.06	0.02	

								Minerals					Vitamins					
	KCAL	H_2O (g)	PRO (g)	CHO (g)	SUGR (g)	DFIB (g)		Na (mg)	Ca (mg)	Mg (mg)	Zn (mg)	Mn (mg)	A (mcg RAE)	C (mg)	B-1 (mg)	NIA (mg)	B-12 (mcg)	
	WT (g)	FAT (g)	SFA (g)	MUFA (g)	PUFA (g)	CHOL (mg)		K (mg)	P (mg)	Fe (mg)	Cu (mg)	Se (mcg)	A (IU)	E (mg ATE)	B-2 (mg)	B-6 (mg)	FOL (mcg DFE)	
	HIS (mg)	ISO (mg)	LEU (mg)	LYS (mg)	MET (mg)	CYS (mg)	TAU (mg)	Cl (mg)	I (mcg)	Mo (mcg)	Cr (mcg)		PANT (mg)	E (IU)	D (IU)	K (mcg)		
	PHE (mg)	TYR (mg)	THR (mg)	TRY (mg)	VAL (mg)	ARG (mg)	CAR (mg)						BIO (mcg)	CHLN (mg)	INOS (mg)			REF
powder, Mead Johnson[8]	44	0.2	0.9	4.6		0.0		12	33	3	0.43		39	5	0.03	0.4	0.13	03804
1 scoop	8	2.3	1.0	0.9	0.4	<1		46	22	0.77	0.032	1.2	129		0.06	0.03		
Follow-Up w/Fe,	20	26.4	0.5	2.6		0.0		8	27	2	0.13		15	2	0.02	0.3	0.06	03805
Carnation - *1 fl oz*	31	0.8	0.4	0.3	0.2	<1		27	18	0.37	0.014	0.2	49		0.02	0.01		
liquid conc, Carnation	41	23.3	1.1	5.4		0.0		16	56	3	0.26		31	3	0.03	0.5	0.13	03900
1 fl oz	31	1.7	0.7	0.5	0.4	1		56	37	0.78	0.031	0.4	103		0.04	0.03		
powder, Carnation	44	0.3	1.1	5.8		0.0		17	60	4	0.28		33	4	0.04	0.6	0.14	03901
1 scoop	9	1.8	0.8	0.6	0.4	1		60	40	0.84	0.034	0.4	111		0.04	0.03		
Gerber, low Fe,	20	26.8	0.4	2.2		0.0		6	16	2	0.20		18	2	0.02	0.2	0.06	03913
Mead Johnson - *1 fl oz*	31	1.1	0.5	0.4	0.2	<1		22	11	0.14	0.015	0.5	60		0.03	0.01		
liquid conc, Mead Johnson	40	23.2	0.9	4.4		0.0		12	31	3	0.40		36	5	0.03	0.4	0.12	03833
1 fl oz	31	2.1	0.9	0.8	0.4	1		44	22	0.28	0.030	1.1	121		0.06	0.02		
powder, Mead Johnson	44	0.2	0.9	4.8		0.0		13	35	4	0.44		40	5	0.04	0.4	0.13	03834
1 scoop	9	2.4	1.0	0.9	0.5	<1		48	24	0.31	0.033	1.2	133		0.06	0.03		
Gerber, soy w/Fe,	20	27.3	0.6	2.0		0.0		7	21	2	0.24		18	2	0.02	0.2	0.06	03835
Mead Johnson - *1 fl oz*	31	1.1	0.5	0.4	0.2	0		24	17	0.37	0.015	0.6	61		0.02	0.01		
liquid conc, Mead Johnson	41	23.3	1.2	4.1		0.0		15	43	4	0.49		37	5	0.03	0.4	0.12	03862
1 fl oz	31	2.2	0.9	0.8	0.4	0		49	34	0.73	0.030	1.1	122		0.04	0.02		
powder, Mead Johnson	46	0.2	1.4	4.7		0.0		17	49	5	0.56		42	6	0.04	0.5	0.14	03865
1 scoop	9	2.4	1.0	0.9	0.5	0		56	39	0.84	0.035	1.3	140		0.04	0.03		
Gerber w/Fe,	20	26.8	0.4	2.2		0.0		6	16	2	0.20		18	2	0.02	0.2	0.06	03863
Mead Johnson - *1 fl oz*	31	1.1	0.5	0.4	0.2	<1		22	11	0.36	0.015	0.5	60		0.03	0.01		
liquid conc, Mead Johnson	40	23.2	0.9	4.4		0.0		12	31	3	0.40		36	5	0.03	0.4	0.12	03828
1 fl oz	31	2.1	0.9	0.8	0.4	1		44	22	0.73	0.030	1.1	121		0.06	0.02		
powder, Mead Johnson	44	0.2	0.9	4.8		0.0		13	35	4	0.44		40	5	0.04	0.4	0.13	03829
1 scoop	9	2.4	1.0	0.9	0.5	<1		48	24	0.80	0.033	1.2	133		0.06	0.03		
Good Start w/Fe,	20	26.7	0.5	2.2		0.0		5	13	1	0.15		18	2	0.01	0.1	0.04	03831
Carnation - *1 fl oz*	31	1.0	0.4	0.3	0.2	2		20	7	0.30	0.016	0.2	61		0.03	0.02		
																		03800

	KCAL WT (g) HIS (mg) PHE (mg)	H₂0 (g) FAT (g) ISO (mg) TYR (mg)	PRO (g) SFA (g) LEU (mg) THR (mg)	CHO (g) MUFA (g) LYS (mg) TRY (mg)	SUGR (g) PUFA (g) MET (mg) VAL (mg)	DFIB (g) CHOL (mg) CYS (mg) ARG (mg)	TAU (mg) CAR (mg)	Na (mg) K (mg) Cl (mg)	Ca (mg) P (mg) I (mcg)	Mg (mg) Fe (mg) Mo (mcg) BIO (mcg)	Zn (mg) Cu (mg) Cr (mcg) CHLN (mg)	Mn (mg) Se (mcg) INOS (mg)	A (mcg RAE) A (IU) PANT (mg)	C (mg) E (mg ATE) E (IU)	B-1 (mg) B-2 (mg) D (IU)	NIA (mg) B-6 (mg) K (mcg)	B-12 (mcg) FOL (mcg DFE) REF
liquid conc, Carnation	40	23.8	1.0	4.4		0.0		10	26	3	0.30		36	3	0.03	0.3	0.09
1 fl oz	31	2.0	0.9	0.6	0.4	4		39	14	0.60	0.031	0.4	119		0.05	0.03	
																	03801
powder, Carnation	45	0.3	1.1	4.9		0.0		10	29	3	0.33		40	4	0.03	0.3	0.10
1 scoop	9	2.3	1.0	0.7	0.5	4		44	17	0.66	0.035	0.9	134		0.06	0.03	
																	03802
Isomil 2, Ross[9]	101	134.8	2.5	10.4				45	137	8	0.76	0.025		9	0.06	1.4	0.46
5 fl oz (150 ml)	~154	5.5						109	91	1.82	0.076	1.8	304	1.0	0.09	0.06	15.2
								63	15				0.8	2	61	11.15	
										5	12	5					RSSP2
Isomil DF, Ross[10]	101	134.8	2.7	10.2				45	106	8	0.76	0.025		9	0.06	1.4	0.46
5 fl oz (150 ml)	~154	5.5						109	76	1.82	0.076	1.8	304	1.0	0.09	0.06	15.2
								63	15				0.8	2	61	11.15	
										5	12	5					RSSP3
Isomil SF w/Fe,	20	26.6	0.5	2.0		0.0		9	21	2	0.15	0.006	18	2	0.01	0.3	0.09
Ross - 1 fl oz	30	1.1	0.4	0.2	0.3	0		22	15	0.36	0.015	0.4	60		0.02	0.01	
										0.2							
																	03847
liquid conc, Ross	40	23.6	1.1	4.0		0.0		18	42	3	0.30	0.012	36	4	0.02	0.5	0.18
1 fl oz	31	2.2	0.9	0.4	0.8	0		43	30	0.72	0.030	0.8	120		0.04	0.02	
										0.3							
																	03848
Isomil w/Fe,	20	26.6	0.5	2.1		0.0		9	21	2	0.15	0.005	18	2	0.01	0.3	0.09
Ross - 1 fl oz	31	1.1	0.4	0.4	0.3	0		22	15	0.36	0.015	0.4	60		0.02	0.01	
										0.2							
																	03841
liquid conc, Ross	40	23.6	1.0	4.1		0.0		18	42	3	0.30	0.010	36	4	0.02	0.5	0.18
1 fl oz	31	2.2	0.7	0.8	0.5	0		43	30	0.72	0.030	0.8	120		0.04	0.02	
										0.3							
																	03842
powder, Ross	45	0.2	1.1	4.6		0.0		20	47	3	0.34	0.013	40	4	0.03	0.6	0.20
1 scoop	9	2.5	0.8	0.9	0.6	0		48	34	0.81	0.034	0.9	135		0.04	0.03	
										0.3							
																	03843
I-Soyalac w/Fe,	20	26.7	0.6	2.0		0.0		9	20	2	0.16		15	2	0.02	0.3	0.06
Carnation - 1 fl oz	31	1.1	0.2	0.2	0.7	0		23	13	0.38	0.023	0.5	63		0.02	0.02	
																	03925
liquid conc, Carnation	41	23.6	1.3	4.1		0.0		17	41	4	0.32		33	5	0.04	0.5	0.13
1 fl oz	31	2.3	0.3	0.5	1.4	0		48	26	0.78	0.048	1.0	129		0.04	0.04	
																	03926
powder, Carnation	22	0.1	0.7	2.2		0.0		9	22	2	0.17		4	3	0.02	0.3	0.07
1 scoop	4.3	1.2	0.2	0.3	0.7	0		26	14	0.42	0.026	0.5	68		0.02	0.02	
																	03928
Kindercal, Mead Johnson[11]	250	200.0	7.1	32.0		0.0		88	240	50	3.00	0.500		58	0.40	4.9	1.40
8 fl oz (240 ml)	~250	10.5						310	200	2.50	0.300	7.5	970	5.9	0.50	0.50	38.0
						15		175	30	13	12.5		3.1	9	125	7.50	
						15				38	63	20					MDJN31
Kindercal TF, Mead Johnson	250	200.0	7.1	32.0		0.0		88	240	50	3.00	0.500		58	0.40	4.9	1.40
8 fl oz (240 ml)	~250	10.5						310	200	2.50	0.300	7.5	970	5.9	0.50	0.50	38.0
						15		175	30	13	12.5		3.1	9	125	7.50	
						15				38	63	20					MDJN30
Lactofree w/Fe,	20	27.1	0.4	2.1		0.0		6	17	2	0.20		18	2	0.02	0.2	0.06
Mead Johnson[12] - 1 fl oz	31	1.1	0.5	0.4	0.2	<1		22	11	0.37	0.015	0.6	61		0.02	0.01	

	KCAL / WT (g) / HIS (mg) / PHE (mg)	H₂0 (g) / FAT (g) / ISO (mg) / TYR (mg)	PRO (g) / SFA (g) / LEU (mg) / THR (mg)	CHO (g) / MUFA (g) / LYS (mg) / TRY (mg)	SUGR (g) / PUFA (g) / MET (mg) / VAL (mg)	DFIB (g) / CHOL (mg) / CYS (mg) / ARG (mg)	TAU (mg) / CAR (mg)	Na (mg) / K (mg) / Cl (mg)	Ca (mg) / P (mg) / I (mcg)	Mg (mg) / Fe (mg) / Mo (mcg)	Zn (mg) / Cu (mg) / Cr (mcg)	Mn (mg) / Se (mcg)	A (mcg RAE) / A (IU) / PANT (mg) / BIO (mcg)	C (mg) / E (mg ATE) / E (IU) / CHLN (mg)	B-1 (mg) / B-2 (mg) / D (IU) / INOS (mg)	NIA (mg) / B-6 (mg) / K (mcg)	B-12 (mcg) / FOL (mcg DFE) / REF
																	03868
liquid conc, Mead Johnson[12]	41	23.3	0.9	4.2		0.0		12	33	3	0.41		37	5	0.03	0.4	0.12
1 fl oz	31	2.2	1.0	0.9	0.4	1		45	22	0.73	0.030	1.1	122		0.04	0.02	
																	03871
powder, Mead Johnson[12]	53	0.1	1.2	5.5		0.0		16	43	4	0.53		47	6	0.04	0.5	0.16
1 scoop	10	2.9	1.2	1.1	0.6	1		58	29	0.95	0.040	1.5	158		0.05	0.03	
																	03869
Lofenalac w/Fe, pwdr, Mead Johnson[13] - *1 scoop*	44	0.3	1.4	5.8		0.0		21	41	5	0.35		41	4	0.03	0.6	0.14
	10	1.7	0.2	0.4	1.0	0		45	31	0.83	0.041	1.0	137		0.04	0.03	
																	03810
prep from pwdr, Mead Johnson[13]	20	26.8	0.7	2.6		0.0		10	19	2	0.16		19	2	0.02	0.3	0.06
1 fl oz	31	0.8	0.1	0.2	0.5	0		20	14	0.38	0.019	0.6	62		0.02	0.01	
																	03811
MSUD, prep from pwdr, Mead Johnson - *5 fl oz (150 ml)*	100	134.0	1.7	13.4				39	103	11	0.78	0.031		8	0.08	1.2	0.31
	~154	4.2						103	56	1.88	0.094	2.8	310	2.1	0.09	0.06	15.6
	51	109			162	46	6	78	7				0.5	3	63	15.60	
	39	109	133	0	90	51							8	13	5		MDJN37
Next Step, Mead Johnson[14]	100	133.0	2.6	11.1				41	120	8	0.90	0.007		9	0.10	1.0	0.25
5 fl oz (150 ml)	~152	5.0						130	84	1.80	0.090	2.8	300	1.3	0.15	0.06	15.0
								86	8				0.5	2	60	8.00	
							3						4	16	5		MDJN38
Next Step Soy, prep from liquid conc, Mead Johnson[15] - *1 fl oz*	20	26.9	0.6	2.0		0.0		7	21	2	0.24	0.005	18	2	0.02	0.2	0.06
	31	1.1	0.5	0.4	0.2	0		24	16	0.36	0.015	0.5	59		0.02	0.01	
													0.1				
																	03932
prep from pwdr, Mead Johnson[15]	20	26.7	0.6	2.4		0.0		9	23	2	0.24	0.005	18	2	0.02	0.2	0.06
1 fl oz	31	0.9	0.4	0.3	0.2	0		30	18	0.36	0.015	0.5	59		0.02	0.02	
													0.1				
																	03930
Nutramigen w/Fe, Mead Johnson[16] - *1 fl oz*	20	27.1	0.6	2.2		0.0		10	19	2	0.20		18	2	0.02	0.2	0.06
	31	1.0	0.4	0.4	0.2	0		22	13	0.36	0.015	0.6	61		0.02	0.01	
																	03813
liquid conc, Mead Johnson[16]	41	23.5	1.2	4.5		0.0		20	39	4	0.41		37	5	0.03	0.4	0.12
1 fl oz	32	2.1	0.9	0.8	0.4	0		45	26	0.74	0.031	1.1	124		0.04	0.02	
																	03816
powder, Mead Johnson[16]	48	0.4	1.3	5.2		0.0		22	44	5	0.47		43	6	0.04	0.5	0.14
1 scoop	10	2.4	1.0	0.9	0.5	0		52	30	0.85	0.036	1.0	142		0.04	0.03	
																	03814
Nutren Junior, van, Nestle *8.3 fl oz (250 ml)*	250	212.0	7.5	31.9				115	250	50	3.80	0.400		25	0.60	5.0	1.50
	~262	10.5						330	200	3.50	0.250	7.5	600	4.7	0.50	0.60	100.0
							20	270	30	8	7.5		2.5	7	140	7.50	
							10						75	75	20		NEST15
Nutren Junior w/fiber, van, Nestle - *8.3 fl oz (250 ml)*	250	211.0	7.5	31.9		1.5		115	250	50	3.80	0.400		25	0.60	5.0	1.50
	~261	10.5						330	200	3.50	0.250	7.5	600	4.7	0.50	0.60	100.0
							20	270	30	8	7.5		2.5	7	140	7.50	
							10						75	75	20		NEST14
PediaSure Enteral Formula, Ross[17] - *8 fl oz (240 ml)*	237	200.0	7.1	26.0				90	230	47	2.80	0.240		24	0.64	4.0	1.40
	~245	11.8	3.3	5.0	2.8			310	190	3.30	0.240	5.4	610	3.6	0.50	0.62	88.0
	88	319	351	657	534	190	17	240	23	9	7.1		2.4	5	120	9.00	
	54	330	323	416	221	180	4						76	71	19		RSSM31

	KCAL / WT(g) / HIS(mg) / PHE(mg)	H₂0(g) / FAT(g) / ISO(mg) / TYR(mg)	PRO(g) / SFA(g) / LEU(mg) / THR(mg)	CHO(g) / MUFA(g) / LYS(mg) / TRY(mg)	SUGR(g) / PUFA(g) / MET(mg) / VAL(mg)	DFIB(g) / CHOL(mg) / CYS(mg) / ARG(mg)	TAU(mg) / CAR(mg)	Na(mg) / K(mg) / Cl(mg)	Ca(mg) / P(mg) / I(mcg)	Mg(mg) / Fe(mg) / Mo(mcg)	Zn(mg) / Cu(mg) / Cr(mcg)	Mn(mg) / Se(mcg)	A(mcg RAE) / A(IU) / PANT(mg) / BIO(mcg)	C(mg) / E(mg ATE) / E(IU) / CHLN(mg)	B-1(mg) / B-2(mg) / D(IU) / INOS(mg)	NIA(mg) / B-6(mg) / K(mcg)	B-12(mcg) / FOL(mcg DFE) / REF
w/fiber, Ross[18] *8 fl oz (240 ml)*	237	200.0	7.1	26.9		1.2		90	230	47	2.80	0.240		24	0.64	4.0	1.40
	~246	11.8	3.3	5.0	2.8			310	190	3.30	0.240	5.4	610	3.6	0.50	0.62	88.0
	88	319	351	657	534	190	17	240	23	9	7.1		2.4	5	120	9.00	
	54	330	323	416	221	180	4						76	71	19		RSSM32
Pediasure w/Fe (child formula), Ross[17] - *1 fl oz*	29	24.9	0.9	3.3		0.0		11	29	6	0.36	0.074	23	3	0.08	0.5	0.18
	31	1.5	0.4	0.6	0.3	1		39	24	0.42	0.029	0.7	76		0.06	0.08	
													0.3				
																	03860
Pediatric EO28, SHS North America[19] - *100 ml*	237		5.9	34.6				47	147	21	1.80	0.240		7	0.13	2.1	0.17
	~106	8.3						220	147	1.80	0.240	3.7	277	1.3	0.15	0.19	14.2
							16	83	14	8	7.1		0.6	2	74	3.60	
							8						5	43	4		SHNA1
Peptamen Junior, Nestle *8.3 fl oz (250 ml)*	250	212.0	7.5	34.4				115	250	50	3.80	0.400		25	0.60	5.0	1.50
	~264	9.6						330	200	3.50	0.250	7.5	600	4.7	0.50	0.60	100.0
							20	270	30	8	7.5		2.5	7	140	7.50	
							10						75	75	20		NEST21
Portagen w/Fe, pwdr, Mead Johnson - *1 scoop*	44	0.3	1.6	5.1		0.0		24	41	9	0.41		104	4	0.07	0.9	0.28
	9	2.2	1.9	0.1	0.2	1		55	31	0.84	0.070	0.2	348		0.08	0.09	
																	03819
prep from pwdr, Mead Johnson *1 fl oz*	20	26.7	0.7	2.3		0.0		11	19	4	0.19		47	2	0.03	0.4	0.13
	31	1.0	0.8	<0.1	0.1	<1		25	14	0.38	0.031	0.1	156		0.04	0.04	
																	03820
Pregestimil w/Fe, pwdr, Mead Johnson - *1 scoop*	44	0.4	1.2	4.5		0.0		17	41	5	0.41		50	5	0.03	0.6	0.14
	9	2.5	1.5	0.4	0.5	0		48	28	0.83	0.041	1.0	167		0.04	0.03	
																	03821
prep from pwdr, Mead Johnson *1 fl oz*	20	26.8	0.6	2.1		0.0		8	19	2	0.19		23	2	0.02	0.3	0.06
	31	1.1	0.7	0.2	0.2	0		22	13	0.38	0.019	0.6	76		0.02	0.01	
																	03822
Prosobee w/Fe, Mead Johnson[20] - *1 fl oz*	20	26.8	0.6	2.0		0.0		7	21	2	0.24		18	2	0.02	0.2	0.06
	31	1.1	0.5	0.4	0.2	0		24	16	0.36	0.015	0.5	60		0.02	0.01	
																	03823
liquid conc, Mead Johnson[20] *1 fl oz*	40	23.2	1.2	4.0		0.0		14	43	4	0.49		36	5	0.03	0.4	0.12
	31	2.1	0.9	0.8	0.4	0		49	34	0.73	0.030	1.1	121		0.04	0.02	
																	03824
powder, Mead Johnson[20] *1 scoop*	44	0.2	1.3	4.5		0.0		16	46	5	0.53		40	5	0.04	0.4	0.13
	9	2.3	1.0	0.9	0.4	0		53	37	0.80	0.034	1.2	133		0.04	0.03	
																	03826
RCF, Ross[21] *5 fl oz (150 ml)*	101	134.8	3.0	10.2				45	106	8	0.76	0.030		9	0.06	1.4	0.46
	~154	5.4						109	76	1.82	0.076	2.1	304	1.0	0.09	0.06	15.2
								63	15				0.8	2	61	11.15	
													5	8	5		RSSP6
Resource Just for Kids, Novartis - *8 fl oz (237 ml)*	237		7.1	26.0				140	270	47	2.80	0.470		24	0.28	4.0	0.57
	~248	11.9						270	190	3.30	0.240	9.5	570		0.36	0.38	88.0
							21	120	28	10	16.0		2.4		78	9.50	
							4						36	95	19		NVAR40
w/fiber, Novartis *8 fl oz (237 ml)*	237		7.1	26.0		1.4		140	270	47	2.80	0.590		24	0.64	4.0	1.40
	~248	11.8						270	190	3.30	0.240	7.1	830	3.6	0.50	0.62	88.0
							21	120	28	8	12.2		2.4	5	120	9.50	
							4						76	95	19		NVAR39
Similac 2, Ross[22] *5 fl oz (150 ml)*	101	134.8	2.1	10.7				24	120	6	0.76	0.005		9	0.10	1.1	0.25
	~154	5.6						106	65	1.82	0.091	1.8	304	2.0	0.15	0.06	15.2

Food / Serving	KCAL / WT(g) / HIS(mg) / PHE(mg)	H₂0(g) / FAT(g) / ISO(mg) / TYR(mg)	PRO(g) / SFA(g) / LEU(mg) / THR(mg)	CHO(g) / MUFA(g) / LYS(mg) / TRY(mg)	SUGR(g) / PUFA(g) / MET(mg) / VAL(mg)	DFIB(g) / CHOL(mg) / CYS(mg) / ARG(mg)	TAU(mg) / CAR(mg)	Na(mg) / K(mg) / Cl(mg)	Ca(mg) / P(mg) / I(mcg)	Mg(mg) / Fe(mg) / Mo(mcg)	Zn(mg) / Cu(mg) / Cr(mcg)	Mn(mg) / Se(mcg)	A(mcg RAE) / A(IU) / PANT(mg) / BIO(mcg)	C(mg) / E(mg ATE) / E(IU) / CHLN(mg)	B-1(mg) / B-2(mg) / D(IU) / INOS(mg)	NIA(mg) / B-6(mg) / K(mcg) / REF	B-12(mcg) / FOL(mcg DFE)
(cont. from prev.)								66	6				0.5	3	61	8.11	
													4	16	5	RSSP7	
Similac Advance, Ross	101	134.8	2.1	10.9				24	79	6	0.76	0.005		9	0.10	1.1	0.25
5 fl oz (150 ml)	~155	5.5						106	43	1.82	0.091	1.8	304	1.0	0.15	0.06	15.2
								66	6				0.5	2	61	8.11	
													4	16	5	RSSP8	
Similac Human Milk Fortifier,	14		1.0	1.8				15	117	7		0.007		25	0.23	3.6	0.64
Ross[23] - 1 packet	4	0.4						63	67	0.40	0.170	0.5	620	2.1	0.42	0.21	23.0
								38						3	120	8.00	
													26	2	4	RSSP15	
Similac, lactose free, w/Fe, Ross[24]	101	134.8	2.2	10.8				30	85	6	0.76	0.005		9	0.10	1.1	0.25
5 fl oz (150 ml)	~154	5.5						108	57	1.82	0.091	1.8	304	2.0	0.15	0.06	15.2
								66	9				0.5	3	61	8.11	
													4	16	4	RSSP14	
Similac, low Fe,	20	27.1	0.4	2.2		0.0		5	16	1	0.15	0.001	18	2	0.02	0.2	0.05
Ross[25] - 1 fl oz	31	1.1	0.4	0.4	0.2	1		21	9	0.04	0.018	0.4	61		0.03	0.01	
													0.1				
																03855	
liquid conc, Ross[25]	40	23.6	0.8	4.3		0.0		10	31	3	0.30	0.002	36	4	0.04	0.4	0.10
1 fl oz	31	2.2	0.8	0.8	0.5	1		42	17	0.09	0.036	0.9	120		0.06	0.02	
													0.2				
																03856	
powder, Ross[25]	46	0.2	0.9	4.8		0.0		11	36	3	0.34	0.002	41	4	0.05	0.5	0.11
1 scoop	9	2.5	0.9	0.9	0.6	1		48	19	0.10	0.041	1.0	137		0.07	0.03	
													0.2				
																03858	
Similac Natural Care,	24	25.8	0.6	2.5		0.0		10	50	3	0.35	0.003	89	9	0.06	1.2	0.13
low Fe, Ross[26] - 1 fl oz	31	1.3	0.8	0.1	0.3	1		30	27	0.09	0.059	0.4	296		0.15	0.06	
													0.5				
																03839	
Similac NeoSure[27]	112	134.3	2.9	11.5				37	118	10	1.34	0.011		17	0.25	2.2	0.45
5 fl oz (150 ml)	~155	6.2						159	69	2.01	0.134	2.6	515	2.7	0.17	0.11	28.0
								84	17				0.9	4	78	12.31	
													10	18	7	RSSP9	
Similac PM 60/40, low Fe,	20	26.7	0.5	2.0		0.0		5	11	1	0.15	0.001	18	2	0.02	0.2	0.05
Ross[28] - 1 fl oz	30	1.1	0.5	0.2	0.4	1		19	5	0.04	0.018	0.4	60		0.03	0.01	
													0.1				
																03836	
powder, Ross[28]	46	0.2	1.0	4.7		0.0		11	26	3	0.35	0.002	42	4	0.05	0.5	0.12
1 scoop	9	2.6	1.1	0.5	0.9	1		40	13	0.10	0.042	0.9	138		0.07	0.03	
													0.2				
																03837	
Similac Special Care 20,	101	134.8	2.7	10.7				44	182	12	1.52	0.012		38	0.25	5.1	0.56
Ross[29] - 5 fl oz (150 ml)	~154	5.5						131	101	0.41	0.253	1.8	1267	2.7	0.63	0.25	37.5
								82	6				1.9	4	152	12.16	
													38	10	6	RSSP10	
w/Fe, Ross[30]	101	134.8	2.7	10.7				44	182	12	1.52	0.012		38	0.25	5.1	0.56
5 fl oz (150 ml)	~154	5.5						131	101	1.82	0.253	1.8	1267	2.7	0.63	0.25	37.5
								82	6				1.9	4	152	12.16	
													38	10	6	RSSP11	
Similac Special Care 24 w/Fe, Ross[30]	122	132.9	3.3	12.9				52	220	15	1.83	0.015		45	0.30	6.1	0.67
5 fl oz (150 ml)	~156	6.6						157	122	2.20	0.305	2.2	1524	3.3	0.76	0.30	45.1
								99	7				2.3	5	183	14.63	
													45	12	7	RSSP12	
Similac w/Fe,	20	26.5	0.4	2.2		0.0		5	16	1	0.15	0.001	18	2	0.02	0.2	0.05
Ross[25] - 1 fl oz	30	1.1	0.4	0.4	0.2	1		21	9	0.36	0.018	0.4	60		0.03	0.01	
													0.1				
																03850	

	KCAL WT (g) HIS (mg) PHE (mg)	H₂0 (g) FAT (g) ISO (mg) TYR (mg)	PRO (g) SFA (g) LEU (mg) THR (mg)	CHO (g) MUFA (g) LYS (mg) TRY (mg)	SUGR (g) PUFA (g) MET (mg) VAL (mg)	DFIB (g) CHOL (mg) CYS (mg) ARG (mg)	Na (mg) K (mg) TAU (mg) CAR (mg)	Ca (mg) P (mg) Cl (mg)	Mg (mg) Fe (mg) I (mcg)	Zn (mg) Cu (mg) Mo (mcg)	Mn (mg) Se (mcg) Cr (mcg)	A (mcg RAE) A (IU) PANT (mcg) BIO (mcg)	C (mg) E (mg ATE) E (IU) CHLN (mg)	B-1 (mg) B-2 (mg) D (IU) INOS (mg)	NIA (mg) B-6 (mg) K (mcg)	B-12 (mcg) FOL (mcg DFE) REF
liquid conc, Ross[25]	40	23.6	0.8	4.3		0.0	10	31	3	0.30	0.002	36	4	0.04	0.4	0.10
1 fl oz	31	2.2	0.8	0.8	0.5	1	42	17	0.72	0.036	0.9	120		0.06	0.02	
												0.2				
																03851
powder, Ross[25]	46	0.2	0.9	4.8		0.0	11	36	3	0.34	0.002	41	4	0.05	0.5	0.11
1 scoop	9	2.5	0.9	0.9	0.6	1	48	19	0.82	0.041	1.0	137		0.07	0.03	
												0.2				
																03853
Vivonex Pediatric, Novartis	200		6.0	31.5			100	243	50	3.00	0.500		25	0.38	5.0	0.75
1 pkt w/water (8.3 fl oz)		5.9					300	200	2.50	0.300	7.5	625	5.0	0.45	0.50	50.0
							20	250	30	19	11.3	1.3	8	125	10.00	
							6					25	50	15		NVAR53

[1] Protein hydrolysate-based infant formula with iron.
[2] Amino acid-based medical formula for infants and toddlers.
[3] Twenty-two calories per fluid ounce infant formula; meets needs of premature infants.
[4] Oral electrolyte maintenance solution made with rice syrup solids; used to maintain fluid and electrolytes in infants and children with diarrhea or vomiting; also used as postoperative fluid and electrolyte therapy.
[5] Prethickened infant formula for first 12 months for infants with uncomplicated regurgitation; thickened with pregelatinized rice starch.
[6] Supplement to be added to mother's milk; increases levels of protein, energy, calcium, phosphorus, sodium, and other nutrients for the needs of the rapidly growing premature infant.
[7] Meets requirements of rapidly growing low-birth weight infant; high protein (whey protein:casein of 60:40); available in low iron and iron-fortified and in 20- and 24- calories per fluid ounce.
[8] Milk-based infant formula with iron for first 12 months.
[9] Soy protein-based infant and toddler formula with iron.
[10] Soy protein-based infant formula for diarrhea.
[11] Lactose-free, isotonic formulation for tube and oral feeding of children 1–10 years of age.
[12] Milk-based, lactose-free, easy-to-digest infant formula for first 12 months.
[13] Hydrolyzed casein formula processed to remove most of the phenylalanine for infants with hyperphenylalanemia including PKU.
[14] Iron-fortified formula for toddlers (1–3 years).

[15] Soy protein-based, iron-fortified formula for toddlers (1–3 years).
[16] Hypoallergenic protein hydrolysate infant formula for first 12 months; galactose-free; gluten-free.
[17] Sodium caseinate and whey protein-based enteral formula for infants and toddlers.
[18] Sodium caseinate and whey protein-based enteral formula with fiber for infants and toddlers.
[19] An elemental medical food formulated to provide complete or supplemental nutritional support for children with severe impairment of the gastrointestinal tract.
[20] Soy protein isolate-based infant formula for first 12 months; milk-free; lactose-free.
[21] Soy protein-based infant formula with iron.
[22] Milk protein-based infant and toddler formula with iron.
[23] Powder added to human milk for preterm infants.
[24] Milk protein-based infant formula with iron.
[25] Milk protein-based infant formula.
[26] Low iron human milk fortifier.
[27] Milk protein-based infant formula with iron; nutrient-rich post-discharge formula.
[28] Milk protein-based, low iron infant formula.
[29] Milk protein-based, low iron premature infant formula.
[30] Milk protein-based premature infant formula.

32.2 MEDICAL FOODS FOR ADULTS

	KCAL WT (g) HIS (mg) PHE (mg)	H₂0 (g) FAT (g) ISO (mg) TYR (mg)	PRO (g) SFA (g) LEU (mg) THR (mg)	CHO (g) MUFA (g) LYS (mg) TRY (mg)	SUGR (g) PUFA (g) MET (mg) VAL (mg)	DFIB (g) CHOL (mg) CYS (mg) ARG (mg)	Na (mg) K (mg) TAU (mg) CAR (mg)	Ca (mg) P (mg) Cl (mg)	Mg (mg) Fe (mg) I (mcg)	Zn (mg) Cu (mg) Mo (mcg)	Mn (mg) Se (mcg) Cr (mcg)	A (mcg RAE) A (IU) PANT (mcg) BIO (mcg)	C (mg) E (mg ATE) E (IU) CHLN (mg)	B-1 (mg) B-2 (mg) D (IU) INOS (mg)	NIA (mg) B-6 (mg) K (mcg)	B-12 (mcg) FOL (mcg DFE) REF
Additions, Nestle[1]	100		6.0	9.0	1.0	0.0	100	0					0			
1 scoop (2 1/3 T)	19	5.0	0.5			0				0.00						
																NEST1
Advera, Ross[2]	303	190.0	14.2	51.2		2.1	250	260	80	3.80	1.300		90	0.75	6.0	12.00
8 fl oz (240 ml)	~248	5.4	1.5	2.1	1.3	<5	670	260	4.50	0.600	14.0	2550	6.0	0.68	0.80	120.0
	99	568	568	1022	980		50	350	30	54	17.0	3.0	9	80	24.00	
				596	966	369	30					90	50	0		RSSM1
AlitraQ, Ross[3]	300	254.0	15.8	49.3		0.0	300	220	80	6.00	1.000		60	0.60	8.0	2.40
1 pkt in wtr (10 fl oz/300 ml)	~324	4.6	2.0	0.4	2.3	0	360	220	4.40	0.400	15.0	1200	6.0	0.68	0.80	80.0
	205	711	758	1264	980		60	390	30	33	24.0	4.0	9	80	16.00	
				901	1343	316	30					120	120	0		RSSM2
Boost Bar, Mead Johnson	190		4.0	29.0	16.0	<1.0	90	150	60	2.30			9	0.23	3.0	0.90
1.6 oz bar	44	7.0	3.5			<5	105	150	1.08	0.200		750	3.0	0.23	0.30	60.0
												1.5	5	60		
												45				MDJN1
Boost Drink, Mead Johnson	240	200.0	10.0	41.0	23.0	0.0	130	330	105	4.50	0.700		60	0.38	5.0	2.10
8 fl oz (240 ml)	~255	4.0	0.5			5	400	310	4.50	0.500	18.0	1250	20.0	0.43	0.70	140.0
								340	38	20	30.0	2.5	30	150	30.00	
												75	50			MDJN2
Boost High Pro Drink, Mead Johnson - *8 fl oz (240 ml)*	240	200.0	15.0	33.0	14.0	0.0	170	330	105	4.50	0.700		60	0.38	5.0	2.10
	~254	6.0	0.5			10	380	310	4.50	0.500	18.0	1250	20.0	0.43	0.70	140.0

	KCAL	H₂0 (g)	PRO (g)	CHO (g)	SUGR (g)	DFIB (g)		Na (mg)	Ca (mg)	Mg (mg)	Zn (mg)	Mn (mg)	A (mcg RAE)	C (mg)	B-1 (mg)	NIA (mg)	B-12 (mcg)
	WT (g)	FAT (g)	SFA (g)	MUFA (g)	PUFA (g)	CHOL (mg)		K (mg)	P (mg)	Fe (mg)	Cu (mg)	Se (mcg)	A (IU)	E (mg ATE)	B-2 (mg)	B-6 (mg)	FOL (mcg DFE)
	HIS (mg)	ISO (mg)	LEU (mg)	LYS (mg)	MET (mg)	CYS (mg)	TAU (mg)	Cl (mg)	I (mcg)	Mo (mcg)	Cr (mcg)		PANT (mg)	E (IU)	D (IU)	K (mg)	
	PHE (mg)	TYR (mg)	THR (mg)	TRY (mg)	VAL (mg)	ARG (mg)	CAR (mg)						BIO (mcg)	CHLN (mg)	INOS (mg)		REF
								320	38	20	30.0		2.5	30	150	30.00	
													75	50			MDJN3
Boost High Pro mix w/nonfat mlk,	290	220.0	21.0	48.0	47.0	0.0		320	590	133	5.00	1.000		22	0.49	7.0	1.93
Md Jhnsn - *54 g pwdr w/8 fl oz mlk*	299	1.0	0.5			14		970	500	6.10	0.700	25.0	1790	6.7	0.54	0.65	146.0
								480	50	33	36.0		3.5	10	133	40.00	
													100				MDJN4
w/water, Mead Johnson	200	240.0	13.0	36.0	35.0	0.0		190	290	105	4.00	1.000		20	0.40	6.8	1.00
54 g powder w/8 fl oz water	299	1.0	0.0			10		560	250	6.00	0.700	18.7	1290	6.7	0.20	0.55	133.0
								220	40	20	32.0		2.7	10	33	30.00	
													90				MDJN5
Boost Plus, Mead Johnson	360	185.0	14.0	45.0	20.0	<1.0		170	330	105	4.50	0.700		60	0.38	5.0	2.10
8 fl oz (240 ml)	~258	14.0	1.5			10		380	310	4.50	0.500	18.0	1250	20.0	0.43	0.70	140.0
								320	38	20	30.0		2.5	30	150	30.00	
													75	50			MDJN6
Boost Pudding, Mead Johnson	240	93.0	7.0	33.0	20.0	0.0		125	250	60	2.70	0.420		36	0.23	3.0	1.30
5 oz	142	9.0	1.0			<5		250	200	2.70	0.300	10.5	750	10.0	0.26	0.42	84.0
								180	23	12	18.0		1.5	15	70	18.40	
													45	25			MDJN7
Boost w/fiber, Mead Johnson	240	200.0	10.0	42.0	16.0	3.0		170	330	105	4.50	0.700		60	0.38	5.0	2.10
8 fl oz (240 ml)	~256	4.0	0.5			5		380	310	4.50	0.500	18.0	1250	20.0	0.43	0.70	140.0
								320	38	20	30.0		2.5	30	150	30.00	
													75	50			MDJN8
Casec powder, Mead Johnson[4]	380		90.0					100	1400								
1 1/3 cup (3.5 oz)	100	2.0						10	800								
																	MDJN9
Choice DM Beverage, Mead	220	200.0	9.0	24.0		3.0		200	330	105	5.00	1.000		60	0.38	5.0	1.50
Johnson - *8 fl oz (240 ml)*	~243	10.0	1.5			0		430	310	4.50	0.500	17.5	1760	30.0	0.43	0.50	100.0
							38	300	38	26	60.0		2.5	45	150	20.00	
							38						75	125	60		MDJN10
Choice DM Nutrition Bar,	140		6.0	19.0		3.0		80	133	50	2.00	0.250		30	0.20	2.7	0.80
Mead Johnson - *1.23 oz bar*	35	4.5	2.5			<5		105	110	3.70	0.300	9.0	730	20.0	0.23	0.27	53.0
								40	20	10	40.0		1.3	30	40	16.00	
													40		40		MDJN14
Choice DM Tube-Feeding Lqd,	250	200.0	10.6	28.0		3.4		200	250	100	5.00	0.750		60	0.38	5.0	1.50
Mead Johnson - *8 fl oz (240 ml)*	~251	12.0	2.1			5		430	250	4.50	0.500	18.0	1250	20.0	0.43	0.50	100.0
							38	300	38	25	50.0		2.5	30	100	30.00	
							38						75	125	60		MDJN15
Compleat, Novartis	265	213.5	10.7	35.0				190	167	67	3.83	0.670		15	0.38	5.0	1.50
8.3 fl oz (250 ml)	~268	9.2						362	183	3.00	0.330	16.7	833	5.0	0.43	0.50	66.7
							3	216	27	50	25.0		1.7	8	67	16.70	
							11						50	50			NVAR2
Comply, Mead Johnson[5]	355	182.0	14.2	43.0				280	280	114	5.70	0.850		43	0.43	5.7	4.30
8 fl oz (240 ml)	~254	14.5						440	280	5.10	0.570	20.0	1420	14.0	0.48	0.80	142.0
							43	400	43	28	34.0		2.8	21	114	34.00	
							43						85	142			MDJN16
Criticare HN, Mead Johnson[6]	250	200.0	9.0	51.0				150	125	50	2.50	0.630		38	0.48	6.3	1.88
8 fl oz (240 ml)	~262	1.2						310	125	2.30	0.250		630	6.3	0.54	0.63	50.0
								250	19				3.1	9	50	31.00	
													38	63			MDJN17
Crucial, Nestle	375	192.0	23.5	33.8				292	250	100	9.00	1.000		250	0.75	7.0	2.00
8.3 fl oz (250 ml)	~267	16.9						468	250	4.50	0.750	25.0	1500	16.7	0.60	1.00	135.0
							38	435	40	55	35.0		3.5	25	100	18.75	
							38						100	113			NEST2
Deliver 2.0, Mead Johnson[7]	470	168.0	17.7	47.0				190	240	95	4.70	0.710		71	0.90	11.8	3.50
8 fl oz (240 ml)	~257	24.0						400	240	4.30	0.470	24.0	1180	11.8	1.02	1.18	95.0
								280	35	59	29.0		5.9	18	95	59.00	
													71	118			MDJN18

	KCAL / WT (g) / HIS (mg) / PHE (mg)	H₂O (g) / FAT (g) / ISO (mg) / TYR (mg)	PRO (g) / SFA (g) / LEU (mg) / THR (mg)	CHO (g) / MUFA (g) / LYS (mg) / TRY (mg)	SUGR (g) / PUFA (g) / MET (mg) / VAL (mg)	DFIB (g) / CHOL (mg) / CYS (mg) / ARG (mg)	— / — / TAU (mg) / CAR (mg)	Na (mg) / K (mg) / Cl (mg) / —	Ca (mg) / P (mg) / I (mcg) / —	Mg (mg) / Fe (mg) / Mo (mcg) / BIO (mcg)	Zn (mg) / Cu (mg) / Cr (mcg) / CHLN (mg)	Mn (mg) / Se (mcg) / — / INOS (mg)	A (mcg RAE) / A (IU) / PANT (mg) / —	C (mg) / E (mg ATE) / E (IU) / —	B-1 (mg) / B-2 (mg) / D (IU) / —	NIA (mg) / B-6 (mg) / K (mcg) / —	B-12 (mcg) / FOL (mcg DFE) / — / REF
Diabetisource, Novartis	250	204.5	12.5	22.5		1.1		250	167	67	3.83	0.830		50	0.38	5.0	1.50
8.3 fl oz (250 ml)	~261	12.2						400	200	3.00	0.330	16.7	1670	5.0	0.43	0.50	100.0
							25	283	25	50	29.2		2.5	8	67	16.70	
							33						75	50	200		NVAR3
Dietsource Sweet n'Free drink	16	240.0	0.0	4.0				50	100		2.25			60		3.0	0.90
mix w/wtr, Novartis - 8 fl oz	~244	0.0				0		28		1.80	0.300			2.0	0.30	0.30	60.0
													1.5	3	60		
																	NVAR4
Enlive! Ross[8]	300	191.0	10.0	65.0	15.0	0.0		65	60	8	3.80	0.900		24	0.38	2.0	1.20
8.1 fl oz (243 ml)	~266	0.0	0.0	0.0	0.0	<5		40	20	2.70	0.300	14.0	1250	6.0	0.34	0.40	80.0
								340	45	34	18.0		0.8	9	60	20.00	
													30				RSSM3
Ensure,	250	200.0	8.8	40.0		0.0		200	300	100	3.80	1.300		30	0.38	5.0	1.50
Ross[9] - *8 fl oz (240 ml)*	~255	6.1	0.5	3.3	1.8	<5		370	300	4.50	0.500	18.0	1250	5.0	0.43	0.50	100.0
								310	38	38	30.0		2.5	8	100	20.00	
													75	100			RSSM14
from powder, Ross[10]	250	200.0	9.0	34.0	13.0	0.0		200	125	50	2.82	0.620		38	0.38	5.0	1.50
1/2 cup w/3/4 cup wtr (8 fl oz)	~252	9.0	1.3	2.2	4.8	<5		370	125	2.25	0.250	9.0	650	3.8	0.43	0.50	100.0
								310	19	19	13.0		2.5	6	50	10.00	
													75	75			RSSM12
Ensure Fiber w/FOS, Ross[11]	250	195.0	9.0	42.0	12.0	3.0		200	350	100	3.80	1.300		30	0.38	5.0	1.50
8 fl oz (240 ml)	~252	6.0	0.5	3.3	1.8	<5		370	300	4.50	0.500	18.0	1250	5.0	0.43	0.50	100.0
								320	38	38	30.0		2.5	8	100	20.00	
													75	100			RSSM4
Ensure High Calcium, Ross[12]	230	203.0	12.0	31.0	19.0	0.0		290	400	100	6.00	1.200		42	0.38	5.0	1.80
8 fl oz (240 ml)	~252	6.0	0.5	3.0	2.0	<5		500	250	4.50	0.500	17.5	1250	10.0	0.42	0.50	120.0
								375	38	38	30.0		2.5	15	140	28.00	
													75	100			RSSM5
Ensure High Protein, Ross[13]	230	203.0	12.0	31.0	19.0	0.0		290	300	100	5.70	1.300		30	0.38	5.0	1.50
8 fl oz (240 ml)	~252	6.0	0.6	3.0	2.0	<5		500	250	4.50	0.500	18.0	1250	8.0	0.43	0.50	100.0
								375	38	38	30.0		2.5	12	100	20.00	
													75	100			RSSM6
Ensure Light, Ross[14]	200	204.0	10.0	33.0	18.0	0.0		200	250	100	3.80	1.300		30	0.38	5.0	1.50
8 fl oz (240 ml)	~251	3.0	0.3	1.9	0.6	<5		370	250	4.50	0.500	18.0	1250	5.0	0.43	0.50	100.0
								310	38	38	30.0		2.5	8	100	20.00	
													75	100			RSSM7
Ensure Nutrition & Energy	230		9.0	35.0	23.0	1.0		135	300	60	3.75	0.800		30	0.38	5.0	0.90
Bars, Ross[15] - *2.12 oz bar*	60	6.0	3.8	1.5	0.7	<5		150	300	3.60	0.500	14.0	1250	5.0	0.42	0.50	60.0
								118	30	38	18.0		2.5	8	80	12.00	
													45	0			RSSM8
Ensure Plus, Ross[16]	360	180.0	13.0	50.1	16.0	0.0		240	200	100	3.80	1.300		30	0.38	5.0	1.50
8 fl oz (240 ml)	~255	11.4	1.0	6.3	3.8	<5		440	200	4.50	0.500	18.0	1250	5.0	0.43	0.50	100.0
								450	38	38	30.0		2.5	8	100	20.00	
													75	100			RSSM11
Ensure Plus HN,	355	182.0	14.8	47.3		0.0		280	250	100	5.70	1.300		75	0.75	10.0	3.00
flvrd, Ross[17] - *8 fl oz (240 ml)*	~256	11.8	2.3	3.0	6.5	<5		430	250	4.50	0.500	18.0	1250	8.0	0.85	1.00	200.0
							38	410	38	38	30.0		5.0	12	100	20.00	
							38						150	150			RSSM9
ready-to-hang, Ross[18]	1500	769.0	62.7	203.6		0.0		1400	1000	400	23.00	5.000		240	3.00	40.0	12.00
33.3 fl oz (1000 ml)	~1085	49.1	7.4	27.7	14.0	<20		1800	1000	18.00	2.000	70.0	8320	30.0	3.40	4.00	800.0
	840	2710	2855	5780	4450	1790	150	1700	150	150	120.0		20.0	45	400	80.00	
	355	3255	3165	3475	2405	1710	150						600	600	0		RSSM10
Ensure pudding, Ross[19]	170	77.0	4.0	27.0	20.0			135	100	40	3.00	0.600		9	0.23	3.0	1.20
4 fl oz (120 ml)	~113	5.0	1.0	3.0	1.0	<5		180	100	2.70	0.200	10.5	500	4.0	0.26	0.30	60.0
								102	45	30	12.0		2.0	6	40	12.00	
													60				RSSM13
Equalyte, Ross[20]	100	972.0	0.0	30.0		0.0		1800	0	0	0.00	0.000					
33.3 fl oz (1000 ml)	~1032	0.0				0		875	0	0.00	0.000	0.0					

								Minerals					Vitamins				
	KCAL	H₂0 (g)	PRO (g)	CHO (g)	SUGR (g)	DFIB (g)		Na (mg)	Ca (mg)	Mg (mg)	Zn (mg)	Mn (mg)	A (mcg RAE)	C (mg)	B-1 (mg)	NIA (mg)	B-12 (mcg)
	WT (g)	FAT (g)	SFA (g)	MUFA (g)	PUFA (g)	CHOL (mg)		K (mg)	P (mg)	Fe (mg)	Cu (mg)	Se (mcg)	A (IU)	E (mg ATE)	B-2 (mg)	B-6 (mg)	FOL (mcg DFE)
	HIS (mg)	ISO (mg)	LEU (mg)	LYS (mg)	MET (mg)	CYS (mg)	TAU (mg)	Cl (mg)	I (mcg)	Mo (mcg)	Cr (mcg)		PANT (mg)	E (IU)	D (IU)	K (mcg)	
	PHE (mg)	TYR (mg)	THR (mg)	TRY (mg)	VAL (mg)	ARG (mg)	CAR (mg)						BIO (mcg)	CHLN (mg)	INOS (mg)		REF
							0	2400	0	0	0.0						
							0								0		RSSM15
f-a-a, Nestle	250	206.0	12.5	44.0				140	200	74	6.00	0.700		85	0.50	7.0	2.00
8.3 fl oz (250 ml)	~266	2.8						375	175	4.50	0.500	9.5	825	5.0	0.60	1.00	135.0
							25	350	38	14	8.5		3.5	8	100	12.50	
							25						100	112			NEST3
Fibersource HN, Novartis	300	203.5	13.4	39.3		2.5		299	257	88	4.82	0.430		50	0.32	4.3	1.29
8.3 fl oz (250 ml)	~266	9.8						509	257	4.24	0.470	17.5	1070	8.6	0.36	0.50	171.0
								225	38	32	28.3		2.1	13	86	20.00	
													64	86			NVAR5
Fibersource Standard,	300	203.5	10.8	41.8		2.5		299	257	88	4.82	0.430		50	0.32	4.3	1.29
Novartis - 8.3 fl oz (250 ml)	~266	9.8						509	236	3.86	0.470	17.5	1070	8.6	0.36	0.50	171.0
								225	38	32	28.3		2.1	13	86	20.00	
													64	86			NVAR6
Forta Drink mix, Ross[21]	77		5.0	13.0		0.3		45	150	40	1.50	0.200		60	0.15	2.0	0.30
.8 oz	23	<1.0						55	100	1.80	0.200		500	2.0	0.17	0.20	40.0
								13	15				1.0	3	40	0.00	
													30	0			RSSM16
Forta Shake mix in whole mlk,	285	214.0	17.0	35.0		0.0		240	550	100	5.25	0.600		15	0.52	5.0	3.00
Ross[22] - 1.4 oz mix in 8 fl oz mlk	284	8.0						810	450	4.50	0.500		1750	5.0	1.20	0.60	100.0
								300	98				3.5	8	220	0.00	
													75				RSSM17
Glucerna, Ross[23]	237	202.0	9.9	22.8		3.4		220	170	67	3.80	0.840		50	0.38	5.0	1.50
8 fl oz (240 ml)	~248	12.9	1.0	9.0	2.0	<5		370	170	3.00	0.340	12.0	1500	5.0	0.43	0.50	100.0
	109	396	465	891	713	277	25	340	25	25	20.0		2.5	8	67	14.00	
	40	495	485	584	327	267	34						75	100	200		RSSM20
Glucerna Shake, Ross	220	200.0	10.0	29.0	7.0	3.0		210	250	100	3.80	1.000		60	0.38	5.0	3.00
8 fl oz (240 ml)	~248	8.5	0.8	6.2	1.5	<5		370	250	4.50	0.500	18.0	1750	20.0	0.43	1.00	200.0
								355	38	38	120.0		2.5	30	100	20.00	
													75	100			RSSM18
Glucerna Snack Bar, Ross	140		6.0	24.0	8.0	4.0		70	250	60	2.30	0.600		60	0.23	3.0	0.90
1 bar	~34	4.0	0.9	2.4	0.5	<5		40	150	2.70	0.300	21.0	750	20.0	0.26	0.30	60.0
								68	23	23	36.0		1.5	30	60	12.00	
													45	100			RSSM19
Glytrol, van, Nestle	250	211.0	11.3	25.0		3.8		185	180	72	3.80	0.750		35	0.50	7.0	2.00
8.3 fl oz (250 ml)	~260	11.9						350	180	3.20	0.380	19.0	1000	5.0	0.60	1.00	100.0
							25	300	30	50	31.0		3.5	8	80	12.50	
							25						75	100	200		NEST4
Immunocal, AmmunoMed	37		9.0	0.1	0.2	0.0		25	60	9				0	0.00	0.0	
1 pkt	~10	<0.1	<0.1	0.0	0.0	<1		30	21	0.93			<1		0.00		
								<1									
																	AMUN1
Impact, Novartis	250	213.3	14.0	32.9				267	200	67	3.75	0.500		20	0.50	5.0	2.00
8.3 fl oz (250 ml)	~268	6.9						350	200	3.00	0.420	25.0	1670	10.0	0.43	0.37	100.0
								333	25	50	25.0		1.7	15	67	16.70	
													50	67			NVAR11
Impact 1.5, Novartis	375	195.0	20.9	35.3				320	240	80	4.50	0.600		24	0.60	6.0	2.40
8.3 fl oz (250 ml)	~269	17.2						420	240	3.60	0.500	30.0	2000	12.0	0.51	0.44	120.0
							72	400	30	60	30.0		2.0	18	80	20.00	
							36						60	80			NVAR7
Impact Glutamine, Novartis	325	201.8	19.5	37.4		2.5		300	300	100	4.88	0.500		65	0.38	5.0	1.50
8.3 fl oz (250 ml)	~270	10.8						450	300	4.50	0.500	17.5	2180	13.0	0.43	0.50	100.0
							35	215	38	19	30.0		2.5	20	100	20.00	
							35						75	125			NVAR8
Impact Recover, Novartis	240	180.0	17.0	26.0		3.0		280	200	68	4.00	0.500		20	0.47	5.0	2.00
62 g pkt w/180 ml wtr (8 oz)	~230	6.6						350	200	3.00	0.400	25.0	1600	10.0	0.40	0.40	100.0
								330	25	50	25.0		1.6	15	68	16.00	
													50	68			NVAR9

	KCAL	H₂0 (g)	PRO (g)	CHO (g)	SUGR (g)	DFIB (g)		Na (mg)	Ca (mg)	Mg (mg)	Zn (mg)	Mn (mg)	A (mcg RAE)	C (mg)	B-1 (mg)	NIA (mg)	B-12 (mcg)
	WT (g)	FAT (g)	SFA (g)	MUFA (g)	PUFA (g)	CHOL (mg)		K (mg)	P (mg)	Fe (mg)	Cu (mg)	Se (mcg)	A (IU)	E (mg ATE)	B-2 (mg)	B-6 (mg)	FOL (mcg DFE)
	HIS (mg)	ISO (mg)	LEU (mg)	LYS (mg)	MET (mg)	CYS (mg)	TAU (mg)	Cl (mg)	I (mcg)	Mo (mcg)	Cr (mcg)		PANT (mg)	E (IU)	D (IU)	K (mcg)	
	PHE (mg)	TYR (mg)	THR (mg)	TRY (mg)	VAL (mg)	ARG (mg)	CAR (mg)						BIO (mcg)	CHLN (mg)	INOS (mg)		REF
Impact w/fiber, Novartis	250	217.0	14.0	33.8		2.5		267	200	67	3.75	0.500		20	0.50	5.0	2.00
8.3 fl oz (250 ml)	~272	6.9						350	200	3.00	0.420	25.0	1670	10.0	0.43	0.37	100.0
								333	25	50	25.0		1.7	15	67	16.70	
													50	67			NVAR10
IntensiCal, Mead Johnson[24]	310	189.0	19.2	35.0				260	270	95	5.00	0.830		177	0.62	8.3	2.50
8 fl oz (240 ml)	~254	9.9						310	260	4.30	0.470	16.6	1780	8.2	0.71	0.83	166.0
							38	350	35	25	28.0		4.1	12	123	18.90	
							38						125	123			MDJN26
Introlite, Ross	530	920.0	22.1	70.6		0.0		930	760	305	18.00	3.800		230	1.80	23.0	6.90
33.3 fl oz (1000 ml)	~1032	18.4	8.9	2.6	6.0	<10		1570	760	14.00	1.600	54.0	3790	23.3	2.00	2.30	455.0
	252	874	1044	1958	1556	597	0	1440	115	115	91.0		12.0	35	305	61.00	
	118	1105	1105	1271	884	593	0						345	455	0		RSSM21
Isocal, Mead Johnson[25]	250	200.0	8.1	32.0				125	150	50	2.50	0.380		38	0.48	6.3	1.88
8 fl oz (240 ml)	~251	10.5						310	125	2.20	0.250	12.5	630	6.3	0.54	0.63	50.0
								250	19	31	15.0		3.1	9	50	31.00	
													38	63			MDJN29
Isocal HN, Mead Johnson[26]	250	200.0	10.4	29.0				220	200	80	4.00	0.600		60	0.75	10.0	3.00
8 fl oz (240 ml)	~251	10.7						380	200	3.60	0.400	14.0	1000	10.0	0.85	1.00	80.0
							30	340	30	20	24.0		5.0	15	80	25.00	
							30						60	100			MDJN28
Isocal HN Plus, Mead Johnson[27]	280	192.0	12.8	37.0				320	240	95	5.00	0.950		57	0.71	9.5	2.80
8 fl oz (240 ml)	~252	9.5						440	240	4.30	0.470	16.6	1180	14.0	0.80	0.95	189.0
							35	350	35	28	28.0		4.7	21	95	18.90	
							35						142	130			MDJN27
Isosource 1.5 Cal, Novartis	375	194.5	16.9	42.0				322	268	107	8.04	0.540		80	0.80	10.7	3.22
8.3 fl oz (250 ml)	~270	16.2						536	268	4.82	0.540	18.8	2680		0.91	1.07	
							27		40	20	32.2		5.4		107	21.40	
							27										NVAR12
Isosource HN, Novartis	300	204.5	13.4	39.9				282	300	88	4.82	0.430		50	0.32	4.3	1.29
8.3 fl oz (250 ml)	~268	9.8						476	300	3.86	0.430	17.5	1070	8.6	0.36	0.50	171.0
								283	38	21	28.3		2.1	13	86	20.00	
													64	86			NVAR13
Isosource Standard, Novartis[28]	300	204.8	10.8	42.5				282	300	88	4.82	0.430		50	0.32	4.3	1.29
8.3 fl oz (250 ml)	~268	9.8						476	279	3.86	0.430	17.5	1070	8.6	0.36	0.50	171.0
								283	38	21	28.3			13	86	20.00	
													64	86			NVAR14
Isosource VHN, Novartis	250	211.8	15.6	32.0		2.5		320	200	80	6.00	0.400		60	0.60	8.0	2.40
8.3 fl oz (250 ml)	~267	7.2						400	200	3.60	0.400	14.0	2000	8.0	0.68	0.80	120.0
							20	340	30	15	24.0		4.0	12	80	16.00	
							20						90	100			NVAR15
Jevity, Ross	250	197.0	10.4	36.5		3.4		220	215	72	4.00	0.900		54	0.41	5.4	1.70
8 fl oz (240 ml)	~253	8.2	2.0	4.2	1.4	<5		370	180	3.20	0.360	13.0	895	5.4	0.46	0.54	110.0
	114	416	489	936	749	291	27	310	27	27	21.0		2.7	8	72	15.00	
	42	520	510	614	343	281	27						81	110	0		RSSM23
Jevity Plus, Ross	285	193.0	13.2	41.1		2.8		320	285	96	5.40	1.200		72	0.54	7.2	2.20
8 fl oz (240 ml)	~257	9.3	2.3	4.8	1.6	<5		440	285	4.30	0.480	17.0	1190	7.3	0.61	0.72	145.0
	145	528	620	1188	950	370	36	360	36	36	29.0		3.6	11	96	20.00	
	53	660	647	779	436	356	36						110	145	0		RSSM22
Lipisorb Liquid, Mead Johnson[29]	320	190.0	13.6	38.0				320	200	80	4.00	0.600		18	0.46	6.0	1.80
8 fl oz (240 ml)	~255	13.4						400	200	3.60	0.400	14.0	1500	6.0	0.52	0.60	120.0
							46	520	30	20	24.0		3.0	9	120	24.00	
							46						90	50			MDJN32
Magnacal Renal, Mead Johnson[30]	470	168.0	17.7	47.0				190	240	47	4.70	0.710		24	0.90	11.8	3.50
8 fl oz (240 ml)	~257	24.0	6.5	12.4				300	189	4.30	0.470	16.6	1180	7.1	1.02	2.40	189.0
							35	280	35	24	28.0		5.9	11	24	28.00	
							35						71	118			MDJN33
MCT Oil, Mead Johnson[31]	115																
1 T	14																

								Minerals					Vitamins				
	KCAL	H₂0 (g)	PRO (g)	CHO (g)	SUGR (g)	DFIB (g)		Na (mg)	Ca (mg)	Mg (mg)	Zn (mg)	Mn (mg)	A (mcg RAE)	C (mg)	B-1 (mg)	NIA (mg)	B-12 (mcg)
	WT (g)	FAT (g)	SFA (g)	MUFA (g)	PUFA (g)	CHOL (mg)		K (mg)	P (mg)	Fe (mg)	Cu (mg)	Se (mcg)	A (IU)	E (mg ATE)	B-2 (mg)	B-6 (mg)	FOL (mcg DFE)
	HIS (mg)	ISO (mg)	LEU (mg)	LYS (mg)	MET (mg)	CYS (mg)	TAU (mg)	Cl (mg)	I (mcg)	Mo (mcg)	Cr (mcg)	PANT (mg)	E (IU)	D (IU)	K (mcg)		
	PHE (mg)	TYR (mg)	THR (mg)	TRY (mg)	VAL (mg)	ARG (mg)	CAR (mg)					BIO (mcg)	CHLN (mg)	INOS (mg)	REF		
																MDJN34	
Microlipid, Mead Johnson[32]	400	40.0															
3 fl oz (89 ml)	~85	45.0															
																MDJN35	
Moducal powder, Mead Johnson[33]	120			32.0													
4 T (1.1 oz)	32																
																MDJN36	
Modulen IBD, Nestle[34]	250	180.0	9.0	27.0				85	222	50	2.30	0.490		23	0.29	2.9	0.80
1.8 oz powder w/6 fl oz water (250 ml)	~231	11.5						300	150	2.70	0.240	8.5	700	3.3	0.32	0.41	60.0
								182	24	18	12.0		1.2	5	100	13.00	
													8	17		NEST7	
Nepro, Ross	475	166.0	16.7	52.8		3.7		200	325	50	5.70	1.300		25	0.60	8.0	2.40
8 fl oz (240 ml)	~259	22.7	1.9	14.9	4.4	<10		250	165	4.50	0.500	24.0	1000	8.0	0.68	2.10	250.0
	199	730	730	1527	1245	481	38	240	38				4.0	12	20	20.00	
	100	830	830	979	564	415	62						120	150	0	RSSM24	
NovaSource 2.0, Novartis[35]	475	165.9	21.3	51.0				190	250	100	3.75	0.500		90	0.38	5.0	1.50
8 fl oz (237 ml)	~259	20.9						360	250	4.50	0.500	17.5	1250	20.0	0.43	0.50	100.0
								284	38	19	30.0		2.5	30	100	20.00	
													75	142		NVAR17	
NovaSource Pulmonary,	375	191.0	18.8	36.4		2.0		322	268	107	8.04	0.540		134	0.80	10.7	3.22
Novartis - 8.3 fl oz (250 ml)	~264	17.0						616	268	4.82	0.540	18.8	2680	71.3	0.91	1.07	161.0
							27	375	40	20	32.2		5.4	107	107	21.40	
							27						121	134		NVAR18	
NovaSource Renal, Novartis	475	168.0	17.4	47.3				210	308	47	5.92	1.180		19	0.59	7.9	2.37
8 fl oz (237 ml)	~257	24.1						192	154	4.26	0.470	23.7	788	7.1	0.69	1.89	237.0
							36	199	38				3.8	11	19	18.90	
							63						118	78		NVAR19	
NuBasics, Nestle	250	213.0	8.8	33.1				219	125	50	2.60	0.500		26	0.40	5.2	1.50
8.3 fl oz (250 ml)	~264	9.2						312	125	2.25	0.250	7.5	750	3.3	0.45	0.75	100.0
							15	300	19	23	7.5		2.6	5	52	9.40	
													75	85		NEST9	
NuBasics Plus, Nestle	375	194.0	13.1	44.1				292	187	75	3.90	0.700		39	0.60	7.8	2.20
8.3 fl oz (250 ml)	~263	16.2						467	187	3.40	0.370	11.2	1125	5.2	0.70	1.10	150.0
							22	435	28	34	11.2		3.9	8	78	14.10	
													112	127		NEST8	
Nutren	250	213.0	10.0	31.8				219	167	67	3.50	0.680		35	0.50	7.0	2.00
1.0, Nestle - 8.3 fl oz (250 ml)	~265	9.5						312	167	3.00	0.350	10.0	1000	4.7	0.60	1.00	135.0
							20	300	25	30	10.0		3.5	7	70	12.50	
							20						100	113		NEST11	
1.0 w/fiber, Nestle	250	210.0	10.0	31.8		3.5		219	167	67	3.50	0.680		35	0.50	7.0	2.00
8.3 fl oz (250 ml)	~262	9.5						312	167	3.00	0.350	10.0	1000	4.7	0.60	1.00	135.0
							20	300	25	30	10.0		3.5	7	70	12.50	
							20						100	113		NEST10	
1.5, Nestle	375	194.0	15.0	42.3				292	250	100	5.00	1.000		53	0.75	10.5	3.00
8.3 fl oz (250 ml)	~269	16.9						468	250	4.50	0.500	15.0	1500	7.0	0.90	1.50	200.0
							30	435	38	45	15.0		5.0	11	105	18.70	
							30						150	168		NEST12	
2.0, van, Nestle	500	175.0	20.0	49.0				325	335	134	7.00	1.300		70	1.00	14.0	4.00
8.3 fl oz (250 ml)	~271	26.5						480	335	6.00	0.700	20.0	2000	9.3	1.20	2.00	270.0
							40	469	50	60	20.0		7.0	14	140	25.00	
							40						200	225		NEST13	
NutriCare milk shake pwdr w/	280		9.0	39.0				193	390					12			
whl mlk, choc/straw/van - 8 fl oz	~270	9.0			36					4.5			1750				
																NTRC1	

Food	KCAL / WT (g) / HIS (mg) / PHE (mg)	H₂0 (g) / FAT (g) / ISO (mg) / TYR (mg)	PRO (g) / SFA (g) / LEU (mg) / THR (mg)	CHO (g) / MUFA (g) / LYS (mg) / TRY (mg)	SUGR (g) / PUFA (g) / MET (mg) / VAL (mg)	DFIB (g) / CHOL (mg) / CYS (mg) / ARG (mg)	TAU (mg) / CAR (mg)	Na (mg) / K (mg) / Cl (mg)	Ca (mg) / P (mg) / I (mcg)	Mg (mg) / Fe (mg) / Mo (mcg)	Zn (mg) / Cu (mg) / Cr (mcg)	Mn (mg) / Se (mcg)	A (mcg RAE) / A (IU) / PANT (mg) / BIO (mcg)	C (mg) / E (mg ATE) / E (IU) / CHLN (mg)	B-1 (mg) / B-2 (mg) / D (IU) / INOS (mg)	NIA (mg) / B-6 (mg) / K (mcg)	B-12 (mcg) / FOL (mcg DFE) / REF
NutriCare nutrl supp pwdr w/ whl mlk, choc/straw/van - *8 fl oz*	280		15.0	36.0				260	47					39			
	~270	9.0			45					6.3			2000				NTRC2
NutriFocus, Ross *8 fl oz (240 ml)*	355	181.0	14.8	50.9		2.5		220	250	100	7.50	0.500		30	0.38	5.0	1.50
	~259	11.7				<5		400	250	4.50	0.500	18.0	2500	5.0	0.43	0.50	100.0
								270	38	19	30.0		2.5	8	100	20.00	
													75	130			RSSM25
NutriHeal, van, Nestle *8.3 fl oz (250 ml)*	250	212.0	15.6	28.2				219	145	50	2.60	0.500		26	0.40	5.2	1.50
	~265	8.3						312	145	2.25	0.250	7.5	750	3.5	0.45	0.75	100.0
							15	300	19	23	7.5		2.6	5	52	9.40	
													75	85			NEST16
NutriHep, Nestle *8.3 fl oz (250 ml)*	375	190.0	10.0	72.5				80	250	100	3.80	1.000		24	0.38	5.0	1.50
	~278	5.3						330	250	4.50	0.500		1250	5.0	0.43	0.50	100.0
							30	375	38				2.5	8	100	30.00	
							30						75	100			NEST17
NutriRenal, van, Nestle *8.3 fl oz (250 ml)*	500	176.0	17.5	51.2				185	350	50	5.00	1.320		22	0.56	6.7	3.00
	~271	26.0						314	175	6.00	0.670	20.0	416	6.7	0.64	2.50	267.0
							40	285	50	25	20.0		3.8	10	25	18.80	
							40						100	163			NEST18
NutriVent, van, Nestle *8.3 fl oz (250 ml)*	375	195.0	17.0	25.0				292	300	120	5.30	1.000		53	0.75	10.5	3.00
	~261	23.7						468	300	4.50	0.530	15.0	1500	7.0	0.90	1.50	203.0
							30	435	38	45	15.0		5.3	11	105	18.70	
							30						150	168			NEST19
Optimental, Ross *8 fl oz (240 ml)*	237	198.0	12.2	32.9				250	250	100	3.80	0.840		50	0.50	6.7	2.00
	~250	6.7	2.7	1.4	2.3			420	250	3.00	0.340	12.0	1950	33.3	0.57	0.67	135.0
								320	38	25	20.0		3.4	50	67	20.00	
													100	100			RSSM26
Osmolite, Ross *8 fl oz (240 ml)*	250	199.0	8.8	35.6				150	125	50	2.90	0.620		38	0.38	5.0	1.50
	~252	8.2	2.0	4.2	1.4	<5		240	125	2.30	0.250	9.0	625	3.8	0.43	0.50	100.0
	100	348	416	780	620	238	19	200	19	19	15.0		2.5	6	50	10.00	
	47	440	440	506	352	236	19						75	75			RSSM29
Osmolite 1 CAL, Ross *8 fl oz (240 ml)*	250	199.0	10.5	33.9				220	180	72	4.10	0.900		54	0.41	5.4	1.70
	~252	8.2	2.0	4.2	1.4	<5		370	180	3.30	0.360	13.0	895	5.4	0.46	0.54	110.0
	120	415	496	930	739	284	27	340	27	27	22.0		2.7	8	72	15.00	
	56	525	525	604	420	282	27						81	110			RSSM28
Osmolite 1.2 CAL, Ross *8 fl oz (240 ml)*	285	195.0	13.2	37.5				320	285	96	5.40	1.200		72	0.54	7.2	2.20
	~255	9.3	2.3	4.8	1.6	<5		430	285	4.30	0.480	17.0	1190	7.3	0.61	0.72	145.0
	145	528	620	1188	950	370	36	370	36	36	29.0		3.6	11	96	20.00	
	53	660	647	779	436	356	36						110	145			RSSM27
Oxepa, Ross *8 fl oz (240 ml)*	355	186.0	14.8	25.0		0.0		310	250	100	5.70	1.300		200	0.75	10.0	3.00
	~248	22.2	7.7	6.0	7.5	10		465	250	4.50	0.500	18.0	2840	50.0	0.85	1.00	200.0
	163	592	696	1332	1066	414	75	400	38	38	30.0		5.0	75	100	24.00	
	59	740	725	873	488	400	43						150	150	0		RSSM30
Peptamen, Nestle *8.3 fl oz (250 ml)*	250	212.0	10.0	31.8				140	200	75	6.00	0.680		85	0.50	7.0	2.00
	~264	9.8						375	175	4.50	0.500	12.5	833	5.0	0.60	1.00	135.0
							25	250	38	30	10.0		3.5	8	100	12.50	
							25						100	113			NEST24
Peptamen 1.5, Nestle *8.3 fl oz (250 ml)*	375	193.0	16.9	47.0				255	250	100	9.00	1.000		128	0.75	10.5	3.00
	~271	14.0						465	250	6.75	0.750	19.0	1250	7.5	0.90	1.50	203.0
							38	435	56	45	15.0		5.3	11	150	18.80	
							38						150	169			NEST20
Peptamen VHP, Nestle *8.3 fl oz (250 ml)*	250	211.0	15.6	26.1				140	200	75	6.00	0.700		85	0.50	7.0	2.00
	~263	9.8						375	175	4.50	0.500	12.5	833	5.0	0.60	1.00	135.0
							25	250	38	30	10.0		3.5	8	100	12.50	
							25						100	113			NEST22
Peptamen w/FOS/inulin, van, Nestle - *8.3 fl oz (250 ml)*	250	211.0	10.0	31.0		1.0		140	200	75	6.00	0.700		85	0.50	7.0	2.00
	~262	9.8						375	175	4.50	0.500	12.0	833	5.0	0.60	1.00	135.0

	KCAL	H₂0 (g)	PRO (g)	CHO (g)	SUGR (g)	DFIB (g)		Na (mg)	Ca (mg)	Mg (mg)	Zn (mg)	Mn (mg)	A (mcg RAE)	C (mg)	B-1 (mg)	NIA (mg)	B-12 (mcg)
	WT (g)	FAT (g)	SFA (g)	MUFA (g)	PUFA (g)	CHOL (mg)		K (mg)	P (mg)	Fe (mg)	Cu (mg)	Se (mcg)	A (IU)	E (mg ATE)	B-2 (mg)	B-6 (mg)	FOL (mcg DFE)
	HIS (mg)	ISO (mg)	LEU (mg)	LYS (mg)	MET (mg)	CYS (mg)	TAU (mg)	Cl (mg)	I (mcg)	Mo (mcg)	Cr (mcg)		PANT (mg)	E (IU)	D (IU)	K (mcg)	
	PHE (mg)	TYR (mg)	THR (mg)	TRY (mg)	VAL (mg)	ARG (mg)	CAR (mg)						BIO (mcg)	CHLN (mg)	INOS (mg)		REF
							25	250	37	30	10.0		3.5	8	100	12.50	
							25						100	113			NEST23
Peptinex, Novartis	237	196.2	11.9	38.6				239	158	63	3.08	0.410		41	0.41	5.4	1.61
8 fl oz (237 ml)	~251	4.0						354	158	2.84	0.320	14.4	790	4.1	0.46	0.54	107.0
							47	196	24	15	24.7		2.7	6	63	12.60	
							24						81	54			NVAR21
Peptinex DT, Novartis	250	207.5	12.5	41.0				425	170	67	3.30	0.330		17	0.40	5.5	1.67
8.3 fl oz (250 ml)	~266	4.3						200	170	3.00	0.330	11.7	830	3.3	0.47	0.55	110.0
							17	200	28	13	20.0		2.8	5	67	13.30	
							17						83	55			NVAR20
Perative, Ross	308	187.0	15.8	42.0		0.0		250	210	83	4.70	1.100		62	0.47	6.2	1.90
8 fl oz (240 ml)	~254	8.8	4.1	2.4	1.9	0		410	210	3.70	0.420	15.0	2060	6.2	0.53	0.62	125.0
	190	632	664	1422	1122	363	31	390	31	31	25.0		3.1	9	83	17.00	
	174	648	664	790	1912	332	31						93	125	0		RSSM33
Phenyl-Free, Mead Johnson[36]	500		16.2	51.0				240	660	66	8.60	0.380		60	1.00	10.0	2.00
16 fl oz (480 ml)	~504	26.0						560	440	9.60	0.860	14.1	1520	6.7	1.00	1.00	100.0
	290	750	1150	2100	1300	360	24	430	76		36.0		3.8	10	380	40.00	
	240	0	1600	1250	970	410							38	60	86		MDJN39
Polycose, Ross	200	70.0	0.0	50.0		0.0		70	20	0	0.00	0.000					
3.3 fl oz (100 ml)	~120	0.0					0	6	3	0.00	0.000	0.0					
							0	140	0	0	0.0						
							0								0		RSSM34
ProBalance, van, Nestle	300	203.0	13.5	39.0		2.5		191	312	100	6.00	1.000		60	0.56	10.0	3.00
8.3 fl oz (250 ml)	~266	10.2						390	250	4.50	0.500	20.0	1000	16.7	0.64	1.00	300.0
							25	324	38	38	25.0		3.8	25	150	20.00	
							25						100	113			NEST25
Product 3200AB, prep, Mead Johnson[37] - *5 fl oz (150 ml)*	100	134.0	3.3	13.0				47	94	11	0.78	0.031		8	0.08	1.2	0.31
	~155	3.9						102	70	1.88	0.094	2.8	310	2.1	0.09	0.06	15.6
	43	172	191	370	360	119	6	70	7				0.5	3	63	15.60	
	13	17	<9	300	122	106							8	13	5		MDJN40
Product 3232A, prep, Mead Johnson - *5 fl oz (150 ml)*	100	127.0	2.8	13.4				43	94	11	0.63	0.031		12	0.08	1.2	0.31
	~148	4.2						109	63	1.88	0.094		380	2.5	0.09	0.06	15.6
	45	137	168	290	240	87	6	86	7				0.5	4	75	18.80	
	45	134	78	210	112	84							8	13	5		MDJN41
Product 80056, prep, Mead Johnson[38] - *5 fl oz (150 ml)*	100	134.0	3.1	12.5				26	94	11	0.78	0.031		8	0.08	1.2	0.31
	~154	3.9						106	52	1.88	0.094	2.8	310	2.1	0.09	0.06	15.6
								63	7				0.5	3	63	15.60	
													8	13	5		MDJN42
ProMod mix, Ross	28	0.6	5.0	0.7		0.0		25	65								
.23 oz scoop	7	0.6						45	33								
	90	335	305	520	450	105											
	120	150	145	285	115	85									0		RSSM35
Promote, Ross	237	198.0	14.8	30.8		0.0		240	285	95	5.70	1.200		82	0.54	7.2	2.20
8 fl oz (240 ml)	~250	6.2	1.5	3.2	1.1	<5		470	285	4.30	0.480	17.0	1720	7.3	0.61	0.72	145.0
	165	607	697	1324	1057	400	36	300	36	36	29.0		3.6	11	95	19.00	
	59	742	715	865	533	399	36						110	145	0		RSSM37
Promote w/fiber, Ross	237	197.0	14.8	32.8		3.4		310	285	95	5.70	1.200		82	0.54	7.2	2.20
8 fl oz (240 ml)	~252	6.7	1.6	3.4	1.2	<5		470	285	4.30	0.480	17.0	1720	7.3	0.61	0.72	145.0
	163	592	696	1332	1066	414	36	300	36	36	29.0		3.6	11	95	19.00	
	59	740	725	873	488	400	36						110	145	0		RSSM36
Protain XL, Mead Johnson[39]	237	200.0	13.5	34.0		2.2		220	189	76	7.10	1.420		57	0.57	7.6	3.50
8 fl oz (240 ml)	~255	7.1						420	189	4.30	0.570	24.0	1660	12.1	0.64	0.76	114.0
							35	320	35	35	35.0		2.8	18	95	28.00	
							35						85	118			MDJN43
Pulmocare, Ross	355	186.0	14.8	25.0		0.0		310	250	100	5.70	1.300		75	0.75	10.0	3.00
8 fl oz (240 ml)	~248	22.1	5.9	9.2	5.5	6		465	250	4.50	0.500	18.0	2840	13.3	0.85	1.00	200.0
	163	592	696	1332	1066	414	36	400	38	38	30.0		5.0	20	100	20.00	
	59	740	725	873	488	400	36						150	150	0		RSSM38

Column key (each food occupies four stacked sub-rows):

- Sub-row 1: KCAL | H₂0 (g) | PRO (g) | CHO (g) | SUGR (g) | DFIB (g) | — | Na (mg) | Ca (mg) | Mg (mg) | Zn (mg) | Mn (mg) | A (mcg RAE) | C (mg) | B-1 (mg) | NIA (mg) | B-12 (mcg)
- Sub-row 2: WT (g) | FAT (g) | SFA (g) | MUFA (g) | PUFA (g) | CHOL (mg) | — | K (mg) | P (mg) | Fe (mg) | Cu (mg) | Se (mcg) | A (IU) | E (mg ATE) | B-2 (mg) | B-6 (mg) | FOL (mcg DFE)
- Sub-row 3: HIS (mg) | ISO (mg) | LEU (mg) | LYS (mg) | MET (mg) | CYS (mg) | TAU (mg) | Cl (mg) | I (mcg) | Mo (mcg) | Cr (mcg) | — | PANT (mg) | E (IU) | D (IU) | K (mcg)
- Sub-row 4: PHE (mg) | TYR (mg) | THR (mg) | TRY (mg) | VAL (mg) | ARG (mg) | CAR (mg) | — | — | — | — | — | BIO (mcg) | CHLN (mg) | INOS (mg) | — | REF

Food	C1	C2	C3	C4	C5	C6	C7	C8	C9	C10	C11	C12	C13	C14	C15	C16	C17
RenalCal, Nestle 8.3 fl oz (250 ml)	500	176.0	8.6	72.6							3.50			15	0.38	5.0	1.50
	~278	20.6										12.5			0.43	1.75	150.0
							25						2.5				
							25						75	100			NEST26
Replete, van, Nestle 8.3 fl oz (250 ml)	250	211.0	15.6	28.3				219	250	100	6.00	1.000		85	0.75	7.0	2.00
	~264	8.5						375	250	4.50	0.500	25.0	1000	10.0	0.60	1.00	135.0
							25	325	40	55	35.0		3.5	15	100	12.50	
							25						100	113			NEST28
Replete w/fiber, van, Nestle 8.3 fl oz (250 ml)	250	209.0	15.6	28.3		3.5		219	250	100	6.00	1.000		85	0.75	7.0	2.00
	~262	8.5						375	250	4.50	0.500	25.0	1000	10.0	0.60	1.00	135.0
							25	325	40	55	35.0		3.5	15	100	12.50	
							25						100	113			NEST27
Resource 2.0, Novartis 8 fl oz (240 ml)	475		21.0	51.0				190	250	100	3.75	0.500		90	0.38	5.0	1.50
	~261	21.0						360	250	4.50	0.500	17.5	1250	20.0	0.43	0.50	100.0
								284	38	19	30.0		2.5	30	100	20.00	
													75	142			NVAR22
Resource Arginaid, Novartis .32 oz pkt	35	0.0		4.0				70						155			
	~9	0.0						10						60.0			
														90			
						4500											NVAR24
Resource Arginaid Extra, Novartis - 8 fl oz (237 ml)	250	197.0	10.5	52.0				<70			15.00	0.400		250	0.30	4.0	1.20
	~260	0.0						<22	850	3.60	0.400		1000		0.34	0.40	80.0
									30				2.0	90	80	16.00	
																	NVAR23
Resource Benefiber mix, Novartis - 1 T pkt	16	0.0	0.0	4.0	0.0	3.0		15						0			
	4	0.0						15									
					5												
																	NVAR25
Resource Benefiber orange/apl drnk, Novartis - 4 fl oz (120 ml)	70		0.0	18.0	14.0	3.0		15						60			
	~124	0.0						108									
																	NVAR26
Resource Dairy Thick, avg for 4 flvrs, Novartis - 8 fl oz (240 ml)	180		8.0	26.0				180	450		5.00						
	~256	5.0				20		370	383				500				
															140		
																	NVAR30
Resource Diabetic, Novartis 8 fl oz (237 ml)	250	200.7	15.0	23.4		3.0		290	260	80	3.00	0.400		100	0.30	4.0	1.20
	~251	11.1						320	260	3.60	0.400	14.0	1200	22.0	0.34	0.40	80.0
							20	220	30	15	24.0		2.0	33	80	16.00	
							25						60	110	200		NVAR31
Resource Egg Nog mix w/whole milk, Novartis - 8 fl oz (240 ml)	290	198.0	15.0	37.0				225		40	0.60			12		5.0	1.20
	~259	9.0				35		600	350	3.60	0.100		1000		0.60	0.10	
									23				0.4		140		
																	NVAR32
Resource Fruit Beverage, Novartis - 8 fl oz (237 ml)	250	196.0	9.0	53.5						1	3.75	0.500		36		5.0	1.50
	~259	0.0							160	2.70	0.300		750		0.43	0.50	
									23				1.5	60		12.00	
																	NVAR33
Resource Health Shake, Novartis - 6 fl oz (180 ml)	300	130.0	9.0	53.0				210	200	60	3.00			12	0.30	4.0	1.20
	~198	6.0				10		160	200	3.60	0.400		1000		0.34	0.40	80.0
									30				2.0		80		
																	NVAR36
no sugar added, Novartis 6 fl oz (180 ml)	300	136.0	12.0	33.0				270	200	60	3.00			12		4.0	1.20
	~194	13.0	2.0			20		350	300	3.60	0.400		1000	4.0	0.34	0.40	80.0
									30				2.0	6	80		
													60				NVAR35
Resource Inst Breakfast mix w/whl mlk, Novartis - 8 fl oz	~289	198.0	15.0	37.0				210	450	140	5.30			21	0.53	7.0	2.10
	~259	9.0				40		620	400	6.30	0.700		1750		0.68	0.70	140.0

								Minerals					Vitamins				
	KCAL	H_2O (g)	PRO (g)	CHO (g)	SUGR (g)	DFIB (g)		Na (mg)	Ca (mg)	Mg (mg)	Zn (mg)	Mn (mg)	A (mcg RAE)	C (mg)	B-1 (mg)	NIA (mg)	B-12 (mcg)
	WT (g)	FAT (g)	SFA (g)	MUFA (g)	PUFA (g)	CHOL (mg)		K (mg)	P (mg)	Fe (mg)	Cu (mg)	Se (mcg)	A (IU)	E (mg ATE)	B-2 (mg)	B-6 (mg)	FOL (mcg DFE)
	HIS (mg)	ISO (mg)	LEU (mg)	LYS (mg)	MET (mg)	CYS (mg)	TAU (mg)	Cl (mg)	I (mcg)	Mo (mcg)	Cr (mcg)		PANT (mg)	E (IU)	D (IU)	K (mcg)	
	PHE (mg)	TYR (mg)	THR (mg)	TRY (mg)	VAL (mg)	ARG (mg)	CAR (mg)			BIO (mcg)	CHLN (mg)	INOS (mg)					REF
(continued from previous page)									53				3.5		140		
										105							NVAR38
Resource Milk Shake mix	~281	<257.0	9.0	41.0				160		80	3.00			12		4.0	1.20
w/whl milk, Novartis - 8 fl oz	~257	9.0				35		410	200	3.60			1000		0.34	0.40	
									30						120		
																	NVAR42
Resource Milk Shake Plus mix	290	198.0	15.0	37.0				355	450	140	5.30			21		7.0	2.10
w/whl mlk, Novartis - 8 fl oz	~259	9.0				40		740	500	6.30			1750	7.3	0.76	0.70	140.0
									53					11	140		
																	NVAR41
Resource Nutritious Jce Drnk,	210	140.0	6.0	46.0				100	200	80	3.00			60	0.30	4.0	1.20
Novartis - 6 fl oz (180 ml)	~192	0.0				0		50	200	3.60	0.400	14.0	1000		0.34	0.40	
									30				2.0		80		
										60							NVAR43
Resource Nutritious Pudding, van,	250	59.0	9.0	35.0				190	200	80	1.50			6	0.30	2.0	0.60
Novartis - 4 oz	113	8.0				5		410	200	1.80	0.220		500	4.0	0.17	0.20	80.0
								280	15				0.9	6	40		
										60							NVAR45
Resource Plus, Novartis	360	181.5	13.0	52.0				310	300	100	6.00	0.500		36	0.60	8.0	2.40
8 fl oz (237 ml)	~258	11.0						460	250	4.50	0.500	17.5	1250	5.0	0.68	0.80	100.0
								340	38	19	30.0		2.5	8	100	20.00	
										75	100						NVAR46
Resource Puree Appeal, dry,	90		7.5	13.5				120	150	24	0.50	0.730				1.2	
Novartis - 3 T	~23	<1.0				0		270	130	1.08	0.120					0.06	36.0
													0.8				
																	NVAR47
Resource Shake, Novartis	270	142.0	9.0	45.0				180		60	3.00			12		4.0	1.20
6 fl oz (180 ml)	~202	6.0				5		300	200	3.60	0.400		750		0.34	0.40	
									30				2.0		80	8.00	
										60							NVAR50
Resource Shake Plus, Novartis	480	157.0	15.0	69.0				200	350	80	5.25			21	0.53	7.0	2.10
8 fl oz (240 ml)	~257	16.0				15		500	350	6.30	0.700		1750	7.0	0.60	0.70	140.0
									53				3.5	11	140		
										105							NVAR48
Resource Shake Thickened,	270	122.0	9.0	45.0				190	200	60	3.00			12		4.0	1.20
Novartis - 6 fl oz (177 ml)	~182	6.0				5		300	200	3.60	0.400		750	4.0	0.34	0.40	80.0
									30				2.0	6	80	8.00	
										60							NVAR49
Resource Standard, Novartis	250	199.1	9.0	40.0				220		100	3.75	0.500		36		5.0	1.50
8 fl oz (237 ml)	~255	6.0						350	250	4.50	0.500	17.5	1000		0.43	0.50	
									38		30.0		2.5		80	20.00	
										60							NVAR51
Respalor, Mead Johnson[40]	355	185.0	17.7	35.0		0.0		300	240	95	5.70	0.950		71	0.71	9.5	2.80
8 fl oz (240 ml)	~254	16.1				5		350	240	4.30	0.470	20.0	1660	13.3	0.80	0.95	189.0
							43	400	35	28	28.0		4.7	20	95	18.90	
							43			142	142						MDJN44
Subdue, Mead Johnson[41]	240	200.0	11.8	30.0				260	260	84	3.80	0.600		36	0.30	4.0	1.80
8 fl oz (240 ml)	~250	8.0				19		380	250	3.60	0.400	21.0	1000	14.0	0.34	0.60	120.0
							24	330	30	49	24.0		2.0	21	120	20.00	
							19			60	83						MDJN46
Subdue Plus, Mead Johnson[42]	355	180.0	18.0	44.0		0.0		280	330	105	3.80	0.500		60	0.38	5.0	1.50
8 fl oz (240 ml)	~254	12.0				30		480	310	4.50	0.500	18.0	1250	20.0	0.43	0.50	100.0
							24	430	38	19	30.0		2.5	30	150	30.00	
							24			75	140						MDJN45
Suplena, Ross	475	169.0	7.1	60.6		0.0		185	330	50	5.60	1.300		25	0.60	8.0	2.40
8 fl oz (240 ml)	~260	22.7	2.1	14.8	4.7	<10		265	175	4.50	0.500	18.0	250	8.0	0.68	2.10	250.0
	78	284	334	639	511	199	38	220	38				4.0	12	20	20.00	
	28	355	348	419	234	192	38			120	150	0					RSSM39

	KCAL WT (g) HIS (mg) PHE (mg)	H₂0 (g) FAT (g) ISO (mg) TYR (mg)	PRO (g) SFA (g) LEU (mg) THR (mg)	CHO (g) MUFA (g) LYS (mg) TRY (mg)	SUGR (g) PUFA (g) MET (mg) VAL (mg)	DFIB (g) CHOL (mg) CYS (mg) ARG (mg)	TAU (mg) CAR (mg)	Na (mg) K (mg) Cl (mg)	Ca (mg) P (mg) I (mcg)	Mg (mg) Fe (mg) Mo (mcg)	Zn (mg) Cu (mg) Cr (mcg)	Mn (mg) Se (mcg)	A (mcg RAE) A (IU) PANT (mg) BIO (mcg)	C (mg) E (mg ATE) E (IU) CHLN (mg)	B-1 (mg) B-2 (mg) D (IU) INOS (mg)	NIA (mg) B-6 (mg) K (mcg)	B-12 (mcg) FOL (mcg DFE) REF
Tolerex pwdr w/water, Novartis - 10 fl oz (300 ml)	300	259.2	6.2	68.0				141		67	2.50	0.330		10		3.3	1.00
	~334	0.4						350	167	3.00	0.330	11.7	833		0.28	0.33	
									27		20.0		1.7		67	13.30	
																	NVAR52
TraumaCal, Mead Johnson[43] 8 fl oz (240 ml)	355	185.0	19.5	34.0				280	177	47	3.50	0.590		35	0.45	5.9	1.77
	~255	16.2						330	177	2.10	0.350		590	5.9	0.51	0.59	47.0
								380	18				3.0	9	47	30.00	
													35	59			MDJN47
TwoCal HN, Ross 8 fl oz (240 ml)	475	166.0	19.9	51.8		0.0		345	250	100	5.70	1.300		75	0.60	8.0	2.40
	~260	21.5	5.5	2.9	12.0	<10		580	250	4.50	0.500	18.0	1250	8.0	0.68	0.80	160.0
	218	792	931	1782	1426	554	38	430	38	38	30.0		4.0	12	100	20.00	
	79	990	970	1168	653	535	38						120	150	0		RSSM40
Ultracal, Mead Johnson[44] 8 fl oz (240 ml)	250	200.0	10.7	34.0		3.4		320	240	95	5.00	0.950		57	0.71	9.5	2.80
	~254	9.3				5		440	240	4.30	0.470	16.6	1180	14.0	0.80	0.95	189.0
							35	350	35	28	28.0		4.7	21	95	18.90	
							35						142	130			MDJN49
Ultracal HN Plus, Mead Johnson[45] - 8 fl oz (240 ml)	280	192.0	12.8	37.0		2.4		320	240	95	5.00	0.950		57	0.71	9.5	2.80
	~252	9.5				9		440	240	4.30	0.470	16.6	1180	14.0	0.80	0.95	189.0
							35	350	35	28	28.0		4.7	21	95	18.90	
							35						142	130			MDJN48
VHC 2.25, van, Nestle 8.3 fl oz (250 ml)	500	168.0	22.5	49.2				300	308	108	15.00	1.020		62	0.88	12.1	3.60
	~271	30.6						433	308	5.63	0.650	18.3	1835	8.2	1.04	1.73	234.0
							40	299	45	40	12.5		6.1	12	122	21.80	
													173	125			NEST29
Vital HN, Ross 1 pkt in 8.6 fl oz wtr (300 ml)	300	260.0	12.5	55.4		0.0		170	200	80	4.50	1.000		60	0.60	8.0	2.40
	332	3.3	1.4	0.4	1.2	6		420	200	3.60	0.400	14.0	1000	6.0	0.68	0.80	160.0
	150	475	588	975	688	275	0	310	30	30	24.0		4.0	9	80	16.00	
	125	550	450	675	625	325	0						120	120	0		RSSM41
Vivonex Plus, Novartis[46] 1 pkt in water (300 ml)	300	255.0	13.5	57.0				183	167	67	3.75	0.330		20	0.50	6.7	2.00
	~328	2.0						317	167	3.00	0.330	11.7	833	3.3	0.57	0.67	133.0
							20	283	27	13	20.0		3.3	5	67	13.30	
							20						100	67			NVAR54
Vivonex RTF, Novartis 8.3 fl oz (250 ml)	250	212.0	12.5	43.8				167	167	67	3.13	0.330		17		5.6	1.67
	~272	2.9						200	167	3.00	0.330	11.7	833	3.3	0.47	0.56	111.0
							17	200	27	13	20.0		2.8	5	67	13.30	
							17						83	55			NVAR55
Vivonex TEN, Novartis[47] 1 pkt in wtr (10 fl oz/300 ml)	300	255.9	11.5	61.7				180	150	60	3.38	0.300		18	0.45	6.0	1.80
	~330	0.8						285	150	2.70	0.300	10.5	750	3.0	0.51	0.60	120.0
							18	255	24	11	18.0		3.0	5	60	12.00	
							18						90	60			NVAR56

[1] Calorie and protein food enhancer that dissolves in hot foods and beverages; ingredients are corn syrup solids, sodium caseinate, canola oil, whey protein isolate, and soy lecithin.

[2] High-calorie, high-protein, low-fat, fiber-fortified formula designed to provide nutritional support for people with HIV or AIDS; supplemental or sole source for oral or tube feeding.

[3] Elemental formula with glutamine for metabolically stressed patients with impaired GI function.

[4] Protein supplement for children or adults.

[5] High-calorie formula for tube feeding.

[6] Ready-to-use high-nitrogen elemental diet.

[7] Nutritionally complete high-calorie, high-nitrogen oral and tube feeding formula.

[8] High-calorie, fat-free clear liquid nutrition for people on clear-liquid, pre- and postsurgical, cancer, bowel-prep, fat-malabsorptive, fat-restricted, low-sodium, or low-cholesterol diet.

[9] Complete, balanced nutrition for supplemental or sole-source oral or tube feeding; 12 flavors.

[10] Reconstituted with water; supplemental or sole-source oral or tube feeding.

[11] Complete, balanced nutrition with fructooligosaccharides, a prebiotic, for supplemental or sole-source oral or tube feeding.

[12] Supplemental oral nutrition for patients who are at risk for fractures, recovering from fractures, or need extra calcium.

[13] Supplemental oral nutrition for people recovering from general surgery or hip fractures or who are at risk for pressure ulcers.

[14] Supplemental oral nutrition for use between or with meals.

[15] For supplemental use between or with meals for people who need extra calories, protein, vitamins, and minerals.

[16] Supplemental oral nutrition to help people gain or maintain healthy weight; 10 flavors.

[17] High-calorie, high-nitrogen liquid nutrition for oral supplementation or tube feeding for people with fluid restrictions or who require volume-limited feedings.

[18] High-calorie, high-nitrogen, low-residue liquid nutrition for tube-fed patients with increased calorie and protein needs or for those with limited volume tolerance; sole-source nutrition via a feeding tube.

[19] Used for people on consistency-modified diets (soft, pureed, or full liquid); for people with swallowing impairments; used with fluid-restricted and volume-limited diets.

[20] Enteral rehydration solution with fructooligosaccharides; replaces fluids and electrolytes lost during diarrhea and vomiting; for oral or tube feeding; not a sole source of nutrition.

	KCAL	H₂0 (g)	PRO (g)	CHO (g)	SUGR (g)	DFIB (g)		Na (mg)	Ca (mg)	Mg (mg)	Zn (mg)	Mn (mg)		A (mcg RAE)	C (mg)	B-1 (mg)	NIA (mg)	B-12 (mcg)
	WT (g)	FAT (g)	SFA (g)	MUFA (g)	PUFA (g)	CHOL (mg)		K (mg)	P (mg)	Fe (mg)	Cu (mg)	Se (mcg)		A (IU)	E (mg ATE)	B-2 (mg)	B-6 (mg)	FOL (mcg DFE)
	HIS (mg)	ISO (mg)	LEU (mg)	LYS (mg)	MET (mg)	CYS (mg)	TAU (mg)	Cl (mg)	I (mcg)	Mo (mcg)	Cr (mcg)			PANT (mg)	E (IU)	D (IU)	K (mcg)	
	PHE (mg)	TYR (mg)	THR (mg)	TRY (mg)	VAL (mg)	ARG (mg)	CAR (mg)							BIO (mcg)	CHLN (mg)	INOS (mg)		REF

[21] High-protein beverage fortified with vitamins and minerals to be used with or between meals; lactose- and gluten-free.

[22] Supplemental oral nutrition that is high in calcium.

[23] Reduced-carbohydrate, modified-fat, fiber-containing formula to improve blood glucose response in people with type 1 and type 2 diabetes and stress-induced hyperglycermia; supplemental or sole-source oral or tube feeding.

[24] Complete elemental nutrition for metabolically stressed patients.

[25] Nutritionally complete, isotonic tube feeding formula.

[26] Nutritionally complete, moderately high-nitrogen, isotonic tube feeding formula.

[27] Moderately high-nitrogen, 1.2 calorie/ml nutritionally complete tube feeding formula.

[28] High-calorie, high-nitrogen, complete liquid formulas with fiber.

[29] Nutritionally complete MCT formulation for patients with fat malabsorption.

[30] Nutritionally complete, high-calorie oral and tube feeding formula.

[31] Medium chain triglycerides containing primarily C8 and C10 saturated fatty acids; for use when long chain fat digestion, absorption, or utilization is impaired.

[32] Fifty percent fat emulsion for special dietary use in oral or tube feeding formulas.

[33] Readily digestible carbohydrate which can be added to foods to increase the caloric content for individuals with increased caloric requirements.

[34] Nutritionally complete, powdered formula for people with inflammatory bowel disease (Crohn's disease and ulcerative colitis); low in n-6 polyunsaturated fatty acids to minimize inflammatory effects; contains transforming growth factor-beta 2 (TGF-B2).

[35] Calorically dense, high-nitrogen, low-sodium, complete liquid formula for management of fluid restriction, elevated nutritional, and wound-healing needs.

[36] Amino acid food formulated without phenylalanine for individuals with hyper-phenylalanemia including PKU.

[37] Hydrolyzed casein formula processed to remove most of the phenylalanine and tyrosine for individuals with type II tyrosinemia or other disorders of tyrosine metabolism.

[38] Protein-free formula base for use with added protein, sodium, potassium, and chloride; for individuals requiring specific mixtures of dietary amino acids or other inborn errors of amino acid metabolism.

[39] Nutritionally complete, high-protein, fiber-containing tube feeding to support wound healing.

[40] Nutritionally complete, high-nitrogen, high-calorie, oral and tube feeding formula for pulmonary patients.

[41] Oral or tube feeding elemental nutrition for patients with impaired gastrointestinal function.

[42] Calorically dense oral or tube feeding elemental nutrition for patients with impaired gastrointestinal function.

[43] Nutritionally complete, high-calorie, high-nitrogen oral or tube feeding formula for metabolically stressed patients.

[44] Nutritionally complete, moderate-nitrogen tube feeding formula with dietary fiber.

[45] Moderately high-nitrogen, 0.5 cal/ml, nutritionally complete tube feeding formula with fiber.

[46] High-nitrogen, very low fat, elemental diet for enteral nutrition.

[47] Very low fat, elemental diet enriched with glutamine to meet nutritional needs of patients with gastrointestinal impairment.

32.3 SPORT, ENERGY, & WEIGHT REDUCTION FOODS

	KCAL	H₂0	PRO	CHO	SUGR	DFIB		Na	Ca	Mg	Zn	Mn		A	C	B-1	NIA	B-12
Clif Bar, choc almond fudge	230		10.0	39.0	20.0	5.0		140	300	120	3.75	0.800			60	0.38	4.0	0.90
2.4 oz bar	68	4.5	1.0			0		230	300	5.40	0.600	17.5	1500	20.0	0.26	0.40	80.0
								22	11	24			2.0	30		20	
													45				CLIF1
Dr. Soy Bar,	180		12.0	29.0	9.0	1.0		190	350	16	15.00				60	1.50	20.0	6.00
choc mint - 1.76 oz bar	50	3.5	2.5			0		80	250	18.00	2.000	0.0	5000	20.0	1.70	2.00	400.0
								150					10.0	30	400		
																	DRSY1
choc peanut	185		11.0	27.0	10.0	1.0		120	350	16	15.00				60	1.50	20.0	6.00
1.76 oz bar	50	4.0	2.5			0		70	400	18.00	2.000	0.0	5000	20.0	1.70	2.00	400.0
								150					10.0	30	400		
																	DRSY2
double choc	180		12.0	27.0	9.0	1.0		170	350	16	15.00				60	1.50	20.0	6.00
1.76 oz bar	50	3.0	2.5			0		80	450	18.00	2.000	0.0	5000	20.0	1.70	2.00	400.0
								150					10.0	30	400		
																	DRSY3
iced oatmeal	180		11.0	26.0	10.0	1.0		190	350	16	15.00				60	1.50	20.0	6.00
1.76 oz bar	50	4.0	2.5			0		65	600	18.00	2.000	0.0	5000	20.0	1.70	2.00	400.0
								150					10.0	30	400		
																	DRSY4
lemon cake	170		11.0	28.0	11.0	1.0		130	350	0	15.00				60	1.50	20.0	6.00
1.76 oz bar	50	2.5	2.0			0		25	350	18.00	2.000	0.0	5000	20.0	1.70	2.00	400.0
													10.0	30	400		
																	DRSY5
yogurt honey peanut	180		11.0	26.0	9.0	1.0		190	350	0	15.00				60	1.50	20.0	6.00
1.76 oz bar	50	4.0	2.5			0		65	600	18.00	2.000	0.0	5000	20.0	1.70	2.00	400.0
													10.0	30	400		
																	DRSY6
Gatorade Energy Bar, avg	255		7.0	46.0	20.0	2.0		170	30						18	0.22	6.0	1.80
all flvrs - 2.29 oz bar	65	5.0	1.0			0				1.98			750	6.0	0.26	0.60	

	KCAL / WT / HIS / PHE	H₂0 (g) / FAT / ISO / TYR	PRO (g) / SFA / LEU / THR	CHO (g) / MUFA / LYS / TRY	SUGR (g) / PUFA / MET / VAL	DFIB (g) / CHOL / CYS / ARG	TAU / CAR	Na (mg) / K / Cl / —	Ca (mg) / P / I / —	Mg (mg) / Fe / Mo / —	Zn (mg) / Cu / Cr / —	Mn (mg) / Se / — / —	A (mcg RAE) / A (IU) / PANT / BIO	C (mg) / E (mg ATE) / E (IU) / CHLN	B-1 (mg) / B-2 / D (IU) / INOS	NIA (mg) / B-6 / K (mcg)	B-12 (mcg) / FOL	REF
(continued)											3.0		9					
																		GTRD1
GeniSoy soy protein bar[1]	229		14.0	33.0	26.8	1.3		171	250	100	3.75			15	0.38	5.0	1.50	
2.2 oz bar	62	4.6	2.8			0		209	250	4.50	0.500	50.0	1250	20.0	0.42	0.50	400.0	
													2.5	30				
																		GENI6
Healthy! soy protein bar, blondie	180		10.0	32.0	21.0	2.0		70	200	60	3.75	0.500		60	0.52	7.0	1.50	
1.76 oz bar	50	2.0	0.0			0			250	1.44	0.500	10.5	2500	20.0	0.60	0.50	140.0	
									38	26			2.5	30	100			
													75					AMNS1
choc	190		10.0	32.0	23.0	2.0		85	200	60	3.75	0.500		60	0.52	7.0	1.50	
1.76 oz bar	50	2.5	1.0			0			250	1.80	0.500	10.5	2500	20.0	0.60	0.50	140.0	
									38	26			2.5	30	100			
													75					AMNS2
chocolate chip	190		10.0	31.0	20.0	2.0		65	200	60	3.75	0.500		60	0.52	7.0	1.50	
1.76 oz bar	50	2.5	0.5			0			250	1.80	0.500	10.5	2500	20.0	0.60	0.50	140.0	
									38	26			2.5	30	100			
													75					AMNS3
peanut butter	190		10.0	32.0	20.0	2.0		105	200	60	3.75	0.500		60	0.52	7.0	1.50	
1.76 oz bar	50	3.0	0.5			0			250	1.44	0.500	10.5	2500	20.0	0.60	0.50	140.0	
									38	26			2.5	30	100			
													75					AMNS4
Luna Bar, choc pecan pie, Clif	180		10.0	24.0	12.0	2.0		125	350	140	5.25	0.700		60	1.50	20.0	6.00	
1.69 oz bar	48	4.5	3.0	1.0	0.5	0		105	350	6.30	0.700	24.5	1250	20.0	1.70	2.00	400.0	
									52	26	42		10.0	30		80		
													300					CLIF2
toasted nuts 'n cranberry, Clif	170		10.0	26.0	12.0	2.0		130	350	140	5.25	0.700		60	1.50	20.0	6.00	
1.69 oz bar	48	3.0	0.0	1.5	1.0	0		100	350	6.30	0.700	24.5	1250	20.0	1.70	2.00	400.0	
									52	26	42		10.0	30		80		
													300					CLIF3
PowerBar, choc	230		10.0	45.0	20.0	3.0		90	300	140	5.25			60	1.50	20.0	6.00	
2.29 oz bar	65	2.0	0.5			0		150	350	6.30	0.700		0	20.0	1.70	2.00	400.0	
											24		10.0	30				
																		PWRB1
SlimFast, all flavors, cnd	220		10.0	40.7	34.7	5.0		220	400	140	2.25	0.700		60	0.52	7.0	2.10	
11 fl oz (325 ml)	336	2.2	0.7	1.2	0.3	5		600	400	2.70		17.5	1750	20.0	0.60	0.70	120.0	
									53				3.5	30	140	20.00		
													105					SLIM6
SlimFast bar, brkfst/lunch bar	145		5.0	19.5	12.5	2.0		73	100	16	3.75			15	0.38	5.0	1.50	
1.2 oz bar	34	5.5	2.8			5		138	100	4.50	0.500		1250	5.0	0.42	0.40	40.0	
									38				2.5	8	80			
													75					SLIM1
on-the-go bar	220		8.0	35.3	22.2	2.0		138	300	140	2.25			21	0.22	7.0	2.10	
2 oz bar	56	5.0	3.4			<5		130	250	2.70		17.5	1750	7.0	0.60	0.70	60.0	
									53				3.5	11	140	20.00		
													105					SLIM2
snack bar	122		0.2	21.2	16.2	0		75	250					8	0.22	3.0	0.90	
1 oz bar	28	4.6	2.3			<1		60	100	2.70			750	3.0	0.26	0.30	60.0	
													1.0	5	60			
													30					SLIM3
SlimFast fruit jce mixable w/ orange jce	220		11.5	44.0	34.0	5.0		210	200	120	4.50	0.700		60	0.60	10.0	2.10	
8 fl oz (240 ml)	244	1.0	0.0	0.0	0.0	5		770	200	6.30	0.200	17.5	750	20.0	0.17	0.70	160.0	
									15				4.0	30	100	20.00		
													150					SLIM4
SlimFast reg powder w/ nonfat mlk	190		13.5	32.0	29.3	2.0		250	450	120	5.25			21	0.52	7.0	2.10	
8 fl oz (240 ml)	244	1.3	0.8	0.0	0.0	9		643	350	6.30	0.200		1250	10.0	0.51	0.70	120.0	
									53				3.5	15	140			
													105					SLIM5

Column key (each food is listed as four stacked data rows matching the four header tiers):

1	KCAL	H₂O (g)	PRO (g)	CHO (g)	SUGR (g)	DFIB (g)	Na (mg)	Ca (mg)	Mg (mg)	Zn (mg)	Mn (mg)	A (mcg RAE)	C (mg)	B-1 (mg)	NIA (mg)	B-12 (mcg)
2	WT (g)	FAT (g)	SFA (g)	MUFA (g)	PUFA (g)	CHOL (mg)	K (mg)	P (mg)	Fe (mg)	Cu (mg)	Se (mcg)	A (IU)	E (mg ATE)	B-2 (mg)	B-6 (mg)	FOL (mcg DFE)
3	HIS (mg)	ISO (mg)	LEU (mg)	LYS (mg)	MET (mg)	CYS/TAU (mg)	Cl (mg)	I (mcg)	Mo (mcg)	Cr (mcg)		PANT (mg)	E (IU)	D (IU)	K (mcg)	
4	PHE (mg)	TYR (mg)	THR (mg)	TRY (mg)	VAL (mg)	ARG/CAR (mg)						BIO (mcg)	CHLN (mg)	INOS (mg)		REF

Minerals = columns c7–c11; Vitamins = columns c12–c16.

SlimFast soy pro pwdr w/ nonfat milk - 8 fl oz (240 ml)

c1	c2	c3	c4	c5	c6	c7	c8	c9	c10	c11	c12	c13	c14	c15	c16
170		15.0	25.5	12.0	5.0	270	600	120	5.25	0.600		60	0.52	7.0	6.00
244	1.8	0.8	0.5	0.5	0	440		6.30	0.200	17.5		20.0	0.60	2.00	200.0
						45	26	42.0			3.5	30	140	20.00	
											105				SLIM8

SlimFast ultra pwdr w/ nonfat mlk - 8 fl oz (240 ml)

c1	c2	c3	c4	c5	c6	c7	c8	c9	c10	c11	c12	c13	c14	c15	c16
201		13.5	36.0	29.3	4.9	244	500	120	5.25	0.700		30	0.52	10.0	3.00
244	1.6	0.9	0.2	0.1	9	635	350	6.30	0.200	17.5	1250	20.0	0.51	0.70	120.0
						53					5.0	30	200	20.00	
											150				SLIM9

SlimFast w/soy pro, all flvrs, cnd - 11 fl oz (325 ml)

c1	c2	c3	c4	c5	c6	c7	c8	c9	c10	c11	c12	c13	c14	c15	c16
220		7.0	46.0	38.5	5.0	170	350	140	2.25	0.700		60	0.52	7.0	2.10
336	1.0	0.0	0.0	0.0	<5	500	400	2.70		17.5	2500	20.0	0.60	0.70	120.0
						53					3.5	30	140	20.00	
											105				SLIM7

Xtreme Bar, carrot cake quake, GeniSoy - 1.6 oz bar

c1	c2	c3	c4	c5	c6	c7	c8	c9	c10	c11	c12	c13	c14	c15	c16
190		9.0	24.0	18.0	1.0	90	150	40	3.75	0.500		15	0.38	5.0	1.50
45	7.0	3.0			0	150	150	4.50			1250		0.42	0.5	100.0
						38					2.5	7.5			
											75				GENI9

peanut butter fix, GeniSoy - 1.6 oz bar

c1	c2	c3	c4	c5	c6	c7	c8	c9	c10	c11	c12	c13	c14	c15	c16
200		9.0	23.0	16.0	2.0	190	200	80	3.75	0.500		15	0.38	5.0	1.50
45	8.0	3.0			0	190	200	4.50			1250		0.42	0.5	100.0
						38					2.5	7.5			
											75				GENI10

raspberry rush, GeniSoy - 1.6 oz bar

c1	c2	c3	c4	c5	c6	c7	c8	c9	c10	c11	c12	c13	c14	c15	c16
190		9.0	24.0	18.0	2.0	90	100	40	3.75	0.500	75	15	0.38	5.0	1.50
45	7.0	3.5			0	190	150	4.50			1250		0.42	0.5	100.0
						38	26				2.5	7.5			
											75				GENI11

rocky roadtrip, GeniSoy - 1.6 oz bar

c1	c2	c3	c4	c5	c6	c7	c8	c9	c10	c11	c12	c13	c14	c15	c16
190		9.0	23.0	16.0	2.0	130	150	60	3.75	0.500		15	0.38	5.0	1.50
45	7.0	3.0			0	180	200	4.50			1250		0.42	0.5	100.0
						38	26				2.5	7.5			
											75				
												7.5			GENI12

¹ Values are averages for 8 flavors, Arctic frost crispy chocolate mint, Dutch crunch sour apple crisp, fair trade Arabica café mocha fudge, New York style blueberry cheesecake, obsession fudge cookies & cream, pure golden honey creamy peanut yogurt, southern style chunky peanut butter fudge, and ultimate chocolate fudge brownie.

SUPPLEMENTARY TABLES FOR THE NUTRIENT CONTENT OF FOODS

Alcohol, Ethyl (Ethanol)

	SERVING SIZE & WEIGHT (g)	ALCOHOL (% by volume)	ALCOHOL (g)	USDA CODE/ SOURCE
BEER, LIGHT				
beer, light (generic)	12 fl oz (354 g)	4.0[1]	11.3	14006
Bud, Ice Light, Anheuser-Busch	12 fl oz (~354 g)	4.1[1]	11.5	ANBU
Bud Light, Anheuser-Busch	12 fl oz (~354 g)	4.2[1]	11.8	ANBU
Busch Light, Anheuser-Busch	12 fl oz (~354 g)	4.2[1]	11.8	ANBU
Coors Light	12 fl oz (354 g)	4.2	11.8[2]	CORS
Keystone Light, Coors	12 fl oz (354 g)	4.2	11.8[2]	CORS
Michelob Golden Draft Light, Anheuser-Busch	12 fl oz (~354 g)	4.1[1]	11.5	ANBU
Michelob Light, Anheuser-Busch	12 fl oz (~354 g)	4.3[1]	12.1	ANBU
Michelob Ultra, Anheuser-Busch	12 fl oz (~354 g)	4.1[1]	11.5	ANBU
Natural Light, Anheuser-Busch	12 fl oz (~354 g)	4.2[1]	11.8	ANBU
BEER, NO ALCOHOL				
Busch NA (no alcohol), Anheuser-Busch	12 fl oz (~354 g)	0.4[1]	1.1	ANBU
Coors NA (no alcohol)	12 fl oz (350 g)	<0.5	<1.4[2]	CORS
Malt beverage, nonalcoholic	12 fl oz (356 g)	0.4[1]	1.1	14305
O'Doul's Amber, Anheuser-Busch	12 fl oz (~354 g)	0.4[1]	1.1	ANBU
O'Doul's, Anheuser-Busch	12 fl oz (~354 g)	0.4[1]	1.1	ANBU
BEER, REGULAR				
beer (generic)	12 fl oz (356 g)		12.8	14003
Bacardi Silver, Anheuser-Busch	12 fl oz (~356 g)	4.8[1]	13.4	ANBU
Bud Dry, Anheuser-Busch	12 fl oz (~356 g)	5.0[1]	14.0	ANBU
Bud Ice, Anheuser-Busch	12 fl oz (~356 g)	5.5[1]	15.4	ANBU
Budweiser, Anheuser-Busch	12 fl oz (~356 g)	4.9[1]	13.7	ANBU
Busch, Anheuser-Busch	12 fl oz (~356 g)	4.6[1]	12.9	ANBU
Busch Ice, Anheuser-Busch	12 fl oz (~356 g)	5.9[1]	16.5	ANBU
Coors Extra Gold	12 fl oz (356 g)	5.0	14.0[2]	CORS
Coors Original	12 fl oz (356 g)	5.0	14.0[2]	CORS
Coors Winterfest	12 fl oz (356 g)	5.6	15.7[2]	CORS
Docs, Anheuser-Busch	12 fl oz (~356 g)	4.8[1]	13.5	ANBU
George Killian's Irish Red	12 fl oz (356 g)	4.9	13.7[2]	CORS
Hurricane, Anheuser-Busch	12 fl oz (~356 g)	5.8[1]	16.3	ANBU
Keystone, Coors	12 fl oz (356 g)	4.4	12.4[2]	CORS
Keystone Ice, Coors	12 fl oz (356 g)	5.9	16.5[2]	CORS
King Cobra, Anheuser-Busch	12 fl oz (~356 g)	5.9[1]	16.5	ANBU
Michelob Amber Bock, Anheuser-Busch	12 fl oz (~356 g)	5.2[1]	14.5	ANBU
Michelob, Anheuser-Busch	12 fl oz (~356 g)	5.0[1]	14.0	ANBU
Michelob Black & Tan, Anheuser-Busch	12 fl oz (~356 g)	5.0[1]	14.0	ANBU
Michelob Golden Draft, Anheuser-Busch	12 fl oz (~356 g)	4.7[1]	13.2	ANBU
Michelob Hefeweizen, Anheuser-Busch	12 fl oz (~356 g)	5.0[1]	14.0	ANBU
Michelob Honey Lager, Anheuser-Busch	12 fl oz (~356 g)	4.9[1]	13.7	ANBU
Natural Ice, Anheuser-Busch	12 fl oz (~356 g)	5.8[1]	16.3	ANBU
Tequiza, Anheuser-Busch	12 fl oz (~356 g)	4.5[1]	12.6	ANBU
Winterfest, Coors	12 fl oz (356 g)	5.6	15.7[2]	CORS
MALT BEVERAGE/ALE				
Blue Moon Belgian White, Coors	12 fl oz (356 g)	5.4	15.2[2]	CORS
Zima, Coors	12 fl oz (356 g)	4.8	13.5[2]	CORS
Zima Citrus, Coors	12 fl oz (356 g)	4.9	13.7[2]	CORS
DISTILLED SPIRITS				
all types, 80 proof	1.5 fl oz (42 g)	39.9[1]	14.0	14037
gin, 90 proof	1.5 fl oz (42 g)	45.3[1]	15.9	14049
rum, 80 proof	1.5 fl oz (42 g)	39.9[1]	14.0	14050
vodka, 80 proof	1.5 fl oz (42 g)	39.9[1]	14.0	14051
whiskey, 86 proof	1.5 fl oz (42 g)	43.0[1]	15.1	14052
LIQUEURS				
coffee, 53 proof	1.5 fl oz (52 g)	32.2[1]	11.3	14414
coffee, 63 proof	1.5 fl oz (52 g)	38.5[1]	13.5	14534
coffee w/cream, 34 proof	1.5 fl oz (47 g)	18.5[1]	6.5	14415
crème de menthe, 72 proof	1.5 fl oz (50 g)	42.5[1]	14.9	14034

	SERVING SIZE & WEIGHT (g)	ALCOHOL (% by volume)	ALCOHOL (g)	USDA CODE/ SOURCE
MIXED DRINKS				
bloody mary (tomato jce, vodka, & lemon jce)	5 fl oz (148 g)	11.9[1]	13.9	Hnd 8-14
bourbon & soda	4 fl oz (116 g)	16.1[1]	15.1	Hnd 8-14
daiquiri (rum, lime jce, & sugar)	2 fl oz (60 g)	29.7[1]	13.9	14010
daiquiri (rum, lime jce, & sugar), cnd	6.8 fl oz (207 g)	12.5[1]	19.9	14009
gin & tonic (tonic water, gin, & lime jce)	7.5 fl oz (225 g)	9.1[1]	16.0	Hnd 8-14
manhattan (whiskey & vermouth)	2 fl oz (57 g)	37.2[1]	17.4	Hnd 8-14
martini (gin & vermouth)	2.5 fl oz (70 g)	38.3[1]	22.4	Hnd 8-14
pina colada (pineapple jce, rum, sugar, & coconut cream)	4.5 fl oz (141 g)	13.3[1]	14.0	14017
pina colada (pineapple jce, rum, sugar, & coconut cream), cnd	6.8 fl oz (222 g)	12.6[1]	20.0	14015
screwdriver (orange jce & vodka)	7 fl oz (213 g)	8.6[1]	14.1	Hnd 8-14
tequila sunrise (orange jce, tequila, lime jce, & grenadine)	5.5 fl oz (172 g)	14.5[1]	18.7	Hnd 8-14
tequila sunrise (orange jce, tequila, lime jce, & grenadine), cnd	6.8 fl oz (211 g)	12.4[1]	19.8	14019
tom collins (club soda, gin, lemon jce, & sugar)	7.5 fl oz (222 g)	9.1[1]	16.0	Hnd 8-14
whiskey sour (lemon jce, whiskey, & sugar)	3 fl oz (90 g)	21.5[1]	15.1	Hnd 8-14
whiskey sour (lemon jce, whiskey, & sugar), cnd	6.8 fl oz (209 g)	12.5[1]	19.9	14027
whiskey sour (lemon jce, whiskey, & sugar), from liquid mix	2 fl oz mix w/1.5 fl oz whiskey (106 g)	18.2[1]	14.9	14029
whiskey sour (lemon jce, whiskey, & sugar), from powdered mix	17 g pkt w/1.5 fl oz water & 1.5 fl oz whiskey (103 g)	21.4[1]	15.0	14025
WINE				
dessert, dry	3.5 fl oz (103 g)	19.3[1]	15.8	14536
dessert, sweet	3.5 fl oz (103 g)	19.3[1]	15.8	14057
table, all types	3.5 fl oz (103 g)	11.7[1]	9.6	14084
table, red	3.5 fl oz (103 g)	11.7[1]	9.6	14096
table, rose	3.5 fl oz (103 g)	11.7[1]	9.6	14104
table, white	3.5 fl oz (103 g)	11.7[1]	9.6	14106
MISCELLANEOUS				
cheese fondue (table wine, swiss cheese, white flour)	1/2 cup (108 g)	0.3[1]	0.3	01163
vanilla extract	1 T (12 g)	38.5[1]	4.5	02052
vanilla extract, imitation w/alcohol	1 T (12 g)	36.8[1]	4.3	02051

[1] Percent alcohol (ethanol) by volume was calculated assuming the weight for ethanol was 23.4 grams per fluid ounce.

[2] Grams of alcohol (ethanol) were calculated assuming the weight for ethanol was 23.4 grams per fluid ounce.

Sources:
ANBU: Anheuser-Busch, St Louis MO.
CORS: Coors Brewing Company, Golden CO.
Hnd 8-14: *Agriculture Handbook No. 8-14, Revised, Composition of Foods, Raw, Processed, Prepared. Beverages,* US Department of Agriculture, Washington DC. May 1986.
USDA Codes: *United States Department of Agriculture Database for Standard Reference,* Release 15 (SR15), 2002. Available at http://www.nal.usda.gov/fnic/foodcomp/Data/SR15/sr15.html.

Amines—Histamine

	HISTAMINE (mg/100 g)	SOURCE		HISTAMINE (mg/100 g)	SOURCE
BEVERAGES			cheese, cheddar, med	14.0	Voight et al, 1974
beer, light	0.6	Souci et al, 2000	cheese, cheddar, mild	19.0	Voight et al, 1974
beer, no alcohol	0.0	Souci et al, 2000	cheese, cheddar, sharp	11.0	Voight et al, 1974
beer, pale	0.5	Souci et al, 2000	cheese, colby	7.0	Voight et al, 1974
beer, pilsener lager	0.0	Souci et al, 2000	cheese, emmental	2.3	Souci et al, 2000
grape jce	tr	Souci et al, 2000	cheese, gouda	7.5	Voight et al, 1974
wine, Hungarian	0.1	Kovacs et al, 1999	cheese, gruyere	6.6	Souci et al, 2000
wine, white (german sekt)	0.7	Souci et al, 2000	cheese, rouquefort	6.5	Souci et al, 2000
			cheese, quark (fresh)	0.0	Souci et al, 2000
CHEESE			cheese, sap-sago	260.0	Voight et al, 1974
cheese, appenzeller, 11% fat	15.0	Souci et al, 2000	cheese, tilsit	27.0	Souci et al, 2000
cheese, appenzeller, 32% fat	17.0	Souci et al, 2000	**CREAMS**		
cheese, blue/Roquefort	50.0	Voight et al, 1974	cream, sour	0.0	Souci et al, 2000
cheese, camembert	7.0	Voight et al, 1974	cream, whipping	0.2	Souci et al, 2000
cheese, cheddar, extra sharp	21.0	Voight et al, 1974	**MEAT & FISH**		
			mackerel	0.0	Souci et al, 2000
			sausage	63.8	Kovacs et al, 1999

	HISTAMINE (mg/100 g)	SOURCE		HISTAMINE (mg/100 g)	SOURCE
MILK & YOGURT			**VEGETABLES**		
buttermilk	0.0	Souci et al, 2000	chives	0.0	Kovacs et al, 1999
milk, whole	0.1	Souci et al, 2000	sauerkraut	7.0	Souci et al, 2000
yogurt, whole milk	0.0	Souci et al, 2000			

Sources:

Kovacs A, L Simon-Sarkadi, K Ganzler. Determination of biogenic amines by capillary electrophoresis. *J Chromatography A* 836:305–313, 1999.

Souci SW, W Fachmann, H Kraut. *Food Composition and Nutrition Tables.* Medpharm GmbH Scientific Publishers, Stuttgart, Germany & CRC Press, Washington DC. 2000.

Voight MN, RR Eitenmiller, PE Koehler, MK Hamdy. Tyramine, histamine, and tryptamine content of cheese. *J Milk Food Technol* 37:377–381, 1974.

Amines—Theobromine

	SERVING SIZE (g)	THEOBROMINE (mg/serving)	THEOBROMINE (mg/100 g)	USDA CODE/SOURCE
BEVERAGES				
carbonated, choc flavor	12 fl oz (369 g)	232	63	14552
carbonated, cola	12 fl oz	0	0	Ahuja and Perloff, 2001
carbonated, diet choc			3	Shively and Tarka, 1984
carbonated, diet crème			3	Shively and Tarka, 1984
coffee, brewed	8 fl oz	0	0	Ahuja and Perloff, 2001
coffee, from inst	8 fl oz	0	0	Ahuja and Perloff, 2001
coffee, inst powder w/cocoa, whitener, & low cal sweetener, decaffeinated	1 t (6 g)	39	606	14204
coffee, inst powder w/sugar, mocha-flavor	2 rd t (12 g)	22	194	14224
tea, brewed, black, 3 min	8 fl oz (237 g)	5	2	14355
tea, from inst	8 fl oz	2		Ahuja and Perloff, 2001
tea, iced, inst powder	1 t (.7 g)	2	293	14366
tea, iced, inst powder, decaffeinated	1 t (.7 g)	0	11	14353
tea, iced, inst powder, lemon flavor	2 rd T (11 g)	14	121	14368
tea, iced, inst powder, lemon flavor w/sugar	3 heaping t (23 g)	2	8	14370
tea, iced, prep from inst powder, lemon flavor w/ Na saccharin	8 fl oz (237 g)	2	1	14376
CANDY				
After Eight Mints, Nestle	5 mints (41 g)	58	142	19153
Baby Ruth, Nestle	.7 oz bar (21 g)	9	44	19111
Baby Ruth, Nestle	2.1 oz bar (60 g)	26	44	19111
Butterfinger, Nestle	.7 oz bar (21 g)	7	34	19069
Butterfinger, Nestle	2.16 oz bar (61 g)	21	34	19069
caramel, choc flavored roll	2.25 oz bar (64 g)	92	144	19076
choc-coated, fondant	1.5 oz patty (43 g)	57	133	19083
choc-coated, peanuts	10 pieces (40 g)	44	109	19126
choc-coated, peanuts, Goobers	1.38 oz pkg (39 g)	43	109	19105
choc-coated, raisins	1/4 cup (45 g)	57	127	19127
choc-coated, raisins, Raisinets	1.58 oz pkg (45 g)	57	127	19149
Chunky, Nestle	1.4 oz piece (40 g)	63	157	19119
Crunch, Nestle	1.55 oz bar (44 g)	69	156	19145
dark choc (semi-sweet)	1.45 oz bar (41 g)	175	426	19081
dark choc (semi-sweet), chips	1 cup/6 oz (168 g)	816	486	19080
dark choc (semi-sweet) chips, Hershey	1/4 cup (1.5 oz)	207	481	Hershey, 2002
dark (sweet) choc	1 oz (28 g)	131	463	Shively and Tarka, 1984
Demet's Turtles, Nestle	6 oz pkg (170 g)	82	48	19158
Fifth Avenue, Hershey	2 oz bar (56 g)	29	51	19098
fudge, choc, homemade	.6 oz piece (17 g)	21	125	19100
fudge, choc marshmallow w/nuts, homemade	.78 oz piece (22 g)	28	129	19301
fudge, homemade, choc w/nuts	.67 oz piece (19 g)	21	108	19101
Hundred Grand, Nestle	1.5 oz bar (43 g)	32	74	19144
Kisses, Hershey	9 pieces (1.55 oz)	91	212	Hershey, 2002
Kit Kat, Hershey	1.5 oz bar (42 g)	45	107	Hershey, 2002
Kit Kat, Hershey	2.8 oz bar (78 g)	92	118	19109
Krackel, Hershey	1.45 oz bar (41 g)	62	151	Hershey, 2002
M&M's Peanut, M&M/Mars	1.74 oz pkg/~25 pieces (49 g)	34	69	19140

	SERVING SIZE (g)	THEOBROMINE (mg/serving)	THEOBROMINE (mg/100 g)	USDA CODE/SOURCE
M&M's Plain, M&M/Mars	1.69 oz pkg/~69 pieces (48 g)	56	116	19141
Mars Almond, M&M/Mars	1.76 oz bar (50 g)	15	29	19115
milk choc	1.55 oz bar (44 g)	74	169	19120
milk choc	1.45 oz bar	69	168	Ahuja and Perloff, 2001
milk choc, chips	1 cup (168 g)	284	169	19120
milk choc, Hershey	1.55 oz bar (43 g)	86	200	Hershey, 2002
milk choc w/almonds	1.55 oz bar (44 g)	70	158	19132
milk choc w/almonds, Hershey	1.45 oz bar (41 g)	66	161	Hershey, 2002
milk choc w/rice cereal	1.55 oz bar (44 g)	68	155	19134
Milky Way, M&M/Mars	.6 oz bar (18 g)	17	92	19135
Milky Way, M&M/Mars	2.1 oz bar (60 g)	55	92	19135
Mounds, Hershey	1.9 oz bar (53 g)	69	130	19142
Mr. Goodbar, Hershey	1.65 oz bar (45 g)	57	127	Hershey, 2002
Mr. Goodbar, Hershey	1.75 oz bar (49 g)	268	547	19143
Oh Henry!, Nestle	2 oz bar (57 g)	38	67	19118
Pot of Gold almond choc bar, Hershey	1.5 oz (43 g)	59	137	Hershey, 2002
Pot of Gold Solitaires, Hershey	1.5 oz (43 g)	62	144	Hershey, 2002
Reese's Peanut Butter Cups, Hershey	2 pieces (46 g)	33	72	Hershey, 2002
Rolo caramels w/milk choc, Hershey	9 pieces (54 g)	35	65	Hershey, 2002
Skor toffee bar, Hershey	1.4 oz bar (39 g)	23	59	Hershey, 2002
Snickers, M&M/Mars	2 oz bar (57 g)	38	67	19155
Special Dark, Hershey	1.45 oz bar (41 g)	195	476	Hershey, 2002
Three Musketeers, M&M/Mars	2.13 oz bar (60 g)	52	87	19159
Twix Cookie Bar, caramel, M&M/Mars	2 bars (58 g)	52	90	19160
Twix Cookie Bar, peanut butter, M&M/Mars	2 bars (58 g)	33	57	19161
Whatchamacallit, Hershey	1.7 oz bar (48 g)	41	86	19162

CEREALS

choc cereal	1 oz (28 g)	22	79	Shively and Tarka, 1984
Cocoa Blasts, Quaker Oats	1 oz (28 g)	7	25	Caudle and Bell, 2000
Cocoa Crispy Rice, Kountry Fresh	1 oz (28 g)	13	45	Caudle and Bell, 2000
Cocoa Crunchies, Kountry Fresh	1 oz (28 g)	19	67	Caudle and Bell, 2000
Cocoa Frosted Flakes, Kellogg	1 oz (28 g)	3	11	Caudle and Bell, 2000
Cocoa Krispies, Kellogg	1 oz (28 g)	17	61	Caudle and Bell, 2000
Cocoa Pebbles, Post	1 oz (28 g)	16	57	Caudle and Bell, 2000
Cocoa Puffs, General Mills	1 oz (28 g)	32	113	Caudle and Bell, 2000
Cookie Crisp, General Mills	1 oz (28 g)	11	38	Caudle and Bell, 2000
Count Chocula, General Mills	1 oz (28 g)	25	87	Caudle and Bell, 2000
Malt-O-Meal, plain/choc, ckd	1 cup (240 g)	17	7	08117
NesQuik, General Mills	1 oz (28 g)	31	108	Caudle and Bell, 2000
Oreo O's, Post	1 oz (28 g)	37	130	Caudle and Bell, 2000
Reese's Peanut Butter Puffs, General Mills	3/4 cup (30 g)	0	1	08194

DESSERTS

brownie, from mix			85	Shively and Tarka, 1984
cake, choc			86	Shively and Tarka, 1984
cookie, choc			106	Shively and Tarka, 1984
cookie, choc chip			71	Shively and Tarka, 1984
cookie, choc chunk pecan, Pepperidge Farm	1 cookie (12 g)	10	83	18159
cookie, choc sandwich	1-1 1/2" dia cookie	47		Ahuja and Perloff, 2001
cookie, choc sandwich w/crème filling	1 cookie (17 g)	4	26	18167
cookie, choc sandwich w/crème filling, choc coated	1 cookie (10 g)	43	430	18166
cookie, choc sandwich w/extra crème filling	1 cookie (13 g)	22	169	18168
cookie, choc wafers	5 wafers (28 g)	63	223	18157
cookie, graham crackers, choc coated	2 1/2" sq cookie (14 g)	51	363	18174
cookie, marshmallow, choc coated	3/4" × 3/4" cookie (13 g)	21	159	18176
cookie, marshmallow pie	3" dia × 3/4" cookie (39 g)	62	159	18176
cookie, mint crème, Snackwell's	1 cookie (25 g)	3	12	18649
doughnut (cake), choc covered			106	Shively and Tarka, 1984
doughnut, cake, choc coated/frosted	3" dia cookie (43 g)	29	68	18249
cupcake, choc			116	Shively and Tarka, 1984
doughnut, choc cake, sugared/glazed	3" dia doughnut (42 g)	9	21	18251
éclair w/custard filling & choc glaze, homemade	5" × 2" × 1 3/4" éclair (100 g)	14	14	18257
frzn dessert, fudge bar			32	Shively and Tarka, 1984
frzn yogurt, nonfat w/low cal sweetener, choc	1 cup (186 g)	197	106	42185
frzn yogurt, soft serve, choc	1/2 cup (72 g)	76	106	19393
granola bar, peanut butter, soft w/choc coating	1.3 oz bar (37 g)	16	42	19026
ice cream bar, choc covered			34	Shively and Tarka, 1984

	SERVING SIZE (g)	THEOBROMINE (mg/serving)	THEOBROMINE (mg/100 g)	USDA CODE/SOURCE
ice cream, choc	1/2 cup (66 g)	41	62	19270
ice cream, choc			51	Shively and Tarka, 1984
ice cream, choc, rich	1 cup (148 g)	92	62	43541
pie, choc			57	Shively and Tarka, 1984
pie, choc cream/crème	1/6 of 8" pie (113 g)	15	13	18310
pie, choc mousse, from mix	1/8 of 9" pie (95 g)	8	8	18312
pie crust, choc wafer, homemade	1/8 of 9" crust (28 g)	46	166	18398
pudding, choc, cnd			131	Shively and Tarka, 1984
pudding, choc, from inst mix w/lowfat milk	1/2 cup (147 g)	57	39	19123
pudding, choc, from inst mix w/whole milk	1/2 cup (147 g)	91	62	19185
pudding, choc, from reg mix w/2% milk	1/2 cup (142 g)	89	63	19190
pudding, choc, from reg mix w/whole milk	1/2 cup (142 g)	88	62	19189
pudding, choc, ready-to-eat	5 oz serving (142 g)	88	62	19183
pudding, rennin dessert, choc, from mix w/ 2% milk	1/2 cup (136 g)	57	42	19213
pudding, rennin dessert, choc, from mix w/ whole milk	1/2 cup (136 g)	57	42	19221
DESSERTS - TOPPINGS				
icing/frosting, choc			131	Shively and Tarka, 1984
icing/frosting, choc, rts	2 T (41 g)	32	79	19226
icing/frosting, from mix, choc made w/butter	1/12 pkg prep (42 g)	61	145	19241
icing/frosting, from mix, choc made w/marg	1/12 pkg prep (42 g)	61	145	19372
syrup, choc	2 T (39 g)	184	471	14181
syrup, choc	1 T	89		Ahuja and Perloff, 2001
syrup, choc, Hershey	2 T (39 g)	69	177	Hershey, 2002
syrup, choc, lite, Hershey	2 T (35 g)	36	104	19345
topping, choc			123	Shively and Tarka, 1984
topping, choc fudge	2 T (38 g)	75	198	19348
topping, choc fudge, Hershey	2 T (37 g)	37	100	Hershey, 2002
FAST FOODS				
brownie	2" sq brownie (60 g)	47	79	21027
cookies, choc chip	1 box (55 g)	46	83	21030
shake, choc	10 fl oz (208 g)	129	62	14346
sundae, hot fudge	1 sundae (158 g)	77	49	21033
shake, choc	12 fl oz (250 g)	155	62	14346
shake, choc	16 fl oz (333 g)	206	62	14346
shake, choc	22 fl oz (458 g)	284	62	14346
MILK BEVERAGES				
choc malted milk, whole milk	8 fl oz (265 g)	74	28	14318
choc malted milk, whole milk w/added nutrients	8 fl oz (265 g)	74	28	14316
choc milk, 1% fat milk	8 fl oz (250 g)	58	23	01104
choc milk, 2% fat milk	8 fl oz (250 g)	58	23	01103
choc milk, 2% fat milk, Hershey	8 fl oz (250 g)	40	16	Hershey, 2002
choc milk, commercial			160	Shively and Tarka, 1984
choc milk, from inst mix	8 fl oz	58		Shively and Tarka, 1984
choc milk, from inst mix w/aspartame	6 fl oz (204 g)	169	83	14423
choc milk, whole milk	8 fl oz (250 g)	58	23	01102
choc milk, whole milk w/choc powder	8 fl oz (266 g)	263	99	14177
choc milk, whole milk w/choc syrup	8 fl oz (282 g)	180	64	14182
cocoa (hot choc), from inst mix	8 fl oz	62		Shively and Tarka, 1984
cocoa (hot choc), homemade	8 fl oz	94		Shively and Tarka, 1984
cocoa (hot choc), homemade w/2% milk	8 fl oz (250 g)	58	23	01105
cocoa (hot choc), prep w/milk from mix	8 fl oz	250		Ahuja and Perloff, 2001
cocoa (hot choc), prep w/water from mix	1 oz pkt in 6 fl oz water (206 g)	173	84	14194
cocoa (hot choc), prep w/water from mix w/ aspartame	1 pkt in 6 fl oz water (192 g)	173	90	14390
milk shake, choc			15	Shively and Tarka, 1984
MILK BEVERAGE MIXES				
choc milk mix	2–3 hp t (22 g)	267	1212	14175
choc milk mix, malted	3 hp t (21 g)	72	345	14317
choc milk mix w/aspartame	.75 oz pkt (21 g)	166	790	14422
cocoa mix	1 oz pkt/3–4 hp t (28 g)	170	606	14192
MISCELLANEOUS				
baking choc (unsweetened)	1 oz square (28 g)	346	1237	19078
baking choc (unsweetened), Hershey	1 oz (28 g)	393	1386	Hershey, 2002

	SERVING SIZE (g)	THEOBROMINE (mg/serving)	THEOBROMINE (mg/100 g)	USDA CODE/SOURCE
baking choc (unsweetened), liquid	1 oz pkt (28 g)	453	1597	19077
baking choc (unsweetened), mexican	1 oz (28 g)	60	210	19124
choc liquor			1220	Shively and Tarka, 1984
cocoa, unsweetened, dry powder	1 T (5 g)	111	2057	19165
cocoa, unsweetened, dry powder, Hershey	1 oz/1/2 cup	737	2600	Hershey, 2002
cocoa, unsweetened, dry powder, natural	1 oz (28 g)	726	2560	Shively and Tarka, 1984
cocoa, unsweetened, dry powder, processed w/alkali	1 T (5 g)	142	2634	19166
cocoa, unsweetened, dry powder, red dutched	1 oz (28 g)	763	2690	Shively and Tarka, 1984

Sources:
Ahuja JKC, BP Perloff. Caffeine and theobromine intakes of children: results from CSFII 1994–96, 1998. *Fam Econ Nutr Rev* 13:47–51, 2001.
Caudle AG, LN Bell. Caffeine and theobromine contents of ready-to-eat chocolate cereals. *J Am Diet Assoc* 100:690–692, 2000.
Hershey website, http://www.hersheys.com/nutrition_consumer/theobromine.shtml (accessed 11 March 2002).
Shively CA, SM Tarka. Methylxanthine composition and consumption patterns of cocoa and chocolate products. *The Methylxanthine Beverages and Foods: Chemistry, Consumption, and Health Effects.* Alan R Liss, Inc, New York NY. 1984.
USDA Codes: *United States Department of Agriculture Database for Standard Reference, Release 15* (SR15), 2002. Available at http://www.nal.usda.gov/fnic/foodcomp/Data/SR15/sr15.html.

Amines—Tryptamine

	TRYPTAMINE (mg/100 g)	SOURCE		TRYPTAMINE (mg/100 g)	SOURCE
BEVERAGES			**GRAINS**		
wine, hungarian	0.01	Kovacs et al, 1999	barley	2.54	Badria, 2002
			rice	4.01	Badria, 2002
CHEESE					
cheese, blue/roquefort	20.0	Voight et al, 1974	**MEAT & FISH**		
cheese, camembert	2.0	Voight et al, 1974	sausage	36.0	Kovacs et al, 1999
cheese, cheddar	0.1	Souci et al, 2000	tuna in oil	0.10	Souci et al, 2000
cheese, cheddar, extra sharp	2.0	Voight et al, 1974			
cheese, cheddar, med	2.0	Voight et al, 1974	**SPICES**		
cheese, cheddar, mild	3.0	Voight et al, 1974	garlic	1.39	Badria, 2002
cheese, cheddar, sharp	4.0	Voight et al, 1974	ginger	3.71	Badria, 2002
cheese, colby	13.0	Voight et al, 1974			
cheese, edam	8.0	Voight et al, 1974	**VEGETABLES**		
cheese, gouda	7.0	Voight et al, 1974	cabbage	0.77	Badria, 2002
cheese, limburger	16.0	Voight et al, 1974	carrot	1.58	Badria, 2002
cheese, mozzarella	10.0	Voight et al, 1974	cauliflower	1.98	Badria, 2002
cheese, muenster	6.0	Voight et al, 1974	chives	0.00	Kovacs et al, 1999
cheese, port-salut	12.0–28.0	Voight et al, 1974	corn	6.17	Badria, 2002
cheese, sap-sago	15.0	Voight et al, 1974	cucumber	1.28	Badria, 2002
cheese, swiss	19.0	Voight et al, 1974	onion	0.92	Badria, 2002
			potato	0.00	Badria, 2002
FRUIT			radish	1.47	Badria, 2002
apple	0.53	Badria, 2002	tomato	0.40	Souci et al, 2000
banana	1.13	Badria, 2002	tomato	0.93	Badria, 2002
orange	0.10	Souci et al, 2000	turnip	2.12	Badria, 2002
pineapple	0.62	Badria, 2002			
pomegranate	0.47	Badria, 2002			
strawberries	0.47	Badria, 2002			

Sources:
Badria FA. Melatonin, serotonin, and tryptamine in some Egyptian food and medicinal plants. *J Medicinal Food* 5:153–157, 2002. faridbadria@yahoo.com
Kovacs A, L Simon-Sarkadi, K Ganzler. Determination of biogenic amines by capillary electrophoresis. *J Chromatography A* 836:305–313, 1999.
Souci SW, W Fachmann, H Kraut. *Food Composition and Nutrition Tables.* Medpharm GmbH Scientific Publishers, Stuttgart, Germany & CRC Press, Washington DC. 2000.
Voight MN, RR Eitenmiller, PE Koehler, MK Hamdy. Tyramine, histamine, and tryptamine content of cheese. *J Milk Food Technol* 37:377–381, 1974.

Amines—Tyramine[1]

BEVERAGES	TYRAMINE (mg/100 g)	SOURCE		TYRAMINE (mg/100 g)	SOURCE
beer, no alcohol	0.12	Souci et al, 2000	cheese, port-salut	12–18	Voight et al, 1974
beer, pilsener (german)	0.14	Souci et al, 2000	cheese, quark (fresh)	0	Souci et al, 2000
wine, hungarian	0.06	Kovacs et al, 1999	cheese, romano	14	Voight et al, 1974
			cheese, sap-sago	52	Voight et al, 1974
CANDY			cheese, stilton	46	Voight et al, 1974
dark choc	0.07	Jalon et al, 1983	cheese, swiss	41	Voight et al, 1974
milk choc	0.03	Jalon et al, 1983	cheese, tilsit	3	Souci et al, 2000
			CREAMS		
CHEESE			cream, sour	0.14	Souci et al, 2000
cheese, appenzeller, 12% fat	5	Souci et al, 2000	cream, whipping	0.17	Souci et al, 2000
cheese, appenzeller, 32% fat	6	Souci et al, 2000	**FRUITS**		
cheese, blue/rouquefort	36	Voight et al, 1974	avocado	2.3	Sullivan and Shulman, 1984
cheese, brick	52	McCabe, 1986	banana	0.7	Souci et al, 2000
cheese, brie	4–26	Voight et al, 1974	orange	1.0	Souci et al, 2000
cheese, camembert	12	Voight et al, 1974	raspberries	5.0	Souci et al, 2000
cheese, cheddar, extra sharp	27	Voight et al, 1974			
cheese, cheddar, med	24	Voight et al, 1974	**MEAT & FISH**		
cheese, cheddar, mild	9	Voight et al, 1974	liver, chicken	10	Souci et al, 2000
cheese, cheddar, processed	11	Voight et al, 1974	liver, ox	27	Souci et al, 2000
cheese, cheddar, sharp	21	Voight et al, 1974	sausage	12	Kovacs et al, 1999
cheese, cheddar, smoked	12	Voight et al, 1974	tuna in oil	0	Souci et al, 2000
cheese, colby	21	Voight et al, 1974	**MILK & YOGURT**		
cheese, cottage	0	Voight et al, 1974	buttermilk	0.22	Souci et al, 2000
cheese, cream	0	McCabe, 1986	yogurt, whole milk	0.13	Souci et al, 2000
cheese, edam	31	Voight et al, 1974			
cheese, emmental	4	Souci et al, 2000	**VEGETABLES**		
cheese, fontinella	10	Voight et al, 1974	chives	0.8	Kovacs et al, 1999
cheese, gjetost	12	Voight et al, 1974	sauerkraut	2.0	Souci et al, 2000
cheese, gouda	29	Voight et al, 1974	tomato	0.4	Souci et al, 2000
cheese, gruyere	52	McCabe, 1986			
cheese, jack	13	Voight et al, 1974	**MISCELLANEOUS**		
cheese, limburger	12	Voight et al, 1974	cocoa powder, sweetened	0.06	Jalon et al, 1983
cheese, mozzarella	16	Voight et al, 1974	soy sauce	0.18	Sullivan and Shulman, 1984
cheese, muenster	14	Voight et al, 1974			
cheese, parmesan	28	Voight et al, 1974			

[1] Tyramine-restricted diets usually exclude cheese, smoked and pickled fish, processed meats, liver, Chianti and vermouth wines, broad beans, meat extracts, yeast extracts, Brewer's yeast, sauerkraut, beer, and ale. Foods that may be used with caution (i.e., in small amounts) include avocado, raspberries, soy sauce, chocolate, red and white wines, port wines, distilled spirits, peanuts, and yogurt and cream from unpasteurized milk.

Sources:
Jalon M, C Santos-Buelga, JC Rivas-Gonzalo, A Marine-Font. Tyramine in cocoa and derivatives. *J Food Sci* 48:545–547, 1983.
Kovacs A, L Simon-Sarkadi, K Ganzler. Determination of biogenic amines by capillary electrophoresis. *J Chromatography A* 836:305–313, 1999.
McCabe BJ. Dietary tyramine and other pressor amines in MAOI regimens: A review. *J Am Diet Assoc* 86:1059–1064, 1986.
Souci SW, W Fachmann, H Kraut. *Food Composition and Nutrition Tables.* Medpharm GmbH Scientific Publishers, Stuttgart, Germany & CRC Press, Washington DC. 2000.
Sullivan EA, KI Shulman. Diet and monoamine oxidase inhibitors: A re-examination. *Can J Psychiatry* 29:707–711, 1984.
Voight MN, RR Eitenmiller, PE Koehler, MK Hamdy. Tyramine, histamine, and tryptamine content of cheese. *J Milk Food Technol* 37:377–381, 1974.

Amino Acids[1] (mg/serving)

	WT (g)	TRY (mg)	THR (mg)	ISO (mg)	LEU (mg)	LYS (mg)	MET (mg)	CYS (mg)	PHE (mg)	TYR (mg)	VAL (mg)	ARG (mg)	HIS (mg)	REF
1. BEVERAGES														
Coffee & Coffee Beverages														
cereal coffee (grain beverage)														
powder—*1 t*	2.3	2	4	5	9	5	2	3	6	4	6	6	3	14236
prep from powder w/water—*1 t*														
powder in 6 fl oz water	180	2	4	5	9	5	2	2	5	4	7	7	2	14237
prep from powder w/whl mlk—*1 t*														
powder in 6 fl oz milk	185	85	278	368	598	481	154	57	296	294	409	224	165	14421
coffee, brewed—*8 fl oz*	237	0	2	5	12	2	0	5	7	5	7	2	5	14209
decaffeinated—*8 fl oz*	237	0	2	5	12	2	0	5	7	5	7	2	5	14201
coffee, inst powder—*1 rd t*	1.5	0	2	3	7	1	0	3	4	2	4	1	2	14214
cappuccino flvr w/sugar—*2 rd t*	14	1	5	6	15	3	1	7	8	5	9	2	5	14228
decaffeinated—*1 rd t*	1.8	1	2	3	8	2	0	3	5	3	5	1	3	14218
french flvr w/sugar—*2 rd t*	12	1	6	7	19	4	1	8	11	7	11	2	7	14229
mocha flvr w/sugar—*2 rd t*	12	6	15	14	25	18	3	6	19	14	22	19	7	14224
w/chicory—*1 rd t*	1.8	0	2	2	6	1	0	3	3	2	4	1	2	14222
coffee, prep from inst powder														
1 rd t in 6 fl oz water	179	0	2	4	9	2	0	4	5	4	5	2	4	14215
decaffeinated—*1 rd t in 6 fl oz water*	179	0	2	4	9	2	0	4	5	4	5	2	4	14219
w/chicory—*1 rd t in 6 fl oz water*	179	0	2	2	5	2	0	2	4	2	4	0	2	14223
Fruit Drinks & Fruit-Flavored Beverages														
grape drink, cnd—*8 fl oz*	250	0	0	0	0	0	0	0	0	0	0	3	0	14277
orange breakfast drink, from frzn conc—*8 fl oz*	250	0	3	3	5	5	3	3	5	3	5	18	3	14427
orange gelatin drink, from powder—*1 pkt in 4 fl oz water*	136	0	122	94	201	261	48	0	144	26	169	521	54	14397
Liqueurs														
coffee w/cream, 34 proof—*1.5 fl oz*	47	19	60	80	129	105	33	12	64	64	88	48	36	14415
Malt Beverages														
beer—*12 fl oz*	356	11	18	18	21	25	4	11	21	53	32	32	18	14003
beer, light—*12 fl oz*	354	11	14	14	18	18	4	7	18	42	25	25	14	14006
Tea														
iced inst powder—*1 t*	0.7	1	0	0	0	0	0	0	0	0	0	0	0	14366
lemon—*2 rd T*	11	8	4	3	3	3	0	4	3	4	3	5	1	14368
lemon w/Na saccharin—*4 T (1/4 cup)*	14	4	2	2	2	2	0	2	2	2	2	3	1	14375
lemon w/sugar—*3 hp t*	23	1	1	1	1	1	0	1	0	1	1	1	0	14370
2. CANDY														
butterscotch—*1 oz (5 pieces)*	28	0	1	1	1	1	0	0	1	1	1	0	0	19070
butterscotch chips—*1 cup*	170	51	163	219	354	287	90	34	175	175	241	131	99	19085
caramels—*2.5 oz (~10 pieces)*	71	43	136	183	296	240	76	28	146	146	202	110	82	19074
choc-coated fondant—*1 large patty (1.5 oz)*	43	12	34	33	51	42	9	10	40	31	51	48	15	19083
choc-coated peanuts—*10 pieces*	40	56	197	224	402	241	84	50	275	222	272	400	107	19126
choc-coated raisins—*1/4 cup*	45	18	71	75	135	91	46	16	84	70	102	77	40	19127
choc flavor roll—*2.25 oz bar*	64	29	88	106	170	139	40	22	93	86	127	84	46	19076
dark choc (semi-sweet) *1.45 oz bar*	41	24	63	62	97	80	16	20	77	60	96	91	27	19081
dark choc (semi-sweet) chips *1 cup (6 oz bag)*	168	106	282	276	432	356	74	87	343	267	427	403	123	19080
fudge, homemade, choc *.6 oz piece*	17	5	15	18	29	24	7	4	18	16	23	17	8	19100
homemade, choc marshmallow w/nuts—*.78 oz piece*	22	9	29	32	55	37	12	8	34	26	41	62	16	19301
homemade, van—*.56 oz piece*	16	2	8	10	17	14	4	2	8	8	11	6	5	19103
marshmallow, miniature *10 pieces*	7	0	2	2	5	5	1	0	3	1	4	10	1	19116b
reg—*1 marshmallow*	7	0	2	2	5	5	1	0	3	1	4	10	1	19116c

	WT (g)	TRY (mg)	THR (mg)	ISO (mg)	LEU (mg)	LYS (mg)	MET (mg)	CYS (mg)	PHE (mg)	TYR (mg)	VAL (mg)	ARG (mg)	HIS (mg)	REF
milk choc—*1.55 oz bar*	44	37	130	162	284	181	65	18	167	139	200	88	47	19120a
milk choc chips—*1 cup*	168	139	497	620	1084	692	249	71	638	533	763	338	178	19120b
milk choc w/almonds—*1.55 oz bar*	44	51	154	190	334	196	70	35	207	161	231	206	70	19132
milk choc w/rice cereal—*1.55 oz bar*	44	33	116	144	254	156	60	22	151	122	180	99	45	19134
peanut bar—*1.6 oz bar*	45	67	234	240	444	245	83	87	354	278	287	818	173	19147
peanut brittle—*1 oz*	28	21	73	75	138	77	26	27	110	86	89	252	53	19148
peanut butter chips—*1 cup*	168	296	1057	1090	2001	1124	279	391	1583	1247	1297	3612	778	19086
sesame crunch—*20 pieces*	35	78	148	154	274	115	118	72	190	150	200	530	106	19154
yogurt chips—*3.5 oz*	100	78	263	352	577	472	150	54	287	285	402	209	158	19079

3. CEREALS & GRAINS, COOKED

	WT (g)	TRY (mg)	THR (mg)	ISO (mg)	LEU (mg)	LYS (mg)	MET (mg)	CYS (mg)	PHE (mg)	TYR (mg)	VAL (mg)	ARG (mg)	HIS (mg)	REF
barley, pearled, ckd—*1 cup*	157	60	121	130	242	132	68	79	199	102	174	177	80	20006
buckwheat groats, roasted, ckd—*1 cup*	168	82	217	213	356	289	74	97	223	104	291	420	133	20010
bulgur, ckd—*1 cup*	182	87	162	207	379	155	87	129	264	164	253	262	129	20013
corn grits, white, reg/quick, enr, ckd—*1 cup*	242	24	131	123	424	97	73	63	169	140	174	172	106	08091
unenr, ckd—*1 cup*	242	24	131	123	424	97	73	63	169	140	174	172	106	08162
corn grits, yellow, reg/quick, enr, ckd—*1 cup*	242	24	131	123	424	97	73	63	169	140	174	172	106	08164
unenr, ckd—*1 cup*	242	24	131	123	424	97	73	63	169	140	174	172	106	08166
couscous, ckd—*1 cup*	157	77	157	231	407	115	93	168	289	157	254	220	121	20029
Cream of Rice, ckd—*1 cup*	244	32	107	37	178	90	63	37	90	120	139	176	63	08101
Cream of Wheat, inst, prep—*1 cup*	241	60	140	193	335	113	82	99	239	140	214	190	101	08107
quick, ckd—*1 cup*	239	50	115	160	275	93	67	81	196	115	177	158	84	08105
reg, ckd—*1 cup*	251	53	120	168	289	98	70	85	206	120	183	166	88	08103
Cream of Wheat Mix & Eat, inst, prep—*1 pkt prep*	142	38	87	121	209	72	51	62	149	88	135	122	62	08109
apple, banana, maple, inst, prep—*1 pkt prep*	150	35	78	107	186	65	47	56	132	78	119	110	57	08111
farina, dry, Malt-O-Meal, enr, ckd—*1 cup*	233	42	89	130	228	65	51	96	163	89	142	123	68	08113
unenr, ckd—*1 cup*	233	42	89	130	228	65	51	96	163	89	142	123	68	08174
millet, ckd—*1 cup*	174	66	197	258	776	117	122	117	322	188	320	212	131	20032
oatmeal, quick/reg, ckd—*1 cup*	234	84	206	248	459	250	112	145	321	206	335	426	145	08121
dry—*1/3 cup (.95 oz)*	27	60	147	177	328	179	80	104	229	147	240	305	103	08120
rice, brown, long grain, ckd—*1 cup*	195	64	185	213	417	193	113	60	259	189	294	382	129	20037
med grain, ckd—*1 cup*	195	59	166	191	372	172	101	55	232	170	265	341	115	20041
rice, white, glutinous, enr, ckd—*1 cup*	174	40	125	151	291	127	82	71	188	117	214	292	82	20055
long grain, enr, ckd—*1 cup*	158	49	152	183	351	153	100	87	228	142	259	354	100	20045
long grain, enr, inst, ckd—*1 cup*	165	40	122	147	281	122	79	69	182	114	208	284	79	20049
long grain, enr, parboiled, ckd—*1 cup*	175	47	144	173	333	145	95	82	214	135	245	334	95	20047
med grain, enr, ckd—*1 cup*	186	52	158	192	366	160	104	91	236	149	270	368	104	20051
short grain, enr, ckd—*1 cup*	186	50	156	190	363	158	104	89	234	147	268	366	104	20053
rice, wild, ckd—*1 cup*	164	80	208	274	453	279	195	77	320	277	380	505	171	20089

4. CEREALS, READY-TO-EAT

	WT (g)	TRY (mg)	THR (mg)	ISO (mg)	LEU (mg)	LYS (mg)	MET (mg)	CYS (mg)	PHE (mg)	TYR (mg)	VAL (mg)	ARG (mg)	HIS (mg)	REF
granola, homemade—*1 cup (4.3 oz)*	122	181	548	659	1074	651	256	307	721	475	813	1338	373	08037
puffed rice—*1 cup (.49 oz)*	14	13	45	47	74	38	26	15	38	50	58	73	27	08156
puffed wheat—*1 cup (.42 oz)*	12	27	54	75	128	49	31	35	91	53	84	85	46	08157

5. CHEESE & CHEESE PRODUCTS

Cheese

	WT (g)	TRY (mg)	THR (mg)	ISO (mg)	LEU (mg)	LYS (mg)	MET (mg)	CYS (mg)	PHE (mg)	TYR (mg)	VAL (mg)	ARG (mg)	HIS (mg)	REF
american processed—*1 oz*	28	90	201	287	548	615	160	40	315	339	371	260	253	01042
blue—*1 oz*	28	87	220	315	537	519	164	30	304	363	436	199	212	01004
brick—*1 oz*	28	91	247	318	628	595	158	37	345	312	412	245	230	01005
brie—*1 oz*	28	90	210	284	540	518	166	32	324	336	375	206	200	01006
camembert—*1 oz*	28	86	201	271	515	494	158	31	309	321	358	196	191	01007
caraway—*1 oz*	28	91	251	438	675	587	185	35	371	340	471	267	248	01008
cheddar—*1 oz*	28	90	248	433	668	580	183	35	367	337	466	263	245	01009a
low fat—*1 oz*	28	80	223	389	601	522	165	31	330	302	419	237	220	01168
low Na—*1 oz*	28	80	223	389	601	522	165	31	330	302	419	237	220	01169
shredded—*1 cup*	113	362	1001	1747	2695	2341	737	141	1481	1358	1879	1063	988	01009b
cheshire—*1 oz*	28	84	233	406	627	545	171	33	345	316	437	247	230	01010
colby—*1 oz*	28	85	237	413	637	554	174	33	350	321	444	251	234	01011

	WT (g)	TRY (mg)	THR (mg)	ISO (mg)	LEU (mg)	LYS (mg)	MET (mg)	CYS (mg)	PHE (mg)	TYR (mg)	VAL (mg)	ARG (mg)	HIS (mg)	REF
cottage cheese, 1% fat—*1 cup*	226	312	1243	1645	2879	2265	843	260	1510	1492	1733	1277	931	01016
2% fat—*1 cup*	226	346	1376	1826	3193	2511	933	287	1675	1654	1923	1417	1033	01015
creamed, large curd—*1 cup*	210	292	1163	1541	2696	2121	790	244	1413	1399	1623	1197	872	01012a
creamed, small curd—*1 cup*	225	313	1247	1652	2889	2273	846	261	1514	1499	1739	1283	934	01012b
creamed w/fruit—*1 cup*	226	249	992	1315	2301	1810	673	208	1207	1193	1385	1022	744	01013
cream cheese—*1 T*	15	10	48	60	110	101	27	10	63	54	66	43	41	01017
edam—*1 oz*	28	99	261	366	720	745	202	71	402	408	507	270	290	01018
feta—*1 oz*	28	56	178	225	391	341	103	23	189	187	298	132	111	01019
fontina—*1 oz*	28	101	262	388	746	652	198	73	419	427	539	234	269	01020
gjetost—*1 oz*	28	38	110	145	278	228	89	16	151	151	214	92	82	01021
goat, hard—*1 oz*	28	90	319	354	737	613	228	39	340	333	588	253	233	01156
semi-soft—*1 oz*	28	64	225	250	521	434	161	27	241	236	416	179	165	01157
soft—*1 oz*	28	55	193	214	447	372	138	24	206	202	357	154	141	01159
gouda—*1 oz*	28	99	260	366	718	743	201	71	401	407	506	269	289	01022
gruyere—*1 oz*	28	118	305	451	869	759	230	85	488	497	628	272	313	01023
limburger—*1 oz*	28	81	207	341	586	469	173	31	312	335	403	195	162	01024
mexican, queso asadero—*1 oz*	28	75	206	343	594	433	166	29	333	297	399	213	194	01166
queso anejo—*1 oz*	28	60	205	295	565	407	151	24	313	333	375	196	190	01165
queso Chihuahua—*1 oz*	28	55	229	301	565	430	170	40	290	285	354	218	167	01167
monterey—*1 oz*	28	88	244	425	656	570	179	34	361	331	458	259	241	01025
mozzarella, part nonfat—*1 oz*	28	95	259	326	662	690	190	40	354	393	425	292	256	01028
part nonfat, low moisture—*1 oz*	28	108	293	369	750	781	214	46	402	445	481	330	289	01029
whole milk—*1 oz*	28	76	207	261	530	552	152	32	284	314	340	234	205	01026
whole milk, low moisture—*1 oz*	28	85	230	290	590	614	169	36	316	350	378	260	228	01027
muenster—*1 oz*	28	92	249	321	633	599	159	37	347	314	415	247	232	01030
neufchatel—*1 oz*	28	25	118	147	270	249	67	24	155	133	164	106	100	01031
parmesan, grated—*1 T*	5	28	77	110	201	192	56	14	112	116	143	77	80	01032
hard—*1 oz*	28	135	369	530	967	926	268	66	538	559	687	369	388	01033
pimento, processed—*1 oz*	28	90	201	286	548	615	160	40	315	339	371	259	253	01043
port du salut—*1 oz*	28	96	245	405	695	556	206	38	370	398	478	232	192	01034
provolone—*1 oz*	28	97	275	305	643	741	192	32	360	426	459	286	312	01035
ricotta, part nonfat—*1/2 cup*	124	157	649	739	1531	1678	352	124	697	739	868	792	575	01037
whole milk—*1/2 cup*	124	155	641	730	1514	1659	348	123	689	730	858	784	569	01036
romano—*1 oz*	28	120	328	472	860	823	239	59	479	497	611	328	345	01038
roquefort (sheep's milk)—*1 oz*	28	85	270	341	592	517	156	35	286	283	452	200	169	01039
swiss—*1 oz*	28	112	291	430	829	724	220	81	465	474	599	260	298	01040
processed—*1 oz*	28	101	225	320	612	687	179	45	352	379	415	290	282	01044
tilsit, whole milk—*1 oz*	28	99	252	416	713	571	211	39	380	408	491	238	197	01041

Cheese Products

	WT (g)	TRY (mg)	THR (mg)	ISO (mg)	LEU (mg)	LYS (mg)	MET (mg)	CYS (mg)	PHE (mg)	TYR (mg)	VAL (mg)	ARG (mg)	HIS (mg)	REF
cheese fondue—*1/2 cup*	108	193	503	744	1434	1253	380	139	806	820	1038	449	515	01163
cheese food,														
american cold pack—*1 oz*	28	80	179	255	487	546	143	35	280	301	330	230	224	01045
american—*1 oz*	28	80	178	254	485	545	142	35	279	300	329	230	224	01046
swiss—*1 oz*	28	89	199	284	543	609	159	39	312	336	368	257	250	01047
cheese sauce, homemade—*2 T*	30	37	107	173	271	232	73	17	145	136	188	105	93	01164
cheese spread, american—*1 oz*	28	67	176	233	498	422	151	29	261	249	382	153	143	01048
mozzarella cheese substitute—*1 oz*	28	42	111	160	259	222	79	14	147	160	190	109	80	01161

6. CREAMS & CREAM SUBSTITUTES

	WT (g)	TRY (mg)	THR (mg)	ISO (mg)	LEU (mg)	LYS (mg)	MET (mg)	CYS (mg)	PHE (mg)	TYR (mg)	VAL (mg)	ARG (mg)	HIS (mg)	REF
creamer, liquid/frzn w/hydg veg oils—*1 T (1/2 fl oz container)*	15	2	6	8	13	10	2	3	8	6	8	12	4	01067
w/lauric acid oils—*1 T (1/2 fl oz container)*	15	2	6	9	15	12	5	1	8	9	11	6	5	01068
creamer, powdered—*1 t*	2	1	4	6	9	8	3	0	5	5	7	4	3	01069
half & half (milk & cream)—*1 T* (1/2 fl oz container)	15	6	20	27	44	35	11	4	21	21	30	16	12	01049
light (coffee/table) cream—*1 T*	15	6	18	24	40	32	10	4	20	20	27	15	11	01050
sour cream, cultured—*1 T*	12	5	17	23	37	30	10	3	18	18	25	14	10	01056
imitation—*1 oz*	28	9	28	41	66	54	20	3	36	38	48	27	20	01074
red fat—*1 T*	15	6	20	27	43	35	11	4	21	21	30	16	12	01055
whipped topping, from mix, prep w/whole milk—*1 T*	4	2	6	9	14	11	4	1	7	7	10	5	4	01071
frzn—*1 T*	4	1	2	3	5	4	2	0	3	3	4	2	1	01073
pressurized—*1 T*	4	1	2	2	4	3	1	0	2	2	3	2	1	01072
whipping cream, heavy fluid—*1 T*	15	4	14	19	30	24	8	3	15	15	21	11	8	01053
light fluid—*1 T*	15	5	15	20	32	26	8	3	16	16	22	12	9	01052
pressurized—*1 T*	3	1	4	6	9	8	2	1	5	5	6	3	3	01054

	WT (g)	TRY (mg)	THR (mg)	ISO (mg)	LEU (mg)	LYS (mg)	MET (mg)	CYS (mg)	PHE (mg)	TYR (mg)	VAL (mg)	ARG (mg)	HIS (mg)	REF
7. DESSERTS														
Brownies & Bars														
brownie—*1 brownie (2 3/4″ × 7/8″)*	56	36	106	125	202	146	63	59	135	93	148	143	57	18151a
Little Debbie—*1 twin wrapped pkg (2 pieces)*	61	39	115	137	220	159	68	64	147	101	161	156	62	18151b
brownie mix, fudge, low fat, Sweet Rewards–*1/18 pkg (1.1 oz)*	32	25	73	85	143	91	42	40	95	69	103	139	44	18154
Cakes & Snack Cakes														
angel food—*1/12 cake (1 oz)*	28	21	69	87	135	102	51	42	94	61	99	85	37	18086
from mix—*1/12 cake of 10″ dia cake*	50	39	130	162	249	190	96	77	172	113	184	158	67	18088
boston cream pie (cake), frzn—*1/6 of 19.5 oz cake*	92	31	86	106	175	125	50	42	109	82	121	104	50	18090
cheesecake, from mix														
1/6 of 17 oz cake	80	51	178	225	371	298	109	57	206	178	251	201	106	18147
no-bake type—*1/8 of 9″ cake*	99	65	207	266	463	359	115	68	261	218	299	200	146	18148
cherry fudge w/choc icing—*1/8 of 20 oz cake*	71	21	74	77	128	105	33	28	70	53	88	79	33	18095
homemade—*1/12 of 9″ dia cake*	95	65	192	228	387	255	110	93	252	187	269	240	114	18101
w/choc icing—*1/8 of 18 oz cake*	64	36	106	123	198	151	54	47	130	99	151	133	56	18096
choc cupcake w/icing, low-fat—*1.5 oz cupcake*	43	26	71	89	143	100	45	41	98	66	104	89	40	18452
choc snack cake, crème-filled w/ icing—*1.8 oz snack cake*	50	24	56	68	117	73	29	33	79	53	82	71	34	18127
coffeecake, cinn w/crumb topping—*1/9 of 20 oz cake*	63	52	143	181	315	164	77	80	204	137	200	195	97	18104
cinn w/crumb topping, from mix—*1/8 of 8″ × 5 3/4″ cake*	56	37	106	137	236	128	67	62	152	104	154	125	69	18108
cream/neufchatel cheese—*1/6 of 16 oz cake*	76	58	198	248	432	305	109	84	268	200	274	227	141	18103
crème filled w/choc icing—*1/6 of 19 oz cake*	90	52	145	183	326	151	83	92	218	139	206	186	101	18105
w/fruit—*1/8 of 14 oz cake*	50	29	83	104	182	94	47	49	125	77	119	127	56	18106
fruitcake—*1 piece (1.5 oz)*	43	18	44	52	89	52	25	27	60	41	62	113	31	18110
gingerbread, from mix, Betty Crocker Classic—*1/8 cake*														
homemade—*1/9 of 8″ sq cake*	74	35	92	112	206	97	59	61	144	93	128	128	64	18116
pineapple upside down, from mix, Betty Crocker Classic—*1/6 cake*														
homemade—*1/9 of 8″ sq cake*	115	49	135	169	304	164	85	76	199	139	192	170	93	18119
pound, fat free—*1 oz*	28	20	60	77	122	89	42	34	81	55	87	72	34	18451
made w/butter—*1/10 of 10.6 oz cake*	30	22	63	78	129	92	40	35	82	59	89	78	37	18120
made w/veg shortening—*1/10 of 10.6 oz cake*	30	21	59	73	121	85	38	33	78	55	83	74	35	18121b
pound snack cake—*2.5 oz snack cake*	71	49	139	173	286	201	89	79	184	131	196	175	82	18121a
shortcake, biscuit-type, homemade *1 oz shortcake*	28	21	52	67	126	55	32	32	85	57	76	67	39	18126
sponge—*1/12 of 16 oz cake*	38	27	81	95	159	113	48	45	100	71	107	100	45	18133
homemade—*1/12 of 16 oz cake*	38	34	117	133	224	159	73	61	142	105	150	154	65	18134
sponge snack cake, crème-filled—*1.5 oz snack cake*	43	19	48	62	105	69	28	25	64	46	69	54	30	18128
white, homemade—*1/12 of 9″ cake*	74	50	141	180	310	178	95	82	208	141	204	174	92	18139
w/coconut icing—*1/12 of 9″ cake*	112	60	176	223	379	228	120	102	255	172	256	239	111	18102
yellow, homemade—*1/12 of 8″ cake*	68	45	130	160	282	167	82	70	181	130	182	162	84	18146
yellow w/choc icing—*1/8 of 18 oz cake*	64	32	93	111	182	134	52	47	118	88	132	118	52	18140
yellow w/van icing—*1/8 of 18 oz cake*	64	29	91	113	186	138	56	43	111	87	127	104	52	18141
Cookies														
animal—*2 oz box (23 pieces)*	57	56	110	150	268	138	66	85	185	112	173	150	80	18150b
anisette sponge—*1 piece*	13	17	61	67	112	88	35	29	66	53	75	79	32	18423b
arrowroot—*1 cookie*	5	5	10	13	24	12	6	7	16	10	15	13	7	18150a
breakfast treat—*1 piece*	24	32	112	124	207	163	64	54	123	98	139	146	60	18423c
butter—*1 oz (5 cookies)*	28	24	60	78	132	86	37	34	84	59	88	73	38	18155
choc chip, 12–17% fat—*1 cookie (2 1/4″ dia)*	10	8	17	23	42	22	10	11	28	18	27	22	12	18158
18–28% fat—*1 cookie (2 1/4″ dia)*	10	7	17	22	40	22	10	10	26	17	26	19	10	18159a
soft type—*1 cookie*	15	8	18	23	40	23	10	10	27	18	27	21	11	18160
choc chip, from refrig dough *1 cookie*	12	8	20	25	44	27	12	12	29	19	29	24	12	18164

	WT (g)	TRY (mg)	THR (mg)	ISO (mg)	LEU (mg)	LYS (mg)	MET (mg)	CYS (mg)	PHE (mg)	TYR (mg)	VAL (mg)	ARG (mg)	HIS (mg)	REF
choc chip, homemade w/butter—1														
cookie (2 1/4″ dia)	16	12	31	36	63	34	17	18	43	30	45	60	20	18378
w/marg—1 cookie (2 1/4″ dia)	16	12	31	36	63	34	17	18	43	30	45	60	20	18165
choc chunk pecan, Pepperidge Farm														
1 cookie	12	9	20	27	48	26	11	11	31	21	31	23	12	18159b
choc sandwich w/crème filling														
1 cookie	17	10	25	26	44	31	9	11	30	22	35	31	12	18167
w/crème filling, choc coated														
1 cookie	10	7	15	18	32	19	7	9	22	15	23	20	9	18166
w/extra crème filling—1 cookie	13	7	15	18	32	18	7	9	22	14	22	20	9	18168
choc wafers—5 wafers (1 oz)	28	27	62	73	125	79	29	36	86	57	90	80	36	18157
coconut macaroon, homemade														
1 cookie (2″ dia)	24	10	34	41	66	49	24	19	45	29	51	73	18	18169
fig bar—1 bar	16	7	18	21	36	22	8	12	23	20	25	19	11	18170b
2 oz pkg (two 3″ bars)	57	26	64	75	128	80	30	42	83	70	88	69	38	18170a
fortune—1 cookie	8	5	10	13	24	13	6	7	16	10	15	13	7	18171
fudge, cake type—1 cookie	21	12	31	37	64	47	15	14	43	28	47	56	18	18156
gingersnap—1 small cookie	7	6	11	15	27	14	7	8	18	11	17	15	8	18172a
1 large (3 1/2″–4″ dia)	32	26	50	68	122	62	30	38	84	51	79	68	36	18172b
graham crackers, choc coated														
1 cracker (2 1/2″ sq)	14	10	28	35	64	32	15	12	42	30	42	30	16	18174
graham crackers, plain/honey														
2 crackers (2 1/2″ sq)	14	13	27	34	67	23	17	21	48	29	40	41	22	18173
ice cream cone, cake/wafer—1 cone	4	4	9	12	22	6	6	7	16	9	14	11	7	18271b
sugar, rolled—1 cone	10	9	21	29	55	15	14	18	39	22	33	28	17	18272
waffle—large waffle cone	29	27	63	87	163	46	41	53	116	64	99	82	50	18271a
ladyfinger—1 ladyfinger	11	15	51	57	95	75	29	25	56	45	64	67	27	18423a
w/lemon jce & rind—1 ladyfinger	11	15	51	57	95	75	29	25	56	45	64	67	27	18175
marshmallow, choc coated—1 small														
cookie (1 3/4″ × 3/4″)	13	5	17	17	29	26	6	6	18	11	22	31	8	18176b
marshmallow pie—1 cookie														
(3″ dia × 3/4″)	39	14	50	50	88	77	19	17	55	32	66	94	23	18176a
molasses—1 large cookie (3 1/2″–4″ dia)	32	26	49	67	121	62	30	38	84	51	78	68	36	18177b
Little Debbie—1 cookie	20	16	31	42	75	39	19	24	53	32	49	42	23	18177a
oatmeal—1 cookie	18	18	31	40	78	43	22	30	53	36	54	66	26	18178
fat-free—2 cookies (1 oz)	28	22	49	61	111	60	30	37	78	49	77	84	37	18456
from refrig dough—1 cookie	12	12	24	30	55	34	16	20	37	26	39	45	17	18183
homemade—1 cookie (2 5/8″ dia)	15	13	35	42	77	41	21	23	53	35	52	59	24	18377
soft type—1 cookie	15	14	29	36	68	41	20	25	45	32	47	56	21	18179
oatmeal raisin, homemade—1 cookie														
(2 5/8″ dia)	15	12	33	38	70	38	20	21	48	32	48	57	23	18184
peanut butter—1 cookie	15	17	48	54	98	57	22	24	73	53	64	128	34	18185
soft type—1 cookie	15	9	26	30	54	30	10	13	40	29	35	69	19	18186
peanut butter, from refrig dough														
1 cookie	12	13	37	43	75	45	17	19	54	39	50	83	25	18188
peanut butter, homemade—1 cookie														
(3″ dia)	20	20	60	68	125	64	30	30	92	66	79	147	43	18189
peanut butter sandwich—1 cookie	14	15	42	48	86	49	18	23	62	45	56	100	29	18190
pecan shortbread—1 cookie (2″ dia)	14	11	20	27	47	25	13	16	33	21	31	39	15	18193
raisin, soft type—1 cookie	15	8	21	25	43	27	13	13	28	19	29	28	14	18191
shortbread—1 cookie (1 5/8″ sq)	8	7	16	20	36	20	10	11	24	15	23	21	10	18192
sugar—1 cookie	15	11	27	35	59	38	17	16	38	26	39	33	17	18204
sugar, from refrig dough—1 cookie	15	10	23	30	51	31	14	16	35	22	34	31	15	18206
sugar, homemade w/marg—1 cookie														
(3″ dia)	14	10	26	32	60	27	17	17	42	27	37	35	19	18208
sugar wafers w/crème filling—8 small														
wafers (1 oz)	28	17	32	44	79	40	20	25	54	33	51	44	23	18209
van sandwich w/crème filling														
1 round cookie (1 3/4″ dia)	10	6	12	17	31	16	8	10	21	13	20	17	9	18210a
1 oval cookie (3 1/8″ long)	15	10	19	26	46	23	11	15	32	19	29	26	14	18210b
van wafers, 12–17% fat—7 wafers (1 oz)	28	19	47	60	102	64	29	31	68	45	68	62	30	18212
18–21% fat—5 wafers (1 oz)	28	17	37	47	85	46	20	26	56	34	54	46	24	18213
Doughnuts														
cake—1 doughnut (3 1/4″ dia)	47	31	82	100	178	109	46	45	109	80	114	102	53	18248
choc coated/frosted—1 doughnut														
(3″ dia)	43	29	80	93	160	111	37	37	101	76	109	110	48	18249
choc, sugared/glazed—1 doughnut														
(3″ dia)	42	24	71	86	142	98	40	38	94	66	98	95	42	18251

	WT (g)	TRY (mg)	THR (mg)	ISO (mg)	LEU (mg)	LYS (mg)	MET (mg)	CYS (mg)	PHE (mg)	TYR (mg)	VAL (mg)	ARG (mg)	HIS (mg)	REF
sugared/glazed—*1 doughnut (3″ dia)*	45	31	85	104	182	115	47	45	110	82	117	107	54	18250
wheat, sugared/glazed—*1 doughnut (3″ dia)*	45	40	98	123	215	128	51	54	133	96	140	132	67	18252
cruller, glazed—*1 cruller (3″ dia)*	41	18	43	54	95	60	23	25	60	41	61	56	28	18253
yeast, glazed—*1 doughnut (3 3/4″ dia)*	60	46	128	160	281	139	68	78	186	120	177	163	86	18255
w/crème filling—*1 oval doughnut (3 1/2″ × 2 1/2″)*	85	66	182	230	407	205	100	108	264	173	256	230	125	18254
w/jelly filling—*1 oval doughnut (3 1/2″ × 2 1/2″)*	85	60	165	207	366	178	89	100	241	156	229	212	112	18256
Frozen Desserts														
ice cream, van, reg (10% fat)—*1/2 cup*	72	23	75	99	161	130	41	15	79	79	110	60	45	19095
van, rich (16% fat)—*1/2 cup*	107	44	148	195	319	265	81	29	159	152	219	144	89	19089
ice cream, low/red cal, light van (1/2 the fat)—*1/2 cup*	66	30	101	134	218	181	55	20	109	105	150	97	61	19088
ice cream, soft serve, french van *1/2 cup*	86	41	145	185	304	255	78	31	151	146	207	148	85	19090
low/red cal, light van (1/2 the fat) *1/2 cup*	88	52	173	229	373	309	96	34	186	180	257	163	103	19096
sherbet, orange—*1/2 cup*	74	10	33	44	71	57	18	7	36	35	49	31	20	19097
Gelatin Desserts														
dry mix, all flvrs, unsweetened *1 oz pkg*	28	0	413	324	687	969	170	0	486	85	583	1852	185	19177b
all flvrs w/aspartame—*.35 oz pkg*	10	0	107	84	177	250	44	0	126	22	151	478	48	19704
all flvrs w/sugar—*3 oz pkg*	85	0	128	100	213	301	53	0	150	26	181	575	58	19172
prep from mix, all flvrs w/aspartame *1/2 cup*	117	0	26	20	43	61	11	0	30	6	36	116	12	19176
all flvrs w/sugar—*1/2 cup*	135	0	31	24	53	74	14	0	36	7	45	142	14	19173
Pastries, Sweet Rolls, Cobblers, Strudels, & Turnovers														
cream puff shell, homemade—*1 shell*	66	73	242	284	474	328	157	131	308	221	320	312	138	18237
croissant—*1 med croissant*	57	56	162	208	355	188	100	98	237	154	234	193	107	18239
apple—*1 med croissant*	57	49	146	185	317	181	86	80	205	139	210	176	95	18240
cheese—*1 med croissant*	57	62	173	232	394	211	107	100	259	172	258	207	121	18241
danish pastry, cinn *1 pastry (4 1/4″ dia)*	65	55	159	202	346	192	90	90	226	151	224	203	104	18244
3.1 oz pastry	88	63	167	214	365	197	106	97	244	167	245	220	112	21016
cream/neufchatel cheese—*1 pastry (4 1/4″ dia)*	71	63	208	263	457	305	124	97	285	208	293	230	146	18245
fruit—*1 pastry (4 1/4″ dia)*	71	45	121	159	283	126	78	84	190	118	179	148	84	18246
lemon—*1 pastry (4 1/4″ dia)*	71	45	121	159	283	126	78	84	190	118	179	148	84	18433
nut—*1 pastry (4 1/4″ dia)*	65	57	155	198	344	176	90	90	219	153	226	280	108	18247
raspberry—*1 pastry (4 1/4″ dia)*	71	45	121	159	283	126	78	84	190	118	179	148	84	18435
eclair w/custard filling & choc glaze, homemade—*1 éclair (5″ long)*	100	80	271	324	532	392	169	127	328	253	365	325	152	18257
puff pastry, frzn—*1 pastry*	40	34	79	110	206	58	52	67	147	82	125	104	63	18211
strudel, apple—*2.5 oz piece*	71	28	84	104	182	109	48	41	107	82	116	96	54	18354
sweet roll, from refrig dough, cinn w/icing—*1 roll*	30	20	48	59	115	42	29	35	80	50	67	65	36	18358
sweet roll, rte, cheese (cream/neufchatel)—*1 roll*	66	51	173	211	366	256	94	74	226	169	234	207	121	18355
cinn raisin—*1 roll*	60	44	127	155	275	146	70	72	180	120	175	170	87	18356
toaster pastry, apple/blueberry/ cherry/strawberry—*1 pastry*	52	30	70	86	170	60	44	51	120	73	99	98	54	18362
toaster pastry, brown sugar cinn *1 pastry*	50	29	73	85	162	69	40	47	107	67	95	87	49	18361
Pies, Pie Crusts, & Pie Fillings														
apple—*1/8 of 9″ pie*	125	33	68	91	161	88	40	50	110	68	105	93	48	18301
homemade—*1/8 of 9″ pie*	155	45	102	129	254	87	65	78	183	112	150	149	82	18302
apple pie filling, cnd—*1/8 can*	74	1	2	2	4	4	1	1	1	1	3	1	1	19312
banana cream, from mix—*1/8 of 9″ pie*	92	42	126	155	262	186	61	46	148	121	167	144	77	18303
homemade—*1/8 of 9″ pie*	144	79	238	292	516	334	132	98	297	242	330	268	167	18304
blueberry—*1/8 of 9″ pie*	125	31	64	86	156	78	39	49	108	64	100	90	46	18305
homemade—*1/8 of 9″ pie*	147	43	107	132	263	84	67	75	187	106	159	166	82	18306
cherry—*1/8 of 9″ pie*	125	35	98	129	216	150	54	39	124	100	149	128	63	18308
homemade—*1/8 of 9″ pie*	180	56	130	158	306	121	77	90	223	135	187	180	103	18309
cherry pie filling, cnd—*1/8 can*	74	1	7	7	10	12	1	1	6	4	9	5	4	19314
choc cream/crème—*1/6 of 8″ pie*	113	38	99	107	186	128	40	47	128	81	141	155	54	18310

	WT (g)	TRY (mg)	THR (mg)	ISO (mg)	LEU (mg)	LYS (mg)	MET (mg)	CYS (mg)	PHE (mg)	TYR (mg)	VAL (mg)	ARG (mg)	HIS (mg)	REF
choc mousse, from mix—1/8 of 9" pie	95	46	132	157	264	191	59	48	158	126	181	159	78	18312
coconut cream—1/6 of 7" pie	64	19	50	66	111	76	28	19	63	52	77	69	33	18313
from mix—1/8 of 9" pie	94	35	103	129	222	149	55	39	122	102	145	112	63	18314
coconut custard—1/6 of 8" pie	104	82	225	297	501	348	126	88	285	233	343	295	146	18316
custard, egg—1/6 of 8" pie	105	75	236	295	478	365	145	104	282	225	331	264	133	18317
lemon meringue—1/6 of 8" pie	113	21	68	75	131	95	34	33	75	61	84	92	38	18320
homemade—1/8 of 9" pie	127	58	182	215	371	230	117	105	246	171	244	243	110	18321
mince, homemade—1/8 of 9" pie	165	45	116	122	246	96	87	84	185	116	158	201	106	18322
peach—1/6 of 8" pie	117	26	67	78	143	75	41	41	95	61	101	77	43	18323
pecan—1/6 of 8" pie	113	73	167	205	338	227	110	106	229	159	235	324	107	18324
homemade—1/8 of 9" pie	122	84	231	272	454	303	153	135	305	217	311	397	142	18325
pie crust, from mix—1/8 of 9" crust	20	15	36	49	92	26	23	30	66	36	56	46	28	18333
pie crust, frzn—1/8 of 9" crust	16	10	20	27	48	25	12	15	33	20	31	27	14	18335
pie crust, homemade—1/8 of 9" crust	23	18	40	51	102	33	26	31	75	45	59	60	33	18336
choc wafer—1/8 of 9" crust	28	21	49	58	99	64	24	27	67	46	72	62	28	18398
graham—1/8 of 9" crust	30	17	36	46	88	33	22	26	62	39	53	53	28	18330
van wafer—1/8 of 9" crust	22	11	28	35	60	39	17	17	39	27	40	35	17	18401
pumpkin—1/6 of 8" pie	109	56	173	223	365	284	100	59	201	178	250	175	102	18326
homemade—1/8 of 9" pie	155	91	279	350	583	428	163	104	339	290	392	308	169	18327
pumpkin pie mix, cnd—1 cup	270	35	84	92	135	159	32	8	95	122	103	157	46	11426
snack pie, fried, cherry—1 snack pie														
(5" × 3 3/4")	128	54	114	154	270	155	67	76	177	115	177	143	79	18444
fruit—1 snack pie (5" × 3 3/4")	128	54	114	154	270	155	67	76	177	115	177	143	79	18319
lemon—1 snack pie (5" × 3 3/4")	128	54	114	154	270	155	67	76	177	115	177	143	79	18445
van cream, homemade—1/8 of 9" pie	126	76	232	287	500	335	130	89	282	238	321	256	147	18328
Puddings & Custards														
banana, from inst mix w/2% milk														
1/2 cup	147	57	184	245	398	322	103	38	197	197	272	147	110	19121
w/whole milk—1/2 cup	147	56	182	243	392	319	101	37	194	194	269	146	109	19319
banana, from reg mix w/2% milk														
1/2 cup	140	57	183	245	398	322	102	38	196	196	272	148	109	19122
w/whole milk—1/2 cup	140	56	182	242	393	318	101	36	195	193	269	146	109	19321
banana, ready-to-eat—5 oz serving	142	44	143	193	315	251	80	30	155	153	214	116	87	19311
choc, from inst mix w/lowfat milk														
1/2 cup	147	65	204	268	434	351	109	44	222	218	306	178	121	19123
w/whole milk—1/2 cup	147	62	194	254	410	332	101	43	210	206	290	169	115	19185
choc, from reg mix w/2% milk														
1/2 cup	142	65	206	267	432	349	108	45	224	217	307	182	119	19190
w/whole milk—1/2 cup	142	62	195	254	409	331	101	43	212	206	291	170	114	19189
choc, ready-to-eat—5 oz serving	142	51	163	210	341	273	84	37	179	172	243	148	94	19183
coconut cream, from inst mix w/2%														
milk—1/2 cup	147	56	182	243	395	318	101	40	197	194	272	169	110	19191
w/whole milk—1/2 cup	147	56	181	241	391	313	100	40	196	191	269	168	109	19323
coconut cream, from reg mix w/2%														
milk—1/2 cup	140	57	183	244	396	318	101	39	197	193	273	172	111	19219
w/whole milk—1/2 cup	140	56	181	241	392	314	101	39	196	192	270	171	109	19325
custard, egg, from mix w/2% milk														
1/2 cup	133	76	263	318	520	432	133	64	247	246	347	221	141	19205
w/whole milk—1/2 cup	133	74	262	315	515	428	132	63	245	243	343	218	140	19170
flan/crème caramel from mix w/2%														
milk—1/2 cup	133	56	180	239	390	315	100	37	193	193	266	145	108	19231
w/whole milk—1/2 cup	133	55	178	237	384	311	98	36	190	190	262	142	106	19232
lemon, from inst mix w/2% milk														
1/2 cup	147	57	184	245	398	322	103	38	197	197	272	147	110	19204
w/whole milk—1/2 cup	147	53	172	232	375	304	96	35	185	185	256	138	104	19331
lemon, from reg mix w/sugar, egg														
yolk, & water—1/2 cup	146	12	54	51	89	79	25	18	44	45	55	72	26	19333
lemon, ready-to-eat—5 oz serving	142	0	3	4	13	3	1	3	6	4	6	6	3	19380
rennin dessert, choc, from mix w/														
2% milk—1/2 cup	136	61	196	257	418	340	106	41	212	208	291	169	116	19213
w/whole milk—1/2 cup	136	60	194	256	412	336	105	41	209	205	287	166	114	19221
rennin dessert, van, from mix w/														
2% milk—1/2 cup	133	57	184	246	399	323	102	39	197	197	273	148	110	19214
w/whole milk—1/2 cup	133	56	182	243	394	319	101	37	194	194	269	145	109	19223
rice, from reg mix w/2% milk														
1/2 cup	144	56	181	243	393	318	101	37	194	194	269	145	108	19208
w/whole milk—1/2 cup	144	56	180	240	389	315	101	36	192	192	265	144	108	19195
rice, ready-to-eat—5 oz serving	142	37	119	159	264	202	68	27	133	129	180	114	72	19193

	WT (g)	TRY (mg)	THR (mg)	ISO (mg)	LEU (mg)	LYS (mg)	MET (mg)	CYS (mg)	PHE (mg)	TYR (mg)	VAL (mg)	ARG (mg)	HIS (mg)	REF
tapioca, from reg mix w/2% milk														
1/2 cup	141	58	183	244	398	321	103	38	196	196	271	149	110	19209
w/whole milk—*1/2 cup*	141	56	182	243	392	317	102	37	193	193	268	147	109	19199
tapioca, ready-to-eat—*5 oz serving*	142	38	121	162	263	212	68	27	131	129	180	104	74	19218
van, from inst mix w/2% milk														
1/2 cup	140	57	185	246	405	323	104	39	199	199	274	150	112	19212
w/whole milk—*1/2 cup*	142	51	166	224	362	294	92	34	179	179	247	133	101	19203
van, from reg mix w/whole milk														
1/2 cup	140	55	175	235	385	307	98	36	189	188	260	141	106	19207
van, ready-to-eat—*4 oz serving*	113	34	112	149	244	195	62	23	120	119	165	90	68	19201
Sauces, Syrups, & Toppings For Desserts														
glaze, homemade—*1/12 recipe yield*	27	2	7	9	15	12	4	1	8	8	11	6	4	19375
icing/frosting, rts, choc—*2 T*	41	7	18	17	27	22	5	5	21	17	27	25	8	19226
coconut nut—*1/12 pkg*	38	12	18	22	36	21	12	13	27	19	28	78	15	19227
van—*2 T*	38	1	2	3	5	3	1	1	2	2	3	2	2	19230
icing/frosting, from mix, choc made														
w/butter—*1/12 pkg prep*	42	7	19	19	30	25	5	5	23	18	29	26	8	19241
choc made w/marg—*1/12 pkg prep*	42	7	19	19	30	25	5	5	23	18	29	26	8	19372
van made w/marg—*1/12 pkg prep*	43	1	5	6	16	5	3	3	6	5	7	6	4	19371
white fluffy made w/water—*1/12 pkg prep*	26	4	17	21	31	26	12	9	22	14	24	24	8	19247
syrup, choc—*2 T (1 fl oz)*	39	10	25	25	39	32	6	8	31	25	37	35	11	14181
topping, butterscotch/caramel—*2 T*	41	8	27	36	59	48	15	5	29	29	40	22	16	19364
topping, choc fudge—*2 T*	38	27	86	83	134	112	27	25	73	61	102	77	33	19348
topping, marshmallow cream—*1 oz*	28	0	10	8	18	21	4	1	11	3	14	40	5	19365
topping, nuts in syrup—*2 T*	41	24	57	72	127	50	36	44	80	56	92	269	46	19367
8. EGGS, EGG DISHES, & EGG SUBSTITUTES														
chicken egg, boiled, hard/soft														
1 large egg	50	77	302	343	538	452	196	146	334	257	384	378	149	01129
dried—*1 T*	5	39	118	151	212	163	78	57	136	100	173	154	58	01134
fried—*1 large egg*	46	76	299	340	532	448	194	144	331	254	380	373	148	01128
omelet, plain—*1 large egg*	61	77	303	344	539	453	196	146	335	257	384	378	149	01130
poached—*1 large egg*	50	76	299	340	532	447	194	145	331	254	379	373	148	01131
raw—*1 large egg*	50	76	300	341	534	449	195	145	332	255	381	375	148	01123
scrambled w/milk—*1 large egg*	61	83	322	371	582	488	207	149	356	279	414	393	161	01132
soufflé, spinach, homemade—*1 cup*	136	166	458	650	994	782	298	143	574	487	719	533	313	11658
chicken egg white, raw—*white of 1 large egg*	33	43	158	196	293	236	119	90	203	135	221	189	78	01124
chicken egg, yolk, raw—*yolk of 1 large egg*	17	33	151	144	250	226	71	51	122	127	159	203	74	01125
duck egg, whole—*1 egg*	70	182	515	419	768	666	403	200	588	429	620	536	224	01138
egg substitute, frzn—*1/4 cup*	60	98	290	396	583	428	232	137	387	274	475	346	154	01142
liquid—*1.5 fl oz*	47	90	260	352	509	370	200	137	360	233	417	368	139	01143
goose egg, whole—*1 egg*	144	406	1148	932	1711	1483	899	445	1310	956	1380	1192	498	01139
quail egg, whole—*1 egg*	9	19	58	73	103	79	38	28	66	49	85	75	28	01140
turkey egg, whole—*1 egg*	79	173	531	675	949	730	349	258	611	450	778	692	261	01141
9. ENTREES & MEALS														
Canned Entrees														
baked beans w/beef—*1 cup (9.4 oz)*	266	205	713	742	1357	1202	277	181	875	484	878	1067	484	16007
w/franks—*1 cup (9.1 oz)*	259	199	723	769	1383	1222	272	192	904	492	894	1106	492	16008
w/pork—*1 cup (8.9 oz)*	253	157	559	587	1063	913	202	144	721	374	696	825	372	16009
chili con carne w/beans—*1 cup (9 oz)*	256	177	614	640	1167	1047	243	156	748	420	753	922	420	16059
cowpeas w/pork—*1 cup (8.5 oz)*	240	82	250	269	504	446	94	72	384	214	314	456	204	16065
Frozen Entrees & Sandwiches														
turkey & gravy—*5 oz pkg*	142	95	372	435	666	787	241	87	331	329	443	582	260	05286
10. FAST FOODS & RESTAURANT FOODS														
Generic Fast Foods														
biscuit, egg—*1 biscuit*	136	143	479	566	938	662	307	248	598	439	636	601	271	21002
egg & bacon—*1 biscuit*	150	216	680	822	1313	1025	422	294	810	594	953	936	431	21003
egg & cheese—*1 biscuit*	146	218	588	781	1244	927	383	266	803	585	937	775	410	21104
egg & ham—*1 biscuit*	192	273	876	1000	1657	1386	540	376	996	735	1083	1190	597	21004
egg & sausage—*1 biscuit*	180	247	787	923	1505	1195	493	335	900	679	1053	1067	497	21005
egg & steak—*1 biscuit*	148	229	747	872	1428	1183	460	296	829	641	980	1014	502	21006

	WT (g)	TRY (mg)	THR (mg)	ISO (mg)	LEU (mg)	LYS (mg)	MET (mg)	CYS (mg)	PHE (mg)	TYR (mg)	VAL (mg)	ARG (mg)	HIS (mg)	REF
grape jce, cnd/bottled—*8 fl oz*	253	0	40	18	30	25	3	0	30	8	25	119	18	09135
from frzn conc, sweetened—*8 fl oz*	250	0	13	5	10	8	0	0	10	3	8	40	5	09137
orange jce, cnd—*8 fl oz*	249	5	17	15	27	20	7	10	17	7	22	100	7	09207
orange jce, raw—*8 fl oz*	248	5	20	20	32	22	7	12	22	10	27	117	7	09206
tangerine jce, cnd, sweetened—*8 fl oz*	249	2	15	12	25	17	5	10	15	7	20	85	5	09223
from frzn conc, sweetened—*8 fl oz*	241	2	12	12	19	14	5	7	12	5	17	70	5	09225
raw—*8 fl oz*	247	2	15	12	25	17	5	10	15	7	20	84	5	09221
tomato jce—*8 fl oz*	243	12	41	36	51	53	10	10	39	24	36	36	29	11540

15. FRUITS

	WT (g)	TRY (mg)	THR (mg)	ISO (mg)	LEU (mg)	LYS (mg)	MET (mg)	CYS (mg)	PHE (mg)	TYR (mg)	VAL (mg)	ARG (mg)	HIS (mg)	REF
apple, boiled w/o skin, cnd														
1 cup slices	171	3	15	17	27	27	5	7	12	9	21	14	7	09005
dried, sulfured—*1 ring*	6	1	2	2	3	3	1	1	2	1	3	2	1	09011
micro ckd w/o skin—*1 cup slices*	170	5	17	19	29	31	5	7	14	9	22	15	7	09006
raw w/skin—*1 med (2 3/4″ dia)*	138	3	10	11	17	17	3	4	7	6	12	8	4	09003
raw w/o skin—*1 med (2 3/4″ dia)*	128	1	6	8	12	12	3	3	5	4	9	6	3	09004
sliced, sweetened—*1 cup slices*	204	4	12	14	22	22	4	4	10	6	16	12	6	09007
applesauce, sweetened, cnd—*1 cup*	255	5	18	18	28	28	5	5	13	8	20	15	8	09020
unsweetened, cnd—*1 cup*	244	5	15	15	24	24	5	5	12	7	20	12	7	09019
apricots, cnd, heavy syrup—														
1 cup whole	258	23	46	41	77	93	8	5	54	31	49	52	21	09028
cnd, jce pack—*1 cup halves*	244	27	56	46	90	107	7	5	63	37	56	59	24	09024
cnd, light syrup—*1 cup halves*	253	23	48	40	78	94	8	5	56	30	48	53	23	09026
cnd, water pack—*1 cup whole*	227	27	57	48	91	109	7	5	64	36	57	61	25	09023
dried, sulfured—*1 cup halves*	130	21	95	82	137	108	20	25	81	51	101	86	61	09032
raw—*1 cup halves (4.4 apricots)*	155	23	73	64	119	150	9	5	81	45	73	70	42	09021
sweetened, frzn—*1 cup*	242	19	58	48	94	119	7	5	63	36	58	53	31	09035
avocado, calif, raw—*1 med*	173	38	121	130	227	173	67	38	125	90	178	109	52	09038
avocado, florida, raw—*1 med*	304	52	161	173	301	228	88	52	164	119	237	143	70	09039
banana chips—*1 oz*	28	8	21	21	44	30	7	11	24	15	29	29	50	19400
raw—*1 med (7–7 7/8″ long)*	118	14	40	39	84	57	13	20	45	28	55	55	96	09040
blueberries, cnd, heavy syrup—*1 cup*	256	8	46	51	100	31	26	18	59	20	69	84	26	09052
raw—*1 cup*	145	4	26	30	58	17	16	10	35	12	41	49	15	09050
sweetened, frzn—*1 cup*	230	5	25	28	53	16	14	9	32	12	39	46	14	09055
carambola (star fruit), raw														
1 med (3 5/8″ dia)	91	4	21	21	36	36	10	0	17	21	24	10	4	09060
crabapples, raw—*1 cup slices*	110	4	15	18	28	28	4	6	12	9	21	14	7	09077
custard apple (bullock's heart),														
raw—*3.5 oz*	100	7	0	0	0	37	4	0	0	0	0	0	0	09086
dates, dried—*1 date*	8	4	4	4	7	5	2	4	4	2	5	5	2	09087
dried fruit bar—*.81 oz bar*	23	5	12	14	28	11	7	8	20	12	17	16	9	19011
elderberries, raw—*1 cup*	145	19	39	39	87	38	20	22	58	74	48	68	22	09088
figs, cnd, heavy syrup—*1 fig w/liquid*	28	1	3	3	5	4	1	2	3	4	4	3	1	09092
dried—*1 fig*	19	5	19	18	25	23	5	10	14	25	22	13	8	09094
raw—*1 med (2 1/4″ dia)*	50	3	12	12	17	15	3	6	9	16	14	9	6	09089
fruit roll—*1 large roll (.74 oz)*	21	2	6	5	11	10	1	2	6	6	7	8	4	19014
grapefruit, cnd, jce pack—*1 cup*	249	5	0	0	0	45	5	0	0	0	0	0	0	09120
cnd, light syrup—*1 cup*	254	5	0	0	0	36	5	0	0	0	0	0	0	09121
pink & red, raw—*1/2 med (3 3/4″ dia)*	123	2	0	0	0	17	2	0	0	0	0	0	0	09112
white, raw—*1/2 med (3 3/4″ dia)*	118	2	0	0	0	21	2	0	0	0	0	0	0	09116
grapes, american (slip skin), raw														
1 cup	92	3	16	5	12	13	19	9	12	10	16	42	21	09131
grapes, european, red/green, seedless,														
raw—*1 cup*	160	5	29	8	22	24	35	18	22	19	29	78	38	09132
grapes, thompson seedless, cnd,														
heavy syrup—*1 cup*	256	5	33	10	26	28	41	20	26	20	33	90	46	09134
guava, raw—*1 med*	90	6	28	27	50	21	5	0	2	9	25	19	6	09139
guava, strawberry, raw—*1 cup*	244	12	54	51	95	39	10	0	2	17	49	37	12	09140
lichis/litchees, dried—*1 fruit*	2	1	0	0	0	4	1	0	0	0	0	0	0	09165
raw—*1 med*	10	1	0	0	0	4	1	0	0	0	0	0	0	09164
lime, raw—*1 med (2″ dia)*	67	2	0	0	0	9	1	0	0	0	0	0	0	09159
longans, dried—*1 oz*	28	0	36	27	57	48	14	0	31	26	61	37	13	09173
raw—*1 med*	3	0	1	1	2	1	0	0	1	1	2	1	0	09172
loquats, raw—*1 med*	16	1	2	2	4	4	1	1	2	2	3	2	1	09174
mammy apple (mamey), raw—*1 med*	846	42	0	0	0	313	51	0	0	0	0	0	0	09175

	WT (g)	TRY (mg)	THR (mg)	ISO (mg)	LEU (mg)	LYS (mg)	MET (mg)	CYS (mg)	PHE (mg)	TYR (mg)	VAL (mg)	ARG (mg)	HIS (mg)	REF
mandarin oranges, cnd, jce pack														
1 cup	249	15	25	42	37	77	32	15	50	25	65	107	27	09219
cnd, light syrup—1 cup	252	10	18	30	28	58	25	13	38	20	48	78	20	09220
mango, raw—1 med	207	17	39	37	64	85	10	0	35	21	54	39	25	09176
orange, all varieties, raw														
1 med (2 5/8″ dia)	131	12	20	33	30	62	26	13	41	21	52	85	24	09200
CA navel, raw—1 med (2 7/8″ dia)	140	14	24	39	36	73	31	15	48	24	62	101	27	09202
CA valencia, raw—1 med (2 5/8″ dia)	121	12	21	34	31	64	27	13	41	22	53	88	24	09201
FL, raw—1 med (2 5/8″ dia)	141	10	16	27	24	49	21	10	32	17	42	69	18	09203
papaya, raw—1 med														
(5 1/8″ long × 3″ dia)	304	24	33	24	49	76	6	0	27	15	30	30	15	09226
peach, cnd, heavy syrup—1 cup	262	3	47	34	68	39	29	10	37	31	66	31	21	09241
cnd, jce pack—1 cup	250	5	63	45	90	50	38	13	50	40	85	40	30	09238
cnd, light syrup—1 cup	251	3	45	33	63	35	28	10	35	30	63	28	20	09240
cnd, water pack—1 cup	244	2	41	32	61	34	27	10	34	27	59	27	20	09237
dried, sulfured—1cup halves	160	16	226	166	326	186	139	46	182	150	315	147	107	09246
raw—1 med (2 1/2″ dia)	98	2	26	20	39	23	17	6	22	18	37	18	13	09236
spiced, cnd, heavy syrup—1 cup	242	2	39	29	56	31	24	7	31	27	56	24	19	09243
sweetened, frzn—1 cup	250	5	60	45	88	50	38	13	50	40	85	40	30	09250
pear, asian, raw—1 pear														
(2 1/2″ long, 2 1/2″ dia)	122	6	16	17	31	21	7	6	16	5	22	11	6	09340
pear, cnd, heavy syrup—1 cup	266	0	13	16	27	19	5	5	13	5	19	8	5	09257
cnd, jce pack—1 cup	248	0	22	25	42	30	10	7	22	7	30	15	10	09254
cnd, light syrup—1 cup	251	0	13	15	25	18	5	5	13	5	18	8	5	09256
cnd, water pack—1 cup	244	0	12	12	22	17	5	5	12	5	17	7	5	09253
dried, sulfured—10 halves	175	0	86	95	165	116	39	32	86	28	116	56	35	09259
raw—1 med	166	0	17	18	33	23	8	7	17	5	23	12	7	09252
persimmon, japanese, dried—1 med	34	8	24	20	34	27	4	10	21	13	24	20	9	09264
raw—1 med (2 1/2″ dia)	168	17	50	42	71	55	8	22	44	27	50	42	20	09263
persimmon, raw—1 med	25	4	10	9	15	11	2	5	9	6	11	9	4	09265
pineapple, cnd, heavy syrup														
1 cup pieces	254	13	23	23	33	41	23	3	23	20	28	30	20	09270
cnd, jce pack—1 cup pieces	249	12	25	25	40	47	27	2	25	25	32	35	22	09268
raw—1 cup pieces	155	8	19	20	29	39	17	3	19	19	25	28	14	09266
plum, cnd, heavy syrup														
1 plum w/liquid	46	0	4	3	5	4	1	1	4	1	4	3	3	09284
cnd, jce pack—1 plum w/liquid	46	0	5	5	6	5	2	1	5	2	6	4	4	09282
raw—1 med (2 1/8″ dia)	66	0	11	11	14	11	4	3	11	4	13	9	9	09279
sapodilla, raw—1 med	170	9	20	26	41	66	5	0	22	24	27	29	27	09313
sapote, raw—1 med	225	52	131	104	189	216	36	0	119	124	173	124	95	09314
soursop, raw—1 cup	225	25	0	0	0	135	16	0	0	0	0	0	0	09315
strawberries, raw—1 cup whole	144	10	27	20	45	36	1	7	26	30	26	37	17	09316
sweetened, frzn—1 cup	255	15	41	31	66	54	3	10	38	43	38	56	26	09319
unsweetened, frzn—1 cup	221	11	29	22	49	38	2	9	27	31	27	40	18	09318
sugar apple, raw—1 med (2 7/8 dia)	155	16	0	0	0	85	11	0	0	0	0	0	0	09321
tamarind, raw—1 cup	120	22	0	0	0	167	17	0	0	0	0	0	0	09322
tangerine, raw—1 med (2 3/8″ dia)	84	5	8	14	13	27	11	6	18	9	23	37	10	09218
watermelon, raw—1 cup pieces	152	11	41	29	27	94	9	3	23	18	24	90	9	09326
16. GRAIN-BASED SNACK FOODS														
cheese puffs/twists—1 oz	28	26	109	102	219	128	42	39	84	72	113	79	51	19008
corn cake—.32 oz cake	9	7	27	28	75	24	16	11	37	29	40	46	20	19419
corn chips—1 oz	28	13	69	66	225	52	38	33	90	74	93	91	56	19003
barbecue—1 oz	28	18	78	78	209	80	38	33	93	76	100	104	56	19004
corn-based cones—1 oz	28	11	61	59	200	46	34	29	80	66	83	81	50	19005
nacho—1 oz	28	16	71	74	212	73	39	29	89	77	98	85	56	19006
corn-based snack, onion flavor—1 oz	28	17	81	80	254	67	43	38	106	87	108	113	65	19007
crisped rice bar w/choc chips														
1 oz bar	28	21	46	56	109	56	29	34	73	55	80	109	32	19010
granola bar, almond, hard														
.85 oz bar	24	34	53	69	140	75	32	55	94	68	97	143	43	19016
granola bar, choc chip, hard														
.85 oz bar	24	32	51	66	132	75	32	53	88	66	95	124	39	19017
soft—1 oz bar	28	25	65	76	140	78	34	42	98	67	105	132	43	19404
soft w/choc coating—1 oz bar	28	20	63	76	133	81	32	18	81	68	97	67	29	19024
granola bar, choc, graham, & marshmallow, soft—1 oz bar	28	24	58	69	128	69	33	39	89	59	94	127	41	19405

	WT (g)	TRY (mg)	THR (mg)	ISO (mg)	LEU (mg)	LYS (mg)	MET (mg)	CYS (mg)	PHE (mg)	TYR (mg)	VAL (mg)	ARG (mg)	HIS (mg)	REF
granola bar, nut & raisin, soft														
1 oz bar	28	28	73	84	152	84	38	45	108	73	111	178	52	19406
granola bar, peanut butter &														
choc chip, soft—*1 oz bar*	28	28	92	97	179	100	37	38	139	109	121	293	66	19027
granola bar, peanut butter, hard														
.85 oz bar	24	31	74	84	163	90	35	48	120	92	109	234	57	19420
soft—*1 oz bar*	28	31	98	105	195	105	41	43	149	117	130	310	72	19021
soft w/choc coating—*1.3 oz bar*	37	46	143	169	297	192	64	45	189	159	205	255	84	19026
granola bar, peanut, hard—*1 oz bar*	28	48	93	113	224	124	51	78	158	118	154	272	73	19019
granola bar, plain, hard—*1 oz bar*	28	50	74	99	203	112	50	85	134	99	142	189	60	19015
soft—*1 oz bar*	28	28	67	82	150	82	36	46	107	70	111	137	46	19020
granola bar, raisin, soft—*1 oz bar*	28	30	72	85	158	84	39	48	110	71	115	164	51	19022
oriental mix, rice-based—*1 oz*	28	54	179	189	347	191	69	71	272	208	223	589	132	19031
popcorn cake—*.35 oz cake*	10	9	36	37	105	31	21	16	49	39	52	58	28	19036
popcorn, caramel—*1 oz*	28	13	42	44	80	79	20	11	43	31	50	66	31	19039
w/peanuts—*1 oz (~2/3 cup)*	28	15	65	64	179	56	31	29	90	73	85	137	51	19038
popcorn, cheese—*1 oz (~2.6 cups)*	28	26	117	113	287	124	53	45	113	98	137	109	71	19040
popcorn, plain, air-popped														
1 oz (~3.5 cups)	28	24	127	121	412	95	71	61	165	137	170	167	103	19034
oil-popped—*1 oz (~2.6 cups)*	28	18	95	90	309	71	53	46	124	102	127	125	77	19035
potato chips—*1 oz*	28	30	71	79	117	119	31	25	87	73	110	90	43	19411
from dried potatoes—*1 oz*	28	13	72	73	109	104	19	21	76	65	97	80	37	19410
potato chips, barbeque—*1 oz*	28	30	90	96	142	140	36	30	94	77	119	106	49	19042
potato chips, cheese—*1 oz*	28	20	102	110	166	155	32	29	109	92	140	112	54	19421
from dried potatoes—*1 oz*	28	18	81	92	143	133	31	23	90	79	115	90	48	19412
potato chips, light—*1 oz*	28	31	73	81	120	122	32	26	89	74	113	92	44	19422
potato chips, reduced fat,														
from dried potatoes—*1 oz*	28	12	69	69	103	99	18	20	72	62	92	76	35	19045
potato chips, sour cream &														
onion—*1 oz*	28	33	119	113	183	161	39	36	76	67	118	72	42	19043
from dried potatoes—*1 oz*	28	20	80	88	136	122	29	21	81	71	106	86	41	19046
pretzels—*10 twists (2.1 oz)*	60	65	155	207	382	133	98	118	272	160	235	209	121	19047
choc coated—*.39 oz pretzel*	11	11	28	32	58	28	14	16	39	26	37	34	18	19048
whole wheat—*2 oz*	57	98	185	235	428	175	101	144	298	187	287	321	147	19050
rice cakes (brown rice)—*.32 oz cake*	9	9	27	31	61	28	17	9	38	28	43	56	19	19051
buckwheat—*.32 oz cake*	9	11	31	32	57	37	14	12	36	21	44	61	20	19052
corn—*.32 oz cake*	9	8	28	30	70	26	16	10	38	29	42	51	20	19413
multigrain—*.32 oz cake*	9	10	27	32	61	28	16	10	38	27	43	56	19	19414
rye—*.32 oz cake*	9	9	26	30	56	28	15	11	36	23	41	50	18	19416
sesame seed—*.32 oz cake*	9	9	25	29	56	26	16	8	35	26	40	54	17	19053
sesame sticks, wheat-based—*1 oz*	28	40	92	118	215	101	54	56	153	99	131	182	73	19418
taro chips—*10 chips (.8 oz)*	23	8	24	19	40	24	7	11	29	20	29	37	12	19524
tortilla chips—*1 oz*	28	14	74	71	243	56	41	36	97	81	100	99	60	19056
nacho—*1 oz*	28	18	79	83	247	81	46	35	105	89	113	108	67	19057
nacho, red fat—*1 oz*	28	19	88	93	277	88	51	39	117	99	125	120	73	19424
ranch—*1 oz*	28	16	80	78	244	69	43	37	100	83	106	108	62	19058
taco flavor—*1 oz*	28	19	82	88	249	84	46	36	108	89	115	112	67	19063

17. GRAIN PRODUCTS

Bagels

	WT (g)	TRY (mg)	THR (mg)	ISO (mg)	LEU (mg)	LYS (mg)	MET (mg)	CYS (mg)	PHE (mg)	TYR (mg)	VAL (mg)	ARG (mg)	HIS (mg)	REF
cinn raisin—*3.7 oz bagel (3 1/2" dia)*	105	120	299	385	705	250	188	221	498	286	445	397	228	18005a
4.6 oz bagel (4 1/2" dia)	131	149	373	481	879	312	234	275	621	356	555	495	284	18005b
egg—*3.7 oz bagel (4" dia)*	105	131	321	432	785	274	200	243	549	323	484	414	243	18003
oat bran—*3.7 oz bagel (4" dia)*	105	145	316	426	795	302	197	266	552	337	506	483	245	18007
plain/onion/poppy seed/														
sesame seed—*3.7 oz bagel (4" dia)*	105	130	316	424	772	264	197	236	545	316	479	403	238	18001

Biscuits

	WT (g)	TRY (mg)	THR (mg)	ISO (mg)	LEU (mg)	LYS (mg)	MET (mg)	CYS (mg)	PHE (mg)	TYR (mg)	VAL (mg)	ARG (mg)	HIS (mg)	REF
mixed grain, refrig dough														
1.6 oz biscuit (2 1/2" dia)	44	33	74	94	187	63	47	58	134	80	110	113	61	18017
plain/buttermilk—*1.8 oz med biscuit*	51	39	90	115	222	85	57	63	157	98	134	125	71	18009
from mix—*1 oz biscuit*	28	25	66	83	154	75	39	37	99	69	95	79	47	18011
from refrig dough, 12–28% fat														
1 oz biscuit (2 1/2" dia)	27	21	48	64	125	36	31	39	93	56	71	70	39	18015
from refrig dough, 2–12% fat														
.7 oz biscuit (2 1/4" dia)	21	20	44	56	113	36	29	35	82	49	66	66	36	18013
homemade—*2.1 oz biscuit (2 1/2" dia)*	60	52	127	164	308	136	79	79	208	139	188	165	97	18016

	WT (g)	TRY (mg)	THR (mg)	ISO (mg)	LEU (mg)	LYS (mg)	MET (mg)	CYS (mg)	PHE (mg)	TYR (mg)	VAL (mg)	ARG (mg)	HIS (mg)	REF
Breads, Quick														
banana, homemade w/marg														
2.1 oz slice	60	32	90	109	196	108	56	54	131	89	125	119	68	18019
boston brown, cnd—*1.6 oz slice*	45	33	73	84	158	70	41	52	105	67	105	115	58	18021
cornbread, from mix—*2.1 oz piece*	60	47	160	186	388	190	98	82	215	161	223	200	109	18023
homemade w/2% milk—*2.3 oz piece*	65	44	168	189	441	192	99	76	215	174	232	203	118	18024
hush puppy, homemade—*.8 oz*														
hush puppy	22	18	61	71	156	68	37	32	84	64	85	77	43	18270
Breads, Yeast														
bread crumbs, dry, grated—*1 cup*	108	161	403	552	945	367	216	234	673	322	677	556	292	18079
seasoned—*1 cup*	120	205	509	703	1208	535	280	282	844	432	868	724	382	18376
cracked wheat—*.9 oz slice*	25	28	65	85	152	61	37	48	105	63	97	87	48	18025
croutons—*1 cup*	30	42	101	137	250	83	63	78	176	101	154	129	77	18242
seasoned—*1 cup*	40	50	130	171	310	138	78	87	210	132	195	161	98	18243
egg—*1.4 oz slice (5″ × 3″ × 1/2″)*	40	45	122	158	277	124	76	83	190	117	177	154	84	18027
french toast, frzn—*2.1 oz piece*	59	55	166	200	345	218	99	84	216	158	224	198	101	18268
homemade w/2% milk—*2.3 oz piece*	65	61	198	244	404	268	122	101	253	183	272	237	116	18269
french/vienna/sourdough														
2.3 oz med slice (4″ × 2 1/2″ × 1 3/4″)	64	65	159	216	394	131	101	123	279	160	244	205	122	18029
irish soda, homemade—*1 oz slice*	28	20	56	66	122	61	39	34	84	56	79	81	45	18032
italian—*1.1 oz slice*														
(4 1/2″ × 3 1/4″ × 3/4″)	30	31	74	100	184	59	47	58	130	74	113	95	56	18033
mixed grain/whole grain/7-grain														
.92 oz slice	26	34	80	101	182	82	43	56	126	74	120	115	58	18035
oat bran—*1.1 oz slice*	30	39	90	120	220	89	54	70	155	97	138	134	68	18037
red cal—*.81 oz slice*	23	24	59	74	130	67	32	31	38	89	84	88	42	18049
oatmeal—*.95 oz slice*	27	31	67	88	164	73	41	56	112	71	106	107	50	18039
red cal—*.81 oz slice*	23	22	54	72	129	60	32	37	88	58	83	75	39	18051
protein/gluten—*.67 oz slice*	19	28	70	89	163	71	38	47	113	69	98	104	51	18043
pumpernickel—*.92 oz slice*	26	25	69	87	157	64	40	49	110	62	103	93	51	18044
raisin—*.92 oz slice*	26	22	58	75	134	52	33	40	94	53	86	94	43	18047
rice bran—*.95 oz slice*	27	29	72	94	168	70	42	51	119	73	109	102	53	18059
rye—*1.1 oz slice*	32	31	82	102	185	75	44	55	132	68	121	104	58	18060
red cal—*.81 oz slice*	23	25	65	82	147	74	36	41	105	66	95	109	48	18053
wheat bran—*1.3 oz slice*	36	40	92	120	217	85	55	69	151	91	139	129	71	18066
wheat germ—*1 oz slice*	28	32	85	108	192	91	48	53	128	82	123	111	60	18068
wheat/wheat berry—*.88 oz slice*	25	30	69	89	161	65	39	50	112	67	102	95	51	18064
red cal—*.81 oz slice*	23	25	63	82	147	60	37	43	102	63	92	78	45	18055
white—*.88 oz slice*	25	24	61	81	145	56	36	44	101	59	90	79	45	18069
homemade w/2% milk														
1.5 oz thick slice	42	41	102	131	242	113	62	62	163	110	149	133	76	18073
homemade w/nonfat milk														
1.6 oz thick slice	44	42	98	125	239	94	62	68	169	107	144	136	77	18071
red cal—*.81 oz slice*	23	24	66	88	151	82	37	35	96	68	96	78	46	18057
whole wheat—*1 oz slice*	28	39	83	105	188	85	43	60	130	81	124	126	63	18075
homemade—*1.6 oz thick slice*	46	56	114	144	264	112	63	86	185	116	173	176	89	18077
Breadsticks														
plain—*35 oz breadstick (7 5/8″ × 5/8″)*	10	14	34	46	84	28	21	26	59	34	52	43	26	18080
Crackers														
cheese crackers—*.5 oz*	14	18	41	59	104	59	27	24	69	48	67	54	34	18214
w/peanut butter filling														
2 crackers w/filling	7	10	28	33	60	31	14	15	44	31	38	67	21	18215
crispbread, rye—*1 crispbread*	10	9	29	32	56	30	12	16	40	17	40	37	18	18216
melba toast														
1 toast (3 3/4″ × 1 3/4″ × 1/8″)	5	7	17	23	42	14	11	13	30	17	26	22	13	18220
rye/pumpernickel—*1 toast*	5	7	18	22	40	17	10	12	28	14	26	23	13	18221
wheat—*1 toast*	5	9	19	24	44	17	11	14	31	19	29	27	14	18222
milk crackers—*1 cracker*	11	11	24	32	60	27	15	17	41	26	37	34	18	18223
round crackers—*.5 oz (~5 crackers)*	14	13	28	36	71	23	18	22	52	31	41	42	23	18229
w/cheese filling—*2 crackers w/filling*	7	8	19	24	45	21	12	13	31	20	28	25	14	18230
w/peanut butter filling														
2 crackers w/filling	7	5	10	14	26	10	7	8	19	11	16	15	8	18231
rusk—*1 rusk*	10	17	51	61	101	68	29	27	67	47	68	65	31	18224

	WT (g)	TRY (mg)	THR (mg)	ISO (mg)	LEU (mg)	LYS (mg)	MET (mg)	CYS (mg)	PHE (mg)	TYR (mg)	VAL (mg)	ARG (mg)	HIS (mg)	REF
rye crackers w/cheese filling														
2 crackers w/filling	7	8	20	25	45	23	11	13	31	19	29	28	15	18225
saltines—5 crackers (.49 oz)	14	17	36	47	88	36	22	28	63	38	54	51	28	18228
fat-free, low-Na—6 saltines (1.1 oz)	30	41	86	113	215	87	54	67	154	93	132	124	67	18457
soda crackers—5 crackers (.5 oz)	14	17	36	47	88	36	22	28	63	38	54	51	28	18425
wheat crackers—.5 oz (~7 thin squares)	14	17	34	44	81	33	19	27	58	35	53	53	27	18232
w/cheese filling—2 crackers w/filling	7	9	21	27	49	24	12	14	33	21	31	29	15	18233
w/peanut butter filling														
2 crackers w/filling	7	11	29	34	64	31	14	17	47	32	40	72	22	18234
whole wheat crackers														
.5 oz (~3.5 crackers)	14	19	36	46	84	34	19	29	59	36	56	58	29	18235
English Muffins														
mixed grain/granola—2.3 oz muffin	66	78	184	238	428	192	104	131	296	185	279	291	133	18260
plain—2 oz muffin	57	52	138	180	315	137	79	91	216	133	201	168	97	18258
raisin cinn/apple cinn—2 oz muffin	57	48	135	168	296	133	82	88	205	126	192	175	99	18262
wheat—2 oz muffin	57	64	152	194	340	154	83	103	235	145	223	205	110	18264
whole wheat—2.3 oz muffin	66	85	187	232	403	204	93	125	275	180	273	275	135	18266
Ethnic Grain Products														
cellophane/long rice noodles, chinese,														
dehydrated—1 cup	140	3	7	10	18	15	3	1	14	7	11	15	7	16082
chow mein noodles—1 cup	45	48	99	145	257	72	59	106	182	99	160	138	76	20113
eggroll wrapper—7″ sq wrapper	32	36	86	118	219	65	56	71	156	87	133	111	67	18368a
indian (navajo) fry bread—5″ dia	90	78	173	220	437	140	113	135	320	192	256	257	141	18031
matzo—1 matzo (1 oz)	28	32	75	104	194	54	49	63	138	77	118	97	60	18217
egg—1 matzo (1 oz)	28	42	108	132	248	109	69	75	175	111	152	152	78	18218
egg & onion—1 matzo (1 oz)	28	34	83	104	197	79	53	60	140	88	119	122	62	18400
whole wheat—1 matzo (1 oz)	28	58	107	137	249	104	57	86	174	108	167	177	87	18219
phyllo dough—1 sheet	19	17	37	47	93	30	24	29	68	41	54	55	30	18338
pita bread, white														
1 large pita (6 1/2″ dia)	60	63	154	209	380	131	96	118	268	154	236	197	117	18041
whole wheat—1 large pita (6 1/2″ dia)	64	95	180	235	429	170	98	146	301	187	282	291	145	18042
rice noodles, ckd—1 cup	176	19	58	69	132	58	37	33	86	53	99	134	37	20134
soba (japanese noodles), ckd—1 cup	114	82	202	222	376	244	82	107	247	120	284	361	136	20115
somen (japanese noodles), ckd—1 cup	176	90	187	273	482	136	109	199	341	185	301	260	143	20117
tortilla, corn—1 med (6″ dia)	24	10	52	50	171	39	29	25	68	57	71	69	42	18363
taco shell—1 med (5″ dia)	13	7	35	34	115	26	20	17	46	38	48	47	29	18360
tortilla, flour—1 med (7–8″ dia)	46	49	113	141	276	98	71	83	200	122	164	164	90	18364
wonton wrapper—3 1/2″ sq wrapper	8	9	21	30	55	16	14	18	39	22	33	28	17	18368b
Muffins														
blueberry, homemade w/2% milk														
2 oz muffin	57	46	125	157	284	150	78	71	185	129	179	158	86	18278
corn—4.9 oz muffin	139	95	314	357	717	388	163	153	413	303	409	443	210	18279
from mix—1 oz muffin	28	23	76	89	185	90	46	39	103	77	106	95	52	18280
homemade w/2% milk—2 oz muffin														
(2 3/4″ × 2″)	57	44	149	173	373	173	89	72	200	154	207	182	104	18282
oat bran—4.9 oz muffin	139	146	292	364	703	385	171	253	481	325	506	656	217	18283
plain, homemade w/2% milk														
2 oz muffin	57	49	132	165	298	159	82	74	195	137	188	165	91	18273
toaster muffin, blueberry, toasted														
1 muffin	31	20	60	68	116	86	22	25	75	53	72	100	38	18386
wheat bran raisin, toasted—1 muffin	34	25	67	74	134	85	32	36	89	61	85	111	46	18388
Pancakes														
buttermilk, homemade—4″ dia pancake	38	31	97	120	207	133	59	46	129	94	138	112	62	18390
plain, from complete mix—4″ pancake	38	22	71	82	169	80	40	36	97	69	98	84	48	18290
from incomplete mix—4″ pancake	38	36	113	143	250	154	68	54	146	111	163	130	71	18292
frzn—4″ pancake	41	25	75	92	171	91	46	41	109	74	107	94	51	18288
homemade—4″ pancake	38	30	90	113	195	122	56	44	121	91	127	106	58	18293
whole wheat, from incomplete mix														
4″ pancake	44	52	139	174	297	193	80	73	184	137	206	190	90	18300
Pasta														
corn pasta, ckd—1 cup	140	27	139	132	451	104	77	66	181	150	186	183	112	20092
egg pasta, homemade, ckd—2 oz	57	38	95	127	218	94	58	82	149	89	141	127	63	20097
refrig, ckd—2 oz	57	37	76	112	198	55	45	82	141	76	124	107	59	20094
homemade pasta w/o egg, ckd—2 oz	57	32	66	96	170	48	39	70	121	66	106	92	51	20098
macaroni, enr, ckd—1 cup	140	85	176	258	456	127	104	188	323	175	284	246	136	20100

	WT (g)	TRY (mg)	THR (mg)	ISO (mg)	LEU (mg)	LYS (mg)	MET (mg)	CYS (mg)	PHE (mg)	TYR (mg)	VAL (mg)	ARG (mg)	HIS (mg)	REF
macaroni, protein-fortified, ckd														
1 cup	115	118	262	367	641	220	148	253	450	253	407	362	194	20102
macaroni, veg, ckd—*1 cup*	134	78	163	235	414	125	94	168	292	161	260	225	123	20106
macaroni, whole wheat, ckd—*1 cup*	140	97	200	290	510	165	120	155	371	195	323	263	175	20108
noodles, egg, & spinach, ckd—*1 cup*	160	107	251	349	582	242	149	213	402	238	390	344	170	20112
noodles, egg, enr, ckd—*1 cup*	160	101	230	323	542	208	139	208	378	219	360	314	158	20110
spaghetti, enr, ckd—*1 cup*	140	85	176	258	456	127	104	188	323	175	284	246	136	20121
spaghetti, protein-fortified, ckd														
1 cup	140	144	319	447	780	267	181	308	547	308	496	441	237	20123
spaghetti, spinach, ckd—*1 cup*	140	81	172	248	437	132	99	176	308	171	274	238	130	20127
spaghetti, whole wheat, ckd—*1 cup*	140	97	200	290	510	165	120	155	371	195	323	263	175	20125
spinach pasta, refrig, ckd—*2 oz*	57	38	90	125	208	86	53	76	144	85	140	123	61	20096
Rolls														
dinner—*1 oz roll (2" sq, 2" high)*	28	28	70	95	169	66	43	50	116	70	106	87	52	18342a
egg—*1.2 oz roll (2 1/2" dia)*	35	39	109	138	240	115	65	70	163	102	155	134	73	18344
homemade w/2% milk														
1.2 oz roll (2 1/2")	35	37	99	124	224	116	61	57	149	103	141	127	69	18396
frankfurter/hot dog														
regular size (1.5 oz)	43	43	106	143	258	95	65	78	179	106	161	133	80	18350b
foot long roll (3 oz)	86	85	216	291	519	203	131	152	358	216	326	267	158	18342b
french—*1.3 oz roll*	38	38	97	128	231	88	58	69	160	95	144	122	71	18349
hamburger—*1.5 oz roll*	43	43	106	143	258	95	65	78	179	106	161	133	80	18350c
mixed grain—1.5 oz roll	43	52	121	154	282	109	69	92	197	114	183	174	91	18351
hard/kaiser—*2 oz roll (3 1/2" dia)*	57	67	162	218	395	138	100	123	279	162	246	205	122	18353
oat bran—*1.2 oz roll*	33	40	90	121	222	89	54	71	157	98	140	135	68	18345
rye—*1.3 oz roll*	36	43	113	143	256	102	62	77	184	94	168	145	81	18346
wheat—*1 oz roll*	28	33	67	90	166	57	41	56	117	69	106	99	54	18347
whole wheat—*1.3 oz roll (2 1/2" dia)*	36	48	94	120	216	96	50	71	148	94	145	147	73	18348
Stuffings & Coatings														
bread stuffing, from mix—*1/2 cup*	100	41	97	120	228	96	57	64	161	101	137	136	74	18082
cornbread stuffing from mix—*1/2 cup*	100	31	95	108	256	85	55	57	145	101	132	128	73	18085
Waffles														
plain, frzn, toasted—*1 waffle (4" sq)*	33	25	64	78	147	64	41	44	102	65	89	88	46	18403
plain, homemade														
1 round waffle (7" dia)	75	74	217	272	473	288	134	109	296	220	307	259	140	18367
18. INFANT, JUNIOR, & TODDLER FOODS														
Baked Products														
teething biscuit—*.4 oz biscuit*	11	21	62	93	161	39	30	17	58	73	97	66	44	03216
Cereals														
barley, dry—*1 T*	2.4	3	9	10	19	9	5	6	16	10	14	14	6	03181
prep w/whole milk—1 oz	28	17	52	66	113	78	29	19	67	56	79	54	32	03681
cereal & egg yolks, junior—*6 oz jar*	170	46	139	170	292	216	87	48	156	143	207	177	77	03198
strained—4 oz jar	113	31	93	113	194	144	58	32	104	95	138	118	51	03197
high protein, dry—*1 T*	2.4	13	35	42	71	57	15	17	45	34	45	67	24	03182
prep w/whole milk—1 oz	28	36	102	127	211	170	47	40	124	102	137	156	67	03682
mixed, dry—*1 T*	2.5	4	10	12	26	10	6	9	17	12	16	18	7	03185
prep w/whole milk—1 oz	28	18	53	68	123	80	30	23	68	60	81	60	34	03685
mixed w/apples & bananas, junior														
6 oz jar	170	22	58	73	146	60	41	44	105	73	99	111	46	03188
mixed w/applesce & bananas,														
strained—4 oz jar	113	15	40	50	99	41	28	31	71	50	67	76	32	03187
mixed w/bananas, dry—*1 T*	2.5	3	9	11	24	12	5	5	14	11	15	13	8	03186
prep w/whole milk—1 oz	28	17	52	66	119	82	29	16	62	57	79	51	35	03686
oatmeal, dry—*1 T*	2	4	9	11	21	11	5	10	11	11	15	21	5	03189
prep w/whole milk—1 oz	28	19	56	72	125	87	31	29	62	62	87	75	32	03689
oatmeal w/applesauce & ban,														
junior—6 oz jar	170	29	78	83	170	92	53	51	114	88	117	160	58	03192
strained—4 oz jar	113	19	52	55	112	60	34	33	75	59	77	105	38	03191
oatmeal w/bananas, dry—*1 T*	2	3	8	10	20	11	5	5	12	10	14	14	7	03190
prep w/whole milk—1 oz	28	18	54	69	120	87	32	19	66	60	83	60	37	03690
rice, dry—*1 T*	2	2	6	6	11	6	4	3	7	6	9	13	4	03194
prep w/whole milk—1 oz	28	15	49	60	101	75	29	15	54	52	72	57	30	03694
rice w/applesce & ban,														
Gerber 2nd Fds—4 oz jar	113	14	45	54	131	77	23	16	66	63	77	45	36	03195b
Heinz Str-2—4.25 oz jar	120	14	48	58	139	82	24	17	70	67	82	48	38	03195a

	WT (g)	TRY (mg)	THR (mg)	ISO (mg)	LEU (mg)	LYS (mg)	MET (mg)	CYS (mg)	PHE (mg)	TYR (mg)	VAL (mg)	ARG (mg)	HIS (mg)	REF
rice w/bananas, dry—*1 T*	2	3	9	9	16	9	5	4	8	7	11	12	5	03212
prep w/whole milk—*1 oz*	28	18	55	68	113	82	30	15	55	54	76	55	33	03712
Desserts														
orange pudding, strained—*4 oz jar*	113	0	51	64	128	102	17	0	47	51	79	96	35	03226
van custard, Bch-Nut Stg 2/														
Gerber 2nd Fds/Heinz Str-2—*4 oz jar*	113	0	67	85	67	129	52	0	82	67	99	70	46	03245
Dinners														
beef & rice, toddler—*6 oz jar*	170	78	340	417	666	639	209	92	335	274	468	575	218	03049
beef lasagna, toddler—*6 oz jar*	170	80	277	350	551	505	139	82	309	224	393	430	173	03043
beef noodle, Bch-Nut Stg 3/														
Gerber 3rd Fds/Heinz Jr-3—*6 oz jar*	170	46	168	235	354	315	90	49	199	158	224	267	126	03287
beef stew, Beech-Nut Table Time														
6 oz jar	170	90	357	418	660	670	241	90	342	270	462	600	218	03052
chicken stew, toddler—*6 oz jar*	170	97	376	437	689	697	190	88	362	292	496	563	218	03072
mac & cheese, junior—*6 oz jar*	170	54	133	221	398	252	153	54	224	209	250	173	105	03090
mac, tom, beef, Beech-Nut Stage 3/														
Gerber 3rd Fds—*6 oz jar*	170	48	153	201	337	253	66	58	190	139	216	226	109	03045
spagh, tom, beef, toddler—*6 oz jar*	170	111	335	456	702	532	177	112	410	313	486	483	240	03051
veg & bacon, Gerber 3rd Fds/														
Heinz Jr-3—*6 oz jar*	170	29	104	139	218	185	63	44	131	97	165	206	68	03060
veg & lamb, Beech-Nut Stage 2/														
Heinz Str-2—*4 oz jar*	113	26	82	102	166	165	34	19	89	70	110	150	52	03066
junior—*6 oz jar*	170	41	131	162	264	262	53	31	141	112	173	240	82	03067
veg & turkey, toddler—*6 oz jar*	170	102	316	423	661	563	150	88	340	296	473	502	194	03086
Meats														
beef, Bch-Nut Stg 1/Gerber 2nd Fds/														
Heinz Str-2—*2.5 oz jar*	71	97	424	439	775	804	297	113	374	322	488	659	328	03002
Gerber 3rd Fds/Heinz Jr-3—*2.5 oz jar*	71	104	451	468	825	856	316	120	398	342	520	701	349	03003
chicken, Beech-Nut Stage 1/Gerber														
2nd Fds/Heinz Str-2—*2.5 oz jar*	71	111	437	458	751	812	261	128	396	312	489	679	295	03012
Gerber 3rd Fds/Heinz Jr-3—*2.5 oz jar*	71	119	469	492	807	872	280	137	425	334	525	730	316	03013
chicken sticks, Gerber Graduates														
2.5 oz jar	71	83	406	518	811	824	229	90	478	353	542	712	328	03014
ham, Gerber 2nd Foods—*2.5 oz jar*	71	98	428	469	789	838	252	121	376	331	508	667	335	03008
junior—*2.5 oz jar*	71	106	466	510	858	911	274	132	409	359	553	726	365	03009
lamb, Bch-Nut Ste 1/Gerber 2nd Fds/														
Heinz Str-2—*2.5 oz jar*	71	99	456	470	790	887	313	138	393	350	507	655	253	03010
junior—*2.5 oz jar*	71	107	492	507	852	958	338	148	425	378	547	707	273	03011
meat sticks, Gerber Graduates														
2.5 oz jar	71	65	413	474	740	734	219	52	431	370	491	618	327	03021
pork, strained—*2.5 oz jar*	71	97	438	483	800	822	283	109	405	362	498	673	317	03007
turkey, Bch-Nut Ste 1/Gerber 2nd Fds/														
Heinz Str-2—*2.5 oz jar*	71	106	449	509	808	841	315	124	419	357	516	645	260	03015
Gerber 3rd Foods—*2.5 oz jar*	71	114	484	548	870	905	339	133	450	384	555	695	279	03016
turkey sticks, Gerber Graduates														
2.5 oz jar	71	72	388	447	760	835	216	87	433	343	462	627	261	03017
veal, Bch-Nut Stg 1/Gerber 2nd Fds/														
Heinz Str-2—*2.5 oz jar*	71	111	400	433	741	770	212	124	371	307	466	637	295	03005
junior—*2.5 oz jar*	71	125	453	489	838	871	239	141	420	347	528	720	333	03006
Vegetables														
beets, Gerber 2nd Fds/Heinz Str-2														
4 oz jar	113	14	36	43	52	38	11	8	20	40	51	34	24	03098
carrots, Beech-Nut Baby's First/														
Gerber 1st Fds—*2.5 oz jar*	71	24	97	107	167	166	28	18	102	84	120	276	53	03121a
Beech-Nut Baby's First/Gerber														
1st Fds/Heinz Beg-1—*2.5 oz jar*	71	8	16	17	23	14	6	4	17	13	21	36	9	03099a
Beech-Nut Stage 1/Gerber 2nd Fds/														
Heinz Str-2—*4 oz jar*	113	12	25	27	36	23	10	7	27	21	34	57	14	03099b
Beech-Nut Stage 3/Gerber 3rd Fds/														
Heinz Jr-3—*6 oz jar*	170	19	39	41	56	36	15	10	43	34	53	88	22	03100
Earth's Best—*4.5 oz jar*	128	14	28	31	41	26	12	8	31	24	38	64	15	03099c
corn, crmd, Bch-Nut Stg 2/														
Grbr 2nd Fds/Heinz Str-2—*4 oz jar*	113	17	59	73	158	92	45	20	55	76	87	68	52	03119
Heinz Jr-3—*6 oz jar*	170	26	88	111	240	139	68	31	83	116	133	102	78	03120
garden veg, strained—*4 oz jar*	113	31	82	97	162	131	49	23	99	107	112	221	51	03283

	WT (g)	TRY (mg)	THR (mg)	ISO (mg)	LEU (mg)	LYS (mg)	MET (mg)	CYS (mg)	PHE (mg)	TYR (mg)	VAL (mg)	ARG (mg)	HIS (mg)	REF
green beans, Bch-Nut Stg 1/Grbr														
2nd Fds/Heinz Str-2—*4 oz jar*	113	17	62	66	96	73	21	12	60	52	80	81	41	03091b
Beech-Nut Stage 3—*6 oz jar*	170	24	87	92	133	100	31	17	83	71	111	112	56	03092
Gerber 1st Fds/Heinz Beg-1														
2.5 oz jar	71	11	39	41	60	46	13	8	38	33	50	51	26	03091a
green beans, crmd, Gerber 3rd														
Fds/Heinz Jr-3—*6 oz jar*	170	26	65	82	133	73	37	19	77	73	99	82	39	03097
mixed veg, junior—*6 oz jar*	170	26	77	95	155	80	36	48	94	88	117	158	53	03282
strained—*4 oz jar*	113	15	43	53	87	45	20	27	53	50	66	89	29	03286
peas, Beech-Nut Stage														
1/Gerber 2nd Fds—*4 oz jar*	113	38	154	171	266	264	45	29	162	134	191	440	85	03121b
spinach, creamed, Gerber 2nd Foods														
4 oz jar	113	41	114	127	250	167	62	35	108	130	171	172	72	03127
squash, Bch-Nut Baby's 1st/Grbr														
1st Fds/Heinz Beg-1—*2.5 oz jar*	71	9	18	23	33	22	7	5	21	20	26	33	11	03104c
Beech-Nut Stage 1/Gerber 2nd Fds/														
Heinz Str-2—*4 oz jar*	113	14	28	37	53	35	11	8	33	32	41	52	18	03104b
Earth's Best—*4.5 oz jar*	128	15	32	42	60	40	13	9	37	36	46	59	20	03104a
Gerber 3rd Foods—*6 oz jar*	170	20	43	56	82	53	19	12	49	48	61	80	27	03105
sweet pot, Bch-Nut Baby's 1st/Grbr														
1st Fds/Heinz Beg-1—*2.5 oz jar*	71	16	38	36	55	31	17	11	44	29	52	38	18	03108c
Beech-Nut Stage 1/Gerber 2nd Fds/														
Heinz Str-2—*4 oz jar*	113	25	61	58	88	50	27	17	70	46	82	61	29	03108b
Beech-Nut Stage 3/Gerber 3rd Fds/														
Heinz Jr-3—*6 oz jar*	170	36	90	85	129	73	39	26	104	68	121	90	43	03109
Earth's Best—*4.5 oz jar*	128	28	69	65	100	56	31	19	79	52	93	69	33	03108a
19. MEATS														
Beef														
Bottom sirloin tri-tip roast, 0″ trim,														
lean & fat, roasted—*3 oz*	85	256	1096	1223	2094	2224	672	255	1028	869	1281	1597	765	23544
lean, roasted—*3 oz*	85	259	1109	1239	2122	2253	681	258	1041	880	1298	1618	774	13985
bottom sirloin tri-tip steak, 0″ trim,														
lean & fat, broiled—*3 oz*	85	275	1176	1313	2249	2388	722	274	1103	932	1376	1715	822	23545
lean, broiled—*3 oz*	85	281	1205	1346	2305	2447	740	280	1131	955	1410	1757	841	13987
breakfast strips, ckd—*3 slices (1.2 oz)*	34	97	402	460	782	816	247	136	383	347	468	657	339	13345
brisket, cured, corned beef, ckd—*3 oz*	85	141	583	667	1134	1183	358	197	556	504	679	954	491	13347
brisket, flat half, 0″ trim, lean & fat,														
braised—*3 oz*	85	290	1131	1165	2048	2156	663	290	1012	870	1260	1637	887	13369
lean, braised—*3 oz*	85	300	1170	1204	2117	2229	686	300	1046	900	1303	1693	917	13370
brisket, flat half, 1/4″ trim, lean & fat,														
braised—*3 oz*	85	239	930	957	1683	1771	545	239	831	716	1035	1346	729	13026
lean, braised—*3 oz*	85	300	1170	1204	2117	2229	686	300	1046	900	1303	1693	917	13028
brisket, point half, 0″ trim, lean & fat,														
braised—*3 oz*	85	224	874	899	1580	1663	512	224	780	672	972	1264	685	13371
lean, braised—*3 oz*	85	267	1041	1072	1884	1984	610	267	931	801	1159	1507	816	13372
brisket, point half, 1/4″ trim, lean &														
fat, braised—*3 oz*	85	211	822	846	1487	1566	482	211	734	632	915	1189	644	13030
lean, braised—*3 oz*	85	267	1041	1072	1884	1984	610	267	931	801	1159	1507	816	13032
brisket, whole (flat & pt hlvs), 0″ trim,														
lean & fat, braised—*3 oz*	85	255	995	1024	1800	1895	583	255	889	765	1108	1439	779	13367
lean, braised—*3 oz*	85	283	1104	1137	1998	2104	648	283	987	850	1230	1598	866	13368
brisket, whole (flat & pt hlvs),														
1/4″ trim, lean & fat, braised—*3 oz*	85	224	873	898	1579	1663	512	224	780	672	972	1262	684	13022
lean, braised—*3 oz*	85	283	1104	1137	1998	2104	648	283	987	850	1230	1598	866	13024
chuck arm pot roast, choice, 0″ trim,														
lean & fat, braised—*3 oz*	85	281	1093	1125	1978	2082	641	281	977	841	1217	1582	857	13374
lean, braised—*3 oz*	85	315	1226	1262	2219	2335	718	315	1096	943	1365	1774	961	13377
chuck arm pot roast, choice, 1/4″ trim,														
lean & fat, braised—*3 oz*	85	257	1001	1031	1812	1908	587	257	895	770	1115	1449	785	13036
chuck arm pot roast, select, 0″ trim,														
lean & fat, braised—*3 oz*	85	286	1118	1151	2023	2129	655	286	1000	860	1245	1618	876	13375
lean, braised—*3 oz*	85	315	1226	1262	2219	2335	718	315	1096	943	1365	1774	961	13378
chuck arm pot roast, select, 1/4″ trim,														
lean & fat, braised—*3 oz*	85	265	1035	1065	1873	1971	607	265	925	796	1153	1498	811	13038
chuck blade roast, choice, 0″ trim,														
lean & fat, braised—*3 oz*	85	257	1001	1031	1812	1908	587	257	895	771	1115	1449	785	13380
lean, braised—*3 oz*	85	296	1153	1187	2087	2196	676	296	1031	887	1284	1669	904	13383

	WT (g)	TRY (mg)	THR (mg)	ISO (mg)	LEU (mg)	LYS (mg)	MET (mg)	CYS (mg)	PHE (mg)	TYR (mg)	VAL (mg)	ARG (mg)	HIS (mg)	REF
chuck blade roast, choice, 1/4" trim,														
lean & fat, braised—3 *oz*	85	249	972	1000	1758	1850	570	249	868	747	1082	1406	762	13052
chuck blade roast, select, 0" trim,														
lean & fat, braised—3 *oz*	85	263	1024	1055	1854	1952	600	263	915	788	1141	1482	803	13381
lean, braised—3 *oz*	85	296	1153	1187	2087	2196	676	296	1031	887	1284	1669	904	13384
chuck blade roast, select, 1/4" trim,														
lean & fat, braised—3 *oz*	85	257	1001	1031	1812	1908	587	257	895	771	1115	1449	785	13054
chuck clod roast, choice, 0" trim,														
lean & fat, roasted—3 *oz*	85	226	965	1075	1842	1955	592	225	904	764	1127	1406	676	23528
lean, roasted—3 *oz*	85	238	1019	1139	1950	2070	626	237	956	808	1193	1486	711	13937
chuck clod roast, choice, 1/4" trim,														
lean & fat, roasted—3 *oz*	85	222	945	1051	1803	1913	579	221	885	748	1103	1377	664	23529
lean, roasted—3 *oz*	85	240	1025	1146	1961	2083	629	238	962	813	1199	1495	715	13938
chuck clod roast, select, 0" trim,														
lean & fat, roasted—3 *oz*	85	251	1071	1195	2048	2173	657	249	1005	849	1252	1561	749	23531
lean, roasted—3 *oz*	85	258	1103	1233	2111	2241	677	257	1035	876	1291	1609	770	13940
chuck clod roast, select, 1/4" trim,														
lean & fat, roasted—3 *oz*	85	224	953	1060	1817	1928	583	223	892	754	1112	1389	670	23532
lean, roasted—3 *oz*	85	246	1051	1174	2010	2134	645	244	986	833	1229	1532	733	13941
chuck clod steak, choice, 0" trim,														
lean & fat, braised—3 *oz*	85	258	1101	1227	2102	2231	675	257	1031	872	1286	1604	770	23533
lean, braised—3 *oz*	85	271	1159	1295	2219	2355	711	269	1088	920	1357	1691	809	13943
chuck clod steak, choice, 1/4" trim,														
lean & fat, braised—3 *oz*	85	244	1039	1154	1980	2100	636	243	972	822	1211	1513	730	23534
lean, braised—3 *oz*	85	272	1164	1301	2226	2363	714	270	1091	923	1362	1697	812	13944
chuck clod steak, select, 0" trim,														
lean & fat, braised—3 *oz*	85	274	1171	1308	2240	2377	719	273	1099	929	1370	1708	818	23536
lean, braised—3 *oz*	85	279	1193	1333	2282	2423	732	277	1119	946	1396	1739	832	13946
chuck clod steak, select, 1/4" trim,														
lean & fat, braised—3 *oz*	85	237	1010	1122	1924	2042	618	236	944	799	1177	1471	711	23537
lean, braised—3 *oz*	85	267	1142	1277	2185	2320	701	265	1072	906	1336	1665	796	13947
chuck, tender steak, choice, 0" trim,														
lean & fat, broiled—3 *oz*	85	236	1011	1130	1934	2053	621	235	949	802	1183	1474	706	23519
lean, broiled—3 *oz*	85	236	1012	1130	1935	2054	621	235	949	802	1183	1474	706	13961
chuck, tender steak, select, 0" trim,														
lean & fat, broiled—3 *oz*	85	239	1024	1144	1959	2080	629	238	961	813	1199	1493	715	23521
lean, broiled—3 *oz*	85	240	1027	1147	1964	2084	630	239	963	814	1201	1497	716	13963
chuck, top blade, choice, 0" trim,														
lean & fat, broiled—3 *oz*	85	236	1012	1130	1935	2054	621	235	949	802	1183	1476	706	23523
lean, broiled—3 *oz*	85	240	1026	1146	1962	2083	630	238	962	813	1200	1495	716	13965
chuck, top blade, select, 0" trim,														
lean & fat, broiled—3 *oz*	85	235	1007	1125	1926	2044	618	235	944	799	1178	1469	704	23525
lean, broiled—3 *oz*	85	240	1028	1148	1966	2087	631	239	964	815	1203	1499	717	13967
flank, choice, 0" trim, lean & fat,														
braised—3 *oz*	85	257	1001	1031	1812	1907	587	257	895	770	1115	1449	785	13066
lean & fat, broiled—3 *oz*	85	252	981	1010	1775	1868	575	252	876	755	1092	1420	769	13067
lean, broiled—3 *oz*	85	258	1006	1034	1819	1915	589	258	898	774	1119	1454	788	13070
ground, 5% fat, crumbles,														
pan-browned—3 *oz*	85	147	978	1086	1932	2065	654	263	951	779	1214	1568	826	23560
loaf, baked—3 *oz piece*	85	138	916	1017	1809	1933	611	246	891	729	1136	1468	774	23561
patty, broiled—3 *oz patty*	85	132	881	979	1741	1861	589	236	858	702	1094	1413	745	23558
patty, pan-broiled—3 *oz patty*	85	130	865	961	1709	1826	578	232	842	689	1074	1386	730	23559
ground, 10% fat, crumbles,														
pan-browned—3 *oz*	85	134	946	1063	1884	2009	631	252	934	753	1186	1548	796	23565
loaf, baked—3 *oz piece*	85	126	885	995	1763	1879	590	236	874	705	1109	1448	745	23566
patty, broiled—3 *oz patty*	85	123	868	976	1729	1844	579	232	858	691	1088	1420	731	23563
patty, pan-broiled—3 *oz patty*	85	119	838	943	1669	1780	558	224	828	667	1051	1371	706	23564
ground, 15% fat, crumbles,														
pan-browned—3 *oz*	85	122	913	1040	1837	1952	607	243	917	726	1157	1529	767	23570
loaf, baked—3 *oz piece*	85	113	854	973	1718	1826	568	227	859	679	1082	1431	717	23571
patty, broiled—3 *oz patty*	85	113	853	973	1718	1825	568	227	858	679	1082	1431	717	23568
patty, pan-broiled—3 *oz patty*	85	108	811	924	1631	1733	539	216	815	644	1028	1358	681	23569
ground, 20% fat, crumbles,														
pan-browned—3 *oz*	85	118	889	1013	1788	1901	592	236	893	707	1127	1489	747	23575
loaf, baked—3 *oz piece*	85	100	822	952	1673	1771	545	218	843	653	1056	1415	688	23576
patty, broiled—3 *oz patty*	85	102	838	972	1706	1806	556	222	859	666	1076	1443	701	23573
patty, pan-broiled—3 *oz patty*	85	95	783	907	1592	1686	519	207	802	621	1005	1347	655	23574

	WT (g)	TRY (mg)	THR (mg)	ISO (mg)	LEU (mg)	LYS (mg)	MET (mg)	CYS (mg)	PHE (mg)	TYR (mg)	VAL (mg)	ARG (mg)	HIS (mg)	REF
ground, 25% fat, crumbles,														
pan-browned—*3 oz*	85	92	844	997	1742	1837	558	223	887	669	1101	1500	704	23580
loaf, baked—*3 oz piece*	85	86	789	932	1628	1716	521	208	829	626	1029	1403	658	23581
patty, broiled—*3 oz patty*	85	89	821	970	1694	1787	542	217	863	651	1071	1459	684	23578
patty, pan-broiled—*3 oz patty*	85	82	753	890	1554	1639	497	199	791	597	983	1339	628	23579
ribs 6–9 (large end), choice, 0″ trim,														
lean & fat, rstd—*3 oz*	85	217	847	871	1532	1612	496	217	757	651	943	1225	664	13386
lean, roasted—*3 oz*	85	262	1023	1052	1850	1947	599	262	914	786	1138	1479	802	13389
ribs 6–9 (large end), choice, 1/4″ trim,														
lean & fat, brld—*3 oz*	85	200	778	801	1408	1482	456	200	695	598	866	1126	610	13103
lean & fat, roasted—*3 oz*	85	213	828	853	1498	1577	485	213	740	637	922	1198	649	13104c
lean, broiled—*3 oz*	85	240	934	962	1691	1780	547	240	836	719	1040	1352	733	13115
lean, roasted—*3 oz*	85	262	1023	1052	1850	1947	599	262	914	786	1138	1479	802	13116
ribs 6–9 (large end), prime, 1/4″ trim,														
lean & fat, brld—*3 oz*	85	193	754	776	1364	1436	442	193	674	580	840	1091	591	13109b
lean & fat, roasted—*3 oz*	85	214	834	859	1510	1589	489	214	745	642	929	1207	654	13110
lean, broiled—*3 oz*	85	235	915	942	1656	1743	536	235	818	704	1018	1323	717	13121
lean, roasted—*3 oz*	85	262	1023	1052	1850	1947	599	262	914	786	1138	1479	802	13122
ribs 6–9 (large end), select, 1/4″ trim,														
lean & fat, brld—*3 oz*	85	213	828	853	1498	1577	485	213	740	637	922	1198	649	13104b
lean & fat, roasted—*3 oz*	85	193	754	776	1364	1436	442	193	674	580	840	1091	591	13109c
lean, broiled—*3 oz*	85	240	934	962	1691	1780	547	240	836	719	1040	1352	733	13118
lean, roasted—*3 oz*	85	262	1023	1052	1850	1947	599	262	914	786	1138	1479	802	13119
ribs 10–12 (small end), choice, 0″ trim,														
lean & fat, brld—*3 oz*	85	235	918	945	1662	1749	538	235	821	706	1023	1329	720	13392
lean, broiled—*3 oz*	85	267	1041	1072	1884	1983	610	267	931	801	1159	1506	816	13395
ribs 10–12 (small end), choice,														
1/4″ trim, lean & fat, brld—*3 oz*	85	224	873	898	1580	1663	512	224	780	672	972	1263	684	13127
lean & fat, roasted—*3 oz*	85	209	816	840	1477	1555	479	209	729	628	909	1181	640	13128
lean, broiled—*3 oz*	85	267	1041	1072	1884	1983	610	267	931	801	1159	1506	816	13139
lean, roasted—*3 oz*	85	256	996	1026	1804	1898	584	256	891	767	1110	1442	781	13140
ribs 10–12 (small end), prime,														
1/4″ trim, lean & fat, brld—*3 oz*	85	227	886	912	1603	1688	519	227	792	682	987	1282	694	13133
lean & fat, roasted—*3 oz*	85	208	813	837	1472	1550	477	208	727	626	906	1177	638	13134
lean, broiled—*3 oz*	85	267	1041	1072	1884	1983	610	267	931	801	1159	1506	816	13145
lean, roasted—*3 oz*	85	254	993	1022	1796	1891	581	254	887	763	1106	1437	778	13146
ribs 10–12 (small end), select, 0″ trim,														
lean & fat, brld—*3 oz*	85	237	925	952	1674	1761	542	237	826	711	1030	1338	725	13393
lean, broiled—*3 oz*	85	267	1041	1072	1884	1983	610	267	931	801	1159	1506	816	13396
ribs 10–12 (small end), select,														
1/4″ trim, lean & fat, brld—*3 oz*	85	227	886	912	1603	1688	519	227	792	682	987	1282	694	13130
lean & fat, roasted—*3 oz*	85	214	834	859	1510	1589	489	214	745	642	929	1207	654	13131
lean, broiled—*3 oz*	85	267	1041	1072	1884	1983	610	267	931	801	1159	1506	816	13142
ribs 6–12 (whole), choice, 1/4″ trim,														
lean & fat, broiled—*3 oz*	85	209	816	840	1476	1554	479	209	729	627	909	1181	639	13075
lean, broiled—*3 oz*	85	251	978	1006	1770	1863	573	251	874	752	1089	1415	767	13087
ribs 6–12 (whole), prime, 1/4″ trim,														
lean & fat, broiled—*3 oz*	85	207	807	830	1459	1536	473	207	721	621	898	1167	632	13081
lean & fat, roasted—*3 oz*	85	212	825	848	1492	1571	483	212	737	634	918	1193	646	13082
lean, broiled—*3 oz*	85	247	966	995	1748	1840	566	247	864	743	1076	1398	757	13093
lean, roasted—*3 oz*	85	259	1010	1040	1828	1924	592	259	903	777	1125	1462	792	13094
ribs 6–12 (whole), select, 1/4″ trim,														
lean & fat, broiled—*3 oz*	85	214	835	859	1511	1590	490	214	746	643	930	1208	655	13078
lean & fat, roasted—*3 oz*	85	218	849	874	1536	1617	497	218	759	653	945	1228	666	13079
lean, broiled—*3 oz*	85	251	978	1006	1769	1862	573	251	874	752	1089	1414	767	13090
lean, roasted—*3 oz*	85	259	1012	1041	1831	1927	593	259	904	779	1126	1464	793	13091
ribs, shortribs, lean & fat, braised—*3 oz*	85	206	801	824	1448	1525	469	206	716	616	892	1159	627	13148
round, bottom, choice, 0″ trim, lean &														
fat, braised—*3 oz*	85	295	1149	1183	2080	2190	674	295	1028	884	1280	1663	901	13401
lean & fat, roasted—*3 oz*	85	270	1055	1085	1909	2009	618	270	943	812	1175	1527	827	13402
lean, braised—*3 oz*	85	301	1173	1207	2122	2234	688	301	1048	902	1306	1697	920	13410
lean, roasted—*3 oz*	85	274	1068	1100	1933	2035	626	274	955	822	1190	1546	837	13411
round, bottom, choice, 1/4″ trim,														
lean & fat, braised—*3 oz*	85	273	1064	1095	1925	2026	624	273	951	819	1185	1539	834	13162
lean & fat, roasted—*3 oz*	85	252	981	1010	1775	1868	575	252	876	755	1092	1420	769	13400
lean, braised—*3 oz*	85	301	1173	1207	2122	2234	688	301	1048	902	1306	1697	920	13170
lean, roasted—*3 oz*	85	274	1068	1100	1933	2035	626	274	955	822	1190	1546	837	13409

	WT (g)	TRY (mg)	THR (mg)	ISO (mg)	LEU (mg)	LYS (mg)	MET (mg)	CYS (mg)	PHE (mg)	TYR (mg)	VAL (mg)	ARG (mg)	HIS (mg)	REF
round, bottom, select, 0″ trim, lean &														
fat, braised—3 *oz*	85	297	1157	1191	2094	2204	678	297	1034	890	1289	1675	907	13404
lean & fat, roasted—3 *oz*	85	272	1062	1093	1921	2022	622	272	949	817	1182	1536	832	13405
lean, braised—3 *oz*	85	301	1173	1207	2122	2234	688	301	1048	902	1306	1697	920	13413
lean, roasted—3 *oz*	85	274	1068	1100	1933	2035	626	274	955	822	1190	1546	837	13414
round, bottom, select, 1/4″ trim,														
lean & fat, braised—3 *oz*	85	275	1072	1103	1940	2042	628	275	958	825	1193	1550	840	13164
lean & fat, roasted—3 *oz*	85	255	995	1023	1799	1894	583	255	889	765	1108	1439	779	13403
lean, braised—3 *oz*	85	301	1173	1207	2122	2234	688	301	1048	902	1306	1697	920	13172
lean, roasted—3 *oz*	85	274	1068	1100	1933	2035	626	274	955	822	1190	1546	837	13412
round, eye of, choice, 0″ trim,														
lean & fat, roasted—3 *oz*	85	275	1069	1101	1935	2037	626	275	956	823	1191	1547	838	13416
lean, roasted—3 *oz*	85	276	1076	1108	1947	2050	631	276	962	828	1199	1557	844	13419
round, eye of, choice, 1/4″ trim,														
lean & fat, roasted—3 *oz*	85	253	988	1017	1788	1881	579	253	883	760	1100	1429	774	13178
lean, roasted—3 *oz*	85	276	1076	1108	1947	2050	631	276	962	828	1199	1557	844	13186
round, eye of, select, 0″ trim,														
lean & fat, roasted—3 *oz*	85	275	1069	1101	1935	2037	626	275	956	823	1191	1547	838	13417
lean, roasted—3 *oz*	85	276	1076	1108	1947	2050	631	276	962	828	1199	1557	844	13420
round, eye of, select, 1/4″ trim,														
lean & fat, roasted—3 *oz*	85	257	1001	1031	1812	1907	587	257	895	770	1115	1449	785	13180
lean, roasted—3 *oz*	85	276	1076	1108	1947	2050	631	276	962	828	1199	1557	844	13188
round, full cut, choice, 1/4″ trim,														
lean & fat, broiled—3 *oz*	85	260	1016	1046	1838	1935	595	260	908	781	1131	1470	796	13152
lean, broiled—3 *oz*	85	278	1085	1116	1963	2066	636	278	969	834	1208	1569	850	13156
round, full cut, select, 1/4″ trim,														
lean & fat, broiled—3 *oz*	85	261	1017	1047	1840	1937	596	261	909	782	1132	1471	797	13154
lean, broiled—3 *oz*	85	279	1086	1118	1965	2069	637	279	971	836	1210	1572	852	13158
round, tip, choice, 0″ trim,														
lean & fat, roasted—3 *oz*	85	266	1040	1069	1880	1980	609	266	929	799	1157	1504	814	13422
lean, roasted—3 *oz*	85	274	1066	1097	1929	2031	625	274	953	820	1187	1543	836	13425
round, tip, choice, 1/4″ trim,														
lean & fat, roasted—3 *oz*	85	252	985	1014	1783	1878	578	252	881	758	1097	1426	773	13194
round, tip, prime, 1/4″ trim,														
lean & fat, roasted—3 *oz*	85	251	979	1007	1771	1865	574	251	875	753	1090	1416	768	13198
lean, roasted—3 *oz*	85	274	1066	1097	1929	2031	625	274	953	820	1187	1543	836	13206
round, tip, select, 0″ trim,														
lean & fat, roasted—3 *oz*	85	269	1046	1077	1893	1992	613	269	935	805	1165	1513	820	13423
lean, roasted—3 *oz*	85	274	1066	1097	1929	2031	625	274	953	820	1187	1543	836	13426
round, tip, select, 1/4″ trim,														
lean, roasted—3 *oz*	85	274	1066	1097	1929	2031	625	274	953	820	1187	1543	836	13204
round, top, choice, 0″ trim,														
lean & fat, braised—3 *oz*	85	339	1323	1361	2393	2519	775	339	1182	1017	1472	1913	1036	13430
lean, braised—3 *oz*	85	344	1341	1380	2427	2555	786	344	1199	1032	1493	1941	1051	13436
round, top, choice, 1/4″ trim,														
lean & fat, braised—3 *oz*	85	320	1247	1284	2256	2375	731	320	1114	959	1388	1804	978	13429
lean & fat, broiled—3 *oz*	85	287	1120	1153	2027	2134	656	287	1001	862	1247	1621	878	13210
lean & fat, panfried—3 *oz*	85	309	1203	1238	2176	2290	705	309	1074	925	1339	1740	943	13211
lean, braised—3 *oz*	85	344	1341	1380	2427	2555	786	344	1199	1032	1493	1941	1051	13435
lean, broiled—3 *oz*	85	302	1176	1211	2129	2241	689	302	1051	905	1310	1703	922	13219
round, top, prime, 1/4″ trim,														
lean & fat, broiled—3 *oz*	85	296	1153	1187	2087	2196	676	296	1030	887	1284	1669	904	13215
lean, broiled—3 *oz*	85	302	1176	1211	2129	2241	689	302	1051	905	1310	1703	922	13224
round, top, select, 0″ trim,														
lean & fat, braised—3 *oz*	85	339	1323	1361	2393	2519	775	339	1182	1017	1472	1913	1036	13432
lean, braised—3 *oz*	85	344	1341	1380	2427	2555	786	344	1199	1032	1493	1941	1051	13438
round, top, select, 1/4″ trim,														
lean & fat, braised—3 *oz*	85	325	1266	1303	2290	2411	742	325	1131	973	1409	1831	992	13431
lean & fat, broiled—3 *oz*	85	287	1120	1153	2027	2134	656	287	1001	862	1247	1621	878	13213
lean, braised—3 *oz*	85	344	1341	1380	2427	2555	786	344	1199	1032	1493	1941	1051	13437
lean, broiled—3 *oz*	85	302	1176	1211	2129	2241	689	302	1051	905	1310	1703	922	13222
shank, crosscuts, choice, 1/4″ trim,														
lean & fat, simmered—3 *oz*	85	292	1139	1173	2062	2170	668	292	1018	876	1269	1648	893	13226
lean, simmered—3 *oz*	85	320	1250	1287	2263	2382	733	320	1118	962	1392	1810	980	13228
short loin porterhse stk, choice,														
1/4″ trim, lean & fat, brld—3 *oz*	85	195	822	909	1561	1655	502	194	766	649	955	1197	582	13230
lean, broiled—3 *oz*	85	230	982	1097	1877	1992	603	228	921	779	1148	1431	684	13232

	WT (g)	TRY (mg)	THR (mg)	ISO (mg)	LEU (mg)	LYS (mg)	MET (mg)	CYS (mg)	PHE (mg)	TYR (mg)	VAL (mg)	ARG (mg)	HIS (mg)	REF
short loin porterhse stk, select,														
1/4″ trim, lean & fat, brld—3 *oz*	85	216	916	1017	1744	1850	560	215	856	725	1068	1335	647	13462
lean, broiled—3 *oz*	85	250	1068	1194	2044	2170	656	248	1002	847	1250	1558	745	13469
short loin T-bone steak, choice,														
1/4″ trim,														
lean & fat, broiled—3 *oz*	85	205	870	963	1653	1754	531	204	812	688	1012	1267	615	13234
lean, broiled—3 *oz*	85	240	1025	1146	1961	2083	629	238	962	813	1199	1495	715	13236
short loin T-bone steak, select,														
1/4″ trim,														
lean & fat, broiled—3 *oz*	85	225	956	1063	1822	1934	585	224	894	757	1115	1393	673	13476
lean, broiled—3 *oz*	85	251	1074	1200	2055	2182	660	250	1008	852	1257	1567	750	13483
short loin, top, choice, 0″ trim,														
lean & fat, broiled—3 *oz*	85	265	1036	1066	1874	1973	607	265	926	796	1153	1499	812	13446
lean, broiled—3 *oz*	85	273	1063	1094	1923	2024	623	273	949	818	1183	1538	833	13449
short loin, top, choice, 1/4″ trim,														
lean & fat, broiled—3 *oz*	85	241	943	970	1705	1795	553	241	842	725	1050	1363	739	13264
lean, broiled—3 *oz*	85	273	1063	1094	1923	2024	623	273	949	818	1183	1538	833	13272
short loin, top, prime, 1/4″ trim,														
lean & fat, broiled—3 *oz*	85	241	943	970	1705	1795	553	241	842	725	1050	1363	739	13268
lean, broiled—3 *oz*	85	273	1063	1094	1923	2024	623	273	949	818	1183	1538	833	13276
short loin, top, select, 0″ trim,														
lean & fat, broiled—3 *oz*	85	267	1043	1073	1886	1986	611	267	932	802	1161	1509	817	13447
lean, broiled—3 *oz*	85	273	1063	1094	1923	2024	623	273	949	818	1183	1538	833	13450
short loin, top, select, 1/4″ trim,														
lean & fat, broiled—3 *oz*	85	247	962	991	1742	1833	564	247	860	740	1072	1392	755	13266
lean, broiled—3 *oz*	85	273	1063	1094	1923	2024	623	273	949	818	1183	1538	833	13274
skirt steak, inside, 0″ trim,														
lean & fat, broiled—3 *oz*	85	240	1026	1145	1961	2082	629	239	962	813	1199	1495	717	23540
lean, broiled—3 *oz*	85	245	1047	1170	2003	2127	643	243	983	830	1226	1527	730	13977
skirt steak, outside, 0″ trim,														
lean & fat, broiled—3 *oz*	85	216	922	1029	1763	1871	566	215	864	731	1079	1345	645	23541
lean, broiled—3 *oz*	85	222	950	1062	1817	1929	583	221	891	753	1112	1385	662	13979
tenderloin, choice, 0″ trim,														
lean & fat, broiled—3 *oz*	85	258	1003	1033	1815	1911	588	258	897	772	1117	1452	786	13440
lean, broiled—3 *oz*	85	269	1049	1080	1898	1998	615	269	938	807	1168	1517	822	13443
tenderloin, choice, 1/4″ trim,														
lean & fat, broiled—3 *oz*	85	239	932	959	1685	1774	546	239	832	717	1037	1347	730	13241
lean & fat, roasted—3 *oz*	85	224	876	903	1586	1670	514	224	784	674	977	1268	688	13242
lean, broiled—3 *oz*	85	269	1049	1080	1898	1998	615	269	938	807	1168	1517	822	13253
lean, roasted—3 *oz*	85	264	1029	1059	1862	1959	603	264	920	791	1146	1488	807	13254
tenderloin, prime, 1/4″ trim,														
lean & fat, broiled—3 *oz*	85	237	925	952	1674	1761	542	237	826	711	1029	1338	725	13247
lean & fat, roasted—3 *oz*	85	225	879	904	1590	1674	515	225	785	676	978	1272	689	13248
lean, broiled—3 *oz*	85	269	1049	1080	1898	1998	615	269	938	807	1168	1517	822	13259
lean, roasted—3 *oz*	85	262	1023	1052	1850	1947	599	262	914	786	1138	1479	802	13260
tenderloin, select, 0″ trim,														
lean & fat, broiled—3 *oz*	85	259	1010	1040	1827	1924	592	259	903	777	1125	1461	791	13441
lean, broiled—3 *oz*	85	269	1049	1080	1898	1998	615	269	938	807	1168	1517	822	13444
tenderloin, select, 1/4″ trim,														
lean & fat, broiled—3 *oz*	85	244	951	978	1720	1811	558	244	850	731	1059	1376	745	13244
lean & fat, roasted—3 *oz*	85	224	876	903	1586	1670	514	224	784	674	977	1268	688	13245
lean, broiled—3 *oz*	85	269	1049	1080	1898	1998	615	269	938	807	1168	1517	822	13256
lean, roasted—3 *oz*	85	264	1029	1059	1862	1959	603	264	920	791	1146	1488	807	13257
top sirloin, choice, 0″ trim,														
lean & fat, broiled—3 *oz*	85	278	1084	1115	1961	2064	635	278	968	834	1207	1568	849	13452
lean, broiled—3 *oz*	85	289	1128	1160	2040	2148	660	289	1008	867	1255	1631	884	13455
top sirloin, choice, 1/4″ trim,														
lean & fat, broiled—3 *oz*	85	263	1025	1055	1855	1952	601	263	916	789	1142	1483	803	13280
lean & fat, panfried—3 *oz*	85	268	1044	1074	1889	1988	612	268	933	803	1162	1510	819	13281
lean, broiled—3 *oz*	85	289	1128	1160	2040	2148	660	289	1008	867	1255	1631	884	13289
lean, panfried—3 *oz*	85	309	1206	1241	2182	2297	706	309	1078	927	1343	1745	945	13290
top sirloin, select, 0″ trim,														
lean & fat, broiled—3 *oz*	85	283	1102	1135	1996	2100	646	283	986	848	1228	1595	864	13453
lean, broiled—3 *oz*	85	289	1128	1160	2040	2148	660	289	1008	867	1255	1631	884	13456
top sirloin, select, 1/4″ trim,														
lean & fat, broiled—3 *oz*	85	267	1040	1070	1881	1981	609	267	929	800	1158	1505	815	13283
lean, broiled—3 *oz*	85	289	1128	1160	2040	2148	660	289	1008	867	1255	1631	884	13292

	WT (g)	TRY (mg)	THR (mg)	ISO (mg)	LEU (mg)	LYS (mg)	MET (mg)	CYS (mg)	PHE (mg)	TYR (mg)	VAL (mg)	ARG (mg)	HIS (mg)	REF
Game														
antelope, roasted—3 oz	85	0	1158	957	2116	2093	712	223	991	869	1114	1647	1191	17145
beaver, roasted—3 oz	85	0	1128	1266	2337	2754	673	0	1204	924	1209	1820	1166	17151
bison, chuck, shoulder clod, lean,														
braised—3 oz	85	217	1303	1386	2463	2664	777	343	1219	977	1545	1955	1052	17333
bison, ground, pan-broiled—3 oz	85	153	916	975	1733	1874	547	241	858	688	1087	1375	740	17331
bison, ribeye steak, lean, broiled														
3 oz	85	190	1136	1209	2148	2322	677	298	1063	852	1346	1704	917	17335b
6.3 oz	179	399	2391	2545	4523	4890	1425	628	2238	1794	2835	3589	1931	17335a
bison, top round, lean, raw—3 oz	85	0	780	799	1472	1478	450	0	709	609	858	1124	502	17266
bison, top sirloin steak, lean,														
broiled—3 oz	85	180	1082	1151	2045	2213	645	284	1012	811	1283	1623	874	17332a
broiled—6.8 oz	194	411	2470	2627	4668	5050	1472	648	2311	1851	2927	3703	1994	17332b
boar, wild, roasted—3 oz	85	323	1131	1162	1955	2371	592	312	962	859	1289	1670	1220	17159
buffalo, water, roasted—3 oz	85	278	1091	1144	1963	1800	571	365	914	915	1213	1429	755	17161
caribou, roasted—3 oz	85	389	1082	1145	2088	2292	565	182	1125	830	1189	1505	1002	17163
deer, all cuts, roasted—3 oz	85	0	1208	1015	2181	2243	633	287	1048	909	1200	1849	1270	17165
deer, ground, pan-broiled—3 oz	85	199	848	963	1707	1822	524	209	848	701	1089	1340	670	17344
deer, loin steak, lean, broiled														
3 oz	85	229	976	1108	1964	2097	603	241	976	808	1254	1543	771	17345
deer, shoulder clod, lean, braised														
3 oz	85	270	1153	1310	2320	2477	711	285	1153	954	1480	1822	911	17346
deer, tenderloin, lean, broiled—3 oz .	85	226	963	1094	1938	2069	595	238	963	796	1237	1522	761	17347
deer, top round steak, lean, broiled														
3 oz	85	240	1023	1163	2060	2199	632	252	1023	847	1314	1618	808	17348b
sep lean, broiled—3.6 oz	102	288	1228	1395	2471	2639	758	303	1228	1016	1577	1941	970	17348a
elk, ground, pan-broiled—3 oz	85	202	910	950	1688	1850	556	223	829	708	1051	1355	698	17339
elk, loin, lean, broiled—3 oz	85	235	1059	1106	1964	2153	647	258	965	824	1223	1576	812	17340a
4 oz steak	114	316	1420	1483	2635	2888	868	347	1294	1105	1640	2114	1089	17340b
elk, roasted—3 oz	85	463	1118	827	2164	2383	616	0	1018	919	906	1762	819	17167
elk, round, lean, broiled—3 oz	85	235	1057	1103	1961	2148	646	258	963	822	1221	1573	810	17341b
6.2 oz steak	176	486	2188	2284	4060	4448	1338	535	1994	1702	2527	3258	1677	17341a
elk, tenderloin, lean, broiled—3 oz	85	234	1051	1097	1949	2136	642	257	957	817	1214	1564	806	17342b
3.2 oz steak	92	253	1137	1188	2110	2312	695	278	1036	884	1314	1693	872	17342a
emu, fan fillet, broiled—3 oz	85	176	762	864	1467	1564	504	192	758	567	885	1196	582	05624
emu, flat fillet, raw—3 oz	85	125	542	615	1044	1113	359	137	540	404	630	851	414	05625
emu, full rump, broiled—3 oz	85	189	820	930	1580	1684	542	207	817	610	953	1289	626	05627
emu, ground, pan-broiled														
3 oz patty	85	160	693	785	1335	1422	458	174	689	516	805	1088	530	05622
emu, inside drum, broiled—3 oz	85	182	789	894	1520	1619	522	199	785	587	916	1238	603	05629
emu, outside drum, raw—3 oz	85	130	563	638	1083	1154	372	142	560	418	654	883	429	05630
emu, oyster, raw—3 oz	85	128	556	630	1070	1141	368	140	553	414	646	873	424	05631
emu, top loin, broiled—3 oz	85	163	708	803	1364	1454	468	179	705	527	823	1112	541	05632
goat, roasted—3 oz	85	343	1097	1165	1919	1714	617	275	800	708	1234	1691	480	17169
horse, roasted—3 oz	85	297	1073	1134	1897	2038	530	334	983	750	1239	1567	919	17171
moose, roasted—3 oz	85	0	1142	1194	2190	2257	637	0	1074	915	1353	1608	836	17173
muskrat, roasted—3 oz	85	0	1051	974	2017	2005	426	0	1056	700	1137	1227	761	17175
ostrich, ground, pan-broiled—3 oz	85	198	975	1056	1806	1963	621	229	917	723	1097	1520	558	05642
ostrich, inside leg, ckd—3 oz	85	220	1081	1171	2003	2178	689	253	1017	802	1218	1686	620	05645
ostrich, inside strip, ckd—3 oz	85	223	1095	1186	2028	2204	698	257	1030	812	1233	1708	627	05647
ostrich, outside strip, ckd—3 oz	85	217	1064	1153	1972	2143	678	249	1001	789	1199	1659	609	05650
ostrich, oyster, ckd—3 oz	85	218	1074	1164	1990	2162	684	252	1011	796	1210	1675	615	05652
ostrich, tip trimmed, ckd—3 oz	85	216	1063	1151	1968	2139	677	249	1000	788	1196	1656	609	05656
ostrich, top loin, ckd—3 oz	85	213	1048	1136	1942	2111	668	246	987	777	1181	1635	600	05658
rabbit, domesticated, roasted—3 oz	85	326	1105	1172	1924	2162	618	310	1014	880	1255	1526	693	17178
stewed—3 oz	85	341	1155	1225	2012	2261	646	325	1060	920	1312	1595	724	17179
rabbit, wild, stewed—3 oz	85	371	1255	1332	2187	2457	702	353	1152	1000	1426	1734	787	17181
squirrel, roasted—3 oz	85	0	996	996	1879	1891	574	0	1012	783	1034	1364	683	17184
Lamb, Domestic US														
foreshank, choice, 1/4″ trim,														
lean & fat, braised—3 oz	85	282	1032	1164	1876	2129	619	288	982	811	1301	1433	764	17008
lean, braised—3 oz	85	308	1128	1272	2050	2328	677	315	1073	886	1422	1566	835	17010
ground, broiled—3 oz	85	246	900	1015	1636	1858	540	251	857	707	1135	1250	666	17225
leg & shoulder, cubed,														
lean, braised—3 oz	85	335	1226	1381	2227	2529	735	342	1166	962	1545	1702	907	17060
lean, broiled—3 oz	85	279	1022	1152	1856	2107	612	285	972	802	1288	1418	756	17061

	WT (g)	TRY (mg)	THR (mg)	ISO (mg)	LEU (mg)	LYS (mg)	MET (mg)	CYS (mg)	PHE (mg)	TYR (mg)	VAL (mg)	ARG (mg)	HIS (mg)	REF
leg, shank half, choice, 1/4″ trim,														
lean & fat, roasted—3 *oz*	85	263	961	1083	1746	1982	576	268	914	755	1211	1334	711	17016
lean, roasted—3 *oz*	85	280	1025	1155	1862	2115	615	286	975	805	1292	1423	758	17018
leg, sirloin half, choice, 1/4″ trim,														
lean & fat, roasted—3 *oz*	85	245	896	1010	1629	1849	537	250	853	704	1130	1244	663	17020
lean, roasted—3 *oz*	85	281	1032	1163	1874	2128	619	287	981	810	1301	1431	763	17022
leg, whole (shank & sirloin), choice,														
1/4″ trim, lean & fat, rstd—3 *oz*	85	254	930	1048	1689	1918	558	259	884	730	1172	1290	688	17012
lean, roasted—3 *oz*	85	281	1029	1160	1871	2124	617	287	979	808	1298	1429	762	17014
loin, choice, 1/4″ trim,														
lean & fat, broiled—3 *oz*	85	250	915	1032	1664	1890	549	255	871	719	1154	1272	677	17024
lean & fat, roasted—3 *oz*	85	224	820	925	1491	1692	492	229	780	644	1034	1139	607	17025
lean, broiled—3 *oz*	85	298	1091	1230	1982	2251	655	304	1038	857	1375	1515	808	17027
lean, roasted—3 *oz*	85	264	967	1091	1758	1996	580	269	921	760	1220	1343	716	17028
rib, choice, 1/4″ trim,														
lean & fat, broiled—3 *oz*	85	210	768	866	1396	1585	461	214	731	604	968	1066	569	17031
lean & fat, roasted—3 *oz*	85	145	528	595	960	1090	317	147	502	415	666	733	391	17029
lean, broiled—3 *oz*	85	230	839	946	1525	1731	503	234	798	659	1057	1165	621	17240
lean, roasted—3 *oz*	85	217	794	895	1442	1638	476	221	755	623	1000	1102	587	17241
shoulder, arm, choice 1/4″ trim,														
lean & fat, braised—3 *oz*	85	302	1106	1246	2009	2281	663	309	1051	869	1394	1535	819	17044
lean & fat, broiled—3 *oz*	85	243	889	1002	1616	1834	533	248	846	698	1121	1234	658	17045
lean & fat, roasted—3 *oz*	85	224	819	924	1490	1692	491	229	779	643	1034	1138	607	17046
lean, braised—3 *oz*	85	353	1293	1458	2349	2667	775	360	1230	1015	1630	1794	957	17048
lean, broiled—3 *oz*	85	275	1008	1136	1832	2080	604	281	959	791	1271	1399	746	17049
lean, roasted—3 *oz*	85	253	927	1044	1683	1911	555	258	881	728	1168	1286	686	17050
shoulder, blade, choice 1/4″ trim,														
lean & fat, braised—3 *oz*	85	283	1037	1170	1885	2140	622	289	987	814	1308	1440	768	17052
lean & fat, broiled—3 *oz*	85	230	840	946	1526	1732	503	234	799	660	1058	1165	621	17053
lean & fat, roasted—3 *oz*	85	221	809	912	1471	1669	485	226	770	636	1020	1124	599	17054
lean, braised—3 *oz*	85	321	1177	1327	2139	2428	706	328	1119	924	1484	1634	871	17056
lean, broiled—3 *oz*	85	253	927	1045	1685	1913	556	258	881	728	1169	1287	686	17057
lean, roasted—3 *oz*	85	245	895	1009	1627	1848	537	250	852	703	1129	1243	663	17058
shldr, whole (arm & blade), choice,														
1/4″ trim, lean & fat, braised—3 *oz*	85	285	1043	1176	1896	2152	626	291	992	819	1315	1448	772	17036
lean & fat, broiled—3 *oz*	85	242	888	1001	1615	1833	533	248	845	698	1120	1233	658	17037
lean & fat, roasted—3 *oz*	85	224	819	923	1488	1690	491	229	779	643	1033	1136	606	17038
lean, braised—3 *oz*	85	326	1193	1346	2169	2462	716	333	1136	938	1505	1657	883	17040
lean, broiled—3 *oz*	85	269	987	1112	1793	2036	592	275	938	774	1244	1369	730	17041
lean, roasted—3 *oz*	85	247	907	1023	1649	1872	544	253	863	712	1144	1260	672	17042
Lamb, Imported From Australia														
foreshank, 1/8″ trim,														
lean & fat, braised—3 *oz*	85	246	899	1017	1638	1860	539	252	856	707	1136	1250	667	17287
lean, braised—3 *oz*	85	273	999	1130	1817	2065	598	281	950	785	1261	1387	740	17289
leg, whole (shank & sirloin), 1/8″ trim,														
lean & fat, roasted—3 *oz*	85	250	914	1034	1663	1889	547	257	869	718	1153	1269	677	17291
lean, roasted—3 *oz*	85	271	992	1122	1805	2050	594	279	944	780	1252	1378	735	17293
loin, 1/8″ trim,														
lean & fat, broiled—3 *oz*	85	253	926	1047	1685	1914	555	260	881	728	1169	1286	687	17311
lean, broiled—3 *oz*	85	264	964	1090	1754	1992	577	270	916	758	1216	1339	715	17313
retail cuts, 1/8″ trim,														
lean & fat, ckd—3 *oz*	85	243	891	1007	1621	1841	534	250	847	700	1124	1238	660	17281
lean, ckd—3 *oz*	85	265	970	1097	1765	2005	581	273	923	763	1224	1348	719	17283
rib, 1/8″ trim, lean & fat, roasted—3 *oz*	85	221	808	914	1471	1669	484	227	768	635	1019	1122	599	17315
lean, roasted—3 *oz*	85	245	894	1012	1628	1850	536	252	851	704	1129	1243	663	17317
shoulder, whole (arm & blade),														
lean & fat, braised—3 *oz*	85	234	856	969	1559	1771	513	241	814	673	1081	1190	635	17319
lean, braised—3 *oz*	85	192	703	795	1279	1454	422	197	669	553	887	977	521	17320
Lamb, Imported From New Zealand														
foreshank, lean & fat, braised—3 *oz*	85	268	981	1106	1783	2025	588	274	933	770	1237	1362	726	17069
lean, braised—3 *oz*	85	305	1119	1261	2033	2309	671	312	1064	879	1411	1553	828	17071
leg, whole (shank & sirloin),														
lean & fat, roasted—3 *oz*	85	247	903	1017	1640	1862	541	252	859	709	1137	1253	668	17073
lean, roasted—3 *oz*	85	275	1007	1135	1830	2077	604	281	958	791	1270	1397	745	17075
loin, lean & fat, broiled—3 *oz*	85	233	853	961	1549	1759	511	238	811	669	1074	1183	631	17077
lean, broiled—3 *oz*	85	292	1066	1202	1938	2200	639	298	1014	837	1344	1480	789	17079

	WT (g)	TRY (mg)	THR (mg)	ISO (mg)	LEU (mg)	LYS (mg)	MET (mg)	CYS (mg)	PHE (mg)	TYR (mg)	VAL (mg)	ARG (mg)	HIS (mg)	REF
retail cuts, trimmed,														
lean & fat, ckd—*3 oz*	85	242	888	1001	1615	1833	533	248	845	698	1120	1233	658	17063
lean, ckd—*3 oz*	85	294	1077	1214	1957	2221	645	300	1024	846	1357	1494	796	17065
rib, lean & fat, roasted—*3 oz*	85	189	690	779	1255	1425	414	193	657	542	870	958	511	17081
lean, roasted—*3 oz*	85	242	888	1001	1615	1833	533	248	845	698	1120	1233	658	17083
shoulder, whole (arm & blade),														
lean & fat, braised—*3 oz*	85	281	1026	1157	1865	2117	615	286	976	806	1294	1425	760	17085
lean, braised—*3 oz*	85	338	1239	1397	2252	2556	743	345	1178	973	1562	1720	917	17087
Pork														
arm, picnic, lean & fat, braised—*3 oz*	85	281	1054	1068	1873	2112	602	293	939	790	1268	1538	891	10075
lean & fat, roasted—*3 oz*	85	232	877	886	1562	1765	499	243	785	655	1059	1301	734	10076
lean, braised—*3 oz*	85	349	1252	1284	2200	2466	726	349	1095	955	1488	1704	1096	10078
lean, roasted—*3 oz*	85	288	1035	1062	1820	2039	600	289	905	791	1230	1410	906	10079
arm, picnic, cured,														
lean & fat, roasted—*3 oz*	85	193	752	732	1362	1469	439	250	740	541	760	1193	581	10168
lean, roasted—*3 oz*	85	254	943	930	1683	1798	560	319	916	695	920	1377	760	10169
backribs, lean & fat, roasted—*3 oz*	85	262	942	966	1655	1855	546	263	823	718	1119	1282	824	10193
bacon, canadian style, cured,														
grilled—*2 slices*	47	113	457	430	802	897	310	142	370	345	454	621	414	10131
unheated—*2 slices*	57	117	473	444	828	926	320	147	382	356	469	642	428	10130
bacon, cured, broiled/panfried														
3 med slices	19	55	222	235	403	430	128	59	223	169	279	354	167	10124a
4.48 oz (yield from 1 lb raw)	127	371	1485	1571	2691	2871	853	396	1491	1126	1862	2363	1114	10124b
bacon, cured, raw—*3 med slices*	68	56	226	239	409	437	130	61	227	171	284	360	169	10123
blade roll, cured, sep lean & fat,														
roasted—*3 oz*	85	176	653	643	1165	1245	388	221	634	482	637	954	526	10171
boston blade (steaks & roasts),														
lean & fat, braised—*3 oz*	85	298	1094	1114	1934	2176	629	304	966	826	1309	1550	938	10081
lean & fat, broiled—*3 oz*	85	276	993	1018	1744	1955	575	277	868	757	1180	1352	869	10082
lean & fat, roasted—*3 oz*	85	241	883	900	1561	1754	508	246	779	667	1056	1247	759	10083
lean, braised—*3 oz*	85	336	1207	1238	2121	2377	700	337	1055	921	1434	1643	1056	10085
lean, broiled—*3 oz*	85	289	1038	1064	1823	2044	602	290	907	792	1233	1413	908	10086
lean, roasted—*3 oz*	85	262	940	964	1652	1851	545	263	822	717	1117	1279	822	10087
breakfast strips, cured,														
ckd—*3 slices (1.2 oz)*	34	95	378	400	685	731	217	101	379	287	474	601	284	10129
raw—*3 slices (2.4 oz)*	68	77	307	324	556	592	176	82	308	233	384	488	230	10128
center loin (chops) w/bone,														
lean & fat, braised—*3 oz*	85	292	1068	1090	1887	2122	615	298	943	808	1278	1505	919	10037
lean & fat, broiled—*3 oz*	85	310	1114	1142	1958	2195	646	311	974	850	1324	1517	975	10038
lean & fat, panfried—*3 oz*	85	312	1143	1165	2020	2271	658	319	1009	865	1367	1612	983	10179
lean, braised—*3 oz*	85	321	1156	1186	2032	2276	671	323	1011	882	1374	1573	1012	10041
lean, broiled—*3 oz*	85	326	1172	1202	2059	2308	679	327	1024	894	1392	1595	1025	10042
lean, panfried—*3 oz*	85	348	1250	1281	2195	2460	724	349	1092	953	1484	1701	1093	10176
center loin (roasts),														
lean & fat, roasted—*3 oz*	85	276	1009	1029	1780	2001	581	281	888	764	1204	1413	870	10039
lean, roasted—*3 oz*	85	298	1069	1097	1879	2105	620	298	935	816	1271	1456	936	10043
center rib (chops) w/bone,														
lean & fat, braised—*3 oz*	85	278	1019	1039	1801	2026	587	284	900	771	1219	1438	876	10045
lean & fat, broiled—*3 oz*	85	301	1102	1123	1946	2187	634	307	972	833	1317	1550	948	10046
lean, braised—*3 oz*	85	306	1100	1128	1934	2167	638	308	962	840	1307	1498	962	10049
lean, broiled—*3 oz*	85	332	1193	1224	2098	2351	692	333	1044	911	1419	1625	1045	10050
lean, panfried—*3 oz*	85	299	1074	1102	1888	2116	623	300	939	819	1277	1463	940	10197
center rib (roasts),														
lean & fat, roasted—*3 oz*	85	288	1053	1075	1857	2087	607	293	927	798	1256	1471	910	10047
lean, roasted—*3 oz*	85	310	1114	1143	1958	2195	646	311	974	851	1324	1517	975	10051
ground, ckd—*3 oz*	85	277	997	1023	1752	1964	578	279	871	761	1185	1357	872	10220
ham, cured (fully ckd ap),														
lean (4% fat), cnd—*3 oz*	85	179	702	677	1222	1351	410	186	606	516	705	973	621	10137
lean (4% fat), cnd, roasted—*3 oz*	85	204	802	774	1398	1545	469	213	694	590	806	1114	711	10138
lean (5% fat), roasted—*3 oz*	85	213	791	780	1412	1509	470	268	768	584	772	1156	638	10134
reg (11% fat), roasted—*3 oz*	85	202	750	740	1338	1430	445	253	728	553	731	1096	604	10136
reg (13% fat), cnd—*3 oz*	85	164	644	621	1122	1239	377	171	557	473	646	893	570	10139
reg (13% fat), cnd, roasted—*3 oz*	85	198	779	751	1357	1499	455	207	672	572	782	1080	689	10140
reg, center slice, lean & fat,														
unheated—*3 oz*	85	206	762	751	1361	1454	452	258	740	563	744	1114	615	10142
whole, lean & fat, roasted—*3 oz*	85	208	800	780	1442	1551	468	268	784	580	800	1240	625	10151
whole, lean & fat, unheated—*3 oz*	85	179	685	669	1237	1330	402	230	672	496	686	1063	536	10150

	WT (g)	TRY (mg)	THR (mg)	ISO (mg)	LEU (mg)	LYS (mg)	MET (mg)	CYS (mg)	PHE (mg)	TYR (mg)	VAL (mg)	ARG (mg)	HIS (mg)	REF
whole, lean, roasted—*3 oz*	85	255	947	933	1690	1805	562	320	920	699	923	1383	763	10153
whole, lean, unheated—*3 oz*	85	228	843	831	1505	1608	501	286	819	622	822	1232	680	10152
ham patties, cured, grilled—*2 oz patty*	60	93	355	349	631	678	211	107	338	262	347	515	291	10147
unheated—*2.3 oz patty*	65	97	370	363	657	706	219	112	352	272	361	536	303	10146
ham steak, extra lean, cured,														
unheated—*3 oz*	85	200	740	729	1319	1409	439	251	718	545	721	1080	596	10149
leg (rump & shank half),														
lean & fat, roasted—*3 oz*	85	275	1018	1035	1804	2032	584	283	903	768	1221	1459	869	10009
lean, roasted—*3 oz*	85	318	1142	1170	2006	2248	662	319	998	871	1356	1554	999	10011
loin blade (chops) w/bone,														
lean & fat, braised—*3 oz*	85	213	813	819	1453	1644	462	225	732	604	985	1225	676	10029
lean & fat, broiled—*3 oz*	85	221	839	847	1495	1691	478	233	752	626	1013	1249	702	10030
lean & fat, panfried—*3 oz*	85	207	795	799	1421	1610	450	220	717	589	964	1208	657	10178
lean, braised—*3 oz*	85	270	972	996	1707	1913	564	271	849	741	1154	1323	850	10033
lean, broiled—*3 oz*	85	274	984	1009	1729	1938	570	275	860	751	1170	1340	861	10034
lean, panfried—*3 oz*	85	267	961	984	1687	1891	557	269	840	733	1141	1307	840	10120
loin blade (roasts),														
lean & fat, roasted—*3 oz*	85	236	891	901	1584	1788	507	247	796	666	1073	1309	750	10031
lean, roasted—*3 oz*	85	287	1033	1059	1815	2033	598	288	903	788	1227	1406	904	10035
loin, whole, lean & fat, braised—*3 oz*	85	286	1045	1066	1843	2071	602	292	920	791	1247	1461	902	10021
lean & fat, broiled—*3 oz*	85	287	1049	1071	1850	2079	605	292	923	796	1252	1465	907	10022
lean & fat, roasted—*3 oz*	85	290	1047	1072	1843	2067	606	292	918	797	1246	1439	912	10023
lean, braised—*3 oz*	85	309	1109	1137	1948	2184	643	309	969	846	1318	1510	970	10025
lean, broiled—*3 oz*	85	309	1109	1137	1948	2184	643	309	969	846	1318	1510	970	10026
lean, roasted—*3 oz*	85	309	1111	1139	1952	2188	644	310	972	847	1320	1512	972	10027
rump, lean & fat, roasted—*3 oz*	85	301	1104	1125	1951	2194	636	308	975	836	1320	1556	949	10013
lean, roasted—*3 oz*	85	334	1201	1232	2110	2365	696	336	1050	916	1426	1635	1051	10015
sausage, fresh, ckd—														
1.1 oz patty (3 7/8"dia, 1/4" thick)	27	42	210	194	356	403	129	53	177	153	213	313	153	07064
sausage w/beef, ckd—														
1.1 oz patty (3 7/8" dia, 1/4" thick)	27	36	150	143	263	294	89	38	129	109	160	230	111	07065
shank, lean & fat, roasted—*3 oz*	85	256	956	970	1697	1915	547	266	851	718	1150	1389	811	10017
lean, roasted—*3 oz*	85	304	1095	1123	1924	2156	635	306	957	836	1301	1491	958	10019
shoulder, whole,														
lean & fat, roasted—*3 oz*	85	236	881	893	1561	1760	504	245	783	661	1057	1273	747	10071
lean, roasted—*3 oz*	85	274	983	1008	1727	1936	570	275	859	751	1168	1339	860	10073
sirloin (chops) w/bone,														
lean & fat, braised—*3 oz*	85	263	967	985	1710	1924	556	269	855	731	1158	1371	830	10053
lean & fat, broiled—*3 oz*	85	277	1017	1037	1799	2023	586	284	899	769	1217	1439	874	10054
lean, braised—*3 oz*	85	292	1048	1074	1841	2064	608	292	916	800	1245	1426	917	10057
lean, broiled—*3 oz*	85	308	1105	1133	1941	2175	641	309	966	843	1312	1504	966	10058
sirloin (roasts),														
lean & fat, roasted—*3 oz*	85	294	1057	1085	1858	2083	613	295	924	807	1256	1439	925	10055
lean, roasted—*3 oz*	85	311	1119	1147	1965	2202	649	312	978	853	1329	1522	978	10059
spareribs, sep lean & fat, braised—*3 oz*	85	314	1128	1157	1982	2221	654	315	986	861	1340	1535	987	10089
tenderloin, lean & fat, broiled—*3 oz*	85	320	1154	1182	2031	2278	668	322	1012	879	1374	1586	1005	10221
lean & fat, roasted—*3 oz*	85	298	1076	1102	1893	2122	623	300	943	819	1280	1475	938	10222
lean, broiled—*3 oz*	85	328	1181	1210	2075	2326	684	330	1032	901	1403	1607	1033	10223
lean, roasted—*3 oz*	85	303	1092	1120	1919	2151	633	305	955	833	1298	1487	955	10061
top loin (chops),														
lean & fat, braised—*3 oz*	85	293	1068	1091	1884	2117	616	298	940	810	1275	1490	924	10063
lean & fat, broiled—*3 oz*	85	324	1163	1193	2043	2290	674	325	1017	887	1381	1583	1017	10064
lean & fat, panfried—*3 oz*	85	305	1114	1136	1964	2207	642	310	980	844	1329	1555	962	10186
lean, braised—*3 oz*	85	314	1128	1157	1982	2222	655	315	986	861	1340	1536	987	10067
lean, broiled—*3 oz*	85	337	1209	1239	2124	2380	701	337	1057	922	1436	1646	1057	10068
lean, panfried—*3 oz*	85	329	1183	1213	2078	2330	686	331	1034	903	1405	1611	1035	10181
top loin (roasts),														
lean & fat, roasted—*3 oz*	85	311	1119	1147	1965	2202	649	312	978	853	1329	1522	978	10065
lean, roasted—*3 oz*	85	326	1174	1204	2062	2311	681	328	1026	895	1394	1598	1027	10069
Veal														
ground, broiled—*3 oz*	85	210	905	1021	1649	1708	484	234	836	660	1145	1219	752	17143
leg (top round),														
lean & fat, braised—*3 oz*	85	311	1343	1514	2446	2533	717	347	1240	980	1699	1808	1116	17095
lean & fat, breaded, panfried—*3 oz*	85	241	996	1138	1837	1822	536	279	960	734	1285	1341	813	17096
lean & fat, panfried—*3 oz*	85	273	1179	1329	2148	2224	630	304	1089	860	1492	1587	979	17097
lean & fat, roasted—*3 oz*	85	238	1029	1159	1874	1940	549	266	950	751	1301	1385	854	17098
lean, braised—*3 oz*	85	316	1363	1537	2484	2571	728	352	1259	995	1725	1835	1132	17100

	WT (g)	TRY (mg)	THR (mg)	ISO (mg)	LEU (mg)	LYS (mg)	MET (mg)	CYS (mg)	PHE (mg)	TYR (mg)	VAL (mg)	ARG (mg)	HIS (mg)	REF
lean, breaded, panfried—*3 oz*	85	251	1038	1185	1912	1900	558	289	998	764	1337	1397	847	17101
lean, pan fried—*3 oz*	85	286	1232	1389	2244	2324	658	318	1138	899	1559	1658	1023	17102
lean, roasted—*3 oz*	85	241	1042	1175	1899	1966	557	269	963	761	1319	1403	866	17103
leg & shoulder, cubed for stew,														
lean, braised—*3 oz*	85	301	1298	1463	2364	2447	693	335	1199	947	1641	1747	1078	17141
loin, lean & fat, braised—*3 oz*	85	260	1121	1264	2043	2114	598	290	1035	818	1418	1509	932	17105
lean & fat, roasted—*3 oz*	85	213	921	1038	1678	1737	492	238	851	672	1165	1240	765	17106
lean, braised—*3 oz*	85	289	1246	1405	2271	2351	666	322	1152	910	1577	1678	1035	17108
lean, roasted—*3 oz*	85	226	978	1102	1781	1844	522	252	903	713	1237	1316	812	17109
rib, lean & fat, braised—*3 oz*	85	279	1204	1357	2194	2272	643	311	1113	879	1524	1622	1000	17111
lean & fat, roasted—*3 oz*	85	207	890	1003	1621	1678	475	230	822	649	1125	1198	740	17112
lean, braised—*3 oz*	85	297	1278	1442	2330	2412	683	331	1182	933	1618	1721	1063	17114
lean, roasted—*3 oz*	85	222	956	1078	1743	1804	511	247	884	698	1210	1288	795	17115
shoulder, arm,														
lean & fat, braised—*3 oz*	85	289	1249	1408	2275	2355	667	323	1153	911	1579	1681	1038	17123
lean & fat, roasted—*3 oz*	85	219	945	1066	1723	1783	505	244	874	690	1196	1273	785	17124
lean, braised—*3 oz*	85	308	1327	1496	2417	2502	709	343	1226	968	1679	1786	1102	17126
lean, roasted—*3 oz*	85	225	971	1094	1768	1830	519	251	897	708	1227	1306	807	17127
shoulder, blade,														
lean & fat, braised—*3 oz*	85	269	1161	1309	2115	2190	621	300	1073	847	1469	1563	965	17129
lean & fat, roasted—*3 oz*	85	217	934	1052	1702	1761	499	241	863	682	1182	1257	776	17130
lean, braised—*3 oz*	85	281	1213	1367	2209	2287	648	314	1120	885	1534	1633	1007	17132
lean, roasted—*3 oz*	85	220	952	1073	1734	1795	508	246	880	694	1204	1282	791	17133
shoulder, whole (arm & blade),														
lean & fat, braised—*3 oz*	85	276	1191	1342	2169	2246	636	308	1100	869	1506	1603	989	17117
lean & fat, roasted—*3 oz*	85	218	940	1060	1713	1774	502	243	869	686	1190	1266	781	17118
lean, braised—*3 oz*	85	290	1250	1409	2278	2359	668	323	1155	913	1582	1684	1039	17120
lean, roasted—*3 oz*	85	222	959	1080	1747	1808	512	247	886	700	1213	1290	796	17121
sirloin, lean & fat, braised—*3 oz*	85	269	1161	1308	2115	2190	620	300	1073	847	1469	1562	965	17135
lean & fat, roasted—*3 oz*	85	216	933	1052	1701	1761	499	241	863	682	1182	1257	776	17136
lean, braised—*3 oz*	85	292	1261	1421	2298	2378	673	326	1165	921	1595	1697	1048	17138
lean, roasted—*3 oz*	85	226	978	1102	1781	1844	522	252	903	713	1237	1316	813	17139
Internal Organs & Other Cuts														
brain, beef, panfried—*3 oz*	85	88	507	414	802	639	222	190	540	379	524	583	272	13319
simmered—*3 oz*	85	77	447	365	706	563	196	167	476	334	462	513	240	13320
brain, lamb, braised—*3 oz*	85	110	478	424	833	684	213	111	514	390	508	719	283	17186
panfried—*3 oz*	85	149	646	574	1127	925	287	150	695	528	687	972	383	17187
brain, pork, braised—*3 oz*	85	132	482	477	899	811	205	182	525	433	587	540	277	10097
brain, veal, braised—*3 oz*	85	98	483	397	753	604	214	102	513	378	464	535	244	17189
panfried—*3 oz*	85	123	609	501	950	762	270	128	648	477	586	675	309	17190
chitterlings, pork, simmered—*3 oz*	85	52	383	357	688	558	165	77	349	322	427	714	183	10099
ears, pork, simmered—*1 ear (3.9 oz)*	111	34	529	405	971	813	142	158	566	354	708	1416	212	10101
feet, pork, cured, pickled—*3 oz*	85	23	310	196	506	495	127	101	333	184	287	862	127	10132
simmered—*3 oz*	85	32	440	277	718	702	179	144	473	261	408	1224	179	10173
heart, beef, simmered—*3 oz*	85	274	1155	1073	2165	2016	626	321	1108	889	1277	1636	673	13322
heart, lamb, braised—*3 oz*	85	230	1001	920	1805	1599	465	178	918	661	1057	1388	485	17192
heart, pork, braised—*1 heart (4.6 oz)*	129	351	1335	1467	2748	2518	779	546	1344	1042	1613	2046	774	10104
heart, veal, braised—*3 oz*	85	264	1095	1186	1944	2131	564	266	1074	812	1295	1537	666	17194
jowl, pork, raw—*3 oz*	85	18	179	143	379	449	81	48	203	88	259	560	61	10105
kidneys, beef, simmered—*3 oz*	85	295	1046	884	1737	1442	451	65	1040	814	1352	1272	565	13324
kidneys, lamb, braised—*3 oz*	85	271	946	800	1509	1303	408	230	931	708	1179	1160	506	17196
kidneys, pork, braised—*3 oz*	85	280	895	1153	1938	1555	463	473	1019	777	1244	1327	519	10107
kidneys, veal, braised—*3 oz*	85	287	1020	951	1811	1488	469	248	1061	858	1183	1379	541	17198
liver, beef, braised—*3 oz*	85	298	949	949	1950	1439	524	318	1104	822	1280	1303	567	13326
panfried—*3 oz*	85	327	1040	1040	2137	1577	574	349	1210	901	1403	1428	621	13327
liver, lamb, braised—*3 oz*	85	302	1124	1119	2122	1405	564	272	1160	927	1431	1457	610	17200
panfried—*3 oz*	85	252	938	935	1773	1174	471	228	969	774	1194	1217	510	17201
liver, pork, braised—*3 oz*	85	311	941	1122	1971	1706	548	417	1083	754	1366	1363	602	10111
liver, veal, braised—*3 oz*	85	193	782	809	1497	829	291	203	889	660	1029	883	401	17203
panfried—*3 oz*	85	265	1077	1114	2060	1141	400	280	1224	910	1415	1216	553	17204
lungs, beef, braised—*3 oz*	85	158	647	827	1273	1229	347	266	705	391	854	1049	527	13329
lungs, lamb, braised—*3 oz*	85	173	621	534	1352	1093	305	265	696	476	931	1017	425	17206
lungs, pork, braised—*3 oz*	85	124	496	564	1095	1029	228	222	587	400	840	734	357	10113
lungs, veal, braised—*3 oz*	85	127	592	660	910	1180	252	136	565	337	677	0	0	17208
pancreas (sweetbread), beef, braised—*3 oz*	85	298	1068	1165	1799	1699	417	295	958	1006	1235	1316	453	13332
pancreas (sweetbread), lamb, braised—*3 oz*	85	248	714	683	1242	1676	280	248	652	466	838	1148	558	17211

	WT (g)	TRY (mg)	THR (mg)	ISO (mg)	LEU (mg)	LYS (mg)	MET (mg)	CYS (mg)	PHE (mg)	TYR (mg)	VAL (mg)	ARG (mg)	HIS (mg)	REF
pancreas (sweetbread), pork,														
braised—*3 oz*	85	531	1089	1272	1811	1670	400	310	1039	1016	1306	1396	469	10116
spleen, beef, braised—*3 oz*	85	222	840	823	1884	1543	393	618	857	608	1284	1236	765	13334
spleen, lamb, braised—*3 oz*	85	248	918	1425	2001	1742	428	288	1022	655	1468	1421	749	17215
spleen, pork, braised—*3 oz*	85	246	959	1070	1960	1791	445	307	1024	672	1304	1308	571	10118
spleen, veal, braised—*3 oz*	85	201	829	940	1300	1515	446	241	727	558	950	0	0	17217
stomach, pork, raw—*3 oz*	85	83	434	476	842	743	245	0	446	350	588	785	209	10119
tail, pork, simmered—*3 oz*	85	87	506	332	809	867	260	187	434	289	434	997	260	10175
thymus (sweetbread), beef,														
braised—*3 oz*	85	143	672	633	1239	1545	258	238	532	386	805	1224	327	13338
thymus (sweetbread), veal,														
braised—*3 oz*	85	240	1262	1584	2034	2375	764	0	1055	0	1486	0	0	17219
tongue, beef, simmered—*3 oz*	85	145	818	809	1404	1449	397	247	776	608	899	1197	487	13340
tongue, lamb, braised—*3 oz*	85	185	829	717	1305	1298	388	201	684	543	878	1208	405	17221
tongue, pork, braised—*3 oz*	85	236	865	934	1642	1675	459	0	849	0	1065	1265	514	10122
tongue, veal, braised—*3 oz*	85	237	884	942	1584	1616	453	218	865	658	1008	1285	501	17223
tripe, beef, raw—*3 oz*	85	97	428	501	806	887	268	143	400	337	521	846	309	13341

20. MEATS, LUNCHEON & SNACK

Frankfurters & Other Luncheon-Type Sausages

	WT (g)	TRY (mg)	THR (mg)	ISO (mg)	LEU (mg)	LYS (mg)	MET (mg)	CYS (mg)	PHE (mg)	TYR (mg)	VAL (mg)	ARG (mg)	HIS (mg)	REF
beef sausage, smoked, ckd														
1.5 oz sausage	43	55	229	262	445	465	141	78	218	198	267	375	193	13357
beerwurst, pork & beef—*2 oz*	56	97	374	382	673	728	217	100	335	284	431	548	301	07931
bockwurst (pork, veal, milk, eggs),														
raw—*3.2 oz sausage*	91	119	545	553	983	1037	337	147	492	402	617	863	399	07006
bratwurst, beef & pork, smoked														
2.3 oz	66	71	307	320	535	596	240	69	267	255	306	505	261	07922
pork, beef, turkey, lite,														
smoked—*2.3 oz*	66	96	373	405	689	721	220	102	343	296	436	564	281	07924
pork, ckd—*3 oz link (4/12 oz pkg)*	85	96	473	437	802	910	291	121	400	345	481	706	345	07013
veal, ckd—*3 oz*	84	119	513	579	935	969	275	133	474	375	649	691	427	07910
brotwurst (pork & beef w/nfdm)														
2.5 oz link (7/lb)	70	92	419	424	756	797	258	114	379	310	473	662	305	07015
chicken, beef & pork sausage,														
skinless, smoked—*1 link*	84	122	475	515	877	917	281	130	436	376	555	718	358	07928
chorizo (pork & beef)														
2.1 oz link (4″ long)	60	167	884	1324	1025	1448	282	166	689	449	548	1016	433	07019
frankfurter, beef—*1.5 oz frank*	43	52	223	249	427	454	137	52	209	177	261	326	156	07022
heated—*1.8 oz frank*	52	65	277	310	530	563	170	64	260	220	324	404	193	07945
frankfurter, beef & pork—*1.6 oz frank*	45	53	209	213	380	409	121	55	189	158	240	318	163	07023
frankfurter, chicken—*1.6 oz frank*	45	46	260	206	461	493	154	59	231	176	241	401	163	07024
frankfurter, meat,														
fat free, Oscar Mayer—*1.8 oz frank*														
heated—*1 frank*	52	55	235	263	449	477	144	55	220	186	275	343	164	07949
unheated—*1 frank*	52	58	246	276	472	501	151	57	231	196	289	359	172	07950
frankfurter, pork—*1 link*	76	114	426	434	761	853	243	118	382	321	515	619	357	07939
frankfurter, pork & beef w/am chs														
(cheesefurter)—*1.5 oz frank*	43	65	232	267	473	499	155	65	241	224	297	361	202	07016
frankfurter, pork & turkey,														
Oscar Mayer—*1.6 oz frank*	45	58	219	241	394	441	132	57	197	181	266	320	167	07240
frankfurter, turkey—*1.6 oz frank*	45	51	307	243	523	557	181	47	266	228	263	419	244	07025
italian sausage, pork, ckd—*2.4 oz link*	67	108	531	490	900	1020	326	135	449	387	539	792	387	07089
sweet—*3 oz link*	84	93	350	368	638	674	203	92	317	276	411	484	280	07914
turkey, smoked—*2 oz*	56	117	458	529	822	948	293	114	413	402	551	724	314	07927
knockwurst/knackwurst														
(pork & beef)—*2.5 oz sausage*	72	99	311	460	629	727	199	162	361	353	460	678	226	07038
polish sausage,														
beef w/chicken, hot—*5 pieces*	55	76	325	336	592	611	208	86	296	244	373	509	244	07915
pork—*8 oz sausage*														
(10″ long, 1 1/4″ dia)	227	313	1342	1387	2443	2520	860	356	1224	1008	1541	2100	1008	07059
pork & beef, smoked—*2.7 oz*	76	81	353	369	616	686	277	80	308	293	353	581	300	07916
pork & beef sausage w/cheddar														
cheese, smoked—*2.7 oz*	77	116	416	477	847	893	277	116	431	400	531	647	362	07917
smoked sausage (smokie),														
pork—*2.4 oz link (4″ long)*	68	147	632	647	1151	1187	405	169	577	475	726	989	475	07074
pork & beef—*2.4 oz link (4″ long)*	68	73	316	330	551	614	248	71	275	262	316	520	269	07075
pork & beef w/flour & nfdm														
2.4 oz link (4″ long)	68	95	389	422	732	734	244	110	367	312	460	591	295	07076

	WT (g)	TRY (mg)	THR (mg)	ISO (mg)	LEU (mg)	LYS (mg)	MET (mg)	CYS (mg)	PHE (mg)	TYR (mg)	VAL (mg)	ARG (mg)	HIS (mg)	REF
pork & beef w/nfdm														
2.4 oz link (4″ long)	68	92	375	411	710	709	234	103	354	307	449	553	282	07077
turkey sausage, breakfast, mild														
2 links (2 oz)	56	117	458	529	822	948	293	114	413	402	551	724	314	07919
hot, smoked—*2 oz*	56	117	458	529	822	948	293	114	413	402	551	724	314	07929
vienna sausage, beef & pork, cnd														
.6 oz sausage (2″ long, 7/8″ dia)	16	17	57	89	128	127	42	28	68	55	92	113	44	07083
Lunch Meats & Spreads														
barbeque loaf—*.8 oz slice*	23	39	157	168	295	303	91	45	147	124	183	224	119	07001
beef, chopped, smoked—*1 oz slice*	28	46	237	232	422	461	137	67	212	171	260	382	164	13358
jellied lunch meat—*1 oz slice*	28	38	208	200	368	409	118	55	188	143	231	368	140	13353
loaf lunch meat—*1 oz slice*	28	29	157	151	278	309	89	42	142	108	174	279	106	07042
sandwich steaks, flaked, chpd														
formed, thinly sliced—*2 oz steak*	56	115	393	402	752	783	219	90	356	293	455	633	298	13342
thin sliced lunch meat														
5 slices (.7 oz)	21	48	247	242	441	482	143	70	221	179	271	399	171	07043
beef pastrami—*1 oz slice*	28	44	182	209	354	370	112	62	174	158	213	298	154	13355
berliner, pork & beef—*.8 oz slice*	23	25	107	112	186	208	84	24	93	89	107	176	91	07004
blood sausage (blood pudding)														
.9 oz slice	25	45	143	80	348	263	50	45	205	85	255	170	178	07005
bologna, beef—*1 oz slice*	28	31	128	146	249	260	78	43	122	111	149	209	108	07007
bologna, beef & pork—*1 oz slice*	28	31	130	128	246	246	71	34	125	99	152	204	82	07008
bologna, pork—*1 oz slice*	28	42	179	186	327	337	115	48	164	135	206	281	135	07010
bologna, pork & turkey, lite—*2 oz*	56	57	200	235	400	372	122	85	225	170	263	352	132	07936
bologna, pork, turkey, & beef—*1 oz*	28	35	143	151	262	287	83	38	133	109	172	254	101	07937
bologna, turkey—*1 oz slice*	28	31	184	145	313	333	108	28	159	137	157	251	146	07011
braunschweiger (pork liver sausage)														
.6 oz slice (2 1/2″ dia, 1/4″ thick)	18	26	96	87	186	164	56	45	100	77	111	138	58	07014
chicken breast, fat-free, mesquite														
flavor, sliced—*2 slices*	42	77	288	341	504	561	184	96	271	221	339	452	201	07932
fat-free, oven-roasted, sliced														
2 slices	42	77	288	341	504	561	184	96	271	221	339	452	201	07933
chicken roll, breast meat,														
oven-roasted—*2 oz*	56	90	334	398	587	654	214	111	315	258	393	520	235	07935
light meat—*2 slices (2 oz)*	57	121	454	537	794	883	289	152	426	348	533	711	316	07017
chicken spread, cnd—*1 oz*	28	55	204	246	360	403	131	66	192	159	241	313	145	07018
corned beef, cnd—*.7 oz slice*	21	52	215	246	418	436	132	73	205	186	250	351	181	13348
jellied loaf—*1 oz slice*	28	46	250	241	444	493	142	67	227	172	278	444	168	07020
ham & cheese loaf—*1 oz slice*	28	58	201	211	379	422	123	66	193	157	225	313	190	07032
Oscar Mayer—*1 oz slice*	28	63	188	219	397	446	123	47	212	205	269	257	188	07211
ham & cheese spread—*1 oz (~2T)*	28	104	191	217	421	413	133	71	216	186	284	250	167	07033
ham, chopped, cnd—*.7 oz slice*	21	38	151	145	262	290	88	40	131	111	151	209	134	07026
packaged—*1 oz slice*	28	58	213	216	385	429	127	72	193	149	224	337	195	07027
ham, minced—*.7 oz slice*	21	33	154	147	264	286	96	40	135	113	157	215	127	07030
ham salad spread—*1 oz (~2T)*	28	25	115	113	203	216	64	14	99	78	125	166	98	07031
ham, sliced, lean (5% fat)—*1 oz slice*	28	65	241	237	430	459	143	81	234	178	235	352	194	07028
reg (11% fat)—*1 oz slice*	28	59	219	216	390	417	130	74	213	161	213	319	176	07029
headcheese (pork)—*1 oz slice*	28	24	125	152	283	271	74	62	170	130	184	321	83	07034
honey loaf (pork & beef)—*1 oz slice*	28	53	191	197	338	376	110	54	169	145	228	262	163	07035
honey roll sausage (beef)—*.8 oz slice*	23	35	179	175	319	349	103	51	160	129	196	289	124	07088
kielbasa/kolbassy (pork & beef														
w/nfdm)—*.9 oz slice*	26	36	112	166	227	263	72	59	130	127	166	245	82	07037
lebanon bologna (beef)—*.8 oz slice*	23	32	99	147	201	232	63	52	115	113	147	217	72	07039
liver cheese (pork liver)—*1.3 oz slice*	38	78	247	240	506	448	130	125	272	177	306	315	149	07040
liver pate, chicken, cnd—*1 oz (2 T)*	28	55	168	206	335	267	95	61	194	137	242	228	97	07053
goose, smoked, cnd—*1 oz (~2T)*	28	45	142	170	288	242	76	43	159	112	201	196	85	07054
truffle flavor—*2 oz*	56	88	318	310	588	469	159	95	326	254	430	501	167	07942
unspecified, cnd—*1 oz (~2T)*	28	44	159	155	294	235	80	48	163	127	215	251	83	07055
liverwurst/liver sausage (pork)														
.6 oz slice (2 1/2″ dia, 1/4″ thick)	18	27	121	118	205	208	51	27	111	65	154	146	81	07041
liverwurst spread—*4 T*	55	83	369	359	626	635	157	82	339	199	471	447	246	07911
luxury loaf (pork)—*1 oz slice*	28	60	246	228	425	463	131	43	201	180	250	328	184	07060
macaroni & cheese loaf,														
chicken, pork, & beef—*1 slice*	38	55	169	206	344	274	101	68	189	144	225	242	123	07940
mortadella (beef & pork)—*.5 oz slice*	15	23	95	106	182	189	59	31	90	80	110	154	78	07050
mother's loaf (pork)—*.7 oz slice*	21	36	127	134	236	247	75	43	120	94	140	191	112	07061

	WT (g)	TRY (mg)	THR (mg)	ISO (mg)	LEU (mg)	LYS (mg)	MET (mg)	CYS (mg)	PHE (mg)	TYR (mg)	VAL (mg)	ARG (mg)	HIS (mg)	REF
olive loaf pork														
1 oz slice	28	29	132	118	244	227	84	40	117	107	142	163	82	07051
pastrami, beef, 98% fat-free														
6 slices	57	89	371	425	722	754	228	126	354	321	433	607	313	07925
peppered loaf (pork & beef)														
1 oz slice	28	53	191	197	338	376	110	54	169	145	228	262	163	07056
pepperoni, pork & beef—.2 oz slice														
(1 3/8″ dia, 1/8″ thick)	6	12	51	54	95	98	32	15	47	40	59	81	40	07057
pickle & pimento loaf pork														
1 oz slice	28	32	146	137	265	251	71	33	123	109	156	186	96	07058
picnic loaf (pork & beef)														
1 oz slice	28	40	184	163	321	334	106	45	150	128	180	249	122	07062
pork & beef loaf, Dutch Brand														
1.3 oz slice	38	55	231	217	412	446	134	62	208	168	255	338	176	07021
pork & beef lunch meat—*2 oz slice*	57	76	310	367	597	675	164	131	291	286	406	527	231	07047
pork & beef luncheon sausage														
.8 oz slice (4″ dia, 1/8″ thick)	23	37	153	181	294	333	81	65	143	141	200	260	114	07090
New England Brand—*.8 oz slice*														
(4″ dia, 1/8″ thick)	23	44	174	175	313	348	103	57	157	123	185	276	150	07091
pork lunch meat, cnd—*.7 oz slice*	21	26	102	120	200	196	70	45	103	80	137	182	75	07045
poultry (chicken/turkey) salad														
spread—*1 oz (~2T)*	28	36	139	164	246	283	90	39	127	115	165	218	97	07067
salami, beef—*.8 oz slice (4″ dia, 1/8″ thick)*	23	26	106	122	207	216	65	36	101	92	124	174	90	07068
salami, beef & pork—*.8 oz slice*														
(4″ dia, 1/8″ thick)	23	26	120	155	214	255	69	45	111	127	154	197	83	07069
salami, beerwurst, beef—*.8 oz slice*														
(4″ dia, 1/8″ thick)	23	26	106	122	207	216	65	36	101	92	124	174	90	07002
pork—*.8 oz slice (4″ dia, 1/8″ thick)*	23	26	130	112	217	237	82	25	104	93	117	186	96	07003
salami, dry/hard,														
pork—*.4 oz slice (3 1/8″ dia, 1/16″ thick)*	10	25	101	108	163	188	47	29	94	69	112	137	61	07071
(3 1/8″ dia, 1/16″ thick)	10	25	101	108	163	188	47	29	94	69	112	137	61	07071
pork & beef—*.4 oz slice*														
(3 1/8″ dia, 1/16″ thick)	10	21	96	97	173	182	59	26	87	71	108	152	70	07072
salami, italian, pork—*1 oz*	28	71	283	304	455	526	132	81	263	192	314	384	172	07926
pork & beef, dry, sliced,														
50% less Na—*5 slices*	28	59	269	272	485	511	166	73	243	199	303	424	196	07941
salami, pork & beef, less Na														
3.5 oz	100	114	521	675	929	1107	301	196	481	552	668	855	359	07913
salami, turkey—*2 slices (2 oz)*	57	103	405	466	722	845	260	105	364	353	484	656	279	07070
sandwich spread, pork & beef														
1 oz (~2T)	28	23	94	94	168	186	55	30	84	66	100	148	78	07073
swisswurst, pork & beef w/swiss														
cheese, smoked—*2.7 oz*	77	116	416	477	847	893	277	116	431	400	531	647	362	07920
thuringer (cervelat), beef & pork														
.8 oz slice	23	33	137	157	267	278	84	46	131	118	160	224	115	07078
turkey breast—*.7 oz slice (3 1/2″ sq)*	21	54	210	246	377	445	137	49	188	187	251	330	147	07079
turkey, ham (cured thigh meat)														
2 slices	57	123	480	561	860	1017	312	112	428	426	573	753	337	07080
turkey pastrami—*2 slices*	57	116	455	523	810	947	292	117	408	396	543	735	313	07052
turkey roll, light & dark meat														
2 slices	57	114	451	518	803	940	291	114	405	392	538	729	311	07082
light meat—*2 slices*	57	117	465	534	827	968	299	117	417	404	555	752	320	07081
Meat-Based Snacks														
bacon & beef sticks—*1 oz*	28	59	269	272	485	511	166	73	243	199	303	424	196	07921
beef, dried—*5 slices (.7 oz)*	21	50	256	250	457	499	148	72	229	185	281	413	177	13350
beef sticks, smoked—*.7 oz stick*	20	37	166	164	295	304	91	58	160	119	190	304	106	19407
pork skins—*1 oz*	28	33	510	387	930	779	134	148	543	337	678	1355	203	19041
barbecue—*1 oz*	28	37	494	384	902	755	133	144	526	332	654	1273	201	19408
summer sausage sticks, pork &														
beef w/cheddar cheese—*1 oz*	28	42	151	174	308	325	101	42	157	146	193	235	132	07918
21. MEAT SUBSTITUTES & SOY PRODUCTS														
Meat Substitutes														
bacon, simulated meat product														
3 strips (.6 oz)	16	26	72	89	146	116	23	28	98	64	95	140	48	16104
meat extender, simulated														
meat product—*1 oz*	28	161	452	559	914	727	146	176	611	400	592	874	299	16106

	WT (g)	TRY (mg)	THR (mg)	ISO (mg)	LEU (mg)	LYS (mg)	MET (mg)	CYS (mg)	PHE (mg)	TYR (mg)	VAL (mg)	ARG (mg)	HIS (mg)	REF
sausage, simulated meat product														
.9 oz link	25	70	196	243	397	316	63	76	265	174	257	380	130	16107b
simulated meat product														
1.3 oz patty	38	106	298	369	603	480	96	116	403	264	391	577	197	16107a
Soy Products														
fuyu (salted & fermented tofu)														
.4 oz block	11	14	37	44	68	59	11	12	44	30	45	60	26	16132
prep w/Ca sulfate—.4 oz block	11	14	37	44	68	59	11	12	44	30	45	60	26	16432
koyadufu (dried tofu), frzn														
.6 oz piece	17	127	333	404	619	537	104	113	397	273	411	542	237	16128
prep w/Ca sulfate, frzn—.6 oz piece	17	127	333	404	619	537	104	113	397	273	411	542	237	16428
miso—1 cup (9.7 oz)	275	393	1757	2230	3105	1815	410	261	1639	996	2041	2054	905	16112
natto—1 cup (6.2 oz)	175	390	1423	1629	2641	2004	364	385	1647	973	1782	1591	896	16113
tempeh—1 cup (5.9 oz)	166	468	1321	1461	2374	1507	289	530	1482	1102	1527	2078	774	16114
tofu, extra firm, prep w/nigari														
1/5 block (3.2 oz)	91	147	387	470	720	623	121	131	460	317	478	630	276	16159
silken, lite, Mori-Nu—1 slice (3 oz)	84	81	200	272	457	360	74	78	305	211	270	443	147	16165
silken, Mori-Nu—1 slice (3 oz)	84	103	260	323	537	416	79	107	361	264	335	447	153	16163
tofu, firm, prep w/Ca sulfate														
1/2 cup (4.4 oz)	126	158	413	501	770	668	130	140	493	339	512	674	295	16126
prep w/Ca sulfate, raw														
1/2 cup (4.4 oz)	126	310	811	985	1511	1309	255	275	968	665	1003	1323	578	16426
prep w/nigari—1/4 block (4.3 oz)	122	242	631	766	1175	1019	198	214	753	517	781	1030	450	16160
silken, lite, Mori-Nu—1 slice (3 oz)	84	80	185	249	421	323	65	66	270	192	240	395	131	16164
silken, Mori-Nu—1 slice (3 oz)	84	71	240	293	492	386	89	84	331	251	323	434	142	16162
tofu, fried—.5 oz piece	13	35	91	111	170	147	29	31	109	75	113	149	65	16129
tofu, okara—1 cup (4.3 oz)	122	61	160	194	298	259	50	54	192	132	198	261	113	16130
tofu prep w/Ca sulfate, fried														
.5 oz piece	13	35	91	111	170	147	29	31	109	75	113	149	65	16429
tofu, soft, prep w/Ca sulfate &														
nigari—1/4 block (4.1 oz)	116	118	311	376	578	500	97	106	370	254	384	506	222	16127b
prep w/Ca sulfate, raw														
1 cup (8.7 oz)	248	253	665	804	1235	1069	208	226	791	543	821	1081	474	16127a
silken, Mori-Nu—1 slice (3 oz)	84	57	181	196	234	286	62	60	255	162	248	322	98	16161
22. MILKS, MILK BEVERAGES, & YOGURT														
Cow Milk														
buttermilk, cultured—8 fl oz	245	88	387	500	806	679	198	76	426	341	595	309	233	01088
buttermilk, dry—1 T	7	34	108	145	235	190	60	22	116	116	161	87	65	01094
condensed, sweetened, cnd—1 fl oz	38	43	136	182	295	238	75	28	145	145	201	109	81	01095
evaporated, nonfat, cnd—1 fl oz	32	34	109	146	237	192	60	22	116	116	162	87	66	01097
evaporated, whole, cnd—1 fl oz	32	31	98	132	213	173	55	20	105	105	146	79	59	01096b
4 fl oz	126	121	387	519	840	680	215	79	415	415	575	311	233	01096a
lowfat, 1% fat—8 fl oz	244	112	364	486	786	637	203	73	388	388	537	290	217	01082
pro fortified—8 fl oz	246	135	435	585	947	768	244	89	467	467	647	349	263	01084
w/nfdm—8 fl oz	245	120	385	517	835	676	213	78	412	412	571	309	230	01083
nonfat—8 fl oz	245	118	377	505	818	662	211	78	404	404	559	301	225	01085
pro fortified—8 fl oz	246	138	440	590	954	772	244	91	470	470	652	352	263	01087
w/nfdm—8 fl oz	245	123	394	529	858	693	221	81	421	421	586	316	238	01086
nonfat, dry—1/4 cup	30	153	490	656	1063	860	272	100	524	524	726	393	294	01091
Ca reduced—1 oz	28	140	449	601	974	788	249	92	480	480	665	360	270	01093
inst—1 1/3 cups (3.2 oz pkt)	91	450	1441	1933	3129	2533	801	296	1542	1542	2138	1157	866	01092
reduced fat, 2% fat—8 fl oz	244	115	366	490	795	644	205	76	393	393	544	295	220	01079
pro fortified—8 fl oz	246	138	438	588	952	770	244	91	470	470	649	352	263	01081
w/nfdm—8 fl oz	245	120	385	517	835	676	213	78	412	412	571	309	230	01080
whole, 3.3% fat—8 fl oz	244	112	364	486	786	637	203	73	388	388	537	290	217	01077
3.7% fat—8 fl oz	244	112	361	483	783	634	200	73	386	386	537	290	217	01078
low sodium—8 fl oz	244	107	342	459	742	600	190	71	366	366	505	273	205	01089
whole, dry—1/4 cup	32	119	380	509	825	668	211	78	407	407	564	305	228	01090
Cow Milk Beverages														
carob flavored mix in whole milk														
8 fl oz	256	113	364	486	786	637	202	74	389	389	538	289	218	14169
choc malted milk, whole milk—8 fl oz	265	125	395	519	848	670	215	93	427	419	578	334	239	14318
choc malted milk, whole milk														
w/added nutrients—8 fl oz	265	111	363	485	784	636	201	74	387	387	535	289	217	14316
choc milk, 1% fat milk—8 fl oz	250	115	365	490	793	643	203	75	390	390	543	293	220	01104
2% fat milk—8 fl oz	250	113	363	485	785	638	203	75	388	388	538	290	218	01103

	WT (g)	TRY (mg)	THR (mg)	ISO (mg)	LEU (mg)	LYS (mg)	MET (mg)	CYS (mg)	PHE (mg)	TYR (mg)	VAL (mg)	ARG (mg)	HIS (mg)	REF
prep from powdered mix														
w/aspartame—*6 fl oz*	204	78	235	298	479	390	114	53	259	247	349	218	133	14423
whole milk—*8 fl oz*	250	113	358	480	778	628	198	73	383	383	530	288	215	01102
whole milk w/choc powder—*8 fl oz*	266	122	388	511	825	668	207	80	418	412	575	325	229	14177
whole milk w/choc syrup—*8 fl oz*	282	121	386	508	823	668	209	82	417	412	572	324	228	14182
cocoa (hot choc), homemade														
2% milk—*8 fl oz*	250	133	415	538	865	703	215	90	453	438	620	370	240	01105
prep w/water from mix														
1 oz pkt in 6 fl oz water	206	43	130	163	262	212	62	29	142	134	192	119	72	14194
eggnog, nonalcoholic—*8 fl oz*	254	137	445	584	937	757	221	97	462	462	643	378	241	01057
mix in whole milk—*8 fl oz*	272	114	370	492	794	645	204	76	392	392	544	299	220	14245
malted milk, whole milk—*8 fl oz*	265	138	427	559	928	702	236	122	472	456	620	382	268	14312
whole milk w/added nutrients														
8 fl oz	265	111	363	485	784	636	201	74	387	387	535	289	217	14310
strawberry flavored milk,														
mix in whole milk—*8 fl oz*	266	112	364	487	787	638	202	74	388	388	537	290	218	14351
Cow Milk Mixes														
choc milk mix—*2–3 hp t*	22	10	24	24	38	31	6	8	30	24	37	35	11	14175
malted—*3 hp t (.7 oz)*	21	12	30	34	61	34	13	20	39	32	41	43	21	14317
w/aspartame—*.75 oz pkt*	21	77	231	292	471	383	112	53	255	242	343	215	131	14422
cocoa mix—*1 oz pkt (3–4 hp t)*	28	42	127	160	258	210	62	29	140	133	188	118	72	14192
eggnog mix, nonalcoholic—*2 rd t*	28	2	6	6	10	8	3	2	5	5	7	8	3	14244
malted milk—*3 hp t (.7 oz)*	21	26	63	73	140	67	34	49	82	68	83	90	49	14311
Cow Milk Yogurt														
lowfat, fruit flavor—*8 oz container*	227	61	454	602	1112	990	325	100	602	556	913	331	272	01122
lowfat, plain—*8 oz container*	227	68	490	649	1201	1069	352	109	649	602	985	359	295	01117
lowfat, van—*8 oz container*	227	64	459	611	1128	1003	329	102	611	565	926	336	277	01119
nonfat, plain—*8 oz container*	227	73	533	711	1310	1167	384	118	711	656	1076	390	322	01118
whole, plain—*8 oz container*	227	45	322	429	795	706	232	73	429	397	651	236	195	01116
Other Mammal Milks														
goat milk—*8 fl oz*	244	107	398	505	766	708	195	112	378	437	586	290	217	01106
human milk—*8 fl oz*	246	42	113	138	234	167	52	47	113	130	155	106	57	01107
indian buffalo milk—*8 fl oz*	244	129	444	495	893	683	237	117	395	447	534	278	190	01108
sheep milk—*8 fl oz*	245	206	657	828	1438	1257	380	86	696	688	1098	485	409	01109
Other (Non-Dairy) Milks														
soy milk—*8 fl oz*	245	105	277	353	590	439	98	115	370	274	345	524	174	16120
23. NUTS & SEEDS														
Nuts & Nut Products														
acorn flour, full-fat—*1 oz*	28	25	81	97	167	131	35	37	92	64	118	162	58	12060
acorns, dried—*1 oz*	28	27	87	105	180	141	38	40	99	69	127	174	63	12059
raw—*1 oz*	28	21	66	80	137	108	29	31	75	52	97	132	48	12058
almond butter—*1 T*	16	43	89	105	188	81	28	43	135	85	124	302	68	12195
almonds, dry roasted—*1 oz (~22 nuts)*	28	56	197	201	428	175	55	82	334	154	233	717	172	12063
honey roasted—*1 oz*	28	79	161	190	339	145	50	79	244	154	225	545	122	12206
oil roasted—*1 oz (22 nuts)*	28	54	190	193	411	168	53	79	321	148	223	690	166	12065
beechnuts, dried—*1 oz*	28	19	62	69	103	103	41	55	73	48	97	124	48	12077
brazilnuts, dried—*1 oz (6–8 nuts)*	28	73	129	168	332	151	284	98	209	128	255	669	113	12078
butternuts, dried—*1 oz (~9 nuts)*	28	102	263	330	616	216	171	136	404	274	431	1361	226	12084
cashew butter—*1 T*	16	44	109	134	236	150	50	52	145	90	191	320	73	12088
cashews, dry roasted—*1 oz*	28	66	166	205	360	229	77	79	221	137	291	487	112	12085
oil roasted—*1 oz (18 nuts)*	28	74	178	204	381	240	94	102	246	131	283	550	118	12086
raw—*1 oz*	28	80	193	221	412	260	101	110	266	142	306	594	128	12087
chestnuts, chinese, boiled &														
steamed—*1 oz*	28	10	32	30	50	44	20	21	36	24	42	83	23	12095
dried—*1 oz*	28	22	76	71	118	104	46	50	87	57	100	196	55	12094
raw—*1 oz*	28	14	47	44	73	64	28	31	53	35	62	120	34	12093
roasted—*1 oz*	28	15	50	47	77	68	30	33	57	38	66	129	36	12096
chestnuts, european,														
boiled & steamed—*1 oz*	28	6	20	22	33	33	13	18	24	15	31	40	15	12101
dried—*1 oz*	28	20	64	71	106	106	42	57	76	50	100	128	50	12099
raw—*1 oz*	28	8	24	27	40	40	16	22	29	19	38	48	19	12097
roasted—*1 oz (3 nuts)*	28	10	32	35	53	53	21	28	38	25	50	64	25	12167
chestnuts, japanese,														
boiled & steamed—*1 oz*	28	3	9	11	14	15	6	7	9	6	14	15	6	12203

	WT (g)	TRY (mg)	THR (mg)	ISO (mg)	LEU (mg)	LYS (mg)	MET (mg)	CYS (mg)	PHE (mg)	TYR (mg)	VAL (mg)	ARG (mg)	HIS (mg)	REF
dried—*1 oz*	28	21	59	72	91	96	35	43	57	42	87	97	37	12175
raw—*1 oz*	28	9	25	31	39	41	15	18	25	18	38	41	16	12202
roasted—*1 oz*	28	12	33	41	52	54	20	24	32	24	49	55	21	12204
coconut cream, raw—*8 fl oz*	240	101	317	341	646	384	163	173	442	269	528	1428	199	12115
sweetened, cnd—*8 fl oz*	296	92	290	314	592	352	148	157	406	246	482	1308	184	12116
coconut, dried—*1 oz*	28	23	70	76	143	85	36	38	98	60	117	316	44	12108
creamed—*1 oz*	28	17	54	58	110	66	28	29	75	46	90	244	34	12177
sweetened, flaked, cnd—*4 oz*	114	44	139	150	284	169	72	75	194	119	231	628	88	12110
sweetened, flaked, packaged—*1 oz*	28	11	33	36	68	41	17	18	46	28	55	151	21	12109
sweetened, shredded—*1 cup*	93	32	98	105	199	118	50	53	136	83	163	440	61	12179
toasted—*1 oz*	28	17	54	58	110	66	28	29	75	46	90	244	34	12114
coconut milk, cnd—*8 fl oz*	226	54	167	179	339	201	86	90	231	140	276	748	104	12118
frzn—*8 fl oz*	240	46	142	151	286	170	72	77	197	120	235	634	89	12176
raw—*8 fl oz*	240	65	199	216	408	242	103	108	278	170	334	902	127	12117
coconut, raw—*1.6 oz piece*														
(2″ × 2″ × 1/2″)	45	18	54	59	111	66	28	30	76	46	91	246	35	12104
coconut water—*8 fl oz*	240	19	62	67	127	77	31	34	89	53	106	283	41	12119
filberts (hazelnuts),														
dried—*1 oz (20 nuts)*	28	54	139	153	298	118	62	78	186	101	196	619	121	12120
dry roasted—*1 oz*	28	54	140	153	299	118	62	78	187	102	197	622	122	12122
ginkgo nuts, cnd—*1 oz (14 nuts)*	28	11	40	31	47	31	8	3	25	9	42	62	15	12129
dried—*1 oz*	28	48	179	140	211	138	37	15	114	41	190	281	68	12128
raw—*1 oz*	28	20	75	59	88	58	15	6	48	17	79	118	29	12127
hickorynuts, dried—*1 oz*														
(~9–10 nuts)	28	39	118	161	288	139	84	76	200	127	204	584	109	12130
macadamia nuts, dry roasted														
1 oz (10–12 nuts)	28	18	102	87	166	5	6	1	183	141	100	386	54	12132
raw—*1 oz (10–12 nuts)*	28	19	104	88	169	5	6	2	186	143	102	393	55	12131
mixed nuts, dry roasted—*1 oz*	28	74	167	208	384	199	64	80	267	189	262	628	134	12135
oil roasted—*1 oz*	28	69	159	203	376	184	95	82	258	183	262	567	132	12137
w/o peanuts, oil roasted—*1 oz*	28	71	159	197	354	191	97	85	230	143	267	557	116	12138
peanut butter, chunk style/crunchy														
2 T	32	75	263	270	499	276	94	99	399	313	323	920	195	16097
creamy/smooth—*2 T*	32	78	276	284	523	290	99	103	418	328	339	965	204	16098
peanut flour, defatted—*1 oz*	28	142	501	514	948	525	179	187	757	594	613	1748	369	16099
lowfat—*1 oz*	28	92	324	333	613	340	116	121	491	385	397	1132	239	16100
peanuts, all types, boiled														
1/2 cup (33 nuts)	28	37	129	133	245	136	46	48	196	154	158	452	95	16088
dry roasted—*1 oz (28 nuts)*	28	64	227	233	430	238	81	85	344	270	278	793	168	16090
oil roasted—*1 cup halves & whole*	144	369	1299	1333	2460	1362	465	487	1966	1542	1591	4537	959	16089
unroasted/raw—*1 oz*	28	70	247	254	468	259	89	93	374	294	303	864	183	16087
peanuts, spanish, oil roasted—*1 oz*	28	76	269	276	508	281	96	101	407	319	329	938	198	16092
unroasted/raw—*1 oz*	28	71	251	258	475	263	90	94	380	298	307	876	185	16091
peanuts, valencia, oil roasted—*1 oz*	28	74	259	266	491	272	93	97	393	308	318	906	192	16094
unroasted/raw—*1 oz*	28	68	241	247	456	252	86	90	364	286	295	840	178	16093
peanuts, virginia, oil roasted—*1 oz*	28	70	248	255	470	260	89	93	375	295	304	866	183	16096
unroasted/raw—*1 oz*	28	69	242	248	457	253	87	90	366	287	296	844	178	16095
pecans, dried—*1 oz (20 halves)*	28	26	86	94	167	80	51	43	119	60	115	330	73	12142
dry roasted—*1 oz*	28	27	89	97	173	83	53	44	123	62	119	342	76	12143
oil roasted—*1 oz*	28	26	86	94	168	81	51	43	120	60	116	331	73	12144
pilinuts, dried—*1 oz (15 nuts)*	28	53	114	135	249	103	111	53	139	107	196	424	71	12145
pine nuts, pignolia, dried														
1 oz (15–16 nuts)	28	85	213	261	484	252	120	122	257	246	347	1307	161	12147
pinyon, dried—*1 oz*	28	41	103	126	234	122	58	59	124	119	167	630	78	12149
pistachios, dried—*1 oz (47 nuts)*	28	76	188	252	435	322	95	100	297	116	347	568	142	12151
dry roasted—*1 oz (47 nuts)*	28	80	196	262	452	335	98	104	309	121	361	590	148	12152
soy nuts, dry roasted—*1 cup*	172	989	2957	3302	5544	4530	918	1097	3554	2575	3399	5282	1837	16111
roasted—*1 cup*	172	881	2632	2939	4933	4032	817	975	3161	2291	3024	4699	1634	16110
trail mix, tropical—*1 oz*	28	21	62	62	101	63	41	32	73	45	83	164	59	19061
w/choc chips—*1 oz*	28	46	140	155	267	164	61	53	192	142	197	419	100	19062
walnuts, black, dried—*1 oz*	28	89	202	270	472	200	131	129	306	207	356	1013	188	12154
english/persian, dried														
1 oz (14 halves)	28	48	167	175	328	119	66	58	199	114	211	638	109	12155
wheat-base formulated nuts,														
flavored—*1 oz*	28	48	155	155	272	248	77	63	164	136	199	275	106	12200
macadamia flavored—*1 oz*	28	39	133	136	239	214	67	52	143	120	174	228	91	12199
unflavored—*1 oz*	28	46	162	155	277	255	78	71	169	136	204	298	110	12140

	WT (g)	TRY (mg)	THR (mg)	ISO (mg)	LEU (mg)	LYS (mg)	MET (mg)	CYS (mg)	PHE (mg)	TYR (mg)	VAL (mg)	ARG (mg)	HIS (mg)	REF
Seeds & Seed Products														
breadfruit seeds, boiled—*1 oz*	28	25	77	89	113	114	19	23	160	109	107	99	41	12003
raw—*1 oz*	28	34	108	124	158	160	27	32	223	152	150	138	58	12001
roasted—*1 oz*	28	29	90	104	132	134	23	27	187	128	125	116	48	12158
cottonseed flour, lowfat—*1 oz*	28	211	516	503	953	708	227	366	869	503	716	1885	440	12008
partially defatted—*1 T*	5	31	76	74	140	104	33	54	128	74	105	277	65	12007
cottonseed kernels, roasted—*1 T*	10	49	121	117	223	165	53	86	203	117	167	440	103	12160
cottonseed meal, partially defatted														
1 oz	28	207	508	495	939	698	223	361	856	495	706	1857	433	12011
lotus seeds, dried—*1 oz (42 seeds)*	28	62	209	214	340	276	75	56	215	105	277	353	120	12013
raw—*1 oz*	28	17	56	57	91	74	20	15	58	28	74	95	32	12205
pumpkin & squash seed kernels,														
dried—*1 oz (142 seeds)*	28	121	253	354	582	513	154	84	342	285	552	1129	191	12014
roasted—*1 oz*	28	162	340	475	782	690	207	113	460	383	742	1517	256	12016
safflower seed kernels, dried—*1 oz*	28	51	164	201	323	150	80	87	226	149	287	490	127	12021
safflower seed meal, partially														
defatted—*1 oz*	28	113	361	442	711	329	175	192	497	327	632	1078	279	12022
sesame butter (tahini),														
from roasted & toasted kernels—*1 T*	15	56	106	110	195	82	84	51	135	107	143	378	75	12166
from unroasted kernels—*1 T*	14	55	104	108	193	81	83	51	133	105	140	373	74	12171
sesame butter paste—*1 T*	16	63	120	124	222	93	96	58	153	121	162	429	85	12169
sesame flour, high fat—*1 oz*	28	189	358	371	660	276	284	174	457	361	481	1278	254	12170
lowfat—*1 oz*	28	307	583	604	1075	450	464	283	744	588	784	2082	413	12033
partially defatted—*1 oz*	28	247	469	486	865	362	373	228	599	473	631	1674	332	12032
sesame meal, partially defatted—*1 oz*	28	104	197	204	364	152	157	96	252	199	265	704	140	12034
sesame seeds, kernels, dried—*1 T*	8	38	94	103	172	66	72	42	122	90	118	266	54	12201
toasted—*1 oz*	28	104	197	204	364	152	157	96	252	199	265	704	140	12029
sesame seeds, whole, dried—*1 T*	9	35	66	69	122	51	53	32	85	67	89	237	47	12023
roasted & toasted—*1 oz*	28	104	197	204	364	152	157	96	252	199	265	704	140	12024
sunflower seed butter—*1 T*	16	48	128	157	229	129	68	62	161	92	182	332	87	12040
sunflower seed flour, partially														
defatted—*1 T*	4	29	78	96	140	79	42	38	99	56	111	203	53	12041
sunflower seed kernels,														
dried—*1 cup w/o hulls*	144	501	1336	1640	2389	1349	711	649	1683	959	1894	3460	910	12036
dry roasted—*1 oz*	28	83	221	271	394	223	118	107	278	158	312	571	150	12037
oil roasted—*1 oz*	28	91	244	299	436	246	130	118	307	175	345	631	166	12038
toasted—*1 oz*	28	74	197	241	351	198	105	95	247	141	278	508	134	12039
watermelon seeds,														
dried—*1 oz (95 large seeds)*	28	109	311	376	602	248	234	123	569	284	436	1371	217	12174
24. POULTRY														
Chicken, Broiler/Fryer Parts														
back w/skin, flour coated & fried														
1/2 back (2.5 oz)	72	226	822	1001	1463	1599	529	272	790	647	973	1235	587	05050
breast w/skin, flour coated & fried														
1/2 breast (3.5 oz)	98	357	1300	1599	2306	2581	845	410	1228	1028	1531	1915	940	05059
roasted—*1/2 breast (3.5 oz)*	98	333	1219	1495	2154	2424	791	382	1146	960	1432	1800	879	05060
stewed—*1/2 breast (3.9 oz)*	110	343	1257	1541	2221	2499	815	395	1181	990	1476	1858	906	05061
breast w/o skin, flour coated & fried														
1/2 breast (3 oz)	86	335	1214	1518	2158	2439	796	368	1142	970	1427	1733	892	05063
roasted—*1/2 breast (3 oz)*	86	311	1127	1409	2002	2266	739	341	1059	900	1324	1609	828	05064
stewed—*1/2 breast (3.4 oz)*	95	322	1163	1454	2066	2339	762	352	1093	929	1365	1661	855	05065
drumstick w/skin, flour coated &														
fried—*1.7 oz drumstick*	49	150	549	672	972	1085	355	174	518	432	646	815	395	05068
roasted—*1.8 oz drumstick*	52	158	583	708	1028	1152	376	186	548	456	684	876	417	05069
stewed—*2 oz drumstick*	57	163	599	730	1057	1187	388	191	563	470	704	897	429	05070
drumstick w/o skin, roasted														
1.6 oz drumstick	44	145	526	657	934	1057	345	159	494	420	617	751	386	05073
leg w/skin, flour coated & fried														
4 oz leg	112	340	1245	1520	2205	2452	804	400	1180	980	1467	1858	893	05077
roasted—*4 oz leg*	114	332	1226	1487	2160	2421	791	393	1153	959	1440	1847	876	05078
stewed—*4.4 oz leg*	125	339	1253	1520	2208	2474	808	401	1178	980	1471	1884	894	05079
leg w/o skin, stewed—*3.6 oz leg*	101	310	1120	1401	1991	2253	734	339	1052	896	1316	1600	823	05083
neck w/skin, flour coated & fried														
1.3 oz neck	36	92	346	403	608	658	218	122	331	264	410	559	237	05086
simmered—*1.3 oz neck*	38	76	295	331	510	557	183	107	278	218	347	500	196	05087
neck w/o skin, simmered—*.63 neck*	18	52	187	233	332	375	122	57	175	149	219	267	137	05090

	WT (g)	TRY (mg)	THR (mg)	ISO (mg)	LEU (mg)	LYS (mg)	MET (mg)	CYS (mg)	PHE (mg)	TYR (mg)	VAL (mg)	ARG (mg)	HIS (mg)	REF
thigh w/skin, flour coated & fried														
2.2 oz thigh	62	187	685	835	1214	1345	442	222	652	539	808	1027	490	05093
roasted—2.2 oz thigh	62	174	643	779	1133	1269	415	206	605	502	755	971	458	05094
stewed—2.4 oz thigh	68	177	654	792	1153	1291	422	211	615	511	768	990	466	05095
thigh w/o skin, roasted—1.8 oz thigh	52	158	570	712	1012	1146	373	173	535	456	669	814	419	05098
wing w/skin, flour coated & fried														
1.1 oz wing	32	90	338	396	592	650	214	116	321	258	398	538	233	05102
roasted—1.2 oz wing	34	98	370	432	645	714	234	126	348	281	435	592	255	05103
stewed—1.4 oz wing	40	98	370	434	646	716	235	125	348	282	435	588	256	05104
Chicken, Broilers/Fryers														
dark meat w/skin, roasted—3 oz	85	246	910	1095	1601	1789	585	296	856	707	1069	1389	645	05037
stewed—3 oz	85	222	824	992	1449	1620	530	267	774	641	968	1255	584	05038
dark meat w/o skin, fried—3 oz	85	289	1038	1299	1850	2075	679	319	983	831	1222	1481	762	05044
roasted—3 oz	85	272	983	1228	1745	1976	643	298	923	785	1153	1403	722	05045
stewed—3 oz	85	258	932	1165	1657	1875	611	282	876	745	1095	1331	685	05046
light & dark meat w/skin,														
batter dipped & fried—3 oz	85	218	784	956	1405	1500	502	264	764	622	935	1171	557	05007
flour coated & fried—3 oz	85	275	1004	1223	1778	1972	648	325	953	789	1183	1501	718	05008
roasted—3 oz	85	259	959	1158	1688	1890	617	309	902	747	1126	1454	682	05009
stewed—3 oz	85	235	867	1048	1527	1709	558	280	815	677	1019	1313	617	05010
light & dark meat w/o skin,														
flour coated & fried—3 oz	85	304	1096	1370	1950	2196	717	334	1034	876	1289	1563	805	05012
roasted—3 oz	85	287	1039	1299	1845	2089	681	315	976	830	1220	1483	763	05013
stewed—3 oz	85	271	980	1225	1741	1970	642	297	921	783	1150	1399	720	05014
light meat w/skin,														
flour coated & fried—3 oz	85	292	1073	1306	1896	2114	693	344	1013	842	1262	1605	768	05031
roasted—3 oz	85	277	1022	1239	1801	2018	660	327	961	799	1200	1539	729	05032
stewed—3 oz	85	250	921	1119	1624	1821	594	295	866	721	1082	1385	658	05033
light meat w/o skin, fried—3 oz	85	326	1178	1472	2094	2366	772	357	1108	942	1384	1681	865	05040
roasted—3 oz	85	307	1109	1387	1971	2232	727	337	1042	887	1303	1584	815	05041
stewed—3 oz	85	286	1037	1296	1842	2086	679	315	974	829	1218	1481	762	05042
Chicken, Roasters														
dark meat w/o skin, roasted—3 oz	85	231	835	1044	1483	1679	547	253	785	667	980	1192	614	05120
light & dark meat w/skin,														
roasted—3 oz	85	226	841	1012	1478	1653	541	272	790	654	988	1280	596	05112
light & dark meat w/o skin,														
roasted—3 oz	85	248	898	1123	1595	1806	589	272	844	717	1054	1283	660	05114
light meat w/o skin, roasted—3 oz	85	269	974	1218	1731	1959	638	295	915	779	1144	1391	716	05118
Chicken, Stewers														
dark meat w/o skin, stewed—3 oz	85	280	1011	1263	1795	2032	662	306	949	808	1187	1443	743	05132
light & dark meat w/skin,														
stewed—3 oz	85	256	946	1146	1667	1867	609	303	889	739	1111	1428	674	05124
light & dark meat w/o skin,														
stewed—3 oz	85	303	1092	1365	1941	2197	716	331	1026	873	1283	1560	802	05126
light meat w/o skin, stewed—3 oz	85	328	1187	1482	2107	2386	777	360	1114	948	1393	1694	871	05130
Chicken, Unspecified Types														
cnd w/broth—5 oz can	142	345	1271	1541	2241	2505	815	422	1196	993	1494	1924	903	05277
Turkey, Roasters														
breast w/skin, roasted—3 oz	85	274	1082	1246	1928	2261	698	269	969	944	1291	1737	747	05218
breast w/o skin, roasted—3 oz	85	190	750	861	1335	1547	480	190	676	648	894	1203	511	05229
dark meat w/skin, roasted—3 oz	85	258	1024	1173	1822	2129	659	261	919	887	1221	1661	704	05208
dark meat w/o skin, roasted—3 oz	85	279	1091	1275	1953	2310	710	255	973	969	1302	1710	765	05212
leg w/skin, roasted														
8.6 oz leg w/o bone	245	779	3067	3545	5473	6431	1982	752	2744	2688	3660	4902	2127	05222
light meat w/skin, roasted—3 oz	85	269	1063	1217	1890	2209	683	271	954	921	1268	1726	730	05206
light meat w/o skin, roasted—3 oz	85	292	1142	1335	2044	2418	743	267	1018	1014	1363	1790	801	05210
skin, roasted—1.2 oz														
(yield from 1 lb of turkey)	34	57	254	229	418	425	142	118	240	162	300	549	137	05204
wing w/skin, roasted														
3.2 oz wing w/o bone	90	262	1053	1173	1855	2134	666	297	951	881	1255	1781	703	05226
Turkey, Young Hen														
dark meat w/skin, roasted—3 oz	85	258	1017	1169	1811	2121	655	255	911	885	1213	1638	701	05240
dark meat w/o skin, roasted—3 oz	85	275	1074	1256	1925	2277	700	252	959	955	1284	1686	754	05244

	WT (g)	TRY (mg)	THR (mg)	ISO (mg)	LEU (mg)	LYS (mg)	MET (mg)	CYS (mg)	PHE (mg)	TYR (mg)	VAL (mg)	ARG (mg)	HIS (mg)	REF
light & dark meat w/skin, roasted—*3 oz*	85	264	1044	1200	1859	2178	672	261	935	909	1245	1680	720	05232
light & dark meat w/o skin, roasted—*3 oz*	85	282	1106	1293	1981	2343	720	258	987	983	1321	1734	776	05234
light meat w/skin, roasted—*3 oz*	85	269	1064	1225	1896	2222	686	266	954	927	1270	1714	734	05238
light meat w/o skin, roasted—*3 oz*	85	289	1131	1321	2025	2394	736	264	1008	1004	1350	1772	793	05242
Turkey, Young Tom														
dark meat w/skin, roasted—*3 oz*	85	277	1085	1267	1942	2298	706	253	967	963	1295	1701	761	05268
dark meat w/o skin, roasted—*3 oz*	85	259	1023	1176	1822	2134	660	258	917	890	1221	1652	706	05264
young tom, light & dark meat w/ skin, roasted—*3 oz*	85	264	1042	1196	1854	2170	671	263	934	904	1243	1683	717	05256
young tom, light & dark meat w/o skin, roasted—*3 oz*	85	283	1110	1298	1988	2352	723	259	990	986	1325	1741	779	05258
young tom, light meat w/skin, roasted—*3 oz*	85	267	1056	1210	1878	2197	679	267	946	915	1259	1707	726	05262
young tom, light meat w/o skin, roasted—*3 oz*	85	288	1130	1321	2024	2394	735	264	1008	1004	1349	1772	792	05266
Turkey, Unspecified Types														
breast w/skin, prebasted, roasted *3 oz*	85	209	822	949	1466	1719	530	208	737	718	982	1321	568	05293
cnd w/broth—*5 oz can*	142	371	1461	1680	2603	3043	939	378	1309	1271	1744	2361	1005	05284
diced, seasoned—*1 oz*	28	58	228	262	405	474	146	59	204	198	272	368	157	05285
ground, ckd—*2.9 oz patty*	82	251	987	1152	1766	2089	643	230	880	876	1178	1547	693	05306
patties, breaded/battered & fried *3.3 oz patty*	94	157	562	673	1049	1091	359	164	556	509	696	858	391	05292
roast, boneless, frzn, seasoned, roasted—*3 oz*	85	206	806	943	1443	1708	524	189	719	717	962	1264	565	05296
sticks, breaded/battered & fried *2.25 oz stick*	64	109	388	465	726	748	248	114	387	351	481	591	269	05300
thigh w/skin, prebasted, roasted *11.1 oz thigh (w/o bone)*	314	659	2587	2996	4619	5423	1670	644	2314	2267	3090	4135	1793	05294
Other Poultry														
cornish game hen, w/skin, roasted—*3 oz*	85	210	779	935	1369	1529	500	253	732	604	914	1190	551	05308
w/o skin, roasted—*3 oz*	85	231	836	1046	1486	1683	548	253	786	669	983	1194	615	05310
duck, w/skin, roasted—*3 oz*	85	197	657	741	1245	1263	404	254	639	544	797	1091	393	05140
w/o skin, roasted—*3 oz*	85	278	853	1025	1686	1708	540	307	836	760	1044	1274	527	05142
goose, w/skin, roasted—*3 oz*	85	282	955	1006	1793	1690	517	332	897	684	1047	1331	595	05147
w/o skin, roasted—*3 oz*	85	343	1052	1265	2080	2108	666	378	1032	938	1289	1572	650	05149
guinea hen, w/o skin, raw—*3 oz*	85	205	741	927	1317	1491	485	224	696	592	870	1058	545	05152
pheasant, w/skin, raw—*3 oz*	85	258	942	1044	1590	1713	547	259	745	615	1046	1200	734	05153
w/o skin, raw—*3 oz*	85	279	1003	1125	1696	1833	583	263	782	657	1109	1218	798	05154
quail, w/o skin, raw—*3 oz*	85	290	927	1009	1586	1619	586	323	802	859	1003	1172	701	05158
squab (pigeon), w/o skin, raw—*3 oz*	85	233	745	812	1276	1302	471	259	645	690	807	943	564	05161
Internal Organs														
giblets, chicken, fried—*3 oz*	85	317	1247	1386	2211	1996	689	371	1258	907	1476	1835	645	05021
simmered—*3 oz*	85	251	996	1102	1756	1603	549	292	995	721	1172	1468	512	05022
giblets, turkey, simmered—*3 oz*	85	261	1023	1138	1819	1658	563	301	1026	745	1216	1503	531	05172
gizzard, chicken, simmered—*3 oz*	85	207	1063	1089	1621	1595	605	303	960	701	1034	1658	465	05024
gizzard, turkey, simmered—*3 oz*	85	224	1153	1181	1757	1729	656	328	1040	761	1120	1797	504	05174
heart, chicken, simmered—*3 oz*	85	287	1017	1203	1958	1882	542	305	1006	804	1272	1440	589	05026
heart, turkey, simmered—*3 oz*	85	292	1030	1220	1983	1907	549	309	1019	815	1289	1459	597	05176
liver, chicken, simmered—*3 oz*	85	292	921	1100	1868	1567	490	278	1030	728	1305	1269	550	05028
liver, duck, raw—*3 oz*	85	224	708	846	1437	1205	377	214	792	561	1004	976	423	05143
liver, goose, raw—*3 oz*	85	196	619	740	1255	1053	330	187	693	490	877	853	370	05150
liver, turkey, simmered—*3 oz*	85	287	906	1082	1839	1542	483	274	1014	717	1284	1249	541	05178
25. SALAD DRESSINGS														
Low & Reduced Calorie														
french—*1 T*	16	0	0	0	0	0	0	0	0	0	0	0	0	04020
italian—*1 T*	15	0	0	0	0	0	0	0	0	0	0	0	0	04021
russian—*1 T*	16	1	4	5	7	5	2	1	4	4	5	6	2	04022
thousand island—*1 T*	15	2	6	7	10	8	3	2	5	5	7	8	3	04023

	WT (g)	TRY (mg)	THR (mg)	ISO (mg)	LEU (mg)	LYS (mg)	MET (mg)	CYS (mg)	PHE (mg)	TYR (mg)	VAL (mg)	ARG (mg)	HIS (mg)	REF
Regular														
blue (bleu) cheese/roquefort—*1 T*	15	11	26	38	65	62	20	4	37	44	52	24	26	04539
french—*1 T*	16	1	5	5	8	6	2	2	4	4	6	7	2	04120
homemade—*1 T*	14	0	0	0	0	0	0	0	0	0	0	0	0	04133
homemade, ckd—*1 T*	16	26	80	105	160	127	48	26	88	78	118	82	44	04134
italian—*1 T*	15	2	6	6	9	7	3	2	5	5	6	7	3	04114
mayonnaise type—*2 T*	15	2	7	8	12	9	3	2	6	6	8	9	3	04018
russian—*1 T*	15	4	13	14	20	16	6	4	11	11	15	17	6	04015
sesame seed—*1 T*	15	7	7	7	12	21	4	0	13	15	10	60	5	04016
thousand island—*1 T*	16	2	8	8	12	10	4	3	6	6	9	10	4	04017
vinegar & oil, homemade—*1 T*	16	0	0	0	0	0	0	0	0	0	0	0	0	04135
26. SAUCES, GRAVIES, & CONDIMENTS														
Condiment Sauces														
catsup (ketchup)—*1 T*	15	2	5	4	6	6	1	1	5	3	5	5	4	11935
mustard (prepared sce)—*1 t*	5	4	8	7	12	10	3	4	7	5	9	12	5	02046
pepper sce, Tabasco—*1 t*	4.7	1	2	2	3	3	1	1	2	1	3	3	1	06169
pepper/hot sce—*1 t*	4.7	0	1	1	1	1	0	0	1	1	1	1	0	06168
soy sauce, made w/soy (tamari)—*1 T*	18	33	73	88	132	132	30	19	96	62	94	73	39	16124
made w/soy & wheat (shoyu)—*1 T*	16	12	33	39	66	47	12	15	44	30	41	57	21	16123
Entrée Sauces														
guava sce—*1 cup*	238	7	29	29	50	21	5	0	2	10	26	19	7	09143
tomato sce, cnd—*1 cup*	245	22	74	64	91	93	17	20	69	44	66	66	51	11549
spanish style—*1 cup*	244	24	81	68	98	100	17	22	73	46	71	71	56	11649
w/herbs & cheese—*1 cup*	244	51	144	171	276	271	68	39	171	146	200	217	122	11555
w/mushrooms—*1 cup*	245	42	105	91	135	181	34	17	96	56	100	103	69	11551
w/tomato pieces—*1 cup*	244	22	73	63	90	93	17	20	68	44	66	66	51	11559
w/onions—*1 cup*	245	39	91	103	120	145	25	44	88	71	83	279	61	11553
w/onions, green peppers, & celery—*1 cup*	250	20	55	53	70	75	13	18	53	35	50	93	38	11557
white sce, med, homemade—*1/2 cup*	125	54	173	233	375	304	96	35	185	185	256	139	104	06166
thick, homemade—*1/2 cup*	125	50	161	216	350	284	89	33	173	173	239	129	98	06167
thin, homemade—*1/2 cup*	125	58	184	248	400	324	103	38	196	196	274	148	111	06165
Olives														
black (manzanillo/mission), cnd														
1 small	3.2	0	1	1	2	1	0	0	1	1	1	2	1	09193a
1 large	4.4	0	1	1	2	1	1	0	1	1	2	3	1	09193b
green (sevailano/ascolano), cnd														
1 jumbo	8	0	2	3	5	3	1	0	3	2	4	6	2	09194b
1 super colossal	15	0	5	5	9	6	2	0	5	4	7	12	4	09194a
Pickles														
pickle, dill—*1 spear*	30	2	5	6	8	8	2	1	5	3	6	12	3	11937a
1 large (4" long)	135	7	23	26	35	35	7	5	23	14	27	54	12	11937b
pickle relish, hamburger—*1/2 cup*	122	9	23	26	37	34	9	9	23	15	27	51	15	11958
pickle relish, hot dog—*1/2 cup*	122	23	57	61	92	84	22	23	56	39	68	118	37	11944
pickle relish, sweet—*1 T*	15	1	2	2	3	2	1	0	2	1	2	3	1	11945
pickle, sour—*1 med (3 3/4" long)*	65	2	6	7	9	9	2	1	6	4	7	14	3	11941
pickle, sweet (gherkin)														
1 small (2 1/2" long)	15	0	2	2	2	2	0	0	2	1	2	4	1	11940a
1 large (3" long)	35	1	4	4	6	5	1	1	4	2	4	8	2	11940b
27. SOUPS														
Condensed														
celery, crm of—*10.8 oz can*	305	46	143	189	302	180	73	46	189	131	217	143	95	06010
cheese—*11 oz can*	312	175	462	783	1245	924	284	109	677	605	924	393	356	06011
chicken, crm of—*10.8 oz can*	305	104	317	415	641	522	195	122	372	287	421	406	223	06016
mushroom, crm of—*10.8 oz can*	305	70	189	235	384	265	95	61	226	183	262	204	113	06043
tomato—*10.8 oz can*	305	49	125	143	241	122	55	67	171	104	162	146	88	06159
Condensed, Prepared With Milk														
asparagus, crm of—*1 cup (8 fl oz)*	248	84	260	340	558	432	144	67	290	270	384	231	159	06201
celery, crm of—*1 cup (8 fl oz)*	248	74	241	322	518	394	131	55	273	248	360	206	149	06210
cheese—*1 cup (8 fl oz)*	251	128	371	567	906	700	218	83	474	444	650	309	256	06211
chicken, crm of—*1 cup (8 fl oz)*	248	99	312	414	657	533	181	87	347	312	444	312	201	06216
clam chowder, new england														
1 cup (8 fl oz)	248	117	350	451	719	605	203	102	374	337	489	407	265	06230

	WT (g)	TRY (mg)	THR (mg)	ISO (mg)	LEU (mg)	LYS (mg)	MET (mg)	CYS (mg)	PHE (mg)	TYR (mg)	VAL (mg)	ARG (mg)	HIS (mg)	REF
mushroom, crm of—*1 cup (8 fl oz)*	248	84	260	340	553	429	141	62	288	270	377	231	156	06243
pea, green—*1 cup (8 fl oz)*	254	130	485	541	1016	831	206	117	572	447	711	853	279	06249
potato, crm of—*1 cup (8 fl oz)*	248	82	243	320	513	402	131	64	278	255	362	221	149	06253
tomato—*1 cup (8 fl oz)*	248	77	233	303	494	370	124	64	265	238	335	206	146	06359
tomato bisque—*1 cup (8 fl oz)*	251	80	248	321	520	409	131	60	271	254	356	211	153	06358
Condensed, Prepared With Water														
asparagus, crm of—*1 cup (8 fl oz)*	244	29	78	98	163	112	41	29	95	76	115	85	49	06401
bean w/franks—*1 cup (8 fl oz)*	250	105	413	488	823	680	125	110	558	298	550	525	260	06406
bean w/pork—*1 cup (8 fl oz)*	253	83	326	385	650	536	99	89	440	235	435	415	205	06404
beef noodle—*1 cup (8 fl oz)*	244	46	154	188	315	261	90	59	195	124	207	198	112	06409
black bean—*1 cup (8 fl oz)*	247	64	249	287	422	415	62	59	311	49	284	331	163	06402
cheese—*1 cup (8 fl oz)*	247	72	190	321	511	380	116	44	279	249	380	163	146	06411
chicken & dumplings—*1 cup (8 fl oz)*	241	53	193	243	407	378	108	72	224	142	277	292	137	06412
chicken, crm of—*1 cup (8 fl oz)*	244	41	129	171	264	215	81	51	154	117	173	166	93	06416
chicken gumbo—*1 cup (8 fl oz)*	244	22	83	100	168	161	46	17	98	68	117	122	59	06417
chicken noodle—*1 cup (8 fl oz)*	241	39	128	159	265	219	77	46	164	106	176	166	94	06419
chicken rice—*1 cup (8 fl oz)*	241	41	142	178	270	251	92	51	152	123	188	234	101	06423
chicken veg—*1 cup (8 fl oz)*	241	31	113	135	231	222	60	24	133	94	159	169	80	06425
chili beef—*1 cup (8 fl oz)*	250	70	275	328	553	455	85	73	373	200	368	350	175	06426
clam chowder, new england *1 cup (8 fl oz)*	244	54	149	183	288	251	90	56	159	127	195	229	137	06430
minestrone—*1 cup (8 fl oz)*	241	31	104	130	236	183	43	34	154	84	178	198	72	06440
mushroom, crm of—*1 cup (8 fl oz)*	244	34	90	112	181	127	44	27	107	88	122	95	54	06443
pea, green—*1 cup (8 fl oz)*	250	73	303	298	623	510	105	80	378	250	443	708	170	06449
pea, split w/ham—*1 cup (8 fl oz)*	253	101	364	435	711	696	139	134	455	319	491	703	215	06451
pepperpot—*1 cup (8 fl oz)*	241	41	195	234	402	311	92	60	234	157	299	494	92	06452
potato, crm of—*1 cup (8 fl oz)*	244	24	61	76	117	83	29	27	83	61	93	76	39	06453
scotch broth—*1 cup (8 fl oz)*	241	43	154	186	316	304	84	34	181	128	217	231	108	06455
stockpot—*1 cup (8 fl oz)*	247	42	151	183	311	299	82	35	178	126	215	227	109	06460
tomato—*1 cup (8 fl oz)*	244	20	51	59	100	51	22	27	71	41	66	61	37	06559
tomato beef w/noodles—*1 cup (8 fl oz)*	244	41	144	171	290	242	83	54	181	115	193	183	102	06461
tomato bisque—*1 cup (8 fl oz)*	247	22	67	77	126	89	30	25	77	59	86	67	44	06558
turkey noodle—*1 cup (8 fl oz)*	244	37	124	151	254	212	73	46	156	102	168	159	90	06465
turkey veg—*1 cup (8 fl oz)*	241	27	96	116	198	190	53	22	113	82	135	145	67	06466
veg beef—*1 cup (8 fl oz)*	244	49	173	210	359	344	95	39	205	146	246	261	122	06471
veg vegetarian—*1 cup (8 fl oz)*	241	14	75	99	147	99	24	24	99	48	99	99	48	06468
veg w/beef broth—*1 cup (8 fl oz)*	241	22	72	92	164	125	31	24	106	58	125	137	51	06472
Ready-To-Serve														
beef, chunky—*1 cup (8 fl oz)*	240	113	466	593	898	929	247	122	482	353	636	610	276	06070
chicken, chunky—*1 cup (8 fl oz)*	240	118	418	528	883	816	233	156	482	312	600	631	298	06015
chicken noodle, chunky *1 cup (8 fl oz)*	240	122	437	552	924	854	245	163	504	326	629	662	312	06018
split pea w/ham, chunky *1 cup (8 fl oz)*	240	110	391	468	766	749	149	144	490	343	526	758	233	06050
turkey, chunky—*1 cup (8 fl oz)*	236	99	404	514	781	809	215	106	418	307	552	531	238	06064
veg, chunky—*1 cup (8 fl oz)*	240	26	108	161	271	190	26	26	161	82	190	190	82	06067
28. SPICES, HERBS, & FLAVORINGS														
basil, ground—*1 T*	4.5	10	26	26	49	28	9	7	33	19	32	30	13	02003
raw—*1 T*	5	2	5	5	10	6	2	1	7	4	6	6	3	02044
caraway seeds—*1 T*	7	17	53	58	85	72	25	23	61	45	73	88	39	02005
chives, freeze-dried—*1/4 cup*	0.8	2	7	7	10	8	2	0	5	5	7	12	3	11615
raw, chopped—*1 T*	3	1	4	4	6	5	1	0	3	3	4	7	2	11156
dill seeds—*1 T*	7	0	40	54	65	73	10	0	47	0	78	88	22	02016
dill weed sprigs, raw—*1 cup*	9	1	6	18	14	22	1	2	6	9	14	13	6	02045
fennel seeds—*1 T*	6	15	36	42	60	45	18	13	39	25	55	41	20	02018
fenugreek seeds—*1 T*	11	43	99	137	193	185	37	41	120	84	121	271	73	02019
garlic powder—*1 T*	8	17	37	52	82	46	27	14	39	17	57	134	25	02020
ginger root, ground—*1 T*	5	3	9	13	19	15	3	2	12	5	19	11	8	02021
raw, sliced—*1/4 cup*	24	3	9	12	18	14	3	2	11	5	18	10	7	11216
mustard seeds, yellow—*1 T*	11	58	120	119	196	167	53	64	117	82	146	193	84	02024
onion, dehydrated flakes—*1/4 cup*	14	18	30	44	44	60	10	22	32	31	29	168	20	11284
powder—*1 T*	7	8	14	21	23	33	6	13	17	16	17	94	10	02026
parsley, freeze-dried—*1/4 cup*	1.4	7	0	0	0	44	3	0	0	0	0	0	0	11625
sprigs, raw—*10 sprigs*	10	5	12	12	20	18	4	1	15	8	17	12	6	11297
peppermint, raw—*2 T*	3.2	2	5	5	9	5	2	1	6	4	6	6	2	02064
poppy seeds—*1 T*	9	23	81	81	134	99	42	41	79	61	116	180	48	02033

	WT (g)	TRY (mg)	THR (mg)	ISO (mg)	LEU (mg)	LYS (mg)	MET (mg)	CYS (mg)	PHE (mg)	TYR (mg)	VAL (mg)	ARG (mg)	HIS (mg)	REF
rosemary, raw—1 T	1.7	1	2	2	4	2	1	1	3	2	3	3	1	02063
shallots, freeze-dried—1/4 cup	3.6	5	17	19	26	22	5	0	14	13	20	32	8	11640
raw, chopped—1 T	10	3	10	11	15	13	3	0	8	7	11	18	4	11677
spearmint, dried—1 T	1.6	5	13	13	24	14	4	4	16	10	16	15	6	02066
raw—2 T	11	6	15	15	27	16	5	4	18	11	18	17	7	02065
thyme, ground—1 T	4.3	8	11	20	18	9	0	0	0	0	22	0	0	02042
raw—1 T	0.8	1	1	2	2	1	0	0	0	0	2	0	0	02049

29. SUGARS, SYRUPS, & OTHER SWEETENERS

honey, strained—1 T	21	1	1	2	2	2	0	1	2	2	2	1	0	19296
jam/preserves—1 T	20	2	5	3	7	6	0	1	4	5	4	6	3	19297
apricot—1 T	20	2	5	3	7	6	0	1	4	5	4	6	3	19719
marmalade, orange—1 T	20	1	1	2	1	3	1	1	2	1	3	4	1	19303
syrup, malt—1 T	24	18	50	50	91	64	26	16	62	41	73	68	32	19352
syrup, pancake/waffle w/butter—1 T	20	0	0	0	0	0	0	0	0	0	0	0	0	19113

30. VEGETABLES & VEGETABLE DISHES

Flower, Stem, & Stalk Vegetables

asparagus, boiled—1/2 cup (6 spears)	90	23	65	86	102	111	23	28	55	37	90	109	36	11012
cnd—1 cup	242	51	145	191	225	244	51	61	123	82	198	242	80	11015
frzn, boiled—1 cup	180	52	148	196	230	252	50	63	126	85	205	248	83	11019
broccoli, boiled—1 med stalk	180	56	175	209	250	270	65	38	162	121	245	279	95	11091
chopped, frzn, boiled—1 cup	184	59	186	223	267	287	68	40	173	129	261	296	101	11093
raw, chopped—1 cup	88	26	80	96	115	124	30	18	74	55	113	128	44	11090
spears, frzn, boiled—1/2 cup	92	29	93	111	133	144	34	20	86	64	131	148	51	11095
cauliflower, boiled—1/2 cup pieces	62	15	42	43	66	61	16	13	41	25	57	55	23	11136
frzn, boiled—1 cup pieces	180	38	106	110	169	155	41	34	104	63	146	140	59	11138
raw—1 cup pieces	100	26	72	75	116	106	28	23	71	43	99	95	40	11135
cauliflower, green, ckd—1/5 head	90	36	99	104	160	147	39	32	97	59	138	131	55	11967
raw—1 cup pieces	64	25	68	72	110	101	27	22	67	41	95	91	38	11965
celery, diced, boiled—1 cup	150	17	36	38	59	48	11	8	36	17	50	36	21	11144
raw—1 med stalk (7.5" long)	40	4	9	9	14	12	2	2	9	4	12	9	5	11143
kohlrabi, sliced, boiled—1 cup	165	18	86	137	117	97	23	12	68	0	87	183	33	11242
leeks, boiled—1 leek	124	7	42	35	64	52	12	17	37	27	38	52	17	11247
raw—1 leek (~1 cup)	89	11	56	46	85	69	16	22	49	36	50	69	22	11246
onion, green/spring (scallion), raw, chopped—1 cup	100	20	72	77	109	91	20	0	59	53	81	132	32	11291
sesbania flower, steamed—1 cup	104	18	53	63	99	59	15	11	64	0	72	64	24	11448

Fruit (Seed-Containing) Vegetables

acorn squash, boiled, mshd—1 cup	245	25	49	64	93	61	20	15	64	56	71	91	32	11484
cubed, baked—1 cup	205	33	68	90	131	84	29	21	90	78	98	127	43	11483
breadfruit, raw—1/4 small	96	0	50	61	62	36	10	9	25	18	45	0	0	09059
butternut squash,														
cubed, baked—1 cup	205	27	55	72	105	68	23	16	72	62	80	103	35	11486
mshd, frzn, boiled—1 cup	240	41	89	115	168	108	36	26	115	98	127	163	55	11488
calabash (white-flowered) gourd,														
cubed, boiled—1 cup	146	4	25	47	51	29	6	0	20	0	38	20	6	11219
chayote, boiled—1 cup pieces	160	13	50	53	93	48	2	0	58	38	75	42	18	11150
crookneck/straightneck squash, raw,														
sliced—1 cup	130	10	30	44	72	68	18	13	43	33	55	52	26	11467
sliced, boiled—1 cup	180	14	40	59	95	90	23	18	58	43	74	68	36	11468
sliced, cnd—1 cup	216	11	32	48	78	73	19	13	48	35	60	56	28	11471
sliced, frzn, boiled—1 cup	192	21	60	88	144	136	35	27	86	65	111	104	54	11474
cucumber, raw w/peel														
1 med 8 1/4" long	301	15	57	63	87	87	18	12	57	33	66	132	30	11205
eggplant (aubergine), boiled—1 cup	99	8	30	36	51	39	9	4	35	22	43	46	19	11210
raw—1 cup	82	7	30	37	52	39	9	5	35	22	43	47	19	11209
green beans (snap beans),														
boiled—1 cup	125	25	103	86	145	114	29	23	86	55	116	95	44	11053
cnd—1 cup	135	16	68	57	96	74	19	15	57	36	77	62	30	11056
frzn, boiled—1 cup	135	22	88	73	123	97	24	19	73	46	99	81	38	11061
hubbard squash,														
boiled, mshd—1 cup	236	50	104	137	198	130	42	31	137	118	151	194	66	11491
cubed, baked—1 cup	205	43	90	119	172	113	37	27	119	103	131	168	57	11490
okra (lady's finger/gumbo),														
boiled—8 pods (3" long)	85	14	52	55	83	64	17	15	52	69	72	66	25	11279
sliced, frzn—1/2 cup	92	16	63	66	100	77	20	18	63	84	87	80	30	11281

	WT (g)	TRY (mg)	THR (mg)	ISO (mg)	LEU (mg)	LYS (mg)	MET (mg)	CYS (mg)	PHE (mg)	TYR (mg)	VAL (mg)	ARG (mg)	HIS (mg)	REF
peppers, ancho, dried—*1 pepper*	17	26	72	63	103	88	24	37	61	42	83	94	39	11978
peppers, chili, green, cnd—*1 cup*	139	14	36	32	53	44	13	19	31	21	42	47	19	11980
peppers, chili, green, hot														
cnd—*1 pepper*	73	9	24	21	34	29	8	12	20	14	28	31	13	11329
raw—*1 pepper*	45	12	33	29	47	40	11	17	28	19	38	43	18	11670
peppers, chili, red, hot														
cnd—*1 pepper*	73	9	24	21	34	29	8	12	20	14	28	31	13	11820
raw—*1 pepper*	45	12	33	29	47	40	11	17	28	19	38	43	18	11819
sun-dried—*1 pepper*	0.5	1	2	2	3	2	1	1	2	1	2	3	1	11962
peppers, hungarian, raw—*1 pepper*	27	3	8	7	11	10	3	4	7	5	9	11	4	11981
peppers, jalapeno, cnd—*1 pepper*	22	3	7	7	11	9	3	4	6	4	9	10	4	11632
raw—*1 pepper*	14	2	7	6	10	9	2	4	6	4	8	9	4	11979
peppers, pimiento, cnd—*1 T*	12	2	5	4	7	6	2	3	4	3	6	6	3	11943
peppers, sweet (bell), green, chpd,														
frzn, boiled—*1 cup pcs*	135	16	47	42	66	57	15	24	39	27	54	61	26	11338
cnd—*1 cup halves*	140	14	41	36	59	50	14	21	35	24	48	53	22	11335
raw—*1 med (2 3/4" long)*	119	13	39	35	55	46	13	20	32	21	44	51	21	11333
sliced, boiled—*1 cup*	135	16	46	41	65	55	15	24	39	26	53	59	26	11334
peppers, sweet (bell), red, chpd,														
frzn, boiled—*1 cup pcs*	135	16	47	42	66	57	15	24	39	27	54	61	26	11918
raw—*1 med (2 3/4" long)*	119	13	39	35	55	46	13	20	32	21	44	51	21	11821
sliced, boiled—*1 cup*	135	16	46	41	65	55	15	24	39	26	53	59	26	11823
peppers, sweet (bell), yellow, raw														
1 large (3 3/4" long)	186	24	69	60	97	82	22	35	58	39	78	89	37	11951
plantain, sliced, ckd—*1 cup*	154	14	32	34	55	57	15	18	42	31	43	102	60	09278
pumpkin, boiled, mshd—*1 cup*	245	22	51	56	83	96	20	5	56	74	61	96	27	11423
cnd—*1 cup*	245	32	78	83	125	147	29	7	86	113	93	145	42	11424
scallop squash, raw, sliced—*1 cup*	130	14	38	56	91	87	22	17	55	42	70	66	34	11475
sliced, boiled—*1 cup*	180	16	45	67	110	103	27	20	65	50	85	79	40	11476
snow peas (edible podded peas),														
boiled—*1 cup*	160	51	184	301	427	376	21	59	168	184	510	251	32	11301
frzn, boiled—*1 cup*	160	54	197	323	458	403	22	64	179	197	547	269	35	11303
raw—*1 cup whole*	63	17	62	101	144	127	7	20	57	62	172	84	11	11300
spaghetti squash, boiled/														
baked—*1 cup*	155	14	28	37	53	34	11	8	37	31	40	51	17	11493
squash, summer (marrow),														
all varieties, raw, sliced—*1 cup*	113	12	32	47	78	73	19	14	46	35	60	57	28	11641
all varieties, sliced, boiled—*1 cup*	180	14	40	59	95	90	23	18	58	43	74	68	36	11642
squash, winter, all varieties, cubed,														
baked—*1 cup*	205	27	55	72	103	68	23	16	72	62	78	100	35	11644
tomato paste, cnd—*6 oz can*	170	43	141	121	173	179	31	36	133	85	128	126	99	11546
tomato puree, cnd—*1 cup*	250	28	95	80	118	123	23	25	88	55	85	83	65	11547
tomato, green, raw—*1 med*	123	11	37	36	54	54	12	20	38	26	38	36	22	11527
tomato, orange, raw—*1 tomato*	111	9	32	30	47	47	11	17	33	22	33	32	20	11695
tomato, red, boiled—*1 cup*	240	19	65	62	94	94	22	34	67	43	65	62	38	11530
raw—*1 med (2 3/5" dia)*	123	7	26	25	38	38	9	14	27	18	27	26	16	11529e
raw, chopped, sliced—*1 cup*	123	7	26	25	38	38	9	14	27	18	27	26	16	11529e
stewed—*1 cup*	101	19	55	65	107	63	24	29	76	41	76	68	36	11660
stewed, cnd—*1 cup*	255	18	59	56	89	89	20	31	64	41	64	56	36	11533
sun-dried—*1 cup*	54	56	193	183	279	280	66	99	198	131	195	185	116	11955
sun-dried, cnd, packed in oil—*1 cup*	110	41	141	133	204	205	48	73	144	96	143	135	85	11956
wedges in tomato jce, cnd—*1 cup*	261	16	52	50	76	76	18	26	55	37	52	50	31	11535
whole, peeled, cnd—*1 cup*	240	17	58	53	82	82	19	29	58	38	58	55	34	11531
tomato, red, cherry, raw—*1 cup*	149	9	31	30	46	46	10	16	33	22	33	31	19	11529a
tomato, red, italian, raw—*1 tomato*	62	4	13	12	19	19	4	7	14	9	14	13	8	11529d
tomato, red, plum, raw—*1 tomato*	62	4	13	12	19	19	4	7	14	9	14	13	8	11529c
tomato, yellow, raw—*1 tomato*	212	15	51	49	76	76	17	28	53	36	53	51	32	11696
waxgourd (chinese preserving melon),														
cubed, boiled—*1 cup*	175	4	0	0	0	16	5	0	0	0	0	0	0	11594
yellow snap beans, boiled—*1 cup*	125	25	103	86	145	114	29	23	86	55	116	95	44	11724
cnd—*1 cup*	135	16	68	57	96	74	19	15	57	36	77	62	30	11932
frzn—*1 cup*	135	22	88	73	123	97	24	19	73	46	99	81	38	11732
zucchini, baby, raw—*1 med*	11	3	7	11	17	17	4	3	11	8	14	13	6	11953
cnd, italian style—*1 cup*	227	20	57	84	136	129	34	25	82	61	104	98	50	11481
raw, sliced—*1 cup*	113	11	32	47	77	72	19	14	46	35	59	55	28	11477
sliced, boiled—*1 cup*	180	11	27	41	67	63	16	13	40	31	52	49	25	11478
sliced, frzn, boiled—*1 cup*	223	22	62	91	149	143	36	27	89	69	116	107	56	11480

	WT (g)	TRY (mg)	THR (mg)	ISO (mg)	LEU (mg)	LYS (mg)	MET (mg)	CYS (mg)	PHE (mg)	TYR (mg)	VAL (mg)	ARG (mg)	HIS (mg)	REF
Leafy Vegetables														
amaranth leaves, boiled—*1 cup*	132	36	112	135	220	144	41	33	150	90	156	137	58	11004
raw—*1 cup*	28	9	28	33	55	36	10	8	37	22	38	34	15	11003
beet greens, boiled—*1/2 cup*	144	58	109	76	166	108	30	35	98	88	109	105	56	11087
brussels sprouts, boiled—*1/2 cup*	78	22	71	78	89	90	19	12	58	0	91	119	44	11099
frzn—*1 cup*	155	62	202	222	254	257	54	36	164	0	259	338	127	11101
cabbage, chinese, pak-choi,														
raw, shredded—*1/2 cup*	70	11	34	60	62	62	6	12	31	20	46	59	18	11116
shredded, boiled—*1 cup*	170	26	87	151	155	158	15	29	78	51	117	148	46	11117
cabbage, chinese, pe-tsai,														
raw, shredded—*1/2 cup*	76	9	30	52	53	54	5	10	27	17	40	51	16	11119
cabbage, chinese, pe-tsai,														
sliced, boiled—*1 cup*	119	18	58	101	105	106	11	20	52	35	79	100	31	11120
cabbage, green, raw, shredded														
1 cup	70	11	34	50	51	47	10	8	32	17	43	57	20	11109
shredded, boiled—*1/2 cup*	75	8	26	38	39	35	8	6	24	13	32	43	15	11110
cabbage, red, raw, shredded—*1 cup*	70	10	34	49	50	46	10	8	31	17	41	55	20	11112
shredded, boiled—*1/2 cup*	75	8	27	40	41	38	8	7	26	14	34	45	16	11113
cabbage, savoy, raw, shredded—*1 cup*	70	14	48	71	72	66	14	12	45	24	60	80	29	11114
shredded, boiled—*1 cup*	145	26	90	132	135	123	26	22	84	45	112	148	54	11115
cabbage, swamp (skunk cabbage),														
chopped, boiled—*1 cup*	98	0	110	81	114	85	34	23	100	63	106	116	36	11504
raw, chopped—*1 cup*	56	0	78	58	82	61	25	16	71	45	76	83	26	11503
celtuce, raw—*12 leaves*	100	6	39	55	52	55	10	10	36	21	46	46	15	11145
chard, swiss, chopped, boiled—*1 cup*	175	32	151	270	236	180	35	0	200	0	200	214	67	11148
chicory greens, raw, chopped—*1 cup*	180	56	85	182	133	121	18	0	74	0	139	223	52	11152
chicory, witloof, raw—*1/2 cup*	45	7	11	24	18	16	2	0	10	0	18	30	7	11151
coleslaw, homemade—*1/2 cup*	60	10	29	37	49	43	11	9	28	20	37	42	17	11159
collards, chopped, boiled—*1 cup*	190	51	141	163	247	192	53	42	143	106	198	205	76	11162
chopped, frzn, boiled—*1 cup*	170	65	179	206	313	240	68	51	179	136	247	258	97	11164
cornsalad, raw—*1 cup*	56	15	42	55	74	57	14	11	51	20	55	51	20	11190
dock (sorrel), boiled—*3.5 oz*	100	0	86	93	152	105	32	0	104	75	121	98	49	11617
raw, chopped—*1 cup*	133	0	125	136	222	153	47	0	152	110	177	144	72	11616
endive, raw, chopped—*1/2 cup*	25	1	13	18	25	16	4	3	13	10	16	16	6	11213
horseradish tree, leafy tips,														
chopped, boiled—*1 cup*	42	34	97	106	186	126	29	33	115	82	144	125	46	11223
jute, potherb, boiled—*1 cup*	87	21	113	152	266	151	44	28	146	101	171	171	76	11232
raw—*1 cup*	28	8	46	62	109	61	18	11	59	41	69	69	31	11231
kale, chopped, boiled—*1 cup*	130	30	111	148	173	148	23	33	126	87	135	138	52	11234
chopped, frzn, boiled—*1 cup*	130	46	165	221	259	221	35	49	190	131	203	205	78	11236
kale, scotch, chopped, boiled—*1 cup*	130	30	111	147	172	147	23	33	126	87	135	137	52	11623
lambsquarters, chopped, boiled														
1 cup	180	52	223	347	481	486	67	122	227	241	310	347	158	11245
lettuce, butterhead, raw, chopped														
1 cup	55	5	32	46	43	46	9	8	30	18	38	39	12	11250
lettuce, iceberg, raw, chopped—*1 cup*	55	4	29	41	39	41	8	8	27	16	34	35	11	11252
lettuce, looseleaf (leaf),														
raw, shredded—*1/2 cup*	28	3	17	24	22	24	4	4	15	9	20	20	6	11253
lettuce, romaine/cos, raw, shredded														
1/2 cup	28	3	21	29	27	29	6	5	19	11	24	25	8	11251
mustard greens, chopped, boiled														
1 cup	140	35	84	115	97	144	29	48	84	167	123	231	56	11271
chopped, frzn, boiled—*1 cup*	150	38	90	125	105	155	32	51	90	180	132	249	62	11273
pumpkin leaves, boiled—*1 cup*	71	25	96	96	195	123	33	19	105	96	111	133	31	11419
purslane, boiled—*1 cup*	115	18	58	61	105	75	16	12	67	28	83	66	26	11428
radicchio, raw, shredded—*1 cup*	40	10	16	34	25	22	3	0	14	0	26	42	10	11952
spinach, boiled—*1 cup*	180	72	229	274	416	328	99	63	241	203	302	302	119	11458
cnd—*1 cup*	214	81	257	308	469	368	111	73	272	227	338	340	133	11461
frzn, boiled—*1/2 cup*	95	40	127	152	232	182	55	36	135	113	168	169	66	11464
raw, chopped—*1 cup*	30	12	37	44	67	52	16	11	39	32	48	49	19	11457
sweet potato leaves, steamed—*1 cup*	64	13	0	0	0	84	32	17	0	0	0	0	0	11506
taro leaves, steamed—*1 cup*	145	38	132	206	310	194	62	51	155	141	203	174	90	11521
turnip greens & turnips, frzn,														
boiled—*1 cup*	163	51	158	165	254	196	67	33	166	108	196	176	73	11577
chopped, boiled—*1 cup*	144	29	91	85	151	107	37	19	101	63	112	104	40	11569
chopped, frzn, boiled—*1 cup*	164	95	302	284	503	358	125	62	338	213	374	344	133	11575
cnd—*1/2 cup*	117	27	87	82	145	103	36	18	97	62	108	99	39	11570
raw, chopped—*1 cup*	55	14	45	43	75	54	19	9	51	32	56	52	20	11568

	WT (g)	TRY (mg)	THR (mg)	ISO (mg)	LEU (mg)	LYS (mg)	MET (mg)	CYS (mg)	PHE (mg)	TYR (mg)	VAL (mg)	ARG (mg)	HIS (mg)	REF
vinespinach, raw—*3.5 oz*	100	28	55	53	101	86	19	27	85	48	65	70	39	11587
watercress, raw, chopped—*1 cup*	34	10	45	32	56	46	7	2	39	21	47	51	14	11591
winged bean leaves, raw—*3.5 oz*	100	116	182	204	359	228	64	75	188	126	245	178	82	11597
Legumes (Beans & Peas)														
adzuki beans, mature, boiled—*1 cup*	230	166	587	690	1454	1304	182	161	915	515	890	1118	455	16002
cnd, sweetened—*1 cup*	296	107	382	447	944	847	118	104	595	334	580	728	296	16003
w/sugar (yokan)—*1 slice*	14	4	16	18	39	35	5	4	24	14	24	30	12	16004
baked beans, cnd, in sweet sce w/pork—*1 cup*	253	159	564	592	1073	921	205	147	726	377	703	832	374	16010
in tomato sce w/pork—*1 cup*	253	154	549	577	1042	896	197	142	706	367	683	807	364	16011
baked beans, homemade—*1 cup*	253	170	577	612	1083	959	218	157	726	392	713	901	387	16005
baked beans, vegetarian, cnd—*1 cup*	254	145	513	538	973	836	183	132	658	343	638	754	338	16006
black beans, mature, boiled—*1 cup*	172	181	642	673	1218	1046	229	165	824	430	798	944	425	16015
black turtle beans, mature, boiled—*1 cup*	185	179	636	668	1208	1040	228	165	818	426	792	938	422	16017
cnd—*1 cup*	240	170	610	638	1154	994	218	158	782	408	756	895	403	16018
broadbeans (fava beans), mature, boiled—*1 cup*	170	122	459	520	972	826	105	165	546	410	575	1193	328	16053
cnd—*1 cup*	256	133	497	566	1052	896	115	179	591	443	622	1293	356	16054
falafel, homemade—*.6 oz patty (2 1/4" dia)*	17	23	84	96	160	146	32	31	120	58	96	218	62	16138
chickpeas (garbanzo beans), boiled—*1 cup*	164	139	540	623	1035	973	190	195	779	361	610	1369	400	16057
cnd—*1 cup*	240	115	442	509	845	794	156	161	636	295	499	1118	326	16058
hummus, homemade—*1 T*	15	7	26	30	55	47	6	9	31	23	33	68	19	16137
cowpeas (blackeye peas), immature, boiled—*1 cup*	165	61	195	281	373	345	74	78	287	215	304	366	170	11192
frzn, boiled—*1 cup*	170	167	537	774	1030	949	206	214	792	592	836	1012	466	11196
cowpeas (blackeye peas), mature, boiled—*1 cup*	172	163	506	540	1018	900	189	146	776	430	633	920	413	16063
cnd—*1 cup*	240	139	432	463	871	770	161	125	665	367	542	787	353	16064
cowpeas, catjang, mature, boiled *1 cup*	171	171	528	564	1065	941	198	154	812	450	662	963	431	16061
cranberry (roman) beans, mature, boiled—*1 cup*	177	196	696	729	1320	1135	248	181	894	466	866	1023	460	16020
cnd—*1 cup*	260	172	606	637	1152	991	216	156	780	406	754	892	400	16021
french beans, mature, boiled—*1 cup*	177	147	526	550	997	857	188	136	674	352	653	773	347	16023
great northern beans, mature, boiled—*1 cup*	177	175	621	651	1177	1012	221	161	798	416	772	913	411	16025
cnd—*1 cup*	262	228	812	852	1541	1326	291	210	1045	545	1011	1195	537	16026
hyacinth beans, immature, boiled—*1 cup*	87	0	108	175	267	177	23	17	57	46	190	175	108	11225
hyacinth beans, mature, boiled *1 cup*	194	132	611	757	1341	1079	126	184	795	565	819	1160	452	16068
kidney beans, mature, all types, boiled—*1 cup*	177	182	646	678	1227	1053	230	166	830	432	804	950	428	16028
all types, cnd—*1 cup*	256	156	561	586	1062	911	200	146	719	374	696	824	371	16029c
CA red, boiled—*1 cup*	256	156	561	586	1062	911	200	146	719	374	696	824	371	16029b
red, boiled—*1 cup*	177	182	646	678	1227	1053	230	166	830	432	804	950	428	16033
red, cnd—*1 cup*	256	159	566	594	1073	922	202	146	727	379	701	832	374	16034
royal red, boiled—*1 cup*	177	198	706	742	1340	1152	253	182	908	473	878	1039	467	16036
lentils, mature, boiled—*1 cup*	198	160	640	772	1295	1247	152	234	881	477	887	1380	503	16070
lima beans, fordhook, frzn, boiled—*1/2 cup*	85	68	218	332	405	341	51	63	254	166	322	345	175	11038
lima beans, immature, baby, frzn, boiled—*1/2 cup*	90	78	254	385	470	395	59	73	295	193	374	401	203	11040
boiled—*1 cup*	170	151	491	745	910	765	116	141	571	372	723	775	393	11032
lima beans, mature, baby, boiled—*1 cup*	182	173	632	770	1263	981	186	162	843	517	881	897	448	16075
large, boiled—*1 cup*	188	173	634	773	1265	983	186	162	844	519	882	899	447	16072
large, cnd—*1 cup*	241	140	513	624	1024	795	149	130	684	419	713	728	364	16073
lupins, mature, boiled—*1 cup*	166	208	951	1154	1960	1381	183	319	1026	971	1079	2771	735	16077
mothbeans, mature, boiled—*1 cup*	177	89	0	687	929	752	133	71	620	0	443	0	466	16079
mung beans, mature, boiled—*1 cup*	202	154	465	600	1099	990	170	125	859	424	735	994	414	16081
mungo beans, mature, boiled—*1 cup*	180	140	472	693	1125	900	198	126	792	421	761	884	380	16084
navy beans, mature, boiled—*1 cup*	182	187	666	699	1265	1087	238	173	855	446	828	981	440	16038
cnd—*1 cup*	262	233	831	870	1575	1355	296	215	1066	555	1032	1221	548	16039

	WT (g)	TRY (mg)	THR (mg)	ISO (mg)	LEU (mg)	LYS (mg)	MET (mg)	CYS (mg)	PHE (mg)	TYR (mg)	VAL (mg)	ARG (mg)	HIS (mg)	REF
peas, green, boiled—*1 cup*	160	59	322	309	512	502	130	51	317	179	371	677	168	11305
cnd—*1 cup*	170	51	281	270	449	440	114	44	277	158	326	593	148	11308
frzn, boiled—*1/2 cup*	80	28	154	148	246	242	62	24	152	86	178	326	81	11313
raw—*1 cup*	145	54	294	283	468	460	119	46	290	165	341	621	155	11304
w/onions, red peppers, & garlic, cnd—*1/2 cup*	114	24	132	127	210	206	54	21	130	74	153	278	70	11310
peas, split, mature, boiled—*1 cup*	196	182	580	674	1172	1180	167	249	753	474	772	1458	398	16086
pigeon peas (red gram), mature, boiled—*1 cup*	168	111	402	412	811	796	128	131	973	282	491	680	405	16102
pink beans, mature, boiled—*1 cup*	169	181	644	676	1222	1051	230	167	828	431	801	948	426	16041
pinto beans, mature, boiled—*1 cup*	171	166	592	621	1122	964	212	152	759	395	735	870	392	16043
cnd—*1 cup*	240	139	492	514	931	802	178	127	631	326	612	725	324	16044
refried beans, cnd—*1 cup*	252	164	582	610	1104	950	209	151	748	391	723	857	386	16103
soybeans, green, boiled—*1 cup*	180	270	886	977	1589	1330	270	203	1006	797	988	1789	598	11451
soybeans, mature, boiled—*1 cup*	172	416	1244	1388	2331	1906	385	461	1495	1084	1429	2221	772	16109
raw—*1 cup*	186	986	2948	3292	5528	4518	915	1094	3543	2567	3387	5266	1830	16108
white beans, mature, boiled—*1 cup*	179	206	732	768	1389	1196	261	190	942	490	911	1078	485	16050
cnd—*1 cup*	262	225	799	838	1517	1305	286	207	1027	534	996	1176	529	16051
small, boiled—*1 cup*	179	190	675	709	1282	1103	242	175	868	453	840	993	448	16046
winged beans, mature, boiled—*1 cup*	172	401	619	771	1311	1121	187	286	750	765	803	991	415	16136
yardlong bean, immature, sliced, boiled—*1 cup*	104	30	98	140	187	173	37	40	145	107	152	184	85	11200
yardlong bean, mature, boiled—*1 cup*	171	174	540	576	1086	959	202	156	828	458	675	982	439	16134
yellow beans, mature, boiled—*1 cup*	177	191	683	717	1296	1113	244	177	878	457	848	1004	451	16048
Sprout & Shoot Vegetables														
alfalfa sprouts, raw—*1 cup*	33	0	44	47	88	71	0	0	0	0	48	0	0	11001
bamboo shoots, boiled—*1 cup*	120	19	60	61	98	95	20	16	64	0	74	68	30	11027
cnd—*1 cup*	131	24	75	76	122	117	26	18	79	0	93	84	37	11028
raw—*1 cup*	151	41	130	133	211	202	45	33	136	0	160	146	63	11026
kidney bean sprouts, boiled—*1 cup*	125	63	254	268	434	344	63	69	304	208	310	329	169	11030
lentil sprouts, stir-fried—*1 cup*	125	0	403	400	771	873	129	410	543	310	489	750	315	11249
mung bean sprouts, boiled—*1 cup*	124	35	72	122	161	153	31	15	107	47	120	181	64	11044
cnd—*1 cup*	125	24	50	84	111	106	21	11	75	33	84	126	45	11626
raw—*1 cup*	104	38	81	137	182	173	35	18	122	54	135	205	73	11043
stir-fried—*1 cup*	124	72	151	257	341	324	66	32	227	100	253	383	135	11045
navy bean sprouts, boiled—*1 cup*	125	93	371	393	635	504	93	100	446	304	454	481	248	11047
pea sprouts, boiled—*1 cup*	125	0	300	276	591	621	111	250	406	205	356	784	271	11317
soy sprouts, raw—*1/2 cup*	35	56	176	203	328	263	48	55	224	167	217	317	122	11452
steamed—*1 cup*	94	97	306	353	571	457	84	96	390	290	377	550	212	11453
stir-fried—*1 cup*	125	199	629	726	1174	940	173	196	801	598	775	1131	435	11454
Tuber & Root Vegetables														
beet (beetroot), sliced, boiled—*1/2 cup*	85	17	42	43	60	51	16	17	41	34	50	37	19	11081
sliced, cnd—*1 cup*	170	19	46	46	66	56	17	19	44	37	54	41	20	11084
sliced, harvard, cnd—*1 cup*	246	25	62	62	86	74	25	25	59	49	71	54	27	11605
sliced, pickled, cnd—*1 cup*	227	20	54	54	77	66	20	23	52	43	64	48	25	11609
burdock root, boiled—*1 cup pieces*	125	10	44	51	55	115	15	10	56	30	58	180	53	11105
carrots, baby, raw—*1 med*	10	1	3	3	4	3	1	1	3	2	4	4	1	11960
raw—*1 large (7 1/2" long)*	72	8	27	30	31	29	5	6	23	14	32	31	12	11124
sliced, boiled—*1/2 cup*	78	9	31	34	36	34	5	7	27	16	36	35	13	11125
sliced, cnd—*1 cup*	146	10	34	37	39	37	6	7	29	18	39	38	15	11128
sliced, frzn—*1 cup*	146	19	63	69	72	67	12	15	54	34	73	72	26	11131
cassava, raw—*1 cup*	206	39	58	56	80	91	23	58	54	35	72	282	41	11134
garlic, raw—*3 cloves*	9	6	14	20	28	25	7	6	16	7	26	57	10	11215
jicama (yambean), boiled—*3.5 oz*	100	0	18	16	25	26	7	6	17	12	22	37	19	11604
raw, sliced—*1 cup*	120	0	22	19	30	31	8	7	20	14	26	44	23	11603
lotus root, raw, sliced—*10 slices (2 1/2" dia)*	81	16	41	44	56	76	18	18	38	23	45	71	31	11254
sliced, boiled—*10 slices (2 1/2" dia)*	89	11	28	29	37	51	12	12	25	15	30	47	20	11255
mountain yam, hawaiian, cubed, steamed—*1 cup*	145	20	88	86	158	97	33	30	116	67	102	209	55	11259
onion, chopped, boiled—*1 cup*	210	42	69	101	101	137	23	50	74	71	65	384	46	11283
chopped, cnd—*1/2 cup*	112	13	22	32	31	44	8	17	24	22	21	122	15	11285
chopped, frzn, boiled—*1/2 cup*	105	12	19	28	28	38	6	15	21	20	19	107	13	11288
raw, chopped—*1 cup*	160	27	45	66	66	88	16	34	48	46	43	250	30	11282
onion rings, breaded, parfried, frzn, heated—*10 med rings (2–3" dia)*	60	42	90	128	210	91	49	65	146	94	130	195	65	11296

	WT (g)	TRY (mg)	THR (mg)	ISO (mg)	LEU (mg)	LYS (mg)	MET (mg)	CYS (mg)	PHE (mg)	TYR (mg)	VAL (mg)	ARG (mg)	HIS (mg)	REF
onions, welsh, raw—*3.5 oz*	100	21	74	81	113	95	21	0	61	55	84	137	33	11293
potato, baked—w/skin—*1 med*														
potato (2 1/4″ dia)	173	67	157	175	260	263	67	54	192	159	244	199	93	11674
w/skin, microwaved														
1 potato (2 1/2″ dia)	202	77	180	200	297	301	79	63	220	184	279	228	109	11675
w/o skin—*1 potato (2 1/3″ × 4 3/4″)*	156	47	111	125	184	186	48	39	136	114	172	140	67	11363
w/o skin, microwaved—*1 potato*														
(2 1/3″ × 4 3/4″)	156	51	119	133	197	200	51	42	145	122	184	151	72	11368
potato, boiled w/o skin														
1 med potato (2 1/4– 3 1/4″ dia)	167	45	104	117	172	174	45	37	127	107	160	132	63	11367
potato, cnd w/o skin—*1 cup*	180	40	92	103	153	155	40	32	113	94	144	117	56	11376
potato, raw w/skin—														
1 potato (2 1/4–3 1/4″ dia)	213	68	160	179	264	268	70	55	196	164	249	202	96	11352
potato, red-skinned, baked w/skin														
1 small (1 3/4–2 1/2″ dia)	138	50	116	128	190	193	50	40	141	117	179	146	69	11358c
baked w/skin—*1 med (2 1/4–3 1/4″ dia)*	173	62	145	161	239	242	62	50	176	147	225	183	87	11358b
baked w/skin—*1 large (3–4 1/4″ dia)*	299	108	251	278	413	419	108	87	305	254	389	317	150	11358a
raw w/skin—*1 potato (2 1/4–3 1/4″ dia)*	213	68	160	179	264	268	70	55	196	164	249	202	96	11355
potato, russet, raw w/skin														
1 potato (2 1/4–3 1/4″ dia)	213	38	117	124	183	215	66	45	383	75	207	192	75	11353
potato, white-skinned,														
baked w/skin—*1 small (1 3/4–2 1/2″ dia)*	138	33	94	92	132	148	43	32	203	69	139	139	47	11357c
baked w/skin—*1 med (2 1/4–3 1/4″ dia)*	173	42	118	116	166	185	54	40	254	87	175	175	59	11357b
baked w/skin—*1 large (3–41/4″ dia)*	299	72	203	200	287	320	93	69	440	150	302	302	102	11357a
raw w/skin—*1 potato (2 1/4″–3 1/4″ dia)*	213	34	117	113	166	181	58	45	320	62	179	177	60	11354
potato pancake, homemade														
1 pancake	76	65	191	217	334	295	107	85	226	178	265	254	106	11672
potato salad, homemade—*1 cup*	250	105	290	353	505	428	165	128	338	260	430	380	155	11414
potatoes au gratin, homemade—*1 cup*	245	172	470	696	1085	933	287	108	622	564	796	497	370	11373
potatoes, cottage fries, frzn, heated														
10 pieces	50	23	78	74	104	92	20	11	74	43	88	82	29	11407
potatoes, fries, extruded,														
frzn,heated—*10 pieces*	50	24	81	77	107	94	20	12	76	45	90	84	30	11409
frzn, heated—*10 pieces*	50	22	65	66	93	82	20	12	68	42	82	72	28	11403
potatoes, hash brown, frzn,														
prep—*1/2 cup*	78	33	112	106	148	131	27	16	105	62	126	116	41	11391
homemade—*1 cup*	156	51	172	162	228	200	42	23	161	95	192	179	64	11370
potatoes, mshd, from flakes														
w/o milk—*1 cup*	210	40	179	204	315	279	67	46	189	172	250	176	97	11379
potatoes, mshd, from granules														
w/milk—*1 cup*	210	38	185	197	300	277	59	53	195	172	254	195	97	11383
potatoes, mshd, homemade														
w/whole milk & butter—*1 cup*	210	61	153	183	277	260	74	48	181	160	235	172	92	11371
potatoes o'brien, frzn, prep—*2/3 cup*	85	29	68	76	111	112	29	26	81	67	102	94	41	11397
homemade—*1 cup*	194	68	173	213	328	279	83	58	206	178	258	211	105	11671
potatoes, scalloped (escalloped),														
homemade—*1 cup*	245	103	282	353	551	470	142	83	331	296	426	289	172	11372
radish, oriental, dried—*1 cup*	116	50	378	399	479	456	87	72	304	174	423	529	173	11432
raw—*1 radish 7″ long*	338	10	85	88	105	101	20	17	68	37	95	118	37	11430
sliced, boiled—*1 cup*	147	6	41	43	51	49	9	7	32	19	46	57	19	11431
radish, red, raw, sliced—*1/2 cup*	58	2	17	17	21	20	4	3	13	8	19	23	8	11429
radish, white icicle, raw, sliced														
1/2 cup	50	3	23	24	29	28	5	5	18	11	26	32	11	11637
rutabaga (swede), cubed, boiled														
1 cup	170	24	85	90	70	71	17	20	58	43	87	270	54	11436
sweet potato, baked w/skin														
1 med (2″ dia, 5″ long)	114	24	98	98	144	97	48	16	117	81	128	91	36	11508
boiled w/o skin, mshd—*1 cup*	328	66	269	269	397	266	134	43	325	223	354	253	102	11510
candied, homemade—														
1 piece (2 1/2″ long & 2″ dia)	105	12	45	46	68	46	22	7	55	38	60	42	18	11659
cnd, mshd—*1 cup*	255	61	250	252	370	247	125	41	303	207	329	235	94	11514
cnd, syrup pack—*1 cup*	196	31	125	125	184	123	63	20	151	104	165	118	47	11647
cnd, vacuum packed														
1 cup pieces	200	40	164	166	242	162	82	26	198	136	216	154	62	11512
cubed, baked, frzn—*1 cup*	176	37	150	151	222	148	74	25	181	123	197	141	56	11517
taro, sliced, ckd—*1 cup*	132	11	32	25	50	30	9	15	37	25	37	48	16	11519
turnip, boiled, mshd—*1 cup*	230	16	46	67	60	64	21	9	32	25	53	44	25	11565a

	WT (g)	TRY (mg)	THR (mg)	ISO (mg)	LEU (mg)	LYS (mg)	MET (mg)	CYS (mg)	PHE (mg)	TYR (mg)	VAL (mg)	ARG (mg)	HIS (mg)	REF
cubed, boiled—*1 cup*	156	11	31	45	41	44	14	6	22	17	36	30	17	11565b
frzn, boiled—*1 cup*	156	23	66	97	89	95	30	14	47	36	80	64	37	11567
yam, cubed, boiled/baked—*1 cup*	136	16	71	68	128	79	27	24	94	53	82	169	45	11602

Vegetable Combinations

	WT (g)	TRY (mg)	THR (mg)	ISO (mg)	LEU (mg)	LYS (mg)	MET (mg)	CYS (mg)	PHE (mg)	TYR (mg)	VAL (mg)	ARG (mg)	HIS (mg)	REF
mixed veg, cnd—*1 cup*	163	42	170	205	280	251	51	39	176	109	220	284	108	11581
frzn—*1/2 cup*	91	26	105	126	173	155	31	24	109	67	136	176	66	11584
peas & carrots, cnd—*1 cup*	255	41	207	201	319	314	79	33	201	115	240	418	107	11318
frzn—*1/2 cup*	80	18	93	90	143	140	35	15	90	51	107	187	48	11323
peas & onions, cnd—*1 cup*	120	29	144	142	229	228	58	26	143	84	166	324	77	11324
frzn, boiled—*1 cup*	180	34	167	164	266	265	67	31	166	97	193	376	88	11327
succotash (corn & lima beans),														
boiled—*1 cup*	192	109	405	549	856	570	131	106	470	332	591	568	309	11496
cnd—*1 cup*	255	74	275	375	584	388	89	71	321	227	403	388	212	11499
frzn, boiled—*1 cup*	170	82	304	413	644	428	99	80	354	250	445	427	233	11502
w/cream style corn, cnd—*1 cup*	266	80	293	396	617	410	93	77	338	239	426	410	223	11497

Other Vegetables

	WT (g)	TRY (mg)	THR (mg)	ISO (mg)	LEU (mg)	LYS (mg)	MET (mg)	CYS (mg)	PHE (mg)	TYR (mg)	VAL (mg)	ARG (mg)	HIS (mg)	REF
corn pudding, homemade—*1 cup*	250	133	495	588	1075	658	293	163	560	455	718	543	288	11656a
corn, yellow, boiled—*1 baby ear*	8	2	11	11	29	11	6	2	12	10	15	11	7	11168c
boiled—*1 ear*	77	18	102	102	276	109	53	21	119	97	147	104	70	11168b
boiled—*1 cup*	164	38	218	218	587	231	113	44	254	207	313	221	149	11168a
cnd—*1 cup*	164	30	172	172	466	184	90	34	200	164	248	175	118	11172
cnd, vacuum pack—*1 cup*	105	18	102	102	273	107	53	21	118	97	145	103	69	11176
cream style, cnd—*1 cup*	256	31	179	179	481	189	92	36	207	169	256	182	123	11174
frzn, boiled—*1/2 cup*	82	27	102	121	221	135	60	34	116	93	148	112	59	11179
w/red & green peppers, cnd—*1 cup*	227	39	211	211	558	225	109	45	243	197	300	216	143	11184
hearts of palm (heart palm),														
cnd—*1 cup*	146	34	142	147	247	133	61	28	143	72	166	260	80	11961
hominy, white, cnd—*1 cup*	165	13	83	96	333	54	51	54	125	92	127	112	74	20030
yellow, cnd—*1 cup*	160	13	80	93	323	53	50	53	122	90	123	109	72	20330
mushrooms, common white,														
boiled—*1 cup pieces*	156	80	158	139	214	354	67	9	137	75	161	173	94	11261
cnd—*1 cup pieces*	156	69	137	120	184	306	58	8	119	66	139	150	81	11264
raw—*1/21/2 cup pieces*	70	46	92	81	125	205	39	5	79	44	93	100	55	11260
mushrooms, crimini, italian, brown,														
raw—*1 piece*	14	8	16	14	21	35	7	1	14	8	16	17	9	11266
mushrooms, enoki, raw—*1 large*	5	3	5	2	7	9	2	0	6	5	4	10	3	11950
mushrooms, portabella, raw														
1 med (3.9 oz)	110	62	124	109	168	277	53	7	107	59	127	135	74	11265
mushrooms, shiitake, ckd														
4 mushrooms	72	3	49	40	67	34	18	19	48	32	48	64	16	11269
dried—*4 mushrooms*	15	5	75	61	102	51	27	29	73	48	73	97	24	11268
nopales (prickly pear), ckd—*1 cup*	149	21	63	77	122	94	24	12	77	45	92	82	39	11964
raw, sliced—*1 cup*	86	12	34	42	66	51	13	7	42	25	51	45	22	11963
seaweed, kelp (kombu/tangle),														
raw—*2 T*	10	5	6	8	8	8	3	10	4	3	7	7	2	11445
seaweed, laver (nori), raw														
2 T (~4 sheets)	10	4	23	26	50	22	15	10	27	25	40	29	14	11446
seaweed, spirulina, dried—*1 cup*	15	139	446	481	742	454	172	99	417	388	527	622	163	11667
raw—*1 oz*	28	27	86	93	143	87	33	19	80	74	101	120	31	11666
seaweed, wakame, raw—*2 T*	10	4	17	9	26	11	6	3	11	5	21	9	2	11669

31. MISCELLANEOUS FOOD INGREDIENTS

	WT (g)	TRY (mg)	THR (mg)	ISO (mg)	LEU (mg)	LYS (mg)	MET (mg)	CYS (mg)	PHE (mg)	TYR (mg)	VAL (mg)	ARG (mg)	HIS (mg)	REF
baking choc (unsweetened)—*1 oz sq*	28	43	114	111	174	144	30	35	138	108	173	163	50	19078
liquid—*1 oz pkt*	28	51	135	132	206	171	35	41	164	128	204	193	59	19077
cocoa, unsweetened powder—*1 T*	5	15	39	38	59	49	10	12	47	37	59	56	17	19165
processed w/alkali—*1 T*	5	14	36	35	55	45	9	11	43	34	54	51	16	19166
cornstarch—*1 cup*	128	1	12	13	46	8	8	8	17	13	18	15	10	20027
gelatin, dry, unsweetened														
1 oz pkt (4 T)	28	0	413	324	687	969	170	0	486	85	583	1852	185	19177a
soy protein concentrate,														
acid wash—*1 oz*	28	234	693	824	1377	1100	228	248	918	644	858	1300	442	16420
alcohol extraction—*1 oz*	28	234	693	824	1377	1100	228	248	918	644	858	1300	442	16121
soy protein isolate—*1 oz*	28	312	878	1191	1899	1492	316	293	1286	902	1147	1868	645	16122
potassium type—*1 oz*	28	312	878	1191	1899	1492	316	293	1286	902	1147	1868	645	16422
ProPlus, Protein Tech														
International—*1 oz*	28	308	924	1176	1988	1512	308	308	1260	924	1232	1820	616	16176

	WT (g)	TRY (mg)	THR (mg)	ISO (mg)	LEU (mg)	LYS (mg)	MET (mg)	CYS (mg)	PHE (mg)	TYR (mg)	VAL (mg)	ARG (mg)	HIS (mg)	REF
Supro, Protein Tech International—*1 oz*	28	308	924	1204	2016	1540	322	322	1288	924	1260	1876	644	16175
tapioca, pearl, dry—*1 cup*	152	5	6	6	9	9	3	6	6	3	8	29	5	20068
whey, acid, dry—*1 cup*	57	137	336	331	636	575	126	120	220	171	330	186	131	01113
fluid—*1 cup*	246	39	93	93	177	160	34	34	62	47	93	52	37	01112
whey, sweet, dry—*1 cup*	145	297	1185	1043	1720	1494	349	367	590	526	1011	544	344	01115
fluid—*1 cup*	246	32	133	116	192	167	39	42	66	59	113	62	39	01114
yeast, bakers, active dry—*.25 oz pkg*	7	34	139	152	214	221	53	36	130	111	164	148	70	18375

[1] TYR = tyrosine, THR = threonine, ISO = isoleucine, LEU = leucine, LYS = lysine, MET = methionine, CYS = cystine, PHE = phenylalanine, TRY = tryptophan, VAL = valine, ARG = arginine, HIS = histidine.

Source:
USDA Codes: *United States Department of Agriculture Database for Standard Reference, Release 15* (SR15), 2002. Available at
http://www.nal.usda.gov/fnic/foodcomp/Data/SR15/sr15.html.

Caffeine

	SERVING SIZE (g)	CAFFEINE (mg/serving)	CAFFEINE (mg/100 g)	USDA CODE/SOURCE
BEVERAGES - ALCOHOLIC				
liqueur, coffee, 53 proof	1.5 fl oz (52 g)	14	26	14414
liqueur, coffee, 63 proof	1.5 fl oz (52 g)	14	26	14534
liqueur, coffee w/cream, 34 proof	1.5 fl oz (47 g)	7	15	14415
BEVERAGES–CARBONATED, LOW CALORIE				
diet cherry cola w/aspartame, Shasta	12 fl oz (355 g)	43	12	SHST
diet cherry cola w/saccharin & aspartame, Shasta	12 fl oz (355 g)	54	15	SHST
Diet Cherry Coke	12 fl oz (355 g)	23	6	COLA
diet choc flavor	12 fl oz (~355 g)	~50	14	CSFII
Diet Coke	12 fl oz (355 g)	31	9	COLA
Diet Coke w/lemon	12 fl oz (355 g)	31	9	COLA
diet cola w/aspartame	12 fl oz (355 g)	50	14	14416
diet cola w/aspartame, caffeine-free, Shasta	12 fl oz (355 g)	<1	<1	SHST
diet cola w/aspartame, Shasta	12 fl oz (355 g)	43	12	SHST
diet cola w/Na saccharin	12 fl oz (355 g)	39	11	14166
diet crème soda	12 fl oz (~355 g)	~4	1	Shively and Tarka, 1984
Diet Dr. Pepper	12 fl oz (~355 g)	54		Bunker and McWilliams, 1979
diet fruit flavor w/caffeine	12 fl oz (~355 g)	~53	15	CSFII
Diet Inca Kola	12 fl oz (355 g)	25	7	COLA
Diet Mello Yello	12 fl oz (355 g)	35	9	COLA
Diet Mr. Pibb	12 fl oz (355 g)	27	8	COLA
diet pepper type	12 fl oz (~355 g)	~50	14	CSFII
Diet RC	12 fl oz (~355 g)	33	~9	Bunker and McWilliams, 1979
Diet-Rite	12 fl oz (~355 g)	32	~9	Bunker and McWilliams, 1979
Tab	12 fl oz (355 g)	31	9	COLA
BEVERAGES–CARBONATED, SUGAR-SWEETENED				
Cherry Coke	12 fl oz (370 g)	23	6	COLA
cherry cola, Shasta	12 fl oz (270 g)	43	12	SHST
choc flavor	12 fl oz (369 g)	7	2	14552
Coca Cola	12 fl oz (370 g)	64		Bunker and McWilliams, 1979
Coca Cola Classic	12 fl oz (370 g)	23	6	COLA
cola	12 fl oz (370 g)	37	10	14400
cola, caffeine-free, Shasta	12 fl oz (370 g)	<1	<1	SHST
cola, Shasta	12 fl oz (370 g)	43	12	SHST
cola w/fruit/van flavor	12 fl oz (~370 g)	~37	10	CSFII

	SERVING SIZE (g)	CAFFEINE (mg/serving)	CAFFEINE (mg/100 g)	USDA CODE/SOURCE
cola w/higher caffeine (Jolt Cola)	12 fl oz (370 g)	100	27	14148
Dr Pepper	12 fl oz (~370 g)	61	~16	Bunker and McWilliams, 1979
fruit flavor w/caffeine	12 fl oz (~370 g)	~56	15	CSFII
Inca Kola	12 fl oz (370 g)	25	7	COLA
lemon-lime w/caffeine	12 fl oz (368 g)	55	15	14144
Mellow Yello	12 fl oz (370 g)	35	9	COLA
Moon Mist	12 fl oz (370 g)	53	14	SHST
Mountain Dew	12 fl oz (~370 g)	55	~15	Bunker and McWilliams, 1979
Mr. Pibb	12 fl oz (370 g)	27	7	COLA
pepper type (Mr. Pibb)	12 fl oz (368 g)	37	10	14153
Pepsi-Cola	12 fl oz (~370 g)	43	~12	Bunker and McWilliams, 1979
Pibb Xtra	12 fl oz (370 g)	27	7	COLA
RC Cola	12 fl oz (~370 g)	34	~9	Bunker and McWilliams, 1979
Red Flash	12 fl oz (370 g)	27	7	COLA
root beer, Barq's	12 fl oz (370 g)	15	4	COLA
Surge	12 fl oz (370 g)	35	9	COLA
BEVERAGES–COFFEE				
café con leche w/sugar	8 fl oz (~245 g)	~66	27	CSFII
café latte	8 fl oz (~240 g)	~50	21	CSFII
cappuccino	4 fl oz (~120 g)	~35	29	CSFII
cappuccino, decaf	4 fl oz (~120 g)	tr	<.5	CSFII
Caramoucha, Planet Java	9.5 fl oz (285 g)	65	23	COLA
coffee, 50% less caffeine, from inst	8 fl oz (~237 g)	~40	17	CSFII
coffee & chicory, from inst	1 rd t in 6 fl oz water (179 g)	38	21	14223
coffee & chicory, from ground	8 fl oz (~237 g)	137	58	CSFII
coffee & chicory, inst powder	1 rd t (6 g)	37	2063	14222
coffee & cocoa, decaf w/whitener, & low cal sweetener, inst powder	1 t (6 g)	1	18	14204
coffee, acid neutralized, from inst	8 fl oz (~237 g)	~69	29	CSFII
coffee, brewed	8 fl oz (237 g)	137	58	14209
coffee, cappuccino-flavor w/sugar, inst powder	2 rd t (14 g)	136	960	14228
coffee, decaf, brewed	8 fl oz (237 g)	2	1	14201
coffee, decaf, from inst	1 rd t in 6 fl oz water (179 g)	2	1	14219
coffee, decaf, inst powder	1 rd t (1.8 g)	2	122	14218
coffee, dripolated	4.8 fl oz (140 g)	146	~104	Bunker and McWilliams, 1979
coffee, french-flavor w/sugar, inst powder	2 rd t (12 g)	49	427	14229
coffee, from inst	8 fl oz (~237 g)	68	~29	Ahuja and Perloff, 2001
coffee, from liquid conc	8 fl oz (~237 g)	~45	19	CSFII
coffee, inst powder	1 rd t (1.5 g)	47	3142	14214
coffee, mocha-flavor w/sugar, inst powder	2 rd t (12 g)	33	290	14224
coffee, percolated	4.8 fl oz (140 g)	110	~79	Bunker and McWilliams, 1979
espresso, decaf	6 fl oz (~178 g)	~2	1	CSFII
espresso, from restaurant	6 fl oz (178 g)	377	212	14210
Javadelic, Planet Java	9.5 fl oz (285 g)	65	23	COLA
Tremble, Planet Java	9.5 fl oz (285 g)	129	45	COLA
BEVERAGES–FRUIT FLAVOR & SPORT				
KMX, blue	8.4 fl oz (252 g)	38	15	COLA
KMX, orange	8.4 fl oz (252 g)	38	15	COLA
mountain berry, Mad River	8 fl oz (250 g)	6	2	COLA
orange carrot medley, Mad River	8 fl oz (250 g)	6	2	COLA
BEVERAGES–TEA				
tea, black, 1 min brew from bag	4.8 fl oz (141 g)	28	~20	Bunker and McWilliams, 1979
tea, black, 3 min brew	8 fl oz (237 g)	47	20	14355
tea, black, 3 min brew, decaf	8 fl oz (237 g)	2	1	14352
tea, black, 4 min brew from bag, Lipton	~6 fl oz (181 g)	38	~21	Groisser, 1978
tea, black, 4 min brew from bag, Red Rose	~6 fl oz (181 ml)	46	~25	Groisser, 1978
tea, black, 4 min brew from bag, Salada	~6 fl oz (181 g)	40	~22	Groisser, 1978
tea, black, 4 min brew from bag, Tetley	~6 fl oz (181 g)	25	~14	Groisser, 1978

	SERVING SIZE (g)	CAFFEINE (mg/serving)	CAFFEINE (mg/100 g)	USDA CODE/SOURCE
tea, black, 4 min brew from bag, Twinings Darjeeling	~6 fl oz (181 g)	65	~36	Groisser, 1978
tea, black, 4 min brew from bag, Twinings English Breakfast	~6 fl oz (181 g)	52	~29	Groisser, 1978
tea, black, 4 min brew from loose tea, Twinings English Breakfast	~6 fl oz (181 g)	77	~43	Groisser, 1978
tea, black, 5 min brew from bag	4.8 fl oz (141 g)	46	~33	Bunker and McWilliams, 1979
tea, black, 5 min brew from loose tea	4.8 fl oz (141 g)	40	~28	Bunker and McWilliams, 1979
tea, black, 6 min brew from loose tea	~6 fl oz (181 g)	95	~52	Anderson et al, 1971
tea, black, brewed from leaves w/ low cal sweetener	8 fl oz (~237 g)	~47	20	CSFII
tea, black, brewed from leaves w/sugar	8 fl oz (~259 g)	~49	19	CSFII
tea, black, decaf	8 fl oz (~237 g)	~2	1	CSFII
tea, black, from frzn conc	8 fl oz (~237 g)	~47	20	CSFII
tea, black, from inst	8 fl oz (~237 g)	25	~11	Ahuja and Perloff, 2001
tea, black, from inst, Lipton	~6 fl oz (181 g)	62	~34	Groisser, 1978
tea, black, from inst, Nestea	~6 fl oz (181 g)	48	~26	Groisser, 1978
tea, black, inst powder	1.5 T (~1 g)	~44	4352	CSFII
tea, black, oolong, 4 min brew from loose tea, Jackson Formosa	~6 fl oz (181 g)	42	~23	Groisser, 1978
tea, black w/low cal sweetener	8 fl oz (~237 g)	~40	17	CSFII
tea, black w/sugar	8 fl oz (~242 g)	~46	19	CSFII
tea, green, 4 min brew from bag, chinese	~6 fl oz (181 g)	36	~20	Groisser, 1978
tea, green, 5 min brew from loose tea	4.8 fl oz (141 g)	35	~25	Bunker and McWilliams, 1979
tea, green, 5 min brew, Japanese	4.8 fl oz (141 g)	20	~14	Bunker and McWilliams, 1979
tea, iced, Cool From Nestea	8 fl oz (237 g)	11	5	COLA
tea, iced, decaf, inst powder	1 t (11 g)	1	169	14353
tea, iced, diet lemon, Nestea	8 fl oz (238 g)	11	5	COLA
tea, iced, diet, Cool From Nestea	8 fl oz (240 g)	7	3	COLA
tea, iced, earl grey, Nestea	8 fl oz (240 g)	33	14	COLA
tea, iced, from inst	8 fl oz (237 g)	31	13	14367
tea, iced, inst powder	1 t (0.7 g)	30	4352	14366
tea, iced, lemon green, Mad River	8 fl oz (240 g)	24	10	COLA
tea, iced, lemon flavor, from inst	8 fl oz (238 g)	26	11	14369
tea, iced, lemon flavor, inst powder	2 rd T (11 g)	203	1794	14368
tea, iced, lemon flavor w/ Na saccharin, from inst	8 fl oz (237 g)	36	15	14376
tea, iced, lemon flavor w/ Na saccharin, inst powder	4 T/1/4 cup (14 g)	323	2240	14375
tea, iced, lemon flavor w/sugar, from inst	8 fl oz (259 g)	28	11	14371
tea, iced, lemon flavor w/sugar, from inst, Lipton	~6 fl oz (181 g)	76	~42	Groisser, 1978
tea, iced, lemon flavor w/sugar, from inst, Nestea	~ 6 fl oz (181 g)	67	~37	Groisser, 1978
tea, iced, lemon flavor w/sugar, inst powder	3 heaping t (23 g)	29	124	14370
tea, iced, lemon/peach/raspberry, Nestea	8 fl oz (240 g)	11	5	COLA
tea, iced, oolong w/honey, Mad River	8 fl oz (240 g)	30	13	COLA
tea, iced, Peach Frrreezer/Raspbrry Cooler, Cool From Nestea	8 fl oz (240 g)	4	2	COLA
tea, iced, red, Mad River	8 fl oz (240 g)	24	10	COLA
tea, iced, unsweetened, Nestea	8 fl oz (240 g)	17	7	COLA
CANDY				
After Eight Mints, Nestle	5 mints (41 g)	8	20	19153
almond choc candies, M&Ms	2 oz (57 g)	6	11	CSFII
almonds, choc covered	1 oz (28 g)	2	8	CSFII
Baby Ruth, Nestle	.7 oz bar (21 g)	1	4	19111
Baby Ruth, Nestle	2.1 oz bar (60 g)	2	4	19111
Bar None	2 oz (57 g)	6	11	CSFII
Butterfinger, Nestle	.7 oz bar (21 g)	1	4	19069
Butterfinger, Nestle	2.16 oz bar (61 g)	2	4	19069
caramel, choc flavored roll	2.25 oz bar (64 g)	3	4	19076
caramels, choc covered	1 oz (28 g)	2	6	CSFII
caramels w/nuts, choc covered	1 oz (28 g)	5	19	CSFII

	SERVING SIZE (g)	CAFFEINE (mg/serving)	CAFFEINE (mg/100 g)	USDA CODE/SOURCE
choc chips, semi-sweet, Hershey	1 T (15 g)	12	80	Hershey, 2002
choc covered fruit	1 oz (28 g)	tr	1	CSFII
choc discs, sugar-coated	1 oz (28 g)	5	18	CSFII
choc flavor roll (Tootsie Roll)	1 oz (28 g)	1	2	CSFII
choc, mexican	1 oz (28 g)	10	35	CSFII
Chunky, Nestle	1.4 oz piece (40 g)	12	29	19119
coconut candy, choc covered	1 oz (28 g)	5	17	CSFII
Cookies 'n'crème white choc, Hershey	1.55 oz bar (43 g)	5	12	Hershey, 2002
Crunch, Nestle	1.55 oz bar (44 g)	11	24	19145
dark choc (semi-sweet)	1.45 oz bar (41 g)	27	66	19081
dark choc (semi-sweet), chips	1 cup/6 oz bag (168 g)	104	62	19080
dark choc (sweet)	1 oz (28 g)	19	68	Shively and Tarka, 1984
Demet's Turtles, Nestle	6 oz pkg (170 g)	7	4	19158
Fifth Avenue, Hershey	2 oz bar (56 g)	3	6	19098
fondant, choc coated	1.5 oz patty (43 g)	3	6	19083
fudge, caramel w/nuts, choc coated	1 oz (28 g)	3	10	CSFII
fudge, choc, choc coated	1 oz (28 g)	5	18	CSFII
fudge, choc, homemade	.6 oz piece (17 g)	4	21	19100
fudge, choc marshmallow w/nuts, homemade	.78 oz piece (22 g)	4	16	19301
fudge, choc w/nuts, homemade	.67 oz piece (19 g)	3	18	19101
gumdrops, choc covered	1 oz (28 g)	2	7	CSFII
honeycombed peanut butter, choc covered	1 oz (28 g)	2	7	CSFII
Hundred (100) Grand, Nestle	1.5 oz bar (43 g)	11	26	19144
Kisses, Hershey	8–9 pieces (1.55 oz/43 g)	11	26	Hershey, 2002
Kit Kat, Hershey	1.5 oz bar (42 g)	6	14	Hershey, 2002
Krackel, Hershey	1.45 oz bar (41 g)	7	17	Hershey, 2002
M&M's Peanut, M&M/Mars	1.74 oz pkg/~25 pieces (49 g)	5	11	19140
M&M's Plain, M&M/Mars	1.69 oz pkg/69 pieces (48 g)	9	18	19141
Mars Almond, M&M/Mars	1.76 oz bar (50 g)	2	4	19115
marshmallow, choc covered	1 oz (28 g)	6	20	CSFII
milk choc	1.55 oz bar (44 g)	11	26	19120
milk choc chips	1 cup (168 g)	44	26	19120
milk choc, Hershey	1.55 oz bar (43 g)	10	23	Hershey, 2002
milk choc w/almonds	1.55 oz bar (44 g)	10	22	19132
milk choc w/almonds, Hershey	1.45 oz bar (41 g)	6	15	Hershey, 2002
milk choc w/crisped rice	1.55 oz bar (44 g)	10	23	19134
milk choc w/fruits & nuts	1 oz (28 g)	7	24	CSFII
milk choc w/peanuts	1 oz (28 g)	6	20	CSFII
Milky Way, dark, M&M/Mars	2.1 oz bar (60 g)	10	17	CSFII
Milky Way, M&M/Mars	.6 oz bar (18 g)	1	8	19135
Milky Way, M&M/Mars	2.1 oz bar (60 g)	5	8	19135
Mounds, Hershey	1.9 oz bar (53 g)	9	17	19142
Mr. Goodbar, Hershey	1.75 oz bar (49 g)	14	29	19143
nougat, choc covered	1 oz (28 g)	2	7	CSFII
nougat w/caramel, choc covered	1 oz (28 g)	2	8	CSFII
Oh Henry!, Nestle	2 oz bar (57 g)	6	10	19118
peanuts, choc coated	10 pieces (40 g)	9	22	19126
peanuts, choc coated, Goobers	1.38 oz pkg (39 g)	9	22	19105
Pot of Gold almond choc bar, Hershey	2.8 oz bar (78 g)	16	21	Hershey, 2002
Pot of Gold Solitaires, Hershey	2.8 oz bar (78 g)	12	15	Hershey, 2002
raisins, choc coated	1/4 cup (45 g)	11	25	19127
raisins, choc coated Raisinets	1.58 oz pkg (45 g)	11	25	19149
Reese's peanut butter chips, Hershey	1 T (15 g)	0	0	Hershey, 2002
Reese's Peanut Butter Cups, Hershey	2 pieces (45 g)	4	9	Hershey, 2002
Reese's Pieces, Hershey	1.63 oz (46 g)	0	0	Hershey, 2002
Rolo caramels w/milk choc, Hershey	9 pieces (54 g)	3	5	19152
Sixlets			18	CSFII
Skor toffee bar, Hershey	1.4 oz (39 g)	3	8	Hershey, 2002
Snickers, M&M/Mars	2 oz bar (57 g)	6	10	19155
Special Dark, Hershey	1.45 oz (41 g)	31	76	Hershey, 2002
Sweet Escapes, caramel & peanut butter, Hershey	1.4 oz (39 g)	3	7	Hershey, 2002
Sweet Escapes, choc toffee, Hershey	1.4 oz (39 g)	8	21	Hershey, 2002

	SERVING SIZE (g)	CAFFEINE (mg/serving)	CAFFEINE (mg/100 g)	USDA CODE/SOURCE
Sweet Escapes, triple choc wafer, Hershey	1.4 oz (39 g)	7	18	Hershey, 2002
Three Musketeers, M&M/Mars	2.13 oz bar (60 g)	7	11	19159
Toberone (milk choc w/honey & almond nougat)	2 oz (56 g)	12	22	CSFII
toffee, choc covered (Heath Bar)	1 oz (28 g)	2	7	CSFII
toffee w/nuts, choc covered	1 oz (28 g)	2	7	CSFII
truffles	1 oz (28 g)	5	19	CSFII
Twix Cookie Bar, caramel, M&M/Mars	2 bars (58 g)	2	3	19160
Twix Cookie Bar, choc fudge, M&M/Mars	2 bars (58 g)	6	10	CSFII
Twix Cookie Bar, peanut butter, M&M/Mars	2 bars (58 g)	5	9	19161
Whatchamacallit, Hershey	1.7 oz bar (48 g)	6	13	19162
white chocolate[1]	1 oz (28 g)	0	0	USDA SR15

CEREALS

cereal w/choc	1 oz (28 g)	3	12	Shively and Tarka, 1984
choc flavor frosted puffed corn	1 oz (28 g)	1	4	CSFII
Cocoa Blasts, Quaker	1 cup (33 g)	7	21	08294
Cocoa Crispy Rice, Kountry Fresh	1 oz (28 g)	1	4	Caudle and Bell, 2000
Cocoa Crunchies, Kountry Fresh	1 oz (28 g)	2	6	Caudle and Bell, 2000
Cocoa Frosted Flakes, Kellogg	1 oz (28 g)	0	1	Caudle and Bell, 2000
Cocoa Krispies, Kellogg's	3/4 cup (31 g)	1	2	08014
Cocoa Pebbles, Post	1 oz (28 g)	1	4	Caudle and Bell, 2000
Cocoa Puffs, General Mills	1 cup (30 g)	1	2	08271
Coco-Roos, Malt-O-Meal	1 oz (28 g)	1	4	CSFII
Cookie Crisp, choc chip/van, General Mills	1 cup (30 g)	1	2	08017
Count Chocula, General Mills	1 cup (30 g)	1	3	08270
Malt-O-Meal, plain/choc, ckd	1 cup (240 g)	2	1	08117
NesQuik, General Mills	1 oz (28 g)	3	10	Caudle and Bell, 2000
Oreo O's, Post	1 oz (28 g)	3	11	Caudle and Bell, 2000
Reese's Peanut Butter Puffs, General Mills	1 oz (28 g)	0	1	Caudle and Bell, 2000
wheat w/choc flavor, ckd w/milk	1 cup (243 g)	2	1	CSFII

DESSERTS

brownie, from mix	1 brownie (~56 g)	7	13	Shively and Tarka, 1984
brownie, Little Debbie	1 twin pkg (61 g)	1	2	18151
cake batter, raw, choc	1 oz (28 g)	3	12	CSFII
cake, choc, from mix	1/8 of 18 oz cake (64 g)	4	7	Shively and Tarka, 1984
cake, pound, choc	1/10 of 10.6 oz cake (~30 g)	~5	15	CSFII
cake, pound, choc, fat free, no cholesterol	1 oz (28 g)	~1	3	CSFII
cake, snack cake, choc crème-filled w/icing	1.8 oz snack cake (~50 g)	~2	3	18127
cake, sponge, choc w/icing	1/12 of 16 oz cake (~38 g)	~5	14	CSFII
cake, sponge, choc w/o icing	1/12 of 16 oz cake (~38 g)	~3	8	CSFII
cheesecake, choc	1/6 oz 17 oz cake (~80 g)	11	14	CSFII
cookie bar w/choc, nuts, & graham crackers	2 bars (~58 g)	~5	9	CSFII
cookie, Caramel Delights, Snackwell's	1 cookie (18 g)	1	8	18650
cookie, choc chip, 12–17% fat	2 1/4" dia cookie (10 g)	1	7	18158
cookie, choc chip, 18–28% fat	2 1/4" dia cookie (10 g)	1	11	18159
cookie, choc chip, homemade w/marg	2 1/4" dia cookie (16 g)	3	16	18165
cookie, choc chip, soft type	1 cookie (15 g)	1	7	18160
cookie, choc chunk pecan, Pepperidge Farm	1 cookie (12 g)	1	11	18159
cookie, choc sandwich w/crème filling	1 cookie (17 g)	<.5	1	18167
cookie, choc sandwich w/crème filling, choc coated	1 cookie (10 g)	1	13	18166
cookie, choc sandwich w/extra crème filling	1 cookie (13 g)	1	5	18168
cookie, choc wafers	5 wafers (28 g)	2	7	18157

	SERVING SIZE (g)	CAFFEINE (mg/serving)	CAFFEINE (mg/100 g)	USDA CODE/SOURCE
cookie, choc w/choc filling	1 cookie (~17 g)	1	4	CSFII
cookie, devil's food, fat free, Snackwell's	1 cookie (16 g)	1	8	18651
cookie, graham crackers, choc coated	2 1/2" sq cookie (14 g)	6	46	18174
cookie, marshmallow, choc coated	1 small cookie (13 g)	1	5	18176
cookie, marshmallow pie	3" dia × 3/4" cookie (39 g)	2	5	18176
cookie, mint crème, Snackwell's	1 cookie (25 g)	42	166	18649
cookie, oatmeal w/choc chips	1 oz cookie (28 g)	3	11	CSFII
cookie, shortbread w/choc filling	1 cookie (~25 g)	~3	12	CSFII
cookie, sugar w/choc icing/filling	1 oz cookie (28 g)	~1	2	CSFII
cookie, van w/caramel, coconut, & choc coating	1 oz cookie (28 g)	~1	2	CSFII
cookie w/peanut butter filling & choc coating	1 oz cookie (28 g)	1	4	CSFII
cupcake, choc w/fruit/crème filling, lowfat	1.5 oz cupcake (43 g)	2	5	CSFII
cupcake, choc w/icing/filling	1.5 oz cupcake (43 g)	2	5	CSFII
cupcake, choc w/icing, low-fat	1.5 oz cupcake (43 g)	1	2	18452
doughnut (cake), choc coated/frosted	3" dia doughnut (43 g)	1	2	18249
doughnut (cake), choc, sugared/glazed	3" dia doughnut (42 g)	<.5	1	18251
doughnut (cake), choc w/choc icing	3" dia doughnut (43 g)	5	12	CSFII
doughnut, choc cream filled	oval doughnut (~85 g)	tr	<.5	CSFII
doughnut (yeast), choc	oval doughnut (~85 g)	~9	10	CSFII
doughnut (yeast), choc covered	oval doughnut ~85 g)	~8	9	CSFII
doughnut (yeast), choc w/choc icing	oval doughnut ~85 g)	~16	19	CSFII
éclair w/custard filling & choc glaze, homemade	1 éclair (100 g)	2	2	18257
frzn dessert, choc	1/2 cup (~72 g)	~1	2	CSFII
frzn dessert, fudge bar	1.75 fl oz bar (51 g)	~1	2	Shively and Tarka, 1984
frzn tofu, choc (Tofutti)	1/2 cup (~72 g)	~5	7	CSFII
frzn yogurt, lowfat/nonfat, choc	1/2 cup (~72 g)	~3	4	CSFII
frzn yogurt, nonfat w/low cal sweetener, choc	1 cup (186 g)	6	3	42185
frzn yogurt, whole fat, choc	1/2 cup (~72 g)	~2	3	CSFII
frzn yogurt, soft serve, choc	1/2 cup (72 g)	2	3	19393
granola bar, peanut butter, soft w/ choc coating	1.3 oz bar (37 g)	2	6	19026
granola bar w/coconut/nuts, choc coated	1 oz bar (28 g)	~1	3	CSFII
ice cream, choc	1/2 cup (66 g)	2	3	19270
ice cream, light, choc	1/2 cup (~67 g)	~1	1	CSFII
ice cream, light, soft serve, choc	1/2 cup (~71 g)	~1	1	CSFII
ice cream, rich, choc	1 cup (148 g)	4	3	43541
pie, choc cream	1/6 of 8" pie (113 g)	~18	16	Shively and Tarka, 1984
pie, choc mousse, from mix	1/8 of 9" pie (95 g)	1	1	18312
pie crust, choc wafer, homemade	1/8 of 9" crust (28 g)	1	5	18398
pudding, choc, from inst mix w/ lowfat milk	1/2 cup (147 g)	1	1	19123
pudding, choc, from inst mix w/ whole milk	1/2 cup (147 g)	3	2	19185
pudding, choc, from reg mix w/ 2% or whole milk	1/2 cup (142 g)	3	2	19190/19189
pudding, choc mousse	1/8 of 9" pie (95 g)	~7	7	CSFII
pudding, choc, rte	5 oz serving (142 g)	7	5	19183
pudding, choc tapioca, rte	5 oz serving (142 g)	10	7	CSFII
pudding, rennin dessert, choc, from mix w/2% milk	1/2 cup (136 g)	1	1	19213
pudding, rennin dessert, choc, from mix w/whole milk	1/2 cup (136 g)	1	1	19221
DESSERTS–TOPPINGS				
icing/frosting, choc, rts	2 T (41 g)	1	2	19226
icing/frosting, from mix, choc made w/butter or marg	1/12 pkg prep (42 g)	2	5	19241/19372
syrup, choc	2 T/1 fl oz (39 g)	5	14	14181
syrup, choc/choc malt, Hershey	2 T (39 g)	7	18	Hershey, 2002
syrup, choc, lite, Hershey	2 T (35 g)	1	3	19345

	SERVING SIZE (g)	CAFFEINE (mg/serving)	CAFFEINE (mg/100 g)	USDA CODE/SOURCE
topping, choc	2 T (~38 g)	4	10	Shively and Tarka, 1984
topping, choc fudge	2 T (38 g)	2	6	19348
topping, choc fudge, Hershey	2 T (37 g)	6	16	Hershey, 2002
FAST FOODS				
brownie	2″ sq brownie (60 g)	1	2	21027
cookies, choc chip	1 box (55 g)	6	11	21030
shake, choc	10 fl oz (208 g)	6	3	14346
sundae, hot fudge	1 sundae (158 g)	2	1	21033
shake, choc	12 fl oz (250 g)	8	3	14346
shake, choc	16 fl oz (333 g)	10	3	14346
shake, choc	22 fl oz (458 g)	14	3	14346
GRAIN PRODUCTS				
croissant, choc	1 med ('57 g)	~11	20	CSFII
muffin, choc	2 oz muffin (57 g)	12	21	CSFII
muffin, choc chip	2 oz muffin (57 g)	3	6	CSFII
pretzel, hard, choc coated	.39 oz pretzel (11 g)	~1	7	CSFII
MILK BEVERAGES & YOGURT				
Cadbury drink	11 fl oz can (~344 g)	6	2	Hershey, 2002
Cadbury drink	15.5 fl oz bottle (484 g)	8	2	Hershey, 2002
choc malted milk, whole milk	8 fl oz (265 g)	8	3	14318
choc malted milk, whole milk w/ added nutrients	8 fl oz (265 g)	5	2	14316
choc milk, 1%/2% fat milk	8 fl oz (250 g)	5	2	01104/01103
choc milk, 2% fat, Hershey	8 fl oz (~250 g)	2	~1	Hershey, 2002
choc milk, from cocoa & sugar mix	8 fl oz (~250 g)	7	~3	Ahuja and Perloff, 2001
choc milk, from mix	8 fl oz (~250 g)	5	~2	Shively and Tarka, 1984
choc milk, from mix w/aspartame	6 fl oz (204 g)	4	2	14423
choc milk, whole milk	8 fl oz (250 g)	5	2	01102
choc milk, whole milk w/choc powder	8 fl oz (266 g)	8	3	14177
choc milk, whole milk w/choc syrup	8 fl oz (282 g)	6	2	14182
cocoa (hot choc)	8 fl oz (250 g)	21	~8	Bunker and McWilliams, 1979
cocoa (hot choc), from mix	8 fl oz (~250 g)	4	~2	Shively and Tarka, 1984
cocoa (hot choc), from mix, prep w/water	1 oz pkt in 6 fl oz water (206 g)	4	2	14194
cocoa (hot choc), from mix w/aspartame, prep w/water	1 pkt in 6 fl oz water (192 g)	6	3	14390
cocoa (hot choc), homemade	8 fl oz (~250 g)	10	~4	Shively and Tarka, 1984
cocoa (hot choc), homemade w/2% milk	8 fl oz (250 g)	5	2	01105
inst breakfast made w/milk/cnd, choc	10 fl oz can (315 g)	9	3	CSFII
yogurt, whole/nonfat, choc	8 oz (227 g)	~5	2	CSFII
MILK BEVERAGE MIXES				
choc milk mix	2–3 hp t (22 g)	8	36	14175
choc milk mix, Hershey	2 T (~16 g)	3	~19	Hershey, 2002
choc milk mix, malted	3 hp t (21 g)	8	37	14317
choc milk mix w/aspartame	.75 oz pkt (21 g)	3	16	14422
cocoa mix	3–4 hp t (28 g)	5	18	14192
cocoa mix, swiss mocha, Hershey Hot Cocoa Collection	35 g pkt	23	66	Hershey, 2002
inst breakfast mix, choc	1.2 oz pkt (35 g)	9	25	CSFII
inst breakfast mix w/low cal sweetener, choc	.72 oz pkt (21 g)	11	52	CSFII
malted milk powder, choc	3 hp t (21 g)	~8	37	CSFII
malted milk powder, fortified, choc	4–5 hp t (21 g)	~6	28	CSFII
MISCELLANEOUS				
baking choc (unsweetened)	1 oz square (28 g)	57	204	19078
baking choc (unsweetened), Hershey	1/2 bar (14 g)	23	164	Hershey, 2002
baking choc (unsweetened), liquid	1 oz pkt (28 g)	13	47	19077
baking choc (unsweetened), mexican	1 oz (28 g)	10	35	19124
choc liquor	1 oz (28 g)	60	214	Shively and Tarka, 1984
cocoa powder, unsweetened	1 T (5 g)	12	230	19165
cocoa powder, unsweetened, Hershey	1 T (5 g)	12	240	Hershey, 2002
cocoa powder, unsweetened, processed w/alkali	1 T (5 g)	4	78	19166

	SERVING SIZE (g)	CAFFEINE (mg/serving)	CAFFEINE (mg/100 g)	USDA CODE/SOURCE
gravy, redeye	1/4 cup (~60 g)	36	60	CSFII
sauce, mole poblana	1/4 cup (~60 g)	3	5	CSFII

[1] The FDA standard (effective January 2004) states that *white chocolate* is the common or usual name of products made from cacao fat, milk solids, nutritive carbohydrate sweeteners, and other safe and suitable ingredients. These products contain no nonfat cacao solids.

Sources:
Ahuja JKC, BP Perloff. Caffeine and theobromine intakes of children: results from CSFII 1994–96, 1998. *Fam Econ Nutr Rev* 13:47–51, 2001.
Anderson W, JG Hollins, PS Bond. The composition of tea infusions examined in relation to the association between mortality and water hardness. *J Hyg Camb* 69:1–13, 1971.
Bunker ML, M McWilliams. Caffeine content of common beverages. *J Am Diet Assoc* 74:28–32, 1979.
Caudle AG, LN Bell. Caffeine and theobromine contents of ready-to-eat chocolate cereals. *J Am Diet Assoc* 100:690–692, 2000.
COLA: The Coca-Cola company, Atlanta GA.
CSFII: United States Department of Agriculture. *Continuing Survey of the Food Intake of Individuals (CSFII) 1994–96, Survey Nutrient Database*, 1998. Data are provided per 100 grams from this source.
Groisser DS. A study of caffeine in tea I. A new spectrophotometric micro-method. II. Concentration of caffeine in various strengths, brands, blends, and types of teas. *Am J Clin Nutr* 31:1727–1731, 1978.
Hershey website, http://www.hersheys.com/nutrition_consumer/caffeine.shtml (11 March 2002).
Shively CA, SM Tarka. Methylxanthine composition and consumption patterns of cocoa and chocolate products. *The Methylxanthine Beverages and Foods: Chemistry, Consumption, and Health Effects.* Alan R Liss, Inc, New York NY. 1984.
SHST: Shasta Sales Incorporated, Columbia SC.
USDA Codes: *United States Department of Agriculture Database for Standard Reference, Release 15* (SR15), 2002. Available at http://www.nal.usda.gov/fnic/foodcomp/Data/SR15/sr15.html.

Carotenoids—Alpha-Carotene, Beta-Carotene, Beta-Cryptoxanthin, Lutein+Zeaxanthin, & Lycopene

	ALPHA-CAROTENE (mcg/100 g)	BETA-CAROTENE (mcg/100 g)	BETA-CRYPTOXANTHIN (mcg/100 g)	LUTEIN+ZEAXANTHIN (mcg/100 g)	LYCOPENE (mcg/100 g)	USDA CODE
CHEESE						
cheese, cheddar	0	85	0	0	0	01009
cheese, cheddar/colby, low fat		307				01168
cheese, cream, low fat	0	0	0			01186
DESSERTS						
cake, pound, fat-free		277				18451
halvah, plain	0	0	0			19117
cookie, oatmeal, fat free		133				18456
ice cream, van	0	19	0	0	0	19095
EGGS						
egg, whole, raw	0	0	0	55	0	01123
ENTREES						
beef stew w/potatoes & carrots, cnd	700	1,780	0	60	302	22502
chicken pot pie w/carrots, potatoes, peas, frzn	242	1,048	27	105	0	22503
green peppers stuffed w/beef, rice, tomato sce, frzn	0	192	0	75	3,092	22511
lasagna w/meat, tomato sce, frzn, ckd	0	170	0	97	7,750	22504
meatloaf w/mshd potatoes, gravy, frzn, ckd	0	110	0	0	930	22501
pasta in tomato sce w/cheese, cnd	0	127	0	0	3,162	22505
pasta w/chicken, carrots, peas, onions, mushrooms in oriental sce, frzn, ckd	365	620	0	312	0	22508
pasta w/shrimp, broccoli, red peppers, yellow zucchini, onion, in lemon pepper sce, frzn, ckd	0	148	0	177	0	22510
pizza, pepperoni, thin crust, frzn	0	264	0	15	4,449	22506
pizza, sausage, pepperoni, mushrooms, peppers, onions, thin crust, frzn	0	170	0	20	2,071	22507
spinach soufflé, frzn, ckd	0	1,300	0	2,727	0	22512
potato, sweet potato, rutabaga, green beans, onions w/beef & sce, frzn	0	352	0	70	285	22509

	ALPHA-CAROTENE (mcg/100 g)	BETA-CAROTENE (mcg/100 g)	BETA-CRYPTOXANTHIN (mcg/100 g)	LUTEIN+ ZEAXANTHIN (mcg/100 g)	LYCOPENE (mcg/100 g)	USDA CODE
FATS, OILS, & SPREADS						
butter	0	158	0	0	0	01001
butter, light, stick		1,164				04601
margarine, unspecified oils	0	485	0	0	0	04132
spread, 0% fat	0	170	0	0	0	04625
spread, stick/tub composite, 60% fat	0	721	0	0	0	04614
FRUIT JUICES						
orange jce, from frzn conc	2	24	99	138	0	09215
orange jce, raw	2	4	15	36		09206
orange jce, raw, all commercial varieties	16	51	122	187	0	09200
orange jce, raw, hybrid varieties	8	39	324	105		—
tangerine jce, from frzn conc		277	2,767			09224
tangerine jce, raw	9	21	115	166		09221
FRUITS						
apple w/peel, raw	30					09003
apricot, cnd, heavy syrup	0	6,640	0	0	65	09357
apricot, raw	0	2,554	0	0	5	09021
avocado, raw	28	53	36			09037
banana, raw	5	21	0	0	0	09040
blueberries, frzn	2					09054
blueberries, raw	0	35				09050
canary melon, raw		53				09180
cantaloupe, raw	27	1,595	0	40	0	09181
cherries, sweet, raw		28				09070
crenshaw melon, raw	15	450	14			09182
durian, raw/frzn	6	23	0			09422
fruit cocktail, cnd, heavy syrup	0	138	52	112	0	09351
grapefruit, pink/red, raw	5	603	12	13	1,462	09112
grapefruit, white, raw	8	14				09116
grapes, red/green, european types, raw		39				09132
kumquats, raw		0				09149
mango, cnd		13,120	1,550			09424
mango, raw	17	445	11			09176
mangosteen, cnd, syrup pack	1	16	9			09177
nectarine, raw	0	101	59			09191
orange, blood, raw	0	120	69			09199
papaya, raw	0	276	761	75	0	09226
passion fruit, yellow, raw	35	525	46			09230
peach, cnd, heavy syrup	0	334	141	33	0	09370
peach, raw	1	97	24	57	0	09236
pear, cnd, heavy syrup		4				09374
pear, raw	6	27				09252
pepino melon, raw	0		0			09426
persimmon, japanese, dried	18	374	156			09264
persimmon, japanese, raw		253	1,447	834	158	09263
persimmon, japanese, raw w/peel	75	349	94			—
pineapple, cnd, jce pack		30				09354
plum, raw		98	16			09279
prickly pear, raw	0	24	3			09287
pummelo, pink, raw	14	320	103			09425
pummelo, raw	0	0	10			09295
rambutan, cnd, syrup pack	0	2	0			09301
raspberries, raw	12	8	0			09302
strawberries, raw	5					09316
tamarind, raw	0	8	0			09322
tangerine, raw	14	71	485	243	0	09218
watermelon, raw	0	295	103	17	4,868	09326
GRAIN FRACTIONS						
barley flour/meal	0	0	0			20130
barley malt flour	0	23	0			20131
cornmeal, yellow, degermed, enr	63	97	0	1,355	0	20022
MEATS & SOY PRODUCTS						
beef liver, raw		621				13325
tofu, firm, prep w/Ca sulfate & MgCl (nigari)	0	0	0			16126

	ALPHA-CAROTENE (mcg/100 g)	BETA-CAROTENE (mcg/100 g)	BETA-CRYPTOXANTHIN (mcg/100 g)	LUTEIN+ ZEAXANTHIN (mcg/100 g)	LYCOPENE (mcg/100 g)	USDA CODE
MILK						
milk, human, mature	0	1		1	3	01107
milk, whole, 3.3% fat	0	8	0	0	0	01077
NUTS & SEEDS						
sunflower seed kernels, oil roasted w/o salt	0	0	0			12038
SAUCES, GRAVIES, CONDIMENTS, & FLAVORINGS						
capers, cnd	0	83	0			02054
gravy, chicken, cnd		386				06119
hoisin sce, rts	0	12	0			06175
horseradish, prep	0	0	0			02055
mole sce, cnd	0	9	0			06137
mole sce, homemade	199	1,282	828			06136
olives, green, cnd/bottled	0	207	4			09195
oyster sce, rts	0	13	0			06176
pepper/hot sce, rts		558				06168
plum sce, rts	0	26	0			06151
salsa, rts		398				06164
tomato catsup	0	730	0	0	17,008	11935
tomato sce, cnd	0	410	0	1	15,916	11549
tomato sce, spaghetti/marinara, rts	0	440	0	160	15,990	06931
SOUPS						
chicken noodle, cnd, cond	151	391				06019
minestrone, cnd, cond	210	920	0	150	1,480	06040
tomato, cnd, cond	0	235	0	90	10,920	06159
veg beef, cnd, cond	489	1,618	0	92	364	06071
vegetarian veg, cnd, cond	410	1,500	0	160	1,930	06068
SPICES & HERBS						
spearmint, dried	0	8,847	650			02066
spearmint, raw	0	2,133	0			02065
thyme, raw		2,851				02049
VEGETABLES						
acorn squash, boiled, mashed	0	490	0	66	0	11484
acorn squash, raw	0	220	0	38	0	11482
arrowroot, raw	0	11	0			11697
asparagus, raw	12	493				11011
balsam pear (bitter gourd), pods, raw	185	190				11024
beans, baked, plain/veg, cnd	147	408				16006
beet greens, boiled		2,560				11087
beet greens, raw	5	3,405				11086
broccoli, boiled	0	1,042	0	2,226	0	11091
broccoli, chopped, frzn		950				11092
broccoli, chopped, frzn, boiled		1,000		830		11093
broccoli, cauliflower, baby carrots w/ butter sce, frzn	333	450	0	142	0	11996
broccoli, raw	1	779	0	2,445	0	11090
broccoli stalk, frzn		270				———
broccoli, chinese, raw	29	968	0			11969
brussels sprouts, boiled	0	465	0	1,290	0	11099
brussels sprouts, frzn		370				11100
brussels sprouts, raw	6	450	0	1,590	0	11098
buttercup squash, raw	24	710				11494
butternut squash, baked	1,130	4,570				11486
butternut squash, raw	834	4,226				11485
cabbage, boiled		90				11110
cabbage, raw	0	65	0	310	0	11109
cabbage, napa, ckd	49	133	0			11970
carrot, baby, raw	4,425	7,275	0	358	0	11960
carrot, boiled	4,109	8,015				11125
carrot, cnd	3,470	5,776	0	0	0	11128
carrot, frzn, boiled	5,542	12,272				11131
carrot, raw	4,649	8,836				11124

	ALPHA-CAROTENE (mcg/100 g)	BETA-CAROTENE (mcg/100 g)	BETA-CRYPTOXANTHIN (mcg/100 g)	LUTEIN+ ZEAXANTHIN (mcg/100 g)	LYCOPENE (mcg/100 g)	USDA CODE
cassava, raw	0	8	0			11134
celery, boiled	0	210	0	250	0	11144
celery, raw	0	150	0	232	0	11143
chayote, fruit, raw	0	0	0			11149
chickpeas, hummus, homemade	0	10	15			16137
chrysanthemum, garland, raw	0	1,320	24			11157
cilantro, raw	72	3,440	404			11971
citronella, raw	0	3	0			11997
collards, boiled	90	4,418	20	8,091	0	11162
collards, frzn		5,510				11163
collards, raw	238	3,323	80			11161
corn, sweet, yellow, boiled				1,800		11168
corn, sweet, yellow, cnd	33	30	0	884	0	11172
corn, sweet, yellow, frzn, boiled	18	50	119			11179
cucumber w/o peel, raw	8	31				11206
cucumber w/peel, raw		138				11205
endive, raw/ckd		960				11213
fava beans, raw	0	196	9			11973
fiddlehead ferns, home cnd	270	1,640				——
fiddlehead ferns, home frzn	280	1,870				——
fiddlehead ferns, raw	331	2,040				11995
grape leaves, cnd	629	2,838	0			11975
grape leaves, raw	0	16,194	4			11974
green (snap) beans, boiled	92	552	0	700	0	11053
green (snap) beans, cnd	0	443	0	660	0	11056
green (snap) beans, frzn		292				11060
green (snap) beans, frzn, boiled	32	167				11061
green (snap) beans, raw	68	377	0	640	0	11052
hubbard squash, raw		820				11489
kale, boiled	0	6,202	0	15,798	0	11234
kale, raw	0	9,226	0	39,550	0	11233
lentils, pink, raw	0	35	0			16144
lettuce, cos/romaine, raw	0	1,272	0	2,635	0	11251
lettuce, iceberg	2	192	0	352	0	11252
lotus root, boiled	0	3	0			11255
mushrooms, black, dried	0	0	0			11999
mushrooms, straw, cnd	0	0	0			11989
okra, boiled	0	170	0	390	0	11279
okra, raw	28	432				11278
onion, spring, raw	6	391				11291
papad urad, dahl, ckd	3	7	0			18465
peas, green, cnd	0	320	0	1,350	0	11308
peas, green, frzn	33	320				11312
peas, green, raw	19	485				11304
pepper, banana, raw	39	184	0			11976
pepper, serrano, raw	18	534	40			11977
pepper, sweet, green, raw	22	198				11333
pepper, sweet, red, boiled	62	2,220				11823
pepper, sweet, red, raw	59	2,379	2,205			11821
pepper, sweet, yellow, raw		120				11951
pinto beans, mature, raw		26				16042
potato w/peel, raw		6				11352
pumpkin, cnd	4,795	6,940	0	0	0	11424
spinach, boiled	0	5,242	0	7,043	0	11458
spinach, cnd		4,820				11461
spinach, frzn		4,940				11463
spinach, raw	0	5,597	0	11,938	0	11457
squash, str infant food	308	1,110	7	3,527	0	03104
summer squash, crookneck/straightneck, raw	0	90	0	290	0	11467
sweet potato, baked in skin	0	9,488	0	0	0	11508
sweet potato, cnd, vacuum pack	0	8,314	0	0	0	11512
sweet potato, frzn		6,220				11516
sweet potato, raw	0	9,180	0	0	0	11507
swiss chard	49	3,954				11147
tomato jce, cnd	0	428	0	60	9,318	11886
tomato paste	29	1,242	0	170	29,330	11887

	ALPHA-CAROTENE (mcg/100 g)	BETA-CAROTENE (mcg/100 g)	BETA-CRYPTOXANTHIN (mcg/100 g)	LUTEIN+ ZEAXANTHIN (mcg/100 g)	LYCOPENE (mcg/100 g)	USDA CODE
tomato puree	0	410	0	90	16,670	11888
tomato, red, boiled	0	300	0	150	4,400	11530
tomato, red, cnd	0	186	0	40	9,708	11531
tomato, red, raw	112	393	0	130	3,025	11529
turnip greens, boiled	0	4,575	0	9,708	0	11569
veg jce cocktail, cnd	210	830	0	80	9,660	11578
wasabi root, raw	0	14	0			11990
yautia (tannier), raw	0	3	0			11991
zucchini, raw	0	410	0	2,125	0	11477

Source:
USDA Codes: *United States Department of Agriculture-University of Minnesota Nutrition Coordinating Center Carotenoid Database for US Foods,* 1998. Available at http://www.nal.usda.gov/fnic/foodcomp/data/car98/car_tble.pdf.

Carotenoids—Zeaxanthin

	ZEAXANTHIN (mcg/100)	USDA CODE		ZEAXANTHIN (mcg/100)	USDA CODE
EGGS			**VEGETABLES**		
egg, whole, raw	23	01123	broccoli, boiled	23	11091
			carrot, baby, raw	23	11960
GRAIN FRACTIONS			celery, boiled	8	11144
cornmeal, degermed, yellow, enr	457	20022	celery, raw	3	11143
			collards, boiled	266	11162
FRUITS & FRUIT JUICES			corn, sweet, yellow, cnd	528	11172
orange, all varieties, raw	74	09200	green (snap) beans, cnd	44	11056
orange jce, from frzn conc	80	09215	kale, boiled	173	11234
peach, cnd, heavy syrup	19	09370	lettuce, cos/romaine, raw	187	11251
peach, raw	6	09236	lettuce, iceberg, raw	70	11252
persimmon, japanese, raw	488	09263	peas, green, cnd	58	11308
tangerine, raw	112	09218	spinach, boiled	179	11458
			spinach, raw	331	11457
			turnip greens, boiled	267	11569

Source:
USDA Codes: *United States Department of Agriculture-Univerity of Minnesota Nutrition Coding Center Carotenoid Database for US Foods,* 1998. Available at http://www.nal.usda.gov/fnic/foodcomp/data/car98/zea_tble.pdf.

Dietary Fiber Components—Lignin & Pectin

	LIGNIN[1] (g/100 g)	PECTIN[2] (g/100 g)	SOURCE
BEVERAGES			
beer		0.20	USDA Agr Hnd
coffee, inst powder		22.2	USDA Agr Hnd
coffee w/mocha flavor & sugar, inst powder		0.87	USDA Agr Hnd
coffee w/mocha flavor & sugar, prep from inst powder		0.10	USDA Agr Hnd
lemonade, from frzn conc		0.10	USDA Agr Hnd
lemonade w/pulp	0.0	0.0	Marlett and Cheung, 1997
orange breakfast drink, from frzn conc		0.10	USDA Agr Hnd
tea, inst powder		4.29	USDA Agr Hnd
whisky sour mix, bottled		0.20	USDA Agr Hnd
whisky sour, prep from bottled mix		0.10	USDA Agr Hnd

	LIGNIN[1] (g/100 g)	PECTIN[2] (g/100 g)	SOURCE
CEREALS & GRAINS, COOKED			
corn/hominy grits, white, ckd	tr	tr	Marlett, 1992
cream of wheat, quick, ckd	0.1	tr	Marlett, 1992
oat bran, not ckd	3.5	0.3	Marlett and Cheung, 1997
oatmeal, reg, ckd	0.5	0.1	Marlett, 1992
rice, white, med grain, ckd	0.1	tr	Marlett, 1992
CEREALS, READY-TO-EAT			
All Bran	4.3	1.0	Marlett, 1992
bran flakes, 40%	1.5	0.7	Marlett, 1992
Corn Chex	1.4	tr	Marlett and Cheung, 1997
corn flakes	0.7	0.1	Marlett, 1992
corn flakes, sugar-frosted	0.4	tr	Marlett and Cheung, 1997
Frosted Miniwheats	1.0	0.2	Marlett, 1992
Golden Grahams	0.4	tr	Marlett and Cheung, 1997
granola	0.4	0.4	Marlett and Cheung, 1997
Grape-Nuts	0.7	tr	Marlett and Cheung, 1997
Grape-Nuts Flakes	0.7	tr	Marlett and Cheung, 1997
Honey Smacks	0.1	0.1	Marlett, 1992
Life	1.8	tr	Marlett and Cheung, 1997
Product 19	1.5	0.2	Marlett, 1992
puffed rice	0.7	tr	Marlett and Cheung, 1997
puffed wheat	0.7	tr	Marlett and Cheung, 1997
Rice Krispies	0.6	0.1	Marlett, 1992
shredded wheat	0.9	0.3	Marlett, 1992
Special K	0.9	0.1	Marlett, 1992
Wheat Chex	0.36	0.36	Marlett and Cheung, 1997
Wheaties	1.4	0.6	Marlett, 1992
Total	1.6	0.1	Marlett, 1992
DESSERTS			
brownie	1.0	tr	Marlett and Cheung, 1997
brownie w/nuts	1.5	tr	Marlett and Cheung, 1997
cake, devil's food	1.0	0.25	Marlett and Cheung, 1997
cake, gingerbread	0.3	tr	Marlett and Cheung, 1997
cake, pound/sponge	0.3	tr	Marlett and Cheung, 1997
cake, yellow	0.1	tr	Marlett, 1992
cherry pie filling, cnd	0.1	0.1	Marlett and Cheung, 1997
cinnamon roll	0.4	0.1	Marlett, 1992
coffeecake	0.2	tr	Marlett and Cheung, 1997
cookies, date	1.7	0.3	Marlett and Cheung, 1997
cookies, fig	1.0	1.7	Marlett and Cheung, 1997
cookies, gingersnaps	0.4	tr	Marlett, 1992
cookies, graham crackers	0.4	0.1	Marlett, 1992
cookies, oatmeal w/o raisins	0.7	tr	Marlett and Cheung, 1997
cookies, oatmeal w/raisins	0.8	tr	Marlett and Cheung, 1997
cookies, peanut	tr	0.4	Marlett and Cheung, 1997
cookies, sugar	tr	tr	Marlett, 1992
cream puff w/o filling	0.6	tr	Marlett and Cheung, 1997
doughnut, glazed	0.5	tr	Marlett and Cheung, 1997
doughnut, jelly	0.15	tr	Marlett and Cheung, 1997
eclair, frzn	0.5	tr	Marlett and Cheung, 1997
ice cream cone, Comet Cup	0.5	tr	Marlett, 1992
pie, apple	0.08	0.17	Marlett and Cheung, 1997
pie, cherry	0.08	0.08	Marlett and Cheung, 1997
pie crust	0.6	tr	Marlett, 1992
pie filling, apple, cnd	tr	0.28	Marlett and Cheung, 1997
pie, pecan	0.2	0.1	Marlett and Cheung, 1997
pie, rhubarb	0.08	0.25	Marlett and Cheung, 1997
pie, strawberry	0.2	0.1	Marlett and Cheung, 1997
sweet roll w/nuts	0.27	0.14	Marlett and Cheung, 1997
sweet roll w/raisins	0.6	tr	Marlett and Cheung, 1997
FRUITS			
apple, frzn, unsweetened		0.47	USDA Agr Hnd
apple, granny smith, raw	0.1	0.8	Marlett, 1992
apple, peeled	0.1	0.5	Marlett and Cheung, 1997
apple, peeled, boiled		0.27	USDA Agr Hnd
apple, peeled, microwave ckd		0.44	USDA Agr Hnd

	LIGNIN[1] (g/100 g)	PECTIN[2] (g/100 g)	SOURCE
apple, peeled, raw		0.38	USDA Agr Hnd
apple, red delicious, peeled, raw	0.1	0.5	Marlett, 1992
apple, red delicious, raw	0.2	0.7	Marlett, 1992
apple, sliced, sweetened, cnd		0.43	USDA Agr Hnd
apple, sweetened, cnd		0.49	USDA Agr Hnd
apple, raw	0.01		Souci et al, 2000
apple, raw		1.07	USDA Agr Hnd
applesauce, cnd	0.1	0.3	Marlett and Cheung, 1997
applesauce, sweetened, cnd		0.30	USDA Agr Hnd
apricot, cnd in syrup	0.1	0.6	Marlett, 1992
apricot, dried	0.7	1.4	Marlett and Cheung, 1997
banana, raw	0.6	0.4	Marlett, 1992
blackberries, frzn	3.0	0.9	Marlett and Cheung, 1997
blueberries, raw	0.9	0.6	Marlett, 1992
cantaloupe, raw	tr	0.3	Marlett, 1992
cherries, tart, cnd	0.2	0.3	Marlett, 1992
cranberry sce, cnd	0.3	0.1	Marlett and Cheung, 1997
currants, black, raw	1.45		Souci et al, 2000
currants, red, raw	0.72		Souci et al, 2000
date, dried	8.0	2.0	Marlett and Cheung, 1997
fig, dried	2.2	2.3	Marlett and Cheung, 1997
fruit cocktail, cnd	0.2	0.1	Marlett and Cheung, 1997
gooseberries, raw	0.23		Souci et al, 2000
grapefruit, pink FL w/membrane, raw	tr	0.7	Marlett, 1992
grapefruit, pink FL w/o membrane, raw	tr	0.3	Marlett, 1992
grapefruit, pink TX w/o membrane, raw	tr	0.1	Marlett, 1992
grapefruit, white FL w/o membrane, raw	tr	0.3	Marlett, 1992
grapes, black/red, raw	0.4	0.2	Marlett and Cheung, 1997
grapes, green, Thompson, raw	0.2	0.3	Marlett, 1992
honeydew melon, raw	tr	0.2	Marlett and Cheung, 1997
kiwifruit, raw		0.42	USDA Agr Hnd
kiwifruit, raw	0.8	0.4	Marlett and Cheung, 1997
lemon, peeled, raw	tr	0.7	Marlett and Cheung, 1997
mandarin orange, cnd	tr	0.1	Marlett and Cheung, 1997
nectarine, raw	0.1	0.3	Marlett, 1992
orange, navel, raw	tr	0.7	Marlett, 1992
orange, FL	tr	0.9	Marlett, 1992
papaya, raw	tr	0.7	Marlett and Cheung, 1997
peach, peeled, raw/cnd	0.1	0.4	Marlett and Cheung, 1997
peach, raw	0.1	0.5	Marlett and Cheung, 1997
pear, bartlett, raw	0.4	0.7	Marlett, 1992
pear, cnd in extra light syrup	0.2	0.3	Marlett, 1992
pineapple, raw/cnd	tr	tr	Marlett and Cheung, 1997
plum, cnd	0.2	0.6	Marlett and Cheung, 1997
plum, prune, raw	0.4	0.7	Marlett and Cheung, 1997
plum, raw	0.2	0.5	Marlett, 1992
prune, dried	1.2	2.4	Marlett and Cheung, 1997
raisins	1.8	0.9	Marlett, 1992
raspberries, raw	2.3	0.5	Marlett and Cheung, 1997
strawberries, raw	0.5	0.5	Marlett, 1992
tangerine, raw	0.1	0.8	Marlett, 1992
watermelon, raw	tr	0.1	Marlett, 1992
GRAIN FRACTIONS			
flour, white wheat	0.2	0.1	Marlett, 1992
oat bran, unckd	3.5	0.4	Marlett, 1992
wheat germ	1.2	0.8	Marlett, 1992
GRAIN PRODUCTS			
biscuit, baking powder	0.1	tr	Marlett, 1992
bread, french	0.1	tr	Marlett, 1992
bread, italian	0.7	0.1	Marlett, 1992
bread, italian w/sesame seeds	1.0	0.1	Marlett, 1992
bread, raisin	0.8	tr	Marlett and Cheung, 1997
bread, rye	0.4	tr	Marlett and Cheung, 1997
bread, white	0.5	0.1	Marlett, 1992
bread, whole wheat	1.4	tr	Marlett and Cheung, 1997
cornbread	0.4	0.1	Marlett, 1992
crackers, cheese w/peanut butter	0.7	tr	Marlett and Cheung, 1997

	LIGNIN[1] (g/100 g)	PECTIN[2] (g/100 g)	SOURCE
crackers, saltines	0.5	tr	Marlett, 1992
crackers, Triscuits	0.7	tr	Marlett and Cheung, 1997
english muffin	0.7	0.1	Marlett, 1992
hush puppy, homemade	0.4	0.2	Marlett and Cheung, 1997
macaroni, ckd	0.7	tr	Marlett, 1992
muffin	0.4	tr	Marlett, 1992
muffin, blueberry	0.75	tr	Marlett and Cheung, 1997
muffin, wheat bran, commercial	0.5	tr	Marlett and Cheung, 1997
muffin, wheat bran, homemade	0.75	tr	Marlett and Cheung, 1997
noodles, egg, ckd	0.4	tr	Marlett, 1992
pancake	0.2	tr	Marlett and Cheung, 1997
pancake, buckwheat	1.7	tr	Marlett and Cheung, 1997
pancake mix	0.6	0.1	Marlett, 1992
popcorn, white/yellow, popped	1.7	tr	Marlett and Cheung, 1997
roll, dinner	0.4	tr	Marlett and Cheung, 1997
roll, hamburger	0.2	tr	Marlett, 1992
roll, hard	1.2	tr	Marlett and Cheung, 1997
roll, submarine	0.9	tr	Marlett and Cheung, 1997
spaghetti, ckd	tr	tr	Marlett, 1992
stuffing, cornbread	0.1	0.1	Marlett and Cheung, 1997
taco shell	0.9	0.3	Marlett, 1992
tortilla, flour	0.3	tr	Marlett, 1992
waffle	0.4	tr	Marlett and Cheung, 1997
NUTS & SEEDS			
almonds	1.9	1.6	Marlett, 1992
almonds, dried		1.36	USDA Agr Hnd
cashews, roasted	1.07	0.7	Marlett and Cheung, 1997
chestnuts, european, raw		1.21	USDA Agr Hnd
chestnuts, roasted		1.21	USDA Agr Hnd
coconut, shredded	0.0	0.3	Marlett, 1992
peanut butter	0.8	1.0	Marlett, 1992
peanuts	0.7	1.2	Marlett, 1992
pumpkin seeds	8.0	tr	Marlett and Cheung, 1997
pecans	1.43	1.07	Marlett and Cheung, 1997
walnuts, english	0.9	0.7	Marlett, 1992
SOUPS & ENTREES			
lasagna w/meat sce, frzn	0.3	0.2	Marlett and Cheung, 1997
soup, crm of mushroom, cnd, prep	0.0	tr	Marlett, 1992
soup, crm of tomato, cnd, prep	0.04	0.04	Marlett and Cheung, 1997
soup, pea, cnd, prep	0.16	0.12	Marlett and Cheung, 1997
soup, veg beef, cnd, prep	0.08	0.08	Marlett and Cheung, 1997
soup, vegetarian veg, cnd, prep	0.1	0.3	Marlett, 1992
VEGETABLES			
artichoke, ckd	0.08	1.0	Marlett and Cheung, 1997
asparagus, raw, ckd	0.1	0.6	Marlett, 1992
asparagus spears, cnd	0.2	0.2	Marlett, 1992
avocado	0.1	1.0	Marlett, 1992
bamboo shoots, cnd	0.1	0.1	Marlett, 1992
bean sprouts, cnd	0.1	0.2	Marlett, 1992
beet greens, ckd	0.14	0.56	Marlett and Cheung, 1997
beets, cnd	tr	0.5	Marlett, 1992
broccoli, chopped/spears, frzn, boiled		1.00	USDA Agr Hnd
broccoli, raw	0.3	0.7	Marlett, 1992
broccoli, raw, ckd	0.3	0.9	Marlett, 1992
brussels sprouts, frzn, boiled		1.40	USDA Agr Hnd
brussels sprouts, frzn, ckd	0.1	1.0	Marlett, 1992
cabbage, green, ckd	0.14	0.7	Marlett and Cheung, 1997
cabbage, raw	tr	0.6	Marlett, 1992
carrot, peeled, raw	0.1	0.8	Marlett, 1992
carrot, raw		1.00	USDA Agr Hnd
cauliflower, raw	0.1	0.6	Marlett, 1992
cauliflower, raw, ckd	tr	0.6	Marlett, 1992
celery, raw	tr	0.6	Marlett, 1992
celery, raw, ckd	tr	0.6	Marlett, 1992
chinese cabbage	tr	0.3	Marlett and Cheung, 1997
collards, frzn, ckd	0.24	1.06	Marlett and Cheung, 1997

	LIGNIN[1] (g/100 g)	PECTIN[2] (g/100 g)	SOURCE
corn, creamed, cnd	0.16	tr	Marlett and Cheung, 1997
corn, sweet, yellow/white, frzn, boiled		0.40	USDA Agr Hnd
corn, whole kernel, cnd	0.5	0.1	Marlett, 1992
corn, whole kernel, frzn	0.3	0.1	Marlett, 1992
cucumber, peeled, raw	tr	0.1	Marlett, 1992
cucumber, raw	0.1	0.2	Marlett, 1992
cucumber, raw	0.03		Souci et al, 2000
eggplant, cnd	0.2	0.6	Marlett and Cheung, 1997
endive, raw	0.4	1.2	Marlett and Cheung, 1997
escarole, raw	0.4	0.4	Marlett and Cheung, 1997
green beans, cut, cnd	0.2	0.4	Marlett, 1992
green beans, french cut, cnd	0.1	0.5	Marlett, 1992
green beans, frzn, boiled		0.90	USDA Agr Hnd
kale, ckd	0.3	1.4	Marlett and Cheung, 1997
kohlrabi, ckd	tr	0.5	Marlett and Cheung, 1997
lettuce, leaf/romaine/iceberg, raw	0.2	0.4	Marlett and Cheung, 1997
mushrooms, cnd	0.1	0.1	Marlett, 1992
mushrooms, cnd	tr	0.3	Marlett and Cheung, 1997
mushrooms, raw	0.3	tr	Marlett and Cheung, 1997
mustard greens, ckd	0.13	1.07	Marlett and Cheung, 1997
okra, frzn, ckd	0.65	0.54	Marlett and Cheung, 1997
onion, green, raw	0.2	0.8	Marlett, 1992
onion rings, frzn, ckd	0.14	0.43	Marlett and Cheung, 1997
onion, yellow, raw	tr	0.5	Marlett, 1992
parsnip, ckd	1.25	1.15	Marlett and Cheung, 1997
peas, green, frzn, boiled		0.60	USDA Agr Hnd
pepper, green, sweet, raw	0.3	0.4	Marlett, 1992
potato, red, boiled	0.13	0.33	Marlett and Cheung, 1997
potato, red, peeled, boiled	tr	0.22	Marlett and Cheung, 1997
potato, white, french fries	0.1	0.4	Marlett, 1992
potato, white, peeled, boiled	tr	0.2	Marlett, 1992
potato, white, baked	0.3	0.3	Marlett, 1992
potato, white, fried (french fries)	tr	0.4	Marlett and Cheung, 1997
potato, white, hash w/corned beef, cnd	0.04	0.13	Marlett and Cheung, 1997
potato, white, salad	tr	0.24	Marlett and Cheung, 1997
potato, white, scalloped, frzn, ckd	tr	0.16	Marlett and Cheung, 1997
pumpkin, cnd	0.2	0.8	Marlett, 1992
radish, red, raw	tr	0.4	Marlett, 1992
rhubarb, ckd w/sugar	0.1	0.2	Marlett and Cheung, 1997
rutabaga, ckd	0.12	0.82	Marlett and Cheung, 1997
sauerkraut, cnd	tr	0.82	Marlett and Cheung, 1997
spinach, boiled		0.80	USDA Agr Hnd
spinach, boiled/cnd	0.3	0.5	Marlett and Cheung, 1997
spinach, frzn, boiled		1.11	USDA Agr Hnd
spinach, raw, chopped		0.79	USDA Agr Hnd
summer squash, all varieties, raw, sliced		0.60	USDA Agr Hnd
summer squash, all varieties, sliced, boiled		0.50	USDA Agr Hnd
summer squash, crookneck, raw, sliced		0.60	USDA Agr Hnd
summer squash, crookneck, sliced, boiled		0.50	USDA Agr Hnd
summer squash, yellow zucchini, ckd/raw	tr	0.25	Marlett and Cheung, 1977
summer squash, zucchini, raw	tr	0.2	Marlett, 1992
sweet potato, cubed, baked, frzn		0.80	USDA Agr Hnd
sweet potato w/peel, baked		0.80	USDA Agr Hnd
swiss chard, ckd	0.23	0.57	Marlett and Cheung, 1997
swede (rutabaga), raw	0.12		Souci et al, 2000
sweet potato, cnd in light syrup	0.1	0.3	Marlett, 1992
tomato, cnd	0.1	0.2	Marlett, 1992
tomato (spaghetti) sce	0.64	0.56	Marlett and Cheung, 1997
turnip greens, frzn	0.1	0.9	Marlett, 1992
waterchestnuts	tr	tr	Marlett and Cheung, 1977
white beans, dry	1.4		Souci et al, 2000
winter squash, acorn/butternut, ckd	tr	0.6	Marlett and Cheung, 1997
winter squash, raw	0.07		Souci et al, 2000

VEGETABLES - LEGUMES

baked beans w/pork, cnd	0.2	0.6	Marlett and Cheung, 1997
black beans, ckd	0.47	0.23	Marlett and Cheung, 1997
black-eyed peas, cnd	0.5	0.3	Marlett, 1992
crowder peas, cnd	0.35	0.35	Marlett and Cheung, 1997

	LIGNIN[1] (g/100 g)	PECTIN[2] (g/100 g)	SOURCE
great northern beans, ckd	0.11	0.8	Marlett and Cheung, 1997
kidney beans, cnd	0.34	0.57	Marlett and Cheung, 1997
lentils, ckd	0.2	0.2	Marlett and Cheung, 1997
lima beans, green, cnd	0.1	0.4	Marlett, 1992
kidney beans, cnd	0.3	0.6	Marlett, 1992
navy beans, ckd	0.11	0.44	Marlett and Cheung, 1997
peas, green, cnd	0.1	0.5	Marlett, 1992
peas, green, frzn	tr	0.7	Marlett, 1992
pigeon peas, cnd	1.04	0.39	Marlett and Cheung, 1997
pork & beans, cnd	0.2	0.6	Marlett, 1992
MISCELLANEOUS			
catsup	0.2	0.3	Marlett, 1992
olives, black	0.6	0.3	Marlett, 1992
olives, green w/pimento	0.4	0.3	Marlett, 1992
pickle, dill	0.1	0.3	Marlett, 1992
pickle relish	tr	tr	Marlett and Cheung, 1997
potato chips	0.0	0.71	Marlett and Cheung, 1997

[1] Lignin is Klason lignin for Marlett, 1992 and Marlett and Cheung, 1997.
[2] Pectin is the sum of soluble and insoluble pectin for Marlett, 1992 and Marlett and Cheung, 1997.

Sources:
Marlett JA. Content and composition of dietary fiber in 117 frequently consumed foods. *J Am Diet Assoc* 92:175–186, 1992.
Marlett JA, T-F Cheung. Database and quick methods of assessing typical dietary fiber intakes using data for 228 commonly consumed foods. *J Am Diet Assoc* 97:1139–1148, 1997.
Souci SW, W Fachmann, H Kraut. *Food Composition and Nutrition Tables.* Medpharm GmbH Scientific Publishers, Stuttgart, Germany & CRC Press, Washington DC. 2000.
United States Department of Agriculture. *Agriculture Handbooks No. 8–9, 8–11, 8–12, 8–14, and 1989 Supplement.* US Government Printing Office, Washington DC, 1982–1989.

Fatty Acids—Omega-3 Fatty Acids[1]

FOOD	SERVING	WEIGHT (g)	OMEGA-3 FATTY ACIDS (g/serving)	SOURCE/USDA CODE
DESSERTS				
pastry, puff, frzn	1 pastry	40	1.035	18211
pie, snack pie, fried, cherry/fruit/lemon	1 snack pie (5″ × 3 3/4″)	128	0.727	18444/18319/18445
topping, nuts in syrup	2 T	41	0.992	19367
Twix Cookie Bar, caramel, M&M/Mars	2.06 oz pkg (2 bars)	58	0.597	19160
EGGS				
goose egg, whole	1 egg	144	0.798	01139
ENTREES				
baked beans w/franks, cnd	1 cup (9.1 oz)	259	0.539	16008
biscuit, egg & bacon	1 biscuit	150	0.534	21003
biscuit, egg & ham	1 biscuit	192	0.501	21004
cheeseburger, reg, double meat, double-decker bun w/lettuce & tomato	1 sandwich	228	0.650	21095
cheeseburger, reg, single meat w/lettuce & tomato	1 sandwich	154	0.551	21091
chicken fillet sandwich	1 sandwich	182	0.959	21102
coleslaw	3/4 cup	99	0.773	21127
corn dog (frank w/corn flour coating)	1 corn dog	175	0.730	21120
fish sandwich w/tartar sce	1 sandwich	158	0.630	21105
fish sandwich w/tartar sce & cheese	1 sandwich	183	0.959	21106
french toast sticks	5 sticks	141	0.646	21024
lamb fat, ckd	3 oz	85	0.952	17006
FATS, OILS, & SPREADS				
cod liver oil	1 T	14	2.684	04589
herring oil	1 T	14	1.613	04590
mayonnaise, reg, soy	1 T	14	0.580	04025
menhaden oil	1 T	14	3.826	04591

FOOD	SERVING	WEIGHT (g)	OMEGA-3 FATTY ACIDS (g/serving)	SOURCE/USDA CODE
mustard oil	1 T	14	0.826	04583
salmon oil	1 T	14	4.802	04593
soy (hydg) & cottonseed oil (for bread)	1 T	13	0.512	04546
soy lecithin	1 T	14	0.698	04531
soy oil	1 T	14	0.925	04044
walnut oil	1 T	14	1.414	04528
wheat germ oil	1 T	14	0.938	04038
FISH & SHELLFISH				
anchovies, raw	3 oz	85	1.256	15001
bass, freshwater, ckd by dry heat	3 oz	85	0.861	15187
bass, freshwater, raw	3 oz	85	0.672	15003
bass, striped, ckd by dry heat	3 oz	85	0.838	15188
bass, striped, raw	3 oz	85	0.654	15004
bluefish, ckd by dry heat	3 oz	85	0.907	15189
bluefish, raw	3 oz	85	0.708	15005
carp, ckd by dry heat	3 oz	85	0.767	15009
carp, raw	3 oz	85	0.598	15008
caviar, black & red, granular	1 T	16	1.086	15012
cisco, smoked	3 oz	85	1.291	15014
crab, alaska king, imitation, made from surimi	3 oz	85	0.536	15138
drum, freshwater, ckd by dry heat	3 oz	85	0.845	15195
drum, freshwater, raw	3 oz	85	0.659	15024
eel, ckd by dry heat	3 oz	85	0.712	15026
eel, raw	3 oz	85	0.555	15025
halibut, atlantic & pacific, ckd by dry heat	3 oz	85	0.569	15037
halibut, greenland, ckd by dry heat	3 oz	85	1.145	15196
halibut, greenland, raw	3 oz	85	0.893	15038
herring, atlantic, ckd by dry heat	3 oz	85	1.884	15040
herring, atlantic, kippered	1 piece (5″ × 1 3/4″ × 1/4″)	40	0.946	15042
herring, atlantic, raw	3 oz	85	1.470	15039
herring, pacific, ckd by dry heat	3 oz	85	2.055	15197
herring, pacific, raw	3 oz	85	1.604	15043
mackerel, atlantic, ckd by dry heat	3 oz	85	1.209	15047
mackerel, atlantic, raw	3 oz	85	2.270	15046
mackerel, jack, cnd	1 cup	190	2.616	15048
mackerel, pacific & jack, ckd by dry heat	3 oz	85	1.760	15201
mackerel, pacific & jack, raw	3 oz	85	1.372	15050
mackerel, spanish, ckd by dry heat	3 oz	85	1.238	15052
mackerel, spanish, raw	3 oz	85	1.255	15051
mussels, blue, ckd by moist heat	3 oz	85	0.736	15165
oysters, eastern, breaded & fried	6 med (3 oz)	88	0.549	15168
oysters, eastern, wild, ckd by moist heat	6 med	42	0.565	15169
oysters, eastern, wild, raw	6 med	84	0.564	15167
oysters, pacific, ckd by moist heat	3 oz	85	1.258	15231
oysters, pacific, raw	3 oz	85	0.629	15171
pomano, florida, raw	3 oz	85	0.655	15068
roe, mixed species, ckd by dry heat	1 oz	28	0.885	15207
roe, mixed species, raw	1 oz	28	0.690	15072
sablefish, ckd by dry heat	3 oz	85	1.806	15208
sablefish, raw	3 oz	85	1.410	15074
sablefish, smoked	3 oz	85	1.856	15075
salmon, atlantic, farmed, ckd by dry heat	3 oz	85	1.921	15237
salmon, atlantic, farmed, raw	3 oz	85	1.704	15236
salmon, atlantic, wild, ckd by dry heat	3 oz	85	2.198	15209
salmon, atlantic, wild, raw	3 oz	85	1.715	15076
salmon, chinook, ckd by dry heat	3 oz	85	1.822	15210
salmon, chinook, raw	3 oz	85	1.421	15078
salmon, chum, ckd by dry heat	3 oz	85	0.807	15211
salmon, chum, cnd w/bone	3 oz	85	1.117	15080
salmon, chum, raw	3 oz	85	0.629	15079
salmon, coho, farmed, ckd by dry heat	3 oz	85	1.152	15239
salmon, coho, farmed, raw	3 oz	85	1.089	15238
salmon, coho, wild, ckd by dry heat	3 oz	85	0.947	15247
salmon, coho, wild, ckd by moist heat	3 oz	85	1.587	15082
salmon, coho, wild, raw	3 oz	85	1.253	15081

FOOD	SERVING	WEIGHT (g)	OMEGA-3 FATTY ACIDS (g/serving)	SOURCE/USDA CODE
salmon, pink, ckd by dry heat	3 oz	85	1.237	15212
salmon, pink, cnd w/bone	3 oz	85	1.493	15084
salmon, pink, raw	3 oz	85	0.965	15083
salmon, red, chunk, cnd w/o skin or bone, Chicken of the Sea	2 oz	57	0.66	CHCK
salmon, sockeye, ckd by dry heat	3 oz	85	1.210	15086
salmon, sockeye, cnd w/bone	3 oz	85	1.125	15087
salmon, sockeye, raw	3 oz	85	1.108	15085
sardines, pacific, cnd in tomato sce	1 sardine	38	0.739	15089
sea bass, ckd by dry heat	3 oz	85	0.730	15092
sea bass, raw	3 oz	85	0.570	15091
shad, american, raw	3 oz	85	2.252	15094
shark, batter-dipped & fried	3 oz	85	0.823	15096
shark, raw	3 oz	85	0.833	15095
shrimp, cnd	3 oz	85	0.521	15152
smelt, rainbow, ckd by dry heat	3 oz	85	0.829	15100
smelt, rainbow, raw	3 oz	85	0.646	15099
spot, ckd by dry heat	3 oz	85	0.840	15216
spot, raw	3 oz	85	0.655	15103
squid, fried	3 oz	85	0.549	15176
sucker, white, ckd by dry heat	3 oz	85	0.660	15217
sucker, white, raw	3 oz	85	0.513	15107
swordfish, ckd by dry heat	3 oz	85	0.898	15111
swordfish, raw	3 oz	85	0.701	15110
tilefish, ckd by dry heat	3 oz	85	0.891	15113
trout, mixed species, ckd by dry heat	3 oz	85	1.165	15219
trout, mixed species, raw	3 oz	85	0.908	15114
trout, rainbow, farmed, ckd by dry heat	3 oz	85	1.051	15241
trout, rainbow, farmed, raw	3 oz	85	0.838	15240
trout, rainbow, wild, ckd by dry heat	3 oz	85	0.999	15116
trout, rainbow, wild, raw	3 oz	85	0.690	15115
tuna, bluefin, ckd by dry heat	3 oz	85	1.414	15118
tuna, bluefin, raw	3 oz	85	1.103	15117
tuna, white, cnd in water, drained	3 oz	85	0.808	15126
whitefish, ckd by dry heat	3 oz	85	1.748	15223
whitefish, raw	3 oz	85	1.363	15130
wolffish, atlantic, ckd by dry heat	3 oz	85	0.735	15224
wolffish, atlantic, raw	3 oz	85	0.574	15134

FLOUR & GRAIN FRACTIONS

FOOD	SERVING	WEIGHT (g)	OMEGA-3 FATTY ACIDS (g/serving)	SOURCE/USDA CODE
soy flour, full fat	1 cup	84	1.158	16115
soy flour, full fat, roasted	1 cup	85	1.239	16116
wheat germ, crude	1 cup	115	0.831	20078
wheat germ, toasted	1 cup	113	0.904	08084

GRAINS & GRAIN PRODUCTS

FOOD	SERVING	WEIGHT (g)	OMEGA-3 FATTY ACIDS (g/serving)	SOURCE/USDA CODE
granola, homemade	1 cup (4.3 oz)	122	0.678	08037
muffin, oat bran	4.9 oz muffin	139	0.637	18283
noodles, chow mein	1 cup	45	0.889	20113
waffle, plain, homemade	1 round waffle (7" dia)	75	0.592	18367

MEATS

FOOD	SERVING	WEIGHT (g)	OMEGA-3 FATTY ACIDS (g/serving)	SOURCE/USDA CODE
lamb, rib, choice, 1/4" trim, lean & fat, roasted	3 oz	85	0.527	17029
pork bacon, cured, broiled/pan fried	4.48 oz (yield from 1 lb raw)	127	1.003	10124b
pork bacon, cured, raw	3 med slices	68	0.510	10123
pork breakfast strips, cured, raw	3 slices (2.4 oz)	68	0.612	10128
pork polish sausage	8 oz sausage	227	0.658	07059
	(10" long, 1 1/4" dia)	227	0.658	07059

MEATS–INTERNAL ORGANS & OTHER CUTS

FOOD	SERVING	WEIGHT (g)	OMEGA-3 FATTY ACIDS (g/serving)	SOURCE/USDA CODE
brain, beef, pan fried	3 oz	85	0.859	13319
brain, beef, simmered	3 oz	85	0.825	13320
brain, lamb, braised	3 oz	85	0.629	17186

FOOD	SERVING	WEIGHT (g)	OMEGA-3 FATTY ACIDS (g/serving)	SOURCE/USDA CODE
brain, lamb, pan fried	3 oz	85	1.369	17187
brain, pork, braised	3 oz	85	0.680	10097
tongue, lamb, braised	3 oz	85	0.519	17221
NUTS				
butternuts, dried	1 oz (~9 nuts)	28	2.472	12084
soy nuts, dry roasted	1 cup	172	2.482	16111
soy nuts, roasted	1 cup	172	2.914	16110
walnuts, black, dried	1 oz	28	0.569	12154
walnuts, english/persian, dried	1 oz (14 halves)	28	2.574	12155
wheat-base formulated nuts, flavored	1 oz	28	0.504	12200
POULTRY–TURKEY				
nuggets/sticks, breaded, Louis Rich	3 pieces (3 oz)	85	0.544	07265
thigh w/skin, prebasted, roasted	11.1 oz thigh (w/o bone)	314	0.534	05294
SALAD DRESSING				
blue (bleu) cheese/roquefort	1 T	15	0.555	04539
russian	1 T	15	0.525	04015
SOUPS				
minestrone, rts, Progresso Healthy Classics	1 cup (8 fl oz)	241	0.877	06206
shark fin, from restaurant	1 cup (8 fl oz)	216	0.570	06180
SOY PRODUCTS				
miso	1 cup (9.7 oz)	275	1.114	16112
natto	1 cup (6.2 oz)	175	1.285	16113
tofu, firm, prep w/Ca sulfate, raw	1/2 cup (4.4 oz)	126	0.733	16426
tofu, firm, prep w/nigari	1/4 block (4.3 oz)	122	0.814	16160
tofu, soft, prep w/Ca sulfate, raw	1 cup (8.7 oz)	248	0.610	16127a
VEGETABLES				
potato salad, homemade	1 cup	250	0.925	11414
soy sprouts, stir-fried	1 cup	125	0.590	11454
spinach, creamed, frzn, Stouffer's	4.4 oz (1/2 pkg)	125	0.664	22602
VEGETABLES–LEGUMES				
french beans, mature, boiled	1 cup	177	0.508	16023
mungo beans, mature, boiled	1 cup	180	0.603	16084
soybeans, green, boiled	1 cup	180	0.637	11451
soybeans, mature, boiled	1 cup	172	1.029	16109
soybeans, mature, raw	1 cup	186	2.474	16108

[1] Omega-3 fatty acids are the sum of available data for alpha-linolenic acid (ALA; 18:3 n-3), eicosapentaenoic acid (EPA; 20:5 n-3), docosapentaenoic acid (DPA; 22:5 n-3), and docosahexaenoic acid (DHA; 22:6 n-3). Values may slightly overestimate omega-3 content because 18:3 values are for undifferentiated fatty acids and may include slight amounts of the n-6 form. Foods containing less than 0.500 g omega-3 fatty acids per serving are not listed.

Source:
USDA Codes: *United States Department of Agriculture Database for Standard Reference, Release 15* (SR-15), 2002. Available at http://www.nal.usda.gov/fnic/foodcomp/Data/SR15/sr15.html.

Fatty Acids—Trans Fatty Acids[1]

	SERVING SIZE	TRANS FATTY ACIDS (g/serving)	TRANS FATTY ACIDS (g/100 g)	SOURCE/ USDA CODE
CANDY				
milk choc w/almond bites, Hershey	17 pieces (39 g)	0.06	0.15	19236
Reese's Bites, Hershey	16 pieces (39 g)	0.02	0.05	19238
Reese's Crunchy Cookie Cups, Hershey	5 miniature pieces (39 g)	0.07	0.17	19242
Reese's Crunchy Cookie Cups, Hershey	1.44 oz pkg/2 cups (40 g)	0.07	0.17	19242
Twizzlers, Cherry Bits, Hershey	4 oz bag/22 pieces (40 g)	0.22	0.54	19067
Whatchamacallit, Hershey	1.7 oz bar (48 g)	0.06	0.12	19162

	SERVING SIZE	TRANS FATTY ACIDS (g/serving)	TRANS FATTY ACIDS (g/100 g)	SOURCE/ USDA CODE
CEREALS, READY-TO-EAT				
corn & oat, fruit flavor, sweetened	1 oz (28 g)	0.35	1.25	Exler et al, 1993
corn & oat, sweetened	1 oz (28 g)	0.10	0.34	Exler et al, 1993
corn flakes	1 oz (28 g)	0.04	0.15	Exler et al, 1993
crisped rice, fruit flavor, sweetened	1 oz (28 g)	0.24	0.84	Exler et al, 1993
wheat & bran flakes, dried fruit, & oat clusters	1 oz (28 g)	0.05	0.19	Exler et al, 1993
wheat & bran flakes, raisins, & nuts	1 oz (28 g)	0.24	0.86	Exler et al, 1993
CHEESE				
cheese, am processed (2 brands)	1 oz (28 g)	0.20	0.73 (0.71/0.74)	Exler et al, 1993
cheese, cheddar	1 oz (28 g)	0.25	0.88	Exler et al, 1993
cheese food, am (2 brands)	1 oz (28 g)	0.20	0.70 (0.64/0.76)	Exler et al, 1993
cheese spread, am (2 brands)	1 oz (28 g)	0.16	0.57 (0.48/0.65)	Exler et al, 1993
DESSERTS				
cake mix, yellow	2 oz (56 g)	0.59	1.06	Exler et al, 1993
cake, pound, cholesterol-free	2 oz (56 g)	3.04	5.43	Exler et al, 1993
cake, pound, fat-free	2 oz (56 g)	0.22	0.40	Exler et al, 1993
cake, yellow w/choc icing	2 oz (56 g)	1.80	3.21	Exler et al, 1993
candy bar w/nougat, caramel, & choc coating	2 oz (56 g)	0.90	1.60	Exler et al, 1993
cheesecake	3 oz (85 g)	0.47	0.55	Exler et al, 1993
chocolate, milk	2 oz (56 g)	0.06	0.10	Exler et al, 1993
cookie bar w/caramel & choc coating	2 oz (56 g)	3.88	6.92	Exler et al, 1993
cookie, choc chip (3 brands)	~3 cookies (30 g)	1.69	5.62 (3.83–9.04)	Exler et al, 1993
cookie, choc w/crème filling (2 brands)	~3 cookies (30 g)	1.67	5.58 (4.87/6.29)	Exler et al, 1993
cookie, van wafers	~7 wafers (28 g)	1.19	4.25	Exler et al, 1993
cookie, van w/crème filling	~3 cookies (30 g)	2.13	7.10	Exler et al, 1993
danish pastry, pecan	2 oz pastry (56 g)	1.19	2.13	Exler et al, 1993
doughnut, cake type, sugared/glazed (5 brands)	1 doughnut (47 g)	1.72	3.67 (0.54–6.92)	Exler et al, 1993
doughnut, yeast, glazed (4 brands)	1 doughnut (60 g)	1.72	2.87 (0.65–6.29)	Exler et al, 1993
granola bar, choc chip, chewy	1 oz bar	0.55	1.96	Exler et al, 1993
ice cream, van (2 brands)	1/2 cup (66 g)	0.27	0.41 (0.38/0.43)	Exler et al, 1993
icing, choc, creamy, rte (3 brands)	2 T (36 g)	1.25	3.48 (3.44–3.52)	Exler et al, 1993
icing, marble, creamy, rte	2 T (36 g)	1.31	3.63	Exler et al, 1993
icing, van, creamy, rte (2 brands)	2 T (36 g)	1.39	3.85 (3.65/4.04)	Exler et al, 1993
snack cake, sponge w/crème filling	1 cake (43 g)	0.29	0.67	Exler et al, 1993
sweet roll, cinn	1 roll (66 g)	1.56	2.36	Exler et al, 1993
FAST FOODS				
french fries (7 brands)	30–40 fries (115 g)	3.43	2.98 (0.99–5.22)	Exler et al, 1993
milk shake, choc (2 brands)	10 fl oz (283 g)	0.11	0.04 (0.00/0.07)	Exler et al, 1993
milk shake, van (2 brands)	10 fl oz (283 g)	0.11	0.04 (0.01/0.07)	Exler et al, 1993
FATS, OILS, & SPREADS				
chicken, fat, raw	1 T (13 g)	0.10	0.74	Exler et al, 1993
lard (3 brands)	1 T (13 g)	0.14	1.07 (0.38–1.56)	Exler et al, 1993
margarine, corn & soy, 80% fat, stick	1 T (14 g)	2.76	19.69	04628
margarine, stick (10 brands)	1 T (14 g)	2.72	19.44 (13.02–64.10)	Exler et al, 1993
margarine, tub (8 brands)	1 T (14 g)	1.07	7.62 (3.05–11.30)	Exler et al, 1993
mayonnaise (2 brands)	1 T (14 g)	0.25	1.82 (0.23/3.4)	Exler et al, 1993
shortening (12 brands)	1 T (13 g)	2.44	18.76 (10.68–32.55)	Exler et al, 1993
shortening, butter flavor	1 T (13 g)	2.71	20.84	Exler et al, 1993
spread (5 brands)	1 T (14 g)	2.18	15.55 (2.79–25.78)	Exler et al, 1993
spread, extra light	1 T (14 g)	0.79	5.66	Exler et al, 1993
spread, fat-free, tub	1 T (15 g)	0.03	0.17	04631
spread, light	1 T (14 g)	1.27	9.09	Exler et al, 1993
spread, soy, 70% fat	1 T (14 g)	2.69	19.23	04629
turkey fat	1 T (13 g)	0.33	2.54	Exler et al, 1993
veg oil, canola (2 brands)	1 T (14 g)	0.03	0.19 (0.16/0.22)	Exler et al, 1993
veg oil, olive	1 T (14 g)	0.01	0.09	Exler et al, 1993
veg oil, sunflower	1 T (14 g)	0.07	0.48	Exler et al, 1993
GRAIN PRODUCTS				
biscuit, from refrig dough	1 biscuit (35 g)	1.42	4.06	Exler et al, 1993
biscuit mix, buttermilk	1 biscuit (35 g)	1.11	3.18	Exler et al, 1993
bread, cracked wheat	1 slice (25 g)	0.25	0.99	Exler et al, 1993

	SERVING SIZE	TRANS FATTY ACIDS (g/serving)	TRANS FATTY ACIDS (g/100 g)	SOURCE/ USDA CODE
breadcrumbs, dry, grated	1 cup (108 g)	0.08	0.07	Exler et al, 1993
bread, rye, seedless	1 slice (32 g)	0.04	0.14	Exler et al, 1993
bread, white, buttertop	1 slice (25 g)	0.21	0.82	Exler et al, 1993
bread, white, firm (3 brands)	1 slice (25 g)	0.19	0.74 (0.11–1.39)	Exler et al, 1993
crackers, cheese	14 crackers (14 g)	1.04	7.43	Exler et al, 1993
crackers, cheese w/peanut butter filling	1 piece (7 g)	0.21	3.01	Exler et al, 1993
crackers, saltines (3 brands)	1 saltine (3 g)	0.08	2.83 (1.52–3.96)	Exler et al, 1993
crackers, snack type (6 brands)	1 cracker (3 g)	0.22	7.47 (5.86–8.41)	Exler et al, 1993
muffin mix, corn	1 oz mix (28 g)	1.00	3.56	Exler et al, 1993
popcorn, lowfat, microwave popped	3.5 cups (28 g)	0.88	3.16	Exler et al, 1993
popcorn, microwave popped (2 brands)	3.5 cups (28 g)	2.11	7.54 (7.41/7.66)	Exler et al, 1993
popcorn, oil popped (2 brands)	2.6 cups (28 g)	2.57	9.19 (6.00/12.37)	Exler et al, 1993
roll, dinner (2 brands)	1 roll (28 g)	0.08	0.30 (0.26/0.33)	Exler et al, 1993
roll, hamburger/frankfurter (2 brands)	1 roll (43 g)	0.30	0.69 (0.09/1.29)	Exler et al, 1993
taco shell, baked	1 med (13 g)	1.04	7.98	Exler et al, 1993
tortilla, wheat flour	7–8" dia (35 g)	0.37	1.06	Exler et al, 1993
INFANT FOODS				
dinner, veg beef, str (2 brands)	4.5 oz jar (128 g)	0.17	0.13 (0.11/0.15)	Exler et al, 1993
MEATS–BEEF, GROUND				
5% fat, crumbles, pan-browned	3 oz (85 g)	0.54	0.64	23560
5% fat, loaf, baked	3 oz piece (85 g)	0.46	0.54	23561
5% fat, patty, broiled	3 oz patty (85 g)	0.47	0.55	23558
5% fat, patty, pan-broiled	3 oz patty (85 g)	0.42	0.50	23559
10% fat, crumbles, pan-browned	3 oz (85 g)	0.65	0.77	23565
10% fat, loaf, baked	3 oz piece (85 g)	0.60	0.71	23566
10% fat, patty, broiled	3 oz patty (85 g)	0.64	0.75	23563
10% fat, patty, pan-broiled	3 oz patty (85 g)	0.58	0.68	23564
15% fat, crumbles, pan-browned	3 oz (85 g)	0.80	0.94	23570
15% fat, loaf, baked	3 oz piece (85 g)	0.75	0.88	23571
15% fat, patty, broiled	3 oz patty (85 g)	0.81	0.95	23568
15% fat, patty, pan-broiled	3 oz patty (85 g)	0.73	0.86	23569
20% fat, crumbles, pan-browned	3 oz (85 g)	0.95	1.12	23575
20% fat, loaf, baked	3 oz piece (85 g)	0.88	1.04	23576
20% fat, patty, broiled	3 oz patty (85 g)	0.97	1.15	23573
20% fat, patty, pan-broiled	3 oz patty (85 g)	0.87	1.02	23574
25% fat, crumbles, pan-browned	3 oz (85 g)	1.11	1.31	23580
25% fat, loaf, baked	3 oz piece (85 g)	1.01	1.18	23581
25% fat, patty, broiled	3 oz patty (85 g)	1.14	1.34	23578
25% fat, patty, pan-broiled	3 oz patty (85 g)	1.00	1.18	23579
MEATS–GAME				
emu, ground, pan-broiled	3 oz patty (85 g)	0.13	0.15	05622
ostrich, ground, pan-broiled	3 oz (85 g)	0.20	0.23	05642
ostrich, top loin, cooked	3 oz (85 g)	0.11	0.13	05658
MEATS–PORK				
pork link sausage, raw	3 oz (85 g)	0.08	0.09	Exler et al, 1993
pork sausage, raw	3 oz (85 g)	0.09	0.11	Exler et al, 1993
MEATS, LUNCHEON				
bologna, beef (2 brands)	1 oz (28 g)	1.62	5.77 (1.53/10.7)	Exler et al, 1993
bologna, pork & beef (2 brands)	1 oz (28 g)	0.05	0.19 (0.16/0.21)	Exler et al, 1993
frankfurter, beef (2 brands)	1 frank (57 g)	0.68	1.20 (0.99/1.40)	Exler et al, 1993
frankfurter, beef, pork, & veal	1 frank (57 g)	0.58	1.01	Exler et al, 1993
frankfurter, pork & beef	1 frank (57 g)	0.10	0.18	Exler et al, 1993
kielbasa, beef, cured	1 oz (28 g)	0.36	1.27	Exler et al, 1993
pepperoni, pork & beef	1 oz (28 g)	0.10	0.36	Exler et al, 1993
MILK & YOGURT				
milk, whole (4 brands)	8 fl oz (244 g)	0.22	0.09 (0.07–0.10)	Exler et al, 1993
yogurt, lowfat (2 brands)	8 fl oz (227 g)	0.07	0.03 (0.02/0.03)	Exler et al, 1993
POULTRY				
chicken, broiler, skin, raw	3 oz (85 g)	0.32	0.38	Exler et al, 1993
turkey breast, raw	3 oz (85 g)	0.03	0.03	Exler et al, 1993

	SERVING SIZE	TRANS FATTY ACIDS (g/serving)	TRANS FATTY ACIDS (g/100 g)	SOURCE/ USDA CODE
turkey burger, ckd	3 oz (85 g)	0.48	0.56	Exler et al, 1993
turkey burger, seasoned, ckd	3 oz (85 g)	0.44	0.52	Exler et al, 1993
turkey, dark meat, raw	3 oz (85 g)	0.02	0.14	Exler et al, 1993
turkey, dark meat, ground, raw	3 oz (85 g)	0.02	0.17	Exler et al, 1993
turkey, ground, raw (9 brands)	3 oz (85 g)	0.25	0.29 (0.15–0.46)	Exler et al, 1993
turkey skin	1 oz (28 g)	0.36	1.28	Exler et al, 1993
SALAD DRESSINGS				
french (2 brands)	1 T (16 g)	0.04	0.24 (0.21/0.27)	Exler et al, 1993
italian (3 brands)	1 T (15 g)	0.05	0.33 (0.19–0.54)	Exler et al, 1993
ranch (3 brands)	1 T (15 g)	0.34	2.28 (0.30–3.71)	Exler et al, 1993
SNACKS				
pork rinds (3 brands)	1 oz (28 g)	0.09	0.33 (0.18–0.58)	Exler et al, 1993
potato chips (12 brands)	1 oz (28 g)	0.50	1.77 (0.00–10.64)	Exler et al, 1993
tortilla chips	1 oz (28 g)	1.15	4.12	Exler et al, 1993
SOUPS				
bouillon cube, beef (3 brands)	1 cube (6 g)	0.08	1.25 (0.23–3.20)	Exler et al, 1993
bouillon cube, chicken (3 brands)	1 cube (5 g)	0.07	1.41 (0.06–3.85)	Exler et al, 1993
VEGETABLES				
potatoes, french fried, frzn (3 brands)	10 pieces (50 g)	1.27	2.53 (1.73–3.38)	Exler et al, 1993

[1] Trans fatty acids are the sum of available data for trans palmitoleic acid (16:1), trans oleic acid (18:1), and trans linoleic acid (18:2).

Sources:
Exler J, L Lemar, and J Smith. *Fat and Fatty Acid Content of Selected Foods Containing Trans-Fatty Acids. Special Purpose Table No. 1.* Available at http://www.nal.usda.gov/fnic/fo.PDF. The data from this source are for foods that were collected between 1989 and 1993. Because the formulations of some products may have changed, the data may not reflect currently available products. These foods do not have code numbers that relate to foods in the main table. Brand names of products were not available; individual data points or averages with ranges are presented. The values were provided per 100 grams of foods, and the amounts in typical serving portions were calculated.
USDA Codes: *United States Department of Agriculture Database for Standard Reference, Release 15* (SR15), 2002. Available at http://www.nal.usda.gov/fnic/foodcomp/Data/SR15/sr15.html.

Flavonoids—Anthocyanidins, Flavan-3-ols, Flavones, Flavonols, & Flavanones

	ANTHOCYANIDINS[1] (mg/100 g)	FLAVAN-3-OLS[2] (mg/100 g)	FLAVONES[3] (mg/100 g)	FLAVONOLS[4] (mg/100 g)	FLAVANONES[5] (mg/100 g)	USDA CODE
BEVERAGES						
beer	0.00	0.00		0.10		14003
chocolate milk, red fat	1.25					01103
coffee, brewed	0.00	0.00		0.10		14209
tea, black, brewed	113.79	0.00		3.86		14355
tea, black, decaffeinated, brewed	53.09			4.42		14352
tea, black, oolong, brewed	45.62	0.00		2.69		99071
tea, green, brewed	133.28	0.34		5.21		99070
tea, green, decaffeinated, brewed	64.96			4.77		99069
tea, green, flavored, brewed	51.03			2.81		99068
tea, green, iced, rtd	11.90			1.56		99343
tea, iced, diet, rtd	16.50			1.17		99342
tea, iced, rtd	27.72			2.27		99341
tea, inst, diet, prep	11.70			0.44		99349
tea, inst, prep, unsweetened	25.70			1.40		14367
tea, inst w/sugar, prep	29.42			1.63		99350
tea leaves, black, dry	10127.85	0.00		371.27		99060
tea leaves, black, decaffeinated, dry	4778.01			398.48		99345
tea leaves, black, oolong, dry	5159.85	.00		3.72		99062
tea leaves, green, dry	12654.68	.34		515.70		99061
tea leaves, green, decaffeinated, dry	4941.38			444.85		99346
wine, berry				1.38		99323
wine, berry, white				0.20		99074
wine, sherry				0.01		99075

	ANTHOCYANIDINS[1] (mg/100 g)	FLAVAN-3-OLS[2] (mg/100 g)	FLAVONES[3] (mg/100 g)	FLAVONOLS[4] (mg/100 g)	FLAVANONES[5] (mg/100 g)	USDA CODE
wine, table, red	9.19	11.90	0.00	1.64		14096
wine, table, white	0.06	1.38	0.00	0.06		14106
CANDY						
chocolate bar, dark		53.49				99321
chocolate bar, milk		13.35				99320
CEREALS, GRAINS, GRAIN FRACTIONS						
barley		3.84				20004
buckwheat				23.09		20008
buckwheat flour, whole groat		3.53		2.72		20011
buckwheat groats, roasted, dry			0.28	5.84		20009
rice, white, long grain, ckd		0.00				20045
FRUIT JUICES						
apple cider		5.49		0.48		99083
apple jce, cnd		0.74	0.00	0.39		09016
black currant jce				3.01		99007
cranberry jce cocktail, bottled		0.19		1.40		14242
cranberry jce, raw		0.92		20.82		99110
crowberry jce, raw				7.37		99066
grapefruit jce, cnd					18.63	09123
grapefruit jce, from frzn conc					31.18	09126
grapefruit jce, pink, raw			0.00	0.00	14.69	09404
grapefruit jce, white, raw			0.00	0.10	24.13	09128
grape jce, cnd/bottled		0.19	0.00	0.99		09135
grape jce, black		0.80				99049
lemon jce, cnd/bottled					26.00	09153
lemon jce, raw			0.00	0.33	18.33	09152
lime jce, raw			0.00	0.51	11.54	09160
lingonberry jce, raw				1.02		99067
orange jce, blood orange, raw			0.00	0.00	14.80	99313
orange jce, chilled					5.08	09209
orange jce, from frzn conc					29.48	09215
orange jce, raw			0.00	0.24	14.98	09206
orange jce, sour orange, raw			0.00	0.00	49.05	99304
pummelo jce, raw			0.65	0.00	29.96	99311
tangerine jce, from frzn conc					25.51	09225
tangerine jce, raw			0.00	0.29	10.78	09221
tangor jce, raw			0.00	0.00	26.77	99306
FRUITS						
apple, raw		9.09	0.00	4.42		09003
applesauce, cnd		6.10	0.00	2.00		09019
apple w/o peel, raw		7.09		1.50		09004
apricot, cnd water pack				0.00	0.00	09023
apricot, raw		11.01	0.00	2.55		09021
avocado, raw		0.56				09037
banana, raw		0.00				09040
bilberries, raw				4.13		99006
bilberry soup				0.60		99065
blackberries, raw		18.74		1.11		09042
blueberries, frzn				5.40		09054
blueberries, raw	112.55	1.11		3.93		09050
bog whortleberries, wild, frzn				25.00		99326
cherries, sour, red, raw	6.64					09063
cherries, sweet, cnd water pack		4.31	0.00	3.20		09365
cherries, sweet, raw	117.42	11.70	0.00	1.25		09070
chokeberries, frzn				8.90		99334
cloudberries, frzn				0.60		99337
cowberries, raw				21.50		99015
cranberries, raw		4.20		18.44		09078
crowberries, frzn				10.10		99339
currants, black European, raw		1.17		13.50		09083
currants, dried		0.00				99073
currants, red, raw		2.44	0.00	0.95		99044
currants, white, raw		0.30		1.95		99045

	ANTHOCYANIDINS[1] (mg/100 g)	FLAVAN-3-OLS[2] (mg/100 g)	FLAVONES[3] (mg/100 g)	FLAVONOLS[4] (mg/100 g)	FLAVANONES[5] (mg/100 g)	USDA CODE
elderberries, raw	749.24			42.00		99018
gooseberries, raw		2.11		3.75		09107
grapefruit, raw				0.90	54.50	99347
grapes, black, raw		20.39	0.00	2.99		99048
grapes, green/white, raw		3.92	0.00	1.32		99047
grapes, red, raw		1.95		3.54		99046
kiwifruit, raw		0.45				09148
lemon w/o peel, raw			1.50	2.29	49.81	09150
lime, raw				0.40	3.40	09159
lingonberries, raw				12.16		99021
mango, raw		1.72				09176
nectarine, raw		2.75				09191
orange, raw		0.00			43.88	99348
						09200
peach, cnd		1.87	0.00	0.00		09370
peach, raw		2.33	0.00	0.00		09236
pear, raw		3.43	0.00	0.72		09252
pear w/o peel, ckd		2.45				99080
pear w/o peel, raw		1.88				99029
pineapple, raw		.00				09266
plum, raw		6.19	0.00	1.20		09279
raisins, seedless		3.68				09298
raspberries, raw	47.60	9.23		0.83		09302
rowanberries, frzn				7.40		99335
strawberries, frzn				0.97		09318
strawberries, raw		4.47	0.00	1.44		09316
tangelo jce, raw			0.00	0.00	118.60	99305
GRAIN PRODUCTS						
bread, whole wheat		0.00				18075
macaroni, enr, ckd		0.00				20100
SOUPS						
soup, tomato, cnd, cond				0.14		06159
SPICES, HERBS, & FLAVORINGS						
basil, raw			0.00	0.00	0.00	02044
capers, cnd				316.33		02054
dill weed, raw			0.00	112.68	0.00	02045
lemon balm leaves, raw			0.00	0.00	0.00	99112
licorice root, raw				0.00		99104
oregano, raw			4.50	0.00	0.00	99115
parsley, dried			13525.95	331.24		02029
parsley, raw			303.24	8.85	0.00	11297
peppermint, raw			20.04	0.00	40.44	02064
rosemary, raw			4.00	0.00	0.00	02063
sage, raw			0.00	0.00	0.00	99116
thyme, raw			56.00	0.00	0.00	02049
tarragon, raw			1.00	26.00	0.00	99117
SWEETENERS						
jam, cherry		1.06				99114
jam, forest fruit		1.64				99113
jam, plum				0.63		99031
jam/preserves, apricot		0.97		0.82		19719
jam, peach				0.58		99027
jam/preserves, strawberry		0.90		1.09		99064
jam, sour orange					11.61	99038
VEGETABLES						
beet, raw		0.00	0.37	0.13		11080
broadbeans, immature, boiled		20.63				11089
broadbeans, immature, raw		49.37	0.00	4.60		11088
broadbeans, mature, cnd		0.00	0.00	0.90		16054
broccoli, boiled				2.44		11091
broccoli, raw		0.00	0.00	9.37		11090
brussels sprouts, raw		0.00	0.34	1.25		11098

	ANTHOCYANIDINS[1] (mg/100 g)	FLAVAN-3-OLS[2] (mg/100 g)	FLAVONES[3] (mg/100 g)	FLAVONOLS[4] (mg/100 g)	FLAVANONES[5] (mg/100 g)	USDA CODE
cabbage, green, raw			0.05	0.13		11109
cabbage, red, raw		0.00	0.07	0.37		11112
carrot, cnd			0.00	0.00		11128
carrot, raw		0.00	0.00	0.07		11124
cauliflower, raw		0.00	0.08	0.28		11135
celeriac, raw			2.41	0.18		11141
celery heart, green, raw			22.60			99118
celery heart, white, raw			2.36			99009
celery, raw			5.92	3.50		11143
chicory greens, raw			0.00	0.00		11152
chicory root, raw		0.00				11154
chinese cabbage (pak-choi/pak-choy), raw		0.00	0.07	0.38		11116
chives, raw			0.15	21.52	0.00	11156
coriander, raw			0.00	5.00	0.00	11165
corn poppy leaves			0.20	30.80		99014
corn, sweet, yellow, raw		0.00				11167
cress, garden, raw			0.00	14.00	0.00	11203
crown daisy leaves, raw			0.01	0.18		99102
cucumber, raw		0.00	0.00	0.10		11205
dock leaves, raw			0.00	102.20		11616
endive, raw		0.00	0.00	4.04		11213
fennel leaves, raw			0.10	86.64		99058
gourd, dishcloth (towelgourd), raw			0.01	0.16		11220
green (snap) beans, cnd			0.00	1.51		11056
green (snap) beans, frzn, ckd				1.51		11061
green (snap) beans, frzn, raw				1.54		11060
green (snap) beans, raw		0.00	0.00	3.14		11052
greens pie (greek dish)			6.60	19.90		99016
hartwort leaves, raw			0.60	38.9		99019
horseradish root, raw			0.90	1.86		99079
kale, chinese, raw			0.01	0.08		99098
kale, cnd			0.00	22.90		99054
kale, raw			0.00	34.45		11233
kidney beans, cnd		2.01				16029
kohlrabi, raw			1.30	2.83		11241
leek, raw		0.00	0.00	3.05		11246
lettuce, butterhead, raw				1.21		11250
lettuce, iceberg, raw		0.00	0.44	2.69		11252
lettuce, looseleaf, raw			0.01	2.01		11253
lovage leaves, raw			0.00	177.00	0.00	99111
marrowfat peas, cnd		9.97				99022
mushrooms, cnd			0.00	0.00		11264
mushrooms, raw		0.00	0.00	0.00		11260
onion, boiled				19.71		11283
onion, raw		0.00	0.00	15.36		11282
onion, red, raw	13.14		0.00	38.76		99055
onion, spring (scallions), raw			0.00	15.79		11291
onion, white, sweet, raw				5.52		99057
parsnip, raw			0.00	0.99		11298
peas, edible podded, raw		0.00				11300
peas, green, cnd			0.00	0.11		11308
peas, green, frzn				0.15		11312
peas, green, frzn, boiled				0.13		11814
peas, green, raw		0.00	0.00	0.00		11304
peppers, ancho, raw			3.36	27.60		99041
peppers, CA, raw			1.13	0.51		99088
peppers, hot chili, green, raw			5.11	16.80		11670
peppers, hot chili, yellow wax, raw			6.93	50.63		99042
peppers, jalapeno, raw			1.34	5.07		11979
peppers, serrano, raw			4.14	15.98		11977
peppers, sweet, green, raw			0.69	0.65		11333
peppers, sweet, red, raw		0.00	0.63	0.00		11821
perilla leaves, raw			0.39	0.96		99105
potato, white, raw		0.00	0.00	0.06		11352
purslane, raw			0.00	0.00		11427
queen anne's lace leaves, raw			46.70	1.70		99032

	ANTHOCYANIDINS[1] (mg/100 g)	FLAVAN-3-OLS[2] (mg/100 g)	FLAVONES[3] (mg/100 g)	FLAVONOLS[4] (mg/100 g)	FLAVANONES[5] (mg/100 g)	USDA CODE
radish, raw			0.00	0.86		11429
rhubarb, ckd		2.35				99052
rhubarb, raw		3.28				09307
rutabaga, raw			3.85	2.78		11435
sauerkraut, cnd			0.00	0.00		11439
spinach, frzn			0.00	0.00		11463
spinach, raw			1.11	4.88		11457
sweetpotato leaves, raw			0.32	30.28		11505
tomato, cherry, raw				2.87		99011
tomato jce, cnd			0.00	1.57		11886
tomato (pasta) sce, rts				0.92		06931
tomato, plum, raw				0.03		99051
tomato puree, cnd				4.20		11547
tomato, red, raw		0.00	0.00	0.64		11529
tomato, yellow, raw				0.25		11696
turnip greens, raw			0.00	5.53		11568
water spinach, raw			0.05	0.21		99107
watercress, raw			0.00	5.00	0.00	11591
yellow beans, raw				3.45		11722
MISCELLANEOUS						
bee pollen				26.09		43201
cocoa powder, unsweetened				20.13		19165
olives, ripe, cnd		0.00				09193
vinegar, cider		5.67		0.68		99351
vinegar, red wine	0.66	2.20				99109
vinegar, white wine		4.20				99108

[1] Anthocyanidins are the sum of available data for cyanidins, delphinidin, malvidin, pelargonidin, peonidin, and petunidin.
[2] Flavan-3-ols are the sum of available data for catechins, epicatechins, theaflavins, and thearubigins.
[3] Flavones are the sum of available data for luteolin and apigenin.
[4] Flavonols are the sum of available data for quercetin, kaempferol, myricetin, and isorhamnetin.
[5] Flavanones are the sum of available data for eriodictyol, hesperetin, and naringenin.
For information on the levels of the individual subcomponents, see the USDA flavonoid database.

Source:
USDA Codes: *USDA Database for the Flavonoid Content of Selected Foods–2003.* Available at http://www.nal.usda.gov/fnic/foodcomp/Data/Flav/flav.html (last modified March 25, 2003).

Flavonoids—Isoflavones (Daidzein, Genistein, & Glycitein)

	DAIDZEIN (mg/100 g)	GENISTEIN (mg/100 g)	GLYCITEIN (mg/100 g)	TOTAL ISOFLAVONES (mg/100 g)	USDA CODE
ADULT FORMULAS W/SOY					
Enrich, Ross	0.14	0.40		0.54	99063
Glucerna Ross	0.02	0.06		0.08	99064
Jevity Isotonic, Ross	0.03	0.31		0.34	99065
BEVERAGES					
soy beverage	2.41	4.60		7.01	99043
soy beverage inst powder	40.07	62.18	10.90	109.51	99018
tea, green, japanese	0.01	0.04		0.05	99107
tea, jasmine, Twinings	0.01	0.03		0.04	99106
tea, lapacho (*Tecoma heptaphylla*)	0.02	0.03		0.05	99020
FLOUR & GRAIN FRACTIONS					
soy flour, defatted	57.47	71.21	7.55	131.19	16117
soy flour, full fat, raw	71.19	96.83	16.18	177.89	16115
soy flour, full fat, roasted	99.27	98.75	16.40	198.95	16116
soy flour, textured	59.62	78.90	20.19	148.61	99080
soy meal, defatted, raw	57.47	68.35		125.82	16119
GRAIN PRODUCTS					
bread, country rye, finland	0.00	0.00		0.00	99010
bread, nine grain	0.01	0.01		0.02	99001

	DAIDZEIN (mg/100 g)	GENISTEIN (mg/100 g)	GLYCITEIN (mg/100 g)	TOTAL ISOFLAVONES (mg/100 g)	USDA CODE
crispbread, rye	0.01	0.01		0.01	18216
granola bar, hard, plain	0.05	0.08		0.13	19015
noodles, soy flat	0.90	3.70	3.90	8.50	99049
INFANT FORMULAS W/SOY					
Enfamil Next Step, dry powder	7.23	14.75	3.00	25.00	03931
Gerber formula w/Fe, dry powder, Mead Johnson	8.08	13.90	3.12	25.09	03863
Prosobee w/Fe, dry powder, Mead Johnson	7.05	14.94	2.95	24.94	03826
Prosobee w/Fe, liquid conc, Mead Johnson	1.10	2.22		6.03	03824
Prosobee w/Fe, rtf, Mead Johnson	1.71	2.18		3.89	03823
Isomil w/Fe, dry powder, Ross	6.03	12.23	2.73	20.99	03843
Isomil w/Fe, recon from powder, Ross	0.78	1.58	0.35	2.71	99112
Isomil w/Fe, rtf, Ross	1.91	2.26		4.17	03841
Nursoy w/Fe, dry powder, Wyeth-Ayerst	5.70	13.55	2.05	26.00	03893
Nursoy w/Fe, liquid conc, Wyeth-Ayerst	1.02	2.82	0.35	4.02	03891
Nursoy w/Fe, rtf, Wyeth-Ayerst	0.75	1.60	0.28	2.63	03890
MEATS					
beef patties w/veg pro, frzn, ckd	0.67	1.09	0.10	1.86	23501
beef patties w/veg pro, frzn, raw	0.35	0.77	0.02	1.14	23506
MEAT SUBSTITUTES					
bacon, meatless	2.80	6.90	2.40	12.10	16104
Big Franks, cnd, Worthington	1.00	2.05	0.30	3.35	22126
Big Franks, cnd, prep, Worthington	1.35	2.00	0.40	3.75	22116
frankfurter, soy, frzn	3.40	8.20	3.40	15.00	99111
Frichick, cnd, ckd	4.35	9.35	0.90	14.60	116173
Frichick, cnd, raw	3.45	7.90	0.85	12.20	16172
Harvest Burger, orig flavor, frzn, Green Giant	2.95	5.28	1.07	9.30	22125
Harvest Burger, orig flavor, prep, Green Giant	2.58	4.68	0.95	8.22	22117
Soylinks, frzn, ckd, Morning Star	0.75	2.70	0.30	3.75	16167
Soylinks, frzn, raw, Morning Star	1.18	2.45	0.30	3.93	16166
NUTS & SEEDS					
soy nuts, dry roasted	52.04	65.88	13.36	128.35	16111
fenugreek seeds	0.01	0.01		0.02	02019
flax seeds, raw	0.00	0.00		0.00	12220
kala chana seeds, mature, raw	0.00	0.64		0.64	99019
peanuts, all types, raw	0.03	0.24		0.26	16087
sunflower seed kernels, dried	0.00	0.00		0.00	12036
SOY-BASED CHEESE, MILK, & YOGURT					
soy cheese, cheddar	1.80	2.25	3.10	7.15	99041
soy cheese, mozzarella	1.10	3.60	3.00	7.70	99054
soy cheese, parmesan	1.50	0.80	4.10	6.40	99056
soy cheese, unspecified	11.24	20.08		31.32	99042
soy curd cheese	9.00	19.20		28.20	43299
soymilk	4.45	6.06	0.56	9.65	16120
soymilk, iced	1.90	2.81		4.71	99014
soymilk skin/film (foo jook/yuba), ckd	18.20	32.50		50.70	99096
soymilk skin/film (foo jook/yuba), raw	79.88	104.80	18.40	193.88	99053
tofu yogurt	5.70	9.40	1.20	16.30	43476
SOY PRODUCTS					
miso	16.13	24.56	2.87	42.55	16112
miso soup mix, dry	24.93	35.46		60.39	99002
natto (boiled, fermented soybeans)	21.85	29.04	8.17	58.93	16113
soy butter, full fat, Worthington	0.22	0.30	0.05	0.57	99105
soy chips	26.71	27.45		54.16	99072
soy fiber	18.80	21.68	7.90	44.43	99045
soy flakes, defatted	36.97	85.69	14.23	125.82	99035
soy flakes, full fat	48.23	79.98	1.57	128.99	99036
soy paste	15.03	15.21	7.70	31.52	99038
soy protein conc, alcohol extraction	6.83	5.33	1.57	12.47	16121
soy protein conc, aqueous wash	43.04	55.59	5.16	102.07	99060
soy protein isolate	33.59	59.62	9.47	97.43	16122
soy sce w/hydrolyzed veg protein	0.10	0.00	0.00	0.10	16125
soy sce w/soy & wheat (shoyu)	0.93	0.82	0.45	1.64	16123
tempeh	17.59	24.85	2.10	43.52	16114

	DAIDZEIN (mg/100 g)	GENISTEIN (mg/100 g)	GLYCITEIN (mg/100 g)	TOTAL ISOFLAVONES (mg/100 g)	USDA CODE
tempeh burger	6.40	19.60	3.00	29.00	99081
tempeh, ckd	19.25	31.55	2.20	53.00	16174
tofu, dried, frzn (koyadofu, kori tofu, tung tou-fu)	25.34	42.15		67.49	16128
tofu, extra firm, prep w/nigari, Azumaya	8.23	12.45	1.95	22.63	99083
tofu, extra firm, steamed, Azumaya	8.00	12.75	1.95	22.70	99084
tofu, fermented	14.30	22.40	2.30	39.00	99034
tofu, firm, ckd, Azumaya	12.80	16.15	2.40	31.35	99085
tofu, firm, prep w/Ca sulfate & nigari	9.44	13.35	2.08	24.74	16126
tofu, firm, silken, Mori-Nu	11.13	15.58	2.40	27.91	16162
tofu, fried (aburage)	17.83	28.00	3.37	48.35	16129
tofu, okara	5.39	6.48	1.64	13.51	16130
tofu, pressed (tau kwa), raw	13.60	13.90	2.00	29.50	99097
tofu, reg, prep w/Ca sulfate, raw	9.02	13.60	1.98	23.61	16427
tofu, salted & fermented (fuyu)	14.29	16.38	5.00	33.17	16132
tofu, soft, prep w/Ca sulfate & nigari	11.99	18.23	2.03	31.10	16127
tofu, soft, silken, vitasoy	8.59	20.65		29.24	99086
VEGETABLE OILS					
canola & soybean	0.00	0.00	0.00	0.00	42299
soybean, salad/cooking	0.00	0.00	0.00	0.00	04044
VEGETABLES					
alfalfa & clover sprouts, raw	0.00	0.00	0.00	0.00	99003
alfalfa sprouts, raw	0.00	0.00	0.00	0.00	11001
black beans, mature, raw	0.00	0.00		0.00	16014
broadbeans (fava beans), fried	0.00	1.29		1.29	99008
broadbeans (fava beans), mature, raw	0.02	0.00		0.03	16052
chickpeas (garbanzo beans, bengal gram), mature, raw	0.04	0.06		0.10	16056
clover sprouts, raw	0.00	0.35		0.35	99009
cowpeas (blackeye, crowder, & southern peas), mature, raw	0.01	0.02		0.03	16062
great northern beans, mature, raw	0.00	0.00		0.00	16024
green (snap) beans, boiled	0.00	0.00		0.00	11053
green(snap) beans, raw	0.00	0.00		0.00	11052
kidney beans, all types, mature, boiled	0.00	0.00		0.00	16028
kidney beans, all types, mature, raw	0.02	0.04		0.06	16027
kidney beans, red, mature, boiled	0.00	0.00		0.00	16033
kidney beans, red, raw	0.01	0.00		0.01	16032
lentils, mature, raw	0.00	0.00		0.01	16069
lima beans, baby, mature, raw	0.00	0.00		0.00	16074
lima beans, large, mature, boiled	0.00	0.00		0.00	16072
lima beans, large, mature, raw	0.02	0.01		0.03	16071
mung beans, mature, raw	0.01	0.18		0.19	16080
mungo beans, mature, raw	0.01	0.01		0.03	16083
navy beans, mature, raw	0.01	0.20		0.21	16037
peas, split, mature, raw	2.42	0.00		2.42	16085
pigeon peas (red gram), mature, raw	0.02	0.54		0.56	16101
pink beans, mature, raw	0.00	0.00		0.00	16040
pinto beans, mature, raw	0.01	0.26		0.27	16042
red beans, mature, raw	0.00	0.31		0.31	99026
soybean sprouts	19.12	21.60		40.71	11452
soybeans, brazilian, raw	20.16	67.47		87.63	99092
soybeans, japanese, raw	34.52	64.78	13.78	118.51	99092
soybeans, korean, raw	72.68	72.31		144.99	99093
soybeans, taiwanese, raw	28.21	31.54		59.75	99040
soybeans, US, green, mature, raw	67.79	72.51	10.88	151.17	99100
soybeans, US, immature, boiled	6.85	6.94		13.79	11451
soybeans, US, immature, raw	9.27	9.84	4.29	20.42	11450
soybeans, US, mature, boiled	26.95	27.71		54.66	16109
soybeans, US, mature, raw, US commodity grade	52.20	91.71	12.07	153.40	99091
soybeans, US, mature, raw, US food quality grade	46.64	73.76	10.88	128.35	16108
white beans, small, mature, raw	0.00	0.74		0.74	16045

Source:
USDA Codes: *United States Department of Agriculture-Iowa State University Database on the Isoflavone Content of Foods,* Release 1.2, 2000. Available at http://www.nal.usda.gov/fnic/foodcomp/data/isoflav/isfl_tbl.pdf.

Flavonoids—Coumesterol, Formononetin, & Biochanin A[1]

	COUMESTEROL (mg/100 g)	FORMONONETIN (mg/100 g)	BIOCHANIN A (mg/100 g)	USDA CODE
BEVERAGES				
tea, green	0.03			99107
tea, jasmine	0.03			99106
tea, lapacho	0.00	0.01	0.03	99020
GRAIN FRACTIONS & PRODUCTS				
bread, nine grain	0.00	0.00	0.00	99001
crispbread, finnish	tr	0.00	0.00	18216
granola bar	tr	0.00	0.00	19015
flour, soy, UK	0.00	0.03	0.07	16115
NUTS & SEEDS				
groundnuts	0.00	0.00	0.01	16095
peanuts	0.00	0.01	0.01	16087
sunflower seeds	tr	0.03	tr	12036
VEGETABLES				
alfalfa sprouts, raw	4.68/0.00	tr/261	0.00/0.00	11001
black gram (urad dahl), dry	0.00	0.00	0.03	16083
broadbeans, dry	0.00	0.02	tr	16052
chickpeas (garbanzo beans), dry	0.00/0.00	0.00/0.14	1.52/1.78	16056
clover sprouts, raw	28.1	2.28	0.44	99009
cowpeas (blackeyed beans), dry	0.00	0.00	1.73/0.00	16062
great northern beans, dry	0.00	0.00	0.60	16024
green (snap) beans, ckd	0.00	tr	tr	11053
green (snap) beans, raw	0.00	0.15	tr	11052
kala chana, dry	6.13	0.00	1.26	99019
kidney beans, ckd	0.00	0.00	0.41	16028
kidney beans, dry	0.00	0.01	tr	16027
kidney beans, red, dry	0.00	0.00	0.01	16032
kidney beans, white, dry	0.00	0.00	0.01	16027
lentils, dry	0.00	0.01	0.00	16069
lima beans, baby, dry	0.00	0.55	0.37	16074
lima beans, large, ckd	0.00	0.01	0.00	16072
lima beans, large, dry	1.48/0.00	tr/0.01	tr/0.00	16071
mung beans, dry	0.00/tr	0.61/0.01	0.00/0.01	16080
navy beans, dry	0.00	0.00	0.00	16037
peas, chinese, ckd	0.00	0.00	9.31	16085
peas, split, round, dry	8.11	0.00	0.00	16085
peas, split, yellow & green, dry	0.00	0.00	0.86/0.00	16085
pigeon peas, dry	tr	0.01	0.10	16101
pink beans, dry	0.00	1.05	0.00	16040
pinto beans, dry	3.61/0.00	tr/0.00	0.56/0.00	16042
soybean sprouts, raw	38.6	0.00		11452
soybeans, dry	0.05	0.07	0.01	16108
white beans, small, dry	0.00	0.82	0.00	16045

[1] Values separated by a slash mark indicate different data from two sources.

Source:
USDA Codes: *United States Department of Agriculture-Iowa State University Database on the Isoflavone Content of Foods,* Release 1.2, 2000. Available at http://www.nal.usda.gov/fnic/foodcomp/data/isoflav/CBF_tbl.pdf.

Glutathione

	GLUTATHIONE (mg/100 g)	SOURCE		GLUTATHIONE (mg/100 g)	SOURCE
FRUITS			cauliflower	9.20	Mills et al, 1997
			celery	0.65	Mills et al, 1997
apple	0.61	Souci et al, 2000	collard greens	2.83	Mills et al, 1997
banana	0.71	Souci et al, 2000	cucumber	1.63	Mills et al, 1997
orange	4.00	Souci et al, 2000	corn	14.14	Mills et al, 1997
orange jce, commercial	0.89	Souci et al, 2000	eggplant	1.63	Mills et al, 1997
pear	1.20	Souci et al, 2000	green beans	4.30	Mills et al, 1997
			kale	3.38	Mills et al, 1997
GRAINS & NUTS			lettuce, iceberg	0.00	Mills et al, 1997
bread, rye	0.65	Souci et al, 2000	mushrooms (*Agaricus bisporus*)	0.98	Souci et al, 2000
corn flour	3.90	Souci et al, 2000	mustard greens	4.92	Mills et al, 1997
peanuts	2.10	Souci et al, 2000	okra	7.99	Mills et al, 1997
			onion, yellow	2.27	Mills et al, 1997
MEAT & MILK			parsley	12.00	Souci et al, 2000
beef muscle	20.00	Souci et al, 2000	pepper, green	4.30	Mills et al, 1997
chicken breast w/skin	9.50	Souci et al, 2000	potato	10.76	Mills et al, 1997
milk, whole	0.33		purslane, chamber-grown, raw	14.81	Simopoulos et al, 1992
			purslane, wild, raw	11.90	Simopoulos et al, 1992
VEGETABLES			radish	4.61	Mills et al, 1997
asparagus stems	18.75	Mills et al, 1997	spinach	13.52	Mills et al, 1997
asparagus tips	28.58	Mills et al, 1997	spinach, raw	9.65	Simopoulos et al, 1992
beet	3.07	Mills et al, 1997	squash, summer, zucchini	6.76	Mills et al, 1997
broccoli flower	25.82	Mills et al, 1997	squash, winter, acorn	5.53	Mills et al, 1997
broccoli stem	9.20	Mills et al, 1997	squash, yellow	8.61	Mills et al, 1997
brussels sprouts	34.42	Mills et al, 1997	sweet potato	6.15	Mills et al, 1997
cabbage core	19.05	Mills et al, 1997	tomato	3.69	Mills et al, 1997
cabbage leaves	2.61	Mills et al, 1997	turnip	2.46	Mills et al, 1997
carrot	1.91	Mills et al, 1997	turnip greens	5.53	Mills et al, 1997

Sources:

Mills BJ, CT Stinson, MC Liu, CA Lang. Glutathione and cyst(e)ine profiles of vegetables using high performance liquid chromatography with dual electrochemical detection. *J Food Comp Anal* 10:90–101, 1997. (Values were converted from micromoles per 100 grams to milligrams per 100 grams by multiplying by 307.33, the molecular weight of glutathione, and dividing by 1000.)

Souci SW, W Fachmann, H Kraut. *Food Composition and Nutrition Tables.* Medpharm GmbH Scientific Publishers, Stuttgart, Germany & CRC Press, Washington DC. 2000.

Simopoulos AP, HA Normal, JE Gillaspy, JA Duke. Common purslane: A source of omega-3 fatty acids and antioxidants. *J Am Coll Nutr* 11:374–382, 1992.

Gluten[1]

GLUTEN-CONTAINING FOODS

barley, malt

bran

breaded/creamed foods (e.g., fish, meat, vegetables)

breads/baked goods prepared from wheat, barley, or rye

bulgur

cereals made from wheat, rye, or barley

couscous (endosperm of durum wheat)

farina

graham flour

gravies prepared with wheat flour, rye, or barley

malt

pasta prepared from wheat, rye, barley, or semolina

rye

salad dressings containing wheat flour, rye, or barley

sauces prepared with wheat flour, rye, or barley

semolina (durum wheat)

soups containing wheat flour, rye, or barley

triticale (wheat-rye hybrid)

wheat (all types), wheat flour, wheat germ, wheat bran, cracked wheat

GLUTEN-FREE FOODS

amaranth

beans, peas, bean flours

breads/baked goods prepared from corn, potato, rice, or soy flours or cornmeal

buckwheat, kasha

cereals prepared from soy, corn, hominy, rice, cornmeal, or quinoa

corn, cornmeal, cornstarch

egg

fish[2]

fruits

gluten-free wheat starch

lima bean flour

meat[2]

millet

milk, cheese, yogurt[3]

nuts, peanut butter

oats, oatmeal[4]

pasta prepared from rice or other gluten-free ingredients

poultry[2]

potato, potato flour

quinoa

rice, rice flour

sorghum

soybeans, soy flour, soy products

tapioca

vegetables[2]

wild rice

---

[1] Celiac disease (also called sprue, nontropical sprue, and celiac sprue) is a genetic disorder of the small intestine caused by intolerance of the protein gluten, which is present in wheat, rye, and barley. Gluten consumption by persons with celiac disease results in immune reactions that damage the lining of the small intestine. A gluten-free diet stops the symptoms and allows for healing of the intestinal damage.

[2] Assumes that the fish, meat, poultry, and vegetables have not been prepared with breading or flour-based sauces.

[3] The coating of some cheeses may contain gluten.

[4] Oats may be contaminated with gluten due to crop rotation and milling with wheat (Pietzak, 2003).

Sources:

Fasano A, C Catassi. Current approaches to diagnosis and treatment of celiac disease: An evolving spectrum. *Gastroenterology* 120:636–651, 2001.

Pietzak MM. Recognizing and managing celiac disease. *Nutrition & the M.D.* 29:1–4, 2003.

Thompson T. Oats and the gluten-free diet. *J Am Diet Assoc* 103:376–379, 2003.

Minerals–Iodine[1]

	IODINE (mcg/100 g)	SOURCE		IODINE (mcg/100 g)	SOURCE
BEVERAGES			**EGGS**		
beer	1	Pennington et al, 1995	egg, fried	52	Pennington et al, 1995
cherry drink, from powder	1	Pennington et al, 1995	egg, raw, Eggland's Best	120	EGLD
coffee, decaf, from inst	0	Pennington et al, 1995	egg, scrambled w/milk	42	Pennington et al, 1995
cola	1	Pennington et al, 1995	egg, soft-boiled	48	Pennington et al, 1995
cola, low cal	1	Pennington et al, 1995	**ENTREES/MEALS**		
lemonade, from frzn conc	1	Pennington et al, 1995	beef & veg stew, homemade	18	Pennington et al, 1995
lemon-lime, carbonated	1	Pennington et al, 1995	chicken, fried w/mashed potatoes, cornbread, veg, frzn dinner	24	Pennington et al, 1995
orange drink, cnd	1	Pennington et al, 1995	chicken noodle casserole, homemade	25	Pennington et al, 1995
tea, brewed	2	Pennington et al, 1995	chili con carne w/beans, cnd	18	Pennington et al, 1995
water, tap	1	Pennington et al, 1995	hamburger, 1/4 lb w/garnish, fast food	20	Pennington et al, 1995
whisky	0	Pennington et al, 1995	lasagna, homemade	33	Pennington et al, 1995
wine, table	1	Pennington et al, 1995	macaroni & cheese, from box mix	34	Pennington et al, 1995
CANDY			pizza, cheese, frzn, heated	95	Pennington et al, 1995
caramels	35	Pennington et al, 1995	pork chow mein, homemade	9	Pennington et al, 1995
milk choc candy	43	Pennington et al, 1995	pot pie, chicken, frzn, heated	39	Pennington et al, 1995
CEREALS & GRAINS, COOKED			spaghetti in tomato sce, cnd	23	Pennington et al, 1995
corn grits, enr, ckd	28	Pennington et al, 1995	spaghetti w/meat sce, homemade	19	Pennington et al, 1995
farina, enr, ckd	8	Pennington et al, 1995	**FATS, OILS, & SPREADS**		
oatmeal, ckd	7	Pennington et al, 1995	butter	3	Pennington et al, 1995
rice, white, enr, ckd	63	Pennington et al, 1995	corn oil	1	Pennington et al, 1995
CEREALS, READY-TO-EAT			margarine, stick type	4	Pennington et al, 1995
corn flakes	93	Pennington et al, 1995	mayonnaise	4	Pennington et al, 1995
crisped rice	66	Pennington et al, 1995	**FISH & SHELLFISH**		
fruit-flavored, sweetened	129	Pennington et al, 1995	cod/haddock fillet, baked	116	Pennington et al, 1995
granola w/raisins	26	Pennington et al, 1995	fish sticks, frzn, heated	63	Pennington et al, 1995
oat ring	48	Pennington et al, 1995	shrimp, breaded & fried, homemade	41	Pennington et al, 1995
raisin bran	19	Pennington et al, 1995	tuna, cnd in oil	20	Pennington et al, 1995
shredded wheat	28	Pennington et al, 1995	**FRUIT JUICES**		
CHEESE			apple jce, cnd/bottled	3	Pennington et al, 1995
cheese, american	46	Pennington et al, 1995	grapefruit jce, from frzn conc	1	Pennington et al, 1995
cheese, cheddar, sharp/mild	43	Pennington et al, 1995	grape jce, cnd/bottled	2	Pennington et al, 1995
cheese, cottage, 4% fat	27	Pennington et al, 1995	orange jce, from frzn conc	1	Pennington et al, 1995
CREAM			pineapple jce, cnd/bottled	1	Pennington et al, 1995
cream, half & half	17	Pennington et al, 1995	prune jce, bottled	1	Pennington et al, 1995
cream substitute, powdered	7	Pennington et al, 1995	**FRUITS**		
DESSERTS & SWEETS			apple, red w/peel, raw	1	Pennington et al, 1995
cake, choc w/choc icing, rte/frzn	23	Pennington et al, 1995	applesauce, sweetened, cnd	0	Pennington et al, 1995
cake, yellow w/white icing, from mix	47	Pennington et al, 1995	avocado, raw	1	Pennington et al, 1995
coffee cake, rte/frzn	29	Pennington et al, 1995	banana, raw	2	Pennington et al, 1995
cookies, choc chip	52	Pennington et al, 1995	cantaloupe, raw	2	Pennington et al, 1995
cookies, choc w/crème filling	76	Pennington et al, 1995	cherries, sweet, raw	0	Pennington et al, 1995
danish/sweet roll, rte/frzn	45	Pennington et al, 1995	fruit cocktail, cnd, heavy syrup	33	Pennington et al, 1995
doughnut, cake type, rte/frzn	25	Pennington et al, 1995	grapefruit, raw	0	Pennington et al, 1995
gelatin dessert, strawberry, from inst mix	12	Pennington et al, 1995	grapes, purple/green, raw	1	Pennington et al, 1995
ice cream, choc	45	Pennington et al, 1995	orange, navel/valencia, raw	1	Pennington et al, 1995
ice cream sandwich	59	Pennington et al, 1995	peach, cnd, heavy syrup	1	Pennington et al, 1995
ice milk, van	30	Pennington et al, 1995	peach, raw	1	Pennington et al, 1995
pie, apple, frzn, heated	44	Pennington et al, 1995	pear, cnd, heavy syrup	1	Pennington et al, 1995
pie, pumpkin, frzn, heated	41	Pennington et al, 1995	pear, raw	1	Pennington et al, 1995
pudding, choc, inst made w/ whole milk	37	Pennington et al, 1995	pineapple, cnd, jce pack	1	Pennington et al, 1995
			plum, purple, raw	1	Pennington et al, 1995
shake, choc, fast food	53	Pennington et al, 1995	prune	30	Pennington et al, 1995
			raisins	3	Pennington et al, 1995
			strawberries, raw	3	Pennington et al, 1995
			watermelon, raw	0	Pennington et al, 1995

	IODINE (mcg/100 g)	SOURCE
GRAIN PRODUCTS		
baguette	10	MAFF1
biscuit, from refrig dough	35	Pennington et al, 1995
bread, brown	6	MAFF1
bread, pumpernickel	<4	MAFF1
bread, rye	49	Pennington et al, 1995
bread, white	91	Pennington et al, 1995
bread, white, standard	4	MAFF1
bread, white, unsliced	4	MAFF1
bread, whole wheat	63	Pennington et al, 1995
cornbread, homemade	68	Pennington et al, 1995
corn chips	30	Pennington et al, 1995
crackers, saltines	148	Pennington et al, 1995
macaroni, enr, boiled	19	Pennington et al, 1995
muffin, blueberry/plain	57	Pennington et al, 1995
noodles, egg, enr, boiled	11	Pennington et al, 1995
popcorn, popped in oil	27	Pennington et al, 1995
roll, white, enr	81	Pennington et al, 1995
scone w/fruit	12	MAFF1
tortilla, flour	75	Pennington et al, 1995
INFANT/JUNIOR FOODS		
cereal, mixed, prep w/whole milk	17	Pennington et al, 1995
cereal, oatmeal w/applesce & bananas	1	Pennington et al, 1995
formula, milk-based, high Fe, rts, cnd	9	Pennington et al, 1995
formula, milk-based, rts, cnd	9	Pennington et al, 1995
fruit, apple jce	3	Pennington et al, 1995
fruit, applesce	1	Pennington et al, 1995
fruit, bananas & pineapple	1	Pennington et al, 1995
fruit, orange jce	2	Pennington et al, 1995
fruit, peaches	1	Pennington et al, 1995
fruit, pears	1	Pennington et al, 1995
fruit, prunes/plums	0	Pennington et al, 1995
dessert, dutch apple/apple betty	1	Pennington et al, 1995
dessert, fruit	0	Pennington et al, 1995
dessert, pudding/custard	9	Pennington et al, 1995
dinner, beef & veg	18	Pennington et al, 1995
dinner, chicken & noodles	8	Pennington et al, 1995
dinner, chicken/turkey & veg	28	Pennington et al, 1995
dinner, ham & veg	8	Pennington et al, 1995
dinner, tomatoes, beef, & macaroni	2	Pennington et al, 1995
dinner, turkey & rice	6	Pennington et al, 1995
dinner, veg w/bacon/ham	2	Pennington et al, 1995
dinner, veg w/beef	1	Pennington et al, 1995
dinner, veg/turkey/chicken	5	Pennington et al, 1995
meat, beef	9	Pennington et al, 1995
meat, chicken/turkey	27	Pennington et al, 1995
meat, pork	7	Pennington et al, 1995
vegetables, carrots	1	Pennington et al, 1995
vegetables, creamed corn	4	Pennington et al, 1995
vegetables, creamed spinach	10	Pennington et al, 1995
vegetables, green beans	1	Pennington et al, 1995
vegetables, mixed	1	Pennington et al, 1995
vegetables, peas	1	Pennington et al, 1995
vegetables, sweet potatoes/yellow squash	1	Pennington et al, 1995
MEATS		
beef/calf liver, panfried	42	Pennington et al, 1995
beef chuck roast, baked	17	Pennington et al, 1995
beef, ground patty, panfried	14	Pennington et al, 1995
beef loin/sirloin steak, panfried	15	Pennington et al, 1995
beef round steak, stewed	18	Pennington et al, 1995
lamb chop, panfried	11	Pennington et al, 1995
meatloaf, baked, homemade	38	Pennington et al, 1995
pork bacon, panfried	16	Pennington et al, 1995

	IODINE (mcg/100 g)	SOURCE
pork chop, panfried	6	Pennington et al, 1995
pork, ham, cured, baked	12	Pennington et al, 1995
pork roast loin, baked	11	Pennington et al, 1995
pork sausage, panfried	21	Pennington et al, 1995
veal cutlet, breaded, panfried	19	Pennington et al, 1995
MEATS—LUNCHEON		
bologna	21	Pennington et al, 1995
frankfurter, boiled	10	Pennington et al, 1995
salami	28	Pennington et al, 1995
MILK & YOGURT		
milk, buttermilk	24	Pennington et al, 1995
milk, choc	24	Pennington et al, 1995
milk, evaporated	38	Pennington et al, 1995
milk, nonfat	21	Pennington et al, 1995
milk, 2% fat	23	Pennington et al, 1995
milk, whole	20	Pennington et al, 1995
yogurt, 2% fat, plain	33	Pennington et al, 1995
yogurt, 2% fat, strawberry	20	Pennington et al, 1995
NUTS & NUT PRODUCTS		
peanut butter, creamy	4	Pennington et al, 1995
peanuts, dry-roasted, salted	6	Pennington et al, 1995
pecans, packaged, unsalted	8	Pennington et al, 1995
soy nuts w/praline coating, GeniSoy	136	GENI
soy nuts, choc covered, GeniSoy	136	GENI
soy nuts, flavored, GeniSoy	136	GENI
soy nuts, unsalted, GeniSoy	136	GENI
POULTRY		
chicken, baked	15	Pennington et al, 1995
chicken, drumstick & breast, breaded, fried, homemade	17	Pennington et al, 1995
turkey breast, baked	40	Pennington et al, 1995
SAUCES & SALAD DRESSINGS		
gravy, brown, from mix	3	Pennington et al, 1995
salad dressing, Italian	1	Pennington et al, 1995
white sce, med, homemade	19	Pennington et al, 1995
SOUPS		
beef bouillon, cond, prep w/water	2	Pennington et al, 1995
chicken noodle, cond, prep w/water	4	Pennington et al, 1995
tomato, cond, prep w/whole milk	11	Pennington et al, 1995
veg beef, cond, prep w/water	3	Pennington et al, 1995
SUGARS, SYRUPS, & SWEETENERS		
honey	38	Pennington et al, 1995
jelly, grape	85	Pennington et al, 1995
sugar, white, granulated	22	Pennington et al, 1995
syrup, pancake	25	Pennington et al, 1995
VEGETABLES		
asparagus, boiled	0	Pennington et al, 1995
beans w/pork, cnd	5	Pennington et al, 1995
beet, cnd	1	Pennington et al, 1995
broccoli, boiled	0	Pennington et al, 1995
cabbage, boiled	0	Pennington et al, 1995
carrot, raw	1	Pennington et al, 1995
cauliflower, boiled	1	Pennington et al, 1995
celery, raw	1	Pennington et al, 1995
coleslaw w/dressing, homemade	4	Pennington et al, 1995
collards, boiled	1	Pennington et al, 1995
corn, boiled	8	Pennington et al, 1995
corn, cnd	8	Pennington et al, 1995
corn, creamed style, cnd	11	Pennington et al, 1995
cowpeas, boiled	26	Pennington et al, 1995

	IODINE (mcg/100 g)	SOURCE		IODINE (mcg/100 g)	SOURCE
cucumber pickle, dill	2	Pennington et al, 1995	potato w/peel, baked	31	Pennington et al, 1995
cucumber, raw	4	Pennington et al, 1995	radish, raw	1	Pennington et al, 1995
green (snap) beans, cnd	2	Pennington et al, 1995	red beans, boiled	21	Pennington et al, 1995
green (snap) beans, boiled	1	Pennington et al, 1995	sauerkraut, cnd	1	Pennington et al, 1995
lettuce, crisphead	0	Pennington et al, 1995	spinach, cnd	5	Pennington et al, 1995
lima beans, immature, frzn, boiled	31	Pennington et al, 1995	spinach, boiled	2	Pennington et al, 1995
lima beans, mature, boiled	9	Pennington et al, 1995	summer squash, boiled	1	Pennington et al, 1995
mixed veg, cnd	2	Pennington et al, 1995	sweet potato w/peel, baked	2	Pennington et al, 1995
mushrooms, cnd	3	Pennington et al, 1995	sweet potato, candied, homemade	15	Pennington et al, 1995
navy beans, boiled	39	Pennington et al, 1995	tomato, cnd	1	Pennington et al, 1995
onion, raw	1	Pennington et al, 1995	tomato jce, cnd	1	Pennington et al, 1995
onion rings, breaded & fried, frzn, heated	30	Pennington et al, 1995	tomato sce, cnd	1	Pennington et al, 1995
			tomato, raw	2	Pennington et al, 1995
peas, green, cnd	4	Pennington et al, 1995	winter squash, hubbard/acorn, boiled	1	Pennington et al, 1995
peas, green, frzn, boiled	4	Pennington et al, 1995			
pepper, sweet, green, raw	1	Pennington et al, 1995	**MISCELLANEOUS**		
pinto beans, boiled	15	Pennington et al, 1995	catsup	5	Pennington et al, 1995
potato, french fries, frzn, heated	29	Pennington et al, 1995	choc powder for milk	10	Pennington et al, 1995
potato, mashed, from inst	51	Pennington et al, 1995	potato chips	5	Pennington et al, 1995
potato, scalloped, homemade	31	Pennington et al, 1995	salt, Lite, Morton	6500[2]	MORT
potato w/o peel, boiled	9	Pennington et al, 1995	salt, Morton	6500[2]	MORT

[1] Foods with high iodine levels may contain erythrosine (a red food dye that is high in iodine) or iodine-containing dough conditioners. Another source of iodine is from iodophor cleaning solutions that are commonly used in the dairy industry.

[2] These products contain 390 mcg of iodine per teaspoon (6 g).

Sources:
EGLD: Eggland's Best, Inc, King of Prussia PA.
GENI: GeniSoy, Fairfield CA.
MAFF1: Ministry of Agriculture, Farms, and Fisheries, UK. Nutrient analysis of Bread and Morning Goods. 20 January 2001.
   (http://www.food.gov.uk/science/surveillance/maffinfo/2000/maff-2000-194) (accessed 20 December 2002).
MORT: Morton Salt, Elgin IL
Pennington JAT, SA Schoen, GD Salmon, B Young, RD Johnson, RW Marts. Composition of core foods of the US food supply, 1982–1991. III. Copper, manganese, selenium, and iodine. *J Food Comp Anal* 8:171–217, 1995.

Minerals—Molybdenum

FOOD	MOLYBDENUM (mcg/100 g)	SOURCE
BEVERAGES		
tea, inst powder	990	Varo et al, 1980d
wine, apple	1	Varo et al, 1980d
wine, red, hungarian	1	Varo et al, 1980d
wine, red, spanish	2	Varo et al, 1980d
wine, white, bordeaux	2	Varo et al, 1980d
CEREALS, RTE		
oats, puffed	20	Varo et al, 1980c
rice, puffed	20	Varo et al, 1980c
CHEESE		
cheese, blue	6	Varo et al, 1980a
cheese, cottage	5	Varo et al, 1980a
cheese, edam, 20%/40% fat	5/6	Varo et al, 1980a
cheese, emmenthal	10	Varo et al, 1980a
cheese, gouda	6	Varo et al, 1980a
cheese, gruyere	10	Varo et al, 1980a
cheese, processed	6	Varo et al, 1980a
cheese, quark	7	Varo et al, 1980a
CREAMS		
cream, coffee	5	Varo et al, 1980a
cream, half & half	5	Varo et al, 1980a
cream, whipping	20	Varo et al, 1980a
ENTREES		
green pea soup	20/10	Varo et al, 1980e
hamburger	20	Varo et al, 1980e
meat balls w/gravy	10	Varo et al, 1980e
meat & cabbage casserole	10	Varo et al, 1980e
FISH & SHELLFISH		
herring, salted	10	Nuurtamo et al, 1980a
mussels, cnd in water	30	Nuurtamo et al, 1980a
salmon, cnd in oil	10	Nuurtamo et al, 1980a
FRUITS		
cloudberries	10	Varo et al, 1980b
cranberries	10	Varo et al, 1980b
currants, black/red	10	Varo et al, 1980b
GRAIN PRODUCTS		
macaroni	20	Varo et al, 1980c
pancake, oven-baked	10	Varo et al, 1980e
rye crisp crackers	20	Varo et al, 1980c
GRAINS & GRAIN FRACTIONS		
rice, parboiled	40	Varo et al, 1980c
rice, whole grain/polished	20	Varo et al, 1980c
soy meal	1000	Varo et al, 1980c
wheat bran	20	Varo et al, 1980c

FOOD	MOLYBDENUM (mcg/100 g)	SOURCE
wheat flour, whole grain	20	Varo et al, 1980c
wheat germ	30	Varo et al, 1980c
MEATS		
beef liver	170	Nuurtamo et al, 1980b
beef (steer) kidney	60	Nuurtamo et al, 1980b
beef (steer) liver	160	Nuurtamo et al, 1980b
liver paste	50	Nuurtamo et al, 1980b
pork kidney	70	Nuurtamo et al, 1980b
pork liver	200	Nuurtamo et al, 1980b
pork, short plate	10	Nuurtamo et al, 1980b
rabbit meat	10	Nuurtamo et al, 1980b
salami, dry	10	Nuurtamo et al, 1980b
sheep liver	70	Nuurtamo et al, 1980b
MILKS		
infant formula, milk-based	10	Varo et al, 1980a
milk, human	1	Varo et al, 1980a
milk, whole	5	Varo et al, 1980a
milk, whole, dry	40	Varo et al, 1980a
VEGETABLES		
cabbage, red, pickled	10	Varo et al, 1980b
green beans	20	Varo et al, 1980b
green beans, frzn	20	Varo et al, 1980b
leek	10	Varo et al, 1980b
mushrooms	20	Varo et al, 1980b
onion, red	30	Varo et al, 1980b
parsley	10	Varo et al, 1980b
parsnip	10	Varo et al, 1980b
peas	20	Varo et al, 1980b
peas, dried	70	Varo et al, 1980b
peas, frzn	20	Varo et al, 1980b
pepper, sweet, red	70	Varo et al, 1980b
sauerkraut	10	Varo et al, 1980b
turnip	10	Varo et al, 1980b
FOOD GROUP		
berries	30	Varo et al, 1980b
fruits	20	Varo et al, 1980b
fruits & berries, all	20	Varo et al, 1980b
fruits & berries, cnd	30	Varo et al, 1980b
vegetables, all	80	Varo et al, 1980b
vegetables, cnd	50	Varo et al, 1980b
vegetables, fruity	320	Varo et al, 1980b
vegetables, leafy	50	Varo et al, 1980b
vegetables, roots	20	Varo et al, 1980b
vegetables, all	80	Varo et al, 1980b
vegetables, cnd	50	Varo et al, 1980b
vegetables, fruity	320	Varo et al, 1980b
vegetables, leafy	50	Varo et al, 1980b
vegetables, roots	20	Varo et al, 1980b

Sources:

Nuurtamo M, P Varo, E Saari, P Koivistoinen. Mineral element composition of Finnish foods. VI. Fish and fish products. *Acta Agriculturae Scandinavica*, Suppl 22:77–87, 1980a.

Nuurtamo M, P Varo, E Saari, P Koivistoinen. Mineral element composition of Finnish foods. V. Meat and meat products. *Acta Agriculturae Scandinavica*, Suppl 22:57–76, 1980b.

Varo P, M Nuurtamo, E Saari, P Koivistoinen. Mineral element composition of Finnish foods. VIII. Dairy products, eggs, and margarine. *Acta Agriculturae Scandinavica*, Suppl 22:115–126, 1980a.

Varo, P, O Lahelma, M Nuurtamo, E Saari, P Koivistoinen. Mineral element composition of Finnish foods. VII. Potato, vegetables, fruits, berries, nuts and mushrooms. *Acta Agriculturae Scandinavica*, Suppl 22:89–113, 1980b.

Varo P, M Nuurtamo, E Saari, P Koivistoinen. Mineral element composition of Finnish foods. IV. Flours and bakery products. *Acta Agriculturae Scandinavica*. Suppl 22:37–55, 1980c.

Varo P, M Nuurtamo, E Saari, P Koivistoinen. Mineral element composition of Finnish foods. IX. Beverages, confectionaires, sugar and condiments. *Acta Agriculturae Scandinavica*, Suppl 22:127–139, 1980d.

Varo P, M Nuurtamo, E Saari, P Koivistoinen. Mineral element composition of Finnish foods. X. Industrial convenience foods, quantity service foods and baby foods. *Acta Agriculturae Scandinavica*, Suppl 22:141–160, 1980e.

Plant Acids—Oxalic Acid

Note: Values from different sources are quite variable perhaps due to the natural variation of oxalic acid in foods and also to different analytical methods for measuring oxalic acid.

	OXALIC ACID (mg/100 g)	SOURCE		OXALIC ACID (mg/100 g)	SOURCE
BEVERAGES			carrot, raw	9.6	Holmes et al, 1995
beer, light	1.6	Souci et al, 2000	carrot, raw	500	USDA
beer, no alcohol	1.2	Souci et al, 2000	cassava, raw	1260	USDA
beer, pilsener, german	1.2	Souci et al, 2000	cauliflower, raw	150	USDA
cola	1.1	Souci et al, 2000	celeriac, raw	6.8	Souci et al, 2000
tea, black, 2 min brew	7.5	Holmes et al, 1995	celery, raw	61.2	Holmes et al, 1995
wine, red	1.4	Souci et al, 2000	celery, raw	190	USDA
wine, white	1.7	Souci et al, 2000	chickpeas, raw	780	Pilac et al, 1971
			chicory, raw	210	USDA
CANDY			chinese cabbage, raw	15	Pilac et al, 1971
dark chocolate, min 40% cocoa	88	Souci et al, 2000	chives, raw	1480	USDA
milk chocolate	56	Souci et al, 2000	collards, raw	450	USDA
nougat crème	36	Souci et al, 2000	coriander, raw	10	USDA
			corn, sweet, raw	10	USDA
FRUITS			cowpeas, white, raw	300	Pilac et al, 1971
apple, raw	0.5	Souci et al, 2000	cucumber, raw	20	USDA
apricot, raw	6.8	Souci et al, 2000	dandelion leaves, raw	25	Souci et al, 2000
banana, raw	73	Pilac et al, 1971	eggplant, raw	190	USDA
bitter melon, raw	90	Pilac et al, 1971	endive, raw	110	USDA
blackberries, raw	12	Souci et al, 2000	fennel leaves, raw	5.0	Souci et al, 2000
carambola, raw	110	Pilac et al, 1971	french beans, raw	44	Souci et al, 2000
cherries, morello, raw	4.7	Souci et al, 2000	garlic, raw	360	USDA
cherries, sweet, raw	7.2	Souci et al, 2000	green (snap) beans, raw	360	USDA
currants, red, raw	9.9	Souci et al, 2000	kale, raw	20	USDA
gooseberries, raw	19	Souci et al, 2000	kidney beans, red, raw	320	Pilac et al, 1971
grapes, raw	8.0	Souci et al, 2000	kidney beans, white, raw	110	Pilac et al, 1971
jackfruit, raw	130	Pilac et al, 1971	kohlrabi, raw	2.8	Souci et al, 2000
mirabelle,[1] raw	11	Souci et al, 2000	lamb's lettuce,[2] raw	38	Souci et al, 2000
mango, raw	36	Souci et al, 2000	lettuce, raw	330	USDA
orange juice	0.4	Holmes et al, 1995	mangold,[3] raw	650	Souci et al, 2000
papaya, raw	40	Pilac et al, 1971	miner's lettuce,[4] raw	14	Schelstraete, Kennedy
pear, raw	6.2	Souci et al, 2000	mungo beans, green, raw	180	Pilac et al, 1971
plum, raw	12	Souci et al, 2000	navy beans, raw	380	Pilac et al, 1971
quince, raw	.33	Silva et al, 2002	okra, raw	50	USDA
raspberries, raw	16	Souci et al, 2000	onion, raw	50	USDA
strawberries, raw	16	Souci et al, 2000	parsley, raw	1700	USDA
tamarind, raw	4600	Pilac et al, 1971	parsnip, raw	40	USDA
			peas, dry pods, raw	2.7	Souci et al, 2000
GRAIN PRODUCTS			peas, green, raw	50	USDA
corn flakes, Kellogg's	1.9	Holmes et al, 1995	pepper, green, raw	40	USDA
Weetabix	76.1	Holmes et al, 1995	potato, flesh & peel, raw	30	Bushway et al, 1984
			potato flesh, raw	30	Bushway et al, 1984
VEGETABLES			potato peel, raw	35	Bushway et al, 1984
amaranth, raw	1090	USDA	purslane, raw	1310	USDA
artichoke, raw	8.8	Souci et al, 2000	radish, raw	480	USDA
asparagus, raw	130	USDA	rhubarb, raw	460	Souci et al, 2000
bamboo shoots, raw	252	Souci et al, 2000	rutabaga, raw	30	USDA
beet, raw	181	Souci et al, 2000	soybean curd	170	Pilac et al, 1971
beet leaves, raw	610	USDA	soybeans, raw	390	Pilac et al, 1971
broccoli, raw	190	USDA	spinach, raw	645	Holmes et al, 1995
brussels sprouts, raw	360	USDA	spinach, raw	970	USDA
cabbage, green, raw	100	USDA	squash, raw	20	USDA
cabbage, red, raw	7.4	Souci et al, 2000	sweet potato, raw	240	USDA
cabbage, savoy, raw	4.9	Souci et al, 2000	taro, raw	36	Souci et al, 2000

	OXALIC ACID (mg/100 g)	SOURCE		OXALIC ACID (mg/100 g)	SOURCE
tomato, raw	5.7	Holmes et al, 1995	watercress, raw	310	USDA
tomato, raw	50	USDA	waxgourd, raw	40	Pilac et al, 1971
turnip, raw	210	USDA	**MISCELLANEOUS**		
turnip greens, raw	50	USDA	cocoa powder	396	Souci et al, 2000
V-8 Juice, Campbell Soup Co	5.8	Holmes et al, 1995	jam, quince	.36	Silva et al, 2002

[1] Mirabelle (*Prunus domestica L, ssp Syriacia B*).
[2] Lamb's lettuce (*Valerianella olitoria*).
[3] Mangold (*Beta vulgaris var.cicla*).
[4] Miner's lettuce (*Montia perfoliata*), a member of the purslane family; fleshy, succulent annual indigenous to the western US; also known as Indian lettuce, Spanish lettuce, Cuban spinach, and, in Europe and the Caribbean Islands, as winter purslane; stem and leaves may be eaten raw or cooked and prepared in the many ways that spinach is used.

Sources:
Bushway RJ, JL Bureau, DF McGann. Determinations of organic acids in potatoes by high performance liquid chromatography. *J Food Sci* 49:75–77, 1984.
Holmes RP, HO Goodman, DG Assimos. Dietary oxalate and its intestinal absorption. *Scanning Microscopy* 9:1109–1120, 1995.
Pilac LM, IC Abdon, EP Mandap. Oxalic acid content and its relation to the calcium present in some Philippine plant foods. *Philippine J Nutr* 24:21–36, 1971.
Schelstraete M, BM Kennedy. Composition of miner's lettuce (*Montia perfoliata*). *J Am Diet Assoc* 77:21–25, 1980.
Souci SW, W Fachmann, H Kraut. *Food Composition and Nutrition Tables*. Medpharm GmbH Scientific Publishers, Stuttgart, Germany & CRC Press, Washington DC. 2000.
Silva BM, PB Andrade, GC Mendes, RM Seabra, MA Ferreira. Study of the organic acids composition of quince (*Cydonia oblonga* Miller) fruit and jam. *J Agric Food Chem* 50:2313–2317, 2002.
USDA: Nutrient Data Laboratory, Agricultural Research Service, United States Department of Agriculture. *Oxalic Acid Content of Selected Vegetables*. Available at http://www.nla.usda.gov/fnic/foodcomp.Data/Other/oxalic.html (accessed 20 February 2002).

Plant Acids—Phytic Acid

	PHYTIC ACID (mg/100 g)	SOURCE		PHYTIC ACID (mg/100 g)	SOURCE
BEVERAGES			**NUTS**		
coffee, brewed from ground roast	5	Harland and Oberleas, 1985	peanut butter	1252	Oberleas and Harland, 1981
			peanuts	1336	Souci et al, 2000
coffee, from inst powder	0	Harland and Oberleas, 1985	peanuts, roasted	175	Oberleas and Harland, 1981
coffee, ground roast	370	Harland and Oberleas, 1985			
coffee, inst powder	200	Harland and Oberleas, 1985	**VEGETABLES**		
tea, brewed	1	Harland and Oberleas, 1985	carrot, raw	9	Oberleas and Harland, 1981
tea, from inst powder	1	Harland and Oberleas, 1985	corn, sweet, yellow, cnd	31	Oberleas and Harland, 1981
tea, inst powder	260	Harland and Oberleas, 1985	green (snap) beans, cnd	91	Oberleas and Harland, 1981
			potato, boiled, peeled	81	Oberleas and Harland, 1981
CEREALS			tomato, cnd	6	Oberleas and Harland, 1981
corn flakes	48	Oberleas and Harland, 1981			
farina, reg, ckd	4	Oberleas and Harland, 1981	**VEGETABLES–LEGUMES**		
granola	625	Oberleas and Harland, 1981	blackeye peas, boiled	995	Reddy et al, 1982
oatmeal, ckd	111	Oberleas and Harland, 1981	blackeye peas, ckd	986	Davies and Warrington, 1986
rice flakes	232	Oberleas and Harland, 1981	blackeye peas, cnd	98	Reddy et al, 1982
wheat flakes	1467	Oberleas and Harland, 1981	blackeye peas, dry	1205	Davies and Warrington, 1986
wheat, shredded	1481	Oberleas and Harland, 1981	blackeye peas, dry	1148	Reddy et al, 1982
			black gram, ground, ckd	888	Davies and Warrington, 1986
FRUITS			black gram, ground, ckd, washed	731	Davies and Warrington, 1986
apple w/peel	63	Oberleas and Harland, 1981			
avocado	17	Souci et al, 2000	black gram, ground, dry	934	Davies and Warrington, 1986
banana	20	Souci et al, 2000	black gram, ground, dry, washed	993	Davies and Warrington, 1986
GRAINS & GRAIN FRACTIONS					
			black gram, whole, dry	794	Davies and Warrington, 1986
barley, whole grain	1070	Souci et al, 2000	black gram, whole, ckd	688	Davies and Warrington, 1986
cornmeal, blue	1870	Kuhnlein et al, 1979	chickpeas, boiled	208	Oberleas and Harland, 1981
cornmeal, pink	1250	Kuhnlein et al, 1979	chickpea flour	788	Davies and Warrington, 1986
cornmeal, white	1740	Kuhnlein et al, 1979	chickpeas, green	280	Souci et al, 2000
corn, whole grain	940	Souci et al, 2000	chickpeas, split, dry	1053	Davies and Warrington, 1986
oats, whole grain	900	Souci et al, 2000	chickpeas, split, ckd	769	Davies and Warrington, 1986
quinoa (pigweed)	541	Souci et al, 2000	chickpeas, whole, ckd	580	Davies and Warrington, 1986
rice, polished, dry	2539	Oberleas and Harland, 1981	chickpeas, whole, dry	560	Davies and Warrington, 1986
wheat bran, crude	3011	Oberleas and Harland, 1981	common mexican beans, ckd	756	Hernandez-Unzon and Ortega-Delgado, 1989
wheat germ	4071	Oberleas and Harland, 1981			
wheat flour, all-purpose	282	Oberleas and Harland, 1981	green gram, ground, ckd	663	Davies and Warrington, 1986
wheat flour, whole	845	Oberleas and Harland, 1981	green gram, ground, ckd, washed	472	Davies and Warrington, 1986
GRAIN PRODUCTS			green gram, ground, dry	863	Davies and Warrington, 1986
bread, brown	169	MAFF1	green gram, ground, dry, washed	871	Davies and Warrington, 1986
bread, pumpernickel	175	MAFF1			
bread, rye	942	Oberleas and Harland, 1981	green gram, whole, ckd	695	Davies and Warrington, 1986
bread, wheat germ	331	MAFF1	green gram, whole, dry	809	Davies and Warrington, 1986
bread, white	69	Oberleas and Harland, 1981	kidney beans, ckd	778	Davies and Warrington, 1986
bread, white, standard	105	MAFF1	kidney beans, dry	893	Davies and Warrington, 1986
bread, whole wheat	390	Oberleas and Harland, 1981	kidney beans, red, dry	1170	Reddy et al, 1982
bread, whole wheat	358	MAFF1	kidney beans, red, boiled	1080	Reddy et al, 1982
chapati flour, dark	695	Davies and Warrington, 1986	kidney beans, red, cnd	260	Reddy et al, 1982
chapati flour, light	578	Davies and Warrington, 1986	lentils, pappadum	673	Davies and Warrington, 1986
chapati flour, whole wheat	669	Davies and Warrington, 1986	lentils, split, ckd	235	Davies and Warrington, 1986
chapati, from dark flour	341	Davies and Warrington, 1986	lentils, split, dry	526	Davies and Warrington, 1986
chapati, from light flour	254	Davies and Warrington, 1986	lentils, whole, ckd	252	Davies and Warrington, 1986
chapati, from whole wheat flour	513	Davies and Warrington, 1986	lentils, whole, dry	495	Davies and Warrington, 1986
			lima beans, dry	1011	Oberleas and Harland, 1981
crackers, saltines	172	Oberleas and Harland, 1981	mung beans, dry	204	Reddy et al, 1982
corn chips	635	Oberleas and Harland, 1981	mung beans, boiled	130	Reddy et al, 1982
macaroni, boiled	81	Oberleas and Harland, 1981	mung beans, cnd	66	Reddy et al, 1982
popcorn, popped, plain	614	Oberleas and Harland, 1981	navy beans, boiled	346	Oberleas and Harland, 1981
roll, whole wheat	285	MAFF1	navy beans, dry	615	Oberleas and Harland, 1981
			peas, green, cnd	28	Oberleas and Harland, 1981

	PHYTIC ACID (mg/100 g)	SOURCE		PHYTIC ACID (mg/100 g)	SOURCE
pink beans, dry	503	Reddy et al, 1982	white beans, dry	800	Souci et al, 2000
pink beans, boiled	370	Reddy et al, 1982			
pink beans, cnd	126	Reddy et al, 1982	**MISCELLANEOUS**		
red gram, ground, ckd	650	Davies and Warrington, 1986	cocoa mix	270	Harland and Oberleas, 1985
red gram, ground, dry	1107	Davies and Warrington, 1986	cocoa powder	1880	Oberleas and Harland, 1981
soybean meal	3441	Mohamed et al, 1991			

Sources:

Davies NT, S Warrington. The phytic acid mineral, trace element, protein, and moisture content of UK Asian immigrant foods. *Human Nutrition: Applied Nutrition* 40A:49–59, 1986.

Harland BF, D Oberleas. Phytate and zinc contents of coffees, cocoas, and teas. *J Food Sci* 50:832–833, 1985.

Hernandez-Unzon HY, ML Ortega-Delgado. Phytic acid in stored common bean seeds (*Phaseolus vulgaris* L.). *Plant Foods for Human Nutrition* 39:209–221, 1989. Kluwer Academic Publishers, The Netherlands.

Kuhnlein HV, DH Calloway, BF Harland. Composition of traditional Hopi foods. *J Am Diet Assoc* 75:37–41, 1979.

MAFF1: Ministry of Agriculture, Farms, and Fisheries, UK. Nutrient analysis of Bread and Morning Goods. 20 January 2001. (http://www.food.gov.uk/science/surveillance/maffinfo/2000/maff-2000-194) (accessed 20 December 2002).

Mohamed AI, T Mebrahtu, M Rangappa. Nutrient composition and anti-nutritional factors in selected vegetable soybean (*Glycine Max* L. Merr.). *Plant Foods for Human Nutrition* 41:89–100, 1991. Kluwer Academic Publishers, The Netherlands.

Oberleas D, BF Harland. Phytate content of foods: Effect on dietary zinc bioavailability. *J Am Diet Assoc* 79:433–436, 1981.

Reddy NR, SK Sathe, DK Salunkhe. Phytates in legumes and cereals. *Advances Food Research* 28:1–92, 1982.

Souci SW, W Fachmann, H Kraut. *Food Composition and Nutrition Tables.* Medpharm GmbH Scientific Publishers, Stuttgart, Germany & CRC Press, Washington DC. 2000.

Plant Acids—Salicylic Acid

	SALICYLIC ACID (mg/100 g)		SALICYLIC ACID (mg/100 g)
BEVERAGES		blueberries, cnd	2.76
		boysenberries, cnd	2.04
ale, draught, stout	0.30	cantaloupe, raw	1.50
brandy	0.40	cherries, sweet	0.85
Coca-Cola	0.25	cherries, sweet, cnd	2.78
coffee, inst powder	0.29	cherries, sour, cnd	0.30
gin	0.40	cranberries, cnd	1.64
hard cider	0.17	cranberry sauce	1.44
liqueur	3.05	currants, black, frzn	3.06
Ovaltine powder	0.00	currants, dried	5.80
port	2.8	currants, red, frzn	5.06
rum	1.02	custard apple, raw	0.21
sherry	0.50	date, dried	4.50
tea, black, bag, Tetley	5.57	date, raw	3.73
tea, black, bag/leaves, Twinings	3.70	fig, cnd	0.25
tea, herbal, bag	0.48	fig, dried	0.64
vodka	0.00	fig, raw	0.18
whiskey	0.00	grapefruit, raw	0.68
wine, cabernet sauvignon	0.86	grapes, cnd	0.16
wine, champagne	1.02	grapes, red, raw	0.94
wine, claret	0.63	grapes, green, raw	1.88
wine, Riesling	0.84	guava, cnd	2.02
wine, rose	0.37	kiwifruit, raw	0.32
wine, vermouth, dry	0.46	lemon, raw	0.18
wine, white, dry	0.10	loganberries, cnd	4.40
		loquat, raw	0.26
CANDY		lychee, cnd	0.36
caramels	0.12	mango, raw	0.11
licorice	8.87	mulberries, raw	0.76
peppermints, Lifesavers	0.86	nectarine, raw	0.49
		orange, raw	2.39
CHEESE, CREAM, & YOGURT		papaya (pawpaw), raw	0.08
cheese, blue vein	0.05	passion fruit (granadilla), raw	0.14
cheese, camembert	0.01	peach, raw	0.58
cheese, cheddar	0.00	peach, cnd	0.68
cheese, cottage	0.00	pear, cnd	0.00
cheese, mozzarella	0.02	pear, raw w/peel	0.27
cream	0.00	pear, raw w/o peel	0.00
yogurt, whole	0.00	persimmon, raw	0.18
		pineapple, raw	2.10
FISH & SHELLFISH		pineapple, cnd	1.36
oysters, raw	0.00	plum, green, raw	0.10
prawn, raw	0.04	plum, red, cnd	1.16
salmon/tuna, cnd	0.00	plum, red prune, cnd	6.87
scallops, raw	0.02	plum, red, raw	0.21
		pomegranate, raw	0.07
FRUIT JUICES		raspberries, frzn	3.88
apple jce	0.19	raspberries, raw	5.14
apricot nectar	0.14	raisins	6.62
grapefruit jce	0.42	raisins, sultana	7.80
grape jce, dark	0.88	strawberries, raw	1.36
grape jce, light	0.18	tamarillo, raw	0.10
orange jce	0.18	tangelo, raw	0.72
peach nectar	0.10	tangerine, raw	0.56
pineapple jce, cnd	0.16	watermelon, raw	0.48
		youngberries, cnd	3.06
FRUITS			
apple, cnd	0.55	**GRAINS & GRAIN FRACTIONS**	
apple, raw, granny smith	0.59		
apple, raw, red varieties	0.46	arrowroot powder	0.00
apricot, cnd	1.42	barley, unpearled, dry	0.00
apricot, raw	2.58	buckwheat grain, dry	0.00
avocado, raw	0.60	cornmeal, dry	0.43
banana	0.00	millet grain, hulled/unhulled, dry	0.00
blackberries, cnd	1.86		

	SALICYLIC ACID (mg/100 g)
oatmeal, dry	0.00
rice grain, brown/white	0.00
rye, rolled, dry	0.00
soy grits, dry	0.00
wheat grain, dry	0.00
MEAT & POULTRY	
beef/lamb/pork, raw	0.00
chicken, raw	0.00
chicken egg white/yolk	0.00
kidney, unspecified, raw	0.00
liver, unspecified, raw	0.05
tripe, unspecified, raw	0.00
NUTS & SEEDS	
almonds, raw	3.00
brazil nuts, raw	0.46
cashews, raw	0.07
coconut, dried	0.26
hazelnuts, raw	0.14
macadamia nuts, raw	0.52
peanut butter	0.23
peanuts, raw	1.12
pecans, raw	0.12
pine nuts, raw	0.51
pistachios, raw	0.55
poppyseeds, dry	0.00
sesame seeds, dry	0.23
sunflower seeds, dry	0.12
walnuts, raw	0.30
SAUCES & CONDIMENTS	
olives, black, cnd	0.34
olives, green, cnd	1.29
pickle, gherkin	6.14
soy sce	0.00
tabasco sce, McIlhenny	0.45
worcestershire sce	64.3
SPICES & HERBS	
allspice	5.20
aniseed	22.8
bay leaves	2.52
basil, ground	3.40
canella	42.6
cardamom	7.70
caraway seeds, ground	2.82
cayenne powder	17.6
celery seed powder	10.1
chili flakes	1.38
chili powder	1.30
cinnamon, ground	15.2
cloves	5.74
coriander leaves, raw	0.20
cumin powder	45.0
curry powder	218.0
dill seed, raw	6.90
dill seed, ground	94.4
fennel, gorund	0.80
fenugreek seeds, ground	12.2
garam masala powder	66.8
ginger root, raw	4.50
mace powder	32.2
mint, raw	9.40
mustard powder	26.0
nutmeg powder	2.40
oregano powder	66.0
paprika, hot powder	203.0

	SALICYLIC ACID (mg/100 g)
paprika, sweet powder	5.70
parsley leaves, raw	0.08
pepper, black	6.20
pepper, white	1.10
pimento powder	4.90
rosemary, ground	68.0
saffron, ground	0.00
sage leaves, dried	21.7
tandori powder	0.00
tarragon, ground	34.8
turmeric, ground	76.4
thyme leaves, dry	183.0
vanilla flavoring, liquid	1.44
SWEETENERS	
honey, liquid	6.30
maple syrup	0.00
molasses, liquid	0.22
sugar, white granulated	0.00
syrup, golden	0.10
VEGETABLES	
alfalfa, raw	0.70
asparagus, cnd	0.32
asparagus, raw	0.14
bamboo shoots	0.00
bean sprouts	0.06
beet, cnd	0.32
beet, raw	0.18
blackeyed peas, dry	0.00
broad beans, raw	0.73
broccoli, raw	0.65
brown beans, dry	0.002
brussels sprouts, raw	0.07
cabbage, green, raw	0.00
cabbage, red, raw	0.08
carrot, raw	0.23
cauliflower, raw	0.16
celery, raw	0.00
chayote (choko), raw	0.01
chickpeas, dry	0.00
chicory, raw	1.02
chives, raw	0.03
corn, sweet, cnd	0.26
corn, sweet, creamed, cnd	0.39
cucumber w/o peel, raw	0.78
eggplant w/o peel, raw	0.30
eggplant w/peel, raw	0.88
endive, raw	1.90
garlic, raw	0.10
horseradish, cnd	0.18
green beans, french, raw	0.11
leek, raw	0.08
lentils, brown/red, dry	0.00
lettuce, raw	0.00
lima beans, dry	0.00
mung beans, dry	0.00
mushrooms, champignon, raw	1.26
mushrooms, common, white, raw	0.24
okra, cnd	0.59
onion, raw	0.16
parsnip, raw	0.45
peas, green, raw	0.04
peas, green, split, dry	0.00
peas, yellow, split, dry	0.02
pepper, green chili, raw	0.64
pepper, green sweet (bell), raw	1.20
pepper, red chili, raw	1.20

	SALICYLIC ACID (mg/100 g)		SALICYLIC ACID (mg/100 g)
pepper, yellow-green chili, raw	0.62	tomato, cnd	0.53
pimientos, red, cnd	0.15	tomato jce	0.13
potato, white w/o peel, raw	0.00	tomato paste	0.81
potato, white w/peel, raw	0.12	tomato, raw	0.13
pumpkin, raw	0.12	tomato sce	1.52
radish, red	1.24	turnip, raw	0.16
rhubarb, raw	0.13	water chestnuts, cnd	2.92
shallot, raw	0.03	watercress, raw	0.84
soybeans, dry	0.00	zucchini, raw	1.04
spinach, frzn	0.16		
spinach, raw	0.58	**MISCELLANEOUS**	
squash, marrow, raw	0.17	carob powder	0.00
squash, winter, raw	0.63	cocoa powder	0.00
sweet potato, white, raw	0.50	tomato soup	0.47
sweet potato, yellow, raw	0.48	vinegar, malt	0.00
swede (rutabaga), raw	0.00	vinegar, white	1.33

Source:
Swain AR, SP Dutton, AS Truswell. Salicylates in foods. *J Am Diet Assoc* 85:950–960, 1985.
Also see: Perry CA, J Dwyer, JA Gelfand, RR Couris, WW McCloskey. Health effects of salicylates in foods and drugs. *Nutr Rev* S2:225–240, 1996 for information on the salicylate content of various drugs and medications.

Plant Sterols—Phytosterols

	PHYTOSTEROLS (mg/100 g)	USDA CODE		PHYTOSTEROLS (mg/100 g)	USDA CODE
CANDY			margarine, soy, stick	219	04080
candy chips, yogurt	24	19079	margarine-butter blend (60% corn oil, 40% butter)	342	04585
caramel, choc flavored roll	14	19076			
peanut brittle	64	19148	mayonnaise, imitation, soy	62	04027
Snickers, M&M/Mars	41	19155	mayonnaise, reg, safflower & soy	347	04026
			mayonnaise, reg, soy	223	04025
CREAMS			sandwich spread	75	04030
creamer, liquid/frzn w/hydg veg oils	13	01067	shortening, beef tallow & cottonseed (for frying)	32	04550
creamer, liquid/frzn w/lauric acid oils	9	01068			
creamer, powdered	32	01069	shortening, coconut (hydg) & palm kernel (for confectionery)	86	04551
sour cream, cultured, imitation	18	01074			
			shortening, lard & veg oil	13	04544
DESSERT TOPPINGS			shortening, palm (for confectionery)	49	04570
glaze, homemade	24	19375	shortening, soy (hydg), 30% linoleic acid (for heavy duty frying)	132	04552
icing/frosting, choc, rts	34	19226			
icing/frosting, from mix, choc made w/marg	29	19372	shortening, soy (hydg) & cottonseed	200	04547
whipped topping, frzn	23	01073	shortening, soy (hydg) & cottonseed (for bread)	200	04546
whipped topping, pressurized	20	01072			
			shortening, soy (hydg) & cottonseed (household)	200	04031
EGGS & EGG SUBSTITUTES					
chicken egg, fried	14	01128	shortening, soy (hydg) & palm (household)	148	04559
chicken egg, omelet, plain	10	01130			
chicken egg, scrambled w/milk	10	01132	spread, corn, 40% fat, stick	270	04107
egg substitutes, frzn	95	01142	spread, soy, 40% fat, stick	106	04110
egg substitutes, liquid	4	01143	spread, soy & cottonseed, 60% fat, soft	159	04106
			spread, soy & palm, 60% fat, stick	159	04526
FAST FOOD			veg oil, almond	266	04529
egg biscuit	13	21002	veg oil, apricot kernel	266	04530
			veg oil, babassu	95	04534
FATS, OILS, SHORTENINGS, & SPREADS			veg oil, cocoa (cacao)	201	04501
			veg oil, coconut	86	04047
margarine, corn, soft	483	04092	veg oil, corn	968	04518
margarine, corn, stick	570	04065	veg oil, cottonseed	324	04502
margarine, liquid	174	04105	veg oil, hazelnut	120	04532
margarine, soy, soft	144	04093	veg oil, olive	221	04053

	PHYTOSTEROLS (mg/100 g)	USDA CODE
veg oil, palm kernel	95	04513
veg oil, peanut	207	04042
veg oil, poppyseed	276	04514
veg oil, rice bran	1190	04037
veg oil, safflower, >70% linoleic acid	444	04510
veg oil, safflower, >70% oleic acid	444	04511
veg oil, sesame	865	04058
veg oil, sheanut	357	04536
veg oil, soy (hydg) & cottonseed	152	04543
veg oil, soy (hydg)	132	04034
veg oil, soy	250	04044
veg oil, sunflower, <60% linoleic acid	100	04060
veg oil, sunflower, >60% linoleic acid	100	04506
veg oil, walnut	176	04528
veg oil, wheat germ	553	04038

FRUITS

apple, raw w/skin	12	09003
apricots, raw	18	09021
banana, raw	16	09040
cantaloupe, raw	10	09181
cherries, sweet, raw	12	09070
figs, raw	31	09089
grapefruit, white, raw	17	09116
grapes, european, red/green, seedless, raw	4	09132
lemon peel	35	09156
loquats, raw	2	09174
orange, CA navel, raw	24	09202
orange peel	34	09216
peach, raw	10	09236
pear, raw	8	09252
persimmon, japanese, raw	4	09263
pineapple, raw	6	09266
plum, raw	7	09279
pomegranate, raw	17	09286
strawberries, raw	12	09316
watermelon, raw	2	09326

GRAIN PRODUCTS & FRACTIONS

amaranth flour	24	20001
biscuit, plain/buttermilk, homemade	30	18016
bread, indian (navajo) fry bread	15	18031
bread (quick), banana, homemade w/marg	34	18019
bread (quick), cornbread, homemade w/2% milk	12	18024
bread (yeast), egg	7	18027
bread (yeast), irish soda, homemade	13	18032
oriental snack mix, rice-based	25	19031
pasta, egg, homemade, ckd	1	20097
pasta, homemade w/o egg, ckd	2	20098
zwieback toast, Gerber	31	03217

MEATS

pork, center loin (chops) w/bone, lean & fat, panfried	2	10179
pork, center loin (chops) w/bone, lean, panfried	3	10176
pork, center rib (chops) w/bone, lean, panfried	3	10197
pork, loin blade (chops) w/bone, lean & fat, panfried	3	10178
pork, loin blade (chops) w/bone, lean, panfried	4	10120
pork, top loin (chops), lean & fat, panfried	2	10186
pork, top loin (chops), lean, panfried	3	10181

	PHYTOSTEROLS (mg/100 g)	USDA CODE
veal, leg (top round), lean & fat, breaded, panfried	3	17096
veal, leg (top round), lean, breaded, panfried	3	17101

MEATS, LUNCHEON

beerwurst, pork & beef	3	07931
frankfurter, pork	1	07939

NUTS & SEEDS

almonds, dry roasted	118	12063
almonds, oil roasted	130	12065
cashews, dry roasted	158	12085
chestnuts, european, raw	22	12097
coconut milk, raw	1	12117
coconut, raw	47	12104
filberts (hazelnuts), dried	96	12120
filberts (hazelnuts), dry roasted	110	12122
macadamia nuts, dry roasted	114	12132
macadamia nuts, raw	116	12131
peanut butter, chunk style/crunchy	102	16097
peanut butter, creamy/smooth	102	16098
peanuts, all types, unroasted/raw	220	16087
pecans, dried	102	12142
pecans, dry roasted	85	12143
pecans, oil roasted	108	12144
pine nuts, pignolia, dried	141	12147
pistachios, dried	214	12151
pistachios, dry roasted	214	12152
sesame seeds, whole, dried	714	12023
sunflower seed kernels, dried	534	12036
trail mix, tropical	80	19061
walnuts, english/persian, dried	72	12155

SALAD DRESSINGS, LOW & REDUCED CALORIE

french	15	04020
italian	25	04021
russian	10	04022
thousand island	27	04023

SALAD DRESSINGS, REGULAR

blue (bleu) cheese/roquefort	130	04539
french	102	04120
french, homemade	176	04133
homemade, ckd	24	04134
italian	121	04114
mayonnaise type	97	04018
russian	127	04015
sesame seed	113	04016
thousand island	97	04017
vinegar & oil, homemade	66	04135

SAUCES & CONDIMENTS

catsup (ketchup)	7	11935
cheese sauce, homemade	11	01164
horseradish (prepared sce)	9	02055
pickle, dill	14	11937
pickle, sour	14	11941
pickle, sweet (gherkin)	14	11940
white sce, med, homemade	29	06166
white sce, thick, homemade	40	06167
white sce, thin, homemade	16	06165

SPICES & HERBS

allspice, ground	61	02001
basil, ground	106	02003
capers, cnd, drained	48	02054

	PHYTOSTEROLS (mg/100 g)	USDA CODE		PHYTOSTEROLS (mg/100 g)	USDA CODE
caraway seeds	76	02005	**VEGETABLES**		
cardamom (cardamon), ground	46	02006	asparagus, boiled	24	11012
celery seeds	60	02007	bamboo shoots, raw	19	11026
chili powder	83	02009	cabbage, green, raw, shredded	11	11109
chives, raw, chopped	9	11156	carrots, raw	12	11124
cinnamon, ground	26	02010	cauliflower, raw	18	11135
cloves, ground	256	02011	celery, diced, boiled	7	11144
coriander (cilantro), seeds	46	02013	celery, raw	6	11143
cumin, seeds	68	02014	celtuce, raw	11	11145
curry powder	72	02015	coriander (cilantro), leaf, fresh	5	11165
dill seeds	124	02016	cucumber, raw w/peel	14	11205
fennel seeds	66	02018	eggplant (aubergine), raw	7	11209
fenugreek seeds	140	02019	grape leaves, raw	21	11974
garlic powder	8	02020	lettuce, iceberg, raw, chopped	10	11252
ginger root, ground	83	02021	lettuce, looseleaf (leaf), raw, shredded	38	11253
ginger root, raw, sliced	15	11216	mung bean sprouts, raw	15	11043
lemon grass (citronella), raw	6	11972	onion, chopped, boiled	18	11283
mace, ground	73	02022	onion, raw, chopped	15	11282
marjoram, dried	60	02023	peppers, banana, raw	3	11976
mustard seeds, yellow	118	02024	peppers, pimiento, cnd	9	11943
nutmeg, ground	62	02025	peppers, serrano, raw	6	11977
onion powder	87	02026	peppers, sweet (bell), green, raw	9	11333
oregano, ground	203	02027	peppers, sweet (bell), green, sliced, boiled	9	11334
paprika	175	02028	peppers, sweet (bell), red, raw	9	11821
parsley sprigs, raw	5	11297	peppers, sweet (bell), red, sliced, boiled	9	11823
pepper, black	92	02030	potato pancake, homemade	28	11672
pepper, red/cayenne	83	02031	potato, raw w/skin, brown-skinned	5	11352
pepper, white	55	02032	potato, raw w/skin, russet	5	11353
peppermint, raw	13	02064	potato, raw w/skin, white-skinned	4	11354
poppy seeds	89	02033	radish, red, raw, sliced	7	11429
poultry seasoning	96	02034	soybeans, green, boiled	50	11451
pumpkin pie spice	71	02035	soybeans, mature, raw	161	16108
rosemary, dried	58	02036	spinach, raw, chopped	9	11457
rosemary, raw	44	02063	tomato, raw, orange	4	11695
sage, ground	244	02038	tomato, raw, red	7	11529
savory, ground	31	02039	tomato, raw, red, cherry/chopped/ sliced/italian/plum	7	11529
shallots, raw, chopped	5	11677			
spearmint, dried	82	02066	tomato, raw, yellow	6	11696
spearmint, raw	10	02065	tomato, red, boiled	9	11530
tarragon, ground	81	02041	tomato, red, stewed	14	11660
thyme, ground	163	02042	turnip greens, raw, chopped	12	11568
turmeric, ground	82	02043			

Source:

USDA Codes: *United States Department of Agriculture Database for Standard Reference, Release 15* (SR-15), 2002. Available at http://www.nal.usda.gov/fnic/foodcomp/Data/SR15/ sr15.html.

Plant Sterols—Beta-Sitosterol, Stigmasterol, & Campesterol

	BETA-SITOSTEROL (mg/100 g)	STIGMASTEROL (mg/100 g)	CAMPESTEROL (mg/100 g)	USDA CODE/ SOURCE
FATS, OILS, & SPREADS				
cocoa butter	138	61	22	Souci et al, 2000
margarine, corn & soy, 80% fat, stick	117	28	41	04628
oil, coconut	48	13	9	Souci et al, 2000
oil, corn	595	51	179	Souci et al, 2000
oil, cottonseed	303	tr	20	Souci et al, 2000
oil, grapeseed	255	36	36	Souci et al, 2000
oil, linseed	206	30	117	Souci et al, 2000
oil, olive	119	1	3	Souci et al, 2000
oil, palm	28	4	7	Souci et al, 2000
oil, palm kernel, refined	53	10	8	Souci et al, 2000
oil, peanut	162	26	29	Souci et al, 2000
oil, poppyseed	173	16	58	Souci et al, 2000
oil, pumpkinseed	6.8	20	19	Souci et al, 2000
oil, canola (rapeseed)	129	3.9	95	Souci et al, 2000
oil, safflower	180	30	46	Souci et al, 2000
oil, sesame seed	430	60	164	Souci et al, 2000
oil, soybean	194	71	65	Souci et al, 2000
oil, sunflower	210	35	32	Souci et al, 2000
oil, walnut	154		9	Souci et al, 2000
oil, wheat germ	1606	19	611	Souci et al, 2000
sheabutter		18		Souci et al, 2000
spread, fat-free, bottle	9	3	1	04632
spread, fat-free, tub	2	1	1	04631
spread, soy, 70% fat	81	25	31	04629
FRUITS				
apple, raw	11		1	Souci et al, 2000
apricot, raw	16		1	Souci et al, 2000
banana, raw	11	3	2	Souci et al, 2000
cantaloupe, raw	8			Souci et al, 2000
cherries, sweet, raw	12			Souci et al, 2000
fig, raw	27	31	1	Souci et al, 2000
grapefruit, raw	13	2	2	Souci et al, 2000
grapes, raw	3			Souci et al, 2000
lemon, raw	8	1	2	Souci et al, 2000
orange, raw	17	2	4	Souci et al, 2000
peach, raw	6	3	1	Souci et al, 2000
pear, raw	7			Souci et al, 2000
pineapple, raw	4		1	Souci et al, 2000
plum, raw	6			Souci et al, 2000
pomegranate, raw	16		tr	Souci et al, 2000
strawberries, raw	10	tr	tr	Souci et al, 2000
watermelon, raw	1			Souci et al, 2000
GRAINS & GRAIN FRACTIONS				
amaranth		2		Souci et al, 2000
buckwheat	164	8	20	Souci et al, 2000
buckwheat flour	16	1	4	Souci et al, 2000
corn, whole grain	120	21	32	Souci et al, 2000
wheat, whole grain	40		27	Souci et al, 2000
NUTS				
almonds, dry roasted	110	4	3	12063
almonds, oil roasted	118	3	9	12065
cashews	130	tr	13	Souci et al, 2000
chestnuts, sweet	18	2	2	Souci et al, 2000
coconut	27	7	3	Souci et al, 2000
filberts (hazelnuts), dried	89	1	6	12120
filberts (hazelnuts), dry roasted	103	1	6	12122
macadamia nuts, dry roasted	107		7	12132
macadamia nuts, raw	108		8	12131
peanuts	142	23	24	Souci et al, 2000
pecans	89	3	5	12142
pecans, dry roasted	78	2	4	12143

	BETA-SITOSTEROL (mg/100 g)	STIGMASTEROL (mg/100 g)	CAMPESTEROL (mg/100 g)	USDA CODE/ SOURCE
pecans, oil roasted	96	5	7	12144
pistachios	90	2	6	Souci et al, 2000
pistachios, dried	198	5	10	12151
pistachios, dry roasted	199	4	10	12152
sunflower seeds, dry	95	15	14	Souci et al, 2000
walnuts	87		6	Souci et al, 2000
walnuts, black, dried	103		5	12154
walnuts, english/persian, dried	64	1	7	12155
VEGETABLES				
asparagus, raw	14	4	1	Souci et al, 2000
brussels sprouts, raw	17		6	Souci et al, 2000
carrot, raw	7	3	1	Souci et al, 2000
cauliflower, raw	12	2	3	Souci et al, 2000
coriander (cilantro), leaf, fresh	2	3		11165
cucumber, raw	14			Souci et al, 2000
eggplant (aubergine), raw	3	2		Souci et al, 2000
grape leaves, raw	20	2		11974
lemon grass (citronella), raw	4	1	1	11972
lettuce, raw	5	4	1	Souci et al, 2000
okra, raw	15	6	3	Souci et al, 2000
onion, raw	12		1	Souci et al, 2000
peas, green, raw	106	10	10	Souci et al, 2000
peppers, banana, raw	2		1	11976
peppers, serrano, raw	3		2	11977
potato, raw	3	1		Souci et al, 2000
pumpkin, raw	12			Souci et al, 2000
radish, raw	6		5	Souci et al, 2000
tomato, raw	3	4	1	Souci et al, 2000

Sources:

Souci SW, W Fachmann, H Kraut. *Food Composition and Nutrition Tables.* Medpharm GmbH Scientific Publishers, Stuttgart, Germany & CRC Press, Washington DC. 2000.

USDA Codes: *United States Department of Agriculture Database for Standard Reference, Release 15* (SR15), 2002. Available at http://www.nal.usda.gov/fnic/foodcomp/ Data.SR15/sr15.html.

Purines

Purine values are the sum of adenine, guanine, xanthine, and hypoxanthine. Purines are normally formed in the body during the metabolism of nucleoproteins. In certain genetic disorders, including gout, uric acid (a metabolite of purines) tends to accumulate and deposit in the toes and in other joints. Drug treatment is generally prescribed for patients with gout; however, dietary restriction of purine-yielding foods may also be advised. Foods that are lowest in purines (0–50 mg/100 g) include fruits, fruit juices, and most vegetables (with a few exceptions); non-whole grain breads, cereals, and other grain products; nuts; milk and cheeses; eggs; beverages (coffee, tea, sodas); fats; and sugars, syrups, and sweets. Foods that are highest in purines (150–825 mg/100 g) include anchovies, brains, beef kidney, game meats, gravies, herring; calf/beef liver, mackerel, meat extracts, sardines, scallops, and sweetbreads. Other foods that are high in purines (50–150 mg/100 g) include several vegetables (asparagus, cauliflower, mushrooms, green peas, spinach); legumes (beans, lentils, peas); whole grain breads and cereals, oatmeal, wheat germ and bran; fresh and saltwater fish, shellfish (crab, lobster, oysters); and meats (beef, lamb, pork, veal), meat soups/broths, and poultry (chicken, duck, turkey).

	PURINES (mg/100 g)	SOURCE[1]		PURINES (mg/100 g)	SOURCE[1]
BEVERAGES			**FISH & SHELLFISH**		
beer, light	14	Souci et al, 2000	anchovies, cnd	321	Clifford and Story, 1976
beer, no alcohol	8	Souci et al, 2000	anchovies, raw	411	Clifford and Story, 1976
beer, pilsener (german)	13	Souci et al, 2000	carp	160	Souci et al, 2000
			caviar	144	Souci et al, 2000
CHEESE & YOGURT			caviar substitute	18	Souci et al, 2000
cheese, brie	7	Souci et al, 2000	clams, cnd	62	Clifford and Story, 1976
cheese, camembert	4	Souci et al, 2000	clams, raw	136	Clifford and Story, 1976
cheese, cheddar	7	Souci et al, 2000	coalfish (saithe)	163	Souci et al, 2000
cheese, cottage	8	Brule et al, 1988	cod	109	Souci et al, 2000
cheese, edam/brie	6	Brule et al, 1988	crayfish	60	Souci et al, 2000
cheese, limburger	32	Souci et al, 2000	eel	139	Souci et al, 2000
cheese, processed	2	Brule et al, 1988	eel, smoked	78	Souci et al, 2000
yogurt, plain	7	Brule et al, 1988	fish, cnd	206	Brule et al, 1988

	PURINES (mg/100 g)	SOURCE[1]
haddock, boiled	95	Brule et al, 1989
haddock, boiled, juice only	23	Brule et al, 1989
haddock, broiled	119/193	Brule et al, 1989, 1992
haddock, raw	102	Brule et al, 1989
halibut, cod, & haddock	125	Brule et al, 1988
herring, cnd	378	Clifford and Story, 1976
herring roe	190	Souci et al, 2000
lobster	118	Souci et al, 2000
mackerel, cnd	246	Clifford and Story, 1976
mackerel, raw	194	Clifford and Story, 1976
mussels	112	Souci et al, 2000
ocean perch (redfish)	241	Souci et al, 2000
oysters, cnd	107	Clifford and Story, 1976
pike	140	Souci et al, 2000
pike perch	110	Souci et al, 2000
plaice	93	Souci et al, 2000
salmon, cnd	88	Clifford and Story, 1976
salmon, raw	250	Clifford and Story, 1976
sardines, cnd	399	Clifford and Story, 1976
sardines, raw	345	Clifford and Story, 1976
scallops	136	Souci et al, 2000
shellfish, unspecified	72	Brule et al, 1988
shrimp, cnd	234	Clifford and Story, 1976
sole	131	Souci et al, 2000
sprat, smoked	840	Souci et al, 2000
squid, raw	135	Clifford and Story, 1976
tench (*Tinca tinca* L)	80	Souci et al, 2000
trout	297	Souci et al, 2000
tuna, cnd	142	Clifford and Story, 1976
whitefish, frzn	129	Brule et al, 1988
whitefish, raw	116	Brule et al, 1988

FRUITS

apple, raw	14	Souci et al, 2000
apricot, dried	73	Souci et al, 2000
avocado, raw	19	Souci et al, 2000
banana, raw	57	Souci et al, 2000
bilberries (huckleberries), raw	22	Souci et al, 2000
cantaloupe, raw	33	Souci et al, 2000
cherries, morello, raw	17	Souci et al, 2000
cherries, sweet, raw	17	Souci et al, 2000
currants, red, raw	17	Souci et al, 2000
date, dried	35	Souci et al, 2000
elderberries, raw	33	Souci et al, 2000
fig, dried	64	Souci et al, 2000
gooseberries, raw	16	Souci et al, 2000
grapes, raw	27	Souci et al, 2000
kiwifruit, raw	19	Souci et al, 2000
orange, raw	19	Souci et al, 2000
peach, raw	21	Souci et al, 2000
pear, raw	12	Souci et al, 2000
pineapple, raw	19	Souci et al, 2000
plum, dried	64	Souci et al, 2000
plum, raw	24	Souci et al, 2000
raisins	107	Souci et al, 2000
raspberries, raw	18	Souci et al, 2000
quince, raw	30	Souci et al, 2000
strawberries, raw	21	Souci et al, 2000

GRAINS & GRAIN FRACTIONS

barley, whole grain w/o husk	94	Souci et al, 2000
millet, shucked grain	62	Souci et al, 2000
oats, whole grain w/o husk	94	Souci et al, 2000
rice, white, ckd	6	Brule et al, 1988
rye, whole grain	51	Souci et al, 2000
wheat flour	12	Brule et al, 1988
wheat, whole grain	51	Souci et al, 2000

	PURINES (mg/100 g)	SOURCE[1]
GRAIN PRODUCTS		
bread, crusty	16	Brule et al, 1988
bread, white	12	Brule et al, 1988
corn cereal	1	Brule et al, 1988
crispbread	60	Souci et al, 2000
pasta w/egg, dry	40	Souci et al, 2000
rolls	21	Souci et al, 2000
waffles/pancakes	4	Brule et al, 1988
MEATS		
beef brisket	90	Souci et al, 2000
beef chuck	120	Souci et al, 2000
beef fillet	110	Souci et al, 2000
beef forerib	120	Souci et al, 2000
beef, ground	90	Brule et al, 1988
beef, roast	125	Brule et al, 1988
beef, roast & stew	109	Brule et al, 1988
beef rump	120	Souci et al, 2000
beef roast (sirloin)	110	Souci et al, 2000
beef shoulder	110	Souci et al, 2000
beef sirloin	125	Brule et al, 1988
beef steak, boiled	108	Brule et al, 1989
beef steak, boiled, juice only	59	Brule et al, 1989
beef steak, broiled	121	Brule et al, 1989
beef steak, raw	106	Brule et al, 1989
lamb roast & chops	128	Brule et al, 1988
pork, cured	86	Brule et al, 1988
pork chop	145	Souci et al, 2000
pork chuck	140	Souci et al, 2000
pork fillet	150	Souci et al, 2000
pork hip bone (hind leg)	120	Souci et al, 2000
pork leg (hind leg)	160	Souci et al, 2000
pork roast/chops	120	Brule et al, 1988
pork sausage	101	Souci et al, 2000
pork shoulder	150	Souci et al, 2000
veal chop, cutlet	140	Souci et al, 2000
veal cutlet	143	Brule et al, 1988
veal knuckle	150	Souci et al, 2000
veal leg	150	Souci et al, 2000
veal neck	150	Souci et al, 2000
veal sausage	91	Souci et al, 2000
veal shoulder	140	Souci et al, 2000
MEATS—GAME		
hare	105	Souci et al, 2000
horse	200	Souci et al, 2000
rabbit	132	Souci et al, 2000
venison, back	105	Souci et al, 2000
venison, leg	138	Souci et al, 2000
MEATS—INTERNAL ORGANS & VARIETY MEATS		
belly, pork	100	Souci et al, 2000
belly, pork, raw, smoked dried	127	Souci et al, 2000
brains, beef	162	Clifford and Story, 1976
brains, calf	92	Souci et al, 2000
brains, ox	75	Souci et al, 2000
brains, pork	83	Souci et al, 2000
heart, beef	171	Clifford and Story, 1976
heart, lamb	171	Clifford and Story, 1976
heart, ox	256	Souci et al, 2000
heart, pork	530	Souci et al, 2000
heart, sheep	241	Souci et al, 2000
kidney, beef	213	Clifford and Story, 1976
kidney, calf	218	Souci et al, 2000
kidney, ox	269	Souci et al, 2000
kidney, pork	334	Souci et al, 2000
kidney, unspecified	231	Brule et al, 1988

	PURINES (mg/100 g)	SOURCE[1]		PURINES (mg/100 g)	SOURCE[1]
liver, beef, boiled	237	Brule et al, 1989	chicken, stewer, thigh, raw	144	Young, 1983
liver, beef, boiled, juice only	49	Brule et al, 1989	chicken, stewer, thigh, stewed	146	Young, 1983
liver, beef, broiled	236/184	Brule et al, 1989, 1992	duck	138	Souci et al, 2000
liver, beef, raw	202	Brule et al, 1989	goose	165	Souci et al, 2000
liver, calf	460	Souci et al, 2000	poultry, unspecified	131	Brule et al, 1988
liver, lamb	147	Clifford and Story, 1976	turkey w/skin	150	Souci et al, 2000
liver, ox	554	Souci et al, 2000			
liver, pork	289	Clifford and Story 1976	**VEGETABLES**		
liver, unspecified	286	Brule et al, 1988	artichoke, raw	78	Souci et al, 2000
lung, calf	147	Souci et al, 2000	asparagus, raw	23	Souci et al, 2000
lung, ox	399	Souci et al, 2000	bamboo shoots, raw	29	Souci et al, 2000
lung, pork	434	Souci et al, 2000	beet, raw	19	Souci et al, 2000
spleen, calf	343	Souci et al, 2000	broccoli, raw	81	Souci et al, 2000
spleen, ox	444	Souci et al, 2000	brussels sprouts, raw	69	Souci et al, 2000
spleen, pork	516	Souci et al, 2000	cabbage, chinese, raw	21	Souci et al, 2000
spleen, sheep	773	Souci et al, 2000	cabbage, red, raw	32	Souci et al, 2000
sweetbread (neck), calf	1260	Souci et al, 2000	cabbage, savoy, raw	37	Souci et al, 2000
tongue, ox	160	Souci et al, 2000	cabbage, white, raw	22	Souci et al, 2000
tongue, pork	136	Souci et al, 2000	carrot, raw	17	Souci et al, 2000
			cauliflower, raw	51	Souci el at, 2000
MEATS—LUNCHEON			celeriac, raw	30	Souci et al, 2000
bierschinken sausage	85	Souci et al, 2000	chicory, raw	12	Souci et al, 2000
black pudding (blutwurst)	55	Souci et al, 2000	chives, raw	67	Souci et al, 2000
cold cuts	70	Brule et al, 1988	corn, raw	52	Souci et al, 2000
corned beef	57	Souci et al, 2000	cress, raw	28	Souci et al, 2000
fleischwurst (sausage)	78	Souci et al, 2000	cucumber, raw	7.3	Souci et al, 2000
frankfurter	89	Souci et al, 2000	eggplant (aubergine), raw	21	Souci et al, 2000
jagdwurst (sausage)	112	Souci et al, 2000	endive, raw	17	Souci et al, 2000
liverwurst (liver sausage)	165	Souci et al, 2000	fennel leaves, raw	14	Souci et al, 2000
luncheon meat	58	Brule et al, 1988	kale, raw	48	Souci et al, 2000
ham, cooked	131	Souci et al, 2000	kohlrabi, raw	25	Souci et al, 2000
mettwurst (sausage)	74	Souci et al, 2000	lamb's lettuce (*Valerianella olitoria* L.), raw	38	Souci et al, 2000
mortadella	96	Souci et al, 2000			
munich weibwurst (sausage)	73	Souci et al, 2000	leek, raw	74	Souci et al, 2000
salami	104	Souci et al, 2000	lettuce, raw	13	Souci et al, 2000
vienna sausage	78	Souci et al, 2000	mushroom (*Agaricus bisporus*), raw	58	Souci et al, 2000
			mushrooms, boletus, dried	488	Souci et al, 2000
NUTS & SEEDS			mushrooms, boletus, raw	92	Souci et al, 2000
almonds	37	Souci et al, 2000	mushrooms, chanterelle, cnd	6	Souci et al, 2000
brazil nuts	23	Souci et al, 2000	mushrooms, chanterelle, raw	17	Souci et al, 2000
hazelnuts	37	Souci et al, 2000	mushrooms, cnd	25	Brule et al, 1988
peanuts	79	Souci et al, 2000	mushrooms, morel, raw	30	Souci et al, 2000
walnuts	25	Souci et al, 2000	mushrooms, oyster, raw	50	Souci et al, 2000
poppy seeds, dry	170	Souci et al, 2000	mushrooms, raw	47	Brule et al, 1988
sesame seeds, dry	62	Souci et al, 2000	onion, raw	13	Souci et al, 2000
sunflower seeds, dry	143	Souci et al, 2000	parsley, raw	57	Souci et al, 2000
			peppers, green, raw	55	Souci et al, 2000
POULTRY			potato, raw	16	Souci et al, 2000
chicken, broiler, breast	131	Young, 1980	potato, ckd w/skin	18	Souci et al, 2000
chicken, broiler, breast, raw	168	Young, 1982	pumpkin, raw	44	Souci et al, 2000
chicken, broiler, breast, roasted	179	Young, 1982	radishes, small (*radicula Pers*), raw	13	Souci et al, 2000
chicken, broiler, drumstick	132	Young, 1980	radish (*niger kerner*), raw	15	Souci et al, 2000
chicken, broiler, gizzard	131	Young, 1980	rhubarb, raw	12	Souci et al, 2000
chicken, broiler, liver	236	Young, 1980	salsify, black (viper's grass), raw	71	Souci et al, 2000
chicken, broiler, neck & back, mech deboned	94	Young, 1980	sauerkraut, raw	16	Souci et al, 2000
			soybean sprouts, raw	80	Souci et al, 2000
chicken, broiler, neck, mech deboned	123	Young, 1980	spinach, raw	57	Souci et al, 2000
chicken, broiler, skin	105	Young, 1980	tomato, raw	11	Souci et al, 2000
chicken, broiler, thigh	127	Young, 1980	zucchini, raw	24	Souci et al, 2000
chicken, broiler, thigh, raw	152	Young, 1982			
chicken, broiler, thigh, roasted	149	Young, 1982	**VEGETABLES—LEGUMES**		
chicken heart	223	Clifford and Story, 1976	chickpeas, dry	56	Clifford and Story, 1976
chicken liver	243	Clifford and Story, 1976	cowpeas, dry	230	Clifford and Story, 1976
chicken, roaster	115	Souci et al, 2000	cranberry beans, dry	75	Clifford and Story, 1976
chicken, stewer, breast, raw	178	Young, 1983	french beans	37	Souci et al, 2000
chicken, stewer, breast, stewed	184	Young, 1983	french beans, dry	45	Souci et al, 2000
chicken, stewer, skin, raw	59	Young, 1983	great northern beans, dry	213	Clifford and Story, 1976
chicken, stewer, skin, stewed	94	Young, 1983	green peas	84	Souci et al, 2000

	PURINES (mg/100 g)	SOURCE[1]		PURINES (mg/100 g)	SOURCE[1]
lentils, dry	222	Clifford and Story, 1976	tofu	68	Souci et al, 2000
lima beans, baby, dry	144	Clifford and Story, 1976	white beans, small, dry	202	Clifford and Story, 1976
lima beans, large, dry	149	Clifford and Story, 1976			
linseed	105	Souci et al, 2000	**MISCELLANEOUS**		
mungo (black gram) beans, dry	222	Souci et al, 2000	cocoa powder	71	Souci et al, 2000
peas, split, dry	195	Clifford and Story, 1976	olives, green, marinated	29	Souci et al, 2000
pinto beans, dry	171	Clifford and Story, 1976	soup w/meat	12	Brule et al, 1988
red beans, dry	162	Clifford and Story, 1976	yeast, bakers, compressed	680	Souci et al, 2000
soybeans, boiled	185	Brule et al, 1992	yeast, brewers, dried	1810	Souci et al, 2000

[1] Values from the sources have been rounded to the nearest whole number. Values from Souci et al, 2000 were provided and expressed here as milligrams of uric acid per 100 grams.

Sources:
Brule D, G Sarwar, L Savoie. Changes in serum and urinary uric acid levels in normal human subjects fed purine-rich foods containing different amounts of adenine and hypoxanthine. *J Am Coll Nutr* 11:353–358, 1992.
Brule D, G Sarwar, L Savoie. Effect of methods of cooking on free and total purine bases in meat and fish. *J Inst Can Sci Technol Aliment* 22:248–251, 1989.
Brule D, G Sarwar, L Savoie. Purine content of selected Canadian food products. *J Food Comp Anal* 1:130–138, 1988.
Clifford AJ, DL Story. Levels of purines in foods and their metabolic effects in rats. *J Nutr* 106:435–442, 1976.
Souci SW, W Fachmann, H Kraut, *Food Composition and Nutrition Tables.* Medpharm GmbH Scientific Publishers, Stuttgart, Germany & CRC Press, Washington DC. 2000.
Young LL. Effect of stewing on purine content of broiler tissues. *J Fd Sci* 48:315–316, 1983.
Young LL. Evaluation of four purine compounds in poultry product. *J Fd Sci* 45:1064–1–67, 1980.
Young LL. Purine content of raw and roasted chicken broiler meat. *J Fd Sci* 47:1374–1375, 1982.

Sugar Alcohols—Mannitol & Sorbitol

	MANNITOL (g/100 g)	SORBITOL (g/100 g)		MANNITOL (g/100 g)	SORBITOL (g/100 g)
BEVERAGES			peach, cnd, jce pack	—	*
beer	—	0.0	peach, dried	—	*
beer, light	—	0.0	peach, raw	—	0.2
			pear, raw	—	2.3
FRUITS & FRUIT JUICES			plum, raw	—	0.6
apple jce, cnd, unsweetened	—	1.0	prune, dried	—	12.0
apple, raw	—	0.3			
apricot, raw	—	0.8	**VEGETABLES**		
cherries, sour, raw	—	1.0	carrot, raw	0.2	—
cherries, sweet, raw	—	2.1	celery, raw	0.1	—
grapes, am, raw	—	0.1	cucumber, raw	0.1	—
nectarine, raw	—	0.6	onion, raw	0.1	—
peach, cnd, jce pack	—	*	radish, red, raw	0.1	—

[1] An asterisk indicates the lack of data for a sugar alcohol known to be present; a dash indicates the lack of data for a sugar that may be present.

Source:
Matthews PH, PR Pehrsson, M Farhat-Sabet. *Sugars Content of Selected Foods: Individual and Total Sugars,* Home Economics Research Report Number 48. September 1987.

Sugars—Galactose, Glucose, Fructose, Lactose, Sucrose, Maltose, & Total Sugars (1987 file)[1]

	SERVING SIZE (WEIGHT)	GAL (g)	GLU (g)	FRU (g)	LAC (g)	SUC (g)	MAL (g)	TOTAL SUGARS (g)
BEVERAGES								
beer	12 fl oz (356 g)	0.0	0.4	0.7	0.0	*	0.4	*
beer cooler	12 fl oz (367 g)	0.0	11.0	14.3	0.0	0.0	—	[25.3]
beer, light	12 fl oz (354 g)	0.0	2.1	*	0.0	*	0.4	*
brandy, cherry	1 1/2 fl oz (42 g)	0.0	6.9	6.8	0.0	0.0	—	13.7
carbonated, all flavors, diet	12 fl oz (355 g)	0.0	0.0	0.0	0.0	0.0	—	0.0
carbonated, cola	12 fl oz (370 g)	0.0	14.8	16.3	0.0	7.8	0.4	39.2
carbonated, ginger ale	12 fl oz (366 g)	0.0	11.3	13.5	0.0	7.0	—	[31.8]
carbonated, lemon-lime	12 fl oz (368 g)	0.0	15.1	22.4	0.0	*	—	[37.5]
carbonated, pepper type	12 fl oz (368 g)	0.0	19.5	16.2	0.0	0.7	—	36.4
carbonated, root beer	12 fl oz (370 g)	0.0	11.8	11.8	0.0	20.7	—	44.0
cappuccino, from dry mix	8 fl oz (256 g)	—	0.3	—	—	9.2	0.0	[9.5]
cherry drink, cnd	8 fl oz (251 g)	0.0	13.1	10.3	0.0	2.0	1.3	26.9
coffee w/mocha, from dry mix	8 fl oz (251 g)	—	0.3	—	0.3	5.8	0.3	[6.5]
citrus drink, from frzn conc	8 fl oz (248 g)	0.0	*	*	0.0	*	—	26.3
lemonade, from frzn conc	8 fl oz (248 g)	0.0	11.4	8.7	0.0	2.7	—	[22.8]
lemonade, from dry mix	8 fl oz (264 g)	0.0	0.0	0.0	0.0	14.5	—	[14.5]
lemonade, from dry mix w/aspartame	8 fl oz (238 g)	0.0	0.0	0.0	0.0	0.0	—	[0.0]
liqueur, coffee	1 1/2 fl oz (52 g)	0.0	1.9	1.9	0.0	15.5	0.9	[20.3]
liqueur, coffee w/cream	1 1/2 fl oz (47 g)	*	*	*	*	8.1	*	*
liqueur, orange	1 1/2 fl oz (50 g)	0.0	0.6	0.0	0.0	13.6	—	[14.2]
orange drink, cnd	8 fl oz (248 g)	0.0	0.0	0.0	0.0	17.9	0.0	17.9
punch, cnd	8 fl oz (248 g)	0.0	8.4	9.2	0.0	9.2	0.0	28.0
punch, from dry mix	8 fl oz (262 g)	0.0	10.7	11.0	0.0	8.9	—	30.4
punch, from frzn conc	8 fl oz (247 g)	0.0	7.2	5.4	0.0	12.6	—	[25.2]
rum	1 1/2 fl oz (42 g)	0.0	—	0.0	0.0	—	—	0.0
sherry, med, dry	2 fl oz (59 g)	0.0	1.1	1.1	0.0	0.0	—	2.1
tea, black, brewed	8 fl oz (240 g)	0.0	0.0	0.0	0.0	0.0	—	0.0
tea, herbal, brewed	8 fl oz (240 g)	0.0	—	—	0.0	—	—	0.0
thirst-quencher beverage, cnd	8 fl oz (241 g)	0.0	5.8	5.1	0.0	3.4	—	14.2
vermouth, dry	1 fl oz (28 g)	0.0	0.5	0.6	0.0	0.4	—	1.5
vermouth, sweet	1 fl oz (30 g)	0.0	1.8	1.8	0.0	1.1	—	4.8
vodka	1 1/2 fl oz (42 g)	0.0	—	—	0.0	—	—	0.0
whiskey sour mix, dry	.56 oz pkt (17 g)	0.0	0.2	0.0	0.0	12.1	0.0	[12.3]
whiskey sour mix, liquid	1 fl oz (32 g)	0.0	2.5	2.6	0.0	1.2	0.7	[7.1]
wine cooler	12 fl oz (355 g)	0.0	13.1	12.8	0.0	9.6	—	[35.5]
wine, red	3 1/2 fl oz (103 g)	0.0	0.1	*	0.0	—	—	*
wine, rose	3 1/2 fl oz (103 g)	0.0	0.8	1.8	0.0	0.0	—	2.6
wine, white	3 1/2 fl oz (103 g)	0.0	0.4	0.3	0.0	0.0	—	0.6
wine w/o alcohol	3 1/2 fl oz (104 g)	0.0	1.9	2.0	0.0	0.0	—	[3.9]
CANDY								
cashew & honey bar	1 oz (28 g)	—	1.8	1.1	0.5	0.4	1.6	[5.4]
chewing gum	1 piece (3 g)	0.0	—	—	—	2.1	0.0	[2.1]
chewing gum, sugarless	1 piece (3 g)	0.0	0.0	0.0	0.0	0.0	0.0	[0.0]
choc-covered caramel & rice cereal	1 oz (28 g)	—	*	*	*	*	*	14.7
choc-covered caramel log	1 oz (28 g)	—	*	*	*	4.8	*	*
choc-covered coconut center & almonds	1 oz (28 g)	—	*	*	*	5.7	*	*
choc-covered crunchy peanut butter	1 oz (28 g)	—	*	*	*	8.4	*	*
choc-covered crunchy peanut butter & almonds	1 oz (28 g)	—	*	*	*	10.1	*	*
choc-covered fondant/discs	1 oz (28 g)	—	*	*	*	12.8	*	*
choc-covered fudge, peanuts, & caramel	1 oz (28 g)	—	*	*	*	6.7	*	*
choc-covered malt nougat & caramel	1 oz (28 g)	—	*	*	*	8.0	*	*
choc-covered malted milk balls	1 oz (28 g)	—	*	*	*	4.1	*	*
choc-covered mint	1 1/2" patty (28 g)	—	*	*	*	22.6	*	*
choc-covered nougat	1 oz (28 g)	*	2.0	0.2	1.0	10.8	2.0	[17.4]
choc-covered nougat & caramel	1 oz (28 g)	—	*	*	*	7.6	*	*
choc-covered nougat, caramel, & almonds	1 oz (28 g)	—	*	*	*	10.3	*	*
choc-covered peanut butter nougat, caramel, & peanuts	1 oz (28 g)	—	1.8	0.1	1.2	7.8	1.8	[12.8]
choc-covered peanuts	1 oz (28 g)	*	*	*	0.3	9.7	—	*
choc-covered wafer cookie bar	1 oz (28 g)	*	*	*	1.4	11.0	—	12.4

	SERVING SIZE (WEIGHT)	GAL (g)	GLU (g)	FRU (g)	LAC (g)	SUC (g)	MAL (g)	TOTAL SUGARS (g)
coconut bar	1 oz (28 g)	—	3.0	0.9	0.0	7.5	0.9	[12.3]
dark choc, semi-sweet	1 oz (28 g)	—	1.3	*	0.0	14.0	0.0	[15.4]
dark choc, sweet	1 oz (28 g)	—	0.0	0.0	0.0	13.7	0.0	[13.7]
fruit & honey bar	1 oz (28 g)	—	2.9	2.2	0.0	1.4	0.7	[7.1]
hard candy	1 oz (28 g)	0.0	*	*	0.0	18.9	—	[18.9]
jelly beans	1 oz (28 g)	0.0	*	*	0.0	16.7	—	*
jelly mints	1 oz (28 g)	0.0	*	*	0.0	16.4	—	*
licorice	1 oz (28 g)	0.0	*	*	0.0	5.5	—	*
milk choc	1 oz (28 g)	0.0	0.1	0.0	2.1	13.3	0.0	14.6
milk choc w/almonds	1 oz (28 g)	*	0.1	0.1	1.7	10.8	0.0	13.8
milk choc w/crisped rice	1 oz (28 g)	*	0.1	0.1	1.8	12.2	—	[14.2]
milk choc w/peanuts	1 oz (28 g)	*	*	*	*	14.9	—	*
nut bar (peanuts, caramel, van fudge)	1 oz (28 g)	—	*	*	—	9.4	—	*
praline, chewy	1 oz (28 g)	—	*	*	—	7.4	—	*
sugar-coated choc & peanut discs	1 oz (28 g)	*	*	*	1.2	12.2	—	[13.4]
sugar-coated choc discs	1 oz (28 g)	*	*	*	1.0	14.6	—	[16.4]
sunflower & honey bar	1 oz (28 g)	—	1.7	1.2	0.4	0.4	2.0	[5.8]
sunflower candy bar	1 oz (28 g)	—	0.1	0.7	0.0	4.1	0.6	[5.5]
taffy, fruit-flavored	1 oz (28 g)	—	3.3	1.0	—	10.6	2.0	18.7
toffee	1 oz (28 g)	—	1.9	1.5	0.7	11.6	—	*
CEREALS & GRAINS, CKD								
amaranth, whole grain, ckd	1 cup (246 g)	0.0	0.2	—	0.0	0.2	*	[0.5]
buckwheat groats, ckd	1 cup (240 g)	0.0	0.5	0.2	0.0	1.0	—	[2.2]
farina, quick/inst, ckd	1 cup (240 g)	0.0	*	*	0.0	0.2	*	*
farina, reg, ckd	1 cup (242 g)	0.0	*	*	0.0	0.0	*	*
millet, proso, ckd	1 cup (240 g)	0.0	*	*	0.0	0.2	*	[0.7]
oatmeal, maple flavor, ckd	1 cup (240 g)	0.0	—	—	0.0	7.2	*	[7.2]
oatmeal, reg/quick, ckd	1 cup (239 g)	0.0	0.0	—	0.0	1.0	*	[1.0]
rice, brown, ckd	1 cup (164 g)	0.0	0.0	*	0.0	0.3	*	0.5
rice, white, ckd	1 cup (152 g)	0.0	0.0	*	0.0	0.2	0.0	[0.3]
rice, white, parboiled, ckd	1 cup (175 g)	0.0	*	*	0.0	0.5	*	*
whole wheat, ckd	1 cup (242 g)	0.0	—	0.0	0.0	0.7	*	[1.0]
wild rice, ckd	1 cup (161 g)	0.0	0.3	0.3	0.0	0.5	*	[1.1]
CEREALS, READY-TO-EAT								
bran flakes	2/3 cup (28 g)	0.0	0.3	0.3	0.0	2.6	0.3	3.4
bran flakes w/raisins	3/4 cup (39 g)	0.0	2.8	3.2	0.0	3.9	0.0	10.4
corn flakes	1 1/8 cups (28 g)	0.0	0.4	0.7	0.0	0.7	0.1	1.9
corn flakes, sugar coated	3/4 cup (28 g)	0.0	0.3	0.3	0.0	10.7	0.0	11.2
granola w/raisins	1/4 cup (28 g)	0.0	1.3	1.3	0.3	4.8	0.0	7.8
oat rings	1 1/4 cups (28 g)	0.0	0.0	0.1	0.0	0.8	0.0	0.8
rice, crispy	1 cup (28 g)	0.0	0.2	0.1	0.0	2.2	0.0	2.5
rice, crispy, sugar coated	3/4 cup (28 g)	0.0	0.2	0.2	0.0	10.7	0.0	11.1
rice, puffed	1 cup (14 g)	0.0	0.0	0.0	0.0	0.0	0.0	0.0
wheat & malted barley flakes	7/8 cup (28 g)	0.0	0.3	0.1	0.0	1.8	1.3	3.5
wheat & malted barley nuggets	1/4 cup (28 g)	0.0	0.2	0.9	0.0	0.0	1.5	2.6
wheat flakes	1 cup (28 g)	0.0	0.2	0.2	0.0	2.3	0.0	[2.8]
wheat, puffed	1 cup (14 g)	0.0	0.0	0.1	0.0	0.1	0.0	0.2
wheat, puffed, sugar coated	7/8 cup (28 g)	0.0	1.0	0.4	0.0	10.8	0.5	12.7
wheat puffed, sugar & honey coated	3/4 cup (28 g)	0.0	3.4	0.3	0.0	12.6	0.0	16.3
wheat, shredded	2/3 cup (28 g)	0.0	0.0	0.0	0.0	0.1	0.0	0.1
wheat, shredded, frosted	4 biscuits (28 g)	0.0	0.0	0.0	0.0	7.0	0.0	7.0
CHEESE								
cheese, am cheese food	1 oz (28 g)	0.0	0.0	0.0	2.7	0.0	—	[2.7]
cheese, cheddar	1 oz (28 g)	0.2	0.0	0.0	0.2	0.0	—	[0.5]
cheese, cottage, creamed, 4% fat	1 cup (225 g)	—	—	0.0	1.4	0.0	—	[1.4]
cheese, cottage, lowfat, <.5% fat	1 cup (145 g)	—	—	0.0	4.6	0.0	—	[4.6]
cheese, cream	1 oz (28 g)	—	—	0.0	0.5	0.0	—	[0.5]
cheese, mozzarella	1 oz (28 g)	—	—	0.0	0.1	0.0	—	[0.1]
cheese, neufchatel	1 oz (28 g)	—	—	0.0	0.3	0.0	—	[0.3]
cheese, ricotta, nonfat milk	1 cup (246 g)	—	—	0.0	3.4	0.0	—	[3.4]
cheese, ricotta, whole milk	1 cup (246 g)	—	—	0.0	3.7	0.0	—	[3.7]
cheese, swiss	1 oz (28 g)	—	0.1	0.0	*	0.1	—	[0.2]
CREAM								
cream, whipping, unwhipped	1 cup (238 g)	—	—	—	6.7	—	—	[6.7]

	SERVING SIZE (WEIGHT)	GAL (g)	GLU (g)	FRU (g)	LAC (g)	SUC (g)	MAL (g)	TOTAL SUGARS (g)
DESSERTS								
cake, fruit	1/12 cake (113 g)	0.0	12.8	12.8	0.0	23.2	0.0	48.7
cake, sponge w/jam filling	1.2 oz cake (32 g)	0.0	2.6	1.2	0.0	11.4	0.0	15.3
cookie, animal crackers	10 cookies (26 g)	0.0	0.5	0.3	0.0	5.1	0.1	5.9
cookie, choc chip	10 small (44 g)	0.0	0.3	0.1	0.8	9.8	0.0	11.0
cookie, choc wafer	.25 oz wafer (7 g)	0.0	0.0	0.1	*	2.6	0.1	2.8
doughnut, cake type	1.8 oz doughnut (50 g)	0.0	1.6	*	0.9	6.0	*	[8.5]
dessert topping, butterscotch	2 T (38 g)	—	*	—	0.5	*	—	*
dessert topping, choc	2 T (38 g)	—	*	—	1.1	*	—	*
gelatin dessert, from mix, orange	1/2 cup (120 g)	0.0	6.0	*	0.0	9.4	—	[15.4]
gelatin dessert, from mix, raspberry	1/2 cup (120 g)	0.0	6.5	*	0.0	4.0	—	[10.4]
gelatin dessert, from mix, strawberry	1/2 cup (120 g)	0.0	1.0	*	0.0	2.2	—	[3.1]
ice cream, choc	1 cup (133 g)	—	*	*	8.8	*	*	[28.7]
ice cream, coffee	1 cup (133 g)	—	*	*	9.2	*	*	[29.1]
ice cream, strawberry	1 cup (133 g)	—	*	*	4.3	*	*	[24.2]
ice cream, vanilla	1 cup (133 g)	—	*	*	9.8	*	*	[29.8]
ice milk, soft serve in cake cone, fast food	1 cone (115 g)	0.0	1.0	0.1	6.6	11.5	0.8	20.0
ice milk, soft serve in sugar cone, fast food	1 cone (93 g)	0.0	0.9	0.4	4.7	11.2	0.6	17.8
icing, carob	1 oz (28 g)	—	1.4	2.3	0.0	7.0	0.0	10.7
icing, choc	1 cup (310 g)	—	11.5	6.5	16.4	133.3	5.0	172.7
icing, other flavors	1 cup (310 g)	—	4.3	2.2	0.0	210.2	3.7	[220.4]
icing, white choc	1 oz (28 g)	—	*	*	2.8	14.9	*	[17.7]
pie, fried apple snack pie	3 oz pie (85 g)	0.0	1.7	2.0	0.2	5.2	0.7	9.8
pie, fried cherry snack pie	3.1 oz pie (88 g)	0.0	5.1	4.6	0.0	*	0.7	10.4
pie, fruit	1/6 pie (149 g)	0.0	8.5	4.2	0.0	32.1	1.3	46.1
pudding, banana, cnd	5 oz can (142 g)	—	*	*	*	16.6	—	*
pudding, butterscotch, cnd	5 oz can (142 g)	—	*	*	*	21.9	—	*
pudding, choc, cnd	5 oz can (142 g)	—	*	*	*	18.9	—	*
pudding, choc fudge, cnd	5 oz can (142 g)	—	*	*	*	20.3	—	*
pudding, coconut cream, refrig	5 oz (142 g)	—	*	*	*	16.2	—	*
pudding, rice, cnd	5 oz can (142 g)	—	*	*	*	14.6	—	*
pudding, tapioca, cnd	5 oz can (142 g)	—	*	*	*	10.8	—	*
pudding, van, cnd	5 oz can (142 g)	—	*	*	*	20.9	—	*
FAST FOODS								
cheeseburger	4.1 oz sandwich (115 g)	—	2.2	2.3	0.2	0.1	1.2	5.9
cheeseburger, double	6.8 oz sandwich (194 g)	—	1.9	2.1	0.2	0.2	1.2	5.6
eggs, scrambled	3.5 oz serving (98 g)	—	0.5	0.1	0.1	0.1	0.1	[0.9]
english muffin w/egg, cheese, canadian bacon	4.9 oz sandwich (138 g)	—	1.0	0.4	0.1	0.1	1.2	2.8
fish sandwich	4.9 oz sandwich (139 g)	—	1.1	1.8	0.3	0.4	1.0	4.6
hamburger	3.6 oz sandwich (102 g)	—	1.7	1.8	0.2	0.1	0.9	4.7
hamburger, 1/4 lb	4 oz sandwich (114 g)	—	1.9	1.9	0.1	0.1	0.9	4.9
pork sausage, ckd	1.9 oz patty (53 g)	*	0.3	*	*	*	*	[0.4]
shake, choc	10 fl oz (291 g)	—	10.5	4.7	14.0	19.5	2.6	51.2
shake, strawberry	10 fl oz (290 g)	—	10.4	5.2	14.2	19.7	4.4	53.9
shake, van	10 fl oz (291 g)	—	9.3	5.2	14.6	19.8	2.9	51.8
sundae, caramel	5.8 oz sundae (165 g)	—	8.2	1.3	8.9	19.5	3.6	41.2
sundae, hot fudge	5.8 oz sundae (164 g)	—	2.5	0.8	9.3	27.9	0.7	41.7
sundae, strawberry	5.8 oz sundae (164 g)	—	10.2	5.6	7.4	20.5	—	44.6
FLOURS & GRAIN FRACTIONS								
cornstarch	1 T (8 g)	0.0	*	*	0.0	*	*	*
cottonseed flour, defatted	1 cup (94 g)	0.0	—	—	0.0	2.2	—	[2.2]
oat bran, raw	1/3 cup (32 g)	0.0	*	*	0.0	0.6	*	0.8
oat bran, ckd	1 cup (232 g)	0.0	—	*	0.0	0.7	*	[0.9]
oat flour	1 cup (104 g)	0.0	0.1	0.0	0.0	0.5	*	0.8
peanut flour, defatted	1 oz (28 g)	—	0.6	0.0	0.0	2.0	*	*
rice bran	1 cup (83 g)	0.0	0.2	0.2	0.0	0.4	*	[0.8]
rice flour	1 cup (128 g)	0.0	*	*	0.0	1.0	—	[1.3]
rye flour	1 cup (106 g)	0.0	0.5	0.3	0.0	*	2.8	[4.9]
sesame flour, defatted	1 oz (28 g)	0.0	0.7	0.5	0.0	0.0	—	[1.2]
soy flour, dehulled, defatted	1 oz (28 g)	2.1	2.3	*	0.0	2.0	0.0	[7.0]
sunflower flour, partially defatted	1 cup (80 g)	0.0	0.0	—	0.0	1.7	—	[2.2]
wheat bran	1/3 cup (28 g)	0.0	0.3	0.2	0.0	3.8	0.4	4.7
wheat bran, crude	2 T (7 g)	0.0	0.0	0.0	0.0	0.1	0.0	0.3
wheat flour, semolina	1 cup (125 g)	0.0	0.4	*	0.0	1.9	*	[2.3]
wheat flour, white	1 cup (125 g)	0.0	0.8	0.4	0.0	0.5	0.0	2.1

	SERVING SIZE (WEIGHT)	GAL (g)	GLU (g)	FRU (g)	LAC (g)	SUC (g)	MAL (g)	TOTAL SUGARS (g)
wheat flour, whole wheat	1 cup (120 g)	0.0	*	*	0.0	0.4	0.1	2.4
wheat germ, crude	1 T (5 g)	0.0	*	*	0.0	0.4	0.0	[0.6]
wheat germ, toasted	1 T (5 g)	0.0	*	*	0.0	0.4	*	[0.6]
FRUIT JUICES								
apple jce, cnd	8 fl oz (248 g)	0.0	6.2	13.9	0.0	4.2	—	27.0
cranberry jce cocktail, bottled	8 fl oz (253 g)	0.0	*	*	0.0	*	—	34.2
fruit cocktail, cnd, jce pack	1 cup (284 g)	—	17.0	17.0	0.0	9.4	—	[43.4]
grapefruit jce, cnd, unsweetened	8 fl oz (247 g)	0.0	*	*	0.0	*	—	18.5
grapefruit jce, raw	8 fl oz (247 g)	0.0	6.7	4.4	0.0	4.4	—	15.6
grape jce, from frzn conc	8 fl oz (250 g)	—	9.0	11.0	0.0	*	—	35.5
lemon jce, raw	8 fl oz (244 g)	0.0	2.4	2.7	0.0	0.7	—	[5.9]
orange jce, from frzn conc	8 fl oz (249 g)	0.0	13.2	11.5	0.0	1.7	—	[26.4]
orange jce, raw	8 fl oz (248 g)	0.0	6.9	7.4	0.0	10.2	—	25.3
pear jce, raw	8 fl oz (250 g)	0.0	4.0	17.8	0.0	*	—	[21.8]
pineapple jce, cnd, unsweetened	8 fl oz (250 g)	0.0	*	*	0.0	*	—	31.2
prune jce, bottled	8 fl oz (256 g)	0.0	14.1	20.2	0.0	—	—	[34.3]
FRUITS								
apple, raw	3 1/4″ dia (138 g)	0.0	3.2	10.5	0.0	4.6	0.1	[18.4]
applesauce, cnd, sweetened	1 cup (255 g)	0.0	11.0	19.1	0.0	12.0	—	[42.1]
apricot, dried	1 cup (130 g)	0.0	26.4	15.9	0.0	8.3	—	[50.6]
apricot, raw	3 apricots (106 g)	0.0	1.7	0.7	0.0	5.5	1.1	9.9
avocado, CA, raw	6.1 oz avocado (173 g)	0.0	0.9	0.3	0.0	0.2	0.0	[1.6]
banana, raw	4 oz banana (114 g)	0.0	4.8	3.1	0.0	7.4	0.0	17.8
blackberries, raw	1 cup (144 g)	0.0	4.5	5.9	0.0	0.6	0.7	11.4
blueberries, raw	1 cup (145 g)	0.0	5.1	5.2	0.0	0.3	0.0	[10.6]
cantaloupe, raw	1/2 melon (267 g)	0.0	3.2	4.8	0.0	14.4	0.0	[23.2]
carambola (star fruit), raw	4.5 oz carambola (127 g)	0.0	3.9	4.1	0.0	1.0	—	[9.0]
cherries, sour, raw	10 cherries (68 g)	0.0	2.9	2.2	0.0	0.3	0.0	[5.5]
cherries, sweet, raw	10 cherries (68 g)	0.0	5.5	4.2	0.0	0.1	0.1	[9.9]
currants, raw	1/2 cup (56 g)	0.0	1.8	2.1	0.0	0.6	0.0	[4.5]
dates, dried	10 dates (83 g)	0.0	*	*	0.0	37.0	—	53.3
figs, dried	10 figs (187 g)	7.7	53.5	48.6	0.0	12.2	—	[124.4]
figs, raw	1 med (50 g)	*	1.8	1.4	0.0	0.2	—	[3.4]
grapefruit, raw	1/2 fruit (120 g)	0.0	1.6	1.4	0.0	4.1	—	7.4
grapes, american	10 grapes (24 g)	—	1.6	1.7	0.0	0.3	0.4	[3.9]
grapes, european	10 grapes (50 g)	0.2	3.2	3.8	0.0	0.2	1.6	[9.1]
guava, raw	3.2 oz guava (90 g)	0.0	1.1	1.7	0.0	0.9	*	5.4
jackfruit, raw	2 oz jackfruit (57 g)	0.0	0.8	0.8	0.0	3.1	—	10.5
kiwifruit, raw	2.7 oz kiwifruit (76 g)	0.0	3.8	3.3	0.0	0.8	—	[8.0]
lemon, raw	2 oz lemon (58 g)	0.0	0.6	0.5	0.0	0.3	—	1.4
lime, raw	2.4 oz lime (67 g)	0.0	0.1	0.1	0.0	0.0	0.0	0.3
mango, raw	7.3 oz mango (207 g)	0.0	1.5	6.0	0.0	20.5	0.0	30.6
nectarine, raw	4.8 oz nectarine (136 g)	0.0	1.6	1.5	0.0	8.4	—	[11.6]
orange, raw	2 5/8″ dia (131 g)	0.0	2.9	3.3	0.0	5.5	0.4	11.7
papaya, raw	10.7 oz papaya (304 g)	0.0	4.3	8.2	0.0	5.5	0.0	[17.9]
passion fruit, raw	.63 oz fruit (18 g)	0.0	0.7	0.6	0.0	0.6	—	2.0
peach, cnd, jce pack	1 cup (248 g)	0.0	16.1	14.6	0.0	8.9	3.5	[43.2]
peach, dried	1 cup (160 g)	0.0	25.3	25.0	0.0	21.1	—	[71.4]
peach, raw	3.1 oz peach (87 g)	0.0	1.0	1.1	0.0	4.9	0.6	[7.6]
pear, cnd, heavy syrup pack	1 cup halves (255 g)	0.0	15.6	15.0	0.0	3.6	4.8	38.8
pear, cnd, jce pack	1 cup halves (248 g)	0.0	8.2	14.4	0.0	1.5	—	24.1
pear, cnd, light syrup pack	1 cup halves (251 g)	0.0	12.1	12.9	0.0	2.8	2.8	30.6
pear, cnd, water pack	1 cup halves (244 g)	0.0	4.6	9.5	0.0	0.7	—	14.9
pear, raw	2 1/2″ dia (166 g)	0.0	3.2	10.6	0.0	3.0	0.7	[17.4]
pineapple, cnd, heavy syrup pack	1 cup (255 g)	0.0	19.1	18.4	0.0	5.6	—	[43.1]
pineapple, cnd, jce pack	1 cup (250 g)	0.0	19.2	16.2	0.0	0.0	—	35.5
pineapple, raw, diced	1 cup (155 g)	0.0	4.5	3.3	0.0	4.8	0.0	18.4
plum, common, raw	2.3 oz plum (66 g)	0.0	1.8	1.2	0.0	2.0	0.0	[5.0]
plum, prune, raw	1 cup halves (165 g)	0.0	5.1	5.4	0.0	8.2	0.5	[19.3]
pomegranate, raw	5.4 oz pomegranate (154 g)	0.0	7.7	7.2	0.0	0.6	0.0	13.7
prune, dried	5 prunes (49 g)	0.0	14.1	7.3	0.0	0.2	—	[21.6]
raisins	1 cup (145 g)	0.0	45.2	49.0	0.0	0.0	*	[94.2]
raspberries, raw	1 cup (123 g)	0.0	4.3	3.9	0.0	3.4	—	[11.7]
strawberries, frzn, unsweetened	1 cup (149 g)	0.0	4.5	4.5	0.0	0.7	—	[9.7]
strawberries, raw	1 cup (149 g)	0.0	3.3	3.7	0.0	1.5	0.1	[8.6]

	SERVING SIZE (WEIGHT)	GAL (g)	GLU (g)	FRU (g)	LAC (g)	SUC (g)	MAL (g)	TOTAL SUGARS (g)
tangelo, raw	4.7 oz tangelo (131 g)	0.0	4.8	—	0.0	4.8	—	[9.7]
watermelon, raw	1/16 melon (482 g)	0.0	7.7	15.9	0.0	17.4	2.4	[43.4]

GRAIN PRODUCTS

biscuit, from mix	1 oz biscuit (28 g)	0.0	0.7	*	0.3	0.3	*	[1.3]
bread, white	.88 oz slice (25 g)	0.0	0.4	0.4	*	*	0.1	1.0
bread, white, toasted	.78 oz slice (22 g)	0.0	0.4	0.4	*	*	0.1	1.0
bread, whole wheat	1 oz slice (28 g)	0.0	0.4	0.6	*	*	0.1	1.1
bread whole wheat, toasted	.88 oz slice (25 g)	0.0	0.4	0.6	*	*	0.1	1.1
cracker, rye	.25 oz cracker (7 g)	0.0	*	0.1	0.0	0.1	*	0.2
english muffin, toasted, buttered	2.2 oz muffin (63 g)	0.0	0.6	0.2	0.1	0.0	1.3	2.4
granola bar	.81 oz bar (23 g)	0.0	0.3	0.3	0.0	4.0	*	[4.5]
noodles, chow mein	1 cup (52 g)	0.0	*	0.1	0.0	0.2	0.3	[0.8]
macaroni/spaghetti, ckd	1 cup (140 g)	0.0	0.4	0.4	0.0	0.4	0.6	[1.8]
macaroni/spaghetti, whole grain, ckd	1 cup (137 g)	0.0	0.3	0.1	0.0	0.1	0.4	[1.1]
popcorn, air-popped	1 cup (7 g)	0.0	*	*	0.0	0.0	*	*
popcorn, caramel coated	1 oz (28 g)	—	0.7	0.2	—	9.6	0.3	11.1
popcorn, oil-popped	1 cup (11 g)	0.0	*	*	0.0	0.1	*	*
roll, hamburger	1.4 oz roll (40 g)	0.0	2.6	*	0.4	*	*	[3.0]
tortilla, corn	7" tortilla (30 g)	0.0	0.0	0.0	0.0	0.1	*	[0.2]

MEAT & POULTRY

beef & pork lunch meat, new england	0.95 oz slice (27 g)	—	0.5	—	—	0.0	—	[0.5]
beef, corned/smoked	3 oz (85 g)	—	0.1	—	—	0.5	—	[0.6]
beef/pork, spiced luncheon loaf	2 slices (57 g)	—	1.7	—	—	0.2	—	[1.9]
bologna, beef	2 slices (46 g)	—	1.1	—	—	0.1	—	[1.2]
frankfurter, beef & pork	1.8 oz frank (51 g)	—	1.0	—	—	0.0	—	[1.0]
ham & cheese luncheon loaf	2 slices (57 g)	*	0.6	—	*	0.0	—	[0.6]
ham, smoked, ckd	3 oz (85 g)	—	0.8	—	—	0.0	—	[0.8]
livercheese, pork	1.3 oz slice (38 g)	—	0.7	—	—	0.0	—	[0.7]
pastrami	2 slices (57 g)	—	0.1	—	—	0.4	—	[0.5]
pork sausage, ckd	.46 oz link (13 g)	—	0.3	—	—	*	—	[0.3]
salami, beef	2 slices (46 g)	—	0.6	—	—	0.0	—	[0.6]
turkey breast, ckd	2 slices (57 g)	—	—	—	—	0.1	—	[0.1]

MILK & YOGURT

milk, acidophilus	8 fl oz (227 g)	1.6	0.0	0.0	5.9	0.0	0.0	[7.5]
milk, buttermilk	8 fl oz (245 g)	0.5	0.0	0.0	9.1	0.0	0.0	11.8
milk, choc made w/choc malt mix	8 fl oz (265 g)	—	*	0.8	10.9	0.5	5.8	18.0
milk, nonfat	8 fl oz (245 g)	0.0	0.0	0.0	10.8	0.0	0.0	[10.8]
milk, nonfat, dry	1/4 cup (30 g)	—	—	0.0	15.1	—	—	[15.1]
milk, whole, 3.4% fat	8 fl oz (244 g)	0.0	0.0	0.0	12.0	0.0	0.0	12.2
yogurt, plain	8 oz (227 g)	3.2	0.0	0.0	8.4	0.0	0.0	11.6
yogurt, strawberry	8 oz (227 g)	2.3	7.7	5.9	7.5	10.0	1.6	34.7

NUTS & SEEDS

almonds, dry-roasted	1 oz (28 g)	0.0	0.1	—	0.0	1.2	0.0	1.5
almonds, oil-roasted	1 oz (28 g)	0.0	0.0	—	0.0	1.4	—	1.5
brazilnuts, oil-roasted	1 oz (28 g)	0.0	0.0	—	0.0	0.7	—	[0.7]
cashews, dry/oil-roasted	1 oz (28 g)	0.0	0.1	—	0.0	1.7	—	[1.8]
chestnuts, italian, raw	1 oz (28 g)	0.0	—	—	0.0	3.0	—	[3.0]
coconut, raw	1.6 oz piece (45 g)	0.0	0.9	0.6	0.0	*	—	1.6
coconut, dried, sweetened, flaked/shredded	1 cup (93 g)	0.0	0.6	0.2	0.0	*	—	32.0
coconut, shredded, toasted	1 oz (28 g)	0.0	—	—	0.0	9.1	—	[10.8]
hazelnuts (filberts), dry-roasted	1 oz (28 g)	*	0.1	—	0.0	0.8	—	[0.9]
hazelnuts (filberts), oil-roasted	1 oz (28 g)	*	0.0	—	0.0	1.3	—	[1.3]
macadamia nuts, oil-roasted	1 oz (28 g)	0.0	0.0	—	0.0	1.7	—	[1.8]
mixed nuts, oil-roasted	1 oz (28 g)	0.0	0.0	—	0.0	1.1	0.0	[1.1]
peanut butter	1 T (16 g)	—	0.2	0.0	0.0	1.1	0.0	[1.2]
peanuts, dried	1 oz (28 g)	—	0.1	0.0	0.0	1.1	0.0	1.2
peanuts, dry-roasted	1 oz (28 g)	—	0.1	0.0	0.0	1.0	0.1	1.3
peanuts, oil, roasted	1 oz (28 g)	—	0.0	0.0	0.0	1.0	0.0	*
peanuts, spanish, dried	1 oz (28 g)	—	0.0	0.0	0.0	1.1	*	*
peanuts, spanish, dry-roasted	1 oz (28 g)	—	0.1	0.0	0.0	1.0	*	*
pecans, dry/oil roasted	1 oz (28 g)	0.0	0.0	—	0.0	1.0	—	[1.0]
pistachio nuts, dried	1 oz (28 g)	0.0	0.1	0.0	0.0	0.4	0.0	1.9
pumpkin seed kernels, dried	1 oz (28 g)	0.0	0.0	—	0.0	0.3	—	[0.3]
safflower seed kernels, dried	1 oz (28 g)	0.0	*	—	0.0	0.4	—	0.4
sesame seeds, dry-roasted	1 T (8 g)	0.0	*	—	0.0	*	—	0.1

	SERVING SIZE (WEIGHT)	GAL (g)	GLU (g)	FRU (g)	LAC (g)	SUC (g)	MAL (g)	TOTAL SUGARS (g)
sunflower seeds, dry-roasted	1 oz (28 g)	0.0	0.0	—	0.0	0.7	—	1.1
sunflower seeds, oil-roasted	1 oz (28 g)	0.0	0.0	—	0.0	0.9	—	1.6
soy nuts, oil-roasted	1 oz (28 g)	—	0.0	0.0	0.0	1.2	0.0	*
walnuts	1 cup (125 g)	0.0	0.0	—	0.0	2.6	—	[2.6]
SALAD DRESSINGS								
salad dressing, caesar	1 T (15 g)	0.0	0.2	0.1	0.0	0.1	0.1	0.4
salad dressing coleslaw	1 T (15 g)	0.0	0.7	0.6	0.0	2.0	0.0	3.2
salad dressing, french, low cal	1 T (16 g)	0.0	1.2	1.1	0.0	0.8	0.0	3.1
salad dressing, russian	1 T (16 g)	0.0	2.8	0.3	0.0	1.0	0.9	5.0
salad dressing, russian, low cal	1 T (15 g)	0.0	2.4	1.8	0.0	0.0	0.0	4.2
SWEETENERS								
choc syrup	2 T (38 g)	—	4.8	2.9	1.9	11.6	1.7	19.7
corn syrup, dark	2 T (42 g)	—	6.3	0.5	0.0	0.9	4.1	[15.5]
corn syrup, high-fructose	2 T (42 g)	—	15.3	15.7	0.0	0.3	*	[31.3]
corn syrup, light	2 T (42 g)	—	8.7	0.9	0.0	*	6.3	[21.5]
honey	1 T (21 g)	0.0	7.1	8.9	0.0	0.3	0.9	[17.2]
maple syrup	2 T (42 g)	0.0	1.0	0.4	0.0	24.8	—	[26.2]
molasses	2 T (40 g)	0.0	4.5	5.2	0.0	13.9	—	[24.0]
molasses, blackstrap	2 T (40 g)	0.0	3.0	3.2	0.0	10.8	—	17.1
pancake syrup	1 T (20 g)	0.0	3.9	1.0	0.0	2.4	2.2	[10.9]
sorghum syrup	1 T (21 g)	0.0	*	*	0.0	7.0	—	13.8
sugar, brown	1 cup (220 g)	0.0	11.4	0.9	0.0	185.5	—	[197.8]
sugar, white, caramelized	1 T (15 g)	0.0	4.8	—	0.0	1.8	0.3	[6.8]
sugar, white, granulated	1 cup (200 g)	0.0	—	—	0.0	193.6	—	193.6
sugar, white, powdered, sifted	1 cup (100 g)	0.0	—	—	0.0	93.0	—	93.0
VEGETABLES								
alfalfa sprouts, raw	1 cup (33 g)	0.0	0.0	0.1	0.0	*	*	*
artichoke, ckd	4.2 oz artichoke (120 g)	0.0	1.0	0.0	0.0	0.4	*	1.3
asparagus, ckd	1.2 cup (90 g)	0.0	0.5	0.7	0.0	0.2	*	1.4
balsam pear, raw	1/2 cup (24 g)	0.0	*	*	0.0	*	*	0.2
beet, raw, sliced	1/2 cup (68 g)	0.0	0.1	0.1	0.0	4.1	*	4.0
borage, raw	1/2 cup (44 g)	0.0	*	*	0.0	*	*	0.4
broadbeans, immature, ckd	1/2 cup (85 g)	0.0	0.1	0.0	0.0	0.2	0.1	0.4
broccoli, raw	1 spear (151 g)	0.0	0.9	1.1	0.0	0.5	*	[3.0]
brussels sprouts, ckd	1 sprout (21 g)	0.0	*	*	0.0	*	*	*
cabbage, green, ckd	1/2 cup (78 g)	0.0	*	*	0.0	*	*	*
cabbage, green, raw, shredded	1/2 cup (35 g)	0.0	0.4	0.3	0.0	0.2	*	1.3
cabbage, red, ckd	1 leaf (22 g)	0.0	0.3	0.2	0.0	0.1	*	0.6
cabbage, red, raw, shredded	1 cup (70 g)	0.0	1.7	1.6	0.0	0.4	*	3.8
cabbage, savoy, raw, shredded	1 cup (70 g)	0.0	*	*	0.0	*	*	2.0
cardoon, raw, shredded	1/2 cup (89 g)	0.0	*	*	0.0	*	*	1.5
carrot, ckd	1/2 cup (78 g)	0.0	0.9	0.8	0.0	2.2	*	3.2
carrot, cnd	1/2 cup (73 g)	0.0	0.6	0.4	0.0	1.3	*	[2.3]
carrot, frzn, ckd	1/2 cup (73 g)	0.0	0.7	0.5	0.0	2.0	0.0	[3.3]
carrot, raw	1 carrot (72 g)	0.0	0.7	0.7	0.0	2.6	*	4.8
cassava root, raw, cubed	1 cup (142 g)	0.0	0.1	0.1	0.0	1.3	0.0	1.7
cauliflower, raw	1/2 cup (50 g)	0.0	0.4	0.4	0.0	0.2	*	1.2
celeriac, raw	1/2 cup (78 g)	0.0	*	*	0.0	*	*	1.6
celery, raw	1 stalk (40 g)	0.0	0.2	0.2	0.0	0.1	*	0.4
celtuce, raw	1 leaf (8 g)	0.0	*	*	0.0	*	*	0.1
chicory greens, raw	1/2 cup (90 g)	0.0	*	*	0.0	0.0	*	0.8
chicory root, raw, chopped	1/2 cup (45 g)	0.0	*	*	0.0	0.4	*	1.1
chinese cabbage, pak-choi, raw	1/2 cup (35 g)	0.0	*	*	0.0	*	*	0.4
chinese cabbage, pe-tsai, raw	1 cup (76 g)	0.0	0.6	0.5	0.0	*	*	1.0
chives, raw, chopped	1 t (1 g)	0.0	0.0	0.0	0.0	0.0	—	0.0
corn, sweet, ckd	1/2 cup (82 g)	0.0	0.4	0.2	0.0	1.2	0.2	[2.1]
corn, sweet, cnd	1/2 cup (82 g)	0.0	0.2	0.2	0.0	2.0	0.0	[2.3]
corn, sweet, frzn, ckd	1/2 cup (82 g)	0.0	0.3	0.2	0.0	1.0	*	[1.5]
cowpeas, immature, raw	1/2 cup (72 g)	0.0	*	*	0.0	*	*	2.2
cucumber, raw, sliced	1/2 cup (52 g)	0.0	0.5	0.5	0.0	0.0	0.0	1.2
dandelion greens, raw	1/2 cup (28 g)	0.0	0.1	0.1	0.0	0.4	*	[0.7]
eggplant, fried, not breaded	1 cup (130 g)	0.0	2.2	2.5	0.0	0.4	*	5.2
endive/escarole, raw, chopped	1/2 cup (25 g)	0.0	*	*	0.0	0.0	*	0.3
garland chrysanthemum, raw	1 stem (14 g)	0.0	0.0	0.0	0.0	0.0	*	*
garlic, raw	1 clove (3 g)	0.0	*	*	0.0	*	*	0.0

	SERVING SIZE (WEIGHT)	GAL (g)	GLU (g)	FRU (g)	LAC (g)	SUC (g)	MAL (g)	TOTAL SUGARS (g)
green (snap) beans, ckd	1/2 cup (62 g)	0.0	0.5	0.6	0.0	0.2	0.1	1.2
green (snap) beans, cnd	1/2 cup (68 g)	0.0	0.4	0.3	0.0	0.1	0.1	[1.1]
green (snap) beans, frzn, ckd	1/2 cup (68 g)	0.0	0.6	0.7	0.0	0.2	0.1	[1.8]
horseradish, raw	14″ stalk (337)	0.0	*	*	0.0	*	*	6.1
jerusalem artichoke, raw, chopped, freshly harvested	1 cup (130 g)	0.0	0.0	0.3	0.0	3.0	0.0	3.2
jerusalem artichoke, raw, chopped, stored	1 cup (143 g)	0.0	0.9	1.1	0.0	10.7	1.0	13.7
kale, raw, chopped	1/2 cup (34 g)	0.0	0.1	0.1	0.0	*	*	0.7
kohlrabi, raw, chopped	1/2 cup (70 g)	0.0	0.9	0.8	0.0	0.4	*	3.2
leek, ckd	1 leek (124 g)	0.0	0.5	0.4	0.0	0.4	*	1.2
lettuce, iceberg, raw	2 leaves (40 g)	0.0	0.3	0.3	0.0	*	*	0.7
lettuce, romaine (cos), raw, shredded	1/2 cup (28 g)	0.0	*	*	0.0	*	*	0.6
mung bean sprouts, raw	1/2 cup (52 g)	0.0	0.5	0.6	0.0	0.1	0.0	1.1
mushrooms, raw	1/2 cup (35 g)	0.0	0.2	0.1	0.0	*	*	[0.7]
mustard greens, raw, chopped	1/2 cup (28 g)	0.0	0.1	0.1	0.0	0.0	*	0.2
okra, raw, sliced	1/2 cup (50 g)	0.0	0.4	0.5	0.0	0.4	*	1.2
onion, raw, chopped	1/2 cup (80 g)	0.0	1.9	0.7	0.0	1.0	*	5.0
onion, spring, raw, chopped	1/2 cup (50 g)	0.0	1.4	*	0.0	0.2	*	1.6
parsley, raw, chopped	1/2 cup (30 g)	0.0	0.0	*	0.0	0.1	*	0.3
parsnip, raw, chopped	1/2 cup (67 g)	0.0	0.1	0.1	0.0	1.7	*	3.2
peas, edible-podded, raw	1/2 cup (72 g)	0.0	*	*	0.0	*	*	2.9
pepper, chili, raw, chopped	1/2 cup (75 g)	0.0	*	*	0.0	*	*	4.0
pepper, sweet, green, raw, chopped	1/2 cup (50 g)	0.0	0.6	0.6	0.0	*	*	1.2
potato, french fried	2.4 oz (68 g)	0.0	0.1	0.1	0.0	0.1	0.0	0.3
potato, hashed brown	1.9 oz (55 g)	0.0	0.1	0.0	0.0	0.1	0.0	0.1
potato peel	2 oz peel (58 g)	0.0	0.2	0.2	0.0	0.3	*	[0.8]
potato w/o peel, baked	1/2 cup (61 g)	0.0	0.2	0.2	0.0	0.1	*	[1.0]
potato w/peel, baked	1 potato (202 g)	0.0	0.8	0.8	0.0	0.6	*	[3.2]
pumpkin, ckd, mashed	1/2 cup (122 g)	0.0	1.6	1.2	0.0	1.2	*	[4.0]
radish, chinese, raw, sliced	1/2 cup (44 g)	0.0	*	*	0.0	*	*	1.1
radish, icicle, raw, sliced	1/2 cup (50 g)	0.0	*	*	0.0	*	*	1.2
radish, red, raw	10 radishes (45 g)	0.0	0.5	0.3	0.0	0.2	*	1.2
rhubarb, raw, diced	1 cup (122 g)	0.0	0.5	0.5	0.0	0.1	*	1.1
rutabaga, raw, cubed	1/2 cup (70 g)	0.0	2.2	1.0	0.0	0.6	*	3.9
salsify, black, raw, sliced	1/2 cup (67 g)	0.0	0.0	0.1	0.0	0.7	*	[0.8]
salsify, raw, sliced	1/2 cup (67 g)	0.0	*	*	0.0	*	*	1.9
shallot, raw, chopped	1 T (10 g)	0.0	*	0.0	0.0	0.2	*	0.3
spinach, ckd	1/2 cup (90 g)	0.0	0.0	0.0	0.0	0.0	*	*
spinach, raw, chopped	1/2 cup (28 g)	0.0	0.0	0.0	0.0	0.0	*	0.1
squash, summer, raw, sliced	1/2 cup (65 g)	0.0	0.6	0.6	0.0	0.1	*	1.4
sweet potato, baked	1/2 cup (88 g)	0.0	*	*	0.0	*	*	9.9
sweet potato, cnd, vacuum pack	1 cup (200 g)	0.0	*	*	0.0	*	*	30.8
swiss chard, chopped, ckd	1/2 cup (88 g)	0.0	0.2	0.2	0.0	0.0	*	0.4
taro, raw, sliced	1/2 cup (52 g)	0.0	*	*	0.0	*	*	0.4
tomato, ckd	1/2 cup (120 g)	0.0	1.6	1.8	0.0	0.0	*	[3.8]
tomato, cnd	1/2 cup (120 g)	0.0	1.2	1.4	0.0	0.0	*	[3.0]
tomato jce, cnd	1/2 cup (122 g)	0.0	1.7	2.3	0.0	0.0	0.0	[4.0]
tomato paste, cnd	1/2 cup (131 g)	0.0	1.4	1.7	0.0	0.0	*	[3.1]
tomato puree, cnd	1 cup (250 g)	0.0	7.2	8.5	0.0	*	*	*
tomato, raw	4.3 oz tomato (123 g)	0.0	1.4	1.7	0.0	0.0	*	3.4
tomato sce, cnd	1/2 cup (122 g)	0.0	2.4	2.2	0.0	*	*	*
turnip, ckd	1/2 cup (78 g)	0.0	*	*	0.0	*	*	*
turnip greens, ckd	1/2 cup (72 g)	0.0	0.1	0.0	0.0	0.0	*	0.1
veg jce, cnd	4 fl oz (121 g)	0.0	1.6	2.3	0.0	0.2	0.0	4.0
waterchestnut, raw	1 nut (12 g)	0.0	*	*	0.0	*	*	0.6
watercress, raw	1 sprig (2 g)	0.0	0.0	0.0	0.0	0.0	*	0.0
waxgourd, raw, cubed	1 cup (132 g)	0.0	0.7	0.7	0.0	0.0	*	[1.4]
yam, ckd	1/2 cup (68 g)	0.0	0.0	0.0	0.0	0.3	0.0	[0.3]
VEGETABLES—LEGUMES								
adzuki beans, ckd	1/2 cup (115 g)	—	*	*	0.0	0.3	0.0	*
baked beans w/franks in tom sce, cnd	1/2 cup (128 g)	—	1.4	1.2	*	2.7	—	[5.9]
baked beans w/pork in sweet sce, cnd	1/2 cup (126 g)	—	2.0	1.8	0.0	5.4	0.0	[10.5]
broadbeans, ckd	1/2 cup (85 g)	0.0	0.1	0.3	0.0	0.3	0.0	[1.5]
chickpeas (garbanzo beans), ckd	1/2 cup (82 g)	0.1	0.1	0.1	0.0	1.0	0.2	[3.9]
common beans, ckd	1/2 cup (88 g)	—	0.0	0.0	0.0	0.4	0.0	[1.9]
cowpeas (blackeyed peas), ckd	1/2 cup (86 g)	0.3	0.0	0..0	0.0	0.9	0.0	[2.8]
lentils, ckd	1/2 cup (99 g)	—	0.0	0.1	0.0	0.5	0.0	[1.8]
lima beans, ckd	1/2 cup (92 g)	—	*	0.2	0.0	0.5	0.0	[2.7]

	SERVING SIZE (WEIGHT)	GAL (g)	GLU (g)	FRU (g)	LAC (g)	SUC (g)	MAL (g)	TOTAL SUGARS (g)
lupins, ckd	1/2 cup (83 g)	—	*	0.0	0.0	0.5	0.0	[2.3]
mung beans, ckd	1/2 cup (96 g)	—	0.0	0.2	0.0	0.3	0.0	[1.9]
peas, green, ckd	1/2 cup (80 g)	0.0	0.2	0.1	0.0	3.8	0.2	[4.7]
peas, green, cnd	1/2 cup (85 g)	0.0	0.0	0.0	0.0	2.6	0.1	[3.0]
peas, green, frzn, ckd	1/2 cup (80 g)	0.0	*	0.1	0.0	3.8	0.2	[4.4]
peas, green, raw	1/2 cup (78 g)	0.0	0.0	0.0	0.0	3.4	0.1	4.4
peas, split, ckd	1/2 cup (98 g)	0.1	*	*	0.0	0.8	0.0	[2.8]
pigeonpeas, ckd	1/2 cup (84 g)	—	*	*	0.0	0.2	0.0	[0.8]
soybeans, ckd	1/2 cup (86 g)	—	0.1	0.2	0.0	0.4	0.0	[2.6]
tofu, raw	1/4 block (116 g)	—	0.0	0.0	0.0	0.0	0.0	[0.5]
winged beans, ckd	1/2 cup (86 g)	—	*	*	0.0	1.7	0.0	[2.2]
MISCELLANEOUS								
baking choc	1 oz (28 g)	—	0.0	0.1	*	0.1	*	[0.2]
carob powder, sweetened	2 T (13 g)	0.0	1.2	0.0	0.0	3.3	—	[4.5]
choc malt mix, dry	4–5 hp t (21 g)	—	*	0.9	1.2	0.7	5.8	[8.5]
cocoa powder	1 oz (28 g)	—	0.0	0.2	*	0.1	*	*
cocoa powder, dutch	1 oz (28 g)	—	0.0	0.2	*	0.1	*	*
sandwich spread (mayo type)	1 T (15 g)	0.0	0.7	0.6	0.0	1.2	0.0	2.5
steak sce	1 T (17 g)	0.0	1.1	0.6	0.0	0.3	0.2	2.2
tomato catsup	1 T (15 g)	0.0	1.1	0.5	0.0	*	*	[1.7]
whey, acid/sweet, fluid	1 cup (246 g)	0.0	0.0	0.0	11.1	0.0	*	[11.1]

[1] Gal = galactose, Glu = glucose, Fru = fructose, Lac = lactose, Suc = sucrose, Mal = maltose. An asterisk indicates the lack of data for a sugar known to be present; a dash indicates the lack of data for a sugar that may be present; 0.0 denotes the absence of the sugar or lack of data for a sugar thought not to be present; brackets around the value for total sugars indicates a calculated value. Some foods contain sugars other than the six presented here.

Source:
Matthews PH, PR Pehrsson, M Farhat-Sabet. *Sugars Content of Selected Foods: Individual and Total Sugars,* Home Economics Research Report Number 48. September 1987.

Sugars—Fructose, Glucose, Sucrose, Maltose, and Total Sugars (2002 file)

	GLUCOSE (g/100 g)	FRUCTOSE (g/100 g)	SUCROSE (g/100 g)	MALTOSE (g/100 g)	TOTAL SUGARS (g/100 g)
CEREALS & GRAINS					
corn grits, inst, ckd	—	0.08	0.20	0.07	0.35
corn grits, quick, ckd	0.09	—	0.20	—	0.29
oatmeal, inst, ckd	—	—	0.78	—	0.78
oatmeal, reg, ckd	—	—	0.13	—	0.13
rice, brown, long grain, ckd	—	—	0.45	—	0.45
rice, white, long grain, ckd	—	—	0.03	—	0.03
FRUITS					
apple, red delicious, raw	1.83	5.60	2.66	—	10.09
avocado, CA haas, raw	0.06	0.10	—	—	0.16
avocado, FL fuerte, raw	2.17	0.25	—	—	2.42
banana, raw	2.43	2.98	5.97	—	11.38
grapefruit, white, raw	1.59	1.66	2.37	0.11	5.73
grapes, thompson seedless, raw	6.07	6.78	0.07	0.06	12.98
guava, raw	0.76	1.80	1.11	—	3.67
mango, raw	0.66	3.80	8.27	—	12.73
nectarine, raw	3.32	3.69	1.11	0.09	8.21
orange, navel, raw	1.88	2.03	4.46	—	8.37
orange juice, from conc	2.03	2.02	4.10	—	8.15
peach, raw	4.52	4.01	0.21	—	8.74
peach, w/o skin, raw	3.52	3.92	3.88	—	11.32
pear, raw	4.20	5.30	1.21	—	10.71
pineapple, raw	2.58	2.83	3.83	—	9.24
plum, raw	5.10	3.28	0.10	0.17	8.65
prunes w/o pits	25.42	12.35	0.15	—	37.92
raisins, seedless	28.10	29.89	0.98	0.18	59.15
watermelon, raw	0.67	2.72	2.87	0.03	6.29

	GLUCOSE (g/100 g)	FRUCTOSE (g/100 g)	SUCROSE (g/100 g)	MALTOSE (g/100 g)	TOTAL SUGARS (g/100 g)
GRAIN FRACTIONS					
cornmeal, yellow, degermed	—	—	0.64	—	0.64
cornstarch	—	—	—	—	0.00
wheat flour, white, all-purpose	—	—	0.22	0.09	0.31
GRAIN PRODUCTS					
bagel, frzn	.82	1.38	—	3.08	5.28
bread, rye, seedless	—	—	—	3.11	3.26[1]
bread, rye w/caraway seed	—	0.34	—	1.71	2.05
bread, wheat, firm	—	0.50	—	1.41	1.91
bread, wheat, soft	0.63	1.00	—	—	1.63
bread, white, red cal, firm	1.04	2.67	2.18	—	5.89
bread, white, red cal, soft	0.41	1.13	—	—	1.54
bread, white, firm	1.88	2.36	—	1.29	5.53
bread, white, soft	0.37	0.73	—	0.25	1.35
bread, whole wheat, firm	2.88	3.82	—	3.38	10.08
bread, whole wheat, soft	3.35	4.41	—	0.20	7.96
roll, hamburger/frankfurter	1.09	1.94	—	—	3.03
spaghetti, ckd	—	—	—	0.47	0.47
tortilla, corn	0.07	0.03	0.28	1.53	1.91
tortilla, wheat flour	—	—	0.71	—	0.71
VEGETABLES					
broccoli, microwaved	0.73	0.89	0.30	—	1.92
broccoli, raw	—	0.28	—	0.42	0.70
cabbage, green, raw	1.64	2.17	0.11	—	3.92
carrot, microwaved	0.47	0.49	6.41	—	7.37
carrot, raw	0.28	0.39	4.19	—	4.86
cauliflower, raw	0.83	1.35	0.30	—	2.48
corn on cob, yellow, from farm	1.39	1.55	3.66	—	6.6
corn on cob, yellow, from grocery	0.64	1.56	0.73	—	2.93
cucumber w/peel, raw	0.67	0.82	—	—	1.49
green beans, microwaved	0.25	1.25	0.91	—	2.41
lettuce, iceberg, raw	0.67	0.91	0.02	0.02	1.62
onion, mature, raw	2.21	1.76	1.38	—	5.35
pepper, sweet, green, raw	0.71	1.04	0.18	—	1.93
potato, fried (french fries), fast food	—	—	0.44	—	0.44
potato, white, baked w/skin	0.15	0.17	0.19	—	0.51
potato, white, boiled w/o skin	0.16	0.11	0.18	0.06	0.51
spinach, raw	0.02	0.51	—	—	0.53
tomato, red, raw	0.49	1.19	—	—	1.68
VEGETABLES—LEGUMES					
beans w/pork & tom sce, cnd	0.87	1.27	2.78	—	4.92
chickpeas, cnd	—	—	0.44	—	0.44
cowpeas, cnd	—	—	0.42	—	0.42
kidney beans, red, cnd	0.23	0.10	3.47	—	3.8
lentils, ckd	—	—	0.39	—	0.39
lima beans, immature, frzn, microwaved	—	0.21	0.56	—	0.77
peas, green, frzn, microwaved	—	—	6.09	—	6.09
peas, split, ckd	—	—	0.65	—	0.65
pinto beans, cnd	—	—	0.54	—	0.54

[1] This product also contains 0.15 g galactose/100 g.

Source:
Li BW, KW Andrews, PR Pehrsson. Individual sugars, soluble, and insoluble dietary fiber contents of 70 high consumption foods. *J Food Comp Anal* 15:715–723, 2002.

Sugars—Raffinose & Stachyose[1]

	RAFFINOSE (g/100 g)	STACHYOSE (g/100 g)		RAFFINOSE (g/100 g)	STACHYOSE (g/100 g)
GRAIN FRACTIONS			lettuce, romaine (cos), raw	0.1	—
amaranth grain	0.3	—	onion, raw	1.4	0.7
cottonseed flour, defatted	9.2	0.8	parsley, raw	0.3	—
millet, proso	0.1	—	parsnip, raw	0.6	0.0
oat bran	0.3	0.2	pepper, sweet, green, raw	0.1	—
oat flour	0.2	0.1	pumpkin, raw	0.1	0.1
rice bran	0.1	—	salsify, black, raw	1.6	1.1
sesame flour, defatted	0.2	0.2	squash, summer, raw	0.1	0.1
sorghum grain	0.1	—	tomato paste	0.0	—
sunflower flour, defatted	3.0	—	**VEGETABLES -LEGUMES**		
soy flour, dehulled, defatted	0.8	4.6	adzuki beans, raw	0.2	3.9
wheat bran	0.1	—	broadbeans, ckd	0.4	0.2
wheat flour, white	0.2	—	broadbeans, raw	0.3	0.9
wheat flour, whole grain	0.2	—	chickpeas (garbanzo beans), ckd	0.4	0.5
NUTS & SEEDS			chickpeas (garbanzo beans), raw	0.7	2.4
peanuts, dried	0.1	0.4	common beans, ckd	0.2	0.7
pistachio nuts, dried	0.6	0.1	common beans, raw	0.3	1.5
			cowpeas (blackeyed peas), raw	0.5	2.4
VEGETABLES			lentils, raw	0.3	1.9
beet, raw	0.1	0.0	lima beans, raw	0.4	2.5
broccoli, raw	0.1	0.2	lupins, raw	0.7	3.7
brussels sprouts, raw	0.2	—	mung beans, ckd	0.3	0.3
cabbage, raw	0.1	0.1	mung beans, raw	0.8	1.4
carrot, raw	0.1	0.1	peas, split, raw	0.7	2.1
cauliflower, raw	—	0.1	pigeonpeas, ckd	0.4	0.4
chicory, raw	1.2	0.3	pigeonpeas, raw	0.7	1.4
corn, sweet, raw	0.2	0.2	soybeans, raw	0.7	3.2
leek, raw	0.1	0.6	winged beans, raw	1.3	2.9

[1] A dash indicates the lack of data for a sugar that may be present.

Source:
Matthews PH, PR Pehrsson, M Farhat-Sabet. *Sugars Content of Selected Foods: Individual and Total Sugars,* Home Economics Research Report Number 48. September 1987.

Vitamins/Vitamin-Like Components—Biotin

	BIOTIN (mcg/100 g)	SOURCE		BIOTIN (mcg/100 g)	SOURCE
BEVERAGES			**CHEESE**		
beer	0.114	Mock et al, 2003	cheese, american	3.1	Mock et al, 2003
Coca-Cola	0.081	Mock et al, 2003	cheese, blue stilton	3.3	MAFF2
punch, red fruit	0.155	Mock et al, 2003	cheese, brie w/o rind	3.6	MAFF2
tea, sweetened	0.142	Mock et al, 2003	cheese, brie, rind only	6.8	MAFF2
wine, white	0.117	Mock et al, 2003	cheese, camembert	7.5	MAFF2
			cheese, cheddar, english white	4.4	MAFF2
			cheese, cheddar, mild	1.4	Mock et al, 2003
CANDY			cheese, cottage, lowfat (1.5–2%)	5.1	MAFF2
dark chocolate	6.0	Souci et al, 2000	cheese, cream	5.1	MAFF2
marzipan	2.0	Souci et al, 2000	cheese, edam	1.5	Souci et al, 2000
milk chocolate	3.0	Souci et al, 2000	cheese, emmental	3.0	Souci et al, 2000
			cheese, goat milk, full fat, soft	5.1	MAFF2
			cheese, gorgonzola	2.0	Souci et al, 2000
CEREALS			cheese, gruyere	1.3	Souci et al, 2000
Cheerios	0.108	Mock et al, 2003	cheese, limburger	8.6	Souci et al, 2000
corn grits, ckd	0.051	Mock et al, 2003	cheese, mozzarella	2.0	Souci et al, 2000
Frosted Flakes	0.138	Mock et al, 2003	cheese, parmesan	3.0	Souci et al, 2000
Golden Grahams	0.146	Mock et al, 2003	cheese, processed, singles	5.6	MAFF2
Kix	0.095	Mock et al, 2003	cheese, provolone	0.117	Mock et al, 2003
oatmeal, ckd	0.191	Mock et al, 2003			

	BIOTIN (mcg/100 g)	SOURCE
CREAM		
cream, min 10% fat	3.4	Souci et al, 2000
cream, sour	3.0	Souci et al, 2000
cream, whipping, min 30% fat	3.4	Souci et al, 2000
DESSERTS		
cake, choc fudge	2.6	MAFF3
cake, van w/icing	0.034	Mock et al, 2003
cheesecake, choc/toffee/caramel	2.1	MAFF3
cookie, choc sandwich	0.143	Mock et al, 2003
cookie, sugar	0.279	Mock et al, 2003
ice cream, choc/choc mint in cone	2.5	MAFF3
ice cream, fat-free	2.2	MAFF3
ice cream, nondairy, choc	2.9	MAFF3
ice cream, soy, nondairy	1.1	MAFF3
ice cream, van	2.2	MAFF3
pavlova/meringue w/fruit & cream	1.3	MAFF3
pie, apple, double crust	0.80	MAFF3
pie, lemon meringue	0.90	MAFF3
pie, oatmeal cream	0.091	Mock et al, 2003
poptart, blueberry	0.033	Mock et al, 2003
profiterole w/choc sce	3.7	MAFF3
pudding, banana	1.02	Mock et al, 2003
sorbet, fruit	0.40	MAFF3
sponge cake w/cream & jam	1.6	MAFF3
tiramisu	2.0	MAFF3
EGGS & EGG SUBSTITUTES		
chicken, egg, white, ckd	5.8	Mock et al, 2003
chicken egg, whole, ckd	21.4	Mock et al, 2003
chicken egg, yolk, ckd	27.2	Mock et al, 2003
hen egg, white, raw (from South Africa)	6.10	Van Niekerk and Van Heerden, 1993
hen egg, whole, raw (from South Africa)	22.0	Van Niekerk and Van Heerden, 1993
hen egg, yolk, raw (from South Africa)	48.0	Van Niekerk and Van Heerden, 1993
egg substitute, Better'n Eggs, Papetti Foods	11.0	PPTT
ENTREES		
chili	0.520	Mock et al, 2003
chili pie w/corn chips	0.059	Mock et al, 2003
macaroni & cheese	0.130	Mock et al, 2003
pizza, cheese	0.109	Mock et al, 2003
pizza, pepperoni	0.212	Mock et al, 2003
soup, beef veg	0.118	Mock et al, 2003
FISH & SHELLFISH		
catfish, breaded, fried	0.744	Mock et al, 2003
clam, soft, raw	2.3	Souci et al, 2000
cod, raw	2.2	Souci et al, 2000
crab, cnd	4.6	Souci et al, 2000
fish sticks, minced, breaded, fried	1.0	Mock et al, 2003
haddock, raw	2.5	Souci et al, 2000
halibut, raw	3.1	Souci et al, 2000
herring, atlantic, raw	450.0	Souci et al, 2000
lobster, raw	4.5	Souci et al, 2000
mackerel, raw	4.3	Souci et al, 2000
oysters, raw	10.0	Souci et al, 2000
salmon, pink, chunk, cnd w/o skin or bone, Chicken of the Sea	4.0	CHCK
salmon, red, chunk, cnd w/o skin or bone, Chicken of the Sea	7.0	CHCK
salmon, pink, cnd in water	5.9	Mock et al, 2003
sardines, cnd in oil	9.1	Souci et al, 2000
scallops, raw	1.1	Souci et al, 2000

	BIOTIN (mcg/100 g)	SOURCE
shrimp, brown, raw	500.0	Souci et al, 2000
smelt, raw	30.0	Souci et al, 2000
trout, raw	4.5	Souci et al, 2000
tuna, chunk light, cnd in canola oil, drained, Chicken of the Sea	2.0	CHCK
tuna, chunk light, cnd in spring water, drained, Chicken of the Sea	2.0	CHCK
tuna, chunk white, cnd in spring water, drained, Chicken of the Sea	2.0	CHCK
tuna, cnd in water	0.682	Mock et al, 2003
tuna, solid light, cnd in olive oil (tonno), drained, Chicken of the Sea	2.0	CHCK
tuna, solid light, cnd in spring water, drained, Chicken of the Sea	2.0	CHCK
tuna, solid white, cnd in canola oil, drained, Chicken of the Sea	2.0	CHCK
tuna, solid white, cnd in spring water, drained, Chicken of the Sea	2.0	CHCK
FRUIT JUICES		
apple jce, cnd	0.052	Mock et al, 2003
grapefruit jce	0.4–3.0	Ranganna et al, 1983
grape jce	1.2	Souci et al, 2000
elderberry jce	0.70	Souci et al, 2000
lemon, CA, jce	0.25	Ranganna et al, 1983
orange jce, cnd	0.413	Mock et al, 2003
orange jce, navel	0.5	Ranganna et al, 1983
orange jce, Valencia	0.79	Ranganna et al, 1983
tangerine juice	0.5	Ranganna et al, 1983
FRUIT		
acerola (west indian cherry), raw	2.5	Souci et al, 2000
apple, raw	0.020	Mock et al, 2003
avocado, raw	0.961	Mock et al, 2003
banana, raw	0.133	Mock et al, 2003
blueberries, raw	1.1	Souci et al, 2000
cherries, sweet, raw	0.4	Souci et al, 2000
currants, black, raw	2.4	Souci et al, 2000
currants, red, raw	2.6	Souci et al, 2000
gooseberries, raw	0.5	Souci et al, 2000
grapes, raw	1.5	Souci et al, 2000
elderberries, black, raw	1.8	Souci et al, 2000
lemon, CA	0.6	Ranganna et al, 1983
lemon, CA, peel	2.5	Ranganna et al, 1983
orange peel, Valencia	5.1	Ranganna et al, 1983
orange, raw	0.049	Mock et al, 2003
orange, raw, Valencia	1.2	Ranganna et al, 1983
peach, cnd	0.2	Souci et al, 2000
peach, raw	1.9	Souci et al, 2000
pear, raw	0.1	Souci et al, 2000
plum, raw	0.1	Souci et al, 2000
raisins	0.391	Mock et al, 2003
raspberries, raw	0.178	Mock et al, 2003
strawberries, raw	1.50	Mock et al, 2003
GRAIN PRODUCTS		
baguette, white	0.5	MAFF1
bread, brown	3.0	MAFF1
bread, wheat germ	1.5	MAFF1
bread, white, grilled (toasted)	1.23	Mock et al, 2003
bread, white, premium	1.0	MAFF1
bread, white, standard	0.6	MAFF1
bread, whole grain	6.3	MAFF1
bread, whole wheat	0.074	Mock et al, 2003
crispbread	7.0	Souci et al, 2000
crackers, saltines	0.290	Mock et al, 2003
crumpet	2.6	MAFF1

	BIOTIN (mcg/100 g)	SOURCE
hush puppies	0.203	Mock et al, 2003
noodles, ckd	0.181	Mock et al, 2003
noodles, ramen oriental	0.101	Mock et al, 2003
pasta w/egg	1.0	Souci et al, 2000
roll, dinner	0.049	Mock et al, 2003
roll, hamburger	0.289	Mock et al, 2003
roll, white, crusty	0.9	MAFF1

GRAINS & GRAIN FRACTIONS

corn flour	6.6	Souci et al, 2000
corn, whole grain	6.0	Souci et al, 2000
oats, rolled	20.0	Souci et al, 2000
oats, whole grain	20.0	Souci et al, 2000
rice, brown, raw	12.0	Souci et al, 2000
rice, white, raw	3.0	Souci et al, 2000
rye, whole grain	5.0	Souci et al, 2000
wheat bran	44.0	Souci et al, 2000
wheat germ	17.0	Souci et al, 2000
wheat flour	2.0	Souci et al, 2000
wheat, whole grain	6.0	Souci et al, 2000

MEAT

beef, corned	2.0	Souci et al, 2000
beef filet, raw	4.6	Souci et al, 2000
beef hamburger patty, ckd	4.5	Mock et al, 2003
beef rump, raw	3.8	Souci et al, 2000
beef, top round, raw	4.6	Souci et al, 2000
mutton brisket, raw	2.0	Souci et al, 2000
mutton leg, raw	6.0	Souci et al, 2000
pork chop, ckd	4.5	Mock et al, 2003
pork hind leg, raw	5.1	Souci et al, 2000

MEAT, INTERNAL ORGANS

brain, calf, raw	6.1	Souci et al, 2000
brain, ox, raw	6.1	Souci et al, 2000
heart, calf, raw	7.3	Souci et al, 2000
heart, ox, raw	7.3	Souci et al, 2000
heart, pork, raw	4.0	Souci et al, 2000
kidney, calf, raw	80.0	Souci et al, 2000
kidney, ox, raw	58.0	Souci et al, 2000
liver, beef, ckd	41.6	Mock et al, 2003
liver, calf, raw	75.0	Souci et al, 2000
liver, ox, raw	100.0	Souci et al, 2000
liver, pork, raw	27.0	Souci et al, 2000
liver, sheep, raw	130.0	Souci et al, 2000
lungs, calf, raw	5.9	Souci et al, 2000
lungs, ox, raw	5.9	Souci et al, 2000
spleen, ox, raw	5.7	Souci et al, 200
tongue, calf, raw	3.3	Souci et al, 2000
tongue, ox, raw	3.3	Souci et al, 2000

MILK & YOGURT

milk, buffalo	0.011	Souci et al, 2000
milk, cow, 2% fat	0.113	Mock et al, 2003
milk, cow, buttermilk	0.002	Souci et al, 2000
milk, cow, choc, lowfat	0.381	Mock et al, 2003
milk, cow, condensed, sweetened	3.8	Souci et al, 2000
milk, cow, nonfat	0.0131	Mock et al, 2003
milk, cow, whole	0.0091	Mock et al, 2003
milk, ewe (sheep)	0.009	Souci et al, 2000
milk, goat	0.004	Souci et al, 2000
milk, human	0.8 mcg/ 100 ml	Hartman and Dryden, 1965
milk, human	0.76 mcg/ 100 ml	Oppe et al, 1977
milk, soy, carob, Edensoy	3.0	EDEN
milk, soy, original, Edensoy	5.0	EDEN
yogurt, plain	0.084	Mock et al, 2003

NUTS & SEEDS

	BIOTIN (mcg/100 g)	SOURCE
almonds, roasted, salted	4.407	Mock et al, 2003
chestnut, sweet (marone)	1.5	Souci et al, 2000
peanuts, roasted, salted	17.5	Mock et al, 2003
pecans, raw	2.00	Mock et al, 2003
soy nuts w/praline coating, GeniSoy	268.0	GENI
soy nuts, choc covered, GeniSoy	268.0	GENI
soy nuts, flavored, GeniSoy	268.0	GENI
soy nuts, unsalted, GeniSoy	268.0	GENI
sunflower seeds, roasted, salted	7.80	Mock et al, 2003
walnuts, raw	2.59	Mock et al, 2003

POULTRY

chicken liver, ckd	187.2	Mock et al, 2003
chicken nuggets, breaded, fried	1.34	Mock et al, 2003
chicken, roaster, raw	2.0	Souci et al, 2000
chicken strips, breaded, fried	0.43	Mock et al, 2003
hot dog, chicken & pork, ckd	3.7	Mock et al, 2003
turkey, deli processed, sliced	0.73	Mock et al, 2003

VEGETABLES

asparagus, cnd	1.7	Souci et al, 2000
asparagus, raw	2.0	Souci et al, 2000
broccoli, raw	0.943	Mock et al, 2003
brussels sprouts	0.4	Souci et al, 2000
cabbage, red, raw	2.0	Souci et al, 2000
cabbage, savoy, raw	0.1	Souci et al, 2000
cabbage, white, raw	3.2	Souci et al, 2000
carrots, cnd	0.622	Mock et al, 2003
cauliflower, raw	0.161	Mock et al, 2003
celery, raw	0.1	Souci et al, 2000
chicory, raw	4.8	Souci et al, 2000
corn, whole kernel, cnd	0.047	Mock et al, 2003
cucumber, raw	0.9	Souci et al, 2000
fennel leaves, raw	2.5	Souci et al, 2000
green beans, cnd	0.007	Mock et al, 2003
kale, raw	0.5	Souci et al, 2000
kohlrabi, raw	2.7	Souci et al, 2000
leek, raw	1.6	Souci et al, 2000
lettuce, raw	1.9	Souci et al, 2000
mungo (black gram) beans, dry	7.5	Souci et al, 2000
mushrooms, cnd	2.16	Mock et al, 2003
onion, raw	3.5	Souci et al, 2000
parsley, raw	0.4	Souci et al, 2000
parsnip, raw	0.1	Souci et al, 2000
peas, dry	19.0	Souci et al, 2000
peas, green, cnd	1.5	Souci et al, 2000
peas w/pods, green, raw	5.3	Souci et al, 2000
potatoes, white, french fries	0.318	Mock et al, 2003
potatoes, white, mashed w/gravy	0.133	Mock et al, 2003
potatoes, white, tator tots	0.062	Mock et al, 2003
pumpkin, raw	0.4	Souci et al, 2000
rutabaga (swede), raw	0.1	Souci et al, 2000
salad, mixed garden	0.285	Mock et al, 2003
soybeans, dry	60.0	Souci et al, 2000
string beans, raw	7.0	Souci et al, 2000
spinach, frzn	0.705	Mock et al, 2003
sweet potato, ckd	1.45	Mock et al, 2003
tomato jce	2.5	Souci et al, 2000
tomato, raw	0.701	Mock et al, 2003
tomato sce w/beef (for spaghetti)	0.060	Mock et al, 2003
turnip, raw	2.0	Souci et al, 2000

MISCELLANEOUS

butter	tr	Souci et al, 2000
cocoa powder	20.0	Souci et al, 2000
ketchup	0.074	Mock et al, 2003

	BIOTIN (mcg/100 g)	SOURCE		BIOTIN (mcg/100 g)	SOURCE
mayonnaise	0.185	Mock et al, 2003	whey, dried powder	43.0	Souci et al, 2000
potato chips, bbq, baked	0.050	Mock et al, 2003	whey, sweet	1.4	Souci et al, 2000
salad dressing, ranch	0.235	Mock et al, 2003	yeast	20.2	Mock et al, 2003

Sources:
CHCK: Chicken of the Sea International, Inc, San Diego CA
EDEN: Eden Foods, Clinton MI
GENI: GeniSoy, Fairfield CA
Hartman AM, LP Dryden. *Vitamins in Milk and Milk Products: A Review.* American Dairy Science Association, Champaign IL, 1965.
MAFF1: Ministry of Agriculture, Farms, and Fisheries, UK. Nutrient analysis of Bread and Morning Goods. 20 January 2001. (http://www.food.gov.uk/science/surveillance/maffinfo/2000/maff-2000-194) (accessed 20 December 2002).
MAFF2: Ministry of Agriculture, Farms, and Fisheries, UK. Nutrient Analysis of Cheese. 25 January 2000 (http://www.food.gov.uk/science/surveillance/maffinfo/2000/maff-2000-196) (accessed 20 December 2002).
MAFF3: Ministry of Agriculture, Farms, and Fisheries, UK. Nutrient Analysis of Ice Creams and Desserts. 23 January 2000 (http://www.food.gov.uk/science/surveillance/maffinfo/2000/maff-2000-195) (accessed 20 December 2002).
Mock DM, C Staggs, B McCabe, W Sealey. Department of Biochemistry and Molecular Biology, UMS, Little Rock AR. personal communication, May 2003.
Oppe TE, D Barltrop, NR Belton, et al. *The Composition of Mature Human Milk,* Dept of Health and Social Security, Report on Health and Social Subjects No. 12. Her Majesty's Stationery Office, London, 1977.
PPTT: Papetti Foods, Gaylord MN
Ranganna S, VS Govindarajan, KVR Ramana. Citrus fruits–Varieties, chemistry, technology, and quality evaluation. Part II. Chemistry, technology, and quality evaluation. A. Chemistry. *Critical Reviews in Food Science and Nutrition.* Vol 18, issue 4. CRC Press, Boca Raton FL. 1983.
Souci SW, W Fachmann, H Kraut. Food Composition and Nutrition Tables. Medpharm GmbH Scientific Publishers, Stuttgart, Germany & CRC Press, Washington DC. 2000.
Van Niekerk PJ, IV Van Heerden. The nutritional composition of South African eggs. *S Afr Med J* 83:842–846, 1993.

Vitamins/Vitamin-Like Components–Choline & Betaine

	CHOLINE (mg/100 g)	TOTAL CHOLINE[1] (mg/100 g)	BETAINE (mg/100 g)	USDA CODE[2]	SOURCE
BEVERAGES					
beer	4.65	9.71	8.65	14003	Zeisel et al, 2003
beer, light	4.07	7.06	6.20	14006	Zeisel et al, 2003
Coca-Cola	0.06	0.67	0.08	14400	Zeisel et al, 2003
coffee	1.89	2.62	0.07	14209	Zeisel et al, 2003
coffee, decaf powder	93.7	101.93	0.65	14219	Zeisel et al, 2003
Diet Coke	——	——	0.06	14416	Zeisel et al, 2003
Orange Crush	——	0.58	0.05	14150	Zeisel et al, 2003
tea, brewed	0.37	0.37	0.90	14355	Zeisel et al, 2003
wine, white	3.56	5.15	0.13	14106	Zeisel et al, 2003
CANDY					
milk choc	9.12	46.11	2.33	19120	Zeisel et al, 2003
Snickers	10.20	40.72	0.98	19155	Zeisel et al, 2003
CEREALS & GRAIN FRACTIONS					
farina w/wheat germ	1.57	3.45	6.09	08105	Zeisel et al, 2003
oat bran, raw	4.41	58.57	31.73	20033	Zeisel et al, 2003
oats	1.25	7.42	2.72	08121	Zeisel et al, 2003
rice, brown	4.66	9.22	0.43	20037	Zeisel et al, 2003
rice, white	0.72	2.08	0.27	20045	Zeisel et al, 2003
wheat bran	50.89	74.39	1339.35	20077	Zeisel et al, 2003
wheat germ, toasted	69.19	152.08	1240.48	08084	Zeisel et al, 2003
CHEESE					
cheese, cottage	3.64	18.42	0.66	01012	Zeisel et al, 2003
cheese, cream	3.58	27.21	0.65	01017	Zeisel et al, 2003
CREAMS					
cream	0.54	2.28	0.08	01069	Zeisel et al, 2003
cream, half & half	3.92	16.82	0.61	01050	Zeisel et al, 2003
cream, sour	4.73	20.33	0.67	01056	Zeisel et al, 2003
DESSERTS					
cake w/icing	4.63	36.38	16.59	18140	Zeisel et al, 2003
cookie, choc chip	8.90	17.05	38.03	18159	Zeisel et al, 2003
danish pastry	8.72	21.84	12.68	18246	Zeisel et al, 2003
frzn yogurt	4.38	23.01	0.77	19293	Zeisel et al, 2003

	CHOLINE (mg/100 g)	TOTAL CHOLINE[1] (mg/100 g)	BETAINE (mg/100 g)	USDA CODE[2]	SOURCE
ice cream	4.78	26.04	0.94	19095	Zeisel et al, 2003
ice cream, van & orange sherbet	1.80	15.59	0.53	——	Zeisel et al, 2003
pie, apple	4.66	7.19	14.57	18301	Zeisel et al, 2003
EGGS					
egg, chicken	.62	251.0	0.53	01123	Zeisel et al, 2003
FAST FOODS					
chicken nuggets	3.87	41.87	15.06	21037	Zeisel et al, 2003
french fries	12.14	22.06	0.66	21138	Zeisel et al, 2003
frankfurter on bun	4.51	30.06	39.39	21118	Zeisel et al, 2003
hamburger	5.66	34.23	29.61	21107	Zeisel et al, 2003
lasagna	5.21	16.98	5.42	——	Zeisel et al, 2003
pizza, cheese	6.68	13.98	23.01	21049	Zeisel et al, 2003
shake, van	4.58	18.21	1.04	14347	Zeisel et al, 2003
taco/burrito	9.55	26.88	13.22	21082	Zeisel et al, 2003
FATS, OILS, & SPREADS					
butter	0.55	18.77	0.24	01001	Zeisel et al, 2003
mayonnaise	0.23	46.02	——	04025	Zeisel et al, 2003
mayonnaise, imit	0.30	14.59	0.31	04027	Zeisel et al, 2003
oil, olive	0.02	0.29	0.10	04053	Zeisel et al, 2003
FISH & SHELLFISH					
cod, atlantic, raw	17.73	83.63	8.58	15016	Zeisel et al, 2003
fish sticks	11.55	28.32	29.32	15027	Zeisel et al, 2003
salmon, raw	8.62	65.45	1.87	15086	Zeisel et al, 2003
shrimp, cnd	5.56	70.60	218.74	15152	Zeisel et al, 2003
FRUIT JUICES					
apple jce	0.71	1.84	0.11	09016	Zeisel et al, 2003
cranberry jce cocktail	0.43	1.13	0.08	14242	Zeisel et al, 2003
lemon, CA, jce	5.5				Ranganna et al, 1983
orange jce	4.16	11.05	0.23	09215	Zeisel et al, 2003
orange, navel, jce	5.6				Ranganna et al, 1983
orange, valencia, jce	8.0				Ranganna et al, 1983
FRUITS					
apple, raw	0.33	3.44	0.9	09003	Zeisel et al, 2003
avocado, raw	8.64	14.18	0.58	09037	Zeisel et al, 2003
banana, raw	3.20	9.76	0.07	09040	Zeisel et al, 2003
blueberries, raw	3.00	6.04	0.16	09050	Zeisel et al, 2003
cantaloupe, raw	4.12	7.58	0.07	09181	Zeisel et al, 2003
grapefruit, raw	3.56	7.53	0.13	09111	Zeisel et al, 2003
grapes, raw	4.80	5.63	0.12	09132	Zeisel et al, 2003
lemon, CA	10.0				Ranganna et al, 1983
lemon, CA, peel	11.0				Ranganna et al, 1983
orange, raw	4.68	8.38	0.11	09200	Zeisel et al, 2003
orange, valencia, raw	11.6				Ranganna et al, 1983
orange, valencia, peel	23.0				Ranganna et al, 1983
peach, cnd	0.43	3.40	0.24	09241	Zeisel et al, 2003
peach, raw	0.78	6.10	0.24	09236	Zeisel et al, 2003
pear, cnd	0.55	1.94	0.23	09257	Zeisel et al, 2003
pear, raw	2.26	5.11	0.14	09252	Zeisel et al, 2003
prune	6.30	9.66	0.39	09288	Zeisel et al, 2003
raisins	9.37	11.14	0.27	09298	Zeisel et al, 2003
strawberries, raw	0.63	5.65	0.14	09316	Zeisel et al, 2003
watermelon, raw	3.08	4.07	0.25	09326	Zeisel et al, 2003
GRAIN/VEG-BASED SNACKS					
corn chips	1.86	12.07	0.10	19003	Zeisel et al, 2003
nachos w/cheese	4.77	26.35	0.62	21078	Zeisel et al, 2003
popcorn	5.17	13.98	0.32	19035	Zeisel et al, 2003
potato chips	4.57	12.07	0.15	19411	Zeisel et al, 2003
pretzel, hard, salted	16.23	38.40	236.45	19047	Zeisel et al, 2003
GRAIN PRODUCTS					
biscuit	6.85	8.89	38.24	18009	Zeisel et al, 2003
bread, wheat	17.98	26.53	201.41	18064	Zeisel et al, 2003

	CHOLINE (mg/100 g)	TOTAL CHOLINE[1] (mg/100 g)	BETAINE (mg/100 g)	USDA CODE[2]	SOURCE
bread, white	6.04	12.17	93.20	18069	Zeisel et al, 2003
cracker, graham	13.15	22.27	172.59	18173	Zeisel et al, 2003
cracker, saltine	12.63	19.59	49.14	18228	Zeisel et al, 2003
cracker, wheat	17.71	31.80	198.71	18232	Zeisel et al, 2003
english muffin	10.26	17.95	95.42	18258	Zeisel et al, 2003
muffin	14.48	43.40	82.12	18273	Zeisel et al, 2003
pancake	5.44	19.21	23.12	18290	Zeisel et al, 2003
tortilla	4.10	13.27	0.34	18363	Zeisel et al, 2003
MEATS					
beef, grnd, 75% lean, broiled	2.22	82.35	7.54	23568	Zeisel et al, 2003
beef, grnd, 85% lean, broiled	2.30	79.32	8.49	23578	Zeisel et al, 2003
beef liver, panfried	56.67	418.22	5.63	13327	Zeisel et al, 2003
beef, trimmed, ckd	3.57	78.15	10.12	13004	Zeisel et al, 2003
pork bacon, ckd	12.06	124.89	3.14	10124	Zeisel et al, 2003
pork loin, ckd	2.19	102.76	1.39	10046	Zeisel et al, 2003
pork sausage	7.39	73.07	2.15	07065	Zeisel et al, 2003
MILK & YOGURT					
milk, cow, 2% fat	2.82	16.40	0.84	01079	Zeisel et al, 2003
milk, cow, nonfat	2.81	16.63	1.70	01085	Zeisel et al, 2003
milk, cow, whole	3.67	14.29	0.54	01077	Zeisel et al, 2003
yogurt, plain	2.32	15.20	0.76	01117	Zeisel et al, 2003
yogurt w/fruit	2.08	14.04	0.74	01121	Zeisel et al, 2003
NUTS					
peanut butter	25.04	63.02	0.70	16098	Zeisel et al, 2003
peanuts	17.59	52.47	0.56	16089	Zeisel et al, 2003
POULTRY					
chicken frankfurter	6.17	51.36	4.53	07024	Zeisel et al, 2003
chicken liver	47.87	290.03	11.43	05028	Zeisel et al, 2003
chicken w/o skin, roasted	5.67	78.74	5.09	05013	Zeisel et al, 2003
chicken w/skin, roasted	5.27	65.83	4.95	05009	Zeisel et al, 2003
SALAD DRESSING					
fat-free	1.49	3.97	1.61	04021	Zeisel et al, 2003
italian, reg	1.62	12.40	0.01	04114	Zeisel et al, 2003
SOUPS					
soup, chicken noodle	3.27	11.22	10.56	06419	Zeisel et al, 2003
soup, clam chowder, new england	1.96	6.89	21.28	06205	Zeisel et al, 2003
VEGETABLES					
beet, cnd	0.40	6.10	296.73	11084	Zeisel et al, 2003
beet, raw	4.12	6.01	114.42	11080	Zeisel et al, 2003
broccoli, raw	8.45	40.06	0.11	11091	Zeisel et al, 2003
brussels sprouts, raw	23.37	40.61	0.13	11101	Zeisel et al, 2003
cabbage, raw	6.87	15.45	0.31	11110	Zeisel et al, 2003
carrot, ckd	0.44	8.77	0.11	11125	Zeisel et al, 2003
carrot, raw	6.82	8.79	0.34	11124	Zeisel et al, 2003
cauliflower, raw	24.53	39.10	0.11	11136	Zeisel et al, 2003
celery, raw	5.25	6.14	0.09	11143	Zeisel et al, 2003
corn, yellow, raw	8.93	21.95	0.15	11179	Zeisel et al, 2003
green (snap) beans, raw	4.00	13.46	0.08	11061	Zeisel et al, 2003
lettuce, iceberg, raw	4.80	6.70	0.08	11252	Zeisel et al, 2003
lettuce, romaine, raw	7.63	9.92	0.08	11251	Zeisel et al, 2003
mushroom, raw	5.93	16.86	9.52	11260	Zeisel et al, 2003
navy beans, dry	14.02	26.93	0.07	16039	Zeisel et al, 2003
onion, raw	4.39	6.10	0.07	11282	Zeisel et al, 2003
peas, raw	2.16	27.51	0.13	11313	Zeisel et al, 2003
pepper, raw	3.62	5.54	0.07	11333	Zeisel et al, 2003
potatoes, french fries, frzn, baked	7.22	20.17	0.28	11403	Zeisel et al, 2003
potatoes, mashed	8.44	14.36	0.38	11657	Zeisel et al, 2003
sauerkraut, cnd	8.68	10.39	0.43	11439	Zeisel et al, 2003
seaweed, kelp, raw	0.10	0.43	0.22	11445	Zeisel et al, 2003
soybeans, raw	47.27	115.87	1.86	16108	Zeisel et al, 2003
spinach, ckd	1.69	24.78	645.06	11458	Zeisel et al, 2003

	CHOLINE (mg/100 g)	TOTAL CHOLINE[1] (mg/100 g)	BETAINE (mg/100 g)	USDA CODE[2]	SOURCE
spinach, raw	2.25	22.08	599.81	11457	Zeisel et al, 2003
squash, summer, yellow, raw	2.08	10.57	0.18	11644	Zeisel et al, 2003
squash, summer, zucchini, raw	0.53	9.36	0.23	11478	Zeisel et al, 2003
tomato, raw	4.40	6.74	0.06	11529	Zeisel et al, 2003
tomato salsa	7.30	11.70	0.22	06164	Zeisel et al, 2003
MISCELLANEOUS					
alfalfa seeds	11.02	14.40	0.35	11001	Zeisel et al, 2003
catsup	6.54	10.53	0.15	11935	Zeisel et al, 2003
mustard seeds	46.21	122.66	1.65	02024	Zeisel et al, 2003
preserves, strawberry	2.57	10.21	0.09	19297	Zeisel et al, 2003
soy sauce	31.01	33.03	35.21	16123	Zeisel et al, 2003
tofu, soft	9.72	27.37	0.36	16127	Zeisel et al, 2003

[1] Total choline is the sum of choline, phosphocholine, glycerophosphocholine, phosphatidylcholine, and sphingomyelin.
[2] These USDA code numbers were provided by Zeisel et al, 2003; however, it is noted that the food descriptions provided in this reference are, in some cases, not as exact or detailed as the USDA food descriptions.

Sources:
Ranganna S, VS Govindarajan, KVR Ramana. Citrus fruits–Varieties, chemistry, technology, and quality evaluation. Part II. Chemistry, technology, and quality evaluation. A. Chemistry. *Critical Reviews in Food Science and Nutrition.* Vol 18, issue 4. CRC Press, Boca Raton FL. 1983.
Zeisel SH, M-H Mar, JC Howe, JM Holden. Concentrations of choline-containing compounds and betaine in common foods. *J Nutr* 133:1302–1307, 2003.

Vitamins/Vitamin-Like Components—Myo-Inositol

	MYO-INOSITOL (mg/100 g)	SOURCE		MYO-INOSITOL (mg/100 g)	SOURCE
BEVERAGES			**CHEESE**		
cocoa mix, inst	31	Clements and Darnell, 1980	cheese, american	7	Clements and Darnell, 1980
coffee, brewed	5	Clements and Darnell, 1980	cheese, cheddar	9	Clements and Darnell, 1980
coffee, inst powder	646	Clements and Darnell, 1980	cheese, cottage, creamed	2	Clements and Darnell, 1980
cola	0	Clements and Darnell, 1980	cheese, cottage, lowfat	1	Clements and Darnell, 1980
Diet Pepsi	1	Clements and Darnell, 1980	cheese, cream	7	Clements and Darnell, 1980
fruit punch, cnd	17	Clements and Darnell, 1980	cheese, mozzarella	5	Clements and Darnell, 1980
ginger ale	<1	Clements and Darnell, 1980	cheese, muenster	3	Clements and Darnell, 1980
grapefruit soda	1	Clements and Darnell, 1980	cheese, parmesan	6	Clements and Darnell, 1980
Kool-Aid powder	<1	Clements and Darnell, 1980	cheese, swiss	5	Clements and Darnell, 1980
lemonade	2	Clements and Darnell, 1980	**CREAMS**		
orange soda, Shasta	1	Clements and Darnell, 1980	cream, sour	76	Clements and Darnell, 1980
raspberry soda	0	Clements and Darnell, 1980	**DESSERTS**		
Seven-Up	0	Clements and Darnell, 1980	cake, angel food	2	Clements and Darnell, 1980
tea, brewed	3	Clements and Darnell, 1980	cake, choc	18	Clements and Darnell, 1980
			cake, lemon	19	Clements and Darnell, 1980
CEREALS & GRAINS, COOKED			cake, strawberry shortcake	69	Clements and Darnell, 1980
barley, ckd	3	Clements and Darnell, 1980	cake, yellow w/sugar icing	5	Clements and Darnell, 1980
corn grits, ckd	10	Clements and Darnell, 1980	cobbler, cherry	30	Clements and Darnell, 1980
cream of wheat, ckd	7	Clements and Darnell, 1980	cookies, graham crackers	10	Clements and Darnell, 1980
oatmeal, regular, ckd	42	Clements and Darnell, 1980	cookies, sugar	34	Clements and Darnell, 1980
oatmeal, quick, ckd	34	Clements and Darnell, 1980	cookies, van wafers	23	Clements and Darnell, 1980
rice, brown, ckd	30	Clements and Darnell, 1980	gelatin dessert	7	Clements and Darnell, 1980
rice, white, ckd	15	Clements and Darnell, 1980	ice cream, van	9	Clements and Darnell, 1980
rice, white, inst, ckd	2	Clements and Darnell, 1980	pie, apple	22	Clements and Darnell, 1980
rice, wild, ckd	27	Clements and Darnell, 1980	pie, choc cream	52	Clements and Darnell, 1980
			pie, lemon	63	Clements and Darnell, 1980
			pie, pecan	64	Clements and Darnell, 1980
CEREALS, READY-TO-EAT			pie, sweet potato	20	Clements and Darnell, 1980
bran flakes, 40%	274	Clements and Darnell, 1980	pudding, cranberry	1	Clements and Darnell, 1980
corn flakes	6	Clements and Darnell, 1980	pudding, lemon	<1	Clements and Darnell, 1980
Cracklin Bran	67	Clements and Darnell, 1980	sherbet	7	Clements and Darnell, 1980
puffed rice	5	Clements and Darnell, 1980	**EGGS**		
puffed wheat	8	Clements and Darnell, 1980	egg, scrambled	8	Clements and Darnell, 1980
raisin bran	107	Clements and Darnell, 1980	egg, white	5	Clements and Darnell, 1980
shredded wheat	35	Clements and Darnell, 1980			
Team Flakes	93	Clements and Darnell, 1980			

	MYO-INOSITOL (mg/100 g)	SOURCE		MYO-INOSITOL (mg/100 g)	SOURCE
egg whole	9	Clements and Darnell, 1980	honeydew melon, raw	46	Clements and Darnell, 1980
egg yolk	34	Clements and Darnell, 1980	kiwifruit, raw	136	Clements and Darnell, 1980
			lemon peel, raw	33	Clements and Darnell, 1980
FISH & SHELLFISH			lemon peel, raw, calif	216	Ranganna et al, 1983
clams	3	Clements and Darnell, 1980	lemon, raw, calif	109	Ranganna et al, 1983
crab	5	Clements and Darnell, 1980	lime, raw	194	Clements and Darnell, 1980
oysters	25	Clements and Darnell, 1980	mandarin oranges, cnd	149	Clements and Darnell, 1980
sardines, cnd	12	Clements and Darnell, 1980	mango, raw	99	Clements and Darnell, 1980
sardines/herring, cnd in oil	20	Clements and Darnell, 1980	nectarine, raw	118	Clements and Darnell, 1980
shrimp, broiled	7	Clements and Darnell, 1980	orange peel, raw, Valencia	257	Ranganna et al, 1983
trout, broiled	11	Clements and Darnell, 1980	orange, raw	307	Clements and Darnell, 1980
tuna, chunk light, cnd in water	9	Clements and Darnell, 1980	orange, raw, Valencia	204	Ranganna et al, 1983
tuna, cnd in oil	11	Clements and Darnell, 1980	papaya, raw	8	Clements and Darnell, 1980
tuna, cnd in water	15	Clements and Darnell, 1980	peach, cling, cnd, water pack	34	Clements and Darnell, 1980
tuna salad	12	Clements and Darnell, 1980	peach, cling, raw	19	Clements and Darnell, 1980
whitefish, broiled	2	Clements and Darnell, 1980	peach, dried	164	Clements and Darnell, 1980
			peach, freestone, raw	58	Clements and Darnell, 1980
FRUIT JUICES			pear, bartlett, cnd, water pack	46	Clements and Darnell, 1980
apple jce, cnd	21	Clements and Darnell, 1980	pear, raw	73	Clements and Darnell, 1980
apple jce, from frzn conc	33	Clements and Darnell, 1980	pineapple, cnd, water pack	16	Clements and Darnell, 1980
apricot nectar, cnd	26	Clements and Darnell, 1980	pineapple, raw	33	Clements and Darnell, 1980
cranapple jce, cnd	1	Clements and Darnell, 1980	plum, purple, raw	11	Clements and Darnell, 1980
cranberry jce cocktail, cnd	7	Clements and Darnell, 1980	plum, red, raw	30	Clements and Darnell, 1980
grapefruit jce, cnd	41	Clements and Darnell, 1980	plum, yellow, raw	<1	Clements and Darnell, 1980
grapefruit jce, from frzn conc	380	Clements and Darnell, 1980	prune, dried	470	Clements and Darnell, 1980
grapefruit jce, squeezed from fruit	88–150	Ranganna et al, 1983	raisins, dried	20	Clements and Darnell, 1980
grape jce, from frzn conc	36	Clements and Darnell, 1980	strawberries, raw	13	Clements and Darnell, 1980
lemon jce, cnd	73	Clements and Darnell, 1980	watermelon, raw	31	Clements and Darnell, 1980
lemon jce, squeezed from fruit	30	Clements and Darnell, 1980			
lemon jce, squeezed from fruit, calif	66	Ranganna et al, 1983	**GRAIN PRODUCTS & SNACKS**		
orange jce, cnd	200	Clements and Darnell, 1980	biscuit	31	Clements and Darnell, 1980
orange jce, from frzn conc	204	Clements and Darnell, 1980	bread, bran, Orowheat	81	Clements and Darnell, 1980
orange jce, squeezed from fruit	35	Clements and Darnell, 1980	bread, French	34	Clements and Darnell, 1980
orange jce, squeezed from fruit, navel	156	Ranganna et al, 1983	bread, mixed whole grain	47	Clements and Darnell, 1980
			bread, pumpernickel	160	Clements and Darnell, 1980
orange jce, squeezed from fruit, valencia	159	Ranganna et al, 1983	bread, Roman Meal	38	Clements and Darnell, 1980
			bread, rye	47	Clements and Darnell, 1980
peach nectar, cnd	1	Clements and Darnell, 1980	bread, rye, cocktail	39	Clements and Darnell, 1980
pineapple jce, cnd	15	Clements and Darnell, 1980	bread, wheat, stone ground	115	Clements and Darnell, 1980
prune jce, cnd	26	Clements and Darnell, 1980	bread, wheat, whole	142	Clements and Darnell, 1980
tangerine jce, squeezed from fruit	135	Ranganna et al, 1983	bread, white	26	Clements and Darnell, 1980
			cornbread	14	Clements and Darnell, 1980
FRUITS			cornbread stuffing	8	Clements and Darnell, 1980
apple, dried, ckd	9	Clements and Darnell, 1980	crackers, Escort	5	Clements and Darnell, 1980
apple, red, delicious, raw	10	Clements and Darnell, 1980	crackers, Cheese Nibs	246	Clements and Darnell, 1980
applesauce, cnd	18	Clements and Darnell, 1980	crackers, Saltines	47	Clements and Darnell, 1980
apple, rome, raw	15	Clements and Darnell, 1980	crackers, soda, salt-free	13	Clements and Darnell, 1980
apple, yellow, delicious, raw	24	Clements and Darnell, 1980	crackers, Wheat Thins	89	Clements and Darnell, 1980
apricot halves, cnd, water pack	52	Clements and Darnell, 1980	french toast made w/egg	8	Clements and Darnell, 1980
blackberries, cnd, water pack	173	Clements and Darnell, 1980	macaroni, ckd	5	Clements and Darnell, 1980
cantaloupe, raw	355	Clements and Darnell, 1980	melba toast	59	Clements and Darnell, 1980
cherries, dark, cnd, water pack	127	Clements and Darnell, 1980	muffin	15	Clements and Darnell, 1980
cherries, black bing, cnd, water pack	59	Clements and Darnell, 1980	noodles, egg, ckd	18	Clements and Darnell, 1980
cherries, red, cnd, water pack	5	Clements and Darnell, 1980	pancake	23	Clements and Darnell, 1980
cherries, red, raw	14	Clements and Darnell, 1980	popcorn, popped	107	Clements and Darnell, 1980
cherries, royal ann, raw	4	Clements and Darnell, 1980	potato chips	73	Clements and Darnell, 1980
cranberries, raw	15	Clements and Darnell, 1980	potato chips, formed, cnd	58	Clements and Darnell, 1980
cranberry sce, cnd	2	Clements and Darnell, 1980	roll, dinner	23	Clements and Darnell, 1980
dates, dried	152	Clements and Darnell, 1980	roll, hamburger	478	Clements and Darnell, 1980
figs, calmyina, dried	91	Clements and Darnell, 1980	roll, hot dog	115	Clements and Darnell, 1980
fruit cocktail, cnd	19	Clements and Darnell, 1980	spaghetti, ckd	31	Clements and Darnell, 1980
grapefruit, raw	199	Clements and Darnell, 1980	waffle	22	Clements and Darnell, 1980
grapefruit sections, cnd	117	Clements and Darnell, 1980			
grapes, green, cnd	7	Clements and Darnell, 1980	**MEATS**		
grapes, green, raw	16	Clements and Darnell, 1980	beef, corned	39	Clements and Darnell, 1980
grapes, purple, raw	15	Clements and Darnell, 1980	beef, hamburger, broiled	8	Clements and Darnell, 1980
			beef liver	64	Clements and Darnell, 1980
			beef, meatloaf	30	Clements and Darnell, 1980

	MYO-INOSITOL (mg/100 g)	SOURCE
beef roast, choice	15	Clements and Darnell, 1980
beef, round, ground, broiled	37	Clements and Darnell, 1980
beef, round steak	15	Clements and Darnell, 1980
beef, sirloin steak	30	Clements and Darnell, 1980
beef tips, braised	7	Clements and Darnell, 1980
lamb chop	37	Clements and Darnell, 1980
pork bacon	23	Clements and Darnell, 1980
pork chop, baked	6	Clements and Darnell, 1980
pork chop, bbq	42	Clements and Darnell, 1980
pork chop, broiled	14	Clements and Darnell, 1980
pork liver	17	Clements and Darnell, 1980
pork roast	30	Clements and Darnell, 1980

MEATS, LUNCHEON

	MYO-INOSITOL (mg/100 g)	SOURCE
beef, corned	19	Clements and Darnell, 1980
bologna	94	Clements and Darnell, 1980
frankfurter	16	Clements and Darnell, 1980
ham, deviled, cnd	4	Clements and Darnell, 1980
ham, spiced	6	Clements and Darnell, 1980
liver cheese	346	Clements and Darnell, 1980
liver loaf	22	Clements and Darnell, 1980
luncheon loaf, spiced	39	Clements and Darnell, 1980
lunch meat, cnd	18	Clements and Darnell, 1980
pastrami	28	Clements and Darnell, 1980
salami	42	Clements and Darnell, 1980
souse	54	Clements and Darnell, 1980
vienna sausage	81	Clements and Darnell, 1980

MILK & YOGURT

	MYO-INOSITOL (mg/100 g)	SOURCE
buttermilk, cultured	1	Clements and Darnell, 1980
milk, choc, lowfat	19	Clements and Darnell, 1980
milk, cond, sweetened	26	Clements and Darnell, 1980
milk, nonfat	4	Clements and Darnell, 1980
milk, whole, 4% fat	4	Clements and Darnell, 1980
yogurt, boysenberry	7	Clements and Darnell, 1980
yogurt, coffee	9	Clements and Darnell, 1980
yogurt, plain	6	Clements and Darnell, 1980
yogurt, raspberry	16	Clements and Darnell, 1980
yogurt, strawberry	16	Clements and Darnell, 1980
yogurt, van	9	Clements and Darnell, 1980

NUTS & SEEDS

	MYO-INOSITOL (mg/100 g)	SOURCE
almonds	278	Clements and Darnell, 1980
cashews	81	Clements and Darnell, 1980
coconut, grated	33	Clements and Darnell, 1980
peanut butter, chunky	128	Clements and Darnell, 1980
peanut butter, creamy	304	Clements and Darnell, 1980
peanuts, ckd	134	Clements and Darnell, 1980
peanuts, raw	133	Clements and Darnell, 1980
sunflower seeds	12	Clements and Darnell, 1980
walnuts	198	Clements and Darnell, 1980

POULTRY

	MYO-INOSITOL (mg/100 g)	SOURCE
chicken, baked	8	Clements and Darnell, 1980
chicken breast	30	Clements and Darnell, 1980
chicken leg, baked	39	Clements and Darnell, 1980
chicken liver	131	Clements and Darnell, 1980
turkey, baked	23	Clements and Darnell, 1980
turkey breast	8	Clements and Darnell, 1980

SALAD DRESSINGS

	MYO-INOSITOL (mg/100 g)	SOURCE
blue cheese	8	Clements and Darnell, 1980
french	7	Clements and Darnell, 1980
low cal, blue cheese (2 brands)	4/40	Clements and Darnell, 1980
low cal, french	8	Clements and Darnell, 1980
low cal, thousand island	8	Clements and Darnell, 1980
oil & vinegar	4	Clements and Darnell, 1980
thousand island	50	Clements and Darnell, 1980

SAUCES & CONDIMENTS

	MYO-INOSITOL (mg/100 g)	SOURCE
catsup	38	Clements and Darnell, 1980
hot sce	25	Clements and Darnell, 1980
olives, black	10	Clements and Darnell, 1980
olives, manzanilla	6	Clements and Darnell, 1980
olives, spanish	2	Clements and Darnell, 1980
pickles, cucumber	30	Clements and Darnell, 1980

SOUPS

	MYO-INOSITOL (mg/100 g)	SOURCE
bouillon cube	41	Clements and Darnell, 1980

SPREADS

	MYO-INOSITOL (mg/100 g)	SOURCE
mayonnaise	4	Clements and Darnell, 1980
mayonnaise, low cal	5	Clements and Darnell, 1980

SWEETENERS

	MYO-INOSITOL (mg/100 g)	SOURCE
honey	33	Clements and Darnell, 1980
syrup, pancake	1	Clements and Darnell, 1980
syrup, table	<1	Clements and Darnell, 1980

VEGETABLES

	MYO-INOSITOL (mg/100 g)	SOURCE
artichoke heart, cnd	116	Clements and Darnell, 1980
artichoke, frzn	80	Clements and Darnell, 1980
artichoke, raw	60	Clements and Darnell, 1980
asparagus, green, frzn	15	Clements and Darnell, 1980
asparagus, green, raw	29	Clements and Darnell, 1980
asparagus, green, spears, cnd	28	Clements and Darnell, 1980
asparagus, white, cnd	38	Clements and Darnell, 1980
avocado, raw	46	Clements and Darnell, 1980
beans, baked w/pork, cnd	86	Clements and Darnell, 1980
beet, cnd	20	Clements and Darnell, 1980
beet, raw	12	Clements and Darnell, 1980
beet, whole small, cnd	8	Clements and Darnell, 1980
broccoli, frzn	11	Clements and Darnell, 1980
broccoli, raw	30	Clements and Darnell, 1980
brussels sprouts, frzn	81	Clements and Darnell, 1980
butter beans, cnd	48	Clements and Darnell, 1980
cabbage, purple, raw	9	Clements and Darnell, 1980
cabbage, savory, raw	70	Clements and Darnell, 1980
cabbage, white, raw	21	Clements and Darnell, 1980
carrot, cnd	52	Clements and Darnell, 1980
carrot, frzn	10	Clements and Darnell, 1980
carrot jce, cnd	1	Clements and Darnell, 1980
carrot, raw	12	Clements and Darnell, 1980
cauliflower, frzn	15	Clements and Darnell, 1980
cauliflower, raw	18	Clements and Darnell, 1980
celery, raw	5	Clements and Darnell, 1980
chinese cabbage, raw	27	Clements and Darnell, 1980
collard greens, cnd	30	Clements and Darnell, 1980
collard greens, frzn	16	Clements and Darnell, 1980
collard greens, raw	64	Clements and Darnell, 1980
corn, white, creamed, cnd	7	Clements and Darnell, 1980
corn, yellow, cnd	24	Clements and Darnell, 1980
corn, yellow, frzn	11	Clements and Darnell, 1980
corn, yellow, creamed, cnd	20	Clements and Darnell, 1980
corn, yellow, creamed, frzn	13	Clements and Darnell, 1980
cowpeas (blackeyed peas), cnd	117	Clements and Darnell, 1980
cowpeas (blackeyed peas), dry	39	Clements and Darnell, 1980
cowpeas (blackeyed peas), raw	116	Clements and Darnell, 1980
crowder peas, frzn	70	Clements and Darnell, 1980
cucumber, raw	15	Clements and Darnell, 1980
eggplant, cnd/raw	84	Clements and Darnell, 1980
eggplant, frzn	44	Clements and Darnell, 1980
endive, raw	11	Clements and Darnell, 1980
great northern beans, cnd	440	Clements and Darnell, 1980
great northern beans, dry	327	Clements and Darnell, 1980
great northern beans, raw	124	Clements and Darnell, 1980
green beans, cnd	51	Clements and Darnell, 1980

	MYO-INOSITOL (mg/100 g)	SOURCE		MYO-INOSITOL (mg/100 g)	SOURCE
green beans, french style, cnd	87	Clements and Darnell, 1980	peas, green, raw	40	Clements and Darnell, 1980
green beans, french style, frzn	55	Clements and Darnell, 1980	peas, purple hull, cnd	98	Clements and Darnell, 1980
green beans, frzn	55	Clements and Darnell, 1980	peas, purple hull, raw	38	Clements and Darnell, 1980
green beans, italian, cnd	35	Clements and Darnell, 1980	peas, split, dry	128	Clements and Darnell, 1980
green beans, pole, frzn	175	Clements and Darnell, 1980	peas, split soup	17	Clements and Darnell, 1980
green beans, raw	105	Clements and Darnell, 1980	pepper, banana, raw	135	Clements and Darnell, 1980
green beans, snap, frzn	49	Clements and Darnell, 1980	pepper, green, bell, frzn	29	Clements and Darnell, 1980
green beans, shelled, raw	193	Clements and Darnell, 1980	pepper, green, bell, raw	57	Clements and Darnell, 1980
hominy, white, cnd	43	Clements and Darnell, 1980	pepper, hot, raw	59	Clements and Darnell, 1980
hominy, yellow, cnd	17	Clements and Darnell, 1980	pepper, jalapeno, cnd	30	Clements and Darnell, 1980
kidney beans, dark red, cnd	249	Clements and Darnell, 1980	pinto beans, cnd	23	Clements and Darnell, 1980
kidney beans, light red, cnd	69	Clements and Darnell, 1980	poke greens, raw	43	Clements and Darnell, 1980
kidney beans, light red, dry	60	Clements and Darnell, 1980	potato, white, au gratin	24	Clements and Darnell, 1980
lentils, dry	45	Clements and Darnell, 1980	potato, white, baked	97	Clements and Darnell, 1980
lettuce, red leaf	22	Clements and Darnell, 1980	potato, white, cnd	47	Clements and Darnell, 1980
lettuce, tossed	18	Clements and Darnell, 1980	potato, white, hash brown	57	Clements and Darnell, 1980
lima beans, baby, green, frzn	42	Clements and Darnell, 1980	potato, white, mashed, from inst	30	Clements and Darnell, 1980
lima beans, green, cnd	146	Clements and Darnell, 1980	potato, white, mashed, homemade	19	Clements and Darnell, 1980
lima beans, green, frzn	48	Clements and Darnell, 1980	pumpkin, cnd	62	Clements and Darnell, 1980
lima beans, green, large, cnd	35	Clements and Darnell, 1980	radish, red, raw	10	Clements and Darnell, 1980
lima beans, green, small, cnd	110	Clements and Darnell, 1980	rutabaga, cnd	252	Clements and Darnell, 1980
lima beans, large, cnd	23	Clements and Darnell, 1980	rutabaga, raw	24	Clements and Darnell, 1980
lima beans, large, dry	33	Clements and Darnell, 1980	romaine, raw	17	Clements and Darnell, 1980
lima beans, small, dry	56	Clements and Darnell, 1980	sauerkraut, cnd	11	Clements and Darnell, 1980
lima beans, speckled, dry	70	Clements and Darnell, 1980	soybeans, dry	88	Clements and Darnell, 1980
lima beans, speckled, frzn	55	Clements and Darnell, 1980	spinach, cnd	25	Clements and Darnell, 1980
mixed vegetables, cnd	5	Clements and Darnell, 1980	spinach, frzn	6	Clements and Darnell, 1980
mixed vegetables, frzn	13	Clements and Darnell, 1980	spinach, raw	8	Clements and Darnell, 1980
mushrooms, raw	9	Clements and Darnell, 1980	squash, acorn, frzn	66	Clements and Darnell, 1980
mushrooms, sliced, cnd	29	Clements and Darnell, 1980	squash, acorn, raw	22	Clements and Darnell, 1980
mushrooms, stems & pieces, cnd	24	Clements and Darnell, 1980	squash, green, raw	17	Clements and Darnell, 1980
mustard greens, cnd	9	Clements and Darnell, 1980	squash, hubbard, raw	66	Clements and Darnell, 1980
mustard greens, frzn	17	Clements and Darnell, 1980	squash, yellow, frzn	25	Clements and Darnell, 1980
mustard greens, raw	23	Clements and Darnell, 1980	squash, yellow, cnd	6	Clements and Darnell, 1980
navy beans, cnd	65	Clements and Darnell, 1980	squash, yellow, raw	32	Clements and Darnell, 1980
navy beans, dry	283	Clements and Darnell, 1980	squash, zucchini, raw	53	Clements and Darnell, 1980
okra, cnd	117	Clements and Darnell, 1980	sweet potato, baked	92	Clements and Darnell, 1980
okra, fried	37	Clements and Darnell, 1980	tomato, cherry, raw	41	Clements and Darnell, 1980
okra, frzn	28	Clements and Darnell, 1980	tomato, chopped, cnd	34	Clements and Darnell, 1980
okra, raw	33	Clements and Darnell, 1980	tomato jce, cnd	48	Clements and Darnell, 1980
onion, green, raw	27	Clements and Darnell, 1980	tomato paste	51	Clements and Darnell, 1980
onion, purple, raw	41	Clements and Darnell, 1980	tomato puree	77	Clements and Darnell, 1980
onion, white, ckd	24	Clements and Darnell, 1980	tomato, raw	54	Clements and Darnell, 1980
onion, white, raw	23	Clements and Darnell, 1980	tomato sce	81	Clements and Darnell, 1980
onion, yellow, ckd	16	Clements and Darnell, 1980	tomato soup	7	Clements and Darnell, 1980
onion, yellow, raw	44	Clements and Darnell, 1980	tomato, whole, cnd	38	Clements and Darnell, 1980
parsley, raw	22	Clements and Darnell, 1980	turnip greens & root, cnd	8	Clements and Darnell, 1980
peas & carrots, frzn	99	Clements and Darnell, 1980	turnip greens, chopped, frzn	8	Clements and Darnell, 1980
peas, field, cnd	48	Clements and Darnell, 1980	turnip greens, cnd	12	Clements and Darnell, 1980
peas, field, frzn	68	Clements and Darnell, 1980	turnip greens, raw	43	Clements and Darnell, 1980
peas, green, large, cnd	235	Clements and Darnell, 1980	V8 Juice, Campbell	29	Clements and Darnell, 1980
peas, green, large, frzn	95	Clements and Darnell, 1980	vegetable soup, cnd/homemade	6	Clements and Darnell, 1980
peas, green, small, cnd	76	Clements and Darnell, 1980	wax beans, cnd	144	Clements and Darnell, 1980
peas, green, small, frzn	85	Clements and Darnell, 1980			

Sources:
Clements RS, B Darnell. Myo-inositol content of common foods: development of a high-myo-inositol diet. *Am J Clin Nutr* 33:1954–1967, 1980.
Ranganna S, VS Govindarajan, KVR Ramana. Citrus fruits–Varieties, chemistry, technology, and quality evaluation. Part II. Chemistry, technology, and quality evaluation. A. Chemistry. *Critical Reviews in Food Science and Nutrition.* Vol 18, issue 4. CRC Press, Boca Raton FL. 1983.

Vitamins/Vitamin-Like Components—Vitamin D₃ (measured in IU)[1]

	SERVING SIZE	VITAMIN D (IU/SERVING)	VITAMIN D (IU/100 g)	SOURCE/ USDA CODE
BEVERAGES				
Smoothies, avg for 4 flavors, Tropicana	11.5 fl oz (345 g)	60	17	TROP
Pulse, women's health formula	16.9 fl oz bottle (~507 g)	400	79	PULS
CANDY				
candy chips, yogurt	3.5 oz (100 g)	49	49	19079
caramel, choc flavored roll	2.25 oz bar (64 g)	11	17	19076
fudge, homemade, choc	.6 oz piece (17 g)	3	16	19100
fudge, homemade, choc w/nuts	.67 oz piece (19 g)	3	14	19101
fudge, homemade, van	.56 oz piece (16 g)	2	15	19103
peanut brittle	1 oz (28 g)	1	3	19148
Snickers, M&M/Mars	2 oz bar (57 g)	0	0	19155
CEREALS				
Alpha-Bits, frosted, Post	1 cup (32 g)	40	125	08325
Alpha-Bits, marshmallow, Post	1 cup (29 g)	40	138	08326
Apple Jacks, Kellogg's	1 cup (30 g)	38	127	08003
Banana Nut Crunch, Post	1 cup (59 g)	40	68	08320
Basic 4, General Mills	1 cup (55 g)	31	57	08262
Blueberry Morning, Post	1 1/4 cups (55 g)	40	73	08321
bran, All-Bran Buds	1/3 cup (30 g)	40	133	08005
bran, All-Bran, Kellogg's	1/2 cup (31 g)	53	170	08001
bran, All-Bran w/extra fiber	1/2 cup (26 g)	55	210	08253
Bran Flakes, Post	3/4 cup (30 g)	40	133	08322
Cheerios, apple cinn, General Mills	3/4 cup (30 g)	40	133	08263
Cheerios, Frosted, General Mills	1 cup (30 g)	40	133	08267
Cheerios, General Mills	1 cup (30 g)	40	133	08013
Cheerios, honey nut, General Mills	1 cup (30 g)	40	133	08045
Cheerios, multi-grain, General Mills	1 cup (30 g)	38	126	08087
Chex, multi-bran, General Mills	1 cup (49 g)	36	73	08345
Chex, rice, General Mills	1 1/4 cups (31 g)	41	133	08064
Chex, wheat, General Mills	1 cup (30 g)	24	80	08082
Cinn Grahams, General Mills	3/4 cup (30 g)	40	133	08139
Cinn Toast Crunch, General Mills	3/4 cup (30 g)	40	133	08272
Cocoa Krispies, Kellogg's	3/4 cup (31 g)	40	130	08014
Cocoa Pebbles, Post	3/4 cup (29 g)	40	138	08323
Cookie Crisp, choc chip/van, Gen Mills	1 cup (30 g)	40	133	08017
Corn Flakes, Country, General Mills	1 cup (30 g)	40	133	08269
Corn Flakes, Kellogg's	1 cup (28 g)	43	152	08020
Corn Flakes, Post Toasties	1 cup (28 g)	40	143	08338
Corn Pops, Kellogg's	1 cup (31 g)	50	162	08068
Cracklin' Oat Bran, Kellogg's	3/4 cup (55 g)	45	82	08023
Cranberry Macadamia Nut, Quaker	1 cup (60 g)	26	43	08400
Crispix, Kellogg's	1 cup (29 g)	40	138	08259
Crispy Rice, Malt-O-Meal	1 cup (33 g)	40	121	08348
Crispy Wheaties 'n Raisins, Gen Mills	1 cup (55 g)	40	73	08026
French Toast Crunch, General Mills	3/4 cup (30 g)	40	133	08086
Froot Loops, Kellogg's	1 cup (30 g)	38	125	08030
Frosted Flakes, Kellogg's	3/4 cup (31 g)	40	129	08069
Frosted Krispies, Kellogg's	3/4 cup (30 g)	42	140	08032
Fruit & Fibre (dates, raisins, walnuts), Post	1 cup (55 g)	40	73	08327
Fruity Pebbles, Post	3/4 cup (27 g)	40	148	08324
Golden Crisp, Post	3/4 cup (27 g)	40	148	08328
Golden Grahams, General Mills	3/4 cup (30 g)	40	133	08035
Granola, low fat, Kellogg's	1/2 cup (49 g)	40	82	08189
Granola, low fat w/raisins, Kellogg's	3/5 cup (60 g)	40	67	08284
Grape Nuts Flakes, Post	3/4 cup (29 g)	40	138	08330
Grape Nuts, Post	1/2 cup (58 g)	40	69	08329
Great Grains, crunchy pecan, Post	3/5 cup (53 g)	40	75	08331
Great Grains, raisin, date, & pecan, Post	3/5 cup (54 g)	40	74	08332
Honey Bunches of Oats, almond, Post	3/4 cup (31 g)	40	129	08334
Honey Bunches of Oats, hny rstd, Post	3/4 cup (30 g)	40	133	08333
Honey Crunch Corn Flakes, Kellogg's	3/4 cup (30 g)	42	140	08309

	SERVING SIZE	VITAMIN D (IU/SERVING)	VITAMIN D (IU/100 g)	SOURCE/ USDA CODE
Honeycomb, Post	1 1/3 cups (29 g)	40	138	08335
Just Right, fruit & nut, Kellogg's	1 cup (60 g)	50	83	08283
Kaboom, General Mills	1 1/4 cups (30 g)	40	133	08278
King Vitaman, Quaker	1 1/2 cups (31 g)	41	133	08047
Kix, berry berry, General Mills	3/4 cup (30 g)	40	133	08274
Kix, General Mills	1 1/3 cups (30 g)	42	141	08048
Lucky Charms, General Mills	1 cup (30 g)	40	133	08050
Marshmallow Mateys, Malt-O-Meal	1 cup (30 g)	40	133	08138
Mueslix, raisin & almond crunch w/dates, Kellogg's	3/5 cup (55 g)	16	29	08286
Natural Cereal, 100% w/oats & honey, Quaker	1/2 cup (51 g)	0	0	08054
Natural Cereal, 100% w/oats, honey, & raisins, Quaker	1/2 cup (51 g)	0	0	08218
Nutrition for Women, golden brown sugar, inst dry, Quaker	1.6 oz pkt (46 g)	140	304	QUAK
Oat Bran Flakes, Common Sense, Kellogg's	3/4 cup (30 g)	42	140	08258
Oreo O's, Post	3/4 cup (27 g)	40	148	08336
Product 19, Kellogg's	1 cup (30 g)	39	131	08058
Raisin Bran Crunch, Kellogg	1 cup (53 g)	40	75	08380
Raisin Bran, Kellogg's	1 cup (59 g)	40	68	08060
Raisin Bran, Post	1 cup (59 g)	40	68	08337
Reese's Peanut Butter Puffs, Gen Mills	3/4 cup (30 g)	40	133	08194
Rice Krispies, Kellogg's	1 1/4 cups (33 g)	41	124	08065
Rice Krispies Treats, Kellogg's	3/4 cup (30 g)	41	135	08288
Smacks, Kellogg's	3/4 cup (27 g)	40	148	08071
Smart Start, Kellogg's	1 cup (50 g)	43	85	08318
Toasty O's, Malt-O-Meal	1 cup (30 g)	40	133	08350
Tootie Fruities, Malt-O-Meal	1 cup (32 g)	40	125	08349
Total, corn, General Mills	1 1/3 cups (30 g)	34	114	08246
Total, General Mills	3/4 cup (30 g)	40	133	08077
Total, raisin bran, General Mills	1 cup (55 g)	40	73	08247
Trix, General Mills	1 cup (30 g)	40	133	08078
Waffle Crisp, Post	1 cup (30 g)	40	133	08344
Wheat Bran Flakes, Kellogg's Complete	3/4 cup (29 g)	40	138	08028
Wheaties, General Mills	1 cup (30 g)	40	133	08089
Wheaties, honey frosted, General Mills	3/4 cup (30 g)	40	133	08266

CHEESE

camembert	1 oz (28 g)	3	12	01007
cheddar	1 oz (28 g)	3	12	01009
cheddar, shredded	1 cup shredded (113 g)	14	12	01009
edam	1 oz (28 g)	10	36	01018
parmesan, hard	1 oz (28 g)	8	28	01033
swiss	1 oz (28 g)	12	44	01040

CREAM

whipping cream, heavy fluid	1 T (15 g)	8	52	01053

DESSERTS

ice cream, van, rich (16% fat)	1/2 cup (107 g)	23	21	19089
pudding, banana, from inst mix w/2% milk	1/2 cup (147 g)	49	33	19121
pudding, banana, from reg mix w/2% milk	1/2 cup (140 g)	49	35	19122
pudding, choc, from inst mix w/lowfat milk	1/2 cup (147 g)	49	33	19123
pudding, flan/crème caramel, from mix, w/2% milk	1/2 cup (133 g)	48	36	19231
pudding, flan/crème caramel, from mix, w/whole milk	1/2 cup (133 g)	48	36	19232
pudding, lemon, from inst mix w/2% milk	1/2 cup (147 g)	49	33	19204
pudding, rennin dessert, choc, from mix w/2% milk	1/2 cup (136 g)	49	36	19213
pudding, rennin dessert, choc, from mix w/whole milk	1/2 cup (136 g)	49	36	19221
pudding, rennin dessert, van, from mix w/2% milk	1/2 cup (133 g)	49	37	19214
pudding, rennin dessert, van, from mix w/whole milk	1/2 cup (133 g)	49	37	19223
pudding, rice, from reg mix w/2% milk	1/2 cup (144 g)	48	34	19208
pudding, rice, from reg mix w/whole milk	1/2 cup (144 g)	48	34	19195
pudding, tapioca, from reg mix w/2% milk	1/2 cup (141 g)	48	34	19209
pudding, tapioca, from reg mix w/whole milk	1/2 cup (141 g)	48	34	19199
pudding, van, from reg mix w/2% milk	1/2 cup (140 g)	49	35	19212

EGGS & EGG SUBSTITUTES

chicken egg whole, raw	1 large egg (50 g)	26	52	01123
chicken egg, yolk, raw	1 large egg yolk (17 g)	25	148	01125
egg substitute, Better'n Eggs, Papetti Foods	1/4 cup (56 g)	24	43	PPTT

	SERVING SIZE	VITAMIN D (IU/SERVING)	VITAMIN D (IU/100 g)	SOURCE/ USDA CODE
egg substitute, Egg Beaters	1/4 cup (61 g)	16	26	EGBT
egg substitute, garden vegetable, Egg Beaters	1/4 cup (61 g)	24	39	EGBT
egg substitute, southwestern, Egg Beaters	1/4 cup (61 g)	24	39	EGBT
FAST FOODS				
eggs, scrambled	2 eggs (94 g)	64	68	21018
english muffin w/egg, cheese, & canadian bacon	1 muffin sandwich (137 g)	44	32	21021
fish sandwich w/tartar sce & cheese	1 sandwich (183 g)	37	20	21106
hamburger, reg, double meat	1 sandwich (176 g)	28	16	21110
hamburger, reg, single meat	1 sandwich (90 g)	11	12	21107
ice milk, van, soft serve w/cone	1 cone (103 g)	8	8	21028
shake, choc	10 fl oz (208 g)	33	16	14346
shake, strawberry	10 fl oz (283 g)	23	8	14428
shake, van	10 fl oz (208 g)	17	8	14347
sundae, caramel	1 sundae (155 g)	12	8	21032
sundae, hot fudge	1 sundae (158 g)	19	12	21033
sundae, strawberry	1 sundae (153 g)	18	12	21034
shake, chocolate	12 fl oz (250 g)	40	16	14346
shake, chocolate	16 fl oz (333 g)	53	16	14346
shake, chocolate	22 fl oz (458 g)	73	16	14346
shake, van	12 fl oz (250 g)	20	8	14347
shake, van	16 fl oz (333 g)	27	8	14347
shake, van	22 fl oz (458 g)	37	8	14347
FATS & OILS				
cod liver oil	1 T (14 g)	1360	10,000	04589
sardine oil	1 T (14 g)	45	332	04594
butter	1 T (14 g)	8	56	01001
FISH & SHELLFISH				
catfish, channel, wild, raw	3 oz (85 g)	425	500	15010
caviar, black & red, granular	1 T (16 g)	37	232	15012
clams, raw	3 oz (85 g)	3	4	15157
cod, atlantic, cnd	3 oz (85 g)	71	84	15017
cod, atlantic, raw	3 oz (85 g)	37	44	15015
flounder/sole (flatfish), raw	3 oz (85 g)	51	60	15028
halibut, greenland, raw	3 oz (85 g)	510	600	15038
herring, atlantic, kippered	1 piece (5″ × 1 3/4″ × 1/4″) (40 g)	48	120	15042
herring, atlantic, pickled	1 piece (1 3/4″ × 7/8″ × 1/2″) (15 g)	102	680	15041
herring, atlantic, raw	3 oz (85 g)	1384	1628	15039
mackerel, atlantic, raw	3 oz (85 g)	306	360	15046
mackerel, jack, cnd	1 cup (190 g)	479	252	15048
oysters, eastern, wild, raw	6 med (84 g)	269	320	15167
salmon, chum, cnd w/bone	3 oz (85 g)	190	224	15080
salmon, pink, cnd w/bone	3 oz (85 g)	530	624	15084
sardines, atlantic, cnd in soy oil	2 sardines (24 g)	65	272	15088
sardines, pacific, cnd in tomato sce	1 sardine (38 g)	182	480	15089
shrimp, raw	3 oz (85 g)	129	152	15149
tuna, light, cnd in oil, drained	3 oz (85 g)	201	236	15119
MEATS, LUNCHEON SAUSAGES				
bockwurst (pork, veal, milk, eggs), raw	3.2 oz sausage (91 g)	10	11	07006
bratwurst, beef & pork, smoked	2.3 oz (66 g)	9	13	07922
bratwurst, pork, beef, turkey, lite, smoked	2.3 oz (66 g)	5	8	07924
bratwurst, pork, ckd	3 oz link (85 g)	37	44	07013
brotwurst (pork & beef w/nfdm)	2.5 oz link (70 g)	8	11	07015
chicken, beef & pork sausage, skinless, smoked	1 link (84 g)	7	8	07928
frankfurter, beef	1.5 oz frank (43 g)	15	36	07022
frankfurter, beef & pork	1.6 oz frank (45 g)	16	36	07023
frankfurter, beef, Oscar Mayer	1.6 oz frank (45 g)	11	24	07241
frankfurter, meat, heated	1 frank (52 g)	16	31	07949
frankfurter, meat, unheated	1 frank (52 g)	16	31	07950
frankfurter, pork & beef w/am cheese (cheesefurter)	1.5 oz frank (43 g)	5	12	07016
frankfurter, pork & turkey, Oscar Mayer	1.6 oz frank (45 g)	3	7	07240
frankfurter, turkey, Butcher Boy Meats	2 oz frank (56 g)	7	12	07269
italian sausage, sweet	3 oz link (84 g)	6	7	07914
italian sausage, turkey, smoked	2 oz (56 g)	4	7	07927
polish sausage, beef w/chicken, hot	5 pieces (55 g)	24	44	07915

	SERVING SIZE	VITAMIN D (IU/SERVING)	VITAMIN D (IU/100 g)	SOURCE/ USDA CODE
polish sausage, pork & beef, smoked	2.7 oz (76 g)	33	44	07916
pork & beef sausage w/cheddar cheese, smoked	2.7 oz (77 g)	9	12	07917
sausage w/beef, ckd	1.1 oz patty (27 g)	8	28	07065
smoked sausage (smokie), pork & beef	2.4 oz link (68 g)	30	44	07075
turkey sausage, breakfast, mild	2 links (2 oz)	4	7	07919
turkey sausage, hot, smoked	2 oz (56 g)	4	7	07929
MEATS, LUNCHEON				
barbeque loaf	.8 oz slice (23 g)	8	36	07001
berliner, pork & beef	.8 oz slice (23 g)	3	13	07004
bologna, beef	1 oz slice (28 g)	8	28	07007
bologna, beef & pork	1 oz slice (28 g)	9	32	07008
bologna, beef, Oscar Mayer	1 oz slice (28 g)	9	32	07201
bologna, pork	1 oz slice (28 g)	16	56	07010
bologna, wisconsin-made ring, Oscar Mayer	2 oz (56 g)	22	40	07206
braunschweiger (pork liver sausage)	.6 oz slice (18 g)	9	48	07014
braunschweiger (pork liver sausage), saren tube, Oscar Mayer	2 oz (56 g)	18	33	07208
braunschweiger (pork liver sausage), sliced, Oscar Mayer	1 oz (28 g)	12	44	07207
ham & cheese loaf	1 oz slice (28 g)	12	44	07032
ham & cheese loaf, Oscar Mayer	1 oz slice (28 g)	12	42	07211
headcheese (pork), Oscar Mayer	1 oz slice (28 g)	13	46	07218
honey loaf (pork & beef)	1 oz slice (28 g)	11	40	07035
honey roll sausage (beef)	.8 oz slice (23 g)	9	40	07088
lebanon bologna (beef)	.8 slice (23 g)	7	32	07039
liver cheese (pork liver), pork fat wrapped, Oscar Mayer	1.3 oz slice (38 g)	19	49	07220
luxury loaf (pork)	1 oz slice (28 g)	8	28	07060
macaroni & cheese loaf, chicken, pork, & beef	1 slice (38 g)	8	20	07940
mother's loaf (pork)	.7 oz slice (21 g)	8	40	07061
olive loaf, pork	1 oz slice (28 g)	12	44	07051
peppered loaf (pork & beef)	1 oz slice (28 g)	9	32	07056
pickle & pimento loaf, pork	1 oz slice (28 g)	12	44	07058
picnic loaf (pork & beef)	1 oz slice (28 g)	13	48	07062
pork & beef loaf, Dutch Brand	1.3 oz slice (38 g)	15	40	07021
salami, beef	.8 oz slice (23 g)	11	48	07068
salami, beerwurst, beef	.8 oz slice (23 g)	8	36	07002
salami, beerwurst, pork	.8 oz slice (23 g)	8	36	07003
salami, dry/hard, Oscar Mayer	3 slices (27 g)	17	62	07230
salami, pork & beef, less sodium	3.5 oz (100 g)	32	32	07913
swisswurst, pork & beef w/swiss cheese, smoked	2.7 oz (77 g)	9	12	07920
thuringer (cervelat/summer sausage), beef & pork	.8 oz slice (23 g)	10	44	07078
thuringer (cervelat/summer sausage), beef, Oscar Mayer	2 slices (46 g)	18	40	07237
thuringer (cervelat/summer sausage), Oscar Mayer	2 slices (46 g)	22	47	07238
MEAT SNACKS				
bacon & beef sticks	1 oz (28 g)	4	13	07921
summer sausage sticks, pork & beef w/cheddar cheese	1 oz (28 g)	3	12	07918
MILK, COW MILK				
choc malted milk, whole milk	8 fl oz (265 g)	98	37	14318
choc malted milk, whole milk w/added nutrients	8 fl oz (265 g)	98	37	14316
choc milk, 1% fat milk	8 fl oz (250 g)	100	40	01104
choc milk, 2% fat milk	8 fl oz (250 g)	100	40	01103
choc milk, whole milk	8 fl oz (250 g)	100	40	01102
evaporated, nonfat, cnd	1 fl oz (32 g)	26	80	01097
lowfat, 1% fat	8 fl oz (244 g)	98	40	01082
lowfat, 1% fat, pro fortified	8 fl oz (246 g)	98	40	01084
lowfat, 1% fat w/nfdm	8 fl oz (245 g)	98	40	01083
malted milk, whole milk	8 fl oz (265 g)	98	37	14312
malted milk, whole milk w/added nutrients	8 fl oz (265 g)	98	37	14310
nonfat	8 fl oz (245 g)	98	40	01085
nonfat, dry	1/4 cup (30 g)	100	332	01091
nonfat, dry, inst	1 1/3 cups (91 g)	400	440	01092
nonfat, pro fortified	8 fl oz (246 g)	98	40	01087
nonfat w/nfdm	8 fl oz (245 g)	98	40	01086
reduced fat, 2% fat	8 fl oz (244 g)	98	40	01079
reduced fat, 2% fat, pro fortified	8 fl oz (246 g)	98	40	01081
reduced fat, 2% fat w/nfdm	8 fl oz (245 g)	98	40	01080

	SERVING SIZE	VITAMIN D (IU/SERVING)	VITAMIN D (IU/100 g)	SOURCE/ USDA CODE
whole, 3.3% fat	8 fl oz (244 g)	98	40	01077
whole, dry	1/4 cup (32 g)	100	312	01090
MILK, COW MILK YOGURT				
lowfat w/vit D, strawberry, Dannon Danimals Drinkable	3.1 fl oz (88 g)	40	45	DANN
lowfat w/vit D, van, Dannon Danimals	4 oz (113 g)	40	35	DANN
lowfat, whpd, orange cream, Dannon	4 oz (113 g)	40	35	DANN
nonfat w/vit A & D, aspartame, & fructose, strawberry, Dannon Light 'n Fit	8 oz (227 g)	100	44	DANN
Milk, Other Mammal Milks				
goat milk	8 fl oz (244 g)	29	12	01106
human milk	8 fl oz (246 g)	10	4	01107
MILK, OTHER (NON-DAIRY) MILKS				
almond milk, choc w/soy protein, Almond Breeze	8 fl oz (245 g)	100	41	BLDM
almond milk, choc, Almond Breeze	8 fl oz (245 g)	100	41	BLDM
almond milk, van w/soy protein, Almond Breeze	8 fl oz (245 g)	100	41	BLDM
almond milk, van, Almond Breeze	8 fl oz (245 g)	100	41	BLDM
soy milk, chai, Silk	8 fl oz (245 g)	80	33	WHWA
soy milk, choc, Silk	8 fl oz (245 g)	120	49	WHWA
soy milk, coffee Silk Soylatee	8 fl oz (245 g)	120	49	WHWA
soy milk, mocha, Silk	8 fl oz (245 g)	80	33	WHWA
soy milk, organic, plain, Silk	8 fl oz (245 g)	120	49	WHWA
soy milk, spice, Silk Soylatte	11 fl oz (337 g)	120	36	WHWA
soy milk, van, Silk	8 fl oz (245 g)	120	49	WHWA
Vitamite 100	8 fl oz	100		DIHL
NUTS				
soy nuts w/praline coating, GeniSoy	1 oz (28 g)	100	357	GENI
soy nuts, choc covered, GeniSoy	1 oz (28 g)	100	357	GENI
soy nuts, flavored, GeniSoy	1 oz (28 g)	100	357	GENI
soy nuts, unsalted, GeniSoy	1 oz (28 g)	100	357	GENI
VEGETABLES				
mushrooms, common white, raw	1/2 cup pieces (70 g)	53	76	11260
mushrooms, shiitake, dried	4 mushrooms (15 g)	249	1660	11268

[1] Vitamin D_3 is cholecalciferol, also known as 7-dehydrocholesterol.

Sources:
BLDM: Blue Diamond Growers, Sacramento CA
DANN: Dannon Company, Tarrytown NY
DIHL: Diehl Specialities International, Defiance OH
EGBT: Egg Beaters, ConAgra foods, Omaha NE
GENI: GeniSoy, Fairfield CA
PPTT: Papetti Foods, Gaylord MN
PULS: Pulse, Baxter International Inc, Deerfield IL
QUAK: Quaker Oats Company, Chicago IL
TROP: Tropicana Products, Inc, Bradenton FL
USDA Codes: *United States Department of Agriculture Database for Standard Reference, Release 15* (SR15), 2002. Available at http://www.nal.usda.gov/fnic/foodcomp/Data/SR15/sr15.html.
WHWA: White Wave, Inc, Boulder CO

Vitamins/Vitamin-Like Components—Vitamin D₃ (measured in mcg)[1]

	VITAMIN D₃ (mcg/100 g)	SOURCE		VITAMIN D₃ (mcg/100 g)	SOURCE
CHEESE			ice cream, van	0.5	MAFF3
cheese, blue stilton	0.2	MAFF2	ice cream, van, premium	0.3	MAFF3
cheese, brie w/o rind	0.2	MAFF2	pavlova/meringue w/fruit & cream	<0.2	MAFF3
cheese, camembert	0.1	MAFF2	pie, apple, double crust	<0.2	MAFF3
cheese, cheddar, english white	0.3	MAFF2	pie, lemon meringue	<0.2	MAFF3
cheese, cream	0.1	MAFF2	profiterole w/choc sce	0.3	MAFF3
cheese, emmental	0.3	MAFF2	tiramisu	<0.2	MAFF3
cheese, mozzarella	0.2	MAFF2			
cheese, parmesan, wedges/grated	0.3	MAFF2	**GRAIN PRODUCTS**		
cheese, port salut/st paulin	0.1	MAFF2	baguette, white	<0.05	MAFF1
cheese spread	0.2	MAFF2	bread, brown	<0.05	MAFF1
			bread, garlic	<0.05	MAFF1
DESSERTS			bread, white, standard	<0.05	MAFF1
cake, choc fudge	0.4	MAFF3	bread, whole grain	<0.05	MAFF1
cake, sponge w/cream & jam	0.4	MAFF3	croissant	0.10	MAFF1
cheesecake, choc/toffee/caramel	0.2	MAFF3	english muffin	<0.05	MAFF1
cheesecake, fruit	0.2	MAFF3	roll, white, cheese-topped	0.06	MAFF1
ice cream, choc/choc mint in cone	1.2	MAFF3	scone w/fruit	<0.05	MAFF1
ice cream dessert, choc/toffee	0.3	MAFF3			

[1] Vitamin D₃ is cholecalciferol, also known as 7-dehydrocholesterol.

Sources:
MAFF1: Ministry of Agriculture, Farms, and Fisheries, UK. Nutrient analysis of Bread and Morning Goods. 20 January 2001. (http://www.food.gov.uk/science/surveillance/maffinfo/2000/maff-2000-194) (accessed 20 December 2002).
MAFF2: Ministry of Agriculture, Farms, and Fisheries, UK. Nutrient Analysis of Cheese. 25 January 2000 (http://www.food.gov.uk/science/surveillance/maffinfo/2000/maff-2000-196) (accessed 20 December 2002).
MAFF3: Ministry of Agriculture, Farms, and Fisheries, UK. Nutrient Analysis of Ice Creams and Desserts. 23 January 2000 (http://www.food.gov.uk/science/surveillance/maffinfo/2000/maff-2000-195) (accessed 20 December 2002).

Vitamins—Vitamin K[1]

	VITAMIN K (mcg/100 g)	USDA CODE		VITAMIN K (mcg/100 g)	USDA CODE
BEVERAGES			puffed rice	0.08	08066
			puffed wheat	2.0	08146
coffee, brewed	10.0	14209	shredded wheat	0.7	08147
cola	tr	14400	Total	0.7	08077
cola, diet	tr	14416			
ginger ale	0.01	14136	**CHEESE & CREAM**		
ginger ale, diet	tr	14166	cheese, cheddar	3.0	01009
lemonade, frzn conc	0.03	14292	cream, sour, cultured	1.0	01056
sake	tr	—			
tea, brewed	0.05	14355	**EGGS, CHICKEN**		
tea, brewed, decaffeinated	0.03	—	egg white, raw	0.01	01124
tea leaves, black	262.0	—	egg yolk, raw	2.0	01125
tea leaves, green	1,428.0	—			
wine, table	tr	14084	**FATS, OILS, & SPREADS**		
			almond oil	7.0	04529
CEREALS & GRAINS, COOKED			butter	7.0	01001
buckwheat, whole groats, ckd	7.0	20011	canola oil	141.0	04582
millet, raw	0.9	20031	corn oil	3.0	04518
oatmeal, inst dry	3.0	08122	margarine, hard stick, mainly soy oil	51.0	04132
rice, white, raw	1.0	20044	mayonnaise	81.0	04025
			olive oil	49.0	04053
CEREALS, READY-TO-EAT			peanut oil	0.7	04042
bran flakes	2.0	08028	safflower oil	11.0	04510
corn flakes	0.04	08020			

	VITAMIN K (mcg/100 g)	USDA CODE		VITAMIN K (mcg/100 g)	USDA CODE
sesame oil	10.0	04058	**MEAT & POULTRY**		
soy oil	193.0	04044	beef, ground, regular, raw	0.5	13309
sunflower oil	9.0	05606	chicken, raw	0.1	05011
walnut oil	15.0	04528	meatloaf	6.0	—
			pork, raw	0.07	10003
FISH & SHELLFISH			turkey, raw	0.02	05167
abalone, mixed species, raw	23.0	15155			
butterfly bream, raw	0.2	—	**MILK & YOGURT**		
clams, mixed species, raw	0.2	15157	milk, choc, lowfat	0.4	01103
eel, mixed species, raw	0.02	15025	milk, nonfat	0.02	01085
mackerel, atlantic, raw	5.0	15046	milk, soy	3.0	16120
octopus, common, raw	0.07	15166	milk, whole, 3.3% fat	0.3	01077
oyster, eastern, wild, raw	0.1	15167	milk, whole, dry	2.0	01090
pacific saury, raw	0.02	—	yogurt, fruit	0.7	01121
salmon, pink, raw	0.4	15083	yogurt, plain, lowfat	0.3	01117
sardines, raw	0.09	—			
shrimp, mixed species, raw	0.03	15149	**NUTS & SEEDS**		
squid, mixed species, raw	0.02	15175	peanut butter, smooth	10.0	16098
top shell, raw	3.0	—	peanuts, raw	0.2	16087
tuna, bluefin, raw	0.03	15117	pistachio nuts, dried	70.0	12151
yellowtail, mixed species, raw	0.08	15135	sesame seeds, dried	8.0	—
			soy nuts, dry roasted	37.0	16111
FRUIT & VEGETABLE JUICES					
apple juice, cnd/bottled	0.1	09016	**SWEETENERS**		
cranberry jce cocktail	tr	14242	fruit spread, assorted flavors	0.5	—
grape jce, cnd/bottled	0.2	09135	honey	0.02	19296
grapefruit jce, cnd	0.2	09123			
orange jce, raw	0.1	09206	**VEGETABLES**		
pineapple jce, cnd	0.7	09273	amaranth leaf, raw	1,140.0	11003
prune jce, cnd	0.6	09294	artichoke, raw	14.0	11007
tomato jce, cnd	4.0	11540	asparagus, raw	40.0	11011
			beet, raw	3.0	11080
FRUITS			broccoli, ckd	270.0	11091
apple peel, green	60.0	—	broccoli, raw	205.0	11090
apple peel, red	20.0	—	brussels sprouts, raw	177.0	11098
apple w/o peel, raw	0.4	09004	brussels sprouts, top leaf	438.0	—
applesauce, cnd	0.5	09019	cabbage, green, raw	145.0	11109
apricot w/peel, cnd, water pack	5.0	09022	cabbage, red, raw	44.0	11112
avocado, raw	40.0	09037	carrot, ckd	18.0	11125
banana, raw	0.5	09040	carrot, raw	5.0	11124
blueberries, cnd, heavy syrup	6.0	09052	cauliflower, ckd	10.0	11136
cranberry sce, cnd	1.0	09081	cauliflower, raw	5.0	11135
fruit cocktail, cnd, water pack	0.8	09096	celery, raw	12.0	11143
grapefruit, raw	0.02	09111	chayote leaf, ckd	270.0	—
grapes, european (adherent skin), raw	3.0	09132	chayote leaf, raw	200.0	—
kiwifruit, raw	25.0	09148	chives, raw	190.0	11156
lemon peel, raw	0.2	09150	chrysanthemum, garland, raw	350.0	11157
melon, unspecified, raw	1.0	09181	coleslaw, fast food	57.0	21127
orange, raw	0.1	09200	coriander leaf, ckd	1,510.0	11165
peach, raw	3.0	09236	coriander leaf, raw	310.0	—
pear, cnd, water pack	0.5	09253	corn, sweet, yellow, raw	0.5	11167
pineapple, raw	0.1	09266	cucumber peel, raw	360.0	—
plum, raw	12.0	09279	cucumber pickle, dill	26.0	11937
			cucumber w/o peel, raw	2.0	—
GRAIN FRACTIONS			cucumber w/peel, raw	19.0	11205
barley flour	1.0	—	eggplant, raw	0.5	11209
rice flour	0.04	20061	endive, raw	231.0	11213
wheat flour, all-purpose	0.6	20081	green (snap) beans, raw	47.0	11052
			kale, leaf, raw	817.0	11233
GRAIN PRODUCTS & SNACKS			leek, raw	14.0	11246
bread, assorted types	3.0	—	lettuce, butterhead, raw	122.0	11250
crackers, graham	0.5	18173	lettuce, leaf, raw	210.0	11253
crackers, saltines	2.0	18228	malabar spinach, raw	22.0	—
potato chips	10.0	19411	mint leaf, ckd	860.0	—
pretzels, hard	1.0	19047	mint leaf, raw	230.0	—
rice cake, brown rice, plain	0.6	19051	mushrooms, raw	0.02	11260
spaghetti, dry	0.2	20120	mustard greens, raw	170.0	11270
			nightshade leaves, ckd	700.0	—

	VITAMIN K (mcg/100 g)	USDA CODE		VITAMIN K (mcg/100 g)	USDA CODE
nightshade leaves, raw	620.0	—	summer squash w/o peel, raw	3.0	11641
onion, raw	2.0	11282	sweet potato, cnd	4.0	11512
onion, spring	207.0	11291	swiss chard, raw	830.0	11147
parsley, ckd	900.0	—	tomato, red, raw	6.0	11529
parsley, raw	540.0	11297	tomato sce, cnd	7.0	11549
parsnips, raw	1.0	11298	tomato sce w/meat for spaghetti	4.0	—
peas, green, ckd	23.0	11305	turnip, cabbage, raw	2.0	—
peas, green, raw	36.0	11304	turnip greens, raw	251.0	11568
pepper, sweet, raw	17.0	11333	turnip, raw	0.09	11564
potato, baked w/peel	4.0	11674	watercress, raw	250.0	11591
potato peel, baked	0.3	11364			
potato, raw w/o peel	0.8	11352	**VEGETABLES—LEGUMES & LEGUME PRODUCTS**		
potatoes, french fries	5.0	11403	chili con carne, fast food	2.0	21042
pumpkin, cnd	16.0	11424	cowpeas, common, raw	5.0	16062
purslane, raw	381.0	11427			
radishes, raw	0.1	11429	kidney beans, raw	19.0	16027
sauerkraut, cnd	25.0	11439	lentils, raw	22.0	16069
seaweed, laver, green	4.0	—	lima beans, raw	6.0	—
seaweed, laver, purple	1,385.0	—	navy beans, raw	2.0	16037
snow (edible podded) peas, raw	25.0	11300	pinto beans, raw	10.0	16042
spinach, stalk, raw	6.0	—	soybean miso	11.0	16112
spinach, raw	400.0	11457	soybeans, raw	47.0	16108
summer squash peel, raw	80.0	—	soybean tofu, regular, raw	2.0	16127

[1] Median values per 100 grams of edible food; tr = trace (<0.005 mcg/100 g). Vitamin K values are listed in Section 32 of the main table for special dietary foods.

Source:
Weihrauch JL, AS Chatra. *Provisional Table on the Vitamin K Content of Foods.* USDA, Agricultural Research Service, Human Nutrition Information Service (HNIA/PT-104). Washington DC. February 1994.

SCIENTIFIC NAMES FOR PLANTS AND ANIMALS USED AS FOODS OR FOOD INGREDIENTS

Scientific Names for Plants and Animals Used as Foods or Food Ingredients[1]

PLANT FOOD	SCIENTIFIC NAME	PLANT FOOD	SCIENTIFIC NAME
acerola	*Malpighia punicifolia*	cardamom/cardamon	*Elettaria cardamonum*
acorn squash	*Cucurbita maxima*	cardoon	*Cynara cardunculus*
acorns	*Quercus* spp	carissa (natal-plum)	*Carissa macrocarpa*
adzuki beans	*Phaseolus angularis*	carob (locust) bean	*Ceratonia siliqua*
alfalfa sprouts	*Medicago sativa*	carrot	*Daucus carota*
allspice	*Pimenta officinalis; P dioica*	casaba melon	*Cucumis melo*
almonds	*Prunus amygdalus; P dulcis*	cashews	*Anacardium occidentale*
amaranth	*Amaranthus* spp	cassava (manioc)	*Manihot utilissima;*
anise/aniseseed	*Pimpinella anisum*		*M esculenta*
apple	*Malus communis; M domestica;*	cauliflower	*Brassica oleracea* var *botrytis*
	M sylvestris; M pumila	celeriac (celery root)	*Apium graveolens* var
apricot	*Prunus armeniaca*		*rapaceum*
arrowroot	*Maranta arundinacea*	celery	*Apium graveolens*
artichoke, globe/french	*Cynara scolymus*	celtuce	*Lactuca sativa*
arugula (garden rocket)	*Eruca sativa*	chard, swiss	*Beta vulgaris* var *cicla*
asparagus	*Asparagus officinalis*	chamomile/camomile	*Anthemis nobilis*
avocado	*Persea americana*	chayote (mirliton)	*Sechium edule*
babassu oil	*Orbignya barbosiana*	cherimoya	*Annona cherimola*
balsam pear (bitter	*Momordica charantia*	cherries, sour	*Prunus cerasus*
melon/gourd)		cherries, sweet	*Prunus avium*
bamboo shoots	*Phyllostachys edulis; P* spp	chervil	*Anthriscus cerefolium*
banana	*Musa nana; M sapientum;*	chestnuts, chinese	*Castanea mollissima*
	M paradisiaca	chestnuts, european	*Castanea sativa*
barley, 6-row/2-row	*Hordeum vulgare; H distichon*	chestnuts, japanese	*Castanea crenata*
basil (sweet basil)	*Ocimum basilicum*	chia seeds	*Salvia colmbariae; S hispanica*
bay leaf (sweet bay/bay)	*Laurus nobilis*	chickpeas (garbanzo beans)	*Cicer arietinum*
beechnuts	*Fagus* spp	chicory (curly endive,	*Cichorium endivia*
beet (beetroot)	*Beta vulgaris* var *Crassa*	radicchio)	
borage	*Borago officinalis*	chicory, whitloof (belgian	*Cichorium intybus* var
blackberries	*Rubus fruticosus; R* spp	endive, whitloof)	*foliosum*
blueberries	*Vaccinium* spp	chives	*Allium schoenoprasum*
boysenberries	*Rubus ursinus* var *loganobaccus*	chrysanthemum	*Chrysanthemum coronarium*
breadfruit	*Artocarpus altilis; A incisus;*	cinnamon	*Cinnamomum zeylanicum;*
	A communis		*C verum; C aromaticum;*
brazil nuts	*Bertholletia excelsa*		*C cassia*
breadnut	*Brosimum alicastrum*	cloud ear fungus	*Auricularia polytricha*
broadbeans (fava beans)	*Vicia faba*	cloves	*Eugenia caryophyllata;*
broccoli	*Brassica oleracea* var *italica*		*E aromatica;*
brussels sprouts	*Brassica oleracea* var *gemmifera*		*Syzygium aromaticum*
buckwheat	*Fagopyrum esculentum*	cocoa (cacao)	*Theobroma cacao*
burdock root	*Arctium lappa*	coconut	*Cocos nucifera*
butterbur (fuki)	*Petasites japonicus*	coffee	*Coffea arabica*
butternut squash	*Cucurbita moschata*	collards	*Brassica oleracea* var *viridis;*
butternuts	*Juglans cinerea*		*B oleracea* var *acephala*
cabbage, chinese	*Brassica chinensis; B rapa*	coriander (cilantro)	*Coriandrum sativum*
(pak-choi, pe-tsai)	var *chinensis*	corn	*Zea mays*
cabbage, green	*Brassica oleracea* var *capitata*	cornsalad (lamb's lettuce)	*Valerianella olitoria;*
cabbage, red	*Brassica oleracea* var		*V locusta* var *olitoria*
	capitata f. rubra	corn, white or yellow	*Zea mays*
cabbage, savoy	*Brassica oleracea* var *sabauda*	cottonseed oil	*Gossypium* spp
cabbage, swamp	*Ipomoea aquatic*	couscous (millet)	*Panicum miliaceum*
calabash gourd	*Lagenaria siceraria*	cowpeas (blackeye peas)	*Vigna unguiculata*
cannellini (white kidney)	*Phaseolus vulgaris*	cowpeas, catjang	*Vigna unguiculata cylindrica*
canola (rapeseed) oil	*Brassica napus; B* spp	crabapples	*Malus* spp
cantaloupe	*Cucumis melo* var *cantalupensis*	cranberries	*Vaccinium oxyoccus;*
capers	*Capparis spinosa*		*V macrocarpon*
carambola (star fruit)	*Averrhoa carambola*	cranberry (roman) beans	*Phaseolus vulgaris*
caraway	*Carum carvi*	crookneck/straightneck squash	*Cucurbita maxima*

PLANT FOOD	SCIENTIFIC NAME	PLANT FOOD	SCIENTIFIC NAME
cucumber	*Cucumis sativus*	leek	*Allium ampeloprasum*
cumin	*Cuminum cyminum*		var *porrum*
currants, black	*Ribes nigrum*	lemon	*Citrus limon*
currants, red	*Ribes rubrum*	lemon grass (citronella)	*Cymbopogon citratus*
currants, white	*Ribes rubrum* var *leucocarpum*	lentils	*Lens esculenta; L culinaris*
currants, zante (dried grapes)	*Vitis vinifera*	lettuce (butterhead, cos	*Lactuca sativa*
custard apple (bullock's heart)	*Annona reticulata*	crisphead, leaf lettuce)	
dandelion greens	*Taraxacum officinale*	lichi/litchee/lychee	*Litchi chinensis*
date	*Phoenix dactylifera*	lima beans	*Phaeseolus lunatus*
dill/dill seeds/dill weed	*Anethum graveolens*	lime	*Citrus aurantifolia*
dishcloth (towel) gourd	*Luffa aegyptiaca*	linseed oil	*Linum usitatissium*
dock (sorrel)	*Rumex* spp; *R acetosa*	loganberries	*Rubus ursinus* var
durian	*Durio zibethinus*		*loganobaccus*
eggplant (aubergine)	*Solanum melongena ovigerum*	longan	*Dimocarpus longan;*
elderberries	*Sambucus* spp		*Euphoria longan*
epazote	*Chenopodium ambrosioides*	loquat	*Eriobotrya japonica*
eppaw/epaw	*Perideridia oregana*	lotus root	*Nelumbo nucifera*
feijoa	*Feijoa sellowiana*	lupins	*Lupinus albus*
fennel	*Foeniculum vulgare;*	macadamia nuts	*Macadamia integrifolia;*
	Nigella sativa		*M tetraphylla*
fennel bulb	*Foeniculum vulgare* var *dulce*	malabar spinach	*Basella rubra; B alba*
fenugreek	*Trigonella foenum-graecum*	mammy apple (mamey)	*Mammea americana*
fiddlehead ferns	*Matteuccia*	mandarin orange	*Citrus nobilis deliciosa*
	struthiopteris	mango	*Mangifera indica*
filberts (hazelnuts)	*Corylus avellana; C maxima*	mangosteen	*Garcinia mangostana*
fig	*Ficus carica*	marjoram	*Origanum majorana;*
flaxseed	*Linum usitatissimum*		*Majorana hortensis*
french (haricot) beans	*Phaseolus vulgaris*	millet	*Panicum miliaceum*
garden cress	*Lepidium sativum*	mothbeans	*Vigna aconitifolia*
garden rocket (arugula)	*Eruca sativa*	mountain yam, hawaiian	*Dioscorea pentaphylla*
garland chrysanthemum	*Chryoanthemum coronarium;*	mulberries	*Morus nigra*
	C spatiosum	mung beans and sprouts	*Phaseolus aureus; Vigna radiata*
garlic	*Allium sativum*	mungo beans	*Vigna mungo*
ginko nuts	*Ginko biloba*	mushrooms, common	*Agaricus bisporus*
ginger	*Zingiber officinale*	white (champignon)	
gooseberries	*Ribes grossularia; Ribes* spp	mushrooms, crimini,	*Agaricus bisporus*
grapefruit	*Citrus paradisi*	italian, brown	
grapes, american	*Vitis* spp	mushrooms, enoki	*Flammulina veluptipes;*
grapes	*Vitis vinifera*		*Collybia veluptipes*
great northern beans	*Phaseolus vulgaris*	mushrooms, oyster	*Pleurotus ostreatus*
green beans (snap beans)	*Phaseolus vulgaris; P coccineus*	mushrooms, portabella	*Agaricus bisporus*
groundcherries	*Physalis* spp	mushroom, shiitake	*Lentinus edodes*
guava	*Psidium guajava*	mushroom, straw	*Volvariella volvacea*
guava, strawberry	*Psidium cattleianum*	mustard seeds, field	*Brassica arvensis*
hearts of palm (palm heart)	*Sabal palmetto*	mustard greens	*Brassica nigra; B juncea;*
hickorynuts	*Carya ovata; C* spp		*Sinapis alba*
hominy	*Zea mays*	mustard spinach	*Brassica rapa* var
honeydew melon	*Cucumis melo*	(tendergreen)	*perviridis*
hops	*Humulus lupulus*	navy beans and sprouts	*Phaseolus vulgaris*
horseradish	*Cochlearia armoracia; Moringa*	nectarine	*Prunus persica* var *nectarina*
	olcifera; Armorica rusticana	new zealand spinach	*Tetragonia tetragonioides*
horseradish tree	*Moringa oleifera*	nigella	*Nigella sativa*
hubbard squash	*Cucurbita maxima*	nopales (prickly pear)	*Nopalea cochenillifera*
hyacinth beans	*Dolichos purpureus; D lablab*	nutmeg	*Myristica fragrans;*
jackfruit	*Artocarpus heterophyllus*		*M officinalis;*
java plum	*Syzygium cumini*		*M moschata;*
jerusalem artichoke	*Helianthus tuberosus*		*M aromatica;*
(sunchoke)			*M amboinensis*
jicama (yambean)	*Pachyrhizus* spp	oats	*Avena sativa*
jujube	*Ziziphus jujuba*	oheloberries	*Vaccinium reticulatum*
jute, potherb	*Corchorus olitorius*	okra (lady's finger/gumbo)	*Hibiscus esculentus*
kale, curly	*Brassica oleracea* var *acephala*	olive	*Olea europaea*
kale, scotch	*Brassica napus* var *pabularia*	onion	*Allium cepa*
kidney beans, red	*Phaeseolus vulgaris*	onion, green (scallions)	*Allium cepa*
kiwifruit	*Actinidia chinensis*	onion, welsh	*Allium fistulosum*
kohlrabi	*Brassica oleracea* var *gongylodes*	orange, bitter (seville)	*Citrus aurantium*
kumquat	*Fortunella* spp	orange, navel or valencia	*Citrus sinensis*
lambsquarters	*Chenopodium album*	oregano	*Origanum vulgare*

PLANT FOOD	SCIENTIFIC NAME	PLANT FOOD	SCIENTIFIC NAME
palm oil	*Elaeis guineensis*	rhubarb	*Rheum rhaponticum;*
papaya (papaw)	*Carica papaya*		*R rhabarbaum*
paprika	*Capsicum anuum;*	rice	*Oryza sativa*
	C tetragonna	rose apple	*Syzygium jambos*
parsley	*Petroselinum crispum;*	roselle	*Hibiscus sabdariffa*
	P hortense; P sativum	rosemary	*Rosmarinus officinalis*
parsnip	*Pastinaca sativa;*	rowan	*Sorbus aucuparia*
	Peucadenum sativa	rutabaga (swede)	*Brassica napus* var *napobrassica*
passion fruit, purple	*Passiflora edulis*	rye	*Secale cereale*
(purple granadilla)		safflower oil	*Carthamus tinctorius*
passion fruit, yellow	*Passiflora laurifolis;*	saffron	*Crocus sativus*
	P laurifolia	sage	*Salvia officinalis; S sclarea;*
peach	*Prunus persica*		*S pratensis*
peanuts	*Arachis hypogaea*	salsify	*Tragopogon porrifolius*
pear	*Pyrus communis*	sapodilla	*Manilkara zapota*
pear, asian	*Pyrus ussuriensis; P pyrifolia*	sapote	*Pouteria sapota*
peas, green	*Pisum sativum*	savory, summer	*Satureja hortensis*
peas, green, sweet	*Pisum sativum* var	savory, winter	*Satureja montana*
	saccharatum	scallop squash	*Cucurbita maxima*
peas, split	*Pisum sativum*	seaweed, agar	*Gelidium corneum;*
pecans	*Carya pecan; C illinoensis*		*Eucheuma* spp
pepeao (jew's ear)	*Auricularia polytricha*	seaweed, irish moss	*Gigartina mamillosa;*
pepper, black	*Piper nigrum*		*Chondrus crispus*
pepper, red (cayenne/chili)	*Capsicum frutescens*	seaweed, kelp	*Laminaria* spp
pepper, white	*Piper nigrum*	(kombu/tangle)	
peppers, ancho, banana,	*Capsicum frutescens;*	seaweed, laver	*Porphyra perforata*
green chili, hungarian,	*C annuum*	seaweed, spirulina	*Spirulina* spp
jalapeno, pasilla,		seaweed, wakame	*Undaria pinnatifida; U* spp
pimento, serrano		sesbania flower	*Sesbania* spp
peppers, hot chili, red,	*Capsicum frutescens*	semolina (wheat)	*Triticum vulgare*
green, or yellow		sesame seeds	*Sesamum indicum; S orientale*
peppers, sweet (bell),	*Capsicum annuum*	sheanuts	*Butyrospermum paradoxum*
green, red, yellow		shallots	*Allium ascalonicum*
peppermint	*Mentha piperita*	shellie (shell) beans	*Phaseolus vulgaris*
persimmon, japanese	*Diospyros kaki*	snow peas (edible podded)	*Pisum sativum*
persimmon, native US	*Diospyros virginiana*	sorghum	*Sorghum vulgare* var
pigeon peas	*Cajanus cajan*		*durra; S bicolor; S* spp
pilinuts, canarytree	*Canarium ovatum*	sorrel (dock)	*Rumex acetosa*
pineapple	*Ananas sativus; A comosus*	soursop	*Annona muricata*
pine nuts, pignolia	*Pinus pinea*	soybeans and sprouts	*Glycine max*
pine nuts, pinyon	*Pinus edulis*	spaghetti squash	*Cucurbita pepo*
pink beans	*Phaseolus vulgaris*	spearmint	*Mentha spicata*
pinto beans	*Phaseolus vulgaris*	spinach	*Spinacia oleracea*
pistachio nuts	*Pistacia vera*	squash, summer (marrow)	*Cucurbita pepo*
pitanga	*Eugenia uniflora*	squash, winter, all varieties	*Cucurbita maxima*
plantain	*Musa paradisiaca*	strawberries	*Fragaria ananassa; F virginiana*
plum	*Prunus domestica; P* spp	sugar apple	*Annona squamosa*
pokeberries/shoots (poke)	*Phytolacca americana*	sugar beet	*Beta vulgaris* var *Crassa*
pomegranate	*Punica granatum*	sugar cane	*Saccharum*
popcorn	*Zea mays* var *everta*		*officinarum*
poppyseeds	*Papaver rhoeas;*	sugar maple	*Acer saccharum*
	P somniferum	sunflower seeds	*Helianthus annuus*
potato	*Solanum tuberosum*	sweet potato	*Ipomoea batatas*
prickly pear	*Opuntia* spp	tamarind	*Tamarindus indica*
prune (dried plum)	*Prunus domestica*	tangerine	*Citrus reticulata*
pummelo	*Citrus grandis*	taro (dasheen)	*Colocasia antiquorum;*
pumpkin	*Cucurbita pepo; Cucurbita* spp		*C esculenta*
pumpkin seeds	*Cucurbita maxima*	taro, tahitian	*Alocasia macrorrhiza*
purslane	*Portulaca oleracea*	tarragon	*Artemisia dracunculus;*
quince	*Cydonia oblonga* var *piriformis*		*Tagetes minuta*
quinoa	*Chenopodium quinoa*	tea	*Camillia sinensis*
radish, red	*Raphanus sativus* var *radicula*	thyme	*Thymus vulgaris*
radish, oriental (daikon)	*Raphanus sativus* var	tomatillo	*Physalis ixocarpa*
	longipinratus	tomato	*Lycopersicom esculentun*
radish, white icicle	*Raphanus sativus* var *radicula*	tree fern	*Cyathea medullaris; C* spp
raisins (dried grapes)	*Vitis vinifera*	triticale	*Triticosecale rimpauli*
rambutan	*Nephelium lappaceum*	turmeric	*Curcuma domestica; C longa*
raspberries	*Rubus idaeus; R* spp	turnip	*Brassica rapa* var *rapifera*

PLANT FOOD	SCIENTIFIC NAME	PLANT FOOD	SCIENTIFIC NAME
vanilla	*Vanilla fragrans; V planifolia*	wheat	*Triticum vulgare; T aestivum*
vinespinach	*Basella alba*	wheat, durum (pasta)	*Triticum durum*
walnuts	*Juglans regina; J nigra*	white beans	*Phaseolus vulgaris*
wasabi root	*Wasabia japonica*	wild rice	*Zizania aquatica; Z spp*
water chestnuts, chinese	*Eleocharis tuberosa;*	winged beans and leaves	*Psophocarpus tetragonolobus*
(matai)	*E dulcis; Scirpus tuberosa*	yam	*Dioscorea batatas; D esculenta;*
	Trapa spp; *Sagittaria sinensis*		*D alata; D spp*
watercress	*Nasturtium officinale;*	yardlong bean	*Vigna unguiculata sesquipedalis*
	N aquaticum	yautia	*Xanthosoma* spp
watermelon	*Citrullus lanatus;*	yellow snap beans	*Phaseolus vulgaris*
	Cucumis citrullus	zucchini, green	*Cucurbita pepo*
waxgourd	*Benincasa hispida*		

ANIMAL FOOD	SCIENTIFIC NAME	PLANT FOOD	SCIENTIFIC NAME
abalone	*Haliotis rufescens*	grouper, black	*Mycteroperca bonaci;*
anchovy	*Engraulis encrasicholus;*		*M microlepis*
	E mordax; E spp	grouper, red	*Epinephelus morio*
antelope	Subfamily *Hippotraginae*	guinea hen	*Numida meleagris*
bass, freshwater, mixed	*Percichthyidae* spp;	haddock	*Melanogrammus aeglefinus*
	Centrarchidae spp	halibut, atlantic	*Hippoglossus hippoglossus*
bass, hybrid striped	*Morone chrysops; M saxatilis*	halibut, greenland	*Reinhardtius hippoglossoides*
bear	*Ursus* spp	halibut, pacific	*Hippoglossus stenolepis*
beaver	*Castor canadensis*	herring, atlantic	*Clupea harengus harengus*
beefalo	⅜ bison *Bison bison;*	herring, pacific	*Clupea harengus pallasi*
	⅝ cow *Bos taurus*	horse	*Equus caballus*
bison	*Bison americanus*	lamb/sheep	*Ovis aries*
bluefish	*Pomatomus saltatrix*	ling	*Molva molva*
boar	*Sus scofa*	lingcod	*Ophiodon elongatus*
buffalo, indian/water	*Bubalus bubalis*	lobster, northern	*Homarus americanus*
burbot	*Lota lota*	mackerel, atlantic	*Scomber Scombrus*
butterfish	*Peprilus triacanthus*	mackerel, jack	*Trachusus synmetricus*
chicken/eggs	*Gallus domesticus*	mackerel, king	*Scombermorus cavalla*
caribou	*Rangifer caribou*	mackerel, pacific	*Scomber japonicus*
carp	*Cypinus carpio*	mackerel, spanish	*Scombermorus maculatus*
catfish, channel, farmed	*Ictalurus punctatus*	menhaden	*Brevoortia* spp
catfish, channel, wild	*Ictalurus punctatus*	milkfish	*Chanos chanos*
cisco	*Coregonus artedii*	monkfish	*Lophius americanus;*
clams, geoduck	*Panopea abrupta*		*L piscatorius*
clams, hardshell	*Mercenaria mercenaria*	moose	*Alces americana*
clams, manila	*Tapes philippinarum*	mullet, striped	*Mugil cephalus*
clams, mixed species	*Lamellibranchia* spp	muskrat	*Ondatra zibethica*
clams, ocean quahog	*Arctica islandica*	mussels, blue	*Mytilus edulis*
clams, softshell	*Mya arenaria*	ocean perch, atlantic	*Sebastes marinus*
clams, surf	*Spisula solidissima*	octopus	*Octopus vulgaris; Octopus* spp
cod, atlantic	*Gadus morhua*	opossum	*Didelphis virginiana;*
cod, pacific	*Gadus macrocephalus*		*Trichosurus* spp
cow (beef, veal, milk)	*Bos taurus*	orange roughy	*Hoplostethus atlanticus*
crab, alaska king	*Paralithodes camtschatica*	ostrich	*Struthio camelus*
crab, blue	*Callinectes sapidus*	oysters, eastern	*Crassostrea virginica*
crab, dungeness	*Cancer magister*	oysters, pacific	*Crassostrea gigas*
crab, queen	*Chionoectes opilio*	perch, mixed species	*Morone americana;*
crayfish	*Procambarus clarkii;*		*Perca flavenscens*
	Astacus spp; *Orconectes*	perch, pacific ocean	*Sebastes* spp
	spp; *Procambarus* spp	perch, white	*Mornoe americana*
croaker, atlantic	*Micropogonias undulatus*	pheasant	*Phasianus colchicus*
cusk	*Brosme brosme*	pig (pork)	*Sus scrofa*
cuttlefish	*Sepia* spp	pike, northern	*Esox lucius*
deer	*Odocoileus* spp	pike, walleye	*Stizostedion vitreum*
drum, freshwater	*Aplodinotus grunniens*	pollock, atlantic	*Pollachius virens; Gadus virens*
duck, domesticated	*Anas platyrhynchos*	pompano	*Trachinotus carolinus*
eel/eel, american	*Anguilla* spp; *A rostrata*	pout, ocean	*Macrozoarces Gadus virens*
elk	*Cervus alces*	quail	*Bonsas umbellus,*
emu	*Dromalus novaehollandiae*		*Colinus virginianus*
flounder, lemon sole	*Pleuronectes americanus*	rabbit, domesticated	*Oryctolagus*
flounder, rock sole	*Pleuronectes bilineatus*		*euniculus*
goat	*Capra* spp	rabbit, wild	*Sylvilagus floridanus*
goose	*Anser anser*	raccoon	*Procyon lotor*

ANIMAL FOOD	SCIENTIFIC NAME	PLANT FOOD	SCIENTIFIC NAME
rockfish, pacific	*Scorpaenidae* family	shrimp, pacific white	*Penaeus vannamei; P stylirostris*
sablefish	*Anoplopoma fimbria*	shrimp, pink	*Pandalus borealis; P jordani*
salmon, atlantic	*Salmo salar*	smelt, rainbow	*Osmerus mordax*
salmon, chinook	*Oncorhynchus tshawytscha*	snapper, mixed species	*Lutjanidae*
salmon, chum	*Oncorhynchus keta*	spiny lobster	*Panulirus* spp; *Jasus* spp
salmon, coho	*Oncorhynchus kisutch*	spot	*Leiostomus xanthuras*
salmon, pink	*Oncorhynchus gorbuscha*	squab (pigeon)	*Columba livia*
salmon, sockeye	*Oncorhynchus nerka*	squid	*Loligoidae pealei; L opalescens;*
sardine, atlantic	*Clupea harengus harengus*		*Illex illecebrosus*
sardine, pacific	*Sardinops* spp	squirrel	*Sciurus vulgaris*
scallops, bay	*Argopecten irradians*	sturgeon, mixed species	*Acipenser* spp
scallops, calico	*Argopecten gibbus*	sucker, white	*Catostomus commersoni*
scallops, queen	*Chlamys opercularis*	sunfish	*Lepomis gibbosus*
scallops, sea	*Placopecten magellanicus*	swordfish	*Xiphias gladius*
scup	*Stenotomus chrysops*	tilefish	*Lopholatilus chamaeleonticeps*
sea bass, mixed species	*Centropristes lateolabrax*	trout, mixed species	*Salmonidae* spp
	japonicus	trout, rainbow	*Salmo gairdneri*
seatrout	*Cynoscion* spp	tuna, albacore	*Thunnus alalunga*
shad, american	*Alosa sapidissima*	tuna, bluefin	*Thunnus thynnus*
shark, mako	*Isurus oxyrinchus*	tuna, skipjack	*Euthynnus pelamis*
shark, mixed species	*Squaliformes*	tuna, yellowfin	*Thunnus albacares*
sheep/lamb	*Ovis aries*	turbot, european	*Scophthalmus maximus*
sheepshead	*Archosargus probatocephalus*	turkey	*Meleagris gallopavo*
shrimp, black tiger	*Penaeus monodon*	whelk	*Buccinidae*
shrimp, gulf, brown	*Penaeus aztecus*	whitefish	*Coregonus clupeaformis*
shrimp, gulf, pink	*Penaeus duorarum*	whiting, mixed species	*Gadidae*
shrimp, gulf, white	*Penaeus setiferus*	yellowtail	*Seriola* spp
shrimp, mixed species	*Penaeidae; Pandalidae*		

[1] The terms generally refer to the genus (upper case) and species (lower case) names. For some foods, the name of the variety (var) is also provided. The abbreviation spp after a genus name means that there are various species of the food. This list is limited to the foods and ingredients included in this 18th Edition of Food Values.

Sources:
Encyclopaedia Britannica. Encyclopaedia Britannica, Inc. Helen Hemingway Benton, Publisher, Chicago IL. 1974.
Hvass E. *Plants that Feed and Serve Us*. Hippocrene Books, NY. 1975 (ISBN 0-88254-158-7).
Kiple KF, KC Ornelas (eds). *The Cambridge World History of Food*. Cambridge University Press, NY. 2000.
Masefield GB, M Wallis, SG Harrison, BE Nicholson. *The Oxford Book of Food Plants*. Oxford University Press, London. 1971.
Nettleton JA. Seafood Nutrition. *Facts, Issues and Marketing of Nutrition in Fish and Shellfish*. Osprey Books, Huntington NY. 1985. ISBN 0-943738-12-1.
Rogers J. *What food Is that? And How Healthy Is It?* Weldon Publishing, Sydney. 1990 (IBSN 1 86302 091 8).
Tiedjeans VA. *The Vegetable Encyclopedia and Gardener's Guide*. Avehel Books, NY. 1943 (MCMXLIII).

Food Name Synonyms and Cross References[1]

FOR THIS NAME . . .	SEE THIS INDEXED NAME	FOR THIS NAME. . .	SEE THIS INDEXED NAME
agar	seaweed, agar	celery root	celeriac
ahi	tuna, yellowfin	cervelat	thuringer (cervelat/
aku	tuna, skipjack		summer sausage)
albacore	tuna, white	cheesefurter	frankfurter, pork &
apple, mammy	mammy apple		beef w/am cheese
artichoke, Jerusalem	jerusalem artichoke	cheese smokie	smoked link sausage
ascolano olives	olives, green		with cheese
	(sevailano/ascolano)	chicken frank	frankfurter, chicken
Asian pear	pear, asian	chicken frankfurter	frankfurter, chicken
asparagus beans	yardlong beans	chicken hot dog	frankfurter, chicken
aubergine	eggplant	Chinese cabbage	cabbage, chinese
au gratin potatoes	potatoes, au gratin	Chinese gooseberry	kiwifruit
awa	milkfish	Chinese parsley	coriander
baked beans	beans, baked	Chinese pears	pears, asian
Barbados cherry	acerola	Chinese preserving melon	waxgourd
basella	winespinach	Chinese waterchestnuts	waterchestnuts, chinese
beans, black	black beans	chinook salmon	salmon, chinook
beans, black turtle soup	black turtle soup beans	chocolate, dark	dark chocolate (semi-sweet)
beans, cranberry	cranberry beans	chocolate, milk	milk chocolate
beans, French	french beans	chocolate syrup	syrup, chocolate
beans, goa	winged beans	chrysanthemum, garland	garland chrysanthemum
beans, great northern	great northern beans	chub	cisco, smoked
beans, hyacinth	hyacinth beans	cilantro	coriander
beans, kidney	kidney beans	citronella	lemon grass
beans, lima	lima beans	Colorado pinyon pines	pine nuts/pinyon nuts
beans, mung	mung beans	confectioner's sugar	powdered sugar
beans, navy	navy beans	corn syrup	syrup, corn
beans, pink	pink beans	cottage fries	potatoes, cottage fries
beans, pinto	pinto beans	cotto salami	salami, beef cotto
beans, Roman	cranberry beans	crème caramel	pudding, flan/crème
beans, shellie	shellie beans		caramel
beans, white, small	white small beans	crowder peas	cowpeas
beans, winged	winged beans	daikon	radishes, oriental
beans, yardlong	yardlong beans	dasheen	taro
beans, yellow	yellow beans	dessert topping	topping (Section 7.10)
beer salami	salami, beerwurst	dogfish	shark, mixed species
beerwurst	salami, beerwurst	edible podded peas	snow peas
beetroot	beet	egg custard	pudding, egg custard
bell peppers	peppers, sweet (bell)	endive, Belgian	chicory, witloof
bengal gram	chickpeas	escalloped potatoes	potatoes, scalloped
bittergourd	balsam pear		(escalloped)
bittermelon	balsam pear	European chestnuts	chestnuts, european
blackeye peas	cowpeas	falafel	broadbeans, falafel
blackstrap molasses	molasses, blackstrap	fava beans	broadbeans
blood pudding	blood sausage	fondant, chocolate coated	chocolate coated fondant
bologna, Lebanon	lebanon bologna	fondu	cheese fondu
bouillon, beef	beef broth/bouillon	Fordhook lima beans	lima beans, fordhook
bouillon, chicken	chicken broth/bouillon	French artichoke	artichoke, globe/French
breakfast sausage	beef sausage;	French fries	potatoes, fries
	pork sausage	fries	potatoes, fries
broth, beef	beef broth/bouillon	frosting	icing/frosting
broth, chicken	chicken broth/bouillon	fruit leather	fruit snack
bullock's heart	custard apple	fry bread	indian (navaho) fry bread
butterbeans	lima beans	fuki	butterbur
cabbage salad	coleslaw	garbanzo beans	chickpeas
cabbage, skunk	cabbage, swamp	genoa salami	salami, genoa
cacao butter	cocoa oil	globe artichoke	artichoke, globe/french
cane syrup	syrup, cane	goa beans	winged beans
cannelloni beans	kidney beans	golden gram	chickpeas
cape gooseberries	groundcherries	goobers/goober peas	peanuts
carambola	star fruit	goosefish	monkfish
cardamon	cardamom	granadilla	passion fruit
catfish, ocean	wolffish	green gram	mung beans
catjang cowpeas	cowpeas, catjang	greenland halibut	halibut, greenland

FOR THIS NAME . . .	SEE THIS INDEXED NAME	FOR THIS NAME . . .	SEE THIS INDEXED NAME
green onion	onion, green/spring	Navel orange	orange, CA, navel
grits	hominy grits	Nestle Crunch	Crunch, Nestle
groundnuts	peanuts	nori	seaweed, laver (nori)
gumbo	okra	nutmeg butter	nutmeg oil
hake	whiting	nut pines	pine nuts/pinyon
ham and cheese roll	ham and cheese loaf/roll	O'Brien potatoes	potatoes, o'brien
hash/hashed browns	potatoes, hashed brown	ocean catfish	wolffish
hazelnuts	filberts	okara	tofu, okara
herring, Atlantic, canned	sardine, atlantic, canned	oranges, Mandarin	mandarin oranges
herring, lake	cisco	Oriental radishes	radishes, oriental
highball	bourbon and water	oyster plant	salsify
hot chocolate	cocoa	Pacific mackerel	mackerel, pacific &
hot dog	frankfurter		jack, mixed species
hot sauce	pepper/hot sce	pak choi	cabbage, Chinese
hummus	chickpeas, hummus	pancake and waffle syrup	syrup, pancake & waffle
ice pop	ice	pastrami, turkey	turkey pastrami
infant formula	See products by brand	pate	liver pate
	name in Section 32.1	pear pods, balsam	balsam pear pods
irish moss	seaweed, irish moss	pectin	fruit pectin
Italian chestnuts	chestnuts, european	penuche	fudge, brown sugar w/nuts
Italian salami	salami, italian	pepeao	jew's ear
Italian stone pines	pine nuts/pignolia	pe-tsai	cabbage, chinese
jack	mackerel, pacific and	pickerel	pike
	jack, mixed species	pigeon	squab
jambolan	java plum	pignolia	pine nuts, pignolia
Japanese pears	pears, asian	pignon	pine nuts, pignolia
Japanese persimmon	persimmon, japanese	pinocchios	pine nuts/pinyon
Kaiser roll	roll, hard/kaiser	pinions	pine nuts/pinyon
kelp	seaweed, kelp	pistache nuts	pistachio nuts
	(kombu/tangle)	pistachia nuts	pistachio nuts
ketchup	catsup	poha	groundcherries
kombu	seaweed, kelp	poke	pokeberry shoots
	(kombu/tangle)	pollack, Alaskan	pollock, walleye
Kool Pop	ice, Kool Pop	popsicle	ice
knackwurst	knockwurst/	porgy	scup
	knackwurst	pork liver sausage	braunschweiger
kolbassy	kielbasa/kolbassy	preserves	jam/preserves
lady's finger	okra	prickly pear [fruit]	prickly pear
lard	pork fat	prickly pear [vegetable]	nopales
laver	seaweed, laver (nori)	Queensland nuts	macadamia nuts
litchis	lichis	Raisinets	chocolate coated raisins,
liver sausage	liverwurst		Raisinets
long rice noodles	chinese noodles	rajah	skate
lox	salmon, chinook, smoked	redfish	ocean perch, atlantic
lychees	lichis	red gram	pigeon peas
mahimahi	dolphinfish	Reese's Peanut Butter	Peanut Butter Cups,
malt syrup	syrup, malt	Cups	Reese's
mamey	mammy apple	relish	pickle relish
mammee apple	mammy apple	rice, wild	wild rice
manioc	cassava	Roman beans	cranberry beans
mango squash	chayote	roughy, orange	orange roughy
manzillo olives	olives, black smoked	salmon, keta	salmon, chum
	(manzillo/mission)	salmon, red	salmon, sockeye
maple syrup	syrup, maple	sausage, blood	blood sausage
marmalade plum	sapote	sausage, liver	liver sausage
marrow	squash, summer	scallion	onion, green/spring
masa harina	corn flour, yellow,	scalloped potatoes	potatoes, scalloped
	masa harina		(escalloped)
mashed potatoes	potatoes, mashed	scrod	cod, atlantic
matai	waterchestnuts, chinese	sea snails	whelks
miriliton	chayote	semi-sweet chocolate	dark chocolate (semi-sweet)
mission olives	olives, black	Sevailano olives	olives, green
	(manzillo/mission)		(sevailano/ascolano)
mousse	pudding, chocolate	shell beans	shellie beans
	mousse	shoyu	soy sauce made w/soy
muffins, English	english muffins		& wheat
muskmelon	cantaloupe	sim-sim	sesame seeds
natal plum	carissa	skipjack tuna	tuna, skipjack
Navaho fry bread	indian (navaho) bread	skunk cabbage	cabbage, swamp

FOR THIS NAME . . .	SEE THIS INDEXED NAME	FOR THIS NAME. . .	SEE THIS INDEXED NAME
snails, sea	whelks	Swiss chard	chard, swiss
snap beans	green beans	tahini	sesame butter
snow peas	peas, edible-podded	tamari	soy sauce made w/soy
sodium chloride	salt	tangerines, canned	mandarin oranges, cnd
sorrel	dock	tangle	seaweed, kelp
southern peas	cowpeas		(kombu/tangle)
soybean curd	tofu	tannier	yautia
Special Dark chocolate	chocolate, dark (semi-	tendergreen	mustard spinach
	sweet), Special Dark	towelgourd	dishcloth gourd
spinach, mustard	mustard spinach	turbot, domestic species	halibut, greenland
spirulina	seaweed, spirulina	turkey frank	frankfurter, turkey
spring onion	onion, green/spring	turkey frankfurter	frankfurter, turkey
sprouts	specific sprouts (e.g.,	turkey hot dog	frankfurter, turkey
	alfalfa sprouts, mung	turtle soup black beans	black turtle soup beans
	bean sprouts)	Valencia orange	orange, CA, valencia
squash seeds	pumpkin & squash seeds	vegetable oyster	salsify
St. John's bread	carob	vegetable pear	chayote
stone pines	pine nuts/pignolia	vegetables, mixed	mixed vegetables
strawberry guava	guava, strawberry	wakame	seaweed, wakame
string beans	green beans	walleye	pollock, walleye
sugar snap peas	snow peas	water convulvolus	swamp cabbage
summer sausage	thuringer (cervelat/	wiener	frankfurter
	summer sausage)	West Indian cherry	acerola
sunchoke	jerusalem artichoke	white-floured gourd	calabash gourd
Surinam cherry	pitanga	witloof chicory	chicory, witloof
swamp cabbage	cabbage, swamp	yambean	jicama
Swede	turnip	yam, mountain, Hawaiian	mountain yam, hawaiian
sweetbread	pancreas; thymus	yellowfin tuna	tuna, yellowfin
sweet chestnuts	chestnuts, european	yokan	adzuki beans w/sugar
sweetsop	sugar apple	York Peppermint Patty	Peppermint Patty, York
smokie	smoked sausage		

[1] To assist users in locating foods in the database. The list provides a food name synonym or a food name with a different arrangement of terms in the left-hand column and the "preferred" food name (i.e., the name used in the 18th edition) in the right-hand column. The preferred food name is listed in the index with the page numbers of its location.

Sources:
Encyclopaedia Britannica. Encyclopaedia Britannica, Inc. Helen Hemingway Benton, Publisher, Chicago IL. 1974.
Hvass E. *Plants that Feed and Serve Us*. Hippocrene Books, NY. 1975 (ISBN 0-88254-158-7).
Kiple KF, KC Ornelas (eds). *The Cambridge World History of Food*. Cambridge University Press, NY. 2000.
Masefield GB, M Wallis, SG Harrison, BE Nicholson. *The Oxford Book of Food Plants*. Oxford University Press, London. 1971.
Nettleton JA. Seafood Nutrition. *Facts, Issues and Marketing of Nutrition in Fish and Shellfish*. Osprey Books, Huntington NY. 1985 (ISBN 0-943738-12-1).
Rogers J. *What food Is that? And How Healthy Is It?* Weldon Publishing, Sydney. 1990 (IBSN 1 86302 091 8).
Tiedjeans VA. *The Vegetable Encyclopedia and Gardener's Guide*. Avehel Books, NY. 1943 (MCMXLIII).

Bibliography for Food Composition Data[1]

Abdel-Aal E_SM, P Hucl. **Amino acid** composition and in vitro protein digestibility of selected **ancient wheats** and their end products. *J Food Comp Anal* 15:737–747, 2002.

Abellan GB. IG de Santiago, AD Marquina, MTO Willanueva. **Macroelements content in nougat**, a traditional Spanish sweet. *J Food Comp Anal* 13:265–273, 2000.

Adindu MN, FF Olayemi, OU Nze-Dike. **Cyanogenic potential of some cassava products** in Port Harcourt markets in Nigeria. *J Food Comp Anal* 16:21–24, 2003.

Aganga AA, JO Amarteifio, N Nkile. Effect of stage of lactation on nutrient composition of **Tswana sheep and goat's milk**. *J Food Comp Anal* 15:533–543, 2002.

Agostoni C, B Carratu, C Boniglia, E Riva, E Sanzini. **Free amino acid content in standard infant formulas: Comparison with human milk**. *J Am Coll Nutr* 19:434–438, 2000.

Agte VV, KV Tarwadi, SA Chiplonkar. **Phytate** degradation during traditional cooking: Significance of the phytic acid profile in **cereal-based vegetarian meals**. *J Food Comp Anal* 12:161–167, 1999.

Agte VV, KV Tarwadi, S Mengale, SA Chiplonkar. Potential of **traditionally cooked green leafy vegetables** as natural sources for supplementation of **eight micronutrients in vegetarian diets**. *J Food Comp Anal* 13:885–891, 2000.

Aguirrezabal M, C Dominguez, JM Zumalacarregui. **Volatile compounds in Spanish paprika**. *J Food Comp Anal* 10:225–232, 1997.

Aigster A, C Sims, S Staples, R Schmidt, SF O'Keefe. Comparison of **cheeses** made from milk having normal and high **oleic fatty acid** composition. *J Food Sci* 65:920–924, 2000.

Akerberg AKE, HGM Lilijeberg, YE Granfeldt, AW Drews, IME Bjorck. An in vitro method, based on chewing, to predict **resistant starch** content in foods allows parallel determination of potentially available starch and **dietary fiber**. *J Nutr* 128:651–660, 1998.

Akpanabiatu, MI, NB Bassey, Eo Udosen, EU Eyong. Evaluation of some **minerals and toxicants in some Nigerian soup meals**. *J Food Comp Anal* 11:292–297, 1998.

Alarcao-E-Silva MLCMM, AEB Leitao, HG Azinheira, MCA Leitao. The **arbutus berry**: Studies on its color and chemical characteristics at two mature stages. *J Food Comp Anal* 14:27–35, 2001

Alegria A, R Barbera, R Farre, MJ Lagarda, JC Lpoez. **Amino acid contents of infant formulas**. *J Food Comp Anal* 12:137–146, 1999.

Allen CM, AM Smith, SK Clinton, SJ Schwartz. **Tomato** consumption increases **lycopene isomer** concentrations in **breast milk** and plasma of lactating women. *J Am Diet Assoc* 102:1257–1262, 2002.

Almazan AM, F Begum, C Johnson. Nutritional quality of **sweetpotato greens** from greenhouse plants. *J Food Comp Anal* 10:246–253, 1997.

Almazan AM, SO Adeyeye. Short communication: **Fat and fatty acid** concentrations in some green vegetables. *J Food Comp Anal* 11:375–380, 1998.

Alttnoz S, S Toptan. Determination of **tartrazine and ponceau-4R** in various food samples by Vierordt's method and ratio spectra first-order derivative UV spectrophotometry. *J Food Comp Anal* 15:667–683, 2002.

Amarteifio JO, D Moholo. The chemical composition of **four legumes consumed in Botswana**. *J Food Comp Anal* 11:329–332, 1998.

American Academy of Pediatrics. The transfer of **drugs and other chemicals into human milk**. *Pediatrics* 108:776–789, 2001.

Amr A, N Hadidi. Effect of cultivar and harvest date on **nitrate (NO3) and nitrite (NO2)** content of selected **vegetables** grown under open field and greenhouse conditions in Jordan. *J Food Comp Anal* 14:59067, 2001.

Anasuya A, S Bapurao, PK Paranjape. **Fluoride and silicon** content of foods from normal and endemic fluorotic areas in India. *J Food Comp Anal* 10:43–48, 1997.

Anderson, JJB, SC Garner. Phytoestrogens and human function. *Nutr Today* 32:232–239, 1997. **(isoflavones and phytoestrogens in legumes)**

Anderson PC, K Hill, DW Gorbet, BV Brodbeck. **Fatty acid and amino acid profiles** of selected **peanut cultivars** and breeding lines. *J Food Comp Anal* 11:100–110, 1998.

Andrade EHA, JGS Maia, MGB Zoghbi. **Aroma volatile constituents of Brazilian varieties of mango fruit**. *J Food Comp Anal* 13:27–34, 2000.

Andrade EHA, MGB Zoghbi, JGS Maia, H Fabricius, F Marx. Chemical characterization of the fruit of *Annona squamosa L.* occurring in the Amazon. *J Food Comp Anal* 14:227–232, 2001.

Andrikopoulos NK, N Kaloperopoulos, A Zerva, U Zerva, M Hassapidou, VM Dapoulas. Evaluation of **cholesterol and other nutrient parameters** of Greek cheese varieties. *J Food Comp Anal* 16:155–167, 2003.

Anzano JM, N Asensio, J Anwar, M C Martinez-Bordenave. **Zinc and manganese** analysis in **maize** by microwave oven digestion and flame atomic absorption spectrometry. *J Food Comp Anal* 13:837–841, 2000.

Arai Y, S Watanabe, M Kimira, K Shimoi, R Mochizuki, N Kinae. Dietary intakes of **flavonols, flavones, and isoflavones** by Japanese women and the inverse correlation between quercetin intake and plasma LDL cholesterol concentration. *J Nutr* 130:2243–2250, 2000. (myricetin, ficetin quercetin, kaemphferol, luteolin, daidzein, and genistein in Japanese foods)

Arnous A, DP Makris, P Kefalas. Correlation of pigment and **flavanol content** with **antioxidant properties** in selected **aged regional wines from Greece**. *J Food Comp Anal* 15:655–665, 2002.

Aro A, E Amaral, H Kesteloot, A Rimestad, M Thamm, G van Poppel. **Trans fatty acids in French fries, soups, and snacks from 14 European countries**: The TRANSFAIR Study. *J Food Comp Anal* 11:170–177, 1998.

Aro A, JM Antoine, L Pizzoferrato, O Reykdal, G van Poppel. **Trans fatty acids in dairy and meat products from 14 European countries**: The TRANSFAIR Study. *J Food Comp Anal* 11:150–160, 1998.

Aro A, J Van Amelsvoort, W Becker, M-A van Erp-Baart, A Kafatos, T Leth, G van Poppel. **Trans fatty acids in dietary fats and oils from 14 European countries**: The TRANSFAIR Study. *J Food Comp Anal* 11:137–149, 1998.

Arogba SS. Comparative analyses of the **moisture isotherms, proximate compositions, physical and functional properties of dried cola nitida and garcinia kola kernels**. *J Food Comp Anal* 13:139–148, 2000.

Arogba SS. **Mango (Mangifera indica) kernel**: Chromatographic analysis of the **tannin**, and stability study of the associated **polyphenol oxidase** activity. *J Food Comp Anal* 13:149–156, 2000.

Ashton BA, GL Ambrosini, GC Marks, PW Harvey, C Bain. Development of a **dietary supplement database**. *Aust NZ J Public Health* 21:699–702, 1997.

Aussenac T, S Laxombe, J Dayde. Quantification of **isoflavones in soybean seeds** by capillary zone elecrophoresis: Effects of variety and environment. *Am J Clin Nutr* 68:1480S–1485S, 1998.

Avallone R, M Plessi, M Baraldi, A Monzani. Determination of chemical composition of **carob** *(Ceratonia siliqua)*: **Protein, fat, carbohydrates, and tannins**. *J Food Comp Anal* 10:166–172, 1997.

Awad AC, et al. **Composition** and functional properties **of cholesterol reduced egg yolk**. *Poult Sci* 76:649–653, 1997.

Ayaz FA, E Bertoft. **Sugar and phenolic acid** composition of stored commercial **oleaster fruits**. *J Food Comp Anal* 14:505–511, 2001.

Ayaz FA, A Kadioglu, M Reunanen, M Var. Note: **Sugar composition in fruits of *Laurocerasus officinalis Roem.* and its three cultivars**. *J Food Comp Anal* 10:82–86, 1997.

Ayaz FA, M Kucukislamoglu, M Reunanen. **Sugar, non-volatile and phenolic acids composition of strawberry tree (*Arbutus unedo L. var. ellipsoidea*) fruits**. *J Food Comp Anal* 13:171–178, 2000.

Badiani A, N Nanni, PP Gatta, B Tolomelli, M Manfredini. Nutrient profile of **horsemeat**. *J Food Comp Anal* 10:254–269, 1997.

Badifu GIO. Effect of processing on **proximate composition**, antinutritional and toxic contents of **kernels from *Cucurbitaceae* species** grown in Nigeria. *J Food Comp Anal* 14:153–161, 2001.

Badmaev V. M Majeed, L Prakash. **Piperine derived from black pepper** increases the plasma levels of coenzyme Q10 following oral supplementation. *J Nutr Biochem* 11:109–113, 2000.

Badria FA. **Melatonin, serotonin, and tryptamine in some Egyptian food** and medicinal plants. *J Medicinal Food* 5:153–158, 2002.

Bales CW, KL Moreno, JR Guyton, PA Yunker, MK McGee, KL Currie, S Brown, M Kuchibhatla, MK Drezner. Comparison of **proximate composition and fatty acid and cholesterol content of lean and typical commerical pork**. *J Am Diet Assoc* 98:1328–1330, 1998.

Baptista JAB, JF de P Tavares, RCB Carvalho. Comparative study and partial characterization of **Azorean green tea polyphenols**. *J Food Comp Anal* 12:273–287, 1999.

Bee G. Dietary conjugated linoleic acids alter adipose tissue and milk lipids of pregnant and lactating sows. *J Nutr* 130:2292–2298, 2000. **(fatty acids in backfat)**

Beecher GR. Nutrient content of **tomatoes and tomato products**. *Proc Soc Exp Biol Med* 218:98–100, 1998.

Behall KM, Dj Scholfield, J Hallfrisch. Effect of **beta-glucan level in oat fiber** extracts on blood lipids in men and women. *J Am Coll Nutr* 16:46–51, 1997.

Belinsky DL, HV Kuhnlein. **Macronutrient, mineral, and fatty acid composition of Canada goose (*Branta Canadensis*)**: An important traditional food resource of the Eastern James Bay Cree of Quebec. *J Food Comp Anal* 13:101–116, 2000.

Blum L, PJ Pelto, GH Pelto, HV Kuhnlein. *Community Assessment of Natural Food Sources of Vitamin A: Guidelines for an Ethnographic Protocol*. International Nutrition Foundation for Developing Countries, 1998. (ISBN 0-9635522-9-5)

Bognar A, J Piekarski. Guidelines for recipe information and calculation of nutrient composition of **prepared foods (dishes)**. *J Food Comp Anal* 13:391–410, 2000.

Booth SL, NM McKeown, AH Lichtenstein, MO Morse, KW Davidson, RJ Wood, C Gundberg. A **hydrogenated form of vitamin K**: Its relative bioavailability and presence in the food supply. *J Food Comp Anal* 13:311–318, 2000.

Booth SL, ME O'Brien/Morse, GE Dallal, KW Davidson, DM Gundberg. Response of vitamin K status to different intakes and sources of **phylloquinone-rich foods**: Comparison of younger and older adults. *Am J Clin Nutr* 70:368–377, 1999.

Booth SL, JW Suttie. Dietary intake and adequacy of **vitamin K**. *J Nutr* 128:785–788, 1998.

Borchers AT, RM Hackman, CL Keen, JS Stern, ME Gershwin. Complementary medicine: a review of immunomodulatory effects of **Chinese herbal medicines**. *Am J Clin Nutr* 66:1303–1312, 1997.

Bos C, C Gaudichon, D Tome. Nutritional and physiological criteria in the assessment of **milk protein quality** for humans. *J Am Coll Nutr* 19:191S–205S, 2000.

Boukaari I, NW Shier, XE Fernandez R, J Frisch, BA Watkins, L Pawloski, AD Fly. **Calcium** analysis of selected **western African foods**. *J Food Comp Anal* 14:37–42, 2001.

Boylan LM, S Hart, KB Porter, JA Driskell. **Vitamin B-6 content of breast milk** and neonatal behavioral functioning. *J Am Diet Assoc* 102:1433–1438, 2002.

Bragagnolo N, DB Rodriguez-Amaya. Comparison of the **cholesterol** content of **Brazilian chicken and quail eggs**. *J Food Comp Anal* 16:147–153.

Brat J, J Pokorny. **Fatty acid composition of margarines and cooking fats available on the Czech market**. *J Food Comp Anal* 13:337–344, 2000.

Bub A, B Watzl, L Abrahamse, H Delincee, S Adam, J Wever, H Muller, G Rechkemmer. Moderate intervention with **carotenoid-rich vegetable products** reduces lipid peroxidation in men. *J Nutr* 130:2200–2206, 2000. (carotenoids in tomato juice, carrot juice, and spinach powder)

Buege DR, BH Ingham, DW Henderson, SH Watters, LL Borchert, PM Crump, EJ Hentges. A nationwide audit of the composition of **pork and chicken cuts** at retail. *J Food Comp Anal* 11:249–261, 1998.

Burns J, PT Gardner, J O'Neil, et al. Relationship among antioxidant activity, vasodilation capacity and **phenolic content of red wines**. *J Agric Food Chem* 48:220–230, 2000.

Burri BJ, et al. Supercritical fluid extraction and reversed-phase liquid chromatography methods for vitamin A and β-carotene heterogeneous distribution of **vitamin A in the liver**. *J Chromatogr A* 21:201–206, 1997.

Califano AN, AE Bevilacqua. Multivariate analysis of the **organic acids content of Gouda type cheese** during ripening. *J Food Comp Anal* 13:949–960, 2000.

Canfield LM, AR Giuliano, Em Neilson, HH Yap, EJ Graver, HA Cui, BM Blashill. **Beta-carotene in breast milk** and serum is increased after a single beta-carotene dose. *Am J Clin Nutr* 66:52–61, 1997.

Carnovale E, S Nicoli. **Changes in fatty acid composition in beef in Italy**. *J Food Comp Anal* 13:505–510, 2000.

Cassens RG. Residual **nitrite in cured meat**. *Food Tech* 51:53–55, 1997.

Castineria A, RM Pena, C Herrero, S Garcia-Martin. Analysis of **organic acids in wine** by capillary electrophoresis with direct UV detection. *J Food Comp Anal* 15:319–331, 2002.

Chaiwanon P, P Puwastein, A Nitithamyong, PP Sirichakwal. **Calcium fortification in soybean milk** and in vitro bioavailability. *J Food Comp Anal* 13:319–327, 2000.

Chavasit V, P Malaivongse, K Judprasong. Study on stability of **iodine in iodated salt** by use of different cooking model conditions. *J Food Comp Anal* 15:265–276, 2002.

Chen, H-Y, DH Pilkington, JB Tharrington, JC Allen. Developing a **dry-cured ham nutritional database**. *J Food Comp Anal* 10:190–204, 1997.

Chen JY, JD Latshaw, HO Lee, DB Min. **Alpha tocopherol content and oxidative stability of egg yolk** as related to dietary alpha tocopherol. *J Food Sci* 63:919–922, 1998.

Chevaux KA, L Jackson, ME Villar, JA Mundt, JF Commisso, GE Adamson, MM McCullough, HH Schmitz, MK Hollenberg. **Proximate, mineral, and procyanidin content** of certain **foods and beverages consumed by the Kuna Amerinds of Panama**. *J Food Comp Anal* 14:553–563, 2001.

Cho S, G Johnson, WO Song. **Folate content of foods**: Comparison between databases compiled before and after new FDA fortification requirements. *J Food Comp Anal* 15:293–307, 2002.

Chow CK. *Fatty Acids in Foods and their Health Implications*. 2nd ed. Marcel Dekker. NY. 1999. (ISBN 0-8247-6782-9).

Christensen NK, AW Sorenson, DG Hendricks, R Munger. **Juniper ash** as a source of **calcium** in the Navajo diet. *J Am Diet Assoc* 98:333–334, 1998. (**Ca, Fe, Mg, K, Cu, Zn, Na, Cr, P, Si, and Al in juniper ash**)

Clausen I, L Ovesen. Proximate contents, losses, and gains of **fat, protein, and water** comparing **raw, hospital- and household-cooked pork cuts**. *J Food Comp Anal* 14:491–503, 2001.

Clinton, SK. **Lycopene**: Chemistry, biology, and implications for human health and disease. *Nutr Rev* 56:35–51, 1998.

Clydesdale FM, SH Chan (eds). First international conference on east-west perspectives on **functional foods**. *Nutr Rev* 54(No 11, Part II):S1-S202, 1996 (40 papers).

Cobiac L, V Droulez, P Leppard, J Lewis. Use of **external fat width** to describe **beef and lamb cuts** in food composition tables. *J Food Comp Anal* 16:133–145, 2003.

Cook JA, DJ VanderJagt, A Pastusyzn, G Mounkaila, RS Glew, M Illson, RH Glew. **Nutrient and chemical composition of 13 wild plant foods of Niger**. *J Food Comp Anal* 13:83–92, 2000.

Cook JA, DJ VanderJagt, A Pastuszyn, G Mounkaila, RH Glew. Nutrient content of **two indigenous plant foods of the Western Sahel**: Balanites aegyptizca and Maerua Crassifolia. *J Food Comp Anal* 11:221–230, 1998.

Cormier A, G Vautour, J Allard. Canada-wide survey of the nutritional composition of **six retail pork cuts**. *J Food Comp Anal* 9:255–268, 1996.

Coward L, M Smith, M Kirk, S Barnes. Chemical modification of **isoflavones in soyfoods** during cooking and processing. *Am J Clin Nutr* 68:1486S–1491S, 1998.

Cressey PJ. **Iodine content of New Zealand dairy products**. *J Food Comp Anal* 16:25–36, 2003

da Costa RSS, M d GT do Carmo, C Saunders, RT Lopes, EGO de Jesus, SM Simabuco. **Trace elements** content of **colostrum milk in Brazil**. *J Food Comp Anal* 15:27033, 2002.

Daniel DR, LD Thompson, LC Hoover. **Nutrition composition of emu** compares favorably with that of other lean meats. *J Am Diet Assoc* 100:836–838, 2000.

Dary O, M Guamuch, P Nestel. Recovery of **retinol in soft-drink beverages** made with fortified unrefined and refined sugar: Implications for national fortification programs. *J Food Comp Anal* 11:212–220, 1998.

De Deckere EAM, O Korver, PM Verschuren, MB Katan. Health aspects of fish and **n-3 polyunsaturated fatty acids from plant and marine origin**. *Eur J Clin Nutr* 52:749–753, 1998.

De Ferrer PAR, A Baroni, ME Sambucetti, NE Lopez, JMC Cernadas. **Lactoferrin levels in term and preterm milk**. *J Am Coll Nutr* 19:370–373, 2000.

Del Prado M, S Villalpando, A Elizondo, M Rodriguez, H Demmelmair, B Koletzko. Contribution of dietary and newly formed **arachidonic acid** to **human milk lipids** in women eating a low-fat diet. *Am J Clin Nutr* 74:242–247, 2001.

De Maria CAB, LC Trugo, LS De Mariz e Miranda. The content of individual **caffeoylquinic acids** in edible **vegetables**. *J Food Comp Anal* 12:289–292, 1999.

De Miguel T, et al. The genus **Rhodosporidium**: A potential source of **beta-carotene**. *Microbiologia* 13:67–70, 1997.

De Vries JHM, PCH Hollman, I van Amersfoort, MR Olthof, MB Katan. **Red wine** is a poor source of bioavailable **flavonols** in men. *J Nutr* 131:745–748, 2001.

De Vries JHM, A Jansen, D Kromhout, P van de Bovenkamp, WA van Staveren, RP Mensink, MB Katan. The **fatty acid and sterol** content of **food composites** of middle-aged men in seven countries. *J Food Comp Anal* 10:115–141, 1997.

Diaz C, JE Conde, C Claverie, E Diaz, JPP Trujillo. Conventional **eno-**

logical parameters of **bottled wines** from the Canary Islands (Spain). *J Food Comp Anal* 16:49–56, 2003.

Dolan SP. SG Capar. Multi-element analysis of food by microwave digestion and inductively coupled plasma-atomic emission spectrometry. *J Food Comp Anal* 15:593–615, 2002. (23 minerals)

Dorea JG. **Magnesium in human milk**. *J Am Coll Nutr* 19:210–219, 2000.

Dorea JG, E Myazaki. **Calcium and phosphorus in milk of Brazilian mothers** using oral contraceptives. *J Am Coll Nutr* 17:642–646, 1998.

dos Santos, EJ, E de Oliveira. Determination of **mineral nutrients and toxic elements in Brazilian soluble coffee** by ICP-AES. *J Food Comp Anal* 14:523–531, 2001.

Dourtoglou VG, DP Makris, F Bois-Dounas, C Zonas. **Trans-resveratrol** concentration in **wines produced in Greece**. *J Food Comp Anal* 12:227–233, 1999.

Dragland S, H Senoo, K Wake, K Holte, R Blomhoff. Several **culinary and medicinal herbs** are important sources of dietary **antioxidants**. *J Nutr* 133:1286–1290, 2003.

Duckett SK, DG Wagner. Effect of cooking on the **fatty acid composition of beef intramuscular lipid**. *J Food Comp Anal* 11:357–362, 1998.

Duke JA. **Wild lettuce**: A bitter herb of biblical proportions. *J Med Food* 3:153–154, 2000.

Eckhoff KM, A Maage. **Iodine** content in **fish** and other food products from **East Africa** analyzed by ICP-MS. *J Food Comp Anal* 10:270–282, 1997.

Edwards AJ, CH Nguyen C-S You, JE Swanson, C Emenhiser, RS Parker. **Alpha- and beta-carotene** from a commercial **carrot puree** are more bioavailable to humans than from **boiled-mashed carrots**, as determined using an extrinsic stable isotope reference method. *J Nutr* 132:159–167, 2002.

Englberger L, W Aalbersberg, MH Fitzgerald, GC Marks, K Chand. **Provitamin A carotenoid** content of different cultivars of edible **pandanas fruit**. *J Food Comp Anal* 16:237–247, 2003.

Englberger L, W Aalbersberg, P Ravi, E Bonnin, GC Marks, MH Fitzgerald, J Elymore. Further analyses of **Micronesian banana, taro, breadfruit, and other foods for provitamin A carotenoids and minerals**. *J Food Comp Anal* 16:219–236, 2003.

Englberger L, J Schierle, GC Marks, MH Fitzgerald. **Micronesian banana, taro**, and other foods: newly recognized sources of **provitamin A and other carotenoids**. *J Food Comp Anal* 16:3–19, 2003.

Ernesto M, AP Cardoso, J Cliff, JH Bradbury. **Cyanogens in cassava flour and roots** and urinary thiocyanate concentration in Mozambique. *J Food Comp Anal* 13:1–12, 2000.

Erney RM, WT Malone, MB Skelding, AA Marcon, KM Kleman-Leyer, ML O'Ryan, G Ruiz-Palacios, MD Hilty, LK Pickering, PA Prieto. Variability of **human milk neutral oligosaccharides** in a diverse population. *J Pediatr Gastroenterol Nutr* 30:181–192, 2000.

Escriche I, C Fuentes, C Gonzalez, A Chiralt. Development of **medium volatility compounds in Manchego-type cheese** as affected by salt content and salting method. *J Food Comp Anal* 13:827–836, 2000.

Fairweather-Tait SH, B Teucher. **Iron and calcium bioavailability of fortified foods** and dietary supplements. *Nutr Rev* 60:360–367, 2002.

Fediuk K, N Hidiroglou, R Madere, HV Kuhnlein. **Vitamin C in Inuit tradition food** and women's diets. *J Food Comp Anal* 15:221–225, 2002.

Feldman EB (ed). The scientific evidence for a beneficial health relationship between **walnuts** and coronary heart disease. *J Nutr* 132:1057S–1102S, 2002.

Fenech M, M Noakes, P Clifton, D Topping. **Aleurone flour** is a rich source of bioavailable **folate** in humans. *J Nutr* 129:1114–1119, 1999.

Fernandez XE, NW Shier, BA Watkins. Effect of alkali saponification, enzymatic hydrolysis and storage time on the total **carotenoid concentration of Costa Rican crude palm oil**. *J Food Comp Anal* 13:179–188, 2000.

Felelon MA, TP Guinee, C Delahuntly, J Murray, F Crowe. Composition and sensory attributes of **retail cheddar cheese with different fat contents**. *J Food Comp Anal* 13:13–26, 2000.

Field RA, RA Deligeersang, G Maiorano, RJ McCormick. **Iron, zinc, and alpha-tocopherol** content of **bovine hemopoietic marrow**. *J Food Comp Anal* 15:19–25, 2002.

Finley JW. The retention and distribution by healthy young men of stable isotopes of **selenium** consumed as selenite, selenate or **hydroponically-grown broccoli** are dependent on the isotopic form. *J Nutr* 129:865–871, 1999.

Finley JW, CD Davis, Y Feng. **Selenium** from high selenium **broccoli** protects rats from colon cancer. *J Nutr* 130:2384–2389, 2000.

Fish WW, P Perkins-Veazie, JK Collins. A quantitative assay for **lycopene** that utilizes reduced volumes of organic solvents. *J Food Comp Anal* 15:309–317, 2002.

Fly, AD, KL Uhlin, JP Wallace. **Major mineral concentrations in human milk** do not change after maximal exercise testing. *Am J Clin Nutr* 68:345–349, 1998.

Forssen KM, MI Jagerstad, K Wigertz, CM Witthoft. **Folates and dairy products**: A critical update. *J Am Coll Nutr* 19:100S–110S, 2000.

Francois P Le, JP Chicot, E Faure, JY Kervella, D Argaud. **Calcium and magnesium** in distributed **water in restaurants** of land forces in France. *J Food Comp Anal* 12:123–127, 1999.

Francois CA, Sl Conner, RC Wander, WE Connor, Acute effects of dietary fatty acids on the **fatty acids of human milk**. *Am J Clin Nutr* 67:301–308, 1998.

Freitas AMC, C Parreira, L Vilas-Boas. The use of an electronic aroma-sensing device to assess **coffee** differentiation–Comparison with SPME gas chromatography–Mass spectrometry **aroma patterns**. *J Food Comp Anal* 14:513–522, 2001.

Fruhbeck G, I Monreal, S Santidrian. Hormonal implications of the hypocholesterolemic effect of intake of **field beans** (*Vicia faba L.*) by young men with hypercholesterolemia. *Am J Clin Nutr* 66:1452–1460, 1997. (composition of field bean flour)

Galan P, J Arnaud, S Czernichow, A-M Delabroise, P Preziosi, S Bertrais, C Franchisseur, M Maurel, A Favier, S Hercberg. Contributions of **mineral waters** to dietary **calcium and magnesium** intake in a French adult population. *J Am Diet Assoc* 102:1658–1662, 2002.

Galdos MEA, M Albrecht-Ruiz, AS Maldonado, JP Minga. **Fat content of Peruvian anchovy** (*Engraulis ringens*), after "El Nino" phenomenon (1998–1999). *J Food Comp Anal* 15:627–631, 2002.

Gallez B, C Baudelet, R Debuyst. **Free radicals in licorice-flavored sweets** can be detected noninvasively using low frequency electron paramagnetic resonance after oral administration to mice. *J Nutr* 130:1831–1833, 2000.

Galvano F, V Galofaro, F Falvano. Occurrence and stability of **aflatoxin M in milk and milk products**: A worldwide review. *J Food Protection* 59:1079–1090, 1996.

Garcia DJ. **Omega-3 long-chain PUFA nutraceuticals**. *Food Tech* 52:44–49, 1998.

Garcia-Lopez PM, M Muzquiz, MA Ruiz-Lopez, JF Zamora-Natera, C Burbano, MM Pedrosa, C Cuadrado, P Garzon-De la Mora. **Chemical composition and fatty acid profile of several Mexican wild lupins**. *J Food Comp Anal* 14:645–651, 2001.

Gatlin LA, MT See, DK Larick, X Lin, J Odle. **Conjugated linoleic acid** in combination with supplemental dietary fat alters **pork fat quality**. *J Nutr* 132:3105–3112, 2002.

Gil-Munoz R, E Gomez-Plaza, A Martinez, JM Lopez-Roca. Evolution of **phenolic compounds** during **wine** fermentation and post-fermentation: Influence of grape temperature. *J Food Comp Anal* 12:259–272, 1999.

Glew RH, SN Okolo, L-T Chuang, Y-S Huang, DJ VanderJagt. **Fatty acid** composition of **fulani 'butter oil' made from cow's milk**. *J Food Comp Anal* 12:235–240, 1999.

Glew RH, DJ VanderJagt, C Lockett, LE Grivetti, GC Smith, A Pastuszyn, M Millson. **Amino acid, fatty acid, and mineral** composition of **24 indigenous plants of Burkina Faso**. *J Food Comp Anal* 10:205–217, 1997.

Gloria MBA, M Izquierdo-Pulido. Levels and significance of **biogenic amines** in **Brazilian beers**. *J Food Comp Anal* 12:129–136, 1999.

Goldbohm RA, HA Brants, KF Hulshof, PA van den Brandt. The contribution of various foods to intake of **vitamin A and carotenoids** in The Netherlands. *Int J Vitam Nutr Res* 68:378–383, 1998.

Granado G, B Olmedilla, J Blanco, E Gil-Martinez, E Rojas-Hidalgo. Variability in the intercomparison of food **carotenoid** content data: A user's point of view. *Crit Rev Food Sci Nutr* 37:621–633, 1997.

Granado F, B Olmedilla, E Gil-Martinez, I Blanco. A fast, reliable and low-cost saponification protocol for analysis of **carotenoids in vegetables**. *J Food Comp Anal* 14:479–489, 2001.

Guerrero JLF, JJG Martinez, MET Isasa. **Mineral nutrient composition of edible wild plants**. *J Food Comp Anal* 11:322–328, 1998.

Guil-Guerrero JL, MM Rebollosos-Fuentes, ME Torija Isasa. **Fatty acids and carotenoids from stinging nettle** (*Urtica dioica L.*). *J Food Comp Anal* 16:111–119, 2003.

Guillemant J, H-T Le, C Accarie, ST du Montcel, A-M Delabroise, MJ Arnaud, S Guillemant. **Mineral water as a source of dietary calcium**: Acute effects on parathyroid function and bone resorption in young men. *Am J Clin Nutr* 71:999–1002, 2000.

Gupta SV, P Khosla. **Pork fat and chicken fat** similarly affect plasma